# BOERICKE'S
# NEW MANUAL
*Of*
# HOMEOPATHIC
# MATERIA MEDICA
*With*
# REPERTORY

*Including Indian Drugs, Nosodes, Uncommon Rare Remedies, Mother Tinctures, Relationships, Sides of the Body, Drug Affinities & List of Abbreviations*


**WILLIAM BOERICKE, M.D.**

*First Professor of Homeopathic Materia Medica and Therapeutics at the University of California; Author of "A Compend of the Principles of Homeopathy"; Translator of the "Sixth Edition of Hahnemann's Organon."*


**THIRD REVISED & AUGMENTED EDITION**

*BASED ON*

**NINTH EDITION**

**B. JAIN PUBLISHERS (P) LTD.**

*USA — EUROPE — INDIA*

**BOERICKE'S NEW MANUAL OF HOMEOPATHIC MATERIA MEDICA WITH REPERTORY**

First Revised & Augmented Edition: 1998
Second Revised & Re-Augmented Edition: 2000
36th Impression: 2015



*Published by Kuldeep Jain for*
**B. JAIN PUBLISHERS (P) LTD.**
1921/10, Chuna Mandi, Paharganj, New Delhi 110 055 (INDIA)
Tel.: +91-11-4567 1000 Fax: +91-11-4567 1010
Email: info@bjain.com Website: **www.bjain.com**

*Printed in India*

ISBN: 978-81-319-0184-7

# PUBLISHER'S NOTE TO THIRD REVISED & AUGUMENTED EDITION

It's always a great honor to bring another edition of Boericke, the ultimate book on Materia Medica, complete in knowledge facilitated with latest updates and changes to accommodate the changing trends and perceptions in homeopathy. It is imperative to state that the last edition, at the beginning of the new millennium was widely appreciated and praised by the homeopathic fraternity for its indepth analysis, modern terminology, dictionary, footnotes, font, print and presentation.

This third revised and augmented edition goes further ahead as the use of the new font and italics accentuate the text and make the contents more comprehensive.

Readers will be delighted to see the insertion of tinctures in this edition as it was something which has been due it's worth for a long time.

Also the 'Rare and Uncommon Remedies' section has been removed as a separate section, but included appropriately along with the related drugs at more relevant places giving a comprehensive account of their viability and use.

To maintain the high standard of the book all abbreviations have been derived from the 'Synthesis Repertory 9.1' in the materia medica and repertory portion, thus making this edition of Boericke more comprehensive and complete in a wholesome manner.

As indeed always, we wish the readers a very happy experience while going through the book which as always has been both enriching and comprehensive in it's whole perspective.

**Kuldeep Jain**
**CEO, B. Jain Publishers**

January 2007,
New Delhi.

# PUBLISHER'S NOTE TO FIRST REVISED & AUGMENTED EDITION

This, latest edition of the *Boericke* comes to you at the beginning of the new millenium with a sincere effort to streamline it in trend with the other advancements in the field of homoeopathy in particular, and medicine in general.

To begin with, an effort has been made to correct all the grammatical errors and to technically upgrade the book in relation to modern terminology. For example, pressure deep in the orbits (glaucoma), without making any changes in the text of the whole book. The modern terminology, confined to brackets throughout the text has been co-related with various source books like, Dictionary of Practical Materia Medica by Dr. J. H. Clarke; 1001 Small Remedies by Dr. F. Schroyens; Handbook of Materia Medica by Dr. T. F. Allen; etc.

This edition has further been facilitated by foot notes given at the bottom of the page, for instance, Pg. 25, throat deafness[1]:- 1—Hearing—impaired—tonsils enlarged (1001 Small Remedies, edited by Dr. F. Schroyens), which further elaborate or explain the corresponding symptom, along with the name of the source book.

All the abbreviations and names of the drugs, in the book and repertory are now, according to the Synthesis, like *Thuya* - *Thuj*.; *Helleb*. - *Hell*.; etc. Also, all the spellings have been corrected according to Dorland's 28th edition, for instance diarrhoea is now diarrhea; anaesthesia is now anesthesia; etc.

The sequence of Mind, Head, Eyes, etc, in the drugs have been arranged according to those in the Kent's Repertory throughout the book to maintain a more orderly and uniform pattern.

*Aluminium silicata* and *Kaolinum* have been merged as one drug as they are one and the same.

In the repertory section of this book, the same pattern has been maintained but the chapters have been re-arranged in accordance to Kent's Repertory to minimise confusion. An Index to the Repertory has been incorporated with the meaning of words along with the correlated page numbers, rendering it more complete and convenient to use.

The previously existing Indian Drugs have been provided with more information and new additions.

A special section on some commonly used Nosodes has been added in this volume along with a re-arranged Rare and Uncommon Remedies, throwing more light on this, comparatively under-studied field of homoeopathy.

And last but not the least, an Index of the drugs, with both common and Latin names, has been introduced in the beginning of this book under Contents with the proper listing of all the chapters as well, to give a head start to the reader in his quest to explore the vast sphere of knowledge that this edition is going to provide.

The Publishers wish to acknowledge to Dr. P. Sivaraman, editor of the first augmented and revised edition and Dr. T. J. Bhagat, B.H.M.S. (Delhi), editor of the second re-augmented edition, for their untiring labour in editing this manual and presenting it in the present shape.

**Kuldeep Jain**
**MD, B. Jain Publishers**

January 2000
New Delhi.

# PREFACE TO THE NINTH EDITION

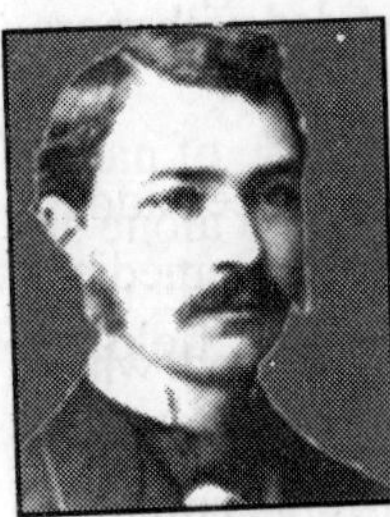

Dr. W. Boericke
The Author

In preparing the ninth edition, I have followed the lines laid out for all the previous editions, namely, to present in a condensed form the homeopathic materia medica for practical use.

The book contains the well known verified characteristic symptoms of all our medicines besides other less important symptoms aiding in the selection of the curative remedy. All the new medicines and essentials of the published clinical experience of the school have been added. In its present compact form, it contains the maximum number of reliable materia medica facts in the minimum space.

I have tried to give a succinct resumé of the symptomatology of every medicine used in homeopathy, including clinical suggestions of several drugs which have not yet been based on provings, thus offering the opportunity to experiment with these and by future provings, discover their distinctive use and enlarge our armamentarium.

I am aware that there is a difference of opinion about the advisability of further introduction of remedies, especially of some which as seem obsolete or to some minds, illusory. But it is not for the compiler to leave out information about any substance that has received the clinical endorsement from a reliable source.

Our materia medica must include all substances which have been proved and which have been used with apparent efficacy. It rests with the individual student to judge for himself the accuracy and reliability of such observation. In this connection, I cannot forego to avail myself of the high authority of that master of homeopathy, Dr. Constantine Hering, who favoured the introduction of all remedies capable of producing reactions in the body that may guide us to their medicinal employment. "Homeopathy is essentially not only many-sided but all-sided." She investigates the action of all substances, whether articles of diet, beverages, condiments, drugs or poisons. She investigates their action on the healthy, the sick, animals and plants. She gives a new interpretation to that ancient, often quoted saying of Paul, "Prove all things—a new meaning, a new application that acts universally." Elimination of the useless may gradually take place with the growth of accurate physiological and pathological knowledge."

Again, imperfectly proved remedies necessitate the use of names of diseases at times instead of the component symptoms that alone are the legitimate guide to the choice of the curative remedy. Here, too, I have Hering, as a pioneer guide for the legitimacy of this method, which he also followed in his great work, the Guiding Symptoms. He said that he used the disease designations not for the purpose of recommending the particular remedy for that disease, but to show the great variety of remedies that may be used for any form of disease when otherwise indicated. For the same reason I have included nosological terms in the symptomatology and the therapeutic index, as this is a practical handbook for every-day service, and an aid for finding the curative remedy ought to be utilized. As Dr. J. Compton Burnett expresses it:

"The fact is, we need any and every way of finding the right remedy; the simple simile, the simple symptomatic simillimum and the farthest reach of all-the pathological simillimum, and I maintain that we are still well within the lines of homeopathy that is expansive, progressive, science fostered and science fostering.'

The dosage needs some apology. It is, of course, suggestive only; more often to be wholly disregarded. I have followed the lines of the earlier homeopathists in this regard, and given what was then considered the usual range of potency, to which I have added my own experience and that of many observing practitioners. Every teacher of materia medica is constantly importuned by students to suggest the potency—something to start with at least.

The book is in no sense a treatise and must not be considered or judged as such. It is as accurate and reliable a compilation and the fullest collection of verified materia medica facts and clinical suggestions as it is possible to obtain with the compass of the volume. It supplements every other work on materia medica, and if used as a ready reminder of the essential facts of our vast symptomatology and as an introduction to the larger books of reference and record of provings, it will fulfill its purpose and prove a useful aid to the student and general practitioner. As such it is again offered with much appreciation of past endorsement to his professional brethren.

I have been aided in seeing this edition through the press by the efficient help of Mr. F.O. Ernesty, who has lightened the labor of making the manuscript more acceptable to the printers, and I desire to express my hearty appreciation of this kind and helpful service.

**William Boericke, M.D.**

San Francisco,
June 1927

## OTHER WORKS OF BOERICKE

Regionals of Boericke
Analogy of Pain

# PREFACE TO THE REPERTORY

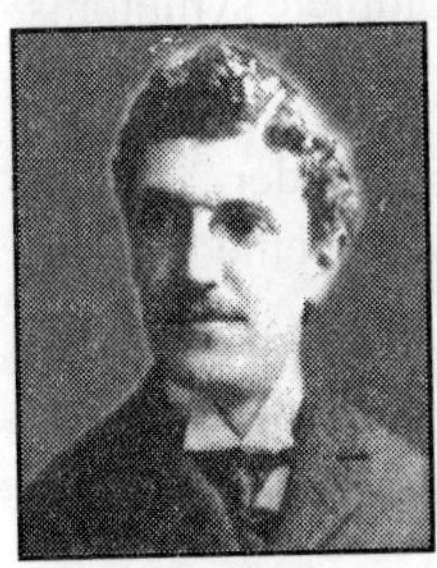

Dr. Oscar. E.Boericke
Compiler of
The Repertory

With the advent of the incomparable ninth edition of the progressive Pocket Materia Medica, its modest companion, the Repertory, had been completely remodelled and brought up to date, by embodying much of the newly incorporated material. Many of the sections have been carefully rewritten, and with appropriate expansion, offer a more trustworthy guide for the selection of the homoeopathic remedy. A few prefatory remarks, pertaining to the practical and expeditious use of the repertorial contents, may assist in clarifying a certain inevitable obscurity of plan.

First, in conformity with established repertorial methods, the *division* of the *sections* in somewhat the old Hahnemannian order is adhered to, and may be stated as follows: Mind; Head; Eyes; Ears; etc.

Secondly, for the purpose of convenience, solely, *headings* and *sub-headings* and specific conditions or symptoms comprised under the latter are arranged in *alphabetical order,* and this is more or less consistently adhered to throughout the entire work. For example, under Mind the headings read, Awkward, Brainfag, Catalepsy, etc.; likewise the heading Delirium embraces its various phases in alphabetical order.

Thirdly, all *headings* when *extensive in scope—e.g. Headache,* are presented under definite captions in the following order: cause, type, location, character of pain, concomitants, nodalities—*i.e.,* aggravations and ameliorations. It is to be observed that some headings include only a few, whereas others include all of these divisions. This method has been resorted to simply to facilitate the task of the use of the repertory.

Fourth, to preserve uniformity, the *technical names of diseases* are bracketed, thereby assuming a subsidiary place, which is in strict accord with the homoeopathic requirement, to prescribe for the symptoms of each specific case, and not for a mere name of a disease. Of course, being a clinical and not a truly symptomatological index (for which the practitioner and student are referred to the monumental works of Kent, Knerr and Clarke) technical terms are often selected as main headings, and when feasible, the more or less complete symptoms constitute the sub-headings.

Fifthly, the *remedies* are arranged in *alphabetical* order, and the *italics* indicate the more frequently verified *clinical* remedy. The abbreviations of the remedies are purely arbitrary and self-explanatory.

A complete alphabetical index, newly added, will surely offer much assistance to the busy practitioner, in the ready reference to the specific information desired.

Lastly, it is only by the persistent use of *one* repertory, that its peculiar and intricate arrangements gradually crystallizes itself in definite outline, in the mind of the student of the same, and thus he attains the ready case and practical insight of the collator, thereby rendering such a clinical bee-line well-nigh in-dispensable in our day of labour-saving devices.

**Oscar E. Boericke, M.D.**

*Philadelphia, Pa.*, June, 1927.

# CONTENTS

## MATERIA MEDICA

(Pharmaceutical or Latin Names)

## REPERTORY

## SOME INDIAN DRUGS

## SOME IMPORTANT NOSODES AND SARCODES



## SOME IMPORTANT MOTHER TINCTURES

## RARE AND UNCOMMON REMEDIES

## LIST OF REMEDIES
(Common Names)

# MATERIA MEDICA

# ABIES CANADENSIS — PINUS CANADENSIS

(Hemlock Spruce) **Abies-c.**

Mucous membranes are affected by *Abies-c.* Gastric symptoms are most marked, a catarrhal condition of the stomach is produced. There are peculiar cravings with chilly sensations that are characteristic, especially in women with uterine displacements, probably due to defective nutrition and debility. Respiration and action of the heart, labored. Wants to lie down all the time; skin cold and clammy, hands cold; very faint. Right lung and liver feel small and hard. Gleet.

**Head:** Feels light headed, tipsy. Irritable.

**Stomach:** Canine hunger with a torpid liver. *Gnawing, hungry, faint feeling* in the epigastrium. Great appetite, craving for meat, pickles, radishes, turnips, antichokes, coarse food. *Tendency to eat far beyond the capacity for digestion* (bulimia). Burning and *distention of the stomach and abdomen with palpitations* (indigestion). Gastritis. Flatulence, disturbing the heart's action. Pain in right shoulder blade and constipation, with burning in the rectum.

**Female:** Uterine displacements. Sore feeling in the fundus of the uterus, relieved by pressure. Prostration; wants to lie down all the time. Feels womb is soft and feeble.[1]

**Fever:** Shivering and chills all over, as if blood was turned into ice water (*Acon.*). Chills run down the back. Sensation of cold water, between the shoulders (*Am-m.*). Skin clammy and sticky. Night sweats (*Chin.*).

**Dose:** First to third potency.

---

[1] Feels womb is soft and feeble, as if it would cause an abortion (Clarke - Dictionary of Practical Materia Medica).

# ABIES NIGRA

(Black Spruce) **Abies-n.**

A powerful and long-acting remedy for various diseases, whenever the characteristic stomach symptoms are present. Most of the symptoms are associated with gastric disturbances. *In dyspeptic problems of the aged,* with functional heart symptoms; also after tea or tobacco. *Constipation.* Pain in the external meatus.

**Head:** Hot, with flushed cheeks. Low spirited. Dull during the day, awake at night. Unable to think.

**Stomach:** *Pain in stomach, always comes on after eating.* Sensation of a painful lump, *as if a hard boiled egg was lodged in the cardiac end of the stomach;* continuous, distressing constriction just above the pit of the stomach, as if everything was knotted up. Total loss of appetite in the morning, but a great craving for food at noon and night. Offensive breath (halitosis). Eructations (dyspepsia).

**Respiratory:** Painful sensation, as if something was lodged in the chest, has to be coughed up; lungs feel compressed. Cannot be fully expanded. Worse coughing; waterbrash succeeds cough. Choking sensation in the throat. Dyspnea worse lying down (orthopnea).

**Heart:** Sharp cutting pain the region of heart. Heart's action is labored and slow; tachycardia, bradycardia.

**Back:** Pain in the small of back.[1] Rheumatic pains and aching in bones.

**Sleep:** Wakeful and restless at night, with hunger. Bad dreams.

**Fever:** Alternate heat and cold; chronic intermittent fever, with pain in the stomach.

**Modalities:** *Worse* after eating.

**Relationship:** Compare: (Lump in stomach—*Chin.; Bry.; Puls.*) also other Conifers—*Thuj., Sabin., Cupressus lawsoniana* (painful indigestion) also *Nux-v., Kali-c.*

**Dose:** First to thirtieth potency.

---

# ABRUS PRECATORIUS—JEQUIRITY

(Crab's Eye Vine) **Abr.**

Epithelioma, lupus, ulcers, granular lids.

---

[1] Pain in the lumbar region (1001 Small Remedies, Edited by Dr. F. Schroyens).

**Eyes:** Purulent conjunctivitis; inflammation spreads to the face and neck. Granular ophthalmia (trachoma). Keratitis.

**Relationship:** Compare: *Jequiritol* (in cases of trachoma and pannus to engraft a new purulent inflammation. The proteid poisons in Jequirity seeds are almost identical in their physiological and toxic properties to those found in snake venom).

**Dose:** Mother tincture diluted locally and 3x internally.

---

## ABROTANUM—ARTEMISIA ABROTANUM

(Southernwood) **Abrot.**

A very useful remedy in *marasmus,* especially of the lower extremities, despite a good appetite. *Metastasis.* Rheumatism, following checked diarrhea. Ill effects of suppressed conditions especially in gouty subjects. *Tuberculous peritonitis. Exudative pleurisy* and other exudative processes. After surgery, for hydrothorax or empyema, a pressing sensation remains. Aggravation of hemorrhoids when rheumatism improves. Epistaxis and hydrocele in boys.

Great weakness after influenza (*Kali-p.*).

**Mind:** Cross, irritable, anxious, depressed.

**Face:** Wrinkled, cold, dry, pale. Blue rings around dull looking eyes. Comedones, with emaciation. Epistaxis. *Angioma of the face.*

**Stomach:** Slimy taste. Appetite good, but emaciation progresses. Food passes undigested (lienteria). Pain in the stomach; worse at night; cutting, gnawing pain. *Stomach feels as if swimming in water;* feels cold. Gnawing hunger and whining. Indigestion, with vomiting of large quantities of offensive fluid.

**Abdomen:** Hard lumps in different parts of the abdomen. *Distended.* Alternate diarrhea and constipation. Hemorrhoids. Frequent urging; bloody stools; worse as rheumatic pains abate. Ascarides. Oozing of blood and moisture from the umbilicus[1]. Sensation as if bowels were sinking.

**Respiratory:** Raw feeling. Impeded respiration. Dry cough following diarrhea. Pain across the chest; severe in the region of heart.

**Back:** Neck very weak, cannot hold head up. Back lame, weak, and painful. Pain in lumbar region extending along the spermatic cord. Pain in the sacrum, with hemorrhoids.

**Extremities:** Pain in the shoulders, arms, *wrists* and *ankles.* Pricking and coldness in fingers and feet (chilblains). *Legs* greatly emaciated. Joints stiff

---

1 especially in new borns (Clarke — Dictionary of Practical Materia Medica).

and lame. Painful contraction of limbs (*Am-m.*).

**Skin:** Eruptions on the face are suppressed, and the skin becomes purplish. Skin flabby and loose. Furuncles. Falling out of hair. Itching chilblains.

**Modalities:** *Worse,* cold air, checked secretions. *Better,* motion.

**Relationship:** Compare: *Scrophularia, Bry., Stel., Benz-ac.,* in gout. *Iod., Nat-m.* in marasmus.

**Dose:** Third to thirtieth potency.

---

# ABSINTHIUM

(Common Wormwood) **Absin.**

A perfect picture an epileptiform seizures is produced by this drug. Nervous tremors precede attack. Sudden and severe giddiness, delirium with hallucinations and loss of consciousness. Nervous excitement and sleeplessness. Cerebral irritation,[1] hysterical and infantile spasms come within the range of this remedy. Poisoning by mushrooms. Chorea. *Tremors.* Nervousness, excitement, and sleeplessness in children.

**Mind:** Hallucinations. Frightful visions. Kleptomania. Loss of memory. Forgets what has happened recently. Wants nothing to do with anybody. Brutal.

**Head:** *Vertigo, with a tendency to fall backward.* General confusion. Wants head low. Pupils dilated unequally. Dull occipital headache (*Gels., Pic-ac.*).

**Face:** Blue (cynosed). *Spasmodic facial twitchings.*

**Mouth:** Jaws fixed. Bites tongue; trembles seizure; feels as if swollen and too large; protruding.

**Throat:** Feels scalded; sensation of a lump.

**Stomach:** Nausea; retching; eructation. Bloated around the waist and *abdomen.* Flatulent colic.

**Urinary:** Constant desire. Very strong odor; deep yellow color (*Kali-p.*).

**Male:** Spermatorrhea, with relaxed enfeebled parts.

**Female:** Darting pain in the right ovary. Premature menopause.

**Heart:** Sensation of weight on the chest. Irregular, tumultuous action of the heart can be heard in the scapular region.

**Extremities:** Pain in limbs. Paralytic symptoms.

**Relationship:** Compare: *Alcoholus, Art-v., Hydr-ac., Cina, Cic.*

**Dose:** First to sixth potency.

---

1 congestion of brain and spine (Clarke - Dictionary of Practical Materia Medica).

# ACALYPHA INDICA

(Indian Nettle) **Acal.**

A drug having a marked action on the alimentary canal and respiratory organs. It is indicated in incipient phthisis, with hard, racking cough, bloody expectoration, arterial hemorrhage, but no febrile disturbance. Very weak in the morning, gains strength during the day. Progressive emaciation. All pathological hemorrhages having *a morning aggravation.*

**Abdomen:** Burning in the intestines. *Spluttering diarrhea with forcible expulsion of noisy flatus,* bearing down pains and tenesmus. Rumbling distention, and griping pain in the abdomen. Rectal hemorrhage; worse in the morning.

**Respiratory:** *Cough dry, hard, followed by hemoptysis;* worse in the morning and at night. Constant and severe pain in the chest. Blood bright red and profuse in the morning; dark and clotted in the afternoon. Pulse, soft and compressible. Burning in the pharynx, esophagus, and stomach.

**Skin:** Jaundiced. Itching and circumscribed furuncle-like swellings.

**Modalities:** *Worse* in the morning.

**Relationship:** Compare: *Mill., Phos., Acet-ac., Kali-n.*

**Dose:** Third to sixth potency.

---

# ACETANILIDUM—ANTIFEBRINUM

**Acetan.**

Depresses heart, respiration and blood pressure, lowers temperature. Cyanosis and collapse. Increased susceptibility to cold. Destroys red blood corpuscles; pallor (anemia).

**Head:** Enlarged sensation. Fainting. Moral depravity.

**Eyes:** Pallor of optic discs, contracted visual field and shrinking of retinal vessel; mydriasis.

**Heart:** Weak, irregular, with blue mucous membranes (cynosed), albuminuria, edema of feet and ankles.

**Relationship**: Compare: *Antip.*

**Dose:** Used as a sedative and antipyretic for various forms of headache and neuralgia in doses of one to three grains. For homeopathic indications, use the third potency.

---

# ACETICUM ACIDUM

(Glacial Acetic Acid) **Acet-ac.**

This drug produces a condition of profound anemia, with dropsy, great debility, frequent fainting, dyspnea, weak heart, vomiting, profuse micturition and sweat. Hemorrhage from any part. Especially indicated in pale, lean people, with lax, flabby muscles. *Wasting and debility. Acet-ac.* has the power to *liquify albuminous and fibrinous deposits.* Epithelial cancer, internally and locally (W. Owens). Sycosis with nodular formations in the joints.[1] Hard chancre. The 1x solution will soften and cause formation of pus.

**Mind:** Irritable, worried about business affairs.

**Head:** Nervous headache, from abuse of narcotics. Blood rushes to the head with delirium. Temporal vessels distended. Pain across the root of tongue.

**Face:** *Pale, waxy, emaciated.* Eyes sunken, surrounded by dark rings. Bright red. Sweaty. Epithelioma of lips. Cheeks hot and flushed. Aching in left temporo-mandebular joint.

**Stomach:** *Salivation. Fermentation* in the stomach. Intense burning thirst. Cold drinks distress. Vomits after every kind of food. Epigastric tenderness. Burning pain, as of an ulcer. Cancer of stomach. Sour belching and vomiting. Burning waterbrash and profuse salivation. Hyperchlorhydria and gastralgia. *Violent burning pains in the stomach and chest, followed by coldness of the skin and cold sweat on the forehead.* Stomach feels as if consumed a lot of vinegar.

**Abdomen:** Feels as if, the abdomen was sinking. Frequent watery stools, worse in the morning. *Tympanitic.* Ascites. Hemorrhage from bowels.

**Urinary:** Large quantities of pale urine. Diabetes, with great thirst and debility (*Ph-ac.*).

**Female:** Excessive catamenia. *Hemorrhages after labor.* Nausea of pregnancy. Breasts painfully enlarged (mastitis), distended with milk. Milk impoverished, bluish, transparent, sour. Anemia is nursing mothers.

**Respiratory:** Hoarse, hissing respiration; *difficulty in breathing; cough when inhaling.* Membranous croup. Irritation of trachea and bronchial tubes. False membrane in the throat (diphtheria). Profuse bronchorrhea. Fibrinous exudation in the throat (gargle).

**Back:** Pain in the back, *relieved only by lying on the abdomen.*

**Extremities:** Emaciation. Edema of feet and legs.

**Fever:** *Hectic, with drenching night sweats. Hyperemic spot on the left cheek. No thirst during fever.* Ebullitions. *Sweat profuse, cold.*

---

1 Phthisis (tubular nodules) in the joints (1001 Small Remedies, Edited by Dr. F. Schroyens).

**Skin:** Pale, waxy, edematous. Burning, dry, hot skin, or bathed in profuse sweat. Decreased sensations on the body surface. Useful after stings, bites, etc. Varicose swellings. Scurvy; *anasarca.* Bruises; sprains.

**Relationship:** *Acet-ac.* is antidotal to all anesthetic vapors. Counteracts sausage poisoning.

Compare: *Ammonium aceticum* (abundant saccharine in urine, patient is bathed in sweat). *Benzoin oderiferum*—Spice wood (*night sweats*). *Ars., Chin., Dig., Liat.* (*general anasarca in heart and* kidney disease, *dropsy,* and chronic diarrhea).

**Dose:** Third to thirtieth potency. Not to be repeated too often, except in croup.

---

# ACONITUM NAPELLUS

(Monkshood) **Acon.**

A state of fear, anxiety; anguish of mind and body. *Physical and mental restlessness,* and fright, are the most characteristic manifestations of *Aconitum. Acute, sudden, and violent invasion, with fever,* calls for it. Does not want to be touched. Sudden and great sinking of strength. *Complaints and tension* caused by exposure to *dry, cold weather,* draught of cold air, checked perspiration, also complaints from *very hot weather,* especially gastro-intestinal disturbances, etc. First remedy in inflammations, inflammatory fevers. Serous membranes and muscular tissues affected markedly. Burning in the internal parts; *tingling, coldness and numbness.* Influenza. *Tension* in arteries;[1] emotional, physical and mental tensions explain many symptoms. When prescribing *Aconitum* remember *Aconitum* causes only functional disturbance, there is no evidence that it can produce tissue changes—its action is brief and *shows no periodicity.* Its sphere is in the beginning of an acute disease and should not be continued after pathological changes come. In hyperemia, congestion, not after exudation has set in. *Influenza* (*Influenzinum).*

**Mind:** *Great fear, anxiety,* and worry accompany every ailment, however trivial. Delirium is characterized by unhappiness, worry, fear, raving, but the patient is rarely unconscious. *Forebodings and fears. Fears death* but believes that he will soon die; predicts the day. *Fears the future,* a crowd, crossing the street. *Restlessness,* tossing about. Tendency to start. Imagination acute, clairvoyance. Pains are intolerable; they drive him crazy. Music is unbearable; makes her sad (*Ambr.*). Thinks his thoughts come from the stomach that parts

---

[1] feels as if circulation was impeded in all vessels (Handbook of Materia Medica by T.F. Allen)

of his body are abnormally thick. Feels as if what had just been done was a dream.

**Head:** Fullness; *heavy,* pulsating, *hot, bursting,* burning, undulating sensation (apoplexy). Intracranial pressure (*Hed.*). Burning headache, sensation as if brain was agitated by boiling water.[1] (*Indg.*). Vertigo; *worse on rising* (*Nux-v., Op.*) and on shaking the head. Sensation as if hair were being pulled or were standing on end especially on the vertex. Nocturnal, furious delirium.

**Eyes:** Red, inflamed (acute conjunctivitis). Feels *dry and hot,* as if sand in them (trachoma). *Lids swollen, hard and red* (blepharitis). Aversion to light (photophobia). Profuse watering after exposure to dry, cold winds, *reflection from snow, after extraction of cinders* and other foreign bodies.

**Ears:** Very *sensitive to noises;* music is unbearable. External ear hot, red, painful, swollen. Otalgia (*Cham.*). Sensation as if a drop of water is in the left ear.

**Nose:** *Smell, acutely sensitive. Pain at the root of the nose.* Coryza; much sneezing; throbbing in the nostrils. Hemorrhage of bright red blood. *Mucous membrane dry, nose stopped up; dry or with scanty watery coryza.*

**Face:** Red, hot, flushed, swollen (mumps). One cheek red, the other pale (*Cham., Ip.*). *On rising, the red face becomes deathly pale, or he becomes dizzy. Tingling* in cheeks with numbness. *Neuralgia, especially of the left side, with restlessness, tingling, and numbness* (trigeminal neuralgia). Pain in jaws.

**Mouth:** Numb, *dry,* and tingling. Tongue swollen; *tip tingles* (glossitis). Teeth sensitive to cold. Constantly moves the lower jaw, as if chewing. *Gums hot and inflamed* (gingivitis). *Tongue coated white* (*Ant-c.*).

**Throat:** *Red, dry, constricted,* numb, prickling, burning, stinging. Tonsils swollen and dry (1st stage of tonsillitis).

**Stomach:** *Vomiting, with fear, heat, profuse sweat and increased micturition.* Thirst for cold water. *Bitter taste* of everything except water. *Intense thirst.* Drinks, vomits, and declares that he will die. Vomiting, bilious, mucoid, bloody and greenish. Pressure in the stomach with dyspnea. Hematemesis. Burning from the stomach to the esophagus.

**Abdomen:** Hot, tense, tympanitic (enteritis). *Sensitive to touch. Colic,* no position relieves. Abdominal symptoms better after warm soup. Burning in the umbilical region.

**Rectum:** Pain with nocturnal itching and stitching pains in the anus. Frequent, small stool with tenesmus; *green, like chopped herbs.* White with red urine. Choleric discharge with collapse, anxiety, and restlessness. Bleeding hemorrhoids (*Ham.*). Watery diarrhea in children (cholera infantum). They cry and complain a lot, are sleepless and restless.

---

[1] Heat and ebullition in the head, as if there was boiling water in the brain. (Clarke — Dictionary of Practical Materia Medica).

**Urinary:** *Scanty, red, hot, painful.* Tenesmus and burning at the neck of the bladder. Burning in the urethra. Urine suppressed, bloody (hematuria). Anxiety always on beginning to micturate. *Retention, with screaming and restlessness, and* handling of genitals. Renal region sensitive (nephritis). Profuse micturition, with profuse perspiration and diarrhea.

**Male:** Crawling and stinging in glans. Bruised pain in the testicles, swollen and hard (orchitis). Frequent erections and emissions. Painful erections.

**Female:** Vagina dry, hot, sensitive. Menses too profuse, with epistaxis, too protracted, late. Frenzy on appearance of menses. *Suppressed from fright, cold,* in plethoric subjects. Ovaries congested and painful. Sharp shooting pain in the womb. *After-pains, with fear and restlessness.*

**Respiratory:** Constant pressure in the left chest; *oppressed breathing* on least motion (asthma). *Hoarse, dry, croupy cough* (bronchitis); loud, labored breathing (pneumonia). Child grasps the throat every time he coughs (whooping cough). Very sensitive to inspired air. *Shortness of breath.* Larynx sensitive. Stitches through the chest (pleurisy, pleurodynia). Cough, dry, short, hacking; *worse at night and after midnight.* Hot feeling in the lungs. Blood comes up with hawking (hemoptysis, phthisis). Tingling in the chest after cough.

**Heart:** *Tachycardia.* Affections of the heart with pain in *the left shoulder.* Stitching pain in the chest (angina pectoris). *Palpitations, with anxiety,* fainting, and *tingling* in fingers. *Pulse full, hard; tense and bounding;* sometimes intermits. Temporal and carotid arteries felt when sitting.

**Back:** Numb, stiff, painful. Crawling and tingling, as if bruised. Stiffness in the nape of neck. Bruised pain between scapulae.

**Extremities:** *Numbness and tingling;* shooting pains; icy coldness and insensibility of hands and feet. Arms feel lame, bruised, heavy, numb. Pain down the left arm (*Cact., Crot-h., Kalm., Tab.*). *Hot hands and cold feet.* Rheumatic inflammation of joints; worse at night; red shiny swelling, very sensitive. Hip joint and thigh feel lame, especially after lying down. Knees unsteady; disposition of the foot to turn (*Aesc.*). Weak and lax ligaments of all joints. Painless cracking of all joints. *Bright red hypothenar eminences on both hands.* Sensation as if drops of water trickled down the thigh.

**Sleep:** Nightmares. Nocturnal ravings. *Anxious dreams.* Sleeplessness, with restlessness and tossing about. (Use thirtieth potency.) Starts in sleep. Long dreams, with anxiety in the chest. Insomnia in the aged.

**Fever:** Cold stage is most marked. Cold sweat and icy coldness of the face. Coldness and heat alternate. Evening chills soon after going to bed. *Cold waves pass through the body. Thirst and restlessness* always present. Chilly, if uncovered or touched. Dry heat, red face. Most valuable febrifuge with mental anxiety, restlessness, etc. Sweat drenching, on parts lain on; relieving all symptoms.

**Skin:** Red, hot, swollen, dry, burning. *Purpura miliaris.* Rash-like measles. Gooseflesh. Formication and numbness. Chilliness and formication down the back. Pruritus relieved by stimulants.

**Modalities:** *Better* in open air; *worse* in a warm room, in the evening and *at night; worse* lying on affected side, from music, from tobacco smoke, dry, cold winds.

**Relationship:** Vinegar in large doses is antidotal to its poisonous effects. Acids, wine, coffee, lemonade, and acid fruits modify its action.

Not indicated in malarial and low fevers or hectic and pyemic conditions, and in inflammations when they localize themselves. *Sulphur* often follows it. Compare *Cham.* and *Coff.* in *intense pain* and sleeplessness.

*Agrostis alba* acts like *Acon.* in fever and inflammations, also *Spiranthes autumnalis.*

Complementary: *Coff., Sulph. Sulphur* may be considered a chronic *Acon.* Often completes a cure begun with *Acon.*

Compare: *Bell., Cham., Coff., Ferr-p.*

*Aconitinum:* (Heavy feeling *as of lead;* pain in the supraorbital nerve; ice cold sensations creep up; symptoms of hydrophobia. Tinnitus aurius, 3x.) *Tingling* sensation.

*Aconitum lycoctonum*—Great yellow wolfsbane: Swelling of glands; Hodgkin's disease. Diarrhea after eating pork. Itching in nose, eyes, anus and vulva. Skin of nose cracked; tastes of blood.

*Aconitum cammarum:* Headache with vertigo and tinnitus. Cataleptic symptoms. Formication of tongue, lips and face.

*Aconitum ferox*—Indian Aconite: More violent in its actions than *Acon.* It is more diuretic and less antipyretic. It has proved valuable in *cardiac dyspnea,* neuralgia, and acute gout. *Dyspnea. Must sit up. Rapid respiration.* Anxiety, with suffocation, as if respiratory muscles are paralysed. Cheyne-Stokes respiration.

*Quebracho* (cardiac dyspnea).

*Achyranthes calea:* A Mexican drug, very similar to *Acon.* in fevers, but has a larger range, also adapted to typhoidal states and intermittent fevers. Muscular rheumatism. A great diaphoretic. Use 6x.

*Eranthis hymnalis*—Winter Aconite: Acts on the solar plexus and works upwards causing dyspnea. Pain in the occiput and neck.

**Dose:** Sixth potency for sensory affections; first to third for congestive conditions. Must be repeated frequently in acute diseases. *Acon.* is a rapid worker. In neuralgias, tincture of the root is often preferable, one drop doses (poisonous), or , the 30th potency, according to the susceptibility of the patient.

---

## ACTAEA SPICATA

(Baneberry) **Act-sp.**

Is a rheumatic remedy, especially of the *small joints;* tearing, tingling pains characterize it. *Wrist rheumatism.* Pulsations over whole body, especially in the liver (hepatitis) and renal region. Cardiovascular spasm. Pains worse from touch and motion.

**Head:** Fearful, starts easily; confused. Ebullition of blood to the head, excited by drinking coffee. Vertigo, tearing headache, better in the open air, throbbing in the brain, pain from the crown to between the eyebrows; heat in the forehead, pain in the left frontal eminence as if the bone was crushed. Itching of scalp alternating with heat. Red tip of nose, fluent coryza.

**Face:** Violent pain in the upper jaw, from the teeth through the malar bones to the temples. Perspiration on face and head.

**Stomach:** Tearing, darting pains in the epigastric region, with vomiting (cancer of stomach). Cramp-like pains in the stomach and epigastrium, with difficult breathing;[1] sense of suffocation. Sudden lassitude after eating.

**Abdomen:** Spasmodic retraction. Sticking pain and distention of hypogastrium.

**Respiratory:** Short, irregular breathing at night, while lying. *Great oppression. Shortness of breath on exposure to cold air.*

**Extremities:** Tearing pain in loins. *Rheumatic pains in small joints,* wrist (*Ulm.*), fingers, *ankles,* toes. *Swelling of joints from slight fatigue. Wrist swollen,* red, worse any motion. Paralytic weakness in the hands. Lame feeling in arms. Pain in knee. Sudden lassitude after talking or eating.

**Relationship:** Compare: *Caul., Cimic., Led.*

**Dose:** Third potency.

---

## ADONIS VERNALIS

(Pheasant's Eye) **Adon.**

A heart medicine, after rheumatism or influenza, or Bright's disease, where the muscles of the heart are in a stage of fatty degeneration, regulates the pulse and increases the power of contractions of the heart, with increased urinary secretions. Most valuable in cardiac dropsy. Low vitality, with a weak heart and slow, weak pulse. Hydrothorax, ascites. Anasarca.

---

1 Difficult inspiration, stiches in epigastric region during deep breathing (pleurisy) (Clarke — Dictionary of Practical Materia Medica).

**Head:** Feels light; aches across the front, from *occiput around the temples to the eyes.* Vertigo on rising, turning the head quickly or on lying down. Tinnitus. Scalp feels tight. Eyes dilated.

**Mouth:** Slimy. Tongue dirty yellow, sore, feels scalded.

**Stomach:** Heavy weight. Gnawing hunger. Faint feeling in the epigastrium. Better outdoors.

**Urinary:** Oily pellicle on urine. Scanty, albuminous.

**Respiratory:** Frequent desire to take a long breath. Sensation of weight on chest.

**Heart:** Mitral and aortic regurgitation. Chronic aortitis. Fatty heart pericarditis. Rheumatic endocarditis (*Kalm.*). *Precordial pain, palpitations, and dyspnea.* Marked venous engorgement. Cardiac asthma (*Queb.*). Fatty heart. Myocarditis, irregular cardiac action, constriction and vertigo. Pulse rapid, irregular.

**Extremities:** Aching in nape. Spine stiff and aching. Edema.

**Sleep:** Restless, with horrible dreams.

**Relationship:** *Adonidinum* is a cardiac tonic and diuretic. Quarter grain daily, or two to five grains of first decimal trituration. Increases arterial pressure and prolongs the diastole, favoring emptying of engorged veins. It is an excellent substitute for *Dig.* and is not cumulative in action.

Compare: *Dig., Crat., Conv., Stroph-h.*

**Dose:** Five to ten drops of the tincture.

---

## ADRENALINUM

(An Internal Secretion of Suprarenal Glands) **Adren.**

*Adrenalin* or *Epinephrin*, the active principle of the medulla of the suprarenal gland (cortical secretion not as yet isolated), is employed as a chemical messenger in the regulation of the activities of the body; in fact, its presence is essential for the activity of the sympathetic nerves. Action of *Adren.* on any part is the same as *the stimulation of sympathetic nerve endings* thereto. Local application (1:1,000 solution) on the mucous membranes promptly induces transient ischemia, seen as *blanching,* persisting several hours after conjunctival instillation. Its action is very prompt, efficient, *evanescent,* owing to rapid oxidation and is practically harmless, *unless* repeated too frequently as in atheroma and myocardial heart lesions (in animals it has been reported). Arteries, heart, suprarenal bodies and the vasomotor system are prominently affected.

The main action of *Adrenalinum* is stimulation of the *sympathetic nerve endings,* notably in the splanchnic area, causing *constriction of the peripheral arterioles,* resulting *in the rise of blood pressure.* This is especially observed in the stomach, and intestines; less in the uterus, and skin; nil in the brain and lungs. Furthermore, it *slows the pulse,* (medullary vagus stimulation), and *strengthens the heart beat* (increased myocardial contractility), resembling *Dig.*; increased glandular activity, glycosuria; depression of the respiratory center; contraction of the muscular tissue is the eye, uterus, vagina; and relaxation of the muscular tissue of the stomach, intestines, and bladder.

**Uses:** Its chief therapeutic use depends on its *vaso-constriction* action; therefore it is a powerful and prompt *astringent* and *hemostatic;* is invaluable *in checking* capillary hemorrhages from *all* parts, where *local* or direct application is feasible; nose, ear, mouth, throat, larynx, stomach, rectum, uterus, bladder. Hemorrhagic conditions not due to defective coagulation of the blood. Complete *bloodlessness,* ischemia, may be induced with impunity. Locally, solutions (1:10,000—1:1,000) sprayed or applied with cotton have been very efficient in bloodless operations of the eye, nose, throat, and larynx.

Congestions of the ethmoidal and sphenoidal sinuses, also hay fever, have been markedly alleviated by a warm spray of Adrenalin chloride, 1:5,000. Here compare, *Hep.* 1x, which will start secretions and so facilitate drainage. Werlhoff's disease, hypodermically, 1:1,000. Externally, it has been used in neuritis, neuralgias, reflex pains, gout, rheumatism, and as an ointment, 1-2 m. of (1:1,000) solution, along the nerve trunk at a point on the skin nearest to origin which can be reached (H.G. Carlton).

Therapeutically, *Adrenalinum* has been suggested in acute congestion of lungs, *asthma,* Grave's and Addison's diseases, arteriosclerosis, chronic aortitis, angina pectoris, hemophilia, chlorosis, hay fever, serum rashes, acute urticaria, etc. Dr. P. Jousset reports success in treating, homeopathically, cases of angina and of aortitis, sub-acute and chronic, when *Adrenalinum* has been prescribed *per os* and in infinitesimal dose. The symptom guiding to this is, *sensation of thoracic constriction with anxiety.* This, with vertigo, nausea and vomiting have been produced by the drug. *Abdominal pain. Shock or heart failure during anesthesia,* it causes a very prompt rise in the blood pressure by its action on the nerve endings in the vessel wall.

**Dose:** Hypodermically, 1-5 m. (1:1,000 solution, as chloride) diluted in water. Internally, 5-30 m. of 1:1,000 solution.

*Caution:* On account of its affinity for oxygen, the drug easily decomposes in watery and dilute acid solutions. The solution must be protected from air and light. It must not be repeated too frequently, owing to cardiac and arterial lesions. For homeopathic use 2x to 6x attenuation.

---

# AESCULUS HIPPOCASTANUM

(Horse Chestnut) **Aesc.**

The action of this drug is most marked on the lower bowel, producing engorged hemorrhoidal veins, with characteristic backache, and absence of actual constipation. Severe pain but little bleeding. General venous stasis, varicose veins in purple color; everything is slowed down, digestion, heart, bowels, etc. Torpor and congestion of the liver and portal system, with constipation. Severe backache rendering the patient unfit for business. Flying pains all over. *Fullness in various parts;* dry, swollen mucous membranes. Throat with hemorrhoidal conditions.[1]

**Head:** Depressed and *irritable.* Head dull, confused, aching as from a cold. Pressure on the forehead, with nausea, followed by stitches in the right hypochondrium. Pain from the occiput to the frontal region, with a bruised sensation of the scalp; worse in the morning. Neuralgic stitches from right to left through the forehead followed by flying pains in the epigastrium. Vertigo when sitting and walking.

**Eyes:** Heavy and hot, with lachrymation, *with enlarged blood vessels.* Eyeballs sore.

**Nose:** Dry; inspired air feels cold, *nasal passages sensitive to it. Coryza,* sneezing. Pressure at the root of the nose. Membrane over turbinate bones distended and boggy, dependent upon hepatic disorders.

**Mouth:** Scalded feeling. Metallic taste. Salivation. Tongue thickly coated, feels as if scalded.

**Throat:** Hot, *dry,* raw, stitching pains radiating to the ears when swallowing. Follicular pharyngitis connected with hepatic congestion. *Veins of the pharynx distended* and tortuous. Throat sensitive to inspired air; feels excoriated and constricted, burns like fire on swallowing, in the afternoon. Early stages of atrophic pharyngitis in dried up, bilious subjects. Hawking of ropy mucus with a sweetish taste. *Laryngitis;* cough *depending on liver disorders.*

**Stomach:** Weight, as of a stone, with gnawing, aching pains; maximum about three hours after meals.

**Abdomen:** Tenderness and fullness in the region of the liver. Dull aching in the liver region and epigastrium. Pain in the umbilical region. Jaundice; throbbing in the hypogastrium and pelvis.

**Rectum:** Dry, aching. *Feels full of small sticks.* Anus raw, sore. Severe pain after stool, with prolapse. *Hemorrhoids,* with sharp shooting pains up the

[1] Follicular inflammation of the posterior wall (Handbook of Materia Medica by T.F. Allen).

back; blind and bleeding; worse during climacteric. Large, hard, dry stools. Mucous membrane seems swollen and obstructs the passage. Irritation caused by ascarides, aids their expulsion. *Burning in the anus with chills up and down the back.*

**Urinary:** Frequent, scanty, dark, muddy, hot. Pain in kidneys, especially left and ureter.

**Male:** Discharge of prostatic fluid during stool (prostatorrhea).

**Female:** *Constant throbbing behind symphysis pubis.* Leucorrhea, with *lameness of the back, across the sacro-iliac articulation;* dark yellow, sticky, corroding; worse after menses.

**Heart:** Feels constricted. Heart's action full and heavy, can feel pulsations all over. Sensation of heat in the chest; pain around the region of heart in hemorrhoidal subjects.

**Back:** Lameness in the neck; aching between the shoulder blades (cervical spondylosis); region of *spine feels weak;* back and legs give out. *Backache affecting sacrum and hips; worse walking or stooping.* When walking, feet turn under. Soles feel sore, tired and swollen. Hands and feet swell, and become red after washing, feel full.

**Extremities:** Aching and soreness in the limbs, in the left acromion process radiating to the arms; finger tips numb.

**Fever:** Chill at 4 p.m. Chills run up and down the back. Fever, 7 p.m. to 12 p.m. Evening fever, skin hot and dry. Sweat profuse and hot with fever.

**Modalities:** *Worse,* in the morning on awaking, and from any motion, *walking;* from moving bowels; after eating, afternoon, standing. *Better,* cool open air.

**Relationship:** *Aesculus glabra*—Ohio buckeye: Proctitis. Very painful, dark purple, external hemorrhoids, with constipation, vertigo and portal congestion. Speech thick, tickling in throat, impaired vision, paresis. *Phytolacca decandra* (throat dry, more often in acute cases). *Negundium americanum*—Boxelder (engorgements of rectum and piles with severe pain, ten drop doses of tincture, every two hours.)

Compare also: *Aloe, Coll., Nux-v., Sulph.*

**Dose:** Tincture to third potency.

---

## AETHIOPS MINERALIS

(Sulphur and Quicksilver, Black Sulphide of Mercury)

**Aethi-m.**

This preparation is of use in *scrofulous* affections, ophthalmia, otorrhea; painful, irritating, scabby eruptions, and hereditary syphilis.

**Skin:** Eruptions. Favus-like, scrofulous, herpetic and eczematous.

**Relationship:** *Aethiops antimonialis*—Hydrargyrum stibiato sulfuratum (often more effective than the above in scrofulous eruptions, glandular swellings, otorrhea and *scrofulous eye affections,* corneal ulcers. Third trituration.)

Compare: *Calc., Sil., Psor.*

**Dose:** The lower triturations, especially the second decimal.

---

## AETHUSA CYNAPIUM

(Fool's Parsley) **Aeth.**

The characteristic symptoms relate mainly to the brain and nervous system, connected with gastro-intestinal disturbance. Anguish, crying, and an expression of uneasiness and discontentment, lead to this remedy, most frequently in diseases of children, during dentition, summer complaints, accompanied by diarrhea, with a *marked inability to digest milk,* and poor circulation. Symptoms set in with *violence.*

**Mind:** Restless, *anxious, crying.* Sees rats, cats, dogs, etc. Unconscious, delirious. *Inability to think, to fix the attention.* Brain fag. Idiocy may alternate with furor and irritability.

**Head:** Feels bound up, or in a vise. *Occipital pain* extending down the spine; better lying down and by pressure. Head symptoms relieved by expelling flatus (*Sang.*) and by stool. *Hair feels pulled. Vertigo with drowsiness, with palpitation; head hot after vertigo ceases.*

**Eyes:** Photophobia; *swelling of Meibomian glands.* Rolling of eyes on falling asleep. *Eyes drawn downward;* pupils dilated (epilepsy). Squinting of eyes downward.

**Ears:** *Feel obstructed.* Sense of something hot escaping from the ears. Hissing sound.

**Nose:** Stopped up with a lot of thick mucus. *Herpetic eruption* on the tip of the nose. Frequent ineffectual desire to sneeze.

**Face:** *Puffed,* red spotted, collapsed. Expression anxious, full of pain; *linea nasalis* marked.

**Mouth:** Dry. Aphthae. Tongue seems too long. Burning and pustules in the throat, with dysphagia.

**Stomach:** *Intolerance of milk;* vomiting as soon as swallowed or in large curds. Hungry after vomiting. *Regurgitation of food about an hour after eating.* Violent vomiting of a white frothy matter. Nausea at the sight of food. Painful contractions of the stomach. Vomiting, *with sweat and great prostration,* accompanied by anxiety and distress, followed by sleepiness. Stomach feels as if turned upside down, with heartburn. Tearing pains in the stomach extending to the esophagus.

**Abdomen:** Cold, internally and externally, with aching pain in bowels. Colic, followed by vomiting, vertigo, and weakness. Tense, inflated, and sensitive. Bubbling sensation around the navel.

**Stool:** Undigested, *thin, greenish,* preceded by colic, tenesmus, and followed by exhaustion and drowsiness. Cholera infantum; child cold, clammy, stupid, with staring eyes and dilated pupils. Obstinate constipation; feels as if action of bowels is lost. Choleraic affections in old age.

**Urinary:** Cutting pain in the bladder, with frequent urging. Pain in kidneys.

**Female:** Lancinating pains in sexual organs. Pimples; itching when warm. Menses watery. Swelling of mammary glands (mastitis), with lancinating pains.

**Respiratory:** Difficult, oppressed, anxious respiration; crampy constriction. Sufferings renders the patient speechless.

**Heart:** Violent palpitations, with vertigo, headache and restlessness. Pulse rapid, hard and small.

**Back and Extremities:** Want of power to stand up or to hold head up. Back feels as if in a vise. Aching in the lumbosacral region Weakness of lower extremities. Fingers and thumbs clenched (epilepsy). Numbness of hands and feet. Violent spasms (convulsions).

**Sleep:** Disturbed by *violent startings;* cold perspiration. Dozing after vomiting or stool. *Child is so exhausted, it falls asleep at once.*

**Fever:** *Great heat; no thirst.* Profuse, cold sweat. *Must be covered during sweat.*

**Skin:** Excoriation of thighs on walking.[1] Easy perspiration. *Surface of body cold and covered with clammy sweat. Lymphatic glands swollen* (lymphadenopathy). Itching *eruptions around joints.* Skin of hands dry and shrunken. Ecchymosis. Anasarca.

**Modalities:** *Worse,* 3 to 4 a. m., and in the evenings; warmth, summers. *Better* in open air and in company.

---

[1] Skin sensitive, rubbing of trousers causes an acute sting (1001 Small Remedies, Edited by Dr. F. Schroyens).

**Relationship**: Compare: *Athamantha oreoselinum* (confused head, vertigo better lying down, *bitter* taste and saliva. Hands and feet icy cold); *Ant., Calc., Ars., Cic.*

Complementary: *Calc.*

**Dose:** Third to thirtieth potency.

---

# AGARICUS MUSCARIUS —AMANITA MUSCARIA

(Toad Stool, Bug Agaric) **Agar.**

This fungus contains several toxic compounds, the best known of which is *Muscarin.* The symptoms of poisoning do not develop at once, usually twelve to fourteen hours elapse before the initial attack. There is no antidote, treatment is entirely symptomatic (Schneider). *Agar.* acts as an intoxicant to the brain, producing more vertigo and delirium than alcohol, followed by profound sopor with lowered reflexes.

Jerking, twitching, trembling, and itching are strong indications. Incipient phthisis; is related to the tubercular diathesis, anemia, *chorea;* twitchings cease during sleep. Various forms of neuralgias and spasmodic affections. Neurotic skin problems are pictured in the symptomatology of this remedy. It corresponds to various forms of cerebral excitement rather than congestion. Thus, is indicated in delirium of fevers, alcoholism (delirium tremens), etc. General paralysis. *Sensation as if pierced by needles of ice.* Sensitive to pressure and cold air. *Violent bearing down pains.* Symptoms appear diagonally like the *right arm and left leg.* Pains are accompanied by sensation of coldness, numbness and tingling.

**Mind:** Sings, talks, but does not answer. *Loquacity.* Aversion to work. Indifference. *Fearless. Delirium* characterized by singing, shouting, and muttering; rhymes and prophesies. Begins with a paroxysm of yawning.

The provings bring out four phases of cerebral excitement:

1. *Slight stimulation*—shown by increased cheerfulness, courage, loquacity, exalted fancy.
2. *More decided intoxication*—great mental excitement and incoherent talking, immoderate gaity alternates with melancholy. Perception of relative size of objects is lost, takes long steps and jumps over small objects as if they were trunks of trees, a small hole appears as a frightful chasm, a spoonful of water, an immense lake. Physical strength is increased, can lift heavy loads. Twitching accompanies all symptoms.

3. *Third stage*—produces a condition of furious or raging delirium, screaming, raving, wants to injure himself, etc.
4. *Fourth stage*—mental depression, languor, indifference, confusion, disinclination to work, etc. We do not get the active cerebral congestion of *Belladonna*, but a general nervous excitement such as is found in delirium tremens, delirium of fevers, etc.

**Head:** *Vertigo from sunlight,* and on walking. Head in constant motion (epilepsy). Falling backward, as if a weight was put on the occiput (meningitis). Lateral headache, as if from a nail (*Coff., Ign.*). Dull headache from prolonged desk work. Icy coldness, *like icy needles,* or splinters. Neuralgia with an icy cold head. Desire to cover the head warmly (*Sil.*). Headache with *epistaxis* or a thick mucoid discharge.

**Eyes:** *Reading difficult, as type seems move, swim.* Vibrating specters. *Diplopia* (*Gels.*), dim and flickering. Asthenopia from prolonged strain, *spasm* of accommodation. *Twitching of lids and eyeballs* (*Cod.*). Margins of lids red; itch, burn and agglutinate (blepharitis). Inner canthi very red.

**Ears:** Burn and itch, as if frozen (frost bite). Twitching of muscles around the ear and *noises* (tinnitus).

**Nose:** *Nervous* nasal disturbances. *Itching* internally and externally. Spasmodic sneezing after coughing; sensitiveness; watery non-inflammatory discharge. Inner angles very red. Fetid, dark, bloody discharge. *Epistaxis in old people.* Sensation of soreness in the nose and mouth.

**Face:** *Facial* muscles feel stiff; *twitch;* face itches and burns. Lancinating, tearing pain in cheeks, as of splinters. Neuralgia, as if cold needles ran through the nerves or sharp pieces of ice touched them.

**Mouth:** Burning and smarting of lips. Herpes labialis . Twitching. Taste sweet. Aphthae at the roof of the mouth. Splinter-like pains in the tongue. Thirsty all the time. Tremulous tongue (*Lach.*). Tongue white.

**Throat:** Stitches along the eustachian tube to the ear. Feels contracted. Small solid balls of phlegm thrown up. Dryness of pharynx, dysphagia. Scratching in the throat; cannot sing a note.

**Stomach:** Empty eructations, tasting of apples. Nervous disturbances, with spasmodic contractions, hiccough. Unnatural hunger. Flatulent distention of the stomach and abdomen. Profuse inodorous flatus. Burning in the stomach, about three hours after a meal, followed by a dull pressure. *Gastric disturbance with sharp pains in the liver region.*

**Abdomen:** Stitching pains in the liver, *spleen* (*Cean.*) and abdomen. Stitches under the short ribs, left side. Diarrhea with much fetid flatus. Fetid stools.

**Urinary:** Stitches in urethra. Sudden and violent urge to micturate. Frequent micturition.

**Female:** Menses, profuse and early. Itching and tearing, pressing pains in genitals and back. Spasmodic dysmenorrhea. Severe *bearing down pains, especially after menopause.* Sexual excitement. Nipples itch, burn. Complaints following parturition and coitus. Leucorrhea, with severe itching.

**Respiratory:** Violent attacks of cough that can be suppressed by effort of will, worse eating, pain in the head while cough lasts. Spasmodic cough at night after falling asleep, *with expectoration of little balls of mucus.* Labored, oppressed breathing. *Cough ends in a sneeze.*

**Heart:** *Irregular, tumultuous palpitations,* after tobacco. Pulse intermittent and irregular. Cardiac region oppressed, as if the thorax was too narrow. Palpitations with hyperemia of the face.

**Back:** Pain, *spine sensitive to touch;* worse in the dorsal region. Lumbago; worse in open air. Crick in the back. *Twitching of cervical muscles.*

**Extremities:** Stiff all over. Pain over the hips. Rheumatism, better motion. Weakness in loins. Uncertain gait. Trembling. *Itching of toes and feet as if frozen or as if from chilblains.* Cramps in the soles. Pain in the shin bone. Neuralgia in locomotor ataxia. Paralysis of lower limbs, with spasmodic condition of arms. Numbness of legs on crossing them. Paralytic pain in the left arm followed by palpitations. Tearing, painful contractions in the calves.

**Sleep:** *Paroxysms of yawning.* Restless from violent itching and burning. On falling asleep, *starts, twitches, and wakes up often.* Vivid dreams. Drowsy during the day. Yawning, followed by involuntary laughter.

**Fever:** Very sensitive to cool air. Violent attacks of heat in the evening. Copious sweat. Burning spots.

**Skin:** *Burning, itching, hyperemia, and swelling, as from frostbites.* Pimples, hard, like flea bites. Miliary eruption, with intolerable itching and burning. Chilblains. Angioneurotic edema; acne, rosacea. Swollen veins (phlebismus) with cold skin. Circumscribed erythematous, papular, pustular and edematous lesions.

**Modalities:** *Worse,* open cold air, after eating, after coitus. In cold weather, before a thunderstorm. *Worse,* pressure on dorsal spine, which causes involuntary laughter. *Better,* moving about slowly.

**Relationship:** Compare: *Muscarinum,* the alkaloid of *Agar.* (has much power over secretions, increasing lachrymal, salivary and hepatic secretions but diminishes renal secretions; probably neurotic in origin, stimulating the terminal fibres of the secretory nerves of all these structures, hence *salivation, lachrymation and excessive perspiration. Atropinum* exactly opposes *Muscarinum.* Resembles *Pilocarpinum* in action). *Amanita verna*—Spring mushroom—a variety of *Agaricus phalloides*—Death cup—active principle is *Phallin,* active like *Muscarinum.* The poison is a toxalbumin, resembling the poison of rattle snake and the poison excreted by the cholera and diphtheria germs. It acts on the red blood corpuscles, dissolving them so that blood escapes into the alimentary canal and the entire system is drained. The amount of this toxic principle is small, even handling of specimens and breathing of spores can be harmful to affect some people. The effects of poison develop slowly. Even 12 to 20 hours after taking it, the patient feels all right, but vertigo, violent cholera-like symptoms with rapid loss of strength and death by the second or third day, preceded by stupor and spasms occur. Fatty degeneration of liver, heart and kidneys, hemorrhages in the lungs, pleura and skin (Dr. J. Schier). Vomiting and purging. Continuous urging to stool, but *no* gastric, abdominal or rectal pain. Intense thirst for cold water, dry skin. Lethargic but mentally clear. *Sharp changes* from rapid to slow and from slow to rapid breathing, extreme collapse, suppressed urine, but *no* cold extremities or cramps). *Agaricus emeticus* (severe vertigo; all symptoms *better, cold water; longing for ice cold water;* gastritis, cold sweat, vomiting, sensation as if stomach was suspended by a string). *Tamus communis* (chilblains and freckles). *Cimic., Cann-i., Hyos., Tarantula hispanica.*

Antidotes: *Absin., Coff., Camph.*

**Dose:** Third to thirtieth and two hundredth potency. In skin affections and brain exhaustions give the lower attenuations

---

## AGAVE AMERICANA

(Century Plant) **Agav-a.**

Indicated in stomach ache, and painful erections in gonorrhea. Strangury. Hydrophobia. Scurvy; countenance pale, gums swollen and bleeding (scorbutic), legs covered with dark purple blotches (ecchymosis, petichea), swollen, painful and hard. Appetite poor; bowels constipated.

**Relationship:** Compare: *Anh., Lyss., Lach.*

**Dose:** Tincture.

---

## AGNUS CASTUS

(The Chaste Tree) **Agn.**

The most effective point of attack of *Agnus castus* on the organism is the sexual organs. It lowers sexual vitality, corresponding with mental depression and loss of nervous energy. It shows this distinctive influence in both sexes, but is more pronounced in men. Premature old age from abuse of sexual power.

History of repeated gonorrhea. A prominent remedy for sprains and strains. *Gnawing itching in all parts, especially eyes.* Tachycardia caused by tobacco in neurotic young men.

**Mind:** Sexual melancholy. Fear of death. *Sadness with impression of speedy death.* Absentminded, forgetful, lack of courage. Illusions of smell, herings, musk. Nervous depression and mental forebodings.

**Eyes:** *Pupils dilated* (*Bell.*). Itching around the eyes; photophobia.

**Nose:** Odor of hering or musk. Aching on the dorsum, better pressure.

**Abdomen:** Splenomegaly, spleen is swollen and sore. Stools soft, recede, difficult. Deep fissures in the anus. Nausea with *sensation as if intestines were pressed downwards;* wants to support bowels (ascites).

**Male:** Yellow discharge from urethra (gonorrhea). No erections. *Impotence. Parts cold, relaxed. Desire gone* (*Sel., Con., Sabal*). Scanty emission without ejaculation. Loss of prostatic fluid on straining (prostatorrhea). Gleety discharge. Testicles, cold, swollen, hard, and painful (orchitis).

**Female:** Scanty menses. Abhorrence of sexual intercourse. Relaxation of genitals, with leucorrhea. *Agalactia;* with sadness. Sterility. Leucorrhea staining yellow; transparent. Hysterical palpitation with epistaxis.

**Relationship:** Compare: *Camph., Lyc., Ph-ac., Sel.*

**Dose:** First to sixth potency.

---

## AGRAPHIS NUTANS

(Bluebell) **Agra.**

Generally, a relaxed condition of the system, prone to take cold on exposure to cold winds.

Catarrhal conditions; obstruction of nostrils. *Adenoids, throat deafness.*[1] *Enlarged tonsils.* Mucoid diarrhea from cold. Chill from cold winds. Throat and ear problems *with a tendency to free discharge from the mucous membranes.* Mutinism of childhood unconnected with deafness.

**Relationship:** Compare: *Hydr., All-c., Calc-p., Sul-i., Calc-i.*

**Dose:** Third potency. Single doses of tincture (Dr. Cooper).

---

[1] Hearing - impaired - tonsils enlarged (1001 Small Remedies, Edited by Dr. F. Schroyens).

# AILANTHUS GLANDULOSA

(Chinese Sumach) **Ail.**

This remedy shows by its peculiar skin symptoms its pronounced power of disorganizing the blood,[1] causing conditions seen in low grade fevers, low types of eruptive diseases, diphtheria, *follicular tonsillitis,* streptococcal infection, gangrene, hemorrhagic diathesis, etc. *The skin appears livid or purplish;* face dark as mahogany, hot; sordes; throat swollen, purple, livid; semi-conscious, delirious (meningitis); weak pulse, general torpor and prostration. Symptoms remarkably similar to malignant scarlatina. Diarrhea, dysentery and *profound prostration* are very marked. *Adynamia* characterizes all its conditions. Lividity, stupor and malignancy. Mucous membranes hemorrhagic and ulcerative (*Lach.; Ars.*).

**Mind:** General stupor with a sighing confused mind. Mental depression.

**Head:** *Headache, frontal* with drowsiness. Passive, congestive headaches.

**Eyes**: *Suffused, dilated eyes;* photophobia.

**Nose:** *Thin, copious, ichorous,* bloody nasal discharge.

**Face**: Dusky.

**Mouth:** *Tongue dry and brown. Teeth covered with sordes.*

**Throat**: Inflamed, edematous, dusky red. *Marked swelling, internally and externally.* Dry, rough, scraping, choking feeling. *Neck tender and swollen.* Hoarse, croupy voice. *Pain during swallowing,* extends to the ears (dysphagia).

**Respiratory:** Hurried breathing; irregular. Dry, hacking cough. Lungs sore and tired.

**Sleep:** Drowsy, restless. Heavy, disturbed, unrefreshing.

**Skin:** Miliary, livid rash, returns annually. Large blisters filled with a dark serum. *Irregular, patchy, livid eruptions,* disappearing on pressure. Cold. Raynaud's disease.

**Relationship:** Antidotes: *Rhus-t., Nux-v.*

Compare: *Am-c., Bapt., Arn., Mur-ac., Lach., Rhus-t.*

**Dose:** First to sixth potency.

---

# ALETRIS FARINOSA

(Stargrass) **Alet.**

An anemic, relaxed condition, especially in females, is protrayed by this remedy. The patient *is tired all the time,* and suffers from prolapsus, leucorrhea, rectal distress, etc. Marked anemia. Chlorotic girls and pregnant women.

---

1 Septicemia, blood poisoning (1001 Small Remedies, Edited by Dr F. Schroyens).

**Mind:** Power and energy weakened. Confused feelings. Cannot concentrate. Fainting, with vertigo.

**Mouth:** Increased, frothy saliva.

**Stomach:** Disgust for food. Least food causes distress. Fainting spells, with vertigo. Vomiting during pregnancy. Nervous dyspepsia. Flatulent colic.

**Rectum:** Loads up with feces, paretic condition. Stool large, hard, difficult accompanied with, great pain.

**Female:** *Premature and profuse menses* (menorrhagia), *with labor- like pains* (dysmenorrhea) (*Bell., Cham., Kali-c., Plat.*). Retarded and scanty flow *(Senec.).* Uterus seems heavy. Prolapse, with pain in the right inguinal region. Leucorrhea due to weakness and anemia. Habitual tendency to abortion. Muscular pains during pregnancy.

**Relationship:** Compare: *Helon., Hydr., Tanac., Chin.*

**Dose:** Tincture to third potency.

---

## ALFALFA

(Medicago Sativa, California Clover, Lucerne) **Alf.**

From its action on the sympathetic nerves, *Alfalfa* favorably influences nutrition, evidenced by the "toning up" of appetite and digestion, resulting in a greatly improved mental and physical vigor, with gain in weight. Disorders characterized by malnutrition are mainly within its therapeutic range, for example, neurasthenia, splanchnic blues, nervousness, insomnia, nervous indigestion, etc. Acts as a fat producer, corrects tissue waste. Deficient lactation. Increases quality and quantity of milk in nursing mothers. Its pronounced urinary action suggests it clinically in diabetes insipidus and phosphaturia; and it is claimed to allay cystitis of prostatic hypertrophy. The rheumatic diathesis seems especially amenable to its action.

**Mind:** It induces mental exhilaration of buoyancy, *i.e.,* a general feeling of well being; clear and bright, so that all blues are dissipated. Dull, drowsy, stupid (*Gels.*); gloomy and irritable, worse during evening.

**Head:** Dull, heavy feeling in the occiput, in and above the eyes, worse towards evening. Pain on the left side of the head. Violent headache.

**Ears:** Stuffed feeling in the eustachian tubes (*Kali-m.*) at night; patulous in the morning.

**Stomach:** Increased thirst. Appetite impaired, but chiefly increased, even to bulimia. Must *eat* frequently, cannot wait for regular meals; hungry in the forenoon (*Sulph.*). Much nibbling of food and craving for sweets.

**Abdomen:** Flatulence with distention. Shifting, flatulent pain along the colon several hours after meals. Frequent, loose, yellow, painful stools, with excoriating flatulence. Chronic appendicitis.

**Urinary:** Kidneys inactive; frequent urging to micturate. Polyuria (*Ph-ac.*). Increased elimination of urea, indican and phosphates.

**Sleep:** Slept better than usual, especially, early morning; it induces a quiet, reposeful and refreshing sleep.

**Relationship:** Compare: *Aven., Dip., Gels., Hydr., Kali-p., Ph-ac.; Zinc.*

**Dose:** The best results are elicited with material doses (5-10) drops of tincture, several times a day. Continue its use until tonic effects ensue.

---

## ALLIUM CEPA

(Red Onion) **All-c.**

A picture of coryza, with *acrid nasal* discharge and laryngeal symptoms, eye secretions *bland;* singers cold, *worse in a warm room* and towards evening; better in open air. Specially adapted to phlegmatic patients; colds in *damp, cold weather.* Neuralgic pains, *like a fine thread,* following amputations or injuries to nerves. Traumatic, chronic neuritis. Burning in the nose, mouth, throat, bladder and skin. Sensation of glowing heat on different parts of the body.

**Head:** Catarrhal headache, mostly in the forehead; *worse in a warm room,* towards evening. Thread-like pains in the face. Headache ceases during menses; returns when flow disappears.

**Eyes:** Red. Intense *burning* (conjunctivitis). *Sensitive to light* (photophobia). Eyes suffused and watery; profuse, *bland* lachrymation, better in open air. Burning in eyelids.

**Ears:** Otalgia, shooting in the eustachian tube.

**Nose:** Sneezing, especially when entering a warm room. *Copious, watery and extremely acrid discharge.* Sensation of a lump at the root of the nose. Hay fever (*Sabad., Sil., Psor.*). Fluent coryza with headache, cough, and hoarseness. Polypus.

**Stomach:** Canine hunger. Pain in the pyloric region. Thirst. Belching. Nausea.

**Abdomen:** Rumbling, offensive flatus. Pain in the left hypogastrium (inguinal hernia). Colic worse sitting, better moving about.

**Rectum:** Diarrhea with very offensive flatus. Stitches in the rectum; itching and rhagades (fissures) in the anus. Glowing heat in the rectum.

**Urinary:** Sensation of weakness in the bladder and urethra. Increased secretion of urine with coryza. Urine red with much pressure and burning in the urethra.

**Respiratory:** *Hoarseness. Hacking cough on inspiring cold air. Tickling in the larynx. Sensation as if larynx is split or torn* (laryngitis). *Oppressed breathing* from pressure in the middle of the chest. Constricted feeling in the region of epiglottis. Pain extending to the ear.

**Extremities:** Lame joints. Ulcers on heel. Painful affections of fingers ground the nails (paronychia). Neuralgia of stump. Bad effects from getting feet wet. Limbs, especially arms, feel sore and tired.

**Sleep:** Yawning with headache and drowsiness. Gaping in deep sleep. Dreams. Wakes up at 2 a.m.

**Modalities:** *Worse,* in the evening, in a warm room. *Better,* in open air, and in a cold room.

**Relationship:** Compare: *Gels., Euphr., Kali-i., Acon., Ip.*

Complementary: *Phos., Thuj., Puls.*

Antidotes: *Arn., Cham., Verat.*

**Dose:** Third potency.

---

## ALLIUM SATIVUM

(Garlic) **All-s.**

Acts directly on the intestinal mucous membrane increasing peristalsis. Colitis, with pathological flora. Has vaso-dilatory properties. Arterial hypotension begins usually in 30 to 45 minutes after twenty to forty drop doses of the tincture.

Adapted to fleshy subjects with dyspepsia and catarrhal affections. High standard of living. Patients who eat a great deal more, *especially meat,* than they drink. *Pain in the hips, pain in psoas and iliac muscles. Pulmonary tuberculosis.*

Cough and expectoration diminishes, temperature becomes normal, weight is gained, and sleep becomes regular. *Hemoptysis.*

**Head:** Heavy; pulsation in temples; catarrhal deafness.

**Mouth:** Sweetish saliva after meals and at night. Sensation of a hair on the tongue or in the throat.

**Stomach:** Voracious appetite. Burning eructations (dyspepsia). Least change in diet causes trouble. Constipation, with constant dull pain in bowels. *Tongue pale, red papillae.*

**Female:** Pain and swelling of breasts. Eruptions in vagina and on breasts and vulva during menses.

**Respiratory:** Constant rattling of mucus in the bronchi. Cough in the morning after leaving the bedroom, with mucoid expectoration, which is tenacious and difficult to raise. Sensitive to cold air. Dilated bronchi, with fetid expectoration. Darting pain in chest.

**Relationship:** *All-s.*, according to Dr. Teste, belongs to the *Bry.* group, including *Lyc.*, *Nux-v.*, *Coloc.*, *Dig.*, and *Ign.* which deeply affect all flesh eating animals and hardly any vegetarians. Hence, they have a special applicability to non-vegetarians rather than to exclusive vegetarians.

Compare: *Caps.*, *Ars.*, *Seneg.*, *Kali-n.*

Complementary: *Ars.*

Antidote: *Lyc.*

**Dose:** Third to sixth potency. In tuberculosis, four to six grammes in moderate state of dessication daily, in divided doses.

---

# ALNUS RUBRA

(Red Alder) **Aln.**

Has some reputation as a remedy for skin affections, glandular enlargements, and indigestion from imperfect secretion of gastric juice. It stimulates nutrition, and thus acts favorably upon strumous disorders, enlarged glands, etc. Ulcerated mucous membranes of the mouth and throat. Fingers covered by crust caused by pustules, disagreeable odor. Indigestion from imperfect secretion of gastric juice.

**Female:** Leucorrhea, with cervical erosions bleeding easily. Amenorrhea, with burning pains from the back to the pubis.

**Skin:** Chronic herpes. Enlarged submaxillary glands. Eczema, prurigo. Purpura hemorrhagica. Poison oak. Use locally.

**Dose:** Tincture to third potency.

---

# ALOE SOCOTRINA

(Socotrine Aloes) **Aloe.**

An excellent remedy to aid in re-establishing physiological equilibrium after over dosing, where disease and drug symptoms are mixed. There is no remedy richer in symptoms of portal congestion and none that has given better clinical results, both for the primary pathological condition and secondary phenomena. Bad effects from sedentary life or habits. Especially suitable to lymphatic and hypochondriacal patients. The rectal symptoms usually determine the choice. Adapted to weary people, aged, phlegmatic, and old beer drinkers. Dissatisfied and angry about himself, alternating with lumbago. Heat internal and external. Has been used successfully in the treatment of consumption by giving the pure juice.

**Head:** Headache alternates with lumbago, with intestinal and uterine affections. Disinclination to mental labor. *Aches above forehead, with heaviness in eyes, must close them partially.* Headache after stool. Dull, pressive pain; worse from heat.

**Eyes:** Compelled to close the eyes during pain in the forehead. Flickering before eyes. Redness of eyes with *yellow* vision. *Pain deep in the orbits.*

**Ears:** Cracking when chewing. Sudden explosion and clashing in left ear.[1] Tinkling as if some thin, metallic globe is in the head.

**Nose:** Coldness of the tip. Epistaxis in the morning on waking up. Full of crusts.

**Face:** Marked redness of lips.

**Mouth:** Taste bitter and sour. Tasteless eructations. Lips cracked and dry.

**Throat:** Thick lumps of tough mucus. Varicose condition of veins in the pharynx. Dry, scrapy feeling.

**Stomach:** Aversion to meat. Longing for juicy things. After eating, flatulence, *pulsation in the rectum,* and sexual irritation. Nausea, with headache. Pain in the pit of stomach from a misstep.

**Abdomen:** Pulsating pain around the navel, worse pressure. Fullness in the region of the liver, pain under the right ribs or in the right hypochondrium. *Abdomen feels full, heavy, hot, bloated.* Weak feeling, as if diarrhea would come on. Great accumulation of flatus, pressing downwards, causes distress in the lower bowels. *Sensation of a plug between symphysis pubis and os coccygis,* with urging to pass stool. Colic before and during stools. Burning, copious flatus.

**Rectum:** Constant bearing down in the rectum; bleeding, sore, and hot; relieved by cold water. Feeling of weakness and loss of power of sphincter ani. *Sense of insecurity of rectum* when passing flatus. Uncertain whether gas or stool will come. Stool passes without an effort, almost unnoticed. Lumpy, watery stool. Jelly-like stools, with soreness of the rectum after stool. *A lot of mucus is passed after stool with proctalgia.* Hemorrhoids protrude like grapes; very sore and tender; better cold water application. *Burning in the anus* and rectum. Constipation, with heavy pressure in the lower part of the abdomen.

[1] As from breaking of glass (Clarke - Dictionary of Practical Materia Medica).

Diarrhea from beer.

**Urinary:** Incontinence in aged, bearing down sensation and enlarged prostate. Scanty and highly colored urine.

**Female:** Bearing down pain in the rectum, worse standing and during menses. Uterus feels heavy, cannot walk much on that account. Labor-like pains in loins; extend down the legs. Climacteric hemorrhage. Menses too early and too profuse (menorrhagia).

**Respiratory:** Winter coughs, with itching. Difficult respiration, with stitches from liver to chest.

**Back:** Pain in the lumbosacral region, worse motion. Stitches through the sacrum. *Lumbago alternating with headache and piles.*

**Extremities:** Lameness in all limbs. *Drawing pains in joints.* Soles pain when walking.

**Modalities:** *Worse,* early morning; summer; heat; in hot, dry weather; after eating or drinking. *Better,* from cold, open air.

**Relationship:** Complementary: *Sulph.*

Compare: *Kali-bi., Lyc., All-s.*

Antidotes: *Op., Sulph.*

**Dose:** Sixth potency and higher. In rectal conditions, a few doses of the third, then wait.

---

## ALSTONIA SCHOLARIS

(Dita Bark) **Alst-s.**

Malarial diseases, with diarrhea, dysentery, anemia, and feeble digestion, are the general conditions suggesting this remedy. Characteristic symptoms are the all gone sensation in the stomach and sinking in the abdomen, with debility. *A tonic after exhausting fevers.*

**Abdomen:** Violent purging and cramps in bowels. Heat and irritation in lower bowels. Camp diarrhea (diarrhea due to contaminated water, as during camps), bloody stool, *dysentery;* diarrhea from bad water and malaria. *Painless watery stools* (*Ph-ac.*). Diarrhea immediately after eating.

**Relationship:** Compare: Similar in action to *Alstonia constricta,* the bitter bark or native quinine of Australia. *Ditainum* (active principle, is anti-periodic, like quinine, but without unpleasant effects). *Cinchona officinalis* (similar in diarrhea, chronic dyspepsia and debility). *Hydr., Ferr cit. et chin.*

**Dose:** Tincture to third potency. Locally, for ulcers and rheumatic pains.

---

# ALUMEN

(Common Potash Alum) **Alumn.**

The clinical application of this remedy points to its bowel symptoms, both in obstinate constipation and in hemorrhage from bowels as in the course of typhoid; *paralytic weakness* of the muscles in all parts of the body. Tendency to *induration* is also marked, a low form of tissue making is favored. Hardening of the tissues of tongue, rectum, uterus, etc., ulcers with indurated bases. Adapted to old people, especially in bronchial catarrhs. *Sensation of dryness and constriction.* Mental paresis; dysphagia especially for *liquids.* Tendency to induration. Scirrhus of the tongue (cancer).

**Head:** *Burning pain as if a weight was put on top of the head, better by pressure* of hand. Vertigo, with weakness in the pit of the stomach. Alopecia.

**Throat:** Throat relaxed. Mucous membrane red and swollen. Cough. Tickling in the throat. Tendency to throat colds. *Enlarged and indurated tonsils.* Burning pain down the esophagus. Complete aphonia. Every cold settles in the throat. Constriction of esophagus.

**Rectum:** *Constipation of the most aggravated kind.* No desire for stool for days. Violent ineffectual urging to stool. No ability to expel stools. *Marble-like masses pass, but rectum still feels full.* Itching after stool. Itching in the anus. Long lasting pain and smarting in rectum after stool; also hemorrhoids. Yellow, like an infant's. Hemorrhage from bowels.

**Female:** Tendency to induration of the neck of the uterus and mammary glands (*Carb-an., Con.*). Chronic yellow vaginal discharge. Chronic gonorrhea, yellow, with little lumps along the urethra. Aphthous patches in the vagina (*Caul.*). Menses watery.

**Respiratory:** Hemoptysis, great weakness of the chest; difficult to expel mucus. Copious, ropy, morning expectoration in old people. Asthma.

**Heart:** Palpitations, *from lying down on the right side.*

**Extremities:** *Weakness of all muscles,* especially arms and legs. Constricted feeling around limbs.

**Skin:** *Ulcers, with indurated bases.* To be thought of in indurated glands, epithelioma, etc., veins become varicosed and bleed. Indurations resulting from long continued, inflammatory irritations. Glands inflame and harden. Alopecia, scrotal eczema and on the dorsum of penis.

**Modalities:** *Worse,* cold except headache, which is relieved by cold.

**Dose:** First to thirtieth potency, the very highest potencies have proved efficacious. Powdered alum, 10 grains, placed on the tongue, is said to arrest an attack of asthma.

# ALUMINA

(Oxide of Aluminum, Argilla) **Alum.**

A very general condition corresponding to this drug is dryness of the mucous membranes and skin, and *a tendency to paretic muscular states.* Old people, with lack of vital heat, or the prematurely old, with debility. Sluggish functions, heaviness, numbness, staggering, and the characteristic constipation find an excellent remedy in *Alumina.* Disposition to colds in the head, and eructations in spare, dry, thin subjects. Delicate children, products of artificial baby foods.

**Mind:** Low spirited; fears loss of reason. Confused about their personal identity. *Hasty, hurried.* Time passes slowly. *Variable mood.* Better as day advances. Suicidal tendency on seeing a knife or blood.

**Head:** Stitching, burning pain in the head, with vertigo, worse in the morning, but relieved by food. Pressure in the forehead, as if from a tight hat. Inability to walk except with eyes open. Throbbing headache, with constipation. Vertigo, with nausea; better after breakfast. Falling hair; scalp itches and is numb.

**Eyes:** Objects look yellow. Eyes feel cold. Lids dry, burn, smart, thickened, aggravation in the morning; chronic conjunctivitis. Ptosis. Strabismus.

**Ears:** Humming; roaring. Eustachian tube feels plugged.

**Nose:** Pain at the root of the nose. Sense of smell diminished. Fluent coryza. Tip of nose *cracked,* nostrils sore, *red;* worse touch. *Scabs with thick yellow mucus.* Tettery redness. *Ozena atrophica sicca.* Membranes distended and boggy.

**Face:** Feels as if an albuminous substance had dried on it. Blood-boils and pimples. Twitchings of the lower jaw. Rush of blood to the face after eating.

**Mouth:** Sore. Bad odor from it (halitosis). Teeth covered with sordes. Gums sore, bleeding. Tensive pain in the articulation of jaw when opening the mouth or chewing.

**Throat:** *Dry,* sore; food cannot pass, esophagus contracted, sensation of a splinter or plug in the throat. Irritable, and relaxed throat. Looks parched and glazed. Clergyman's sore throat in thin subjects. Thick, tenacious mucus drops from posterior nares. Constant inclination to clear the throat.

**Stomach:** Abnormal cravings, chalk, charcoal, dry food, tea-grounds. Heartburn; feels constricted. Aversion to meat (*Graph., Arn., Puls.*). *Potatoes disagree.* No desire to eat. *Can swallow, but small morsels at a time.* Constriction of the esophagus.

**Abdomen:** Colic, like painter's colic. Pressing in both groins towards sexual organs. *Left sided abdominal complaints.*

**Stool:** *Hard,* dry, knotty stools; *no desire.* Rectum sore, dry, inflamed, bleeding. Itching and burning in the anus. *Even a soft stool is passed with difficulty. Great straining.* Constipation in infants (*Coll., Psor., Paraf.*) and old people from an inactive rectum, and in women with very sedentary habits. Diarrhea on micturating. *Evacuation preceded by painful urging long before stool, and then straining at stool.*

**Urinary:** Muscles of bladder paretic, *must strain at stool in order to micturate.* Pain in kidneys, with mental confusion. Frequent desire to micturate in old people. Difficult starting.

**Male:** Excessive desire. Involuntary emissions when straining at stool. Prostatic discharge.

**Female:** Menses too early, short, *scanty, pale, followed by great exhaustion* (*Carb-an., Cocc.*). Leucorrhea *acrid, profuse,* transparent, *ropy,* with burning; worse during daytime, and after menses. Relieved by washing with cold water.

**Respiratory:** Cough soon after waking in the morning. Hoarseness, aphonia, tickling in the larynx; wheezing, rattling respiration. Cough on talking or singing, *in the morning.* Chest feels constricted. Condiments produce cough. Talking aggravates soreness of chest.

**Back:** Stitches. Gnawing pain, as if from a hot iron. Pain along the cord, with paralytic weakness.

**Extremities:** Pain in the arms and fingers, as if hot iron had penetrated. Arms feel paralyzed. Legs fall asleep, *especially when sitting with legs crossed. Staggers on walking* (locomotor ataxia). *Heels feel numb.* Soles tender; on stepping, feel soft and swollen. Pain in shoulder and upper arm. Gnawing beneath finger nails. *Brittle nails.* Inability to walk, except when eyes are open or in daytime. Spinal degenerations and paralysis of lower limbs.

**Sleep:** Restless; anxious and confused dreams. Sleepy in the morning.

**Skin:** Chapped, dry tettery. Brittle nails. *Intolerable itching when getting warm in bed.* Must scratch till it bleeds; then becomes painful. Brittle skin on fingers.

**Modalities:** *Worse,* periodically; in the afternoon; from potatoes. *Worse,* in the morning on waking up; in a warm room. *Better,* in open air; from cold washing; in the evening and on alternate days. *Better,* damp weather.

**Relationship:** Compare: *Aluminium chloridum* (pains of locomotor ataxia. Lower triturations in water). *Slag—Aluminium-silico-sulpho-calcite 3x* (anal itching, piles, constipation, flatulent distention); *Sec., Lath., Plb. Aluminium aceticum* solution (externally a lotion for putrid wounds and skin infections. Arrests hemorrhage from inertia of uterus. Parenchymatous hemorrhage from various organs 2-3% solution. Hemorrhage following tonsillectomy is controlled by rinsing out the nasopharynx with a 10% solution).

Complementary: *Bry.*

Antidotes: *Ip., Cham.*

**Dose:** Sixth to thirtieth and higher. Action slow to develop.

---

## ALUMINA SILICATA

(Andalasite Rock—Alumina 63, Silica 37 parts)

**Alum-sil.**

Deep acting remedy for chronic complaints of brain, spine, and nerves. Constriction is a marked general symptom, especially of the orifices. Venous distention. Weakness, especially spinal. Aching and burning in the spine. Formication, numbness, pain in all the limbs. Epileptiform convulsion. Coldness during pains.

**Head:** Congestion of brain. Constriction of the scalp. Pain in the head, better heat, perspiration.

**Eyes:** Pain in the eyes; flickering before the eyes.

**Nose:** Frequent coryzas. Swelling and ulceration of the nose (ozena). Itching and burning. Discharge *yellow. Sore, scabby,* stopped up.

**Respiratory:** Catarrh, pain, raw feeling. Sensation of great weakness in the chest. Stitching pains. Spasmodic cough with purulent viscid expectoration. *Soreness of the chest,* along the trachea; cannot stand percussion. Gray sputum. Capillary bronchitis. Larynx and chest sore. Membranous croup extends to the trachea.

**Extremities:** Heaviness, jerking, numbness, aching and pains.

**Skin:** Formication along the course of nerves, veins feel full and distended. Sore to touch and pressure.

**Modalities:** *Worse,* cold air, after eating, standing. *Better,* warmth, fasting, resting in bed.

**Dose:** Higher potencies.

---

## AMBRA GRISEA

(Ambergis—A Morbid Secretion of the Whale) **Ambr.**

Suitable to excitable, nervous children and thin, nervous patients. Extreme *nervous hypersensitiveness.* External numbness of the entire body in the morning with weakness. Nervous, bilious temperament. Thin, scrawny women. Adapted to hysterical subjects, or those suffering from spinal irritation, with convulsive cough, eructation, etc. Also for patients *weakened by age* or overwork, who are anemic and sleepless. A great remedy for the aged, with impairment of all functions, weakness, coldness and *numbness,* usually of single parts, fingers, arms, etc. One sided complaints call for it. *Music aggravates symptoms.* Ebullitions and pulsations after walking in open air.

**Mind:** Dread of people, and desire to be alone. Cannot do anything in presence of others. Intensely shy, blushes easily. *Music causes weeping.* Despair, loathing of life. Fantastic illusions. Bashful. Loss of love for life. Restless, excited, very loquacious. Time passes slowly. Thinking, difficult in the morning with old people. Dwells upon unpleasant things.

**Head:** Slow comprehension. Vertigo, with weakness in the head and stomach. Pressure on the front part of head with mental depression. *Tearing pains in the upper half of brain. Senile dizziness.* Rush of blood to the head, when listening to music. *Hearing impaired.* Epistaxis, especially in the morning. Profuse bleeding from teeth. Hair falls out.

**Stomach:** Eructations, with violent, convulsive cough. Acid eructations, like heartburn. *Distention of stomach and abdomen* after midnight. Sensation of coldness in the abdomen.

**Urinary:** Pain in the bladder and rectum at the same time. Burning at the urethral and anal orifice. *Sensation in the urethra as if a few drops passed out.* Burning and itching in the urethra while micturating. *Urine turbid, even during emission,* forming a brown sediment.

**Male:** Voluptuous itching of scrotum. Parts externally numb; burn internally. Violent erections without any voluptuous sensations.

**Female:** Nymphomania. *Itching in the pudendum* (pruritus vulva), *with soreness and swelling.* Menses too early. Profuse, bluish leucorrhea. Worse at night. *Discharge of blood between periods, at every little accident.*

**Respiratory:** Asthmatic breathing with eructations of gas. *Nervous, spasmodic cough,* with hoarseness and *eructations,* on waking in the morning; worse in presence of people. Tickling in the throat, larynx and trachea, chest oppressed, gets out of breath when coughing. *Hollow, spasmodic, barking cough, coming deep from the chest.* Choking when hawking up phlegm.

**Heart:** *Palpitations, with pressure on the chest as if from a lump lodged there, or as if the chest was obstructed.* Conscious of the pulse. Palpitations in open air with a pale face.

**Extremities:** *Cramps in hands* and fingers, worse grasping anything. Cramps in legs.

**Sleep:** *Cannot sleep from worry; must get up.* Anxious dreams. Coldness of the body and twitching of limbs, during sleep.

**Skin:** Itching and soreness, especially around genitals. Numbness of skin. Arms "go to sleep."

**Modalities:** *Worse,* music; presence of strangers; *from any unusual thing;* morning, warm room. *Better,* slow motion; in air; lying on painful part; cold drinks.

**Relationship:** Do not confound with *Amber—Succinum. q.v. Moschus* frequently follows advantageously.

Compare: *Oleum succinum* (hiccough). *Sumb., Castm., Asaf., Croc.*

**Dose:** Second and third potencies; may be repeated with advantage.

---

## AMBROSIA ARTEMISIAEFOLIA

(Rag-weed) **Ambro.**

A remedy for hay fever, *lachrymation* and *intolerable itching of the eye lids.* Some forms of whooping cough. Respiratory tract in its entire length is obstructed. *Several types of diarrhea,* especially during summer months, also dysentery.

**Eyes:** Smart and burn. Lachrymation.

**Nose:** Watery coryza; sneezing: *Epistaxis.* Stuffed up feeling in the nose and head. Irritation of the trachea and bronchial tubes, with asthmatic attacks (*Aral., Eucal.*). Wheezy cough.

**Relationship**: Compare in hay fever: *Sabad., Wye., Succ-ac., Ars-i., Arund.*

**Dose:** Tincture to third potency; 10 drops in water during and after an epistaxis. In hay fever, high potencies.

---

## AMMONIACUM GUMMI—DOREMA AMMONIACUM

(Gum Ammoniac) **Ammc.**

A remedy for the aged and feeble, especially in chronic bronchitis. Ill-humor. Sensitive to cold. Sensation of burning and scratching in the neck and esophagus.

**Head:** Catarrhal headache due to closure of frontal sinuses.

**Eyes:** Dim sight (amblyopia). Stars and fiery points float before the eyes. Easily fatigued from reading (aesthenopia).

**Throat:** Throat dry; worse inhaling fresh air. Sensation of fullness in the back of the throat and gullet with nausea, burning and scraping sensation. Immediately after eating, sensation as if something was stuck in the esophagus, which incites efforts to swallow.

**Respiratory:** *Difficult breathing* (asthma). Chronic bronchial catarrh (bronchitis). Large accumulation of purulent discharges and feeble expectoration; worse in cold weather. Mucus tough and hard.

Heart beats stronger, extends to the pit of stomach. Coarse rattling in the chest of old people.

**Relationship:** Antidotes: *Bry., Arn.*

Compare: *Seneg., Ant-t., Bals-p.*

**Dose:** Third trituration.

---

## AMMONIUM BENZOICUM

(Benzoate of Ammonia) **Am-be.**

A remedy for albuminuria, especially in patients with gouty diathesis. Gout, with deposits in joints. Urinary incontinence, in the aged.

**Head:** Heavy, stupid.

**Face:** Bloated, swollen eyelids. Swelling under the tongue like a ranula.

**Urinary:** Smoky, scanty urine. Albuminous with large deposits.

**Back:** Pain across the sacrum, with an urgency to pass stools. Soreness in the region of right kidney.

**Relationship:** Compare: *Ter., Benz-ac., Ammonia salts, Caust.*

In albuminuria compare: *Kalm., Helon., Merc-c., Berb., Canth.*

**Dose:** Second trituration.

---

## AMMONIUM BROMATUM

(Bromide of Ammonia) **Am-br.**

Indicated in chronic laryngeal and pharyngeal catarrh, neuralgic headaches, and obesity. Constrictive pains in the head, chest, legs, etc. Irritable feeling under the finger nails; relieved only by biting them.

**Head:** Cerebral congestion. Sensation of a band above the ears. Sneezing; thick nasal discharge.

**Eyes:** Edges of lids red and swollen, also Meibomian glands (chalazion). Eyeballs feel large; pain around the eyes radiates to the head (ciliary neuralgia).

**Throat:** Smarting in the mouth. Tickling in the throat, *with an inclination to dry, spasmodic cough, especially at night.* Burning in fauces. White, sticky, mucus. Chronic speakers catarrh.

**Respiratory:** Sudden, short cough, strangling. Tickling in trachea and bronchial tubes. Wakes up at 3 a. m. due to cough. Feels suffocated; continuous cough, when lying down at night; sharp pain in the lungs. Whooping cough, dry, spasmodic cough on lying down.

**Relationship:** *Hyos., Con., Arg-n., Kali-bi.*

**Dose:** First potency.

---

# AMMONIUM CARBONICUM

(Carbonate of Ammonia) **Am-c.**

The diseased conditions met by this remedy are such that are often found in rather stout women who are always tired and weary, take cold easily, suffer from cholera-like symptoms before menses, lead a sedentary life, have a slow reaction generally and are disposed to the frequent use of a smelling bottle. Too frequent and profuse menses. Mucous membranes of the respiratory organs are especially affected. Fat patients with weak hearts, wheezing, feel suffocated. Very sensitive to cold air. Great aversion to water; cannot bear to touch it. Malignant scarlatina, with somnolence, swollen glands, dark red sore throat, faintly developed eruptions. Uremia. *Heaviness in all organs.* Uncleanliness in bodily habits. Swelling of parts, glands, etc. Acid secretions. Prostration from trifles.

**Mind:** Forgetful, ill humored, gloomy during *stormy weather. Uncleanliness.* Talking and hearing others talk, affects greatly. Sad, lachrimose, unreasonable.

**Head:** Pulsating forehead; better, by pressure and in a warm room. Shocks through the head.

**Eyes:** Burning in eyes with an aversion to light (photophobia). Eye strain (*Nat- m.*). Asthenopia. Sore canthi.

**Ears:** Hardness of hearing. Shocks through ears, eyes, and nose, when gnashing teeth.

**Nose:** Sharp, watery discharge. Burning. *Stoppage at night, with long continuous coryza. Cannot breathe through the nose. Snuffles* in children. *Epistaxis after washing and after eating.* Ozena, blows bloody mucus from the nose. Tip of nose congested.

**Face:** Tetters around mouth. Boils and pustules, during menses. Corners of mouth sore, cracked, and burn.

**Mouth:** Great dryness of mouth and throat. Toothache. *Pressing teeth together sends shocks through the head, eyes and ears.* Vesicles on the tongue. Taste sour; metallic. Cracking of jaw on chewing.

**Throat:** Enlarged tonsils and glands of neck. Burning pain down the throat. Tendency to gangrenous ulceration of tonsils. Diphtheria *when nose is stopped up.*

**Stomach:** Pain in the pit of the stomach, with heartburn, nausea, waterbrash, and chilliness. Great appetite, but easily satisfied. Flatulent dyspepsia.

**Abdomen:** Noise and pain in the abdomen. Flatulent hernia.

**Rectum:** Stools difficult, hard, and knotty. *Bleeding piles; worse during menses.* Itching in the anus. Protruding piles, worse after stool, better lying down.

**Urinary:** Frequent desire; involuntary at night. Tenesmus of bladder. Urine white, sandy, bloody, copious, turbid and fetid.

**Male:** Itching and pain in the scrotum and spermatic cords. Erection without desire. Seminal emissions.

**Female:** Itching, swelling and burning of pudendum. Leucorrhea burning, acrid, watery. Aversion to the other sex. Menses too *frequent, profuse,* early (menorrhagia), copious, clotted, black; colicky pains (dysmenorrhea), with hard, difficult stool and *fatigue,* especially of thighs; yawning and chilliness.

**Respiratory:** Hoarseness. Cough every morning around three o'clock, with dyspnea, palpitations, burning in the chest; worse ascending. Chest feels tired. Emphysema. *Oppression during breathing;* worse after any effort, and on entering *a warm room,* or ascending even a few steps (asthma). Asthenic *pneumonia.* Slow labored, stertorous breathing; bubbling sound (rattling). Winter catarrh, with slimy sputum and specks of blood (hemoptysis). Pulmonary edema.

**Heart:** Audible palpitations with fear, cold sweat, lachrymation, inability to speak, loud breathing and trembling hands. *Heart weak,* awakens with difficult breathing and palpitations.

**Extremities:** Tearing in joints relieved by heat of bed; inclination to stretch limbs. Hands cold and blue; distended veins. Fingers swell when arm is hanging down. Panaritium, deep seated periosteal pain. Cramps in calves and soles. Big toe painful and swollen (gout). Felons in the beginning. Heel painful on standing. Tearing in ankles and bones of feet, better when warm in bed.

**Sleep:** Sleepiness during the day. Starts from sleep, stranglulated.

**Skin:** Violent itching and burning blisters. Scarlet rash. Miliary rash.

Malignant scarlatina. Faintly developed eruptions from defective vitality. Erysipelas in the aged, with mental symptoms. Eczema in the bends of extremities, between legs, around the anus and genitals.

**Modalities:** *Worse,* evenings, from cold, wet weather, wet applications, washing, between 3 to 4 a. m. and during menses. *Better,* lying on painful side and on stomach; in dry weather.

**Relationship:** Inimical to *Lach.,* similar in action.

Antidotes: *Arn., Camph.*

Compare: *Rhus-t., Mur-ac., Ant-t.*

Of use in poisoning by charcoal fumes.

**Dose:** Lower potencies deteriorate with age. Sixth potency best for general use.

---

## AMMONIUM CAUSTICUM

(Hydrate of Ammonia, Ammonia Water) **Am-caust.**

This is a powerful cardiac stimulant. Useful in *syncope,* thrombosis, hemorrhage, snake bites, chloroform narcosis; may be given by inhalation.

The edema and ulceration of mucous membranes produced by this powerful drug, have been utilized as the guiding symptoms for its use; hence in membranous croup with burning in esophagus. Aphonia (see *Causticum*).

**Respiratory:** Difficult respiration. Accumulation of mucus with incessant coughing. *Loss of voice. Burning rawness in the throat.* Spasm of the glottis with suffocation; patient gasps for breath. Pain in esophagus on breathing deeply. Scraping and burning in the throat and esophagus. Uvula covered with white mucus. Nasal diphtheria, with burning, excoriating discharge.

**Extremities:** *Excessive exhaustion* and muscular debility. Rheumatism of shoulders. Skin hot and dry.

**Dose:** First to third potency; also five to ten minims, well diluted with water.

---

## AMMONIUM IODATUM

(Iodide of Ammonia) **Am-i.**

Indicated when iodine has but partially relieved its cases of laryngitis and bronchitis, catarrhal pneumonia, edema of lungs.

**Head:** Dull headache, especially in young people, stupid expression on the face, heavy; vertigo, Meniere's disease.

**Relationship:** Compare: *Ammonium tartaricum* (dry hacking cough after every cold).

**Dose:** Second and third trituration.

---

## AMMONIUM MURIATICUM

(Sal Ammoniac) **Am-m.**

A state of prostration bordering on a typhoid state is produced by this remedy. All mucus secretions are increased and retained. It is especially adapted to fat and sluggish patients who have respiratory problems. Cough associated with catarrh and liver affections. Tendency to irregular circulation, blood seems to be in a constant turmoil, pulsations, etc. Many groups of symptoms are accompanied by cough *and profuse glairy secretions.* Periods of aggravation are peculiarly divided according to the bodily region affected; thus the head and chest symptoms are worse in the mornings, the abdominal, in the afternoon, pain in the limbs, skin and febrile symptoms, in the evenings. "Boiling" sensation.

**Mind:** Melancholy, apprehension; from internal grief. *Desire to cry,* but cannot. Consequences of grief.

**Head:** Hair falls out, with itching and dandruff. Feels full, compressed; worse mornings.

**Eyes:** Mist before eyes, optical illusions in incipient cataract; capsular cataract.

**Nose:** Free, *acrid, hot, watery discharge* corroding the lip. Sneezing. Nose sore to touch; ulcerative pain in the nostrils. *Loss of smell* (anosmia). *Obstructed, stuffy feeling;* constant and unavailing efforts to blow it out. Itchy.

**Face:** Inflammation, eruptions on the face. Faceache.[1] Mouth and lips sore and excoriated.

**Throat:** Throbbing in, and swelling of tonsils, can scarcely swallow. Tonsillitis. Sore spot behind uvula, relieved by eating. Internal and external swelling of throat *with viscid phlegm.* So tough, that it cannot be hawked up. Stricture of esophagus.

**Stomach:** Thirst for lemonade, regurgitation of food, bitter waterbrash. Nausea. Gnawing in stomach. Epigastric pain immediately after eating. Cancer of stomach.

---

1 Sensation of tearing in the zygomatic bone (T.F. Allen — Handbook of Materia Medica).

**Abdomen:** Stitches in the region of spleen, especially in the morning, with difficulty in respiration. Pain around the navel. Abdominal symptoms appear during pregnancy. Chronic congestion of liver. Excessive fatty deposit around the abdomen. Much flatus. Strained feeling in groin.

**Rectum:** Itching and hemorrhoids, soreness with pustules. Hard, *crumbly* stool, or covered with glairy mucus. Stinging in perineum. Green mucoid stools alternate with constipation. During and after stool, burning and smarting in the rectum. Hemorrhoids after suppressed leucorrhea.

**Female:** Menses too early, too free, dark, clotted; *flow more at night* (menorrhagia). Pain as if sprained, in the left side of abdomen, during pregnancy. Diarrhea, greenish mucoid stools, and pain around the navel *during menses.* Leucorrhea, like white of an egg (*Alum., Borx., Calc-p.*); with pain around the navel; brown, slimy *after every passage of urine.*

**Respiratory:** *Hoarseness and burning in larynx.* Dry, hacking, scraping cough; worse lying on the back or on the right side. Stitches in the chest. Cough loose in the afternoon, with profuse expectoration and rattling of mucus. Oppression of chest. Burning in small spots in the chest. Scanty expectoration. Cough with profuse salivation.

**Back:** *Icy coldness between shoulders;* not relieved by a warm covering, followed by itching. Bruised pain in coccyx; backache, as if in a vise when sitting.

**Extremities:** Pain as from ulcerations on the finger tips. Shooting and tearing *pains in the tips of the fingers* and toes. Ulcerative pain in heels. *Contraction of hamstring tendons.* Sciatica, *worse sitting, better lying.* Neuralgic pain in amputated limbs. Offensive sweaty feet. Pain in feet during menses.

**Fever:** *Chills during the evenings after lying down* and on awakening, without thirst. Palms and soles hot. Sub-acute, low fever due to unhealthy climate. Lowest potencies.

**Skin:** Itching, generally in the evenings. Blisters on various parts. Intense burning better, cold applications.

**Modalities:** *Better,* open air. *Worse,* head and chest symptoms in the morning; abdominal symptoms in the afternoon.

**Relationship:** Antidotes: *Coff., Nux-v., Caust.*

Compare: *Calc., Seneg., Caust.*

**Dose:** Third to sixth potency.

---

## AMMONIUM PHOSPHORICUM

(Phosphate of Ammonia) **Am-p.**

A remedy for chronic gout, patients with uric acid diathesis; indicated in bronchitis and *nodosities in the joints* of the fingers and at the back of the hands. Facial paralysis. Pain in shoulder joint. Tightness around the chest. Heaviness of limbs, unsteady, tottering gait. Coldness from least draft of air.

**Head:** Sneezing with an excessive running discharge from the nose and eyes, *only in the morning.*

**Urinary:** Rose colored sediment in urine.

**Respiratory:** Deep rough cough with greenish expectoration.

**Dose:** Third decimal trituration.

---

## AMMONIUM PICRICUM

(Picrate of Ammonia) **Am-pic.**

A remedy for malarial fever, neuralgias and so called bilious headaches. Pain in the occiput and mastoid region. Whooping cough.

**Head:** Periodical neuralgia *on right side of occiput;* boring pain extends to the ear, orbit and jaw. Vertigo on rising. Periodic bilious headaches (*Sang.*).

**Dose:** Third trituration.

---

## AMMONIUM VALERIANICUM

(Valerianate of Ammonia) **Am-val.**

A remedy for nervous, hysterical people, suffering from neuralgia, headache and insomnia. Great nervous erethism is always present.

**Heart:** Pain in the cardiac region. Functional disturbances, tachycardia.

**Dose:** Lower triturations.

---

## AMPELOPSIS QUINQUEFOLIA

(Virginia Creeper) **Ampe-qu.**

Renal dropsies, hydrocele, and chronic hoarseness in scrofulous patients have been benefited by this drug. Choleraic symptoms. Generally worse around 6 p. m. Dilated pupils.

Left costal region sore and sensitive. Elbow joints pain, back sore. Soreness of all limbs. Vomiting, purging with tenesmus. Rumbling in the abdomen.

**Dose:** Second to third potency.

---

## AMYGDALUS PERSICA

(Peach Tree) **Amgd-p.**

A very valuable remedy in vomiting of various kinds; *morning sickness.* Irritation of eyes. Ischuria and hematuria. Hemorrhage from the bladder.

Gastric irritation in children; no form of food is tolerated. Loss of smell and taste. Gastric and intestinal irritation, tongue is elongated and pointed, tip and edges are red (glossitis). Constant nausea and vomiting

**Relationship:** Compare: *Amygdala amara*—Bitter almond (pain in the tonsils, throat dark (hyperemic), dysphagia, vomiting, cough with a sore chest).

**Dose:** Fresh infusion or mother tincture.

---

## AMYLENUM NITROSUM

(Amyl Nitrite) **Aml-ns.**

On inhaling this drug, it rapidly dilates all the arterioles and capillaries, produces heat, and throbbing in the head with flushing of the face. Superficial arterial hyperemia. Palpitations of the heart and similar conditions are readily cured by it, especially flushings and other discomforts at climacteric. *Hiccough and yawning.* Often relieves epileptic convulsions temporarily. Seasickness.

**Head:** *Anxiety,* as if something might happen; *must have fresh air. Surging of blood to the head and face;* sensation as if the blood would burst through the skin, with heat and redness. *Hot flushes, followed by sweat at climacteric.* Ears hyperemic. Throbbing.

**Throat:** Constriction; collar seems too tight.

**Female:** After-pains; hemorrhage associated with facial flushes. *Climacteric headache and flushes of heat, with anxiety and palpitations.*

**Respiration:** Dyspnea feels asthmatic. Great oppression and fullness of chest; spasmodic, suffocative cough.

**Heart:** Precordial anxiety. *Tumultuous action of heart.* Pain and constriction around the heart (angina pectoris). Fluttering on the slightest excitement.

**Extremities:** *Constant stretching for hours.* Veins of hands dilated; pulsations felt at the finger tips.

**Fever:** Hot flushes; sometimes followed by a cold and clammy skin and profuse sweat. Throbbing throughout the body. *Abnormal sweat after influenza.*

**Relationship:** Compare: *Glon., Lach.*

Antidotes: *Cact., Stry., Ergot.*

**Dose:** Third potency.

**Non-homeopathic Uses:** For *palliation*, in all conditions where the blood vessels are spasmodically *contracted,* as in angina pectoris, epileptic seizure, migraine, accompanied by coldness, pallor, etc. Also in paroxysms of asthma, chloroform asphyxia, inhalation of *Aml-ns.* will give immediate relief. For this non-homeopathic application, two to five minims (put up in pearls) dropped on a handkerchief and inhaled, may be required.

---

# ANACARDIUM ORIENTALE

(Marking Nut) **Anac.**

The *Anacardium* patient is found mostly among the neurasthenics; they have a type of nervous dyspepsia, relieved by food, *impaired memory,* depression, and irritability with diminution of senses (smell, sight, hearing). Syphilitic patients often suffer with these conditions. Intermittency of symptoms. Fear of examination in students. Weakening of all senses, sight, hearing, etc. Aversion to work; lacks self confidence; irresistible desire to swear and curse. *Sensation of a plug* in various parts—eyes, rectum, bladder, etc., also *of a band.* Empty feeling in the stomach; *eating temporarily relieves all discomfort.* This is a sure indication, often verified. Its skin symptoms are similar to *Rhus-t,* and it has often proved to be a valuable antidote to Poison oak.

**Mind:** Fixed ideas. Hallucinations; *thinks he is possessed by two people or wills.* Anxiety when walking, feels as if pursued. Profound melancholy and hypochondriasis, with a *tendency to use violent language. Brain fag. Impaired memory. Absent mindedness. Very easily offended.* Malicious; seems bent on wickedness. Lack of confidence in himself or others. Suspicious (*Hyos.*). Clairaudient, hears voices far away or of the dead. Senile dementia. Absence of all moral restraint.

**Head:** Vertigo. Pressing pain, *as if from a plug;* worse after mental exertion, in the forehead; occiput, temples, vertex; *better during a meal.* Itching and little boils on scalp.

**Eyes:** Pressure, a plug like sensation in the orbit. Blurred vision. *Objects appear too far away.*

**Ears:** Pressing in the ears as if from a plug. Hard of hearing.

**Nose:** Frequent sneezing. *Sense of smell perverted.* Coryza with palpitation, especially in the aged.

**Face:** Blue rings around the eyes. Face pale.

**Mouth:** Painful vesicles; fetid odor (halitosis). Tongue feels swollen, impeding speech and motion, with saliva in the mouth. Burning around the lips, as if from pepper.

**Stomach:** Weak digestion, with fullness and distention. *Empty feeling in the stomach.* Eructation, nausea, vomiting. *Eating relieves the Anacardium dyspepsia.* Apt to choke when eating or drinking. Swallows food and drinks hastily.

**Abdomen:** *Pain as if a plug was pressed into the intestines.* Rumbling, pinching, and griping.

**Rectum:** Bowels inactive. *Ineffectual desire; rectum seems powerless, as if plugged up;* spasmodic constriction of the sphincter ani; even soft stool passes with difficulty. *Itching in the anus; moisture from rectum.* Hemorrhage during stool. Painful hemorrhoids.

**Male:** Voluptuous itching; increased desire; seminal emissions without dreams. Prostatic discharge during stool.

**Female:** Leucorrhea, with soreness and itching. Menses scanty.

**Respiratory:** Pressure on the chest, as if from a plug. Oppression of chest, with internal heat and anxiety, driving him into the open air. Cough excited by talking, in children, after a fit of temper. Cough after eating with vomiting of food and pain in the occiput.

**Heart:** Palpitations, with a weak memory, and coryza in the aged; stitches in the heart region. Rheumatic pericarditis with double stitches.[1]

**Back:** Dull pressure in the shoulders, as if from a weight. Stiffness of the nape of neck.

**Extremities:** Neuralgia in the thumb. Paralytic weakness. Knees feel paralyzed or bandaged. Cramps in calves. Pressure, as if from a plug in the glutei muscles. Warts on the palms. Fingers swollen with vesicular eruption.

**Sleep:** Spells of sleeplessness lasting for several nights. Anxious dreams.

**Skin:** *Intense itching,* eczema, with mental irritability; vesicular eruption; swelling, urticaria; eruption like that of Poison oak (*Xero., Grin., Crot-t.*). Lichen planus; neurotic eczema. Warts on hands. Ulcers on forearm.

---

1 Stiches through the cardiac region, one stitch is quickly followed by another and then there is a long gap (T. F. Allen — Handbook of Materia Medica).

**Modalities:** *Worse,* on application of hot water. *Better,* from eating. When lying on side, from rubbing.

**Relationship:** Antidote: *Grin., Coff., Jug-c., Rhus-t., Eucal.*

Compare: *Anacardium occidentale* — Cashewnut (erysipelas, vesicular facial eruptions, anaesthetic variety of leprosy; warts, corns, ulcers, cracking of skin on soles of feet). *Rhus-t., Cypr., Chel., Xero.*

*Plat.* follows well. *Cereus serpentinus* (swearing).

**Dose:** Sixth to two hundredth potency.

---

# ANAGALLIS ARVENSIS

(Scarlet Pimpernel) **Anag.**

Marked action on the skin, characterized by severe itching and tingling everywhere. Favors expulsion of splinters. An old medicine for hydrophobia and dropsy. Possesses power of softening flesh and destroying warts.

**Head:** Great hilarity; headache over supra-orbital ridges, with rumbling in bowels and eructations; better from coffee. Sick headache. Pain in facial muscles.

**Urinary:** Irritation of the urethra, inclining to coition.[1] Burning pain on micturating with agglutination of orifice (gonorrhea). Urine passes in several streams; presses to micturate.

**Extremities:** Rheumatic and gouty pains. Pain in shoulder and arm. Cramps in the balls of thumbs and fingers.

**Skin:** *Itching;* dry, bran-like eruption, especially *on hands and fingers. Palms* especially affected. Vesicles in groups (ringworm). Ulcers and swellings on joints.

**Relationship:** *Anag.* contains *Saponin q. v.*

Compare: *Cycl., Primula obconica.*

**Dose:** First to third potency.

---

# ANANTHERUM MURICATUM

(Cuscus—An East Indian Grass) **Anan.**

A skin remedy of high order.

---

[1] Burning in urethra before and during erection. Ceases during coitus (T. F. Allen — Handbook of Materia Medica).

Painful swelling of various parts, proceeding towards suppuration. Glandular inflammation.

**Head:** State of drunkeness and staggering (Clarke). Pain pierces the brain like pointed arrows. Worse in the afternoon. Herpes, ulcers and tumors on scalp.

**Face:** Wart-like growths on the eyebrows. Boils and tumors on the tip of the nose. Ulcers and herpes on the face.

**Mouth:** Tongue fissured, as if cut on the edges. Copious salivation. Speech difficult, stammering.

**Urinary:** Turbid, thick, full of mucus. *Constant urging.* Bladder cannot hold even the smallest quantity. Involuntary. Cystitis.

**Male:** Chancre-like sores (syphilis).

**Female:** Chancre-like sores. Scirrhus-like swelling in the cervix. Breasts swollen, indurated, nipples excoriated.

**Skin:** Diseased and deformed nails. Offensive foot sweat. *Abscesses, boils, ulcers.* Erysipelas. Pruritus, herpes.

**Relationship:** Compare: *Staph., Merc., Thuj.*

**Dose:** Third potency.

---

## ANEMOPSIS CALIFORNICA

(Yerba Mansa—A Household Herb) **Anemps.**

A remedy for mucous membranes. Chronic forms of inflammation of the Schneiderian membrane with considerable relaxation and profuse discharge. Of chief value in *catarrhal states,* with a full, stuffy sensation in the head and throat. Useful in cuts, bruises and sprains; as a diuretic and in malaria. Not yet proven, but found useful in profuse mucus or serous discharges; in nasal and pharyngeal catarrh, diarrhea and urethritis. Recommended in heart disease, as a relaxing agent when unduly excited. Flatulence; promotes digestion.

**Relationship:** Compare *Pip-m.*

**Dose:** Tincture internally and locally as a spray.

---

## ANGUSTURA VERA

(Bark of Galipea Cusparia) **Ang.**

Rheumatic and paralytic complaints, great difficulty in walking. Crackling in all joints.

Intense craving for coffee is a characteristic symptom. Caries of long bones. Paralysis. Tetanus. Stiffness of muscles and joints. *Oversensitiveness.*

Principal action is on spinal motor nerves and mucous membranes.

**Head:** Oversensitive. Headache, with heat of face. Cramp-like pains in the cheek bones and in the masseters, as if fatigued by chewing too much. Drawing in facial muscles. Pain in the temporal muscles, when opening the jaws. Pain in articulation of jaw. Cramp-like pain in the zygomatic arch.

**Stomach:** Bitter taste. *Irresistible desire for coffee.* Pain from navel to the sternum. Atonic dyspepsia. Belching, with cough (*Ambr.*).

**Abdomen:** Diarrhea and colic. Tenesmus with soft stools; chronic diarrhea, with debility and loss of flesh. Burning in the anus.

**Back:** Itching along the spine. Pain in cervical vertebrae (cervical spondylosis). Drawing in the neck. Pain in the spine, at the nape of the neck and sacrum, worse on pressure. Twitching and jerking along the back (tetnus). Bends backward (opisthotonus).

**Extremities:** Stiffness and tension of muscles and joints. Pain in the limbs on walking. Arms tired and heavy. Caries of long bones. Coldness of fingers. *Pain in knees* (osteoarthritis). Crackling in joints.

**Skin:** Caries, very painful ulcers which affect the bone.

**Relationship:** Compare: *Nux-v., Ruta; Merc., Brucea antidysenterica*: Bark of *Nux vomica* or *Angustura falsa* (tetanic spasms with undisturbed consciousness, worse noise, liquids, paralyzed lower extremities, worse least touch, *cries for fear of being touched.* Painful jerking of legs; cramp-like pain in the knees; rigid and lame limbs of paralytics. For pain, during the passage of a calculus).

**Dose:** Sixth potency.

---

## ANHALONIUM LEWINII

(Mescal Button) **Anh.**

*Mescal* is a strong intoxicating spirit distilled from *Pulque fuerte.* Pulque is made from the *Agave americana* of Mexico, locally known as *Maguey,* it is the national beverage of Mexico. Indians call it Peyote. It weakens the heart and produces insanity. Its most striking effect appears in the *auditory nerve* for it makes "each note on the piano, a center of melody which seems to be surrounded by a halo of color pulsating to the rhythm of music"[1] (Hom. World).

---

1 Noises or touch perceived by a colored vision (O. A. Julian — Homeopathic Materia Medica).

Causes a form of intoxication accompanied by wonderful visions, remarkably beautiful and varied kaleidoscopic changes, and a sensation of increased physical ability. Also visions of monsters and various gruesome figures. A cardiac tonic and respiratory stimulant. Hysteria and insomnia. A remedy for brain fag, delirium, migraine, hallucinations, with brilliantly colored visions. Motor incoordination. Extreme muscular depression; increased patellar reflex. Paraplegia.

**Mind:** Loss of conception of time. Difficult enunciation. Distrust and resentment. Lazy contentment.

**Head:** Aches with disturbed vision. Vertigo, brain fag.

**Eyes:** Sees fantastic, brilliant, moving colored objects. Pupils dilated. *Polychrome spectra.*

**Ears:** Exaggerated reverberation of ordinary sounds.

**Relationship:** Compare: *Agave americana.* The intoxication of *Anh.* is similar to that of *Cannabis indica* and *Oenanthe crocata.*

**Dose:** Tincture.

---

## ANILINUM

(Coal Tar Product—Amidobenzene) **Anil.**

Marked giddiness and pain in the head; *face has a purple hue.* Pain in the penis (balanitis) and scrotum with swelling. *Tumors in the urinary passages.* Profound anemia with discoloration of skin, blue lips, anorexia, gastric disturbances. Swelling of skin.

**Relationship:** Compare: *Ars., Antip.*

---

## ANTHEMIS NOBILIS

(Roman Chamomile) **Anth.**

This remedy is akin to the ordinary *Chamomilla.* Gastric disturbance with coldness. Sensitive to cold air and cold things.

**Abdomen:** Aching in the region of liver; griping and *chilliness inside the abdomen,* radiating to the legs. Itching in the anus, with white, putty-like stools.

**Urinary:** Bladder feels distended. Pain along the spermatic cord, which feels full, as if varicosed. Frequent micturition.

**Respiration:** Coryza with increased lachrymation, sneezing, and discharge of clear water from the nose. Symptoms worse indoors. Constriction and rawness of the throat. Cough, tickling; worse in a warm room.

**Skin:** Itching of the soles, as if from chilblains. Gooseflesh.

**Dose:** Use the third potency.

---

## ANTHRACINUM

(Anthrax Poison) **Anthraci.**

This nosode has proven to be a great remedy in epidemic of splenic diseases in domestic animals, and in septic inflammations, *carbuncles* and *malignant ulcers. In boils* and boil like eruptions, and acne. Terrible burning. Induration of cellular tissue, abscess, bubo, and inflammation of connective tissue in which a purulent focus exists.

**Tissues**: Hemorrhages, black, thick, tar-like, rapidly decomposing, from any orifice. Glands swollen, *cellular tissues edematous and indurated.* Septicemia. Ulceration, sloughing and *intolerable burning.* Erysipelas. Black and blue blisters. Dissecting wounds. Insect stings. Bad effects from inhaling foul odors. Gangrenous parotitis. *Succession of boils.* Gangrene. Foul secretions.

**Relationship:** Similar to *Ars.*, which it often follows.

Compare: *Pyrog., Lach., Crot-h., Hippoz., Echi., Sil.* follows well. In the treatment of carbuncles, remember the prescription of the prophet Isaiah for King Hezekiah's carbuncle *i.e.,* the pulp of a fig placed on a poultice and applied.

Compare: *Tarent-c.*

**Dose:** Thirtieth potency.

---

## ANTHRAKOKALI

(Anthracite Coal Dissolved in Boiling Caustic Potash)

**Anthraco.**

Useful in skin affections, scabies, prurigo, chronic herpes, cracks and ulcerations. Papular eruptions with a vesicular tendency, especially on the scrotum, also on the hands, tibia, shoulders and dorsum of feet. Intense thirst. Chronic rheumatism. Bilious attacks, vomiting of bile, tympanic distention of abdomen.

**Dose:** Low triturations.

# ANTIMONIUM ARSENICOSUM

(Arsenite of Antimony) **Ant-ar.**

Found useful in *emphysema with excessive dyspnea* and cough, increased mucoid secretion. Worse on eating and lying down. Catarrhal pneumonia associated with influenza. Myocarditis and cardiac weakness. Pleurisy, especially of the left side, *with exudation*, pericarditis, and effusion. Sense of weakness. Inflammation of eyes and edema of face.

**Dose:** Third trituration.

---

# ANTIMONIUM CRUDUM

(Black Sulphide of Antimony) **Ant-c.**

For homeopathic employment, the mental symptoms, and those of the gastric sphere, determine its choice. *Excessive irritability and fretfulness,* with a *thickly coated, white tongue,* are the true guiding symptoms for many forms of diseases calling for this remedy. All the conditions are aggravated by *heat and by cold bathing.* Cannot bear heat of sun. Tendency to grow fat. Absence of pain, where it could be expected, is noticeable. Gout with gastric symptoms.

**Mind:** Very concerned about his fate. Cross and contradictive; whatever is done fails to give satisfaction. Sulky; does not wish to speak. Peevish; vexed without a cause. *Child cannot bear to be touched or looked at.* Angry at every little attention. Sentimental mood.

**Head:** Aching, worse in the vertex, on ascending, *from bathing, from a disordered stomach,* especially from eating candy or drinking acid wines. Suppressed eruptions. Heaviness of the forehead with vertigo; nausea, and epistaxis. Headache with great loss of hair.

**Eyes:** Dull, sunken, red, itch, inflamed, agglutinated. *Canthi raw and fissured. Chronic blepharitis.* Pustules on the cornea and lids.

**Ears:** Redness; swelling; pain in the eustachian tube. Ringing and deafness. Moist eruptions around the ear.

**Nose:** Nostrils *chapped and covered with crusts. Eczema of nostrils, sore, cracked and scurfy.*

**Face:** Pimples, pustules, and boils on the face. *Yellow crusty eruptions on cheeks* and chin. Sallow and haggard looking face.

**Mouth:** *Cracks at the corners of the mouth.* Dry lips. Saltish saliva. Slimy mucus. *Tongue coated thick white, as if white washed.* Gums detach from teeth; bleed easily (scorbutic). Toothache in hollow teeth. Rawness of palate, with expectoration of much mucus. *Canker sores.* Pappy taste. No thirst. Subacute eczema around the mouth.

**Throat:** Thick, yellowish mucus from posterior nares. Hawking in open air. Laryngitis. Rough voice from over use.

**Stomach:** *Loss of appetite. Desire for acids, pickles.* Thirst in the evening and at night. *Eructations tasting of the ingesta* (dyspepsia). Heartburn, nausea, vomiting. After nursing, the child vomits milk as curds, refuses to nurse afterwards, and is very cross. Gastric and intestinal complaints from bread and pastry, acids, sour wine, cold bathing, overheating, hot weather. *Constant belching.* Gouty metastasis to stomach and bowels. Sweetish waterbrash. *Bloating after eating.*

**Stool:** Anal itching. *Diarrhea alternates with constipation,* especially in old people. Diarrhea after acids, sour wine, baths, overeating; slimy, flatulent stools. Mucoid piles, continuous *oozing of mucus. Hard lumps mixed with watery discharge. Catarrhal proctitis.* Stools composed entirely of mucus.

**Urinary:** Frequent, with burning, and backache; turbid and foul odor.

**Male:** Eruptions on the scrotum and around the genitals. Impotence. Atrophy of penis and testicles.

**Female**: Excited; parts itch. Before menses, toothache; menses too early and profuse (menorrhagia). Menses suppressed from cold bathing, with sensation of pressure in the pelvis and tenderness in the ovarian region. Leucorrhea watery; acrid, lumpy.

**Respiratory:** Cough worse *coming into a warm room,* with a burning sensation in the chest, *itching of chest,* oppression. Aphonia from becoming overheated. *Voice harsh and badly pitched.*

**Back:** Itching and pain in the neck and back.

**Extremities:** Twitching of muscles (chorea). Jerks in arms. *Arthritic pain in fingers.* Nails brittle; grow out of shape. Horny warts on hands and soles. Weakness and shaking of hands when writing, followed by offensive flatulence. *Feet very tender;* covered with large horny corns. Inflamed corns. Pain in the heels (callosities).

**Sleep:** *Continuous drowsiness in old people.*

**Fever:** Chilly, even in a warm room. Intermittent with disgust, nausea, vomiting, eructations, coated tongue, diarrhea. Hot sweat.

**Skin:** Eczema with gastric derangements. Pimples, vesicles, and pustules. Sensitive to cold bathing. Thick, hard, honey colored scabs. *Urticaria;* measle-like eruption. Itching when warm in bed. Dry skin. *Warts* (*Thuj., Sabin., Caust.*). Dry gangrene. Scaly, pustular eruptions with burning and itching, worse at night.

**Modalities:** *Worse* in the evening, from heat, acids, wine, water, and washing. Wet poultices. *Better* in the open air, during rest. Moist warmth.

**Relationship:** Compare: *Antimonium chloridum* — Butter of Antimony (a remedy for cancer. Mucous membranes destroyed. Abrasions. Skin cold and clammy. Great prostration of strength. Dose: third trituration).

*Antimonium iodatum* (uterine hyperplasia; humid asthma. Pneumonia and bronchitis; loss of strength, and appetite, yellowish skin, sweaty, dull and drowsy. In sub-acute and chronic colds which have extended downwards and have affected the bronchial tubes as a hard, croupy cough with a decided wheeze and an inability to raise the sputum, especially in the aged and weak patients (Bacmeister). Stage of resolution in pneumonia, slow and delayed).

Compare: *Kermes mineral— Stibium sulphuratum rubrum* (bronchitis.) Also *Puls., Ip., Sulph.*

Complementary: *Sulph.*

Antidote: *Hep.*

**Dose:** Third to sixth potency.

---

## ANTIMONIUM SULPHURATUM AURATUM

(Golden Sulphuret of Antimony) **Ant-s-aur.**

A remarkable remedy for many forms of chronic nasal and bronchial catarrh. Acne. Amaurosis.

**Nose and Throat:** *Epistaxis on washing.* Increased secretions from the nose and throat. Rough and scrapy feeling. Anosmia. Metallic, styptic taste.

**Respiratory:** Tickling in the larynx. *Increased mucus* which fills up the bronchi. Respiration difficult, pressure in bronchi, with constriction. Tough mucus in bronchi and larynx. Dry hard cough. Congestion in the upper lobe of left lung. Winter coughs, patient is sore all over. Pneumonia, hepatization stage when resolution fails to take place.

**Skin:** Acne (pustular variety). Itching of hands and feet.

**Dose:** Second or third trituration.

---

## ANTIMONIUM TARTARICUM

(Tartar Emetic, Tartrate of Antimony and Potash) **Ant-t.**

Has many symptoms in common with *Antimonium crudum,* but has its own characteristic simptoms. Clinically, its therapeutic application has been confined, largely to the treatment of respiratory diseases, *rattling of mucus with little expectoration* has been a guiding symptom. *Drowsiness, debility and sweat* are characteristic to the drug. Gastric affections of drunkards and gouty subjects. *Cholera morbus.* Sensation of coldness in blood vessels. *Bilharziasis. Ant-t.* is homeopathic to dysuria, strangury, hematuria, albuminuria, catarrh of bladder and urethra (cystitis, urethritis), burning in the rectum, bloody mucus stools, etc. *Ant-t.* acts indirectly on the parasites by stimulating the oxidizing action of the protective substance. Side effects following injection for bilharziasis. *Chills, contractures* and pain in muscles. Trembling of the whole body, great prostration and faintness. Lumbago. Warts on glans penis.

**Mind:** Great despondency. Fear of being alone, muttering delirium and stupor. Child whines on being touched.

**Head:** Vertigo alternates with drowsiness. Vertigo, with dullness and confusion. Band-like sensation over the forehead. Headache as if a band is compressing the head (*Nit-ac.*).

**Face:** Cold, blue, *pale; covered with cold sweat. Incessant quivering of chin and lower jaw* (*Gels.*). Face pale and sunken.

**Mouth:** *Tongue coated, pasty, thick white,* with red edges. Red and dry, especially in the center. Brown.

**Stomach:** Difficult deglutition of liquids. Vomiting in any position, except when lying on the right side. *Nausea, retching and vomiting,* especially after food, with deathly faintness and prostration. *Thirst for cold water, little and often. Desire for apples, fruits, and acids generally.* Nausea produces fear; with pressure in the precordial region, followed by headache with yawning, lachrymation and vomiting.

**Abdomen:** Spasmodic colic, much flatus. Pressure in the abdomen, especially on bending forward. Cholera morbus. Diarrhea in eruptive diseases.

**Urinary:** Burning in urethra during and after micturition. Last drops bloody with pain in the bladder. Frequent urging. Catarrh of bladder and urethra. Stricture. Orchitis.

**Respiratory:** Hoarseness. *Great rattling of mucus, but very little is expectorated.* Velvety feeling in the chest. Burning sensation in the chest, which ascends to the throat. Rapid, short, difficult breathing; seems as if he would suffocate (asthma); must sit up. Emphysema in the aged. *Coughing and gaping consecutively.* Bronchial tubes overloaded with mucus. Cough excited by eating, with pain in the chest and larynx (bronchitis); pneumonia. *Edema and impending paralysis of lungs.* Palpitations, with uncomfortable hot, feeling. Pulse rapid, weak, trembling. Dizziness, with cough. Dyspnea relieved by eructations. Cough and dyspnea better by lying on the right side (opposite *Badiaga*), whooping cough.

**Back:** *Violent pain in the sacro-lumbar region.* Slightest effort to move may cause retching and cold clammy sweat. *Sensation of a heavy weight on the coccyx, dragging downward all the time.* Twitching of muscles; limbs tremulous.

**Sleep:** *Great drowsiness.* On falling asleep, electric-like shocks. Irresistible inclination to sleep with nearly all complaints.

**Fever:** Coldness, trembling, and chilliness. Intense heat. Copious perspiration. Cold, clammy sweat, with faintness. Intermittent fever with lethargic condition.

**Skin:** Pustular eruption, leaving a bluish-red mark. Smallpox. Warts.

**Modalities:** *Worse,* in the evening; from lying down at night; from warmth; in damp cold weather; from all sour things and milk. *Better,* from sitting erect; from eructation and expectoration.

**Relationship:** Antidotes: *Puls., Sep.*

Compare: *Kali-s., Ip.*

**Dose:** Second and sixth trituration. The lower potencies sometimes aggravate.

---

## ANTIPYRINUM

(Phenazone—A Coal-tar Derivative) **Antip.**

*Antipyrinum* is one of the drugs that induces leucocytosis, similar to ergotin, salicylates, and tuberculin. Acts especially on the vasomotor centers, causing dilation of capillaries of the skin and consequently circumscribed patches of hyperemia and swelling. In large doses, causes profuse perspiration, dizziness, cyanosis, and somnolence, albumin and blood in urine. Acute erythema multiforme.

**Mind:** Fear of becoming insane; nervous anxiety; *hallucinations of sight and hearing.*

**Head:** Throbbing headache; *sensation of constriction.* Flashes of heat. *Pain below the ears with otalgia.*

**Eyes:** Puffiness of lids. Conjunctiva red and edematous, *with lachrymation.* Red spots (*Apis.*).

**Ears:** Otalgia, buzzing. *Tinnitus.*

**Face:** Edema and puffiness; hyperemic.

**Mouth:** Swelling of lips. Burning in the mouth and gums. Ulceration of lips and tongue; vesicles and bullae. Small lump in the cheek. Tongue swollen. Bloody saliva. Toothache along the lower jaw.

**Throat:** Pain on swallowing. Expectoration of fetid pus. Abscess, white false membrane. Sensation of burning.

**Stomach:** Nausea and vomiting; burning and pain.

**Urinary:** Diminished. Penis black.

**Female:** Itching and burning in vagina. Menses suppressed. Watery leucorrhea.

**Respiratory:** Fluent coryza. Nasal mucous membrane swollen. Dull pain in frontal sinus. Aphonia. Oppression and dyspnea. Cheyne-Stokes respiration.

**Heart:** Faintness, with sensation as if the heart stopped. Throbbing throughout the body. Rapid, weak, irregular pulse.

**Nervous System:** Epileptiform seizures. Contractures. Trembling and cramps. Crawling and numbness. *General prostration.*

**Skin:** *Erythema,* eczema, pemphigus. *Intense pruritus. Urticaria,* appearing and disappearing suddenly, with internal coldness. Angioneurotic edema. Dark blotches on the skin of penis, sometimes with edema.

**Dose:** Second decimal potency.

---

## APIS MELLIFICA

(The Honey-bee) **Apis**

Acts on cellular tissues causing edema of skin and mucous membranes.

The very characteristic effects of a bee sting furnish, unerring indications for its employment in disease. Swelling or puffing up of various parts, *edema,* red rosy hue, stinging pains, soreness, intolerance of heat and slightest touch, and afternoon aggravation are some of the general guiding symptoms. Erysipelatous inflammations, dropsical effusions and anasarca, acute inflammation of kidneys and other parenchymatous tissues are characteristic pathological states corresponding to *Apis. Apis* acts especially on the outer parts, skin, coatings of inner organs, serous membranes, etc. It produces serous inflammation with effusions in the membranes, of brain, heart, pleura, etc. Extreme sensitiveness to touch and general soreness is marked. *Constricted* sensations. Sensation of stiffness and as if something is torn off from inside the body. Marked prostration.

**Mind:** Apathy, indifference, and unconsciousness. *Awkward; drops things readily.* Stupor, with sharp cries and starts suddenly. Stupor alternating with erotic mania. Sensation of dying. Listless; cannot think clearly. Jealous, fidgety, hard to please. Sudden shrill, piercing screams. *Whining. Tearful.* Jealousy, fright, rage, vexation, grief. Cannot concentrate when attempting to read or study.

**Head:** Brain feels *very tired.* Vertigo with sneezing, worse on lying down or closing the eyes. Heat, throbbing, pressing pains, better on pressure, and worse on motion. Sudden stabbing pain. Dull, heavy sensation in the occiput, as if from a blow, extending to the neck (better on pressure), accompanied with sexual excitement. Bores head into pillow and screams out.[1]

**Eyes:** Lids *swollen,* red, *edematous,* everted, inflamed; burn and sting (blepharitis). Conjunctiva bright red, puffy (conjunctivitis). *Lachrymation, hot.* Photophobia. *Sudden piercing pains* (optic neuritis). Pain around the orbits. *Serous exudation, edema, and sharp pains. Suppurative inflammation of eyes.* Keratitis with *intense chemosis of ocular conjunctiva.* Staphyloma of cornea following suppurative inflammation. *Styes,* prevents their recurrence.

**Ears:** External ear red, inflamed, sore; stinging pains.

**Nose:** Coldness of the tip of the nose. *Red, swollen* inflamed, with sharp pains.

**Face:** Swollen, red, with piercing pain. Waxy, pale, edematous. Erysipelas with stinging, burning edema. Extends from right to left.

**Mouth:** Tongue fiery red, swollen, sore, and raw, with vesicles (glossitis). Scalding in the mouth and throat. Tongue feels scalded, red hot, trembling. Gums swollen. Lips swollen, especially upper. Membrane of mouth and throat glossy, as if varnished. *Red, shining, and puffy,* like erysipelas. Cancer of the tongue.

**Throat:** Constricted, stinging pains. *Uvula swollen,* sac like. Throat swollen, inside and out; tonsils swollen, *puffy, fiery red* (tonsillitis). Ulcers on tonsils (quinsy). *Fiery red margin* around a leathery membrane (diphtheria). Sensation of a fishbone in the throat.

**Stomach:** Sore feeling. *Thirstless.* Vomiting of food. *Craving for milk* (*Rhus-t.*).

**Abdomen:** *Sore, bruised* on pressure, when sneezing. *Extremely tender.* Dropsy of the abdomen (ascitis). Peritonitis. Swelling in right groin (inguinal hernia).

**Stool:** Involuntary stools on every motion; *anus seems open.* Bloody, painless. Anus feels raw. Hemorrhoids, with stinging pain, after confinement. Diarrhea watery, yellow; *cholera infantum type.* Cannot micturate without passing stool. Dark, fetid, worse after eating. Constipation; feels as if something would break on straining.

**Urinary:** Burning and soreness when micturating. Suppressed, loaded

---

1 Especially in meningitis and tubercular hydrocephalus (T. F. Allen—Handbook of Materia Media).

with casts; frequent and involuntary; stinging pain and strangury; *scanty, high colored.* Incontinence. *Last few drops* burn and smart.

**Female:** Edema of labia; relieved by cold water. Soreness and stinging pains; ovaritis; worse in *right* ovary. Menses suppressed, with cerebral and head symptoms, especially in young girls. Dysmenorrhea, with severe ovarian pains. Metrorrhagia profuse, with heaviness of the abdomen, faintness and stinging pain. Sense of tightness. Bearing down, as if menses were to appear. Ovarian tumors (cysts), metritis with stinging pains. Great tenderness in the abdomen, over the uterine region.

**Respiratory:** Hoarseness; *dyspnea,* breathing hurried and difficult. Edema of larynx (laryngitis). Feels as *if he could not draw another breath* (pleurisy). Suffocation; short, dry cough, suprasternal. Hydrothorax.

**Extremities:** Edematous. Synovitis. Felons in the beginning. Knee swollen, shiny, sensitive, sore, with stinging pain. Feet swollen and stiff. Feels too large. Rheumatic pain in the back and limbs. Tired, bruised feeling. Numbness of hands and finger tips. Hives with intolerable itching. Edematous swellings (cellulitis, erysipelas).

**Sleep:** Very *drowsy.* Dreams full of care and toil. Screams and *sudden starting during sleep.*

**Fever:** *Afternoon chill, with thirst; worse on motion and heat.* External heat, with a smothering sensation. Sweat stage absent or very slight, with sleepiness. Sleeps *after* the fever paroxysm. After perspiration, nettle rash, with shuddering.

**Skin:** Swellings after bites; *sore, sensitive.* Stinging. Erysipelas, with sensitiveness and swelling, rosy hue. Carbuncles, with burning, stinging pain (*Ars., Anthraci.*). Sudden puffing up of the whole body (cellulitis).

**Modalities:** *Worse,* heat in any form; *touch;* pressure; late in the afternoon; after sleeping; in closed and heated rooms. Right side. *Better,* in open air, uncovering, and cold bathing.

**Relationship:** Complementary: *Nat-m.,* the "chronic," *Apis;* also *Bar- c.,* if lymphatics are involved.

Inimical: *Rhus-t.*

Compare: *Apium virus* (auto-toxemia, with pus products); *Zinc., Canth., Vesp., Lach.*

**Dose:** Tincture to thirtieth potency. In edematous conditions, the *lower* potencies are used. Sometimes action is slow; thus several days elapse before it's action is seen and then the quantity of urine is increased. *Apium virus*, sixth trituration.

---

## APIUM GRAVEOLENS

(Common Celery) **Ap-g.**

Contains a soporific active principle. Obstinate retention of urine, throbbing headaches and heartburn, have been produced by celery. Swelling, of throat, face, and hands. Rheumatic pain in muscles of neck and sacrum. Growing pains. Hungry for apples. Dysmenorrhea, with sharp, short pains, better flexing legs.

**Head:** Depressed; energetic; fidgety; cannot sleep from thinking. Headache; better eating. Eyeballs feel sunken. Itching in eyes. Itching and smarting in inner canthus of left eye.

**Abdomen:** Sore; sharp sticking pain as if stool would come; diarrhea, sharp pains in the left iliac region going over to the right side. Nausea increases with pains.

**Female:** Sharp sticking pains in both ovarian regions, especially left, better bending over, by lying on the left side, *with legs flexed;* nipples tender.

**Respiratory:** Tickling, dry cough. *Intense constriction over the sternum,* with a drawing feeling through the back on lying down. Throat swollen, dyspnea.

**Sleep:** Unrefreshed; sleepless. Awake between 1 to 3 a. m. Eating does not help sleep. Not fatigued from loss of sleep.

**Skin:** Itchy blotches; burning, creeping sensation. Profuse discharge from granulating ulcers. Urticaria with shuddering.

**Dose:** First to thirtieth potency.

---

## APOCYNUM ANDROSAEMIFOLIUM

(Dogbane) **Apoc-a.**

The rheumatic symptoms of this remedy promise highly curative results. Pain is of a wandering nature, with stiffness and drawing. Everything smells and tastes like honey. Worms. Trembling and prostration. Swollen sensations.

**Extremities:** Pain in all joints. Pain in toes and soles. Swelling of hands and feet. Profuse sweat, with sensation of violent heat in soles. Tingling pain in toes. Cramps in soles (*Sulph.*).

**Dose:** Tincture and first potency.

---

# APOCYNUM CANNABINUM

(Indian Hemp) **Apoc.**

Increases secretions of mucous and serous membranes; acts on cellular tissues, producing edema and dropsy, and on the skin causing diaphoresis. Acute hydrocephalus. A diminished frequency of pulse is a prime indication. This is one of our most efficient remedies in *dropsies,* ascites, anasarca, hydrothorax, hydrocephalus, and in urinary problems, especially suppression and strangury. Indicated in digestive complaints of Bright's disease with nausea, vomiting, drowsiness and difficult breathing. Dropsy is characterized by great thirst and gastric irritability. Arrhythmia. *Mitral and tricuspid regurgitation. Acute alcoholism.* Relaxation of sphincters.

**Mind:** Bewildered. Low spirited.

**Nose:** Long continued sneezing. Snuffles in children (*Samb.*). Chronic nasal catarrh with tendency to acute stuffiness and dull, sluggish memory. Dull headache. Takes cold easily, nostrils become congested and blocked up easily.

**Stomach:** Nausea, with drowsiness. Thirst on walking. *Excessive vomiting.* Food or water is immediately ejected. Dull, heavy, sick feeling. Oppression in the epigastrium and chest, impeding respiration (*Lob.*). Sensation of sinking in the stomach. Abdomen bloated. Ascites.

**Stool:** *Watery stools,* flatulent, with soreness of the anus; worse after eating; sensation as if the sphincter was open and the stools ran right out.

**Urinary:** Bladder, distended. Turbid, hot urine, with thick mucus and burning in urethra, after micturition. Little expulsive power. Dribbling. Strangury. *Renal dropsy* (hydronephrosis).

**Female:** Amenorrhea, with bloating of abdomen; metrorrhagia with nausea; fainting, vital depression. Hemorrhages (menorrhagia) at change of life (menopause). Blood expelled in large clots.

**Respiratory:** Short, dry cough. *Respiration short and unsatisfactory.* Sighing. Oppression in the epigastrium and chest.

**Heart:** Tricuspid regurgitation; rapid and feeble, irregular cardiac action, low arterial tension, pulsating jugulars, general cyanosis and anasarca.

**Sleep:** Great restlessness with little sleep.

**Modalities:** *Worse,* cold weather; cold drinks; uncovering.

**Relationship:** *Cymarinum* (the active principle of *Apoc.*,) lowers pulse rate and increases blood pressure. *Strophanthus* (extreme cardiac depression with intense gastric disturbance; dropsy). *Aralia hispida*—Wild elder (a valuable diuretic. Useful in dropsy of the cavities, due to hepatic or renal disease with constipation. Urinary disorders, especially with dropsy. Scudder advises a dose of five to thirty drops in sweetened cream of tartar solution). *Apis, Ars., Dig., Hell.*

**Dose:** Tincture (ten drops, three times daily) and in acute alcoholism, 1 dram of decoction in 4 oz. water.

---

# APOMORPHINUM HYPOCHLORICUM

(Alkaloid from Decomposition of Morphine by Hydrochloric Acid)

**Apom.**

The chief power of this drug lies in the speedy and effective vomiting that it produces, which becomes a strong guiding symptom for its homeopathic use. The vomiting is preceded by nausea, lassitude and increased secretion of sweat, saliva, mucus and tears. Pneumonia with vomiting. *Alcoholism,* with constant nausea, constipation, insomnia.

**Head:** Vertigo. Dilated pupils. Feels hot, all over the body, especially in the head.

**Stomach:** Empty retching and headache; heartburn; pain between shoulder blades. Reflex vomiting of pregnancy. *Seasickness. Nausea and vomiting.* Violent inclination to vomit.

**Non-homeopathic Uses:** The hypodermic injection of one sixteenth of a grain will cause full emesis within five to fifteen minutes in an adult without developing any other direct action apparently. Do not use in opium poisoning. *Apom.* hypodermically, one-thirtieth grain or less, acts as a safe and sure hypnotic. Acts well even in delirium. Sleep comes on in half an hour.

**Dose:** Third to sixth potency.

---

# AQUILEGIA VULGARIS

(Columbine)

**Aqui.**

A remedy for hysteria. Globus and clavus hystericus. Women at climaxis, with bilious vomiting especially in the morning. *Sleeplessness.* Nervous trembling of the body; sensitive to light and noise. Dysmenorrhea in young girls.

**Female:** Menses scanty; dull, painful, pressure in the right lumbar region, increasing at night.

**Dose:** First potency.

---

# ARAGALLUS LAMBERTI

(White Locoweed, Rattle Weed) **Arag.**

Acts principally on the nervous system, producing a bewildered, confused state. Symptoms of incoordination and paralysis. Locomotor ataxia. Tired in the morning.

**Mind:** Great depression; worse in the morning or in the evening. Cannot study. Cross, irritable, restless. *Bewildered.* Mental confusion and apathy. Desires to be alone. Difficulty in concentrating the mind, absent minded. Lack of ambition. Defective expression in writing. Restlessness and aimless wandering. Must concentrate on his walking.

**Eyes:** Diplopia. Burning in eyes.

**Face:** Cracking of lower lip.

**Throat:** Aches. Feels full. Sore with nausea. Pharynx dark, swollen, glazed (pharyngitis).

**Respiratory:** Weight on chest, in the region of ensiform cartilage. Constriction with a sensation of a wide band across the chest. Soreness of the chest under the sternum. Oppression.

**Extremities:** Weakness of limbs. Pain in left sciatic nerve. Cramps in the muscles, in front of the leg while walking.

**Relationship:** Compare: *Astragalus Lamberti* or *Oxyt.*, a variety of Locoweed; also *Bar-c.*

**Dose:** Sixth and two hundredth potencies.

---

# ARALIA RACEMOSA

(American Spikenard) **Aral.**

This is a remedy for asthmatic conditions, with *cough aggravated on lying down.* Drenching sweat during sleep. Extremely sensitive to draughts. Diarrhea, prolapse of rectum. Aching in the rectum extending upwards; worse lying on the side lain upon.

**Nose:** The least current of air causes sneezing and *copious watery, excoriating nasal discharge, with a salty acrid taste.*

**Female:** Menses suppressed; leucorrhea foul smelling, acrid, with pressing down pain. Lochia suppressed, with tympanites.

**Respiratory:** *Dry cough coming on after first sleep,* (around the middle of the night). *Asthma on lying down at night* with spasmodic cough; worse after first sleep, with tickling in the throat. Constriction of chest; *sensation of* *a foreign body in the throat.* Obstruction worse in spring. Hay fever; *frequent sneezing.* Rawness and burning behind the sternum.

**Modalities:** Worse around 11 p. m. (cough).

**Relationship:** Compare: *Pecten jacobaeus* — Scallop (humid asthma. Quick, labored breathing. Constriction of chest, especially right side. Asthma preceded by coryza and burning in the throat and the chest. Attack ends with copious expectoration of tough, frothy mucus. Worse at night). *Ars-i., Naphtin., All-c., Rosa, Sabad., Sin-n.*

**Dose:** Tincture to third potency.

---

# ARANEA DIADEMA

(Papal-cross Spider) **Aran.**

All spider poisons powerfuly affect the nervous system (see *Tarentula hispanica, Mygale lasiodora*, etc.).

All symptoms of *Aran.* are characterized by *periodicity, coldness* and a great susceptibility to dampness. It is the remedy for the constitution favorable to malarial poisoning, every damp place or weather favors chilliness. Patient feels cold to the very bones. Coldness, not relieved by anything. *Sensation as if parts were enlarged and heavier.* Wakes up at night with hands feeling twice their natural size. Spleen swollen (splenomegaly). *Hydrogenoid constitution, i.e.,* abnormal sensitivity to dampness and coldness, inability to live near fresh water lakes, rivers, etc., or in damp, chilly places (*Nat-s., Thuj.*).

**Head:** Pain in the right trigeminal nerve from periphery inwards. Confusion; *better by smoking in open air.*

**Eyes:** Heat and flickering in eyes; worse in damp weather.

**Mouth:** Sudden violent pain in teeth at night, immediately after lying down.

**Stomach:** Cramps after eating little; epigastrium tender on applying pressure.

**Abdomen:** Splenomegaly. Colic returns at the same hour everyday. Heaviness in the lower abdomen, as of a stone. Diarrhea.

**Female:** *Menses too early, too copious* (menorrhagia). Distension of the abdomen. Lumbo-abdominal neuralgia.[1]

**Chest:** Pain along the course of intercostal nerve, from the nerve endings to the spine. Bright red hemorrhage from lungs (hemoptysis) (*Mill., Ferr-p.*).

---

[1] Spasms commencing in the stomach (Clarke: Dictionary of Practical Materia Medica).

**Extremities:** Bone pain in extremities. Pain in *os calcis. Sensation of swelling,* and of parts going to sleep.

**Sleep:** Restless wakes up frequently as if hands and forearms were swollen and heavy.

**Fever:** *Coldness, with pain in long bones,* sensation of a stone in the abdomen at the same hour daily. *Chilly day and night;* always worse during rain.

**Modalities:** *Worse,* damp weather; late in the afternoon, and at midnight. *Better,* smoking tobacco.

**Relationship:** *Tela aranearum* — Spider's web (cardiac sleeplessness[1], increased muscular energy. Excitement and nervous agitation in febrile states. Dry asthma, harassing coughs; periodic headaches with *extreme nervous erethism. Obstinate intemittent fever.* Acts immediately on the arterial system, pulse full, strong, compressible. Lowers pulse rate frequency. Marked periodical diseases, hectic, broken down patients. Symptoms come on *suddenly* with cool, *clammy* skin. Numbness of hands and legs when at rest. *Continuous chills*).

*Aranea scinencia* — Grey spider (constant twitchings under the eyelids. Sleepiness. Worse in a warm room). *Helo., Cedr., Ars.*

**Dose:** Tincture to thirtieth potency.

---

## ARBUTUS ANDRACHNE

(Strawberry Tree) **Arb.**

A remedy for eczema associated with gouty and rheumatic symptoms. Arthritis; especially larger joints. Urine rendered more clear. Lumbago. Symptoms shift from skin to joints. Vesical symptoms.

**Relationship:** *Arbin., Led., Bry., Kalm.*

**Dose:** Tincture to third potency.

---

## ARECA CATECHU

(Betel Nut) **Arec.**

Of use in helminthiasis. Its alkaloid, *Arecolinum brom-hydricum* contracts the pupil, acting more promptly and energetically than *Eserinum* but the action

---

1 Rapidly lowers the frequency of pulse rate. In some, it produces a calm and delightful state of feeling, followed by a disposition to sleep. (Clarke — Dictionary of Practical Materia Medica).

is of a shorter duration. Serviceable in glaucoma. Acts also as a salivatory like *Pilocarpinum.* Also increases the amplitude of pulsations in the heart and promotes the contractibility of the intestines.[1]

## ARGEMONE MEXICANA

(Prickly Poppy) **Arge.**

Colicky cramps and spasm of bowels. Painful neuro-muscular conditions, preventing sleep. Rheumatic disease associated with Bright's disease (D. MacFarlan).

**Head:** Throbbing headache in eyes and temples. Head hot.

**Throat**: Very dry pain on swallowing.

**Stomach:** Feels sick, feels like vomiting. Griping in the pit of the stomach. No appetite. Belching and passing gas.

**Urinary:** Passes scanty urine. Changing color.

**Female:** Menses suppressed. Diminished sexual desire with weakness.

**Extremities:** Left knee stiff and painful (osteoarthritis). Feet swollen.

**Modalities:** *Worse* at noon (weakness).

**Dose:** Sixth potency. Fresh juice is applied on ulcers and warts.

## ARGENTUM METALLICUM

(Silver) **Arg-met.**

Emaciation, a gradual drying up, desire for fresh air, dyspnea, sensation of expansion and left sided pains are characteristic. The chief action is centered on the articulations and their component elements, bones, cartilages, and ligaments. Exostosis. Here the small blood vessels, close or wither and carious affections result. The symptoms come on insidiously, lingeringly, but progressively. The larynx is also a special center of action for this drug.

**Mind:** Hurried feeling; time passes slowly; melancholy.

**Head:** Dull paroxysmal neuralgia over the left side (migraine), gradually increasing and ceasing suddenly. Scalp very tender to touch. Vertigo, with an intoxicated feeling, on looking at running water. *Head feels empty, hollow* (brain fag).

[1] Hence acts as a tineafuge (tapeworm) (Clarke — Dictionary of Practical Materia Medica).

**Eyes:** Eyelids red and thick (blepharitis). Pain between the left eye and frontal eminence.

**Nose:** Exhausting coryza with sneezing.

**Face:** Pain in the facial bones.

**Throat:** Raw, hawking, gray, *jelly like mucus.* Throat sore on coughing. *Profuse and easy* expectoration in the morning.

**Urinary:** Diuresis. Urine *profuse, turbid with a* sweet odor. Frequent micturition. Polyuria.

**Male:** Crushed pain in testicles. *Seminal emissions, without excitement.* Frequent micturition with burning.

**Female:** Ovaries feel too large. Bearing down pain. Prolapse of uterus. *Eroded, spongy cervix. Leucorrhea* foul, excoriating. Palliative in scirrhus of uterus. Pain in the left ovary. *Climacteric hemorrhage.* Sore feeling throughout the abdomen; worse by jarring. Uterine disease with pain in joints and limbs.

**Respiratory:** *Hoarseness.* Aphonia. Raw, sore feeling when coughing. Total loss of voice in professional singers. Larynx feels sore and raw (laryngitis). *Easy expectoration, looks like boiled starch. Sensation of a raw spot near the supra-sternal fossa. Worse from use of voice. Cough on laughing.* Hectic fever at noon. Must hem and hawk on reading aloud. *Great weakness of the chest;* worse on the left side. Alteration in timbre of voice. Pain in left lower ribs.

**Back:** Severe backache; must walk bent, with oppression of chest.

**Extremities:** Rheumatic affections of joints, especially elbow and knee. Legs weak and trembling, worse descending stairs. Involuntary contractions of fingers, partial paralysis of forearm; Writer's cramp. *Swelling of ankles.*

**Modalities:** *Worse* from touch, towards noon. *Better* in open air; cough at night when lying down (opposite *Hyos.*).

**Relationship:** Antidotes: *Merc., Puls.*

Compare: *Sel., Alum., Plat., Stann., Ampelopsis quinquefolia* (chronic hoarseness in scrofulous patients).

**Dose:** Sixth trituration and higher. Not to be repeated frequently.

---

## ARGENTUM NITRICUM

(Nitrate of Silver) **Arg-n.**

In this drug the neurotic effects are very marked, many brain and spinal symptoms present themselves which give certain indications for its homeopathic employment. Symptoms of incoordination, loss of control and want of balance everywhere, mentally and physically; *trembling* in affected parts. Is an irritant of mucous membranes, producing violent inflammation of the throat, and marked gastroenteritis. Characteristic symptoms of this drug are, great *desire for sweets,* splinter-like pains, and free mucopurulent discharge from the inflamed and ulcerated mucous membranes. Sensation as if a part was expanding and other errors of perception are also characteristic. Withered up and dried constitutions present a favorable field for its action, especially when associated with unusual or long continuous mental exertion. Head symptoms often determine the choice of this remedy. Pains increase and decrease gradually. Flatulent state. A prematurely aged look. Explosive belching, especially in neurotics. Upper abdominal affections brought on by undue mental exertion. Paraplegia, myelitis and disseminated sclerosis of brain and cord. *Intolerance of heat.* Sensation of a sudden pinch (Dudgeon). Destroys red blood corpuscles, producing anemia.

**Mind:** Thinks his understanding will and must fail. Fearful and *nervous;* impulse to jump out of a window. Faintish and tremulous. *Melancholic;* apprehensive of serious disease. *Time passes slowly* (*Cann-i.*). Memory weak. Errors in perception. *Impulsive; wants to do things in a hurry* (*Lil-t.*). *Peculiar mental impulses.* Fears and anxieties. Hidden irrational motives for actions.

**Head:** *Headache with coldness and trembling.* Emotional disturbances cause appearance of hemi-cranial attacks. Migraine; bones of head feel as if separated. Sense of *expansion.*[1] Brain fag, with general debility and trembling. Headache from mental exertion, from dancing. *Vertigo,* with buzzing in the ears and with nervous affections. Aching in the frontal eminence, with *an enlarged feeling in the corresponding eye.* Boring pain; *better on tight bandaging and pressure.* Itching of scalp.

**Eyes:** Inner canthi *swollen and red.* Spots before the eye. Blurred vision (amblyopia). Photophobia in a warm room. *Purulent ophthalmia.* Great swelling of conjunctiva (chemosis); *discharge abundant and purulent.* Chronic ulceration on margin of lids; sore, thick, swollen (blepharitis). Unable to keep eyes steadily fixed. Eye strain from sewing (hypermetropia); worse in a warm room. Aching, tired feeling in the eyes, better on closing or pressing upon them. Useful in restoring power to the weakened ciliary muscles. Paretic condition of ciliary muscle. Acute granular conjunctivitis. Cornea opaque (leucoma). Corneal ulcer. Pterygium.

**Nose:** Anosmia. Itching. Ulcers on the septum. Coryza, with chilliness, lachrymation and headache.

**Face:** Sunken, old, pale and bluish. Old man's look; tight drawing of skin over bones.

[1] Convulsions — epileptic — aura (before epileptic convulsions) — expansion of body, sensation of — cause — from nervousness (1001 Small Remedies, Edited by Dr. F. Schroyens).

**Mouth:** Gums tender and bleed easily (scorbutic). Tongue has prominent papillae; tip is red and painful (glossitis). Pain in sound teeth. Taste coppery, like ink. Canker sores.

**Throat:** Abundan *thick mucus* in the throat and mouth causes hawking. Raw, rough and sore. *Sensation of a splinter in the throat* on swallowing. Throat dark red. Catarrh in smokers, with tickling due to sensation of a hair in the throat. *Feels strangulated.*

**Stomach:** *Belching* accompanies most gastric ailments. Nausea, retching, vomiting of glairy mucus. Flatulence; *painful swelling in the pit of the stomach.* Painful spot over stomach that radiates to all parts of the abdomen. Gnawing ulcerating pain; burning and constriction. Ineffectual efforts at eructation. *Great craving for sweets.* Gastritis in drunkards. Ulcerative pains on the left side, under the ribs. Trembling and throbbing in stomach. Enormous distention. Gastric ulcers *with radiating pain.* Desire for cheese and salt.

**Abdomen:** Colic, *with flatulent distention.* Stitchy, ulcerative pain on the left side of stomach, below the short ribs.

**Stool:** Watery, noisy, flatulent; *green, like chopped spinach,* with shreddy mucus and enormous distention of abdomen; very offensive. Diarrhea immediately after eating or drinking. *Fluids go right through him;* after sweets; after any emotion with flatulence. Itching in the anus.

**Urinary:** Urine passes unconsciously, day and night (enuresis). Urethra inflamed, with pain, burning, itching; pain as from a splinter (urethritis). Urine scanty and dark. Emission of a few drops after having finished. Divided stream. Early stage of gonorrhea; profuse discharge and terrible cutting pains; hematuria.

**Male:** Impotence. Erection fails when coition is attempted. Cancer-like ulcers. Desire wanting. Genitals shrivelled. Dysparunia.

**Female:** Gastralgia at the beginning of menses. Intense spasm of chest muscles. Orgasms at night. Nervous erethism at menopause. Leucorrhea profuse, with cervical erosion. Bleeding easily. Uterine hemorrhage, two weeks after menses (metrorrhagia). Painful affections of left ovary.

**Respiratory:** *High notes cause cough.* Chronic hoarseness. Suffocative cough, as if from a hair in the throat. Dyspnea.

**Chest**: Feels as if a bar was around it. Palpitations, pulse irregular and intermittent; worse lying on *right side* (*Alumn.*). Painful spots in the chest. Angina pectoris, nocturnal aggravation. Many people in a room seem to take away his breath.

**Back:** Severe pain. Spine sensitive with nocturnal pain (*Ox-ac.*), paraplegia; posterior spinal sclerosis.

**Extremities:** Cannot walk with eyes closed. Trembling, with general debility. Paralysis, with mental and abdominal symptoms. Rigidity of *calves.*

Debility especially in calves. Walks and stands unsteadily, especially when unobserved (locomotor ataxia). Numbness of arms. Post-diphtheritic paralysis (after *Gels.*).

**Sleep:** Sleeplessness, from fanciful imagination; horrible dreams of snakes, and of sexual gratification. Drowsy stupor.

**Fever:** Chills with nausea. Chilly when uncovered, yet feels smothered if wrapped up.

**Skin:** Brown, tense, and hard. Drawing sensation in skin, as from a spider web, or from an albuminous substance, withered and dried up. Irregular blotches.

**Modalities:** *Worse,* warmth in any form; at night; from cold food; *sweets;* after eating; at menstrual period; from emotions, *left side. Better,* from eructations; fresh air; *cold;* pressure.

**Relationship:** Antidote: *Nat-m.*

Compare: *Ars., Merc., Phos., Puls., Argentum cyanatum* (angina pectoris, asthma, spasm of esophagus);

*Argentum iodatum* (throat disorders, hoarseness, glands affected).

*Protargol* (gonorrhea after acute stage, 2 percent solution; syphilitic mucoid patches, chancres and chancroids, 10 percent solution applied twice a day; ophthalmia neonatorum, 2 drops of 10 percent solution).

*Argentum phosphoricum* (an excellent diuretic in dropsy).

*Argentum oxydatum* (chlorosis with menorrhagia and diarrhea).

**Dose:** Third to thirtieth potency.

Best as an aqueous solution, 1 is to 9, 2 or 3 drop doses. This solution in water is preferable to lower triturations; unless fresh, it readily decomposes into the oxide.

---

## ARISTOLOCHIA MILHOMENS

(Brazilian Snake Root) **Arist-m.**

Stitching pain in various parts. Pain in heels, burning in anus and frequent irritation. Flatulence. Pain in the back and extremities. Stiffness of legs. Pain in tendo-Achillis. Itching and swelling around the malleoli.

**Relationship:** Compare: *Aristolochia serpentaria*—Virginia snake root (symptoms of intestinal tract; colliquative diarrhea, meteorism. Flatulent dyspepsia. Cerebral congestion. Distention and cutting pains in the abdomen. Symptoms like those of Poison oak).

**Dose:** Lower potencies.

# ARNICA MONTANA

(Leopard's Bane) **Arn.**

Produces conditions upon the system quite similar to those resulting from injuries, falls, blows, contusions. Tinnitus aurium. *Putrid phenomena.* Septic conditions; prophylactic for purulent infection. Apoplexy, red, full face.

It is especially suited to cases when any injury, however remote, seems to have caused the present problem. *After traumatic injuries,* overuse of any organ, strains. *Arnica* is disposed to cerebral congestion. Acts best in plethoric, dark haired people of rigid muscles, with a nervous, sanguine nature, but it acts feebly in debilitated people with impoverished blood. Cardiac dropsy with dyspnea. A muscular tonic. Traumatism of grief, remorse or sudden realization of financial loss. Limbs and body ache, as if beaten; joints as if sprained. Bed feels too hard. Marked effect on the blood. Affects the venous system inducing stasis. Ecchymosis and hemorrhages. Relaxed blood vessels, black and blue spots (purpura). Tendency to hemorrhage and states of low grade fever. Tendency to tissue degeneration, septic conditions, abscesses that do not mature. *Sore, lame, bruised feeling.* Neuralgias originating by the disturbances in the pneumo-gastric nerve. Rheumatism of muscular and tendinous tissue, especially of the back and shoulders. Aversion to tobacco. *Influenza.* Thrombosis. Hematocele.

**Mind:** Fears touch, or the approach of anyone. Unconscious; when spoken to, answers correctly, but relapses. Indifference; inability to perform continuous active work; morose, delirious. Nervous; cannot bear pain; the whole body is oversensitive. Says that nothing is the matter with him. Wants to be left alone. Agrophobia (fear of space). After mental strain or shock.

**Head:** *Hot, with a cold body;* confused; sensitiveness of the brain, with sharp, pinching pains (meningitis). Scalp feels contracted. Cold spot on the forehead. Chronic vertigo; objects whirl about especially when walking.

**Eyes:** Diplopia from traumatism, muscular paralysis, retinal hemorrhage. Bruised, sore feeling in the eyes after intricate work. Must keep eyes open. Dizzy on closing them. Feel tired and weary after sight seeing, moving pictures, etc. (aesthenopia).

**Ears:** Noises in the ear caused by rush of blood to the head. Shooting in and around the ears. Bleeding from ears. Dullness of hearing after concussion. Pain in cartilages of ears, as if bruised.

**Nose:** Epistaxis after every fit of coughing, dark fluid blood. Nose feels sore; *cold.*

**Face:** Sunken; very red. Heat in lips. Herpes on the face.

**Mouth:** *Fetid breath* (halitosis). Dry and thirsty. Bitter taste (*Coloc.*).

*Taste as if from bad eggs.* Soreness of gums after tooth extraction (*Sep.*). Empyema of maxillary sinus.

**Stomach:** Longing for vinegar. Distaste for milk and meat. Canine hunger. Hematemesis. Pain in the stomach while eating. Repletion with loathing[1] Oppressive gases pass upward and downward. Pressure as if from a stone. *Feels as if the stomach was pressing against the spine. Fetid* vomiting.

**Abdomen:** Stitches under the false ribs. Distended; offensive flatus. Sharp thrusts through the abdomen.

**Stool:** *Straining with tènesmus in diarrhea. Offensive,* brown, *bloody,* putrid, involuntary. Looks like brown yeast. Must lie down after every stool. Diarrhea of consumption; worse lying on left side. Dysenteric stools with muscular pain.

**Urinary:** Urine retained from over exertion. Dark brick-red sediment. Cystitis with very painful micturition (dysuria).

**Female:** Bruised parts after labor. Violent after-pains. Uterine hemorrhage from mechanical injury, after coition. Sore nipples. Mastitis after injury. Feels as if the fetus was lying crosswise.

**Respiratory:** Cough depending on cardiac lesion, paroxysmal, at night, during sleep, worse exercise. Acute tonsillitis, swelling of soft palate and uvula. Pneumonia; approaching paralysis. Hoarseness from over use of voice. Raw, sore feeling in the morning. Cough produced by weeping and lamenting. Dry, from tickling, low down in the trachea. Bloody expectoration. Dyspnea with hemoptysis. All bones and cartilages of the chest are painful. *Violent spasmodic cough, with facial herpes.* Whooping cough, child cries before coughing. *Pleurodynia* (*Ran-b., Cimic.*).

**Heart:** *Angina pectoris;* pain especially severe in the left elbow. Stitches in the heart region. Pulse feeble and irregular. Cardiac dropsy with distressing dyspnea. Extremities distended (edematous), feel bruised and sore. Fatty heart and hypertrophy.

**Extremities:** Gout. Great fear of being touched or approached. Pain in the back and limbs, as if bruised or beaten. Sprained and dislocated feeling. Soreness after overexertion. Everything on which he lies seems too hard. Deathly coldness of the forearm. Cannot walk erect, on account of the bruised pain in the pelvic region (pelvic hematocele). Rheumatism begins low down and ascends (*Led.*).

**Sleep:** Sleepless and restless when overtired. Comatose drowsiness; awakens with a hot head; dreams of death, mutilated bodies, anxious and terrible. Horrors in the night. Involuntary stools during sleep.

---

[1] Well fed with a loathing for food — principally milk, meat, broth and tobacco (Clarke — Dictionary of Practical Materia Medica).

**Fever:** Febrile symptoms closely related to typhoid. Shivering all over the body. Heat and redness of the head, while rest of the body is cold. Internal heat; hands and feet cold. Sour sweat at night.

**Skin:** Black and blue. Itching, burning, eruption of small pimples. *Crops of small boils* (*Ichth., Sil.*). Ecchymosis. Bed sores. Acne indurata, characterized by *symmetry in distribution.*

**Modalities:** *Worse,* least touch, motion, rest, wine, damp cold. *Better, lying down,* or *lying with head low.*

**Relationship:** Antidotes: *Camph.*

*Vitex trifolia* — Indian arnica (sprains and pains, headache in temples, pain in joints, abdomen, and testicles).

Complementary: *Acon., Ip.*

Compare: *Acon., Bapt., Bell-p., Ham., Rhus-t., Hyper.*

**Dose:** Third to thirtieth potency. Locally, the tincture, but should never be applied *hot* or when abrasions or cuts are present.

---

# ARSENICUM ALBUM

(Arsenious Acid, Arsenic Trioxide) **Ars.**

Acts profoundly on every organ and tissue. Its clear cut characteristic symptoms and correspondence to several severe types of disease make its homeopathic employment constant and certain. Its general symptoms alone, often lead to its successful application. Among these, the all prevailing debility, exhaustion *and restlessness* with *nocturnal aggravation,* are most important. *Great exhaustion after the slightest exertion.* This, with the peculiar irritability of fibre, gives the characteristic *irritable weakness. Burning pains.* Unquenchable thirst. Burning relieved by heat. *Seaside complaints* (*Nat-m., Aqua marina*). Injurious effects of fruits, especially the more watery ones. Easens and quitens the last moments of life when given in a high potency. *Fear, fright and worry.* Green discharges. Infantile kala-azar (Dr. Neatby).

*Ars.* should be thought of in ailments from alcoholism, *ptomaine poisoning,* stings, dissecting wounds, chewing tobacco and ill effects from decayed food or animal matter. Odor of discharges is *putrid.* Complaints return annually. Anemia and chlorosis. Degenerative changes. Gradual loss of weight from impaired nutrition. Reduces the refractive index of blood serum (also *Chin.* and *Ferr-p.*). Maintains the system under the stress of malignancy regardless of location. Malarial cachexia. *Septic infections and low vitality.*

**Mind:** *Great anguish and restlessness. Changes place continuously. Fears,* of death, of being left alone. Great fear, with cold sweat. feels it is useless to take medicine. Suicidal. Hallucinations of smell and sight. Despair drives him from place to place. Miserly, malicious, selfish, lacks courage. General sensibility increased (*Hep.*). Sensitive to disorder and confusion.

**Head:** Headaches relieved by cold, other symptoms are aggravated by cold. Periodical burning pains, with *restlessness;* with a cold skin. Hemicrania (migraine), with an icy feeling on the scalp and great weakness. Head sensitive, in open air. Delirium tremens; cursing and raving; vicious. Head is in constant motion. Scalp *itches* intolerably; circular patches of bare spots (tinea capitis), rough, dirty, sensitive, and covered with dry scales; nocturnal burning and itching; dandruff. Scalp very sensitive; cannot brush hair.

**Eyes:** *Burning in eyes, with acrid lachrymation.* Lids red, ulcerated, scabby, scaly, granulated (blepharitis). Edema *around* the eyes. External inflammation, with extreme pain; *burning, hot,* and excoriating lachrymation. Corneal ulcers. *Intense photophobia;* better external warmth. Ciliary neuralgia, with fine burning pain.

**Ears:** Skin raw and burning within. *Thin, excoriating, offensive* otorrhea. Roaring in ears, during a paroxysm of pain.

**Nose:** *Thin, watery, excoriating* discharge. Nose feels *stopped up.* Sneezing *without* relief. Hay fever and coryza; worse in the open air; better indoors. *Burning* and bleeding. Acne of nose.. Lupus.

**Face:** Swollen, pale, yellow, *cachectic,* sunken, cold, and covered with sweat (*Acet-ac.*). Expression of agony. Tearing, *needle-like* pains; burning. Lips black, livid. Angry, circumscribed flushes of cheeks.

**Mouth:** Unhealthy, easily bleeding gums. Ulceration of mouth (apthae) with dryness and burning heat (cancrum oris). Epithelioma of lips. Tongue dry, clean, and red (glossitis); stitching and burning pains in the tongue, ulcerated with a blue color. Bloody saliva. Neuralgia of teeth; teeth feel long and very sore; worse after midnight; better warmth. Metallic taste. *Gulping up of burning water*[1].

**Throat:** Swollen, edematous, constricted, *burning,* unable to swallow. Diphtheritic membrane, looks dry and wrinkled.

**Stomach:** *Cannot bear the sight or smell of food. Great thirst; drinks much, but little at a time.* Nausea, retching, vomiting after eating or drinking. Anxiety in the pit of the stomach. *Burning pain.* Craves acids and coffee. Heartburn; gulping up of acid and bitter substances which seem to excoriate the throat. Long lasting eructations. Vomiting of blood, bile, green mucus, or brown-black mixed with blood. Stomach extremely irritable; seems raw, as if torn (gastric ulcer). Gastralgia from slightest food or drink. Dyspepsia from vinegar, acids, ice cream, ice water, tobacco. Terrible fear and dyspnea, with

[1] Regurgitation of acrid matter (Clarke — Dictionary of Practical Materia Medica).

gastralgia; also faintness, icy coldness and great exhaustion. Malignant symptoms. Everything swallowed seems to lodge in the esophagus, which seems closed, as if nothing would pass. *Ill effects of a vegetable diet, melons,* and *watery fruits generally.* Craves milk.

**Abdomen:** Gnawing, burning pains like coals of fire; relieved by heat. *Liver and spleen enlarged and painful.* Ascites and anasarca. Abdomen swollen and painful (peritonitis). Pain as if from a wound in the abdomen on coughing.

**Rectum:** Painful, spasmodic protrusion of rectum (prolapse). Tenesmus. *Burning* pain and pressure in rectum and anus. Hemorrhoids burn like fire; relieved by heat. Skin excoriated around the anus.

**Stool:** *Small, offensive, dark, with marked prostration. Worse at night, and after eating and drinking;* from chilling the stomach, alcoholic abuse and spoiled meat. Dysentery, dark, bloody and very offensive. Cholera, with intense agony, prostration, and burning thirst. Body cold as ice (*Verat.*).

**Urinary:** Urine scanty, burning, involuntary. Bladder feels as if paralyzed. *Albuminous.* Epithelial cells; cylindrical clots of fibrin and globules of pus and blood. After micturating, feeling of weakness in the abdomen. Bright's disease. Diabetes.

**Female:** Menses too profuse and too soon. Burning in ovarian region. Leucorrhea, acrid, burning, offensive, thin. Pain as if from red-hot wires; worse least exertion; causes great fatigue; better in a warm room. *Menorrhagia.* Stitching pains in the pelvis extending down the thighs. Endometritis.

**Respiratory:** Unable to lie down; fears suffocation (hydrothorax). Air passages constricted. Asthma worse midnight. Burning in the chest. Suffocative catarrh. Cough worse after midnight; worse lying on back. Expectoration scanty, *frothy. Darting pain through the upper third of right lung* (pneumonia). Wheezing respiration. Hemoptysis with pain between the shoulders; burning heat all over. Cough dry, as if from sulphur fumes; *after drinking.* Pleurisy.

**Heart:** Palpitations, pain, dyspnea, faintness. Irritable heart in smokers and tobacco chewers. *Pulse more rapid in the morning* (*Sulph.*). Dilatation. Cyanosis. Fatty degeneration. Angina pectoris, with pain in the neck and occiput.

**Back:** Weakness in the small of back (lumbosacral region). Drawing in of the shoulders. Pain and burning in the back (*Ox-ac.*).

**Extremities:** Trembling, twitching, spasms, weakness, heaviness, uneasiness. Cramps in calves. Swelling of feet. Sciatica. Burning pains. Peripheral neuritis. Diabetic gangrene. Ulcers on the heel (*All-c., Lam.*). Paralysis of the lower limbs with atrophy.

**Sleep:** Disturbed, anxious, restless. Head must be raised by pillows. Suffocative fits during sleep. Sleeps with hands over the head. Dreams are full of care and fear. Drowsiness, sleeping sickness.

**Fever:** High temperature. *Periodicity marked with adynamia.* Septic fevers. *Intermittent* fevers. *Paroxysms incomplete, with marked exhaustion. Hay fever.* Cold sweats. Typhoid, not too early, often prescribed after *Rhus-t.* Complete exhaustion. Delirium; worse after midnight. Great restlessness. Great heat around 3 a. m. Sordes.

**Skin:** Itching, burning, swellings, edema; eruptions, papular, *dry, rough, scaly; worse cold* and scratching. Malignant pustules. Ulcers with an offensive discharge. Anthrax. Poisoned wounds. Urticaria, with burning and restlessness. *Psoriasis.* Scirrhus. Icy coldness of the body. Epithelioma of the skin. Gangrenous inflammations.

**Modalities:** *Worse,* wet weather, after midnight, from cold (except headache), cold drinks or food, seashore, right side. *Better* from heat, from head elevated, warm drinks.

**Relationship:** Complementary: *Rhus-t., Carb-v., Phos., Thuj., Sec.* Antidotal to lead poisoning.

Antidotes: *Op., Carb-v., Chin., Hep., Nux-v.*

Chemical antidotes: Charcoal; Hydrated peroxide of iron; Lime water.

Compare: *Arsenicum stibiatum* 3x (chest inflammations in children, restlessness with thirst and prostration, loose mucoid, cough, oppression, hurried respiration, crepts and rales). *Cenchris contortrix; Iod., Phos., Chin., Verat., Carb-v., Kali-p. Epilobium palustre* (intractable diarrhea of typhoid). *Hoang nan. Atoxyl:* Sodium arseniate 3x, sleeping sickness; commencing optic atrophy. *Levico water*-containing *Ars.*, iron and copper of South Tyrol (chronic and dyscratic skin diseases, chorea minor and spasms in scrofulous and anemic children. Favors assimilation and increases nutrition. Debility and skin diseases, especially after the use of higher potencies where progress seems suspended. Dose: Ten drops in a wine glass of warm water, 3 times a day after meals. Burnett). *Sarcolacticum acidum* (influenza with violent vomiting).

**Dose:** Third to thirtieth potency. The very highest potencies often yield brilliant results.

Low attenuations in gastric, intestinal, and kidney diseases; higher in neuralgias, nervous diseases, and skin. But if only surface conditions call for it, give the lowest potencies, 2x to 3x trituration. Repeated doses advisable.

---

# ARSENICUM BROMATUM

(Bromide of Arsenic) **Ars-br.**

Has proven to be a great anti-psoric and anti-syphilitic remedy. Herpetic eruptions, syphilitic excrescences, glandular tumors and indurations, carcinoma, locomotor ataxia, obstinate intermittent fever and diabetes are all greatly influenced by this preparation.

**Face:** *Acne rosacea,* with violet papules on the nose; worse in the spring. *Acne* in young people.

**Dose:** Tincture, two to four drops daily in water. In diabetes, three drops, three times a day in a glass of water.

---

# ARSENICUM HYDROGENISATUM

(Arseniuretted Hydrogen) **Ars-h.**

The general action of *Ars.* is more accentuated in this. Anemia. Anxiety; despair. *Hematuria,* with general disorganization of blood. Hemorrhages from mucous membranes. Urine suppressed, followed by vomiting. Prepuce and glans covered with pustules and round superficial ulcers. Collapse. Coldness; prostration. Sudden weakness and nausea. Skin becomes dark brown.

**Head:** Violent vertigo on going upstairs.

**Eyes:** Sunken; broad, blue circles around.

**Nose:** Violent sneezing. Nose cold. Must be wrapped up in warm clothes.

**Mouth:** Tongue enlarged; deep, irregular ulcer; nodular swelling. Mouth hot and dry; little thirst.

**Dose:** Third potency.

---

# ARSENICUM IODATUM

(Iodide of Arsenic) **Ars-i.**

It is preferred in persistently irritating, corrosive discharges. The discharge irritates the membrane from which it flows and *over* which it flows. The discharge may be fetid, watery, and the mucous membrane is always red, angry, swollen; itches and burns. Influenza, *hay fever,* old nasal catarrhs, and catarrh of the middle ear. Swelling of tissues within the nose. Hypertrophied condition of the eustachian tube with deafness. Senile heart, myocarditis and fatty degeneration. Pulse shotty. Chronic aortitis. Epithelioma of the lip. Cancer of the breast after ulceration has set in.

It seems probable that in *Ars-i.*, we have a remedy very closely allied to the manifestations of tuberculosis. In the early stages of tuberculosis, even though there is an afternoon rise in temperature, *Ars-i.* is very effective. It will be indicated by profound prostration, rapid irritable pulse, recurring fever and sweats, emaciation, and a tendency to diarrhea. Chronic pneumonia, with lung abscess. Hectic; debility; night sweats.

This remedy is also to be remembered in phthisis with hoarse, racking cough and profuse purulent expectoration, attended with cardiac weakness, emaciation and general debility; in chronic, watery diarrhea in phthisical subjects; in cases of emaciation with a good appetite; in amenorrhea, with anaemic palpitations and dyspnea. In chronic pneumonia, when an abscess is about to form. Great emaciation. Arteriosclerosis, myocardial degeneration and senile heart. Threatened pyemia (*Pyrog., Methyl.*).

**Head:** *Vertigo,* with tremulous feeling, especially in the aged.

**Eyes:** Scrofulous ophthalmia.

**Ears:** Otitis media, with fetid, corrosive otorrhea. Thickening of tympanum.

**Nose:** *Thin, watery, irritating, excoriating discharge from anterior and posterior nares; sneezing.* Hay fever. Irritation and tingling in the nose, constant desire to sneeze (*Pollantinum*). *Chronic nasal catarrh;* swollen nose; profuse, thick, yellow discharge; ulcers; *membrane sore and excoriated* (ozena). Aggravation by sneezing.

**Throat:** Burning in the pharynx. Tonsils swollen. Thick membrane from fauces to lips. Breath fetid, glandular involvement. Diphtheria. Chronic follicular pharyngitis.

**Stomach:** Pain and pyrosis. Vomiting an hour after eating food. Nausea distressing. Pain in the epigastrium. Intense thirst; water is immediately ejected.

**Respiratory:** Slight hacking cough, with dry and stopped up nostrils. Pleuritis exudativa. Chronic bronchitis. Pulmonary tuberculosis. Pneumonia that fails to clear up. Broncho-pneumonia after influenza. Cough dry, with little or difficult expectoration. Aphonia.

**Fever:** Recurrent fever and sweats. *Drenching nightsweats.* Pulse rapid, feeble, weak, irregular. Chilly, cannot endure cold.

**Skin:** Dry, scaly, itchy. *Marked exfoliation of skin in the form of large scales,* leaving a raw exuding surface beneath. *Ichthyosis. Enlarged scrofulous glands. Venereal bubo.* Debilitating night sweats. Eczema of the beard; watery, oozing, itching; worse, washing. Emaciation. Psoriasis. Acne hard, shotty with an indurated base and pustule at the apex.

**Relationship:** Compare: *Tub., Ant-i.* In hay fever, compare: *Aral., Naphtin., Rosa, Sangin-n.*

**Dose:** Second and third trituration. Ought to be prepared fresh and protected from light. Should be continued for some time. Clinically, it has been found advisable in tuberculosis, begin with 4x and gradually go lower to the second x trituration, 5 grains, 3 times a day.

---

## ARSENICUM METALLICUM

(Metallic Arsenic) **Ars-met.**

Arouses latent syphilis. Periodicity is very marked; symptoms recur every two and three weeks. Weakness. Swollen sensation in parts.

**Mind:** Low spirited, weak memory. *Desire to be alone.* Annoyed by visions, which make her cry.

**Head:** Head feels too large. Left sided headache extending to the left eye and ear (migraine). Headache worse stooping and lying down. Edematous swelling of forehead.

**Eyes:** Watery, burn with coryza. Eyes weak, daylight and gas light aggravate. Lids swollen.

**Face:** Red bloated with itching and burning.

**Mouth:** Tongue is coated white, and shows imprint of teeth. Mouth sore and ulcerated.

**Abdomen:** Soreness in the region of the liver, pain radiates to the shoulders and spine. Pain in the region of spleen, extending to the groin. Pain in the breast extends to the hip and spleen. Diarrhea, burning watery stools which relieves the abdominal pain.

**Dose:** Sixth potency.

---

## ARSENICUM SULFURATUM FLAVUM— ARSENIC TRISULPH.

**Ars-s-f.**

Sensation of needle pricks from within outwards in the chest especially right side also on the forehead. Sticking pain behind the ear. Difficult respiration. Skin chafed around the genitals.

Leucoderma and squamous syphilides. Sciatica and pain around the knee.

**Relationship:** *Arsenicum sulphuratum rubrum* (influenza with intense catarrhal symptoms, great prostration and high temperature, purulent discharges, psoriasis, acne and sciatica. Chilly, even in front of a fire. Itching in various parts. Pellagra).

**Dose:** Third trituration.

---

# ARTEMISIA VULGARIS

(Mugwort) **Art-v.**

Has some reputation as a remedy for epileptic condition, and convulsive diseases of childhood and in girls at puberty. Locally and internally it is injurious to eyes. *Petit mal.* Epilepsy without aura; after fright and other violent emotions; after masturbation. Several convulsions, close together. Somnambulism. Gets up at night and works, remembers nothing in the morning (*Kali-p.*).

**Head:** Drawn back by spasmodic twitchings. Mouth drawn to the left. Congestion of brain (hydrocephalus).

**Eyes:** *Colored light produces dizziness.* Pain and blurring of vision; better, rubbing; worse, using the eyes.

**Female:** Profuse menses. Violent uterine contractions. Spasms during menses (dysmenorrhea).

**Fever:** Profuse sweat, *smelling like garlic.*

**Relationship:** Compare: *Absin., Cina, Cic.*

**Dose:** First to third potency. Said to act better when given with wine.

---

# ARUM DRACONTIUM

(Green Dragon) **Arum-d.**

A remedy for pharyngitis with a sore, raw and tender throat.

**Head:** Heavy.

**Ears**: Shooting pain in ears; aching pain, behind right ear.

**Throat:** Dry, sore, worse swallowing. Raw and tender. Continuous disposition to clear throat. Croupy, hoarse cough with a sore throat.

**Urinary:** Irresistible desire to pass urine, burns and smarts.

**Respiratory:** Hoarseness; excess of mucus in the larynx. Asthmatic at night. Expectoration thick, heavy.

**Relationship:** *Arum italicum* (brain fag, with headache in the occipital region). *Arum maculatum* (inflammation and ulceration of mucous membranes. Nasal irritation with polypus).

**Dose:** First potency.

---

## ARUM TRIPHYLLUM

(Jack in the Pulpit) **Arum-t.**

*Arum maculatum, italicum, dracontium, have the same action as Arum triphyllum.* They all contain an irritant poison, causing inflammation of mucous surfaces and destruction of tissues. *Acridity* is the keynote of action characteristic to *Arum-t.*

**Head:** Bores head into the pillow (meningitis). Headache from too warm clothing, hot coffee.

**Eyes:** Quivering of upper eyelids, especially left.

**Nose:** Soreness of nostrils. *Acrid, excoriating discharge,* producing raw sores. *Nose obstructed; must breathe through the mouth. Boring in the nose.* Coryza; discharge blood streaked, watery. Nose completely stopped, with fluent, acrid discharge. Hay fever, with pain over root of nose. Large scabs high up on the right side of nose. Face feels chapped, as if from cold wind; feels hot. *Constant picking at nose till it bleeds.*

**Mouth:** *Raw feeling of the roof and palate.* Lips and soft palate sore and burning. Lips chapped and burning. *Corners of mouth, sore and cracked.* Tongue red, sore; whole mouth is raw. Picking lips until they bleed. Saliva profuse, acrid, corroding.

**Throat:** Swelling of sub-maxillary glands. *Constricted and swollen; burns;* raw. Constant hawking. *Hoarseness.* Expectoration of much mucus. Lungs feel sore. Clergyman's sore throat. Voice uncertain, uncontrollable. Worse, talking, singing. Diphtheria.

**Skin:** Scarlet rash; *raw, bloody surfaces* anywhere. Impetigo contagiosa.

**Modalities:** *Worse, northwest wind;* lying down.

**Relationship:** Compare, *Am-c., Ail., All-c.*

Antidotes: *Buttermilk; Acet-ac., Puls.*

**Dose:** Third to thirtieth potency.

---

## ARUNDO MAURITANICA

(Reed) **Arund.**

A remedy for catarrhal states. Hay fever.

**Head:** Itching; falling off of hair; roots of hair painful. Pustules. Pain in the occiput, extends to the right ciliary region. Deep seated pain on the sides of the head.

**Ears:** Burning and itching in auditory canals. Eczema behind the ears.

**Nose:** Hay fever begins with burning and *itching of the palate* and conjunctiva. *Annoying itch in the nostrils and the roof of the mouth* (*Wye.*). Coryza; loss of smell (anosmia) (*Nat-m.*). Sneezing, *itching of nostrils.*

**Mouth:** Burning and itching; bleeding from gums. Ulcers and exfoliations in the commissures. Fissures on tongue.

**Stomach:** Coldness in stomach. Longing for acids.

**Abdomen:** Movement as if from something alive. Flatulent pain in the pubic region.

**Stool:** Greenish. Burning is the anus. Diarrhea in nursing children (*Cham., Calc-p.*).

**Urinary:** Urine burning. Red sediment (*Lyc.*).

**Male:** Pain in spermatic cord after embrace.

**Female:** Menses too early and profuse (menorrhagia). Neuralgic pains from face to the shoulders and pubis. Desire with vaginal pruritus.

**Respiratory:** Dyspnea; cough; bluish expectoration. Burning and pain in nipples.

**Extremities:** Itching, burning; edema of hands and feet. Burning and swelling of soles. Copious and offensive foot sweat.

**Skin:** Eczema; itching and crawling, especially on the chest, upper extremities. Fissures in fingers and heels.

**Relationship:** Compare: *Anthoxanthum*—Sweet vernal grass (a popular medicine for hay fever and coryza). *Lolium, All-c., Sabad., Sil.*

**Dose:** Third to sixth potency.

---

# ASA FOETIDA

(Gum of the Stinkasand) **Asaf.**

The flatulence and spasmodic contraction of stomach and esophagus with reverse peristalsis are the most marked symptoms. In its selection, its relation to the hysterical and hypochondriacal patients, must be borne in mind. Besides these superficial symptoms, it has been found to favorably affect deep ulcerations, caries of bones, especially in a syphilitic organism; here *extreme sensitiveness,* intense throbbing and nocturnal pains, act as a guide for its use.

**Head:** Irritable; complains of her problems; sensitive. Boring above eyebrows. *Pressive pain from within outwards.*

**Eyes:** Orbital neuralgia; better, pressure and rest. Iritis and intraocular inflammations with boring, and throbbing pains at night. Stitches under the left frontal eminences. Boring pains in and around the eyes. Syphilitic iritis. Superficial corneal ulcer with digging pains; worse at night.

**Ears:** Offensive otorrhea, with boring pains in the mastoid bone. Mastoid disease (caries) with pain in the temporal region with *a pushing out sensation.* Offensive, purulent discharge.

**Nose:** Syphilitic ozena, with very offensive purulent discharge. *Caries of nasal bones* (*Aur.*).

**Throat:** *Globus hystericus.* Ball rises in the throat. Sensation as if the peristaltic motion was reversed and the esophagus was being driven from the stomach to the throat.

**Stomach:** Great difficulty in bringing up wind. *Flatulence and regurgitation of liquids.* Hysterical flatulence. Great distention. Sensation of emptiness and weakness with distention and throbbing in the stomach and abdomen. Forcible eructation of gas. *Pulsations in the pit of the stomach.* Violent gastralgia; cutting and burning in the stomach and in the region of diaphragm. Gurgling and rolling of wind which escapes afterwards with a loud and difficult eructation.

**Rectum:** Distended, griping, with hunger. Obstinate constipation. Pain in perineum, as if something dull was pressed out. *Diarrhea, extremely offensive with meteorism* and regurgitation of food.

**Female:** Mammae turgid with milk in the unimpregnated. *Deficient milk* with oversensitiveness.

**Chest:** *Spasmodic tightness,* as if the lungs cannot be fully expanded (asthma). Palpitations, more like tremors.

**Bones:** Darting pain and caries in bones. Periosteum painful, swollen, enlarged. Ulcers, affecting bones; thin, ichorous pus (osteo- myetitis).

**Skin:** Itching, better scratching; ulcers painful on edges. Suppressed skin symptoms produce nervous disorders.

**Modalities:** *Worse* at night, from touch, left side, during rest, warm applications. *Better,* open air, from motion, pressure.

**Relationship:** Antidotes: *Chin., Merc.*

Compare: *Mosch., Chin., Merc., Aur.*

**Dose:** Second to sixth potency.

---

# ASARUM EUROPAEUM

(European Snakeroot) **Asar.**

A remedy for nervous affections, loss of energy, with excessive *erethism. Scratching on silk, linen or paper unbearable.* Pain and spasmodic muscular actions. Nervous deafness and asthenopia. Cold shivers from any emotion. Feels, as if parts were pressed together. Tension and contractive sensations. *Always feels cold.*

**Mind:** Thoughts vanish, with drawing pressure in the forehead. *Sensibility increased, even from mere imagination*[1].

**Head:** Compressive pain. Tension in scalp; hair painful (*Chin.*).

**Eyes:** Feel stiff; burn; feel cold. Better, in cold air or when water is applied; worse, sunlight and wind. Darting pains in the eyes after surgery. Asthenopia.

**Ears:** Sensation as if plugged up. Catarrh with deafness. Heat of external ear. Noises.

**Nose:** Coryza, with sneezing.

**Stomach:** Loss of appetite, flatulence, eructations, and vomiting. *Desire for alcoholic drinks.* Smoking tobacco, tastes bitter. Nausea; worse after eating. Clean tongue. Great faintness. Accumulation of cold, watery saliva.

**Rectum:** *Strings* of odorless, yellow mucus pass from the bowels. Diarrhea of tough mucus. *Undigested stools.* Prolapse.

**Female:** Menses too early, long lasting, black. Violent pain in small of back (lumbosacral region). Tenacious, yellow leucorrhea.

**Respiratory:** Nervous, hacking cough. Short respiration.

**Back:** Paralytic pain in the muscles of the nape of neck. Weakness, with staggering.

**Fever:** Chilliness, single parts get icy cold. Easily excited perspiration.

**Modalities:** *Worse,* in cold dry weather; penetrating sounds. *Better,* from washing; in damp and wet weather.

**Relationship:** *Asarum canadense*—Wild ginger (colds, followed by amenorrhea and gastroenteritis. Suppressed colds).

Compare: *Ip.,* especially in diarrhea; *Sil., Nux-v., Chin.*

**Dose:** Third to sixth potency.

---

## ASCLEPIAS SYRIACA (CORNUTI)

(Silkweed) **Asc-c.**

Seems to act especially on the nervous system and urinary organs. A remedy for dropsy, hepatic, renal, cardiac and post-scarlatinal; causes diaphoresis and augments the urinary secretion. Acute rheumatic inflammation of large joints. Intermittent, pressing down uterine pains.

**Head:** Sensation as *if a sharp instrument was thrust from one temple to the other.* Constriction across the forehead. Nervous headache, after suppressed perspiration, followed by *increased urine, with high specific gravity.* Headache

1 Hypersensitivity of nerves - only the thought of someone touching him makes him horrified and he looses control over his present thoughts (Clarke — Dictionary of Practical Meteria Medica).

from retention of effete matters in system.

**Relationship:** Compare: *Asclepias vincetoxicum*—Swallow-wart—*Cynanchum* (a gastro-intestinal irritant, producing vomiting and purgation. Useful in dropsy, diabetes with great thirst and profuse micturition).

**Dose:** Tincture.

## ASCLEPIAS TUBEROSA

(Pleurisy-root) **Asc-t.**

Its action on the chest muscles is most marked and has been verified. Sick headache, with flatulence. Dyspepsia. Bronchitis and pleurisy come within its range. Catarrhal states from cold and damp weather. Irritation of larynx with huskiness; influenza, with pleuritic pain.

**Stomach:** Fullness, pressure, weight. Flatulence after meals. Sensitive to tobacco.

**Rectum:** *Catarrhal dysentery, with rheumatic pains all over the body.* Stools smell like rotten eggs.

**Respiratory:** Respiration painful, especially at the base of the left lung. Dry cough; throat constricted; causes pain in the head and abdomen. Pain in the chest; shooting downward from the left nipple. A general eliminative remedy, acting specially on the sudoriparous glands. Chest pains are relieved by bending forward. Intercostal spaces near the sternum, tender. Lancinating pain between shoulders. Catarrh, with frontal headache, and sticky yellow discharge.

**Extremities:** Rheumatic joints with a sensation as if the adhesions world break on bending.

**Relationship:** Compare: *Asclepias incarnata*—Swamp milk weed (chronic gastric catarrh and leucorrhea. Dropsy with dyspnea). *Periploca graeca*—One of the Asclepiades (cardiac tonic, acts on the circulation and respiratory centre, accelerating respiration in a ratio disproportionate to the pulse). *Bry., Dulc.*

**Dose:** Tincture and first potency.

## ASIMINA TRILOBA

(American Papaw, Carica Papaya) **Asim.**

Produces a series of symptoms very similar to scarlet fever; sore throat, fever, vomiting, scarlet eruptions; tonsils and submaxillary glands enlarged, with diarrhea. Fauces red and swollen, face swollen. Desire for ice cold things. *Hoarseness.* Languid, drowsy, irritable.

Acne. Itching in the evening on undressing.

**Relationship:** Compare: *Caps., Bell.*

**Dose:** 1x, 3x trituration.

---

## ASPARAGUS OFFICINALIS

(Common Garden Asparagus) **Aspar.**

Its marked and immediate action on the urine secretion is well known. It causes weakness and cardiac depression with dropsy. Rheumatic pains. Especially around the left shoulder and heart.

**Head:** Confused. Coryza, with profuse, thin fluid. Aching in the forehead and root of the nose. Migraine-like morning headaches with scotoma. Throat feels rough, with hawking of copious, tenacious mucus from the throat.

**Urinary:** Frequent, with fine stitches at the orifice; burning; peculiar odor. Cystitis, with pus, mucus and tenesmus. Lithiasis.

**Heart:** *Palpitations, with oppression of chest.* Pulse intermits, weak, pain around the left shoulder and heart, associated with bladder disturbances. Great oppression in breathing. Hydrothorax.

**Extremities:** Rheumatic pains in the back, especially near the shoulder and limbs. Pain at the acromion process of the left scapula, under the clavicle and down the arm, with a feeble pulse.

**Relationship:** Antidotes: *Acon., Apis.*

Compare: *Althaea officinalis*—Marshmallow (contains asparagin; irritable bladder, throat and bronchi). *Physalis alkekengi, Dig., Sars., Spig.*

**Dose:** Sixth potency.

---

## ASPIDOSPERMA QUEBRACHO

(Quebracho) **Queb.**

*Digitalis* of the lungs (Hale), stimulates the respiratory centres, increasing the oxidation of blood and excretion of carbonic acid. Pulmonary stenosis. Thrombosis of the pulmonary artery. Uremic dyspnea. An effective remedy in many cases of asthma. "Want of breath" during exertion is the guiding symptom. *Cardiac asthma.*

**Relationship:** Compare: *Coca, Ars., Coff., Catalpa bignonodes* (difficult respiration).

**Dose:** First trituration or tincture, or Aspidospermin hydrochloride. 1 grain of 1x trituration. Every hour for a few doses.

---

# ASTACUS FLUVIATILIS —CANCER ASTACUS

(Crawfish)

**Astac.**

Skin symptoms most important. *Urticaria.*

**Fever:** Chilliness inside; very sensitive to air, worse uncovering; violent fever, with headache.

**Skin:** Nettle rash all over the body. Itching. Crusta lactea, with enlarged lymphatic glands. Erysipelas and *liver affections with nettle rash.* Swelling of cervical glands. Jaundice.

**Relationship:** Compare: *Bombyx processonea*—Caterpillar: Itching of whole body (urticaria). *Apis, Rhus-t., Nat-m., Homar.*

**Dose:** Third to thirtieth potency.

---

# ASTERIAS RUBENS

(Red Starfish)

**Aster.**

A remedy for sycotic diathesis; flabby, lymphatic constitution, with *a red* face. Lancinating pains. Nervous disturbances, neuralgias, chorea and hysteria come within the range of this remedy. Has been used for cancer of the breast, and has an unquestioned influence over cancerous disease. Excitement in both sexes.

**Head:** Cannot bear contradiction. Shocks in the brain; throbbing; *heat in the head, as if surrounded by hot air.*

**Face:** Red. Pimples on the sides of the nose, chin and mouth. *Disposition to pimples at adolescene.*

**Stool:** Constipation. Ineffectual desire. Stool like olives. Diarrhea, watery brown, gushing out in a jet.

**Female:** Colic and other sufferings cease with appearance of flow. Breasts swell and pain; worse left side. Ulceration with sharp pains, piercing the scapulae. Pain radiates to the left arm and fingers, worse motion. Excitement of sexual instinct with nervous agitation.

Nodes and indurations of mammary gland, dull aching, neuralgic pain in this region (*Con.*).

**Chest:** Breasts swollen, indurated (mastitis). Neuralgia of the left breast and arm (*Brom.*). Pain under the sternum and in muscles of precordial region. *Left breast feels as if pulled inward* and pain extends to the inner arm and tip of little finger. Numbness of the hand and fingers of the left side. *Cancer of mammae, even in the ulcerative stage. Acute, lancinating pain. Axillary glands swollen, hard and knotted.*

**Nervous System:** Gait unsteady; muscles refuse to obey will. Epilepsy; preceded by twitching all over the body.

**Skin:** Without pliability and elasticity. Itchy spots. Ulcers, with a fetid ichor. Acne. Psoriasis and herpes zoster worse left arm and chest. Enlarged axillary glands, worse, at night and in damp weather.

**Modalities:** *Worse,* coffee, night; cold damp weather, left side.

**Relationship:** Antidotes: *Plb., Zinc.*

Compare: *Con., Carb-v., Ars., Cund.*

Incompatible: *Nux-v., Coff.*

**Dose:** Sixth potency.

---

# ASTRAGALUS MOLLISSIMUS

(Purple or Woolly Locoweed) **Astra-mo.**

Affects animals like the effects of alcohol, tobacco and morphine on a man. First stage, period of hallucination or mania with defective eyesight during which the animal performs all sorts of antics. After acquiring a taste for the plant, it refuses every other kind of food. Second stage brings emaciation, sunken eyeballs, lusterless hair and feeble movements—after a few months it dies from starvation (U. S. Dept. Agriculture). Irregularities in gait, paralytic affections. Loss of muscular co-ordination.

**Head:** Fullness in the right temple and upper jaw. Pain over the left eyebrow. Pain extends to the facial bones. Dizzy. Pressive pains in temples. Pain and pressure in maxillae.

**Stomach:** Weakness and emptiness. Burning in the esophagus and stomach.

**Extremities:** Purring sensation in the right foot, on the outer side, from the heel to the toe. Icy coldness of left calf.

**Relationship:** Compare: *Aragallus lamberti*—White loco weed—Rattleweed; *Bar-c., Oxyt.*

**Dose:** Sixth potency.

---

# AURUM METALLICUM

(Metallic Gold) **Aur.**

Given full play, *Aur.* develops in the organism, by attacking the blood, glands and bones, conditions bearing a striking resemblance to mercurial and syphilitic infections; and it is for such deteriorations of the body fluids and alterations in the tissues, that *Aur.* assumes great importance as a remedy. Like the victim of syphilis, mental states of great depression are produced by it. Hopeless, despondent and *a great desire to commit suicide.* Every opportunity is sought for self destruction. Exostosis, caries, nocturnal bone pains, especially cranial, nasal, and palatine. Glands swollen in scrofulous subjects. Palpitation and congestions. Ascites often in conjunction with heart affections. Frequently indicated in secondary syphilis and in effects of mercury. This use of gold as an anti-venereal and anti-scrofulous remedy is very old, but it has been well forgotten by the old school till it was rediscovered and placed, on its scientific basis, by homeopathy, and now it can never be lost again. When syphilis is implanted on the scrofulous constitution, we have one of the most intractable morbid conditions, and gold seems to be especially suited to the vile combination. *Ennui.* Ozena; sexual hyperesthesia. *Arteriosclerosis,* high blood pressure; nocturnal paroxysms of pain behind the sternum. Sclerosis of liver, arterial system, brain. Pining boys; low spirited, lifeless, weak memory.

**Mind:** Feeling of self condemnation and utter worthlessness. Profound despondency, with increased blood pressure, a thorough *disgust for life,* and thoughts of suicide. *Talks of commiting suicide.* Great fear of death. Peevish and vehement at least contradiction. Anthropophobia. Mental derangements. Constant, rapid questioning without waiting for a reply. Cannot do things fast enough. *Oversensitiveness (Staph.) to noise,* excitement, confusion.

**Head:** *Violent pain in the head; worse at night,* outward pressure. Roaring in the head. Vertigo. Tearing pain through the brain, extending to the forehead. Pain in the bones extending to the face (exostosis). Congestion of head. Boils on scalp.

**Eyes:** *Extreme photophobia.* Great soreness around the eyes and in the eyeballs. Diplopia; *upper half of objects invisible* (hemiopia). Feel tense (glaucoma). Sees fiery objects. Violent pain in bones around the eye (*Asaf.*). Interstitial keratitis. *Vascular cornea. Sticking pains inward.* Trachoma with pannus.

**Ears:** Caries of ossicula and mastoid. *Obstinate fetid otorrhea* after scarlatina. External meatus bathed in pus. Chronic nerve deafness; labyrinthine disease due to syphilis.

**Nose:** *Ulcerated, painful,* swollen, obstructed. Inflammation of the nose;

caries; fetid discharge, purulent, bloody (ozena). Boring pains in the nose; worse at night. *Putrid smell* from nose. Sensitive to smells (*Carb-ac.*). Horrible odor from the nose and mouth. Knobby tip of nose.

**Face:** Tearing in zygoma. Mastoid and other facial bones inflamed.

**Mouth:** Halitosis in girls at puberty. Taste, putrid or bitter. Ulceration of gums.

**Throat:** Stitches when swallowing; pain in glands. Caries of the palate.

**Stomach:** Appetite and thirst increased, with qualmishness. Swelling in the epigastrium. Burning in the stomach with hot eructations.

**Abdomen:** Right hypochondrium hot and painful. Incarcerated flatus. Swelling and suppuration of inguinal glands.

**Rectum:** Constipation, stools hard and knotty. Nocturnal diarrhea, with burning in rectum.

**Urinary:** Urine turbid, like buttermilk, with thick sediment. Painful retention.

**Male:** Pain and *swelling in testicles* (orchitis). Chronic induration of testicles. Violent erections. *Atrophy of testicles in boys.* Hydrocele.

**Female:** Great sensitiveness of the vagina. Uterus enlarged and prolapsed. Sterility; vaginismus.

**Respiratory:** Dyspnea at night. Frequent, deep breathing; stitches in the sternum.

**Heart:** *Sensation as if the heart stopped beating* for two or three seconds, immediately followed by a tumultuous rebound, with sinking in the epigastrium. Palpitations. Pulse *rapid, feeble, irregular.* Hypertrophy. *High blood pressure*: valvular lesions of arteriosclerotic nature (*Aur. 30*).

**Bones:** Destruction of bones, like in secondary syphilis. Pain in bones of head, lumps under the scalp, exostosis with nocturnal pains in bones. Caries of nasal, palatine and mastoid bones. Soreness of affected bones, better in the open air, worse at night.

**Extremities:** All the blood seems to rush from the head to the lower limbs. Dropsy of lower limbs. Orgasm, as if blood was boiling in all veins. Paralytic, tearing pains in joints. Knees weak.

**Sleep:** Sleepless. Sobs aloud in sleep. Frightful dreams.

**Modalities:** *Worse,* in cold weather, when getting cold. Many complaints come on only in winters; from sunset to sunrise.

**Relationship:** Compare: *Aurum arsenicum* (chronic aortitis; lupus, phthisis, syphilitic headaches; also in anemia and chlorosis. It causes rapid increase of appetite).

*Aurum bromatum* (in headaches with neurasthenia, migraine, terrors, valvular diseases).

*Aurum muriaticum* (burning, yellow, acrid leucorrhea; heart symptoms, glandular affections; warts on the tongue and genitals; sclerotic and exudative degeneration of the nervous system. Multiple sclerosis. Morvan's disease. Second trituration. *Aur-m.* is a sycotic remedy, causing suppressed discharges to reappear. Valuable in climacteric hemorrhages from the womb. Diseases of frontal sinus. Stitching pain on the left side of the forehead. Weariness, aversion to all work. Drawing feeling in stomach. Cancer of tongue, hard as leather; induration after glossitis).

*Aurum muriaticum kalinatum:* Double chloride of potassium and gold (in uterine induration and hemorrhage).

*Aurum iodatum* (chronic pericarditis, valvular diseases, arteriosclerosis, ozena, lupus, osteitis, ovarian cysts, myomata uteri, are pathological lesions, that offer a favorable ground for the action of this powerful drug. *Senile paresis*).

*Aurum sulphuratum* (paralysis agitans; constant nodding of the head; affections of mammae; swelling, pain, cracked nipples with lancinating pains).

Also, *Asaf.* (in caries of bones of ears and nose), *Syph., Kali-i., Hep., Merc., Mez., Nit-ac., Phos.*

Antidotes: *Bell., Chin., Cupr., Merc.*

**Dose:** Third to thirtieth potency. Latter potency especially in high blood pressure.

---

# AURUM MURIATICUM NATRONATUM

(Sodium Chloroaurate) **Aur-m-n.**

This remedy has a very pronounced effect on the female organs and most of its clinical application has been based thereon. Has more power over uterine tumors than any other remedy (Burnett). Psoriasis syphilitica. Periosteal swelling of the lower jaw. Swelling of testicle (orchitis). High blood pressure due to disturbed function of nervous mechanism. Arteriosclerosis. Syphilitic ataxia.

Burning; stitches, and induration of the tongue. Old cases of rheumatism and gouty pains. Hepatic cirrhosis. Interstitial nephritis.

**Female:** Indurated cervix. Palpitations in young girls. Coldness in the abdomen. Chronic metritis and prolapse. Uterus fills up the whole pelvis. Ulceration on the neck of the womb and vagina. Leucorrhea, with spasmodic contraction of vagina. Ovaries indurated. Ovarian dropsy. Sub-involution. Ossified uterus.

**Dose:** Second and third trituration.

---

# AVENA SATIVA

(Common Oat) **Aven.**

Has a selective action on the brain and nervous system, favorably influencing their nutritive function.

Nervous exhaustion, sexual debility and the morphine habit call for this remedy in rather material dosage. Best tonic for debility after exhausting diseases. Nervous tremors in the aged; chorea, paralysis agitans, epilepsy. Post-diphtheritic paralysis. Rheumatism of heart. *Colds.* Acute coryza (20 drop doses in hot water, hourly for a few doses). Alcoholism. Sleeplessness, especially in alcoholics. Bad effects of *morphine* habit. Nervous states in many female problems.

**Mind:** Inability to keep the mind on any one subject.

**Head:** Nervous headache at menstrual period, with burning on top of the head. Occipital headache, with phosphaturia.

**Male:** Spermatorrhea: impotency; after too much indulgence.

**Female:** Amenorrhea and dysmenorrhea, with weak circulation.

**Extremities:** Numbness of limbs, as if paralyzed. Strength of hands diminished.

**Relationship:** Compare: *Alf.* (general tonic similar to *Aven.*—also in scanty and suppressed urine).

**Dose:** Tincture, ten to twenty drop doses, preferably in hot water.

---

# AZADIRACHTA INDICA

(Melia azadirachta, Nim, Margosa) **Aza.**

An afternoon fever and rheumatic pains in various parts are caused by this remedy. Pain in the sternum and ribs, in the back, shoulders and extremities; heat, pricking and aching in hands, especially palms, fingers, and toes.

**Head:** Forgetful; giddy on rising; headaches, scalp sensitive.

**Eyes:** Burn, pain in right eyeball.

**Fever:** Slight chill, afternoon fever; glowing heat in the face, hands and feet; copious sweat on the upper part of body.

**Relationship:** Compare: *Cedron, Nat-m., Ars.*

**Dose:** 6, 30 and 200 potencies.

---

# BACILLINUM BURNETT

(A Maceration of a Typical Tuberculous Lung—
Introduced by Dr. Burnett) **Bac.**

Has been employed successfully in the treatment of tuberculosis; its effects are seen in the sputum, which becomes decreased, more aerated and less purulent. Many forms of chronic non-tubercular diseases are influenced favorably by *Bacillinum*, especially when bronchorrhea and dyspnea are present. Respiratory pyorrhea.[1] *The patient expectorates less.*

*Bacillinum* is especially indicated in lungs of old people, with chronic catarrhal condition and enfeebled pulmonary circulation, attacks of suffocation at night with difficult cough. Suffocative catarrh. Tubercular meningitis. Favors falling off of tartar on teeth. Constant disposition to take cold.

**Head**: Irritable, depressed. Severe, deep seated headache, sensation of a tight loop around the head. Ringworm. Eczema of eyelids.

**Abdomen:** Abdominal pains, enlarged glands in groins, tabes mesenterica. Sudden diarrhea before breakfast. Obstinate constipation, with offensive flatus.

**Respiratory:** *Oppression. Catarrhal dyspnea. Humid asthma. Bubbling rales and muco-purulent expectoration.* Note: this muco-purulent expectoration in bronchitic patients is equally poly-bacillary; it is a mixture of diverse species and hence *Bacillinum* is truly indicated (Cartier). Often relieves congestion of the lungs, thus paving way for other remedies in tuberculosis.

**Skin:** *Ringworm;* pityriasis. Eczema of eyelids. Glands of neck enlarged and tender.

**Modalities:** Worse, night and early morning; cold air.

**Relationship:** *Ant-i., Lach., Ars-i., Myos-a., Lev.*, 5-10 drops, follows as an intercurrent remedy where there is severe debility (Burnett).

Complementary: *Calc-p., Kali-c.*

Compare: Its effects seem to be identical to that of *Koch's Tuberculinum*. Both are useful in the tubercular diathesis before phthisis has developed. In the *early stages* of tubercular diseases of glands, joints, skin and bones. *Psor.* seems to be its chronic equivalent. *Bacillinum testium* (acts especially on the lower half of the body).

**Dose:** The dose is important. Should not be given below the thirtieth, and should not repeated frequently. One dose a week is often sufficient to bring about a reaction. It is *rapid in action,* and good results ought to be seen soon, otherwise there is no need of repetition.

---

[1] Excessive muco-purulent bronchial secretion threatening to occlude the lungs (Clarke — Dictionary of Practical Materia Medica).

# BADIAGA

(Fresh Water Sponge) **Bad.**

Soreness of muscles and integuments; worse motion and friction of clothes, with sensitiveness to cold. Glands swollen. General paresis. Basedow's disease. Lues (syphilis), bubo, roseola.

**Head:** Sensation of enlargement and fullness. Pain in the forehead and temple, *extending to eyeballs,* worse in the afternoon. Blueness under the eyes. *Dandruff;* scalp sore, dry, tetter like. Dull, dizzy feeling in the head. *Coryza,* sneezing, watery discharge, with asthmatic breathing and suffocative cough. Influenza. Slight sounds are greatly accentuated.

**Eyes:** Twitching of *left* upper lid; eyeballs tender; aching in the eyeballs. Intermittent sore pain in eyeball, coming on at 3 p.m.

**Stomach:** Mouth hot. Marked thirst. Lancinating pain in the pit of the stomach extending to the vertebra and scapula.

**Female:** Metorrhagia; worse at night, with sensation of enlargement of head (*Arg-n.*). Cancer of breast (*Aster., Con., Carb-an., Plb-i.*).

**Respiratory:** Cough; worse in the afternoon, better in a warm room. Mucus *flies out of the mouth and nostrils.* Whooping cough, with thick yellow expectoration; flies out. Hay fever, with asthmatic breathing. Pleuritic stitches in chest, neck and back.

**Heart:** Indescribable bad feeling around the heart with soreness and pain, flying stitches all over.

**Back:** Stitches in the nape, scapulae. Pain in the lumbosacral region, hips and lower limbs. Very stiff neck. *Muscles and skin sore,* as if beaten.

**Skin:** Sore to touch. *Freckles. Rhagades.*

**Modalities:** *Worse* by cold. *Better,* by heat.

**Relationship:** Compare: *Merc.* similar but opposite modalities. *Spong., Kali-i., Phyt., Con.*

Complementary: *Sulph., Merc., Iod.*

**Dose:** First to sixth attenuation.

---

# BALSAMUM PERUVIANUM

(Peruvian Balsam from Myroxylon Pereirae) **Bals-p.**

Useful in bronchial catarrh, with copious, purulent expectoration. *Debility; hectic fever.*

**Nose:** Profuse, thick discharge. Eczema, with ulceration. Chronic, fetid, nasal catarrh.

**Stomach:** Vomiting of food and mucus. Catarrh of stomach.

**Urinary:** Urine scanty; with a lot of mucoid sediment. Catarrh of the bladder (cystitis) (*Chim.*).

**Respiratory:** Bronchitis and phthisis, *with muco-purulent, thick, creamy expectoration.* Loud rales in chest (*Kali-s., Ant- t.*). Very loose cough. Hectic fever and night sweats with an irritating, short cough and scanty expectoration.

**Relationship:** *Balsamum tolutanum*—the Balsam of Myroxylon toluifera (chronic bronchitis with profuse expectoration). *Oleum caryophyllatum*—Oil of cloves—in *profuse* septic expectoration—3 to 5 minims in milk or capsules.).

**Dose:** First attenuation. In hectic: 6x.

**Non-homeopathic Uses:** Locally, as a stimulant to raw surfaces in indolent ulcers, scabies, cracked nipples, rhagades, itch. Promotes granulation, removes fetor. A one percent solution in alcohol or ether may be used with the atomizer in respiratory affections. Internally, as an expectorant, in chronic bronchitis. Dose, 5 to 15 M., made into an emulsion with mucilage or yolk of egg.

---

# BAPTISIA TINCTORIA

(Wild Indigo) **Bapt.**

The symptoms of this drug are of an asthenic type, simulating low fevers, *septic conditions* of the blood, malarial poisoning and extreme prostration. Indescribable sick feeling. *Great muscular soreness and putrid phenomena are always present.* All the secretions are offensive—breath, stool, urine, sweat, etc. Epidemic influenza. Chronic intestinal toxemias in children with fetid stools and eructations.

*Bapt.* in low dilutions produces a form of antibodies to the bacillus. typhosus, viz., the agglutinins (*Mellon.*). Thus it raises the natural body resistance to the invasion of bacillary intoxication, which produces the typhoid syndrome. Typhoid carriers. After inoculation with anti-typhoid serum. Intermittent pulse, especially in the aged.

**Mind:** Wild, wandering feeling. Inability to think. Mental confusion. Ideas confused. Illusion of a divided personality. *Thinks he is broken or double, and tosses about in bed trying to get pieces together* (*Caj.*). Delirium, wandering, muttering. Perfect indifference. Falls asleep while being spoken to. Melancholia, with stupor.

**Head:** Confused, feels as if swimming. Vertigo; pressure at the root of the nose. Skin of forehead feels tight; seems drawn to the back of the head. Feels too large, *heavy, numb.* Soreness of eyeballs. Brain feels sore. Stupor; falls asleep while being spoken to. Early deafness in typhoid conditions. Eyelids heavy.

**Face:** *Besotted look.* Dark red. Pain at the root of the nose. Muscles of jaw rigid (lockjaw).

**Mouth:** Taste flat, bitter. Teeth and gums sore, ulcerated. *Breath fetid* (halitosis). *Tongue feels burned;* yellowish-brown; edges red and shining (glossitis). Dry and brown in the center, with dry and glistening edges; surface cracked and sore (stomatitis). *Can swallow liquids only;* least solid food gags.

**Throat:** Dark red tonsils and soft palate (hyperemic). *Constric*tion, *contraction of esophagus* (*Caj.*). Great difficulty in swallowing solid food. Painless sore throat, and offensive discharge. *Contraction at the cardiac orifice.*

**Stomach:** Can swallow only liquids, vomiting due to spasm, of esophagus. Enteric fever (typhoid). No appetite. Constant desire for water. *Sinking feeling in the stomach.* Pain in the episgastric region. Sensation of a hard substance (*Abies-n.*). All symptoms worse from beer (*Kali-bi.*). Cardiac orifice contracts convulsively with ulcerative inflammation of stomach (gastric ulcer) and bowels (ulcerative colitis).

**Adomen:** Right side markedly affected. Distended and rumbling. Soreness over region of gall bladder, with diarrhea.

**Stool**: *Very offensive, thin, dark, bloody.* Dysentery in old people. Soreness of abdomen, in the region of liver.

**Female:** Threatened miscarriage from mental depression, shock, night watching, low fevers. Menses too early, too profuse (menorrhagia). Lochia acrid, fetid. Puerperal fever.

**Respiratory:** Lungs feel compressed, breathing difficult; seeks an open window. Fears going to sleep on account of nightmare and *sense of suffocation.* Constriction of chest.

**Back and Extremities:** Neck tired. Stiffness and pain, aching and drawing in arms and legs. Pain in sacrum, around hips and legs. *Sore and bruised.* Decubitus.

**Sleep:** Sleepless and restless. Nightmares and frightful dreams. Cannot get herself together, feels scattered over the bed. Falls asleep while answering a question.

**Fever:** Chills, with rheumatic pains and soreness all over the body. Heat all over, with occasional chills. Chill around 11 a.m. *Adynamic fevers.* Typhus fever. Shipboard fever.

**Skin:** Livid spots all over the body and limbs. Burning and heat in skin (*Ars.*). Putrid ulcers with stupor,low delirium and prostration.

**Modalities:** *Worse;* humid heat; fog; indoors.

**Relationship:** Compare: *Bry.* and *Ars.* may be needed to complete the favorable reaction. *Ail.* differs, being more painful. *Bapt.* more painless. *Rhus-t., Mur-ac., Ars., Bry., Arn., Echi., Pyrog.*

*Baptisia confusia* (pain in right jaw and oppression in left hypochondrium, producing dyspnea and a necessity to assume an erect position).

**Dose:** Tincture to twelfth attenuation. Has a rather short action.

---

## BAROSMA CRENULATUM

(Buchu) **Baros.**

Marked specific effect on genito-urinary system; *mucopurulent discharges.* Irritable bladder, with cystitis; prostatic disorders. Gravel. Leucorrhea.

**Relationship:** Compare: *Cop., Thuj., Pop., Chim.* See *Diosma linearis.*

**Dose:** Tincture or tea from leaves.

---

## BARYTA ACETICA

(Acetate of Barium) **Bar-act.**

Produces paralysis beginning in the extremities and spreading upward. Senile pruritis.

**Mind:** Forgetful; wavering long between opposite resolutions. Lack of self confidence.

**Face:** Sensation of a cobweb on the face.

**Extremities:** Drawing pain going down the left leg. Crawling, with burning stitches. *Paralysis.* Lumbago and rheumatic pain in muscles and joints.

**Dose:** Second and third trituration in repeated dosage.

---

## BARYTA CARBONICA

(Carbonate of Baryta) **Bar-c.**

Specially indicated in *infancy* and *old age.* This remedy aids scrofulous children, especially if they are backward mentally and physically, are dwarfish, do not grow and develop, have scrofulous ophthalmia, a swollen abdomen, take cold easily and *always have swollen tonsils.* People subjected to quinsy, which is prone to suppuration; gums bleed easily. Diseases of old men when degenerative changes begin, cardiac, vascular and cerebral, who have a hypertrophied prostate or indurated testes, are very sensitive to cold, have offensive foot sweats and are very weak and weary, must sit, lie down or lean on something. Very averse to meeting strangers. Catarrh of posterior nares with frequent epistaxis. Often useful in the dyspepsias of the young who have masturbated and who suffer from seminal emissions, together with cardiac irritability and palpitations. Affects glandular structures, and is useful in general degenerative changes, especially in the coats of arteries, *aneurism,* and senility. *Bar-c.* is a cardiovascular poison acting on the muscular coats of the heart and vessels. Arterial fibrosis. Blood vessels soften and degenerate, become distended, aneurisms rupture and apoplexies result.

**Mind:** Loss of memory, mental weakness. Irresolute. Looses confidence in himself. Senile dementia. Confusion. *Bashful.* Aversion to strangers. Childish; grief over trifles.

**Head:** Vertigo; stitches, when standing in the sun, extending through the head. Brain feels loose. Hair fall out. Confusion. *Wens.*

**Eyes:** Alternate dilatation and contraction of pupils (meningitis). Photophobia. Gauze before eyes. Cataract (*Calc., Phos., Sil.*).

**Ears:** Hardness of hearing. *Crackling noise. Glands around the ears painful and swollen.* Reverberation on blowing the nose.

**Nose:** Dry; sneezing; *coryza, with swelling of upper lip and nose.* Sensation of smoke in nose. Discharge of thick, yellow mucus. Frequent epistaxis. Scabs around alae of nose.

**Face:** Pale, puffed; sensation of a cobweb (*Alumina*). Upper lip swollen.

**Mouth:** Wakes up with a dry mouth. Gums bleed and retract (scorbutic). Toothache before menses. Mouth filled with inflamed vesicles (stomatitis), foul taste. Paralysis of tongue. Smarting, burning pain on the tip of the tongue. Dribbling of saliva at dawn. Spasm of esophagus when food enters.

**Throat:** Submaxillary glands and tonsils swollen. *Takes cold easily, with stitches and smarting pain. Quinsy. Suppurating tonsils after every cold.* Tonsils inflamed, with swollen veins. Smarting pain when swallowing; worse empty swallowing. Sensation of a plug in the pharynx. Can only swallow liquids. Spasm of esophagus as soon as food enters the esophagus, causes gagging and choking (*Merc-c., Graph.*). Throat problems from over use of voice. Stinging pain in tonsils, pharynx or larynx.

**Stomach:** Waterbrash, hiccough, and eructation, which relieves pressure, as if from a stone. Hungry, but refuses food. Pain and weight in the stomach immediately after a meal, with epigastric tenderness (*Kali-c.*). Worse after warm food. Gastric weakness in the aged with possible malignancy present.

**Abdomen:** *Hard and tense, distended.* Colicky. Enlarged mesenteric glands. Pain in the abdomen on swallowing food. Habitual colic, with hunger, but food is refused.

**Rectum:** Constipation, with hard, knotty stools. Hemorrhoids protrude on micturating . Crawling in rectum. Oozing from the anus.

**Urinary:** Every time patient micturates, his piles protrude. Urging to micturate. Burning in urethra during micturition.

**Male:** Diminished desire and premature impotence. Enlarged prostate. Testicles indurated.

**Female:** Before menses, pain in stomach and lumbosacral region. Menses scanty.

**Respiratory:** Dry, suffocative cough, especially in old people, full of mucus but lacking strength to expectorate, worse every change of weather (*Seneg.*). Larynx feels as if smoke is inhaled. Chronic aphonia. Stitches in chest; worse inspiration (pleurisy). Lungs feel full of smoke.

**Heart:** Palpitations and distress in region of heart. Aneurism (*Lyc.*). Accelerates the heart's action at first, blood pressure increases, contraction of blood vessels. Palpitations when lying on the left side, especially when thinking of it; pulse full and hard. Cardiac symptoms after suppressed foot sweat.

**Back:** *Swollen glands in the nape of the occiput.* Fatty tumors around the neck. Bruised pain between scapulae. Stiffness in sacrum. Weakness of spine.

**Extremities:** Pain in the axillary glands. Cold, clammy feet (*Calc.*). *Fetid foot sweats.* Numbness of limbs. Numb feeling from knees to scrotum; disappears when sitting down. Toes and soles sore; soles painful when walking. Pain in joints; burning pain in lower limbs.

**Sleep:** Talking in sleep; wakes up frequently; feels too hot. Twitching during sleep.

**Modalities:** *Worse,* while thinking of symptoms; from washing; lying on painful side. *Better,* walking in open air.

**Relationship:** Compare: *Dig., Rad-br., Arag., Oxyt., Astrag.*

Complementary: *Dulc., Sil., Psor.*

Incompatible: *Calc.*

Antidote for poisonous doses: *Epsom salts.*

**Dose:** Third to thirtieth potency, the latter removes the predisposition to quinsy. *Bar-c.* is slow in action, bears repetition.

---

# BARYTA IODATA

(Iodide of Baryta) **Bar-i.**

Acts on the lymphatic system, *increased leucocytosis. Quinsy. Indurated glands, especially tonsils and breasts.* Strumous ophthalmia, with tumefaction of cervical glands and stunted growth. Tumors.

**Relationship:** Compare: *Acon-l.* (swelling of cervical, axillary and mammary glands). *Lapis, Con., Merc., Carb-an.*

**Dose:** Second and third trituration.

---

# BARYTA MURIATICA

(Barium Chloride) **Bar-m.**

The different salts of *Baryta* are indicated in organic lesions of the aged who are dwarfish, both mentally and physically. Arteriosclerosis and cerebral affections. Headaches, but without an acute crisis, in the aged, heaviness rather than pain. Vertigo, due to cerebral anemia and noises in the ears (tinnitus). Acts on the lower alimentary canal, especially on the rectum; on muscles and joints, producing stiffness and weakness as if from overwalking. White blood corpuscles increased (leucocytosis; leukemia). Hypertension and vascular degeneration. Increased tension of pulse. Arteriosclerosis (*Aur., Sec.*) with a high systolic pressure and a comparatively low diastolic tension is attended by cerebral and cardiac symptoms.

This remedy has induration and *narrowing of the cardiac orifice with pain* immediately after eating and epigastric tenderness, which has been repeatedly verified. Also of use in *aneurism* and chronic hypertrophy of the tonsils. Nymphomania and satyriasis. Convulsions. In every form of mania when the sexual desire is increased. *Icy coldness of the body with paralysis.* Multiple sclerosis of brain and cord. *Voluntary muscular power lost, but perfectly sensible.* Paresis after influenza and diphtheria. General feeling of lassitude in the morning, especially weakness in the legs with muscular stiffness. Children who go around with their mouth open and who talk through the nose. Stupid appearing, hard of hearing.

**Ears:** Whizzing and buzzing. Noises on chewing, swallowing or sneezing. Otalgia; better sipping cold water. Parotids swollen (mumps). Offensive otorrhea. Middle ear inflates on blowing the nose.

**Throat**: Dysphagia. *Tonsils enlarged.* Paresis of pharynx and eustachian tubes, with sneezing and tinnitus. Tubes feel too wide open.

**Stomach:** *All gone feeling in the epigastrium* is a good guiding symptom for it in chronic affections. Retching and vomiting. Sensation of heat ascending to the head.

**Abdomen**: Throbbing (*Sel.*); *induration* of pancreas (pancreatitis); abdominal aneurism. Inguinal glands swollen. Spasmodic pain in rectum.

**Urinary**: *Great increase in uric acid,* diminution of chlorides in urine.

**Respiratory**: *Bronchial affections in old people* with cardiac dilation.

*Facilitates expectoration.* Great accumulation and rattling of mucus with difficult expectoration. Arteriosclerosis of the lung, thus indicated in senile asthma, modifies the arterial tension.

**Relationship**: Compare in sclerotic degenerations, especially of spinal cord, liver, and heart. *Plb. and Plb-i.* Also *Aur-m.* (which often accomplishes more in sclerotic and exudative degenerations than any other remedies. Multiple sclerosis, fulgurating pains, tremors, Morvan's disease, hypertrophy of fingers).

**Dose**: Third trituration. Bears repetition of dosage well.

---

# BELLADONNA

(Deadly Nightshade) **Bell.**

*Belladonna* acts on every part of the nervous system, producing active congestion, furious excitement, perverted special senses, twitching, convulsions and pain. It has a marked action on the vascular system, skin and glands. *Belladonna* is always associated with hot, red skin, flushed face, glaring eyes, throbbing carotids, an excited mental state, hyperesthesia of all senses, delirium, restless sleep, convulsive movements, dryness of mouth and throat with an aversion to water and *neuralgic pains* that come and go suddenly (*Oxyt.*). *Heat, redness, throbbing and burning. A great remedy for children.* Epileptic spasms followed by nausea and vomiting. *Scarlet fever,* is also prophylactic for it, the thirtieth potency is used for it. *Exophthalmic goitre.* Corresponds to the symptoms of "air sickness" in aviators. Can be given as a preventive. *No thirst, anxiety or fear. Belladonna* stands for *violence* of attack and *suddenness* of onset. *Bell.* is indicated in extreme thyroid toxemia. Use 1x (Beebe).

**Mind:** Patient lives in a world of his own, engrossed in spectres and visions and is oblivious to the surrounding realities. While the retina is insensible to actual objects, a host of visual hallucinations throng him from within. He is acutely alive and crazed by a flood of *subjective* visual impressions and fantastic illusions. Hallucinations; sees monsters, hideous faces. Delirium; frightful images; *furious;* rages, bites, strikes; *desire to escape.* Loss of consciousness. Disinclined to talk. Perversity, with tears. *Acuteness of all senses.* Changeable temperament.

**Head:** Vertigo, with falling to the left side or backwards. Sensitive to least contact. Severe throbbing and heat. Palpitations reverberate in the head with labored breathing. Pain; fullness, *especially in the forehead,* occiput and temples. Headache from suppressed catarrhal flow. Sudden outcries. *Pain worse light, noise, jar, lying down and in the afternoon;* better by pressure and in a semi-erect posture. Boring of head into the pillow; drawn backward and rolls from side to side (meningitis, hydrocephalus). Constant moaning. Hair splits; is dry and comes out. Headache worse on the right side and on lying down; ill effects, colds, etc., from having a hair cut.

**Eyes:** Throbbing deep in the eyes on lying down. *Pupils dilated* (*Agn.*). Eyes feel swollen and protruding, *staring, brilliant;* conjunctiva red; *dry,* burns; photophobia; shooting pain in the eyes (conjunctivitis). Exophthalmos. Ocular illusions; fiery appearance. *Diplopia,* squinting, spasm of lids. Sensation as if eyes were half closed. Eyelids swollen. Fundus congested.

**Ears:** Tearing pain in middle and external ear. Humming noises. Membrana tympani bulges and injected. Parotid gland swollen (mumps, parotiditis). Sensitive to loud tones. Hearing, very acute. *Otitis media. Pain, causes delirium. Child cries out in sleep;* throbbing and beating (throbbing) pain deep in the ears, synchronous with the heart beat. Hematoma auris. Acute and sub-acute conditions of the eustachian tube. Autophony—hears one's own voice in the ear.

**Nose:** Imaginary odors. Tingling in the tip of the nose. Red and swollen. *Epistaxis,* with a red face. Coryza; mucus mixed with blood.

**Face:** Red, *bluish-red,* hot, swollen, shiny; convulsive motion of the muscles of face (epilepsy). Upper lip edematous. Facial neuralgia with twitching muscles and a flushed face.

**Mouth:** Dry. Throbbing pain in teeth. Gumboil. Tongue red on edges. Strawberry tongue. *Grinding of teeth.* Tongue swollen and painful (glossitis). Stammering.

**Throat:** Dry, as if glazed; angry looking congestion (*Gins.*)*; red, worse on the right side.* Tonsils enlarged (tonsillitis); *throat feels constricted; difficult deglutition;* worse, liquids. Sensation of a lump. Esophagus dry; feels contracted. *Spasms* in throat. Continuous inclination to swallow. Scraping sensation. Muscles of deglutition very sensitive. Hypertrophy of the mucous membrane.

**Stomach:** Loss of appetite. Averse to meat and milk. Spasmodic pain in the epigastrium. Constriction; pain extends to the spine. Nausea and vomiting. *Great thirst for cold water.* Spasms of stomach. Empty retching. Abhorrence of liquids. Spasmodic hiccough. *Dreads drinking.* Uncontrollable vomiting.

**Abdomen:** Distended, hot. Transverse colon protrudes like a pad. Tender, swollen. Pain as if clutched by a hand; worse, jar, pressure. Cutting pain across; stitches on the left side of the abdomen, when coughing, sneezing, or touching it. Extreme sensitiveness to touch, to bed-clothes, etc. (*Lach.*).

**Stool:** Thin, green, dysenteric; in lumps like chalk. Shuddering during stool. Stinging pain in rectum; spasmodic stricture. Piles more sensitive with backache. Prolapsus ani (*Ign., Podo.*).

**Urinary:** *Retention.* Acute urinary infections. Sensation of motion in the bladder, as of a worm. Urine scanty, with tenesmus; *dark and turbid,* loaded with phosphates. Vesical region sensitive (cystitis). Incontinence, continuous dripping. *Frequent and profuse.* Hematuria where no pathological condition can be found. Prostatic hypertrophy.

**Male:** Testicles hard, drawn up, inflamed (orchitis). Nocturnal sweat on genitals. Flow of prostatic fluid. Desire diminished.

**Female:** Sensitive, forcing downwards, *as if all the viscera would protrude* (prolapse). Dryness and heat of vagina. Dragging pain around the loins. Pain in sacrum. Menses increased; *bright red, too early, too profuse* (menorrhagia). *Hemorrhage hot.* Cutting pain from hip to hip (dysmenorrhea). *Menses and lochia very offensive and hot.* Labor pains come and go suddenly. *Mastitis,* pain, throbbing, redness, streaks radiate from the nipple. Breasts feel heavy; are hard and red. Tumors of breast, pain worse lying down. Offensive smelling hemorrhages, hot gushes of blood. Diminished lochia.

**Respiratory:** Dryness of the nose, fauces, larynx, and trachea. *Tickling, short, dry cough; worse at night* (bronchitis). Larynx feels sore. Respiration oppressed, quick, unequal. Cheyne-Stokes respiration (*Cocain., Op.*). *Hoarseness;* aphonia. Painless hoarseness. Cough with pain in the left hip. Barking cough, whooping cough with pain in the stomach before the attack and hemoptysis. Stitches in chest when coughing (pneumonia). *Larynx, very painful;* feels as if a foreign body was in it, with cough (laryngitis). *High, piping voice. Moaning at every breath.*

**Heart:** Violent palpitations, reverberating in the head with labored breathing. Palpitations from least exertion. Throbbing throughout the body. Dichrotism. Heart seem too large. Rapid but weak pulse.

**Back:** Stiff neck. *Swelling in the glands of the neck.* Pain in the nape, as if it would break (cervical spondylosis). Pressure maximum in the dorsal region. Lumbago, with pain in hips and thighs.

**Extremities:** Shooting pains along the limbs. Joints swollen, red, shining with red streaks radiating. Tottering gait. Shifting rheumatic pains. Phlegmasia alba dolens. Jerking in the limbs. Spasms. Involuntary limping. *Cold extremities.*

**Sleep:** Restless, crying out, gritting of teeth. Kept awake by pulsations of blood vessels. Screams out in sleep. Sleeplessness with drowsiness. *Starting on closing the eyes or during sleep.* Sleeps with hands under the head (*Ars., Plat.*).

**Fever:** A high feverish state, with comparative absense of toxemia. *Burning, pungent, steaming heat.* Feet icy cold. Superficial blood vessels, distended. Perspiration dry, only on the head. *No thirst with fever.*

**Skin:** Dry and *hot;* swollen, sensitive; burns, scarlet, smooth (cellulitis). Eruption like scarlatina, suddenly spreading. Erythema; pustules on the face.

*Glands swollen, tender,* red. *Boils.* Acne rosacea. Suppurative wounds. *Alternate redness and paleness of the skin.* Induration after inflammations. Erysipelas.

**Modalities:** *Worse,* touch, jar, noise, draught, after noon, lying down. *Better,* semi-erect position.

**Relationship:** Compare: *Sanguisorba officinalis* 2x-6x, a member of the Rosaceae family (*profuse, long lasting* menses (menorrhagia), especially in nervous patients with congestive symptoms of head and limbs. Passive hemorrhages at climacteric. Chronic metritis. Hemorrhage from lungs. Varices and ulcers). *Mandragora officinarum* —(Mandrake), a narcotic of the ancients—Restless excitability and physical weakness. Desire for sleep. Has antiperiodic properties like *Chin.* and *Aran.* Useful in epilepsy and hydrophobia, also *Cetonia aurata* (A. E. Lavine). *Hyos.* (less fever, more agitation); *Stram.* (more sensorial excitement, frenzy); *Hoitzia coccinea*—A Mexican drug, similar in action to *Bell.* (useful in fever, scarlatinal eruption, measles, urticaria, etc. High fever with red eruptions. Dry mouth and throat, red face, injected eyes, delirium). *Calc.* is often required after *Bell., Atropinum.* Alkaloid of *Belladonna* covers the neurotic sphere more (great *dryness of the throat,* almost impossible to swallow. Chronic stomach affections, with great pain and vomiting of all food. Peritonitis. All kinds of illusions of sight. Everything appears large *(Platina opposite). Hypochlorhydria;* pyrosis. Motes over everything. On reading, *words run together;* diplopia, *all objects seem elongated.* Eustachian tube and tympanic congestion. Affinity for the pancreas. Paroxysms of gastric pain; ovarian neuralgia).

**Non-homeopathic Uses:** *Atropinum* and its salts are used for ophthalmic purposes, to dilate the pupil and paralyze accommodation.

Given internally or hypodermically, it is antagonistic to *Opium* and *Morphinum*. *Physostigma* and *Prussic acid.* Narcotic poisons and mushroom poisoning. Renal colic 1-200 of a grain hypodermically.

*Atropin* injected subcutaneously in doses from a milligram upwards for intestinal obstruction threatening life.

Hypodermically, 1-80 gr.; night sweats in phthisis.

*Atropia* 1-20 gr. is antagonistic to 1 gr. *Morphine.*

Also used as a local anesthetic, antispasmodic, and to dry up secretions, milk, etc.

Dose: *Atropinum sulphuricum,* 1-120 to 1-60 grain.

Antidotes to *Belladonna*: *Camph., Coff., Op., Acon.*

Complementary: *Calc.,* especially in semi-chronic and constitutional diseases.

Incompatible: *Acet-ac.*

**Dose:** First to thirtieth potency and higher. Must be repeated frequently in acute diseases.

# BELLIS PERENNIS

(Daisy)

**Bell-p.**

It acts upon the muscular fibers of the blood vessels. Marked muscular soreness. Lameness, as if sprained. Venous congestion, due to mechanical causes. First remedy for injuries to the deeper tissues, after major surgical work. Results of injuries to nerves with intense soreness and intolerance to cold bathing. After gout, debility of limbs.

Traumatism of the pelvic organs and, auto-traumatism express the conditions calling for this remedy; ill effects from masturbation. Excellent remedy for sprains and bruises. Complaints due to cold food or drink when the body is heated, and in affections due to cold wind. Externally, in nevi. Acne. *Boils all over. Sore, bruised feeling in the pelvic region.* Exudations, stasis, swelling come within the range of this remedy. Rheumatic symptoms. Does not vitiate the secretions. "It is a princely remedy for old laborers, especially gardeners" (Burnett).

**Head:** Vertigo in elderly people. Headache from occiput to the top of the head. Forehead feels contracted. *Bruised soreness.* Itching around the scalp and over the back, worse from a hot bath and bed.

**Abdomen:** *Soreness of the abdominal wall and uterus.* Stitches in spleen; sore, enlarged (splenomegaly). Yellow, painless diarrhea, foul odor, worse at night. Bloated; rumbling in bowels.

**Female:** Breasts and uterus engorged. Varicose veins during pregnancy. *During pregnancy inability to walk.* Abdominal muscles lame. *Uterus feels sore, as if squeezed.*

**Extremities:** Joints sore, muscular soreness (rheumatism). Itching on back and flexor surfaces of thighs. Pain down the anterior portion of thighs. Wrist feels contracted as if from an elastic band around the joint. Sprains with great soreness. *Railway spine.*

**Sleep:** Wakes up early in the morning and cannot get to sleep again.

**Skin:** *Boils.* Ecchymosis, swelling, very sensitive to touch. Venous congestion due to mechanical causes. Varicose veins with bruised, sore feeling. Exudations and swellings. Acne.

**Modalities:** *Worse, left side;* hot bath and warmth of bed; before storms; cold bathing; cold wind.

**Relationship:** Compare: *Arn., Ars., Staph., Ham., Bry., Vanad.* (degenerative states).

**Dose:** Tincture to third potency.

# BENZOLUM—COAL NAPHTHA

(Benzol, $C_6H_6$) **Benzol.**

The most striking fact in the proving of *Benzol.* seems to be the influence it has on the circulatory system. It causes a slowing of the pulse stream, which in guinea pigs brought about the formation of infarcts. In the human provers it resulted in a *decrease of red, and increase of white cells* (R. F. Rabe, M.D.).

It ought to be of use in leukemia. Eye symptoms striking. Hallucinations; epileptiform attacks, coma and anesthesia.

**Head:** Sense of falling through the bed and floor. Pains from below upward. Tired and nervous. Frontal headache exending to the root of the nose. Dizzy. Pressing feeling in the head. Right sided headache.

**Eyes:** Illusions of vision with wide open eyes. Twitching of lids. Photophobia, objects blurred. Aching in eyes and lids. Marked dilation of pupils. Failure to react to light, particularly daylight.

**Nose:** Profuse, fluent coryza, especially in the afternoon. Violent sneezing.

**Male:** Swelling of the right testicle (orchitis). Severe pain in testicles. Itching of scrotum. Profuse micturition.

**Extremities:** Heavy limbs, cold legs, exaggerated knee jerk. Pains from below upward.

**Skin:** Eruptions like measles. Perspiration on side not lain on. Itching all over the back.

**Modalities:** *Worse* at night. Worse right side.

**Relationship:** Compare: *Benzinum*—Petroleum ether—not as pure a compound as benzene (*benzol*). It is the same, but with a mixture of hydrocarbons. It seems to exercise a special influence on the nervous system and on the blood. Oxyhemoglobinemia. Physical weakness, cramps, exaggeration of knee jerks, nausea, vomiting, dizziness, *heaviness* and coldness of limbs. Tremors of eyelids and tongue. *Benzinum dinitricum*—D. N. B. (the most obvious results of poisoning by skin absorption are changes in the red blood corpuscles and liver degeneration; in amblyopia, color blindness, retinitis. Field of vision contracted. Black urine). *Benzinum nitricum* (dark,black blood, coagulates with difficulty; venous hyperemia of the brain and general venous engorgement. Burning taste in mouth. Blue lips, tongue, skin, nails and conjunctiva (cynosed). Cold skin, pulse small, weak, breathing slow and irregular, unconsciousness, symptoms of apoplectic coma. *Rolling of eyeballs in their vertical axis; pupils dilated.* Nystagmus. Respiration very slow, difficult, sighing). *Trinitrotoluenum* (T.N.T.), Trotyl—is a high explosive, obtained by nitrating toluene—a product of coal tar distillation. When the skin or hair is exposed to T. N. T. a characteristic yellow or tawny-orange stain is produced, which lasts for several weeks. Indicated in graver forms of anemia (pernicious) and jaundice. Produces fatal toxic jaundice.

**Dose:** Sixth potency.

# BENZOICUM ACIDUM

(Benzoic Acid) **Benz-ac.**

The most marked characteristic pertains to the odor and the color of urine. It has a marked action on metabolism. It produces and cures symptoms of a uric acid diathesis, with highly colored and very offensive urine; gouty symptoms. Renal insufficiency. Child wants to be nursed in the arms, will not be laid down. Pains suddenly change their locality. Antisycotic. Gouty and asthmatic.

**Mind:** Prone to dwell on unpleasant things of the past. Omits words in writing. Depression.

**Head:** Vertigo inclination to fall sideways. Throbbing in temporal arteries, causes puffing around the ears. Cold sweat on forehead. Wens.

**Ears:** Noises on swallowing. Swelling behind the ears (*Caps.*).

**Nose:** Itching in septum. Pain in the nasal bones.

**Face:** Copper colored spots. Red, with little blisters. Circumscribed redness of cheeks.

**Mouth:** Ulceration of the tongue (apthae). Prickling, puckered constriction of the mouth, bluish and bleeding gums.

**Stomach:** Sweat while eating; pressure in stomach, sensation of a lump.

**Abdomen:** Cutting around the navel. Stitching in the liver region.

**Rectum:** Stitches and *constricted* feeling. Puckering constriction of rectum. Itching and warty elevations around the anus.

**Stool:** Frothy, *offensive, liquid,* light colored, like soapsuds, bowel movements mostly windy.

**Urinary:** Repulsive odor; changeable color; brown, acrid. *Enuresis;* dribbling, *offensive urine of old men.* Excess of uric acid. Vesical catarrh from suppressed gonorrhea. Cystitis.

**Respiratory:** Hoarse in the morning. Asthmatic cough; worse night; lying on the right side. Chest very tender. Pain in the region of the heart. Expectoration, of green mucus.

**Back:** Pressure on the spinal column. Coldness of the sacrum. Dull pain in the region of kidneys; worse, wine.

**Extremities:** Joints crack on motion. Tearing with stitches. *Pain in tendo-Achillis.* Rheumatic gout; nodes very painful. Gouty deposits. Ganglion; swelling of the wrist. Pain and swelling in knees. Bunion of great toe. Tearing pains in the great toe.

**Fever:** Cold hands, feet, back, knees. Chills; cold sweat. Internal heat on awakening.

**Skin:** Red spots. Itching in spots.

**Modalities:** *Worse,* in open air; by uncovering.

**Relationship:** Useful after *Colch.* fails in gout; after *Cop.* in gonorrhea.

Compare: *Nit-ac., Am-be., Sabin., Tropaeolum majus*—Garden nasturtium *(fetid urine).*

Antidote: *Cop.*

Incompatible: *Wine.*

**Dose:** Third to sixth potency.

---

# BERBERIS AQUIFOLIUM—MAHONIA

(Mountain Grape) **Berb-a.**

A remedy for skin, chronic catarrhal affections, and secondary syphilis. Hepatic torpor, lassitude and other evidences of incomplete metamorphosis; stimulates all glands and improves nutrition.

**Head:** Sensation of a band just above the ears. Bilious headache. "Scald head" (thick crusts). Scaly eczema.

**Face:** Acne. Blotches and pimples. Clears the complexion.

**Stomach:** Tongue thickly coated, yellowish-brown; feels blistered. Burning in the stomach. Nausea and hunger after eating.

**Urinary:** Stitching, crampy pains; thick mucus, and bright red, mealy sediment[1].

**Skin:** *Pimply, dry, rough, scaly.* Eruptions on the *scalp extending to the face* and neck. Tumor of breast, with pain. Psoriasis. Acne. Dry eczema. Pruritus. Glandular induration.

**Relationship:** *Carb-ac., Euon., Berb., Hydr.*

**Dose:** Tincture in rather material doses.

---

# BERBERIS VULGARIS

(Barberry) **Berb.**

Rapid change of symptoms—pain changes in regard to place and character, thirst alternates with thirstlessness, hunger, loss of appetite, etc. Acts forcibly on the venous system, producing pelvic engorgements and hemorrhoids.

Hepatic, and rheumatic affections, particularly with urinary, hemorrhoidal and menstrual complaints.

---

1 Turbid urine with abundant, mucoid and clayey sediment which is bright red in color (Clarke — Dictionary of Practical Materia Medica).

Old gouty constitutions. Pain in the region of kidneys is most marked; hence it is useful in renal and bladder problems, gall stones, and cystitis. It causes inflammation of kidneys (nephritis), with hematuria. Pains may be felt all over the body, emanating from the lumbar region. It also has a marked action on the liver, promoting the flow of bile. Often called in arthritic affections with urinary disturbances. Wandering, *radiating* pain. Acts well in fleshy people with good livers but with little endurance. Spinal irritation. All *Berb.* pains radiate, are not worse by pressure, but worse in various attitudes, especially standing and during active exercise.

**Head:** Listless, apathetic, indifferent. Puffy sensation, feels as if the head is becoming larger. Vertigo with attacks of fainting. Frontal headache. Chills in the back and occiput. Tearing pains in the auricle and gouty concretions. Sensation *of a tight cap pressing upon the whole scalp.*

**Nose:** Dry; obstinate catarrh of left nostril. Crawling sensation in the nostrils.

**Face:** Pale, sickly. Sunken cheeks and eyes, with bluish circles.

**Mouth:** Sticky sensation. Diminished saliva. Sticky, frothy saliva, like cotton (*Nux-m.*). Tongue feels scalded; vesicles on the tongue.

**Stomach:** *Nausea before breakfast.* Heartburn.

**Abdomen:** Stitches in the region of gall bladder; worse, pressure, extending to the stomach. Catarrh of the gall bladder (cholecystitis) with constipation and yellow complexion (jaundice). Stitching pains in front of the kidneys extending to the liver, spleen, stomach, groins and Poupart's ligament. Sticking pain, deep in the ilium.

**Stool:** Constant urging to stool. Diarrhea painless, clay colored, burning and smarting in anus and perineum. Tearing around the anus. *Fistula in ano.*

**Urinary:** Burning pains. Sensation as if some urine remained after micturating. Urine with thick *mucus and bright red,* mealy sediment.[1] Bubbling, sore sensation in kidneys. Pain in the bladder region. *Pain in the thighs and loins on micturating.* Frequent micturition; urethra burns when not micturating (urethritis).

**Male:** Neuralgia of spermatic cord and testicles. Smarting, burning, stitching in the testicles, prepuce and scrotum.

**Female:** Pinching constriction in mons veneris, vaginismus, contraction and tenderness in the vagina. Burning and soreness in vagina. Desire diminished, cutting pain during coition (dysparunia). Menses scanty, gray mucus with pain in kidneys and chilliness, pain extends down the thighs. Leucorrhea, grayish mucus, with painful urinary symptoms. Neuralgia of ovaries and vagina.

---

[1] Red, bran-like sediment (Clarke — Dictionary of Practical Materia Medica).

**Respiratory:** Hoarseness; polyp in the larynx. Tearing stitches in the chest and region of heart.

**Back:** Stitches in the neck and back; worse, respiration. Sticking pain in the region of kidneys radiating around the abdomen, to the hips and groins. Numb, bruised sensation. Stitches from kidneys to the bladder. Tearing, sticking pain with stiffness, making rising difficult, involving hips, nates, limbs, with numbness. Lumbago (*Rhus-t., Ant-t.*). Metatarsus and metacarpus feel sprained. Post-operative pain in the lumbar region; soreness with sharp pain following the course of circumflex iliac nerve to the bladder with frequent micturition.

**Extremities:** Rheumatic paralytic pain in the shoulders, arms, hands and fingers, legs and feet. *Neuralgia under the finger nails,* with swelling in finger joints. Sensation of coldness on the outside of thighs. Heels painful, as if ulcerated. Stitching between the metatarsal bones as if from a nail when standing. Pain in the balls of feet on stepping. Intense weariness and lameness of legs after walking a short distance.

**Fever:** Cold sensations in various parts, as if spattered with cold water. Warmth in the lower part of back, hips, and thighs.

**Skin:** Flat warts. *Itching,* burning and smarting; *worse, scratching;* better, cold applications. Small pustules all over the body. Eczema of *anus* and *hands. Circumscribed pigmentation* following eczematous inflammation.

**Modalities:** *Worse,* motion, *standing.* It brings on, or increases, urinary complaints.

**Relationship:** Compare: *Ipomoea bona-nox—Convo-d.*—Morning glory (pain in the left lumbar muscles on stooping. Kidney disorders with pain in the back. Marked abdominal flatulence. Aching on top of the right shoulder; renal colic; aching in the lumbar region and extremities), *Aloe, Lyc., Nux-v., Sars. Xanthorrhoea arborea* (severe pain in kidneys, cystitis and gravel. Pain from the ureters to the bladder and testicles; pain in the lumbar region returns from least chill or dampness). *Xanthorrhiza apifolia*—Shrub yellow root—contains Berberine. Dilatation of stomach and intestines, atony, enlarged spleen.

Antidotes: *Camph., Bell.*

**Dose:** Tincture to sixth potency.

---

## BETA VULGARIS AQUATICA

(Beetroot) **Beta**

Influences chronic catarrhal states and tuberculosis. The salt *Betainum muriaticum* obtained from the Beetroot itself seems to be best adapted to phthisical patients. Children yield very quickly to the action of this remedy. 2x trituration used generally.

---

# BETONICA AQUATICA

(Betony Wood) **Beto.**

Produces pains in various parts.

**Head:** Stitches in the right temple. Inability to concentrate.

**Abdomen:** Pain in the abdomen, hepatic region and transverse colon, also in the gall bladder, right inguinal region and spermatic cords.

**Extremities:** Shooting pain at the back of both the wrist joints. Wrist drop. Pain in the right popliteal space extending down the leg, which feels paralyzed.

**Dose:** 3x and above.

---

# BISMUTHUM

(Precipitated Sub-nitrate of Bismuth) **Bism.**

Irritation and catarrhal inflammation of the alimentary canal, is the chief action of this drug.

**Mind:** Solitude is unbearable. *Desire for company.* Complains about his condition. *Anguish.* Discontented.

**Head:** Headache alternates with gastralgia. Neuralgic pain, as if torn by pincers; involves the face and teeth; worse, eating; better, cold; alternates with gastralgia. Cutting pains or pressure above the right orbit, extending to the occiput. Pressure in the occiput; worse, motion; with heaviness.

**Mouth:** *Gums swollen* (scorbutic). Toothache; better, cold water in the mouth (*Coff.*). Tongue white. Swollen. Black, gangrenous looking wedges on the dorsum and sides of tongue. Profuse salivation, teeth loose. Thirst for cold drinks. Tongue coated white; sweetish, metallic taste.

**Stomach:** Vomits, with convulsive gagging and pain. *Water is vomited as soon as it reaches the stomach.* Eructation after drinking. Vomits all fluids. *Burning; sensation of a load.* Will eat for several days; then vomits. Slow digestion, with *fetid eructations.* Gastralgia; pain from the stomach to the spine. Gastritis. *Better, cold drinks,* but vomiting when stomach becomes full. Inexpressible pain in stomach; must bend backwards. Pressure as if from a load on one spot, alternating with burning, crampy pain and pyrosis.

**Stool:** Painless diarrhea with great thirst and frequent micturition and vomiting (cholera). Pinching in lower abdomen with rumbling.

**Chest:** Pinching in the middle of the diaphragm, extending transversely through the chest. Angina pectoris; pain around the heart, extending to the left arm and fingers.

**Extremities:** Cramps in hands and feet. Tearing in the wrist. Paralytic weakness, especially of the right arm. Tearing in the tips of fingers, under the nails (*Berb.*). Itching erosions near the tibia and the dorsum of feet near the joints. Cold limbs.

**Sleep:** Restless on account of voluptuous dreams. Sleepy in the morning, a few hours after eating.

**Relationship:** Antidotes: *Nux-v., Caps., Calc.*

Compare: *Ant., Ars., Bell., Kreos.*

**Dose:** First to sixth potency.

---

# BLATTA AMERICANA

(Cockroach) **Blatta-a.**

Ascites. Various forms of dropsy. Yellow complexion (jaundice). Extreme weariness. Pain in the urethra on micturating (urethritis). Weariness on going upstairs.

**Dose:** Sixth potency.

---

# BLATTA ORIENTALIS

(Indian Cockroach) **Blatta-o.**

A remedy for asthma. Especially when associated with bronchitis. Indicated after *Ars.,* when it is insufficient.

Cough with *dyspnea* in bronchitis and phthisis. Acts best in stout and corpulent patients. Much pus-like mucus.

**Dose:** Lowest potencies during an attack. After the spasm, for the remaining cough, use the higher. Stop with improvement to prevent aggravation.

---

# BOLETUS LARICIS—POLYPORUS OFFICINALE

(White Agaric) **Bol-la.**

Quotidian intermittent fever. Sweat is light, and without relief. Night sweat in phthisis.

**Head:** Feels light and hollow with deep frontal headache. Thick, yellow coating of tongue; teeth indented. Constant nausea.

**Fever:** Chilliness along the spine with frequent hot flushes. Yawns and stretches when chilly. Severe aching in shoulders, joints and lumbosacral region. *Profuse perspiration at night,* with hectic chills and fever.

**Skin:** Hot and dry, especially the palms. Itching more between the scapulae and on the forearms.

**Relationship**: Compare: *Agaricinum,* active constituent of *Polyporus officinale* (phthisical and other enervating night sweats 1-4 to 1-2 gr. doses; also in chorea, in dilatation of heart with pulmonary emphysema, fatty degeneration, profuse perspiration and erythema). *Boletus luridus* (violent pain in the epigastrium, urticaria tuberosa). *Boletus satanus* (dysentery, vomiting, great debility, cold extremities, spasm of extremities and face).

**Dose:** First attenuation.

---

# BORAX VENETA

(Borate of Sodium) **Borx.**

Gastro-intestinal irritation. Salivation, nausea, vomiting, colic, diarrhea, collapse, albuminuria, casts and vesical spasm. Delirium, visual changes, hematuria, and skin eruptions have all been observed from over dosing.

*Dread of downward motion* in nearly all complaints. For homeopathic purposes, the peculiar nervous symptoms are very characteristic and have frequently been verified, especially in the therapeutics of children. Of much value in epilepsy. Aphthous ulceration of mucous membranes.

**Mind:** Extreme anxiety, especially from motion which has a downward direction, rocking, being carried downstairs, and when laid down. Anxious expression on the face during the downward motion, patient starts and throws up hands when laying him down, as if afraid of falling. Excessively nervous; easily frightened. *Sensitive to sudden noises.* Violent fright from retort of gun, even at a distance. Fear of thunder.

**Head:** Aches, with nausea and trembling of the whole body. Hair tangled at tips, cannot be separated as in plica polonica (*Vinc.*).

**Eyes:** Lashes turn inward (entropion). Visions of bright waves. Eyelids inflamed, lids cut against eyeball (blepharitis).

**Ears:** *Very sensitive to the slightest noise;* not disturbed so much by louder ones.

**Nose**: Red nose in young women (*Nat-c.*). Red and shiny swelling, with throbbing and a tensive sensation. Tip swollen and ulcerated. Dry crusts.

**Face**: Pale, earthy, with an expression of suffering. Swollen with pimples on the nose and lips. Sensation of cobwebs.

**Mouth**: *Aphthae.* White fungus-like growth (candidiasis). Mouth hot and tender; ulcers bleed on touch and eating. Painful gum-boil. Crying when nursing. Taste bitter (*Bry., Puls., Cupr.*). Taste of a "cellar mould."

**Stomach and Abdomen:** Distention after eating; vomiting. Gastralgia depending upon uterine disturbance. Pain as if diarrhea would result.

**Stool**: *Loose, pappy, offensive in children.* Diarrhea, offensive, preceded by colic; mucous stools, with an aphthous sore mouth.

**Urinary:** Hot, smarting pain in the orifice. Pungent smell. Child afraid to micturate, screams before micturating (*Sars.*). Small red particles on the diaper.

**Female**: Labor-like pains with frequent eructations. *Galactorrhea* (*Calc., Con., Bell.*). While nursing, pain in *the opposite breast.* Leucorrhea like white of eggs, with a sensation as if warm water was flowing. Menses *too soon, profuse,* with griping pain, nausea and pain in the stomach extending to the lumbosacral region. *Membranous dysmenorrhea.* Sterility. Favors easy conception. Sensation of distention in clitoris with sticking. Pains.Pruritus vulva and eczema.

**Respiratory**: Hacking and violent cough; expectoration with a mouldy taste and smell. *Stitches in the chest* on inspiration and cough. Cough with a mouldy taste, breath smells mouldy. Pleurodynia, worse upper part of right chest. Breathing arrested when lying; is obliged to jump and catch breath, which causes pain on the right side. Out of breath on going up stairs.

**Extremities**: Sensation of cobwebs on the hands. Itching in finger joints and hands. Throbbing pain at the tip of the thumb. *Stitches in the sole.* Pain in the heel. Burning pain in great toe (gout); inflammation of balls of toes. Eczema of toes and fingers with loss of nails.

**Sleep:** Voluptuous dreams. Cannot sleep on account of heat, especially in the head. Cries out in sleep, as if frightened (*Bell.*).

**Skin**: *Psoriasis.* Erysipelas on the face. Itching on the dorsum of the finger joints. Unhealthy skin; slight injuries suppurate. Herpes (*Rhus-t.*). Erysipelatous inflammation with swelling and tension. Chilblains relieved in the open air. Trade eruptions on fingers and hands, itching and stinging. Ends of hair become tangled.

**Modalities:** *Worse,* downward motion, noise, smoking, warm weather, after menses.

*Better,* pressure, evening, cold weather.

**Relationship:** Acetic acid, vinegar, and wine are incompatible.

Antidotes: *Cham., Coff.*

Compare: *Calc., Bry., Sanic., Sul-ac.*

**Dose:** First to third trituration. In skin diseases continue its use for several weeks. Locally in pruritus pudendi. A piece of borax, the size of a pea, dissolved in the mouth, acts magically in restoring the voice, in cases of sudden hoarseness brought on by cold, and frequently for an hour or so, it renders the voice silvery and clear.

---

# BORICUM ACIDUM

(Boracic Acid) **Bor-ac.**

Used as an antiseptic disinfectant, since it arrests fermentation and putrefaction.

Pain in the region of ureters, with a frequent urging to micturate. *Coldness* (*Helo.*). *Diabetes,* Tongue dry, red, and cracked. Cold saliva.

**Female:** Climacteric flushings (*Lach., Aml-ns.*). Vagina cold, as if packed with ice. Frequent micturition with burning and tenesmus.

**Skin:** Multiform erythema of the trunk and upper extremities. Exfoliating dermatitis. Edema of tissues around the eyes.

**Non-homeopathic Uses:** When the diplococcus of Weichselbaum is present in the sputum of pharyngitis or bronchitis, pneumonia with tenacious sputum, hacking cough and pain, five grain doses, six times daily. A solution of *Bor-ac.,* as an injection, in chronic cystitis or a teaspoonful to a glass of hot milk, is taken internally. Boro-glyceride in solution (1:40) is a powerful antiseptic. *Styes,* 15 gr. to 1 oz. water externally. As a dusting powder on ulcerated surfaces. In cystitis, as an irrigating fluid.

**Dose:** Third trituration.

---

# BOTHROPS LANCIOLATUS — LACHESIS LANCIOLATUS

(Yellow Viper) **Both.**

Its venom is very coagulating (also *Lach.*). We should expect to find under these remedies the symptomatology of thrombosis, also thrombotic phenomena like hemiplegia, aphasia, inability to articulate etc. (Linn J. Boyd).

Broken down, hemorrhagic constitutions; septic states. Great lassitude and sluggishness; hemorrhages from every orifice of the body; black spots. Hemiplegia with aphasia. Inability to articulate, without any affection of the tongue. Nervous trembling. Pain in the right big toe. Diagonal course of symptoms. Pulmonary congestion.

**Eyes:** Amaurosis; blindness from hemorrhage into the retina, Hemeralopia, day blindness, can hardly see her way after sunrise; conjunctivial hemorrhage.

**Face:** Swollen and puffy. Besotted expression.

**Throat:** Red, dry, constricted; dysphagia, cannot pass liquids.

**Stomach:** Epigastric distress. Black vomiting. Intense hematemesis. Tympanitis and bloody stools.

**Skin:** Swollen, livid, cold with hemorrhagic infiltration. Gangrene. Lymphatics swollen. Anthrax. Malignant erysipelas.

**Modalities:** *Worse,* right side.

**Relationship:** Compare: *Toxicophis pugnax*—Moccasin snake (pain and fever *recur* annually after a bite from this snake and sometimes change location with disappearance of first symptoms. An unusual dryness of the skin follows the bite. Edematous swellings and periodical neuralgia. Pain travels from one part to another). Other snake poisons, notably *Lach.*

*Trachinus draso*—Stingfish (intolerable pains, swelling, acute blood poisoning, gangrene).

**Dose:** Sixth to thirtieth potency.

---

## BOTULINUM

(Toxin of Bacillus Botulinum) **Botul.**

Food poisoning from canned spinach produced a clinical picture suggested in bulbar paresis.

Eye symptoms, ptosis, diplopia, blurred vision.

Difficulty in swallowing and breathing, choking sensation; weakness and uncertainty in walking, "blind staggers," dizziness, thickening of speech. Cramps in the stomach.

Mask-like expression of face, due to weakness of facial muscles. Severe constipation.

**Dose:** Higher potencies.

---

## BOVISTA LYCOPERDON

(Puff Ball) **Bov.**

Has a marked effect on the skin, producing eruptions like eczema, also upon the circulation, predisposing to hemorrhages; marked languor and lassitude. Adapted to stammering children, old maids with palpitation and "tettery" patients. Stage of numbness and tingling in multiple neuritis. Asphyxia due to charcoal fumes.

**Mind:** *Enlarged sensation* (*Arg-n.*). Awkward; *everything falls from the* *hands*. Sensitive.

**Head:** Sensation *as if the head was enlarging,* especially the occiput. Distensive headache; worse early morning, open air, lying down. Discharge from the nose *stringy,* tough. Dull, bruised pain in the brain. *Stammering* (*Stram., Merc.*). Scalp itches; worse, warmth; sensitive; must scratch until sore.

**Face:** Scurf and crusts about the nostrils and corners of the mouth. Lips chapped. Bleeding of nose and gums. Cheeks and lips feel swollen. *Acne* worse in summer; due to use of cosmetics.

**Stomach:** Sensation of a lump of ice in the stomach. Intolerant of tight clothing around the waist.

**Abdomen:** *Colic* with red urine (hematuria); *relieved by eating.* Must bend double. Pain around the umbilicus. Stitches through the perineum radiating towards the rectum and genitals.

**Rectum**: Chronic diarrhea in old people; worse at night and early morning.

**Female:** *Diarrhea before and during menses.* Menses too early and profuse (menorrhagia); *worse at night.* Voluptuous sensation. Leucorrhea acrid, thick, tough, greenish, follows menses. *Cannot bear tight clothing around the waist* (*Lach.*). *Traces of menses between menstruation.* Soreness in pubes during menses. Metrorrhagia. Panovarian cysts.

**Extremities:** Great weakness of all joints; clumsy with hands, drops things from hands. Weariness of hands and feet. Sweat in axillae; *smells of onion. Tip of coccyx itches intolerably.* Moist eczema on the back of the hand. Itching in feet and legs. Edema in joints after fracture.

**Skin:** Blunt instruments leave deep impression on the skin. *Urticaria on excitement* with rheumatic lameness, palpitations and diarrhea (*Dulc.*). Itching on getting warm. Eczema, moist; formation of thick crusts. Pimples cover the entire body; scurvy; herpetic eruptions. Pruritus ani. Urticaria on waking up in the morning, worse from bathing. Pellagra.

**Relationship:** *Bov.* antidotes tar applications. Suffocation from gas. After *Rhus-t.* in chronic urticaria.

Compare: *Calc., Rhus-t., Sep., Cic.*

**Dose:** Third to sixth potency.

---

## BRACHYGLOTTIS REPENS

(Puka-puka) **Brach.**

*Fluttering sensation* (*Calad.*). Kidney and bladder symptoms predominate. *Bright's disease.* Produces symptoms of albuminuria. Itching in ears and nostrils. Oppression of chest. Writer's cramp.

**Abdomen:** Sensation as if something was rolling around. Fluttering in the region of ovary.

**Urinary:** Pressure in the neck of the bladder; urging to micturate. Sense of swashing in the bladder. Soreness in urethra; sensation as if urine cannot be retained. Urine contains mucus, corpuscles, epithelium, albumen and casts.

**Extremities:** Cramp in fingers, thumb and wrist when writing, soreness extending along flexor carpi ulnaris (Writer's cramps).

**Relationship:** Compare: *Apis, Helon., Merc-c., Plb.*

**Dose:** Third potency.

---

# BROMIUM

(Bromine) **Brom.**

Most marked effects are seen in the respiratory symptoms, especially in the larynx and trachea. It seems to especially affect scrofulous children with enlarged glands. *Blond type.* Enlarged parotid and goitre. Tendency to spasmodic attacks. *Left sided mumps.* Sense of suffocation; excoriating discharges, profuse sweats and great weakness. Complaints from being over heated. *Tendency to infiltrate glands, become hard, but seldom suppurate.*

**Mind:** Delusion that strange people are looking over the patient's shoulder and that she would see some one on turning. Quarrelsome.

**Head:** Migraine of the left side; worse stooping, especially after drinking milk. Headache; worse heat of sun (sunstroke) and by rapid motion. Sharp pain through the eyes. Dizzy when crossing a stream of water.

**Nose:** Coryza, with corrosive soreness of nose. Stoppage of right nostril. Pressure at the root of the nose. *Tickling, smarting, as from cobwebs.* Fan-like motion of alae (*Lyc.*). Epistaxis relieving the chest symptoms.

**Throat:** Throat feels raw in the evening, with hoarseness. Tonsils, pain on swallowing, deep red, with a network of dilated blood vessels. Tickling in the trachea during inspiration. Hoarseness coming on from being overheated.

**Stomach and Abdomen:** Severe burning extending from the tongue to the stomach. Pressure as of a stone. Gastralgia; better eating. Tympanitic distention of the abdomen. Painful hemorrhoids, with black stools (malena).

**Male:** Swelling of testicles. Indurated, with pains worse on slight jar (orchitis).

**Female:** Swelling of ovaries. Menses too early; too profuse, with membranous shreds (menorrhagia, dysmenorrhea). Low spirited before menses. Tumor in breasts, with stitching pains; worse left side. Stitching pains from the breast to the axillae. Sharp shooting pains in the left breast, worse, pressure.

**Respiratory:** Whooping cough (use persistently for about ten days). *Dry cough, with hoarseness* and burning pain *behind the sternum. Spasmodic cough, with rattling of mucus* in the larynx; suffocative. *Hoarseness. Croup* after febrile symptoms have subsided. Difficult and painful breathing. Violent, cramping pain in chest. Chest pains run upward. *Cold sensation when inspiring.* Every inspiration provokes cough. *Laryngeal diphtheria,* membrane begins in the larynx and spreads upwards. Spasmodic constriction. Asthma; difficulty in getting air *into* the lungs (*Chlorum,* in expelling). Better at sea, in seafaring men when they come on land. Hypertrophy of the heart from gymnastics (*Rhus-t.*). Fibrinous bronchitis, great dyspnea (emphysema). Bronchial tubes feel filled with smoke.

**Sleep:** Full of dreams and anguish; jerking and starting during sleep, full of fantasies and illusions; difficult to go to sleep at night, cannot sleep enough in the morning; trembling and weakness on awaking.

**Skin:** Acne, pimples and pustules. Boils on arms and face. *Glands stony hard, especially* in *the lower jaw* and throat. Hard goitre (*Spong.*). Gangrene.

**Modalities:** *Worse*, from evening till midnight and when sitting in a warm room; warm damp weather, when at rest and lying on the left side, *Better,* from any motion; exercise; at sea.

**Relationship:** Antidotes: *Am-c., Camph.* Salt inhibits the action of *Brom.*

Compare: *Con., Spong., Iod., Aster., Arg-n.* Avoid milk when taking *Brom. Hydrobromicum acidum* (throat dry and puckering; constriction in the pharynx and chest; waves of heat over the face and neck; pulsating tinnitus with great nervous irritability (Houghton); vertigo, palpitations; arms heavy; seems as if parts do not belong to him. Seems to have a specific effect on the inferior cervical ganglion, increasing the tonic action of the sympathetic nerves, thus promoting vaso-constriction. Relieves headache, tinnitus and vertigo, especially in vaso-motor stomach disturbance. Dose, 20 minims).

**Dose:** First to third attenuation. Must be prepared fresh, as it is liable to rapid deterioration.

---

## BRYONIA ALBA

(Wild Hops) **Bry.**

Acts on all serous membranes and the viscera they contain. Aching in every muscle. The general character *of the pain produced is stitching, tearing; worse by motion, better rest.* These characteristic stitching pains, greatly aggravated by any motion, are found everywhere, especially in the chest; worse pressure. *Mucous membranes are all dry.* The *Bry.* patient is irritable, has vertigo from raising the head, pressive headache; dry, parched lips, mouth; excessive thirst, bitter taste, sensitive epigastrium, and sensation of a stone in the stomach; stools large, dry, hard; dry cough; rheumatic pains and swellings; dropsical effusions into the synovial and serous membranes.

*Bry.* especially affects the constitution of a robust, firm fibered, dark complexioned person with a tendency to leaness and irritability. It prefers the right side, evening, open air, and warm weather after cold days to manifest its action to the maximum.

Children don't like to be carried or raised. *Physical weakness,* all-pervading apathy. Complaints apt to develop slowly.

**Mind:** Exceedingly *irritable;* everything puts him out of humor. Delirium; wants to go home; *talks of business.*

**Head:** Vertigo, nausea, faintness on rising, confusion. *Bursting, splitting headache,* as if everything would be pressed out; as if hit by a hammer from within; worse from motion, stooping, opening the eyes (meningitis). Headache seated in the occiput. Drawing in bones towards the zygoma. Headache and pain in the eyeballs worse on motion. Frontal headache, frontal sinuses involved (sinusitis).

**Eyes:** Pressing, crushing, aching pain. Glaucoma. Sore to touch and when moving them.

**Ears:** Aural vertigo (Meniere's disease) (*Aur., Nat-sal., Sil., Chin.*). Roaring, buzzing (tinnitus).

**Nose:** *Frequent epistaxis when menses should appear.* Also in the morning,relieving the headache. Coryza with shooting and aching in the forehead. Swelling of the tip of the nose, feels as if it would ulcerate when touched.

**Mouth:** *Lips parched, dry, cracked. Dryness of the mouth, tongue, and throat, with excessive thirst.* Tongue coated yellowish, dark brown; heavily white in gastric derangements. Bitter taste (*Nux-v., Coloc.*). Burning in the lower lip of old smokers. Lip swollen, dry, black and cracked.

**Throat:** Dryness, sticking pain on swallowing, scraped and constricted (*Bell.*). Tough mucus in the larynx and trachea, loosened only after much hawking; worse coming into a warm room.

**Stomach:** *Nausea and faintness on rising up.* Abnormal hunger, loss of taste. Thirst for a large draught. Vomiting of bile and water immediately after eating. Worse, warm drinks, which are vomited. *Stomach, especially the epigastrium are sensitive to touch. Pressure in stomach after eating, as of a stone.* Soreness in the stomach when coughing. Dyspeptic ailments during summer heat.

**Abdomen:** Liver region swollen, sore, tensive (hepatomegaly). Burning pain, *stitches; worse, pressure, coughing, breathing.* Tenderness of the abdominal walls (peritonitis).

**Stool:** Constipation; stools hard, dry, as if burnt; seem too large. Stools brown, thick, bloody; *worse in the morning, from moving,* in hot weather, after being heated, from cold drinks, every spell of hot weather.

**Urinary:** Red, brown, like beer; scanty, hot (nephritis).

**Female:** Menses too early, too profuse (menorrhagia); worse from motion, with tearing pains in the legs; *suppressed, with vicarious discharge or splitting headache.* Stitching pains in the ovaries on taking a deep inspiration; very sensitive to touch. Pain in right ovary as if torn, extending to the thigh (*Lil-t., Croc.*). Milk fever. Pain in breasts at the menstrual period. *Breasts hot, painful and hard* (mastitis). Abscess of mammae. Frequent epistaxis at the appearance of menses. Menstrual irregularities, with gastric symptoms. Ovaritis. *Intermenstrual pain, with great abdominal and pelvic soreness* (*Ham.*).

**Respiratory:** Soreness in the larynx and trachea. Hoarseness; worse in open air. Dry, hacking cough from irritation in the upper trachea. Cough, dry at night; *must sit up; worse after eating or drinking,* vomiting, *with stitches in the chest* and expectoration of rust colored sputa (hemoptysis). Frequent desire to take a long breath; *must* expand lungs. Difficult, quick respiration; worse every movement; caused by stitches in the chest (pleurisy). Cough, with a sensation as if the chest would fly to pieces; presses the hand upon the sternum; must support the chest. Croupous and pleuro-pneumonia. Expectoration of a brick shade, tough and falls like lumps of jelly. Tough mucus in the trachea, loosened only after much hawking. *Coming into a warm room excites cough* (*Nat-c.*). Heaviness beneath the sternum extending towards the right shoulder. Cough *worse* by going into a warm *room.* Stitches in the cardiac region. Angina pectoris (use tincture).

**Back:** Painful stiffness in the nape of neck. *Stitches and stiffness in the lumbar region.* From hard water and sudden changes of weather.

**Extremities:** Knees stiff and painful (arthritis). Hot swelling of feet. *Joints red, swollen, hot,* with stitches and tearing; worse on least movement. Every spot is painful on pressure. Constant motion of the left arm and leg (*Hell.*).

**Sleep:** Drowsy; starting when falling asleep. Delirium; busy with business matters and what he had read.

**Fever:** Pulse full, hard, tense, and quick. Chills with external coldness, dry cough, stitches. Internal heat. Sour sweat after slight exertion. Easy, profuse perspiration. Rheumatic fever and typhoid marked by gastro-hepatic complications.

**Skin:** Yellow; pale, swollen, dropsical; hot and painful. Seborrhea. *Hair very greasy.*

**Modalities:** *Worse,* warmth, any motion, morning, eating, hot weather, exertion, touch. Cannot sit up; gets faint and sick. *Better,* lying on *the painful side, pressure, rest, cold things.*

**Relationship:** Complementary: *Upa* when *Bry.* fails. *Rhus-t., Alum. Illecebrum verticillatum*—A Mexican drug (fever with catarrhal symptoms, gastric and typhoid fever symptoms).

Antidotes: *Acon., Cham., Nux-v.*

Compare: *Asc-t., Tub., Kali-m., Ptel.*

**Dose:** First to twelfth attenuation.

---

## BUFO RANA

(Poison of the Toad) **Bufo**

Acts on the nervous system and skin. Uterine symptoms marked. Lymphangitis of septic origin. Symptoms of paralysis agitans. Striking rheumatic symptoms.

Arouses the lowest passions. Causes a desire for intoxicating drink, and produces impotence.

Of use in feeble minded children. Prematurely senile. Epileptic symptoms. Convulsive seizures occur during sleep at night. More or less connected with derangements of the sexual sphere, seem to come within the range of this remedy. Injuries of the fingers; pain runs in streaks up the arms.

**Mind:** Anxious about health. Sad, restless. Propensity to bite. Howling; impatient; nervous; imbecile. *Desire for solitude. Feeble minded.*

**Head:** Sensation as if hot vapor rose to the top of the head. Numbness of brain. Face bathed in sweat. Epistaxis with a flushed face and pain in the forehead, better epistaxis.

**Eyes:** Cannot bear sight of brilliant objects. Little blisters form on the eye.

**Ears:** Music is unbearable (*Ambr.*). Every little noise distresses.

**Male:** Involuntary emissions; *impotence,* discharge too quick, spasms during coition. *Buboes.* Disposition to handle organs (*Hyos., Zinc.*). Effects of onanism.

**Female:** Menses too early and copious (menorrhagia), clots and bloody discharge at other times (metrorrhagia); watery leucorrhea. Excitement with epileptic attacks. Epilepsy at time of menses. Induration in mammary glands. Palliative in cancer of the mammae. Burning in ovaries and uterus. Ulceration of the cervix. Offensive bloody discharge. Pains run into the legs. Bloody milk. Milkleg (phlegmasia alba dolens). Veins swollen. Tumors and polypi of the womb.

**Heart:** Feels too large. Palpitations. Constriction around the heart. Sensation of heart swimming in water.

**Extremities:** Pain in loins, numbness of limbs, cramps, staggering gait, feels as if a peg was driven into the joints; swelling of bones.

**Skin:** Panaritium; pain runs up the arm. Patches of skin lose sensation (leprosy). Pustules, suppuration from every slight injury. Pemphigus. Bullae which open and leave a raw surface, exuding an ichorous fluid. Blisters on palms and soles. Itching and burning. Carbuncle.

**Modalities:** *Worse,* in a warm room, on awakening. *Better,* from bathing or cold air; from putting feet in hot water.

**Relationship:** Compare: *Bar-c., Aster., Salam.* (epilepsy and softening of brain).

Antidotes: *Lach., Seneg.*

Complementary: *Salam.*

**Dose:** Sixth potency and higher.

---

# BUTYRICUM ACIDUM

(A Volatile Acid Obtained Chiefly from Butter) **But-ac.**

**Head:** Worries over trifles; impulsive thoughts of suicide; constant state of fear and nervousness. Headache makes him apprehensive about trifles; worse going upstairs or on rapid motion. Dull, hazy ache of head.

**Stomach:** Poor appetite. Flatulent stomach and bowels. Cramps in the pit of the stomach,worse at night. Stomach feels heavy and overloaded.

**Abdomen:** Cramps in the abdomen, below the umbilicus. Bowels irregular, stools accompanied by pain and straining.

**Back:** Tired feeling and dull pain in the lumbosacral region, worse walking. Pain in the ankles extending up the back of leg. Pain low down in the back and extremities.

**Sleep:** Pronounced sleeplessness; dreams of a serious nature.

**Skin:** Perspiration on slightest exertion. *Profuse foot sweat.* Crumbling of finger nails.

**Modalities:** *Worse,* at night, fast walking, going upstairs.

**Dose:** Third attenuation.

---

# CACTUS GRANDIFLORUS—SELENICEREUS SPINULOSUS

(Night Blooming Cereus) **Cact.**

Acts on the circular muscular fibres, hence constrictions. The heart and arteries at once respond to the influence of *Cact.* producing very characteristic *constrictions,* as of an iron band. This sensation is found in various places like the esophagus, bladder, etc. The mental symptoms produced correspond to those found in heart affections, sadness and melancholy. *Hemorrhage, constrictions, periodicity,* and *spasmodic pain. The* whole body feels caged, as if each wire is being twisted tighter. Atheromatous arteries and a weak heart. Congestions; irregular distribution of blood. *Favors formation of clots speedily.* Great periodicity. Toxic goitre with cardiac symptoms. *Cact.* is pulseless, panting and prostrated.

**Mind:** Melancholy, taciturn, sad, ill-humored. Fear of death. Screams with pain. Anxiety.

**Head:** Headache if obliged to pass the dinner hour (*Ars., Lach., Lyc.*). *Sensation of weight on the vertex.* Right sided pulsating pain. *Congestive headaches,* periodical, threatening apoplexy. Blood vessels of the head, distended. Feels as if the head was compressed in a vise. Pulsations in the ears. Dim sight. *Right sided prosopalgia,* constricting pains, returns at the same hour daily (*Cedr.*).

**Nose:**Profuse epistaxis. Fluent coryza.

**Throat:** Constriction of esophagus. Dryness of the tongue, as if burnt; needs a lot of liquid to get food down. Suffocative constriction of the throat, with full, throbbing carotids in angina pectoris.

**Stomach:** *Constriction,* pulsation, or heaviness in the stomach. Vomiting of blood (hematemesis).

**Stool:** Hard, black stools (malena). Diarrhea in the morning. Hemorrhoids swollen and painful. Sensation of great weight in the anus. Hemorrhage from bowels in malarial fevers with heart symptoms.

**Urinary:** Constriction in the neck of bladder, causing retention of urine. Hemorrhage from bladder. Clots of blood in the urethra. Constant micturition.

**Female:** Constriction in the uterine region and ovaries. Dysmenorrhea; pulsating pain in the uterus and ovaries. Vaginismus. Menses early, dark, pitch-like (*Cocc., Mag-c.*)*;* ceases on lying down, with heart symptoms.

**Respiratory:** Oppressed breathing as if from a weight on the chest. *Constriction in the chest, as if bound, hindering respiration.* Inflammation of diaphragm. Hemoptysis with convulsive, spasmodic cough. Diaphragmitis, with great difficulty in breathing.

**Heart:** Constriction of the heart, as if from an iron band. *Endocarditis with mitral insufficiency together with violent and rapid action.* Acts best in the incipiency of cardiac incompetence. Weakness of the heart in arteriosclerosis. Tobacco heart. Violent palpitations; *worse lying on the left side, at approach of menses.* Angina pectoris, with suffocation, cold sweat, and an ever present iron band feeling. Pain in the apex, shooting down the left arm. Palpitations, with vertigo, dyspnea, flatulence and pain shooting down the left arm. *Constriction;* very acute pains and stitches in the heart; pulse feeble, irregular, quick, without strength. Endocardial murmurs, excessive impulse, increased precordial dullness, enlarged ventricle. Low blood pressure.

**Extremities:** Edema of the hands and feet. Hands soft; feet enlarged. Numbness of the left arm. Icy cold hands. Restless legs.

**Sleep:** Sleepless on account of pulsations in different parts of the body. Frightful dreams.

**Fever:** Fever every day at the same hour. Coldness in the back with icy cold hands. Intermittent fever; paroxysms around midday (11 a. m.), incomplete in their stages; accompanied by hemorrhages. Coldness predominates; cold sweat, with great anguish. Persistent *subnormal* temperature.

**Modalities:** *Worse,* around noon, lying on the left side; walking, going upstairs, 11 a. m. and 11 p. m. *Better,* open air.

**Relationship:** Antidotes: *Acon., Camph., Chin.*

Compare: *Dig., Spig., Conv., Kalm., Naja, Magn-gr.*

**Dose:** Tincture (best made from flowers), to third attenuation. Higher in nervous palpitations.

---

## CADMIUM SULPHURATUM

(Cadmic Sulphate) **Cadm-s.**

Its pathogenesis gives symptoms corresponding to very low forms of disease, as in cholera, *yellow fever,* where, with exhaustion, vomiting, and *extreme prostration,* the disease runs deathward. Important gastric symptoms. Carcinoma ventriculi; persistent vomiting.

The attack is especially upon the stomach. Patients must keep quiet. *Chilliness and coldness* even when near the fire.

**Head:** Unconscious. Vertigo; room and bed seem to spin around. Hammering in the head. Heat in the head.

**Eyes:** *Corneal opacity* (leucoma). Blue circle around the eyes. One pupil dilated (meningitis). Night blindness (nyctalopia).

**Nose:** *Ozena.* Tightness at the root. Nose obstructed; *polypus.* Caries of the nasal bones. Boils on the nose. Nostrils ulcerated.

**Face:** Distortion of the mouth. Trembling of the jaw. *Facial paralysis;* more on the left side (Bell's palsy, after apoplexy).

**Mouth:** Dysphagia. Esophagus constricted (*Bapt.*). Salty belching. Intense nausea with pain and coldness. Stringy, offensive exudations on the mucous membranes. Salty taste.

**Throat:** Sore throat, constant tickling; gagging and nausea, worse deep breathing; chilliness and aching.

**Stomach:** Soreness in the pit of the stomach on pressure. Violent *nausea;* retching. *Black vomit.* Vomiting of mucus, bile, blood with great prostration and great tenderness over the stomach. Burning and cutting pains in the stomach. Carcinoma, helps persistent vomiting. Coffee ground vomiting (hematemesis).

**Abdomen:** Sore, tender, tympanitic. Region of liver sore. Coldness. Black, offensive clots of blood from bowels. Pain in abdomen with vomiting. Tenderness and tympanites.

**Stool:** Bloody, black, and offensive. Gelatinous, yellowish-green; semi-fluid, with urinary suppression.

**Urinary:** Rawness and soreness in the urethra (urethritis), urine mixed with pus and blood (pyuria, hematuria).

**Heart:** Palpitations, with constriction of the chest.

**Sleep:** Stops breathing on going to sleep. Wakes up suffocated. Fears to go to sleep again. Protracted sleeplessness.

**Fever:** *Icy coldness* (*Camph., Verat., Helo.*). *Yellow fever* (*Crot-h., Carb-v.*).

**Skin:** Blue, yellow, sallow, scaly, cracking. Itching; better scratching. Chloasma, yellowish stains on the nose and cheeks; worse exposure to sun and wind. Chilblains.

**Modalities:** *Worse,* walking or carrying burdens; after sleep; from open air, stimulants. *Better,* eating and rest.

**Relationship:** Compare: *Cadm-o., Cadm-br.* (pain and burning in the stomach, and vomiting); *Cadm-i.* (itching in anus and rectum during the day only; constipation, frequent desire, tenesmus, abdomen bloated); *Zinc.*, *Ars.*, *Carb-v., Verat.*

**Dose:** Third to thirtieth potency.

## CAHINCA

(Brazilian Plant—Chiococca) **Cain.**

This remedy has been found useful in dropsical affections. Its urinary symptoms are well marked. Albuminuria with dyspnea on lying down at night. Ascites and anasarca, with dry skin.

**Urinary:** Constant desire to micturate. Polyuria while travelling. Urine fiery. Burning pain in urethra, especially in the glandular portion.

**Male:** Drawing in of testicles and spermatic cord. Pain worse during passage of pungent smelling urine.

**Back:** Pain in region of kidneys; better lying bent backward. General fatigue.

**Relationship:** Compare: *Apoc., Ars., Coff.,* (similar botanically and in relieving effects of fatigue).

**Dose:** Third potency or lower.

---

## CAJUPUTUM—OLEUM WITTNEBIANUM

(Cajuput Oil) **Caj.**

Acts like oil of cloves. A remedy for *flatulence* and affections of the tongue. *Sense of enlargement.* Causes copious diaphoresis. Retrocedent gout. Neuralgic affections not inflammatory. Nervous dyspnea.

**Head:** Feels very enlarged. As if he could not get himself together (*Bapt.*).

**Mouth:** Persistent sensation of choking. *Spasmodic stricture of esophagus.* Constricted sensation on swallowing solid food. *Tongue feels swollen,* fills the whole mouth.

**Stomach:** *Hiccough,* on the slightest provocation.

**Abdomen:** *Flatulent colic;* tympanites (*Ter.*). Nervous distention of bowels. Urine smells like cat's urine. Spasmodic cholera.

**Modalities:** *Worse,* around 5 a. m., at night.

**Relationship:** Compare: *Bov., Nux-m., Asaf., Ign., Bapt.*

**Dose:** First to third potency (5 drops of oil).

---

## CALADIUM SEGUINUM

(American Arum) **Calad.**

This remedy has a marked action on the genital organs, and on pruritus of this region. Coldness of single parts with an inclination to lie down, aggravation on lying on the left side. Slightest noise startles from sleep. *Dread of motion.* Modifies craving for tobacco. Tobacco heart. Asthmatic complaints.

**Head:** Headaches and mental states of smokers. Very forgetful, does not know about the occurrence of things. Confused headache with pain in the shoulder, pressure in the eyes and forehead; extremely sensitive to noise, throbbing in the ears.

**Stomach:** Gnawing in the stomach at the orifice, which prevents deep breathing. Eructations. *Stomach feels full of dry food; sensation of fluttering.* Acrid vomiting, thirstless, tolerates only warm drinks. Sighing respiration.

**Male:** *Pruritus.* Glans very red (balanitis). Organs seem larger, puffed, relaxed, cold sweating; skin of scrotum is thick. Erections when half asleep; cease when fully awake. *Impotence;* relaxation of penis during excitement. No emission and no orgasm during embrace.

**Female:** *Pruritus of the vulva* (*Ambr., Kreos.*) and vagina during pregnancy (Hydrogen peroxide 1:12 locally). Voluptuousness (nymphomania). Cramping pains in the uterus at night.

**Respiratory:** Larynx seems constricted. Breathing impeded. Catarrhal asthma; mucus not readily raised. Patient afraid to go to sleep.

**Skin:** Sweet sweat, attracts flies. Insect bites burn and itch intensely. Itching rash alternates with asthma. *Burning sensation* and erysipelatous inflammation.

**Modalities**: *Better,* after sweat, after sleeping in the daytime. *Worse,* motion.

**Relationship**: Incompatible: *Arum-t.*

Complementary: *Nit-ac.*

Compare: *Caps., Phos., Caust., Sel., Lyc. Tribulus terrestris* (sexual weakness, emissions, prostatic enlargement).

**Dose**: Third to sixth attenuation.

---

## CALCAREA ACETICA

(Acetate of Lime) **Calc-act.**

Has had brilliant clinical results in inflammations of the mucous membranes characterized by a *membranous exudation;* otherwise it's action and application is like *Calc.* Cancer pains.

**Head:** Vertigo in open air. *Senses obscure while reading. Migraine,* with great coldness in the head and sour taste.

**Female:** Membranous dysmenorrhea (*Borx.*).

**Respiratory:** Rattling expiration. *Cough loose with expectoration of large pieces* like casts of bronchial tubes. Breathing difficult; better bending shoulders backward. Constrictive, anxious sensation in the chest.

**Relationship:** Compare: *Brom., Borx.,* also *Calc-ox.* in excruciating pains of open cancer.

**Dose**: Third trituration.

---

# CALCAREA ARSENICOSA

(Arsenite of Lime) **Calc-ar.**

Epilepsy with rush of blood to the head before an attack; aura felt in the region of heart; flying sensation. Complaints in fat women around climacteric. Chronic malaria. Infantile hepatosplenomegaly. *Nephritis,* with great sensitivenss in the kidney region. Complaints in drunkards after abstaining (*Carb-s.*). Fleshy women at climacteric, *slightest emotions causes palpitations.* Dyspnea, with a feeble heart. *Chilliness.* Albuminuria. Dropsy. Affections of the spleen and mesenteric glands. Hemoglobin and red corpuscles are low.

**Mind**: Anger, anxiety. Desire for company. Confusion, delusions, illusions. Great depression.

**Head:** Violent rush of blood to the head with vertigo. Pain in the head, *better by lying on the painful side.* Weekly headache. Benumbing headache mostly around the ears.

**Stomach:** Region of stomach distended. Hepatosplenomegaly in children. Pancreatic disease; relieves burning pain in cancer of pancreas. Belching with saliva and palpitations.

**Urinary**: *Kidney region sensitive to pressure.* Albuminuria, passes urine every hour.

**Female**: Offensive, bloody leucorrhea. Cancer of the uterus; burning pain in the uterus and vagina.

**Heart**: Constriction and pain in the region of heart, suffocative feeling, *palpitations,* oppression, throbbing and pain in the back extending to the arms.

**Back**: Pain and stiffness near the nape of neck..Severe backache, throbbing, drives him out of the bed.

**Extremities**: Removes inflammatory products in veins of lower extremities. Weariness and lameness of lower limbs.

**Modalities**: *Worse* from slight exertion.

**Dose**: Third trituration.

---

# CALCAREA CARBONICA—OSTREARUM

(Carbonate of Lime) **Calc.**

This great Hahnemannian anti-psoric is a constitutional remedy *par excellence.* Its chief action is centered in the vegetative sphere, impaired nutrition being the keynote of its action, the glands, skin and bones being instrumental in the changes wrought. Increased local and general perspiration, swelling of glands, scrofulous and rachitic conditions generally offer numerous opportunities for the exhibition of *Calc.* Incipient phthisis (*Ars-i., Tub.*). It covers the tickling cough, fleeting chest pains, nausea, acidity and dislike for fat. Gets out of breath easily. *A jaded state, mental or physical, due to overwork. Abscesses in deep muscles; polypi and exostosis.* Pituitary and thyroid disfunction.

Raises blood coagulability (*Stront-c.*). Is a definite stimulant to the periosteum. Is a hemostatic and gives this power probably to the gelatin injections.

Easy relapses, interrupted convalescence. Scrofulous constitutions who take cold easily with increased mucoid secretions, children who grow fat, are large bellied with a large head, pale skin, chalky look, and the so-called leuco-phlegmatic temperament; affections caused by working in water. Great sensitiveness to cold; partial sweats.[1] Children crave eggs, eat dirt and other indigestible things; are prone to diarrhea. *Calc.* patient is fat, fair, flabby, perspiring, cold, damp and sour.

**Mind:** *Apprehensive;* worse towards the evening; *fears loss of reason, misfortune,* contagious diseases. *Forgetful,* confused, low spirited. Anxiety with palpitations. Obstinacy; slight mental effort produces a hot head. Averse to work or exertion.

**Head:** Sense of weight on top of the head. Headache, with cold hands and feet. Vertigo on ascending and on turning the head. Headache from overlifting, from mental exertion, with nausea. Head feels hot and heavy with a pale face. *Icy coldness in, and on the head,* especially right side. Open fontanelles; head enlarged (hydrocephalus); *much perspiration, wets the pillow.* Itching of the scalp. Scratches the head on waking.

**Eyes:** Sensitive to light (photophobia). Lachrymation in open air and early in the morning. *Spots and ulcers on the cornea.* Lachrymal ducts close on exposure to cold. Eyes fatigue easily (aesthenopia) . Far sighted (hypermetropia). Itching of lids, swollen, scurfy (blepharitis) . *Chronic dilatation of pupils.* Cataract. Dimness of vision, as if looking through mist. Lachrymal fistula; scrofulous ophthalmia.

1 Chiefly on chest and head (Clarke — Dictionary of Practical Materia Medica).

**Ears:** Throbbing; cracking in ears; stitches; pulsating pain as if something would press out. Deafness from working in water. Polypi which bleed easily. Scrofulous inflammation *with muco-purulent otorrhea and enlarged glands.* Perversion of hearing; hardness of hearing. Eruptions on and behind the ear (*Petr.*). Cracking noises in the ear. Sensitive to cold around the ears and neck.

**Nose:** Dry *nostrils, sore, ulcerated.* Stoppage of nose, with fetid, yellow discharge (ozena). Offensive odor in the nose. *Polypi;* swelling at the root of the nose. Epistaxis. Coryza. *Takes cold at every change of weather.* Catarrhal symptoms with hunger; coryza alternates with colic.

**Face:** Swelling of the upper lip. Pale, with deep seated eyes, surrounded by dark rings. Crusta lactea; itching, burning after washing. Submaxillary glands swollen. Goitre. Itching pimples in the whiskers. Pain from the right mental foramen, along the lower jaw, to the ear.

**Mouth:** Persistent *sour taste.* Mouth fills with sour water (waterbrash). Dryness of the tongue at night. Bleeding from gums. Difficult and delayed dentition. Toothache; excited by a current of air, anything cold or hot. Burning pain at the tip of the tongue; worse, from taking anything warm.

**Throat:** *Swelling of tonsils* and submaxillary glands; stitches on swallowing. Hawking up of mucus. Dysphagia. *Goitre.* Parotid fistula.

**Stomach:** Aversion to meat, boiled things; *craving for indigestible things—chalk, coal, pencils;* also for eggs, salt and sweets. Milk disagrees. *Frequent sour eructations; sour vomiting. Dislikes fat. Loss of appetite when overworked.* Heartburn and loud belching. Cramps in the stomach; worse, pressure, cold water. Ravenous hunger. Swelling over the pit of stomach, like a saucer turned bottom up. Repugnance to hot food. Pain in the epigastric region on touch. Thirst; longing for *cold* drinks. Aggravation while eating. Hyperchlorhydria (*Phos.*).

**Abdomen:** Sensitive to slightest pressure (peritonitis). Liver region painful when stooping. Cutting in the abdomen; swollen abdomen. Incarcerated flatulence. *Inguinal and mesenteric glands swollen* and painful. Cannot bear tight clothes around the waist. *Distention* with hardness. *Gall stone colic.* Increase of fat in the abdomen. Umbilical hernia. Trembling; weakness, as if sprained. Children are late in learning to walk.

**Rectum:** Crawling and constriction in rectum. Stools large and hard (*Bry.*); whitish, watery, *sour.* Prolapsus ani with burning, stinging hemorrhoids. Diarrhea of undigested food (lienteria), fetid, with a ravenous appetite. *Diarrhea in children.* Constipation; stool at first hard, then pasty, then liquid.

**Urinary:** Urine dark, brown, sour, fetid, abundant with white sediment, bloody (hematuria). Irritable bladder. Enuresis (use 30th, also *Tub. 1M.*).

**Male:** *Frequent emissions.* Increased desire. Semen emitted too soon. Coition followed by weakness and irritability.

**Female:** Before menses, headache, colic, chilliness and leucorrhea. Cutting pains in the uterus during menstruation (dysmenorrhea). Menses *too early, too profuse, too long* with vertigo, toothache and *cold, damp feet* (menorrhagia); the least excitement causes their return (metrorrhagia). Uterus easily displaced. Leucorrhea, *milky* (*Sep.*). Burning and itching of parts before and after menstruation; in little girls. Increased sexual desire (nymphomania); easy conception. Hot swelling of breasts. Breast tender and swollen before menses. Milk too abundant; disagreeable to the child. Deficient lactation, with distended breasts in lymphatic women. Increased sweat around the external genitals. Sterility with copious menses. Uterine polypi.

**Respiratory:** Tickling cough troublesome at night, dry and free expectoration in the morning; cough when playing the piano, or by eating. Persistent, irritating cough from arsenical wall paper (Clarke). Extreme dyspnea. *Painless hoarseness;* worse in the morning. Expectoration only during the day; thick, yellow, sour mucus. Bloody expectoration (hemoptysis, phthisis); with a sour sensation in the chest. *Suffocating spells;* tightness, burning and soreness in the chest; *worse going upstairs* or on the slightest ascent, must sit down. Sharp pains in the chest from before backwards. *Chest very sensitive to touch percussion or pressure.* Longing for fresh air. Scanty, salty expectoration (*Lyc.*).

**Heart:** Palpitations at night and after eating. Palpitations with sensation of coldness; restless oppression of the chest; after suppressed eruptions.

**Back:** Pain as if sprained; can scarcely rise; from overlifting. Pain between the shoulder blades, impeded breathing. Rheumatism in the lumbar region; weakness in the lumbosacral region. Curvature of dorsal vertebrae. Nape of neck stiff and rigid (cervical spondylosis). *Renal colic.*

**Extremities:** Rheumatoid pains, as after exposure to water. Sharp sticking pains as if parts were wrenched or sprained. *Cold, damp* feet; feels as if damp stockings were worn. Cold knees, cramps in calves. Sour foot sweat. Weakness of extremities. Swelling of joints, especially knee. Burning in soles. Sweat of hands. Arthritic nodosities. *Soles of feet raw.* Feet feel cold and dead at night. Old sprains. Tearing in the muscles.

**Sleep:** Ideas crowding in her mind prevent sleep. Horrid visions when opening the eyes. Starts at every noise; fears that she will go crazy. Drowsy in the early part of the evening. Wakes up frequently at night. *Same disagreeable idea always arouses from a light slumber.* Night terrors (*Kali-p.*). Dreams of the dead.

**Fever:** *Chills at 2* p. m. *begins internally in the stomach region. Fever* *with sweat.* Pulse full and frequent. Chills and heat. Partial sweats; *night sweats, especially on head,* neck and chest. Hectic fever. Heat at night during menstruation with restless sleep. *Sweat over the head in children, so much so that the pillow becomes wet.*

**Skin:** Unhealthy; readily ulcerating; flaccid. Small wounds do not heal readily. Glands swollen. Nettle rash; better in cold air. Warts on the face and hands. *Petechial eruptions.* Chilblains. Boils.

**Modalities:** *Worse,* from exertion, mental or physical; ascending; *cold* in every form; water, washing, moist air, wet weather; during full moon; standing. *Better,* dry climate and weather; lying on the painful side. Sneezing (relieves pain in the head and nape).

**Relationship:** Antidotes: *Camph., Ip., Nit-ac., Nux-v.*

Complementary: *Bell., Rhus-t., Lyc., Sil.*

*Calc.* is useful after *Sulphur* where the pupils remain dilated. When *Puls.* fails in school girls.

Incompatible: *Bry., Sulphur* should not be given *after Calc.*

Compare: *Aqua calcarea*—Lime water (½ teaspoonful in milk; as an injection for Oxyuris vermicularis), and *Calcarea causticum*—Slaked lime (pain in back and heels, jaws and malar bones; also symptoms of influenza). *Calcarea bromata* (removes inflammatory products from uterus; children of lax fibre, nervous and irritable, with gastric and cerebral irritation. *Tendency to brain diseases.* Insomnia and cerebral congestion. Give lx trituration). *Sulph.* (differs in being worse by heat, hot feet, etc.).

*Calcarea calcinata*—Calcinated oyster shell: A remedy for warts. Use 3d trituration. *Ova tosta*—Toasted eggshells (*backache and leucorrhea.* sensation as if the back was broken in two; tired feeling. Also effective in controlling suffering from cancer).

*Calcarea lactica* (anemia, hemophilia, urticaria, where the coagulability of blood is diminished; nervous headache with edema of eyelids, lips or hands; 15 grains, three times a day, but low potencies often equally effective).

*Calcarea lactica phosphorica* (5 grains, 3 times a day in cyclic vomiting and migraine).

*Calcarea muriatica*—*Calcium chloratum:* Rademacher's liquor (l part to 2 of distilled water, of which take 15 drops in half a cup of water, five times daily. Boils. *Prurigo capitis. Vomiting of all food and drink,* with gastric pain. Impetigo, glandular swellings, angioneurotic edema. Pleurisy with effusion. Eczema in infants).

*Calcarea picrica* (peri-follicular inflammation; a remedy of prime importance in *recurring of chronic boils,* particularly when located on parts thinly covered with muscle tissue, as on shin bones, coccyx, *auditory canal,* dry, scurfy accumulation and exfoliation of epithelial scales, etc., styes, phlyctenules. Use 3x trituration).

Compare also with *Calc.*, *Lyc.*, *Sil.*, *Puls.*, *Cham.*

**Dose:** Sixth trituration. Thirtieth and higher potencies. Should not be repeated too frequently in elderly people.

---

# CALCAREA FLUORICA—FLUOR SPAR.

(Fluoride of Lime) **Calc-f.**

A powerful tissue remedy for hard, stony glands, varicose and enlarged veins and malnutrition of bones. Hard knots in the female breast. Goitre. Congenital, hereditary syphilis. *Induration threatening to suppurate.* Many cases of cataract have undoubtedly been influenced favorably by it. Congenital syphilis manifesting itself as ulceration of mouth and throat, caries and necrosis with boring pains and heat in parts. Arteriosclerosis; threatened apoplexy. Tuberculosis. Used after surgery, tendency to adhesions is reduced.

**Mind:** Great depression; groundless fears of financial ruin.

**Head:** Creaking noise in the head. Blood tumors (aneurysms) in newborn infants. Hard excrescences on the scalp (exostosis). Ulcers on the scalp with callous, hard edges.

**Eyes:** Flickering and sparks before the eyes, spots on the cornea; conjunctivitis; cataract. *Strumous phlyctenular keratitis. Subcutaneous palpebral cysts.*

**Ears:** Calcareous deposits on tympanum; sclerosis of ossicula and petrous portion of temporal bone with deafness, ringing and roaring. *Chronic suppuration of the middle ear* (otorrhea).

**Nose:** Cold in the head; stuffy cold; dry coryza; ozena. Copious, offensive, thick, greenish, lumpy, yellow nasal catarrh. Atrophic rhinitis, especially when crusts are prominent.

**Face:** Hard swelling on the cheek, with pain or toothache, hard swelling on jaw bone.

**Mouth:** Gum-boil, with a hard swelling on the jaw. Cracked appearance of the tongue, with or without pain. Induration of the tongue, hardening after inflammation. Unnatural looseness of the teeth, with or without pain; teeth become loose in their sockets (scorbutic). Toothache, with pain if any food touches the tooth.

**Throat:** Follicular sore throat; plugs of mucus are continuously forming in the crypts of the tonsils (follicular tonsillitis). Pain and burning in the throat;

better by warm drinks; worse, cold drinks. Hypertrophy of Luschka's tonsil. Relaxed uvula, tickling referred to the larynx.

**Stomach:** Vomiting in infants. Vomiting of undigested food. Hiccough (*Caj., Sul-ac.*). Flatulence. Weakness and daintiness of appetite, nausea and distress after eating in young children who are overtaxed by studies. *Acute indigestion from fatigue* and brain fag; much flatulence.

**Rectum:** Diarrhea in gouty subjects. Anal fissure, an intensely sore crack near the lower end of the bowel. Itching in the anus as from pin-worms. Bleeding hemorrhoids. Internal or blind piles frequently, with pain in the back, generally far down the sacrum and constipation. Marked wind in the lower bowels. Worse, pregnancy.

**Male:** Hydrocele; indurations of the testicles.

**Respiratory:** Hoarseness. *Croup.* Cough with expectoration of tiny lumps of yellow mucus, with a tickling sensation and irritation on lying down. Spasmodic cough. *Calc-f.* removes fibroid deposits around the endocardium and restores normal endocardial structure (Eli G. Jones, M. D.).

**Circulatory System:** Chief remedy for vascular tumors with dilated blood vessels and for *varicose or enlarged veins.* Aneurism. Valvular disease. When the tuberculous toxins attack the heart and blood vessels.

**Back:** Chronic *lumbago;* aggravated when beginning to move and ameliorated on continuous motion. Osseous tumors (exostosis). *Rachitic enlargement of the femur in infants.* Pain in the lower part of back with burning.

**Extremities:** Ganglia or encysted tumors at the back of the wrist. Gouty enlargements in the joints of the fingers. Exostoses on fingers. Chronic synovitis of knee joint.

**Sleep:** Vivid dreams, with sense of impending danger. Unrefreshing sleep.

**Skin:** Marked whiteness of skin[1]. Scar tissue; adhesions after surgery. Chaps and cracks. Fissures or cracks on the palms of the hands or hard skin. Anal fissures. Suppurations with callous, hard edges. Whitlow. Indolent, fistulous ulcers secreting thick, yellow pus. Hard, elevated edges of the ulcer, surrounding skin purple and swollen. Knots, kernels, hardened glands in the female breast. *Swellings or indurated enlargements* having their seat in the fasciae and capsular ligaments of joints or in the tendons. *Indurations of stony hardness.*

**Modalities:** *Worse,* during rest, changes of weather. *Better,* heat, warm applications.

**Relationship:** Compare: *Con., Lap-a., Bar-m., Hecla, Rhus-t., Natrium cacodylicum* (tumors).

---

[1] Discoloration - white - spots (1001 Small Remedies, Edited by Dr. F. Schroyens).

*Calcarea sulphurata - stibiata* (acts as a hemostatic and absorptive in uterine myoma).

*Mangifera indica* (varicose veins).

**Dose:** Third to twelfth trituration. A 'chronic' remedy. Needs some time before manifesting its effects. Should not be repeated too frequently.

---

## CALCAREA IODATA

(Iodide of Lime) **Calc-i.**

It is in the treatment of scrofulous affections, especially enlarged glands, tonsils, etc., that this remedy has gained marked beneficial results. Thyroid enlargements (goitre) which occur around puberty. Flabby children, subject to colds. Secretions inclined to be profuse and yellow. Adenoids. Uterine fibroids. *Croup.*

**Head:** Headache while riding against cold wind. Light headed.

**Nose:** Catarrh; worse at the root of the nose; sneezing; very little sensation. Polypi of nose and ear.

**Throat:** Enlarged tonsils with filled, little crypts (follicular tonsillitis).

**Respiratory:** Chronic cough. Pain in the chest, difficulty in breathing after syphilis and mercurialization (Grauvogl). Hectic fever; green, purulent expectoration. Croup. *Pneumonia.*

**Skin:** *Indolent ulcers, accompanying varicose veins.* Easy perspiration. Copper colored and papulous eruptions, tinea, favus, crusta lactea, swelling of the glands (Hodgkin's disease), skin cracked, falling out of hair.

**Relationship:** Compare: *Agraphis nutans*—Bluebell (adenoids with enlarged tonsils). Here *Sul-i.* follows both *Agra.* and *Calc-i. Acon-l.* (swelling of glands, Hodgkin's disease).

Compare also: *Calc-f., Sil., Merc-i.*

**Dose:** Second and third trituration.

---

## CALCAREA PHOSPHORICA

(Phosphate of Lime) **Calc-p.**

One of the most important tissue remedies, and while it has many symptoms in common with *Calc.,* there are some differences and it has characteristic features of its own. It is especially indicated in tardy dentition and in problems incident to that period, bone diseases, non-union of fractured bones and anemias after acute diseases and chronic wasting diseases. *Anemic children who are peevish, flabby, have cold extremities and feeble digestion.* It has a special affinity where bones form sutures or symphyses and all its symptoms are worse from any change of weather. *Numbness and crawling* are characteristic sensations, tendency to perspiration and glandular enlargement are symptoms it shares with the carbonate. Scrophulosis, chlorosis and phthisis.

**Mind:** Peevish, forgetful; after grief and vexation (*Ign., Ph-ac.*). Always wants to go somewhere.

**Head:** Headache, *worse near the region of sutures, from change of weather*, in school children around the pubertal age. Fontanelles remain open too long. Cranial bones soft and thin. Defective hearing. Headache, with abdominal flatulence (sick headache). Head hot, with smarting in the roots of hair.

**Eyes:** Diffused opacity in the cornea following an abscess.

**Mouth:** Swollen tonsils; cannot open mouth without pain. Complaints during dentition; teeth develop slowly; rapid decay of teeth. *Adenoid growth.*

**Stomach:** Infant wants to nurse all the time and vomits easily. *Craving for bacon, ham, salted or smoked meats. Severe flatulence.* Great hunger with thirst, flatulence temporarily relieved by sour eructations. Heartburn. Easy vomiting in children.

**Abdomen:** Colicky pain in abdomen on attempting to eat. *Sunken and flabby.* Colic, soreness and burning around the navel.

**Stool:** Bleeding after hard stools. Diarrhea from juicy fruits or cider; during dentition. Green, slimy, *hot,* sputtering, undigested, *with fetid flatus* (cholera infantum). Fistula in ano, alternating with chest symptoms.

**Urinary:** Increased urine, with a sensation of weakness. Pain in the region of kidneys (Bright's disease), when lifting or blowing the nose..

**Female:** Menses too early, excessive and bright in girls (menorrhagia). If late, blood is dark; sometimes, first bright, then dark with *violent backache,* during lactation with sexual excitement. Nymphomania, with aching, pressing pains, or weakness in the uterine region (*Plat.*). After prolonged nursing. Leucorrhea, like *white of egg.* Worse morning. Child refuses breast; milk tastes salty. Prolapse in debilitated women.

**Respiratory:** Involuntary sighing. Chest sore. Suffocative cough; better lying down. Hoarseness. Pain through the lower left lung (phthisis - calcified nodes).

**Back:** Rheumatic pain from draught of air, with stiffness and dullness in the head. Soreness in the sacro-iliac symphyses as if broken (*Aesc.*).

**Extremities:** Stiffness and pain *with a cold, numb feeling,* worse change of weather. Crawling and coldness. Buttocks, back and limbs asleep. Pains in joints and bones[1]. Weary when going upstairs.

**Modalities:** *Worse,* exposure to damp, cold weather, melting snow. *Better, in summer;* warm, dry atmosphere.

**Relationship:** Complementary: *Ruta; Hep.*

Compare: *Calcarea hypophosporosa* (is preferred when it seems necessary to furnish the patient with liberal doses of phosphorus as a consequence of continuous abscesses which reduce the vitality. Give first and second decimal triturations. Loss of appetite, rapid debility, night sweats; acne pustulosa—pallor of skin, habitually *cold extremities.* Phthisis—diarrhea and cough; acute pains in the chest. Mesenteric tuberculosis. Bleeding from lungs; angina pectoris; asthma; affection of arteries. Veins stand out like whipcords. Attacks of pain occurring two hours after meals (relieved by a cup of milk or light food). *Cheiranthus cheiri* (effects of cutting wisdom teeth). *Calcarea renalis—Lapis renalis* (arthritic nodosities. Rigg's disease; lessens tendency to accumulation of tartar on teeth; gravel and renal calculi). *Conchiolinum*—Mater perlarum—Mother of pearl (osteitis; has a wide range of action in bone affections, especially when the growing ends are affected. *Petechiae). Sil., Psor., Sulph.*

**Dose:** First to third trituration. Higher potencies often more effective.

---

## CALCAREA SILICATA

(Silicate of Lime) **Calc-sil.**

A deep, long acting medicine for complaints which come on slowly and reach their final development after long periods. Hydrogenoid constitution (*Nat*-s.). Very sensitive to *cold. Patient is weak, emaciated, cold and chilly, but worse from being overheated;* generally sensitive. Atrophy in children.

**Mind:** Absent minded, irritable, irresolute, lacks self confidence. *Fearful.*

**Head:** Vertigo, head cold, especially the vertex; catarrh of the nose and posterior nares, discharge thick, yellow, hard crusts. Corneal exudation.

**Stomach:** Sensation of coldness, especially when empty. Sinking sensation in the pit. Great thirst. Flatulence and distention after eating. Vomiting and eructations.

**Female:** Uterus heavy, prolapsed. Leucorrhea, painful with irregular menses. Flow between periods (metrorrhagia).

**Respiratory:** Sensitive to cold air. Difficult respiration. Chronic irritation

[1] due to arthritic nodosities (1001 Small Remedies, Edited by Dr. F. Schroyens)

of air passages. Copious, yellowish green mucus. Cough with coldness, weakness, emaciation, sensitiveness and peevishness, worse from cold air. Pain in the chest walls.

**Skin:** Itching, burning, cold and blue, very sensitive. Pimples, comedones, wens. Psoric eruptions.

**Relationship:** Compare: *Ars., Tub., Bar-c., Iod.*

**Dose:** All potencies from the lowest to highest.

---

## CALCAREA SULPHURICA

(Sulphate of Lime, Plaster of Paris) **Calc-s.**

Eczema and torpid glandular swellings. Cystic tumors. Fibroids. Suppurative processes come within the range of this remedy, after pus has found a vent. *Mucus discharges are yellow, thick and lumpy.* Lupus vulgaris.

**Head:** Scald head of children, if there is purulent discharge, or yellow, purulent crusts (crusta lactea).

**Eyes:** *Inflammation of the eyes, with discharge of thick, yellow matter* (opthalmia with purulent discharge). Sees only half an object (hemiopia). Cornea smoky. Ophthalmia neonatorum.

**Ears:** Deafness, with discharge of matter from the middle ear, sometimes mixed with blood (otorrhea). Pimples around the ear.

**Nose:** Cold in the head with thick, *yellowish, purulent secretion,* frequently tinged with blood (sinusitis). One sided discharge from the nose. *Yellowish discharge* from the posterior nares (post-nasal drip). Edges of nostrils sore.

**Face:** *Pimples and pustules on the face.* Herpes.

**Mouth:** Inside of lips sore. Tongue flabby, resembling a layer of dried clay. Sour, soapy, acrid taste. Yellow coating at the base.

**Throat:** Last stage of ulcerated sore throat, with discharge of yellow matter. Suppurating stage of tonsillitis, when the abscess is discharging.

**Abdomen:** Pain in the liver region on the right side of pelvis, followed by weakness, nausea and pain in the stomach.

**Stool:** Purulent diarrhea mixed with blood (dysentery). Diarrhea after maple sugar and from change in weather. Pus like slimy discharge from the bowels. *Painful abscesses around the anus* in cases of fistula.

**Female:** Menses late, long lasting with headache, twitching and great weakness.

**Respiratory:** Cough with purulent, sanious sputa and hectic fever. Empyema, pus formation in the lungs or pleural cavities. Purulent, sanious expectoration. Catarrh, with thick, lumpy, whitish yellow or pus like secretion (pneumonia - third stage, emphysema).

**Extremities:** *Burning and itching in the soles.*

**Fever:** Hectic fever, caused by formation of pus. With cough and burning in soles.

**Skin:** Cuts, wounds, bruises, etc., unhealthy, discharging pus; they do not heal readily. Yellow, purulent crusts or discharges. Purulent exudations in or upon the skin. Skin affections with yellowish scabs. Many little matterless pimples under the hair, bleeding when scratched. Dry eczema in children.

**Relationship:** Compare: *Hep., Sil.*

**Dose:** Second and third trituration. The twelfth potency has been found effective in lupus.

---

## CALENDULA OFFICINALIS

(Marigold) **Calen.**

The most remarkable healing agent applied locally. Useful for open wounds, parts that will not heal, ulcers, etc. Promotes healthy granulations and rapid healing by first intention. Hemostatic after tooth extraction. Deafness. Catarrhal conditions. Neuroma. Constitutional tendency to erysipelas. Pain is excessive and out of proportion to the injury. *Great disposition to take cold, especially in damp weather.* Paralysis after apoplexy. In cancer, as an intercurrent remedy. Has a remarkable power to produce local exudations and helps to make acrid discharges healthy and free. Cold hands.

**Head:** Extremely nervous; easily frightened; tearing headache; weight on the brain. Pain in the right side of neck. Lacerated *scalp* wounds.

**Eyes:** Injuries to the eyes which tend to suppurate; after surgery; blenorrhea of lachrymal sac.

**Ears:** Deafness; worse in *damp* surroundings and with eczematous conditions. Hears best on a train, and distant sounds.

**Nose:** Coryza in one nostril; with profuse, green discharge.

**Face:** Submaxillary glands swollen, painful to touch.

**Stomach:** Hunger immediately after nursing. Bulimia. *Heartburn with horripilations.* Nausea in chest. Vomiting. Sinking sensation. Epigastric *distention.*

**Female:** *Warts on the os externum.* Menses suppressed, with cough. Chronic endocervicitis. Uterine hypertrophy, sensation of weight and fullness in the pelvis; stretching and dragging in the groins; pain on sudden movement. Os lower than natural (prolapse). Menorrhagia.

**Respiratory:** Cough, with green expectoration, hoarseness; with distention of the inguinal ring.

**Fever:** *Coldness, great sensitiveness to open air;* shuddering in the back, skin feels warm to touch. Heat in the evening.

**Skin:** *Yellow;* goose flesh. Promotes favorable cicatrization, with least amount of suppuration. Slough, proud flesh and raised edges. Superficial burns and scalds. Erysipelas (use topically).

**Modalities:** *Worse,* in damp, *heavy, cloudy* weather.

**Relationship:** Compare: *Ham., Hyper., Symph., Arn.*

Compare in deafness: *Ferr-pic., Kali-i., Calc., Mag-c., Graph.*

Antidote: *Chel., Rheum.*

Complementary: *Hep.*

**Dose:** Locally. *Aqueous Calen.* (Marigold) for all wounds, the greatest healing agent. Also as an injection in leucorrhea; internally, tincture to third potency. For burns, sores, fissures and abrasions, etc., use *Calendula cerate.*

---

## CALOTROPIS GIGANTEA

(Akanda) **Calo.**

Has been used with marked success in the treatment of *syphilis* following mercury; also in elephantiasis, leprosy and acute dysentery. Pneumonic phthisis. Tuberculosis.

Increases the circulation in the skin; has powerful effects as a sudorific. In secondary symptoms of syphilis, where mercury has been used but cannot be pushed safely any farther, it rapidly recruits the constitution, heals the ulcers and blotches from the skin and perfects the cure. *Primary anemia of syphilis. Heat in the stomach* is a good guiding symptom. *Obesity,* while flesh decreases, muscles become harder and firmer.

**Relationship:** Compare: *Merc., Kali-i., Berb-a., Sars.,* Ip.

**Dose:** Tincture, one to five drops, three times a day.

---

## CALTHA PALUSTRIS

(Cowslip) **Calth.**

Pain in the abdomen, vomiting, headache, singing noises in the ears, dysuria and diarrhea. Anasarca.

**Skin:** Pemphigus. Bullae are surrounded by a ring. Severe itching. Face very swollen, especially around the eyes. Itching eruptions on the thighs. Pustules. *Uterine cancer.*

**Dose:** Tincture.

---

# CAMPHORA OFFICINALIS

(Camphor) **Camph.**

Hahnemann says, "The action of this substance is very puzzling and difficult even in the healthy organism because its *primary action,* very frequently alternates and becomes intermixed with the vital reactions (after effects) of the organism. On this account, it is often difficult to determine what belongs to the vital reactions of the body and *what, to the alternating effects due to the primary action of Camphor."*

Pictures a state of collapse. *Icy coldness* of the whole body; sudden sinking of strength; pulse small and weak. After surgery, if temperature is subnormal, low blood pressure, 3 doses of *Camph.* 1x, at15 minute intervals. This condition is met with in cholera, and it is here that *Camph.* has achieved classical fame. *First stages of a cold with chilliness and sneezing.* Subsultus and extreme restlessness. Crackling in joints. Epileptiform convulsions. *Camph.* has a direct relationship to muscles and fascia. In local rheumatic affections during cold climates, it is necessary. Distention of veins. As a heart stimulant for emergency use, *Camph.* is the most satisfactory remedy. Drop doses on sugar, as often as every five minutes.

A characteristic of *Camph.* is that the patient *will not be covered,* not withstanding the icy coldness of the body. One of the main remedies in shock. *Pain better while thinking of it.* Very sensitive to cold and touch. Sequelae of measles. *Violent convulsions,* with wandering and hysterical excitement. Tetanic spasms. Scrofulous children and irritable, weak blondes are especially affected.

**Head:** Vertigo, tendency to unconsciousness, feeling as if he would die. Influenza; headache with catarrhal symptoms, sneezing, etc. Beating pain in the cerebellum. Cold sweat. *Nose cold and pinched.* Tongue cold, flabby, trembling. *Fleeting stitches in the temporal region and orbits.* Head sore. *Occipital throbbing, synchronous with the pulse.*

**Eyes:** Fixed, staring; pupils dilated. Sensation as if all objects were too bright and glittering (delusion).

**Nose:** Stopped; sneezing. Fluent coryza on sudden change of weather. Cold and pinched. *Persistent epistaxis,* especially with goose flesh state of skin.

**Face:** Pale, haggard, *anxious,* distorted; *bluish,* cold. Cold sweat.

**Stomach:** Pressive pain in the pit of the stomach. *Coldness,* followed by burning.

**Stool:** Blackish; involuntary. *Asiatic cholera* with cramps in the calves, coldness of the body, anguish, great weakness, *collapse,* tongue and mouth cold.

**Urinary:** Burning and *strangury* with tenesmus of the neck of the bladder. Retention with full bladder.

**Male:** Desire increased. Chordee. *Priapism.* Nocturnal emissions.

**Respiratory:** Precordial distress. Suffocative dyspnea. Asthma. Violent, dry, hacking cough. Palpitations. *Breath cold.* Suspended respiration.

**Extremities:** Rheumatic pain between shoulders. Difficulty in motion. Numbness, tingling and *coldness.* Cracking in joints. Cramps in calves. Icy cold feet, ache as if sprained.

**Sleep:** *Insomnia,* with cold limbs. Subsultus and extreme restlessness.

**Fever:** Pulse small, weak, slow. *Icy coldness of the whole body.* Cold perspiration. *Congestive chill. Tongue cold,* flabby, trembling.

**Skin:** *Cold,* pale, blue (cynosed), livid. Cannot bear to be covered (*Sec.*).

**Modalities:** *Worse,* motion, night, contact, cold air. *Better,* warmth.

**Relationship:** *Camph.* antidotes or modifies the action of nearly every vegetable medicine—tobacco, opium, worm medicines, etc. *Luffa actangula* (entire body ice cold with restlessness and anxiety; burning thirst). *Camphoricum acidum* (a prophylactic against catheter fever, cystitis; 15 grains, three times a day; also for prevention of night sweats).

Incompatible: *Kali-n.*

Complementary: *Canth.*

Antidotes: *Op., Nit-s-d., Phos.*

Compare: *Carb-v., Cupr., Ars., Verat.*

**Dose:** Tincture, in drop doses, repeated frequently, or smelling of spirits of *Camph.* Potencies are equally effective.

---

## CAMPHORA MONO-BROMATA

(Monobromide of Camphor) **Camph-mbr.**

*Nervous excitability* is the guiding condition. Suppression of milk. Nocturnal emissions. Painful erections. Paralysis agitans. Cholera infantum and infantile convulsions. Intensifies the action of quinine and renders it more permanent.

**Mind:** Directions appear reversed, i.e., north seems south, and east seems west. Hysteria; weeping and laughing alternately. Trance- like state.

**Dose:** Second trituration.

# CANCHALAGUA

(Erythraea Venusta, Centaury) **Canch.**

Used extensively as a fever remedy and bitter tonic (*Gentiana*), antimalarial and antiseptic. Of use in severe types of intermittent fever, in hot countries; also in influenza. Sore, as if bruised all over. Sensation of drops falling from and upon different spots.

**Head:** Congested. Scalp feels tight; head feels as if bound.

**Eyes:** Burning in the eyes.

**Ears:** Buzzing in the ears (tinnitus).

**Fever:** Chill all over; worse in bed, at night. Sensitive to cold trade winds on the Pacific coast. General sore and bruised feeling; nausea and retching.

**Skin:** Wrinkled like a washerwoman's. Scalp feels tight, as if drawn together by India rubber.

**Dose:** Tincture, in drop doses. Must be made from the fresh plant. Its medicinal properties are lost in the dry plant.

---

# CANNABIS INDICA

(Hashish) **Cann-i.**

Inhibits the higher faculties and stimulates the imagination to a remarkable degree without any marked stimulation of the lower or animal instinct. A condition of *intense exaltation* in which all perceptions and conceptions, all sensations and emotions are exaggerated to the utmost degree.

Subconscious or *dual nature state.* Apparently under the control of the second self, but, the original self, prevents the performance of acts which are under the domination of the second self. Apparently the two natures cannot act independently, one acting as a check upon the other. (Effects of one dram doses by Dr. Albert Schneider.)

The experimenter feels ever and anon that he is distinct from the subject of hashish dream and can think rationally.

Produces the most remarkable hallucinations and imaginations, *exaggeration in the duration of time and extent of space, being most characteristic.* Conception of time, space and place is gone. Extremely happy and contented, nothing troubles. Ideas crowd upon each other. Has a great soothing influence in many nervous disorders like epilepsy, mania, dementia, delirium tremens and irritable reflexes. Exophthalmic goitre. Catalepsy.

**Mind:** Excessive loquacity; *exuberance of spirits. Time seems too long; seconds seem like ages; a few rods, an immense distance.* Constantly theorizing.

Anxious depression; constant fear of becoming insane. Mania, must move constantly. *Very forgetful; cannot finish a sentence.* Is lost in delicious thoughts. *Uncontrollable laughter.* Delirium tremens. Clairvoyance. Emotional excitement; rapid change of mood. Cannot realize her identity, chronic vertigo as if floating in air.

**Head:** Feels *as if the top of the head was opening and shutting and as if calvarium was being lifted.* Shocks through the brain (*Aloe, Coca*). Uremic headache. Throbbing and weight on the occiput. Headache with flatulence. *Involuntary shaking of head* (epilepsy, delirium tremens). Migraine, attack preceded by unusual excitement and loquacity.

**Eyes:** Fixed. Letters run together when reading. Clairvoyance. Spectral illusions without terror.

**Ears:** Throbbing, buzzing, and ringing (tinnitus). Noises like boiling water. Extreme sensitiveness to noise.

**Face:** Expression drowsy and stupid. Lips glued together. *Grinding of teeth in sleep.* Mouth and lips dry. Saliva thick, frothy, and sticky.

**Stomach:** Increased appetite. Pain at the cardiac orifice; pressure. Distention. Pyloric spasm. Sensation of tension in the abdominal vessels—feels distended, as if bursting

**Rectum:** Sensation in anus as if sitting on a ball.

**Urinary:** Urine loaded with slimy mucus. Must strain; *dribbling;* has to wait for some time before the urine flows. Stitches and burning in the urethra. Dull pain in the region of the right kidney (nephritis).

**Male:** After sexual intercourse, *backache.* Oozing of white, glairy mucus from glans (gonorrhea). Satyriasis. Prolonged thrill. Chordee. Sensation of swelling in the perineum or near the anus, as if sitting on a ball.

**Female:** Menses *profuse,* dark, painful, without clots. Backache during menses. Uterine colic, with great nervous agitation and sleeplessness. Sterility (*Borx.*). Dysmenorrhea with sexual desire (nymphomania).

**Respiratory:** Humid asthma. Chest oppressed with deep, labored breathing.

**Heart:** Palpitations wake him up. Piercing pain, with great oppression. *Pulse very slow (Dig., Kalm., Apoc.).*

**Extremities:** *Pain across the shoulders and spine; must stoop; cannot walk erect.* Thrilling through arms, hands and from knees down. *Paralysis of the lower extremities.* Pain in soles and calves; sharp pains in the knees and ankles; *very exhausted after a short walk.*

**Sleep:** Very sleepy, but unable to do so. Obstinate and intractable forms of insomnia. Catalepsy. Dreams of dead bodies; prophetic. Nightmares.

**Modalities:** *Worse,* morning; from coffee, liquor and tobacco; lying on the right side. *Better* from fresh air, cold water, rest.

**Relationship:** *Bell., Hyos., Stram., Lach., Agar., Anh.* (time sense disordered; time periods enormously overestimated, thus, minutes seem hours, etc.).

**Dose:** Tincture and low attenuations.

---

# CANNABIS SATIVA

(Hemp) **Cann-s.**

Seems to affect the urinary, sexual and respiratory organs specially. It has characteristic sensations of, dripping water. Great fatigue, as if from over exertion; weary after meals. Choking on swallowing; things go down the wrong way. Stuttering. Confusion of thought and speech. Wavering speech, hasty, incoherent.

**Head:** Lectophobia. Vertigo; sensation of water dropping on the head. Pressure at the root of nose.

**Eyes:** *Corneal opacity* (leucoma). Cataract from nervous disturbances, abuse of alcohol and tobacco; patient feels as if approaching blindness (amaurosis). Misty sight (cataract). Pressure from the back of the eyes, forward. Gonorrheal ophthalmia. Eyeballs ache. Scrofulous eye problems (*Sulph., Calc.*).

**Urinary:** Retained, with obstinate constipation. Painful urging. Urine in split stream. Stitches in the urethra. Inflamed sensation, with soreness to touch (urethritis). *Burning while micturating, extending to the bladder.* Urine scalding, with spasmodic closure of sphincter. Gonorrhea, acute stage; urethra very sensitive. Walks with legs apart. Dragging in the testicles. Zigzag pain along the urethra. Sexual over excitement. Urethral caruncle (*Eucal.*), phimosis. Stoppage of urethra by mucus and pus.

**Female:** Amenorrhea when physical powers have been overtaxed with constipation.

**Respiratory:** Oppressed breathing and palpitation; *must stand up.* Weight on chest; rattling, wheezing, breathing. Cough, with green viscid, bloody expectoration.

**Heart:** Sensation as if drops were falling from the heart. Painful strokes and tension with palpitations. Pericarditis.

**Extremities:** Contraction of fingers after a sprain. Dislocation of patella on going upstairs. Feet feel heavy on going upstairs. Paralytic tearing pains. Affections in the ball of the foot and in the under part of toes.

**Sleep:** Frightful dreams. More tired in the morning. Sleepy during the day.

**Modalities:** *Worse,* lying down; going upstairs.

**Relationship:** Antidotes: *Camph., Lemon juice.*

Compare: *Hedysarum ildefonsianum*—Brazilian Burdock (gonorrhea and inflammation of penis; balanitis); *Canth., Apis, Cop., Thuj., Kali-n.*

**Dose:** Tincture to third attenuation. In stuttering, the 30th.

---

# CANTHARIS VESICATORIA

(Spanish Fly) **Canth.**

This powerful drug produces a furious disturbance in the animal economy, attacking the urinary and sexual organs perverting their function, setting up violent inflammations and causing a frenzied delirium, simulating symptoms of hydrophobia (*Anag.*). Puerperal convulsions. Produces a very violent inflammation of the entire gastro-intestinal canal, especially the lower bowel. Oversensitiveness of all parts. Irritation. *Raw, burning pains.* Hemorrhages. *Intolerable, constant urging to micturate* is very characteristic. Gastric, hepatic and abdominal complaints *that are aggravated by drinking coffee.* Gastric derangements of pregnancy. *Dysuria,* with other complaints. Increases secretion of mucous membranes, tenacious mucus. The inflammations *Canth.* produces (bladder, kidneys, ovaries, meninges, pleuritic and pericardial membranes) are usually associated with bladder irritation.

**Mind:** Furious delirium. Anxious restlessness, ending in rage. Crying, barking; worse touching the larynx or drinking water. Constantly attempts to do something, but accomplishes nothing. *Acute mania,* generally of a sexual type; amorous frenzy; fiery sexual desire (erotomania). Paroxysms of rage, crying, barking. *Sudden* loss of consciousness with a red face.

**Head:** Burning sensation in the brain (meningitis). Sensation as if boiling water is in the brain. Vertigo; worse, open air.

**Eyes:** Yellow vision (*Santin.*). *Fiery, sparkling, staring look.* Burning in the eyes (conjunctivitis).

**Ears:** Sensation as if wind was coming out from the ear; or hot air. Bones around the ear painful (*Caps.*).

**Face:** Pale, wretched, death-like appearance. Itching vesicles on the face, burning when touched. Erysipelas on the face with burning, biting heat with urinary symptoms. Hot and red.

**Throat:** Tongue covered with vesicles; deeply furred; edges red. *Burning in the mouth, pharynx, and throat;* vesicles in the mouth (stomatitis). *Great difficulty in swallowing liquids.* Very *tenacious* mucus (*Kali-bi.*). Violent spasms reproduced on touching the larynx. Inflammation of the throat; as if on fire. Constriction; aphthous ulceration (*Hydrin-m., Nit-ac.*). Scalding sensation. Burnt, after taking very hot food.

**Stomach:** Burning sensation in the esophagus and stomach (*Carb-v.*). Disgust for everything—drink, food, tobacco. Burning thirst with aversion to all fluids. Very sensitive, *violent burning.* Vomiting of blood streaked membrane[1] and violent retching. *Aggravation from drinking coffee;* drinking the smallest quantity increases pain in the bladder and is vomited. Thirst unquenchable.

**Stool:** *Shivering with burning.* Dysentery; mucoid stools, *like scrapings of intestines.* Bloody, with *burning* and *tenesmus, shuddering after stool.*

**Urinary:** *Intolerable urging* and tenesmus. Nephritis with hematuria. Violent paroxysms with cutting and burning in the entire renal region with painful urging to micturate; bloody urine passes in *drops.* Intolerable tenesmus; cutting before, during, and after urine. *Urine scalds and is passed drop by drop. Constant desire to micturate.* Membranous scales looking like bran in water. Urine jelly-like, shreddy.

**Male:** *Strong desire;* painful erections. Pain in glans (balanitis) (*Prun., Pareir.*). Priapism in gonorrhea.

**Female:** Retained placenta (*Sep.*), with dysuria. Expels moles, dead fetuses, membranes, etc. *Nymphomania* (*Plat., Hyos., Lach., Stram.*). Puerperal metritis with cystitis. Menses too early and too profuse (menorrhagia); black swelling of vulva with irritation. Constant discharge from the uterus; worse false step. Burning pain in ovaries; extremely sensitive (ovarian cysts). Pain in os coccyx, lancinating and tearing.

**Respiratory:** Pleurisy, as soon as effusion has taken place, *with exudation.* Intense dyspnea; palpitations; frequent dry cough. *Tendency to syncope.* Short, hacking cough, blood streaked *tenacious* mucus (hemoptysis). Burning pains. Voice low; weak feeling. Stitches in the chest (*Bry., Kali-c., Squil.*).

**Heart:** Palpitation; pulse feeble, irregular; tendency to syncope. *Pericarditis with effusion.*

**Back:** Pain in the loins, with an incessant desire to micturate.

**Extremities:** Tearing in limbs. Ulcerative pain in soles; cannot step.

**Fever:** Cold hands and feet; cold sweat. Soles burn. Chill, as if water was poured over him.

**Skin:** Dermatitis venenata with bleb formation. Secondary eczema around scrotum and genitals, following excessive perspiration. Tendency to gangrene. Eruptions with mealy scales (bran-like scales). *Vesicular eruptions* with burning and itching. Sunburn. *Burns, scalds* with rawness and smarting, relieved by cold applications, followed by undue inflammation. *Erysipelas, of* vesicular type with great restlessness. Burning in soles of feet at night.

---

[1] Membranous flakes (a morbid secretion of the alimentary canal) a cylinderical mass, apparently the inner membrane of the gullet. Vomiting of bloody mucus also (Handbook of Materia Medica by T.F. Allen).

**Modalities:** *Worse,* from touch, or approach, micturating, drinking cold water or coffee. *Better,* rubbing.

**Relationship:** Antidotes: *Acon., Camph., Puls.*

Compare: *Cantharidinum* (glomerular nephritis). The immediate pharmacological action of *Cantharidinum* is irritability of the capillaries, rendering the passage of nutritive fluids through them less difficult. This is most marked in the capillaries of the kidneys. The increase of blood sugar coincident with glomerular nephritis appears to be a valuable observation. *Versicaria communis* (urinary and kidney remedy. Smarting, burning sensation along the urethra and in the bladder with a frequent desire to void urine, often with strangury. Cystitis, irritable bladder. Tincture, 5-10 drop doses). *Fuschinum* coloring substance used in adulteration of wine (cortical nephritis with albuminuria, 6th-30th potency. Redness of ears, mouth, swollen gums; deep, red urine; red, profuse diarrhea, with severe abdominal pains). *Androsace lactea* (urinary problems, diuretic; dropsy). *Apis, Ars., Merc*-c.

Complementary: *Camph.*

**Dose:** Sixth to thirtieth potency. Bears repeated doses well. Locally, in burns and eczema, lx and 2x, in water, or as cerate.

---

# CAPSICUM ANNUUM

(Cayenne Pepper) **Caps.**

Seems to especially suit people of lax fibre, weak; diminished vital heat. A relaxed, plethoric, sluggish, cold remedy. Not much of a reactive force. Such people are fat, indolent, opposed to physical exertion, averse to go outside their routine and, get homesick easily. *General uncleanliness of the body.* Abstainers from accustomed alcoholism. It affects the mucous membranes, producing a sensation of *constriction.* Inflammation of the petrous bone. Burning pains and general chilliness. Older people who have exhausted their vitality, especially by mental work, and poor living; blear eyed appearance; who do not react. Fear of the slightest draught. Marked tendency to suppuration, in every inflammatory process. Prostration and feeble digestion in alcoholics. Myalgia, aching and jerking of muscles.

**Mind:** Excessive peevishness. *Homesickness,* with sleeplessness and a disposition to suicide. Wants to be lelt alone. Peppery disposition. *Delirium tremens.*

**Head:** Bursting headache (meningitis); worse, coughing. Hot face. Red cheeks. Face red, though cold (*Asaf.*).

**Ears:** Burning and stinging in ears. *Swelling and pain behind the ears.*

*Inflammation of the mastoid. Tenderness over the petrous bone;* extremely sore and tender to touch (caries) (*Onos.*). Otorrhea and mastoid disease before suppuration.

**Mouth:** Herpes labialis (apply one drop of the mother tincture). *Stomatitis.* Disagreeable smell from the mouth. *Fetid odor from mouth* (halitosis).

**Throat:** *Hot feeling in the fauces.* Subacute inflammation of the eustachian tube with great pain. *Pain and dryness in the throat* extending to the ears. *Sore throat in smokers and drinkers.* Smarting in the throat; constriction. Burning constriction worse between acts of deglutition. Inflamed uvula and palate; swollen and relaxed.

**Stomach:** Burning at the tip of the tongue. Atonic dyspepsia. Much flatulence, especially in debilitated subjects. Intense craving for stimulants. Vomiting, sinking at the pit of the stomach. *Marked thirst; but drinking causes shuddering.*

**Stool:** *Bloody mucus with burning and tenesmus* (dysentery); drawing pains in the back after stool. *Thirsty after stool with shivering. Bleeding piles,* with soreness in the anus. Stinging pain during stool.

**Urinary:** Strangury, frequent, almost ineffectual urging. *Burning in the orifice.* Comes first in drops, then in spurts; neck of bladder spasmodically contracted. Ectropion of the meatus.

**Male:** *Coldness of the scrotum* with impotency, atrophied testicles, loss of sensibility in testicles with softening and dwindling. Gonorrhea, with chordee, excessive burning, pain in prostate.

**Female:** Climacteric disturbances with burning on the tip of the tongue (*Lath.*). Uterine hemorrhage near menopause, with nausea. Sticking sensation in the left ovarian region.

**Respiratory:** *Constriction* of the chest; arrests breathing. Hoarseness. Pain at the apex of the heart or in the rib region, worse touch. Dry, hacking cough, expelling an offensive breath from the lungs. Dyspnea. Sensation as if the chest and head would fly into pieces. Explosive cough. Threatened gangrene of lungs. *Pain in distant parts on coughing*—bladder, legs, ears, etc.

**Extremities:** Pain from hips to feet. Sciatica, worse bending backward; *Worse, coughing.* Tensive pain in the knee.

**Fever:** Coldness, with ill humor. *Shivering after drinking.* Chills begin in the back; better, heat. Must have some hot things on the back. Thirst before chill.

**Modalities:** *Better,* while eating, from heat. *Worse,* open air, uncovering, draughts.

**Relationship:** Antidote: *Cina, Calad.*

Compare: *Puls., Lyc., Bell., Centaurea tagana* (surging of blood; homesickness; intermittent fever).

**Dose:** Third to sixth attenuation. In delirium tremens, dram doses of tincture in milk or tincture of orange peel.

---

## CARBO ANIMALIS

(Animal Charcoal) **Carb-an.**

Seems to be especially adapted to scrofulous and venous constitutions, old people, and after debilitating diseases, with feeble circulation and lowered vitality. *Glands are indurated,* veins distended (varices), skin blue. *Stitch remaining after pleurisy.* Easily strained from lifting. Weakness in nursing women. Ulceration and decomposition. All its secretions are offensive. Causes local congestions *without* heat.

**Mind:** Desire to be alone, sad and reflective, *avoids conversation.* Anxiety at night with orgasm of blood.

**Head:** Headache, as if head had been blown to pieces. Rush of blood with confusion. Sensation as if something lay above the eyes so that she cannot look up. Bluish cheeks and lips (cynosis). Vertigo followed by epistaxis. Nose swollen, tip bluish, small tumor on it. Hearing confused; *cannot tell direction of sound.*

**Stomach:** Eating tires the patient. Weak, empty feeling in the stomach. Burning and gripping. *Weak digestion. Flatulence.* Ptomaine poisoning. Repugnance to fatty food. Sour water from the mouth. Pyrosis.

**Female:** Nausea of pregnancy; worse at night. Lochia offensive (*Kreos., Rhus-t., Sec.*). Menses too early, frequent, long lasting (menorrhagia), *followed by great exhaustion,* so weak, can hardly speak (*Cocc.*), flow only in the morning (*Borx., Sep.*). Burning in the vagina and labia. Darting in the breast; *painful indurations* in the breast, especially right. Cancer of uterus, burning pain extending down the thighs.

**Respiratory:** Pleurisy, like typhoid in character, and remaining stitch. Ulceration of lungs, with a feeling of coldness in the chest. Cough with discharge of greenish pus.

**Extremities:** Pain in the coccyx; burns when touched. Ankles turn easily. Straining and over lifting produce great debility. Joints weak. Easy dislocation. Pain in the hip joints at night. *Night sweat,* fetid and profuse. Wrist pain.

**Skin:** Spongy ulcers, copper colored eruption. Acne rosacea. Chilblains, worse in the evening, in bed and from cold. Verruca on hands and face of old people, with a bluish color of extremities. *Glands indurated,* swollen, painful in the neck, axillae, groin, mammae; pains lancinating, cutting, burning (*Con., Merc-i-f.*). Burning, rawness and fissures; moisture. *Bubo.*

**Modalities:** *Worse,* after shaving, loss of animal fluids.

**Relationship:** In the Carbon group, all have putrid discharges and exhalations. All act on the skin, causing intertrigo and excoriations. Glandular enlargements and catarrhal states, flatulence and asphyxiation.

*Carboneum tetrachloridum* is said to cause fatty liver (*Phos., Ars., Chlf.*). Paralysis of interosseus muscles of feet and hands. Wonderful clinical results in the treatment of hookworm disease. See *Thymolum.*

Complementary: *Calc-p.*

Antidotes: *Ars., Nux-v.*

Compare: *Bad., Sep., Sulph., Plb-i.*

**Dose:** Third to thirtieth potency. The third trituration for insufflation in aural polypi.

---

# CARBO VEGETABILIS

(Vegetable Charcoal) **Carb-v.**

Disintegration and *imperfect oxidation* is the keynote of this remedy. The typical *Carb-v.* patient is sluggish, fat, lazy and has a tendency to chronicity in his complaints. Blood seems to stagnate in the capillaries causing blueness, coldness, and ecchymosis. Body becomes blue, icy cold (cynosis). Bacteria find a rich soil in the nearly lifeless blood stream, sepsis and typhoidal state ensues.

A lowered vital power from loss of fluids; after drugging; after other diseases; in old people with venous congestions; states of collapse in cholera, typhoid; these are some of the conditions offering special inducements to the action of *Carb-v*. The patient may be almost lifeless, but the head is hot; coldness, breath cool, pulse imperceptible, oppressed and a quickened respiration. Must have air, must be fanned hard, must have all the windows open. This is the typical state of *Carb-v*. The patient faints easily, is worn out, and must have fresh air. Hemorrhage from any mucous surface. Very debilitated. Patient seems to be too weak to hold out. *People who have never fully recovered from the effects of some previous illness.* Sense of weight, on the head (occiput), eyes and eyelids, before the ears, in the stomach, and elsewhere in the body; putrid (septic) condition of all its affections, coupled with a burning sensation. General venous stasis, bluish skin and cold limbs.

**Mind:** Aversion to darkness. Fear of ghosts. Sudden loss of memory.

**Head:** *Aches from any over indulgence.* Hair feels sore, *falls off easily;* scalp itches when getting warm in bed. Hat pressed upon the head like a heavy weight. Head feels heavy, constricted. Vertigo with nausea and tinnitus. Pimples on the forehead and face.

**Eyes:** Vision of black floating spots. Asthenopia. Burning in the eyes. Muscles painful.

**Ears:** Otorrhea following exanthematous diseases. Ears dry. Malformation of cerumen with exfoliation of dermoid layer of meatus.

**Nose:** *Epistaxis, daily attacks after straining with a pale face.* Tip of the nose red and scabby, itching around nostrils. Varicose veins on the nose. Eruptions in the corner of alae nasi. Coryza with cough, especially in moist, warm weather. Ineffectual efforts to sneeze.

**Face:** Puffy, cyanotic. Pale, hippocratic, cold with cold sweat; blue (*Cupr.*, *Op.*). Mottled cheeks and red nose.

**Mouth:** Tongue coated white or yellowish-brown, *covered with aphthae.* Teeth very sensitive when chewing; gums retracted and bleed easily (scurvy). Blood oozing from gums when cleaning teeth. Pyorrhea.

**Stomach:** *Eructations, heaviness, fullness, and sleepiness;* tense from flatulence, with pain; worse lying down. Eructations after eating and drinking. Temporary relief from belching. Rancid, sour, or putrid eructations. Waterbrash, asthmatic breathing from flatulence. Nausea in the morning. Burning in the stomach, extending to the back, extends along the spine. *Contractive pains extending to the chest, with distention of abdomen.* Faint, all gone feeling in the stomach, not relieved by eating. Crampy pains, forcing the patient to bend double. Distress comes on half an hour after eating. Sensitiveness of the epigastric region. *Digestion slow; food putrefies* before it digests. Gastralgia in nursing women with excessive flatulence, sour, rancid belching. Aversion to milk, meat, and *fatty things. The simplest food distresses.* Epigastric region very sensitive.

**Abdomen:** Pain as if from lifting a weight; colic from riding in a carriage; excessive discharge of fetid flatus. Cannot bear tight clothing around the waist and abdomen. Ailments accompanying intestinal fistulae. *Abdomen greatly distended;* better, passing wind. *Flatulent colic.* Pain in the liver.

**Rectum:** Flatus hot, moist, offensive. Itching, gnawing and burning in the rectum. *Acrid, corrosive moisture from rectum.* A musty, glutinous moisture exudes. Soreness, itching moisture in the perineum at night. Discharge of blood from the rectum. Burning in the anus, burning varices (*Mur-ac.*). Painful diarrhea in old people. Frequent, involuntary, cadaverous smelling stools, followed by burning. White hemorrhoids; excoriation of the anus. *Bluish,* burning piles; *pain* after stool.

**Male:** Discharge of prostatic fluid with stool. Itching and moisture on the thigh, near the scrotum.

**Female:** Premature and copious menses; pale blood. Vulva swollen; aphthae; varices on the pudenda. Leucorrhea before menses, thick, greenish, milky, excoriating (*Kreos.*). During menstruation, burning in hands and soles.

**Respiratory:** Cough with itching in the larynx; spasmodic with gagging and vomiting of mucus. Whooping cough, especially in the beginning stage. Deep, rough voice, failing on the slightest exertion. *Hoarseness; worse, evenings,* talking; evening oppression of breathing, sore and raw chest. Wheezing and rattling of mucus in the chest. Occasional spells of long coughing attacks. *Cough with burning in the chest;* worse in the evening, in the open air, after eating and talking. Spasmodic cough, bluish face, offensive expectoration, neglected pneumonia. Breath cold; *must be fanned.* Hemorrhage from lungs. *Asthma in the aged with blue skin* (cynosis).

**Extremities:** Heavy, stiff; feel paralyzed; *limbs, go to sleep;* want of muscular energy; joints weak. Pain in shins. Cramps in soles; feet numb and sweaty. *Cold, from knees down.* Toes, red, swollen (chilblains). Burning pain in bones and limbs.

**Fever:** Coldness, with thirst. Chill begins in the forearm. Burning in various places. Perspiration on eating. Hectic fever, exhausting sweats.

**Skin:** *Blue, cold, ecchymosed.* Marbled with venous over- distention. Itching; worse in the evening, when warm in bed. Moist skin; *hot perspiration;* senile gangrene beginning in toes; bed sores; bleed easily. Falling of hair from a general weakened condition. Indolent ulcers, burning pain. Ichorous, offensive discharge; tendency to gangrene at the margins. Purpura. *Varicose ulcers,* carbuncles (*Ars., Anthraci.*).

**Modalities:** *Worse,* evening; night and open air; cold; from fat food, butter, coffee, milk, warm damp weather; *wine. Better,* from eructation, *from fanning,* cold.

**Relationship:** Antidotes: *Spiritus nitri dulcis; Camph., Ambr., Ars.*

Compare: *Carboneum*—Lampblack (spasms commencing in the tongue, extending down the trachea and extremities. Tingling sensation). *Lyc., Ars., Chin.*

Complementary: *Kali-c., Dros.*

**Dose:** First to third trituration in stomach disorders. Thirtieth potency and higher in chronic conditions and in collapse.

---

## CARBOLICUM ACIDUM

(Phenol, Carbolic Acid) **Carb-ac.**

*Carbolicum acidum* is a powerful irritant and anesthetic. A languid, foul, painless destructive remedy. Stupor, paralysis of sensation and motion, feeble pulse and depressed breathing, death due to paralysis of respiratory centres. Acts primarily on the central nervous system. *Increased olfactory sensibility.*

Produces mental and physical languor, disinclination to study with headache, sensation of a band around the head. Very marked *acuteness of smell* is a strong guiding symptom. Stomach symptoms are also important. Pains are terrible; come and go suddenly. Physical exertion brings on abscesses somewhere. Putrid discharges (*Bapt.*). Scarlet fever, with marked tendency to destruction of tissues internally and a fetid odor. Spasmodic cough. Arthritis (see Dose).

**Head:** Disinclined to mental work. Tight feeling, as if compressed by a rubber band (hydrocephalus) (*Gels., Berb-a.*). Orbital neuralgia over the right eye. Headache, better by green tea; while smoking.

**Nose:** *Smell, very acute.* Putrid discharge. Ozena with fetor and ulceration. Influenza and resulting debility.

**Throat:** Ulcerated patches on the inside of lips and cheeks (stomatitis). *Burning in the mouth, extending to the* stomach. Fauces red, and covered with exudation. Uvula white and shrivelled. *Putrid discharge.* Almost impossible to swallow. *Diphtheria, fetid breath, regurgitation* on swallowing liquids, but little pain (*Bapt.*). Face dusky red; white around the mouth and nose. Rapid sinking of vital forces.

**Stomach:** Appetite lost. *Desire for stimulants and tobacco.* Constant belching, nausea, *vomiting,* dark olive green. Heat rises up the esophagus. Flatulent distention of the stomach and abdomen. Painful flatulence often marked in one part of the bowel. *Fermentative dyspepsia* with bad taste and breath.

**Stool:** Constipation with *very offensive breath* (halitosis). Bloody, like scrapings of intestines. Great tenesmus. Diarrhea; stools thin, black, putrid.

**Urinary:** Almost black. Diabetes. Irritable bladder in old men with frequent micturition at night, probably prostatic in nature (use 1x).

**Female:** Discharges always offensive (*Nit-ac., Nux-v., Sep.*). Pustules around the vulva containing bloody pus. Agonizing backache across the loins, dragging down the thighs. Pain in the left ovary; worse walking in open air. Cervical erosions, fetid, acrid discharge. Leucorrhea in children (*Cann-s., Merc., Puls., Sep.*). Puerperal fever with offensive discharge. Irritating leucorrhea, causing itching and burning (*Kreos.*).

**Extremities:** Cramps in the fore part of the leg, close to the tibia *during walking.* Gnawing pains in the shin bones. Arthritis.

**Skin:** Itching vesicles with burning pain. Burns tend to ulcerate.

**Relationship:** Compare: *Chrysarobinum* (locally *in ringworm* of the scalp, 5-10 percent in glycerine and alcohol. Equal parts). *Ars., Kreos., Carb-v., Guano australis* (violent headache as if from a band around the head. Itching in the nostrils, back, thighs, genitals. Symptoms like hay fever).

Antidote: *Alcohol, Vinegar, Chalk, Iod.* Glauber's salt in watery solution. Incompatible: *Glycerine* and *vegetable oils.*

**Dose:** Third to thirtieth potency. Phenol in arthritis, according to Goodno. Must be absolutely pure. Crystals solution (25%) in equal parts of water and glycerine, dose 20 minims well diluted 3 times daily (Bartlett).

---

## CARBONEUM HYDROGENISATUM

(Carburetted Hydrogen) **Carbn-h.**

Symptoms resemble an apopletic attack. Spasm as in lockjaw (tetnus). Trismus. Involuntary stools and urine.

**Mind:** Stupefaction. Extraordinary sensation of contentment. All thoughts appear in a moment, as if seen in an inner mirror.

**Eyes:** Lids half closed (ptosis). Oscillation of eyeballs (nystagmus). Pupils insensible to light (apoplexy, convulsions).

---

## CARBONEUM OXYGENISATUM

(Carbonous Oxide) **Carbn-o.**

Herpes zoster, pemphigus and trismus are produced by this drug. Coldness, *sleepiness,* loss of consciousness are marked. Vertigo.

**Head:** Cerebral congestion; hallucinations of vision, hearing and touch. Inclination to turn in a circle. *Jaws firmly clenched.* Trismus. Heaviness of the head. Sticking pain in the temples. Roaring in ears.

**Eyes:** Ocular paralysis, hemianopsia, disturbed pupilary reaction, optic neuritis and atrophy, subconjunctival and retinal hemorrhages.

**Sleep:** Deep. *Prolonged;* sleepiness for several days.

**Skin:** Anesthesia; vesication along course of nerves; *herpes zoster;* pemphigus with large and small vesicles. Hand icy cold.

**Dose:** First attenuation.

---

## CARBONEUM SULPHURATUM

(Alcohol Sulphuris, Bisulphide of Carbon) **Carbn-s.**

This drug has a deep and disorganizing action. Has a wide range of action judging from the symptomatology. Very useful in patients broken down by abuse of alcohol. Sensitive patients, worse cold, wasted muscles and skin. Mucous membranes anesthetic. Special affinity for eyes. Chronic rheumatism, sensitive and cold. Lack of vital heat. Diarrhea every four to six weeks. Paralysis with intense congestion of nerve centres. Tabes. Sensory difficulties in limbs.

*Impotence,* sciatica come within the therapeutic sphere of this remedy. Chronic plumbism. *Diminished sensibility* of arms, hands and feet. Peripheral neuritis.

**Mind:** Irritable, anxious, intolerant; *stupor.* Sluggishness of the mind. Hallucinations of sight and hearing. Changeable mood. Dementia alternating with excitement.

**Head:** Headache and dizziness. Aches, as if wearing a tight cap. Ears feel obstructed. *Noises in the head.* Ulceration of the lips, anesthesia of mouth and tongue.

**Eyes:** Myopia, asthenopia, and dischromotopsia, cloudiness and atrophy of the optic disc. Central scotoma for red and green light not for white light. Optic neuritis advancing toward atrophy. Arteries and veins congested. Retinal congestion; optic disc pale. Everything seems in a fog (amblyopia). Vision greatly impaired (amaurosis). Color blindness.

**Ears:** Hearing impaired. Buzzing and singing noises like an aeolian harp. *Tinnitus aurium. Meniere's disease.*

**Abdomen:** Pain with *wandering swellings* as from flatus. Distention with soreness and rumbling.

**Male:** Desire lost, parts atrophied. Frequent, profuse emissions.

**Extremities:** Herpes on the dorsal surface of hands. Sore, bruised limbs; anesthesia of arms and hands. Cramps in the limbs. Lightening- like pains, with cramps. Fingers swollen, *insensible,* rigid, stiff. Gait unsteady, tottering; worse in dark. Feet insensible. *Sciatica. Flying pains, returning regularly* for a long time. Pain in the lower limbs with cramps and formication. *Neuritis.* Progresive muscular atrophy.

**Sleep:** Deep morning sleep with anxious, vexatious dreams.

**Skin:** Anesthesia; burning; itching; ulcers; small wounds fester. Useful in restraining the growth of cancer. Furunculosis. Chronic skin diseases with much itching.

**Modalities:** *Better,* in open air. *Worse,* after breakfast; bathing. Sensitive to warm, damp, weather.

**Relationship:** Compare: *Potass xantate* (similar in action. Acts on the cortical substance; loss of memory, marked blood degeneration; impotence and senility). *Tub., Rad., Carb-v., Sulph., Caust., Sal-ac., Chin.* In eye symptoms compare: *Ben-d. Thyreoidinum* (progressive diminution of sight with central scotoma).

**Dose:** First attenuation. Locally in facial neuralgia and sciatica.

# CARCINOSINUM

(A Nosode From Carcinoma) **Carc.**

It is claimed that *Carcinosinum* acts favorably and modifies all cases in which either a history of carcinoma can be elicited, or symptoms of the disease itself exist (J. H. Clarke, M. D.).

Carcinoma of the mammary glands with great pain and induration of glands; of uterus, with offensive discharges, hemorrhage and pain are greatly relieved.

Indigestion, accumulation of gas in the stomach and bowels; rheumatism, cancerous cachexia.

**Mind:** Intellectual torpor. Thinks with difficulty; indifference; apathy. Worse by conversation. Tendency to suicide. Dislikes consolation. Children have great fear, sensitive to reprimands (*Med.*), but is sympathetic to others (*Phos*).

**Relationship:** Compare: *Bufo; Con., Phyt., Ast-r.*

**Dose:** Thirtieth and 200th potency, a dose at night or less frequently.

---

# CARDUUS MARIANUS

(St. Mary's Thistle) **Card-m.**

The action of this drug is centered on the liver and portal system causing soreness, pain and jaundice. Has specific relation to the vascular system. Abuse of alcoholic beverages, especially beer. *Varicose veins* and ulcers. Diseases in miners, associated with asthma. Dropsical conditions due to pelvic congestion and hepatic disease. Disturbs sugar metabolism. Influenza, when liver is affected. Debility. Hemorrhages, especially connected with hepatic disease.

**Mind:** Despondency; forgetful, apathetic.

**Head:** Sensation of contraction above the eyebrows. Dull heavy, stupid with a foul tongue[1]. Vertigo, with a tendency to fall forward. Burning and pressure in the eyes. Epistaxis.

**Stomach:** Taste bitter. Aversion to salt meat. Appetite small; tongue furred; *nausea; retching; vomiting of green, acrid fluid.* Stitches on the left side of stomach, near the spleen (*Cean.*). Gallstones with hepatomegaly.

**Abdomen:** Pain in the liver region. Left lobe very sensitive. Fullness and soreness with a moist skin. Constipation; *stools hard, difficult, knotty;* alternates with diarrhea. Stools bright yellow. Swelling of the gall bladder with painful tenderness, gall stones. Hyperemia of the liver with jaundice. Cirrhosis with dropsy.

---

1 With a disposition to anger (T. F. Allen, Handbook of Materia Medica).

**Rectum:** Hemorrhagic piles, prolapse of rectum, burning pain in the anus and rectum, hard and knotty, clayey stools. Profuse diarrhea due to rectal cancer. 10 drop doses (Wapler).

**Urinary:** Urine cloudy; golden colored (jaundice).

**Chest:** Stitching pains in the lower, right ribs and front (pleurisy); worse, moving, walking, etc. *Asthmatic respiration.* Pain in chest, going to the shoulders, back, loins and abdomen with an urge to micturate.

**Extremities:** Pain in the hip joint, spreading through the buttocks and down the thigh, *worse from stooping* (sciatica). Difficulty on rising (arthritis). Weakness felt in the feet, especially after sitting.

**Relationship:** Compare: *Carduus benedictus* (strong action on the eyes, and sensation of contraction in many parts; stomach symptoms similar); *Chel., Chion., Merc., Podo., Bry., Aloe.*

**Dose:** Tincture and lower potencies.

---

# CARLSBAD AQUA

(The Waters of the Sprudel Springs) **Carl.**

Famous for its action on the liver and in the treatment of obesity, diabetes and gout. In homeopathic potencies useful in weakness of all organs, constipation, great liability to take cold. Periodicity, effects repeated after two to four weeks (*Ox-ac., Sulph.*). *Flashes of heat all* over. Itching in various parts.

**Mind:** Discouraged and anxious about domestic duties.

**Head:** Aches, with swollen temporal veins (*Sang.*); better, motion, in open air.

**Face:** Yellow; sallow; red and hot; pain in the zygomatic process; feels as if cobwebs were on it.

**Mouth:** Tongue coated white. Offensive smell from the mouth. Furry sensation. Sour or salty taste.

**Stomach:** Hiccough and yawning. Heartburn (*Carb-v.*).

**Rectum:** *Feces held back.* Stools slow and passed after much abdominal pressure. Burning in the rectum and anus. Bleeding piles.

**Urinary:** Stream *weak and slow;* only passed by pressing abdominal muscles.

**Relationship:** Compare: *Nat-s., Nux-v.*

**Dose:** Lower potencies.

---

## CASCARA SAGRADA—RHAMNUS PURSHIANA

(Sacred Bark) **Cas-s.**

Introduced as a palliative for constipation (non-homeopathic), fifteen drops of fluid extract, restores normal function by its tonic effects, but it has a wider sphere of action as careful provings will show. Chronic indigestion, cirrhosis and jaundice. Hemorrhoids and constipation. Gastric headache. Broad, flabby tongue; halitosis.

**Urinary:** Must wait for a minute before flow starts, then first part comes as drops.

**Extremities:** *Rheumatism of muscles and joints, with obstinate constipation.*

**Relationship:** Compare: *Hydr., Nux-v., Rhamnus californica* (tincture for constipation; tympanites, appendicitis, and especially rheumatism).

**Dose:** Tincture to sixth potency.

## CASCARILLA

(Sweet Bark) **Casc.**

Acts on the digestive tract; constipation. Aversion to the smell of tobacco. *Inclination to vomit* very marked.

**Stomach:** Hunger after meals. Desire for hot drinks. *Nausea and vomiting.* Pain in the stomach as if from a shock. Pressing colic.

**Rectum:** Constipation; stools hard, covered with mucus (*Graph.*). Bright blood with stool. Diarrhea alternating with hard, lumpy stools, with backache and lassitude, preceded by griping. Gnawing pain high up in the rectum.

**Dose:** First to third potency.

## CASTANEA VESCA

(Chestnut Leaves) **Castn-v.**

A useful remedy in *whooping cough,* especially in the early stage, with dry, ringing, violent, spasmodic cough. Desire for warm drinks. Very thirsty. Loss of appetite. Diarrhea. Thick urine.

Lumbago, weak back, can hardly straighten up.

**Relationship:** Compare: *Pertussinum* (whooping cough when symptoms return again after being allayed). *Dros., Meph., Naphtin., Am-br.*

**Dose:** Tincture.

## CASTOR EQUI

(Rudimentary Thumb-nail of the Horse) **Castor-eq.**

General action on the thickening of the skin and epithelium. *Psoriasis linguae.* The clinical experience of Hering and his fellow-provers has shown this to be a highly useful remedy in *cracked and ulcerated nipples.* Affects the female organs principally. Acts on the nails and bones; pain in the right tibia and coccyx. Warts on the forehead and breast. Chapped hands.

**Chest:** Cracked, sore nipples, excessively tender. Swelling of mammae (mastitis). Violent itching in breasts; areola reddened.

**Relationship:** Compare: *Graph., Hipp., Calc-ox.*

**Dose:** Sixth and twelfth potency.

---

## CASTOREUM CANADENSE

(The Beaver) **Castm.**

A great remedy for hysteria. Prostration marked.

Hysterical symptoms. Day blindness; cannot endure light. Nervous women who do not recover fully, but are continuously irritable and suffer from debilitating sweats. Spasmodic affections after debilitating diseases. Constant yawning. Restless sleep with frightful dreams and starts.

**Mouth :** Tongue swollen. Rounded elevation, size of a pea in the center, with a drawing sensation from the center to the hyoid bone.

**Female:** Dysmenorrhea; blood discharged in drops with tenesmus. Pain commences in the middle of the thighs. Amenorrhea with painful tympanites.

**Fever:** Predominant chilliness. Attacks of chilliness with icy coldness of the back.

**Relationship:** Compare: *Ambr., Mosch., Mur-ac., Valer.*

Antidote: *Colch.*

**Dose:** Tincture and lower potencies.

---

## CATARIA NEPETA

(Catnip) **Catar.**

Children's remedy for *colic,* also for nervous headache and hysteria, abdominal complaints, pain, flexing of thighs, twisting of body, crying. Similar to *Chamomilla* and *Mag-p.*

**Dose:** 5 to 10 drops of the tincture.

## CAULOPHYLLUM THALICTROIDES

(Blue Cohosh) **Caul.**

This is a woman's remedy. Want of tonicity in the womb. During labor, when the pains are deficient and the patient is exhausted and fretful. Besides, it has a special affinity for the smaller joints. *Thrush,* locally and internally.

**Stomach:** *Cardialgia, spasms of the stomach.* Dyspepsia with spasmodic symptoms.

**Female:** Extraordinary rigidity of the os (*Bell., Gels., Verat-v.*). Spasmodic and severe pains, which fly in all directions; shivering, without progress; false pains. Revives labor pains and furthers progress of labor. After pains. Leucorrhea with moth spots on the forehead. Habitual abortion from uterine debility (*Helon., Puls., Sabin.*). Needle- like pains in the cervix. Dysmenorrhea, with pains flying to other parts of the body. Lochia protracted; great atony. Menses and leucorrhea profuse.

**Extremities:** Severe drawing, erratic pain and stiffness in small joints, fingers, toes, ankles, etc. (rheumatism). Aching in wrists. Cutting pains on closing the hands. Erratic pains, changing place every few minutes.

**Skin:** Discoloration of the skin in women with menstrual and uterine disorders.

**Relationship:** Incompatible: *Coff.*

Compare: *Viol-o.* (rheumatic carpal and metacarpal joints); *Cimic., Sep., Puls., Gels.*

**Dose:** Tincture to third attenuation.

---

## CAUSTICUM

(Hahnemann's Tinctura Acris Sine Kali) **Caust.**

Manifests its action mainly in chronic rheumatic, arthritic and paralytic affections, indicated by the tearing, drawing pains in the muscular and fibrous tissues with deformities of the joints; progressive loss of muscular strength, tendinous contractures. Broken down seniles. In catarrhal affections of the air passages, seems to choose dark complexioned and rigid fibred persons. Restlessness at night, with tearing pains in the joints and bones, and faint-like sinking of strength. This weakness progresses until we have a gradually appearing paralysis. Local paralysis of vocal cords, muscles of deglutition, tongue, eyelids, face, bladder and extremities. Children are slow to walk. The skin of a *Causticum* patient is *dirty, white,* sallow with warts, especially on the face. Emaciation due to disease, worry, etc., of long standing. *Burning, rawness and soreness* are characteristic.

**Mind:** Child does not want to go to bed alone. Least thing makes it cry. Sad, hopeless. *Intensely sympathetic.* Ailments from long lasting grief, sudden emotions. Thinking of complaints, aggravates, especially hemorrhoids.

**Head:** Sensation of an empty space between the forehead and brain. Pain in the right frontal eminence.

**Eyes:** Cataract with motor disturbances. Inflammation of eyelids; ulceration (ulcerative blepharitis). Sparks and dark spots before the eyes. *Ptosis* (*Gels.*). Vision impaired, as if a film was before the eyes (amaurosis, cataract). Paralysis of ocular muscles after exposure to cold.

**Ears:** Ringing, roaring, pulsating noises with deafness; words and steps re-echo; chronic otitis media; accumulation of ear wax.

**Nose:** *Coryza, with hoarseness.* Scaly nose. Nostrils ulcerated. *Pimples and warts.*

**Face:** Paralysis of the right side. Warts. Pain in the facial bones. Dental fistula. Pain in the jaws with difficulty in opening the mouth.

**Mouth:** Bites inside of cheek when chewing. Paralysis of the tongue with indistinct speech. Rheumatism of articulation of lower jaw (temporo-mandibular joint). Gums bleed easily.

**Stomach:** Greasy taste. Aversion to sweets. Feels as if lime was burned in the stomach. Worse after eating fresh meat; smoked meat agrees. Sensation of a ball rising in the throat. Acid dyspepsia.

**Stool:** Soft and small, size of goose-quill (*Phos.*). Hard, tough, covered with mucus; shines like grease; small shaped; expelled after much straining, or only on standing. Pruritus. Partial paralysis of rectum. Rectum sore and burns. Fistula and large piles.

**Urinary:** Involuntary when coughing, sneezing (*Puls.*). Expelled very slowly, and sometimes retained. Involuntary during first sleep at night (nocturnal enuresis); also from the slightest excitement. *Retention* after surgery. Loss of sensibility on passing urine.

**Female:** *Uterine inertia during labor.* Menses cease at night; *flow only during the day* (*Cycl., Puls.*). Leucorrhea at night, with great weakness (*Nat-m.*). Menses delayed, late (*Con., Graph., Puls.*).

**Respiratory:** *Hoarseness* with pain in the chest; *aphonia.* Larynx sore (laryngitis). *Cough, with raw soreness of the chest.* Expectoration scanty; *must be swallowed.* Cough *with pain in the hip,* especially left, worse in the evening; *better, drinking cold water;* worse, warmth of bed. Sore streak down the trachea. Mucus under the sternum, which he cannot *quite reach.* Pain in the chest, with palpitations. Cannot lie down at night. Voice re-echoes. Own voice roars in the ears and distresses. Difficulty in the voice of singers and public speakers (Royal).

**Back:** Stiffness between the shoulders. Dull pain in the nape of the neck.

**Extremities:** Left sided sciatica, with numbness. Paralysis of single parts.

Dull, tearing pain in the hands and arms. Heaviness and weakness. Tearing pain in joints. Unsteadiness of *the muscles of forearm* and hand. Numbness; loss of sensation in the hands. *Contracted tendons.* Weak ankles. Cannot walk without suffering. *Rheumatic tearing pains in the limbs; better by warmth, especially heat of bed.* Burning in joints. Slow in learning to walk. Unsteady walking and easy falling. *Restless legs at night.* Cracking and tension in knees (arthritis deformans); stiffness in the hollow of knee. Itching on the dorsum of feet.

**Sleep:** Very drowsy; can hardly keep awake. Nocturnal sleeplessness with dry heat, inquietude.

**Skin:** Soreness in the folds of skin, behind the ears, between thighs. *Warts* large, jagged, bleeding easily, on tips of fingers and nose. Old burns that do not get well, and ill effects of burns. Pain in burns. Cicatrices freshen up; old injuries reopen. Skin prone to intertrigo during dentition.

**Modalities:** *Worse,* dry, cold winds, in clear fine weather, cold air; from motion of carriage. *Better, in damp, wet weather; warmth.* Heat of bed.

**Relationship:** According to the careful investigations of Dr. Wagner of Basel, *Causticum* corresponds to *Ammonium causticum* 4x. *Causticum* does not agree with *Phosphorus*; the remedies should not be used after each other. *Diphtherotoxinum* follows, *Causticum* in chronic bronchitis.

Antidote: Paralysis from lead poisoning.

Complementary: *Carb-v., Petros.*

Compare: *Rhus-t., Ars., Am-ph.* (facial paralysis).

**Dose:** Third to thirtieth attenuation. In chronic ailments and especially in paralytic states, higher potencies once or twice a week.

---

# CEANOTHUS AMERICANUS

(New Jersey Tea) **Cean.**

This remedy seems to possess a specific relation to the spleen. Ague cake of malaria. A left sided remedy generally. Anemic patients where liver and spleen are at fault. Chronic bronchitis with profuse secretion. Marked blood pressure, reducing power. Active hemostatic, materially reducing the clotting of blood.

**Abdomen:** Enormous enlargement of the spleen (splenomegaly). *Splenitis; pain radiates up the left side.* Deep seated pain in the left hypochondrium, hypertrophy of spleen. Leukemia. Violent dyspnea. Menses profuse and yellow, weakening leucorrhea. Unable to lie on the left side. Pain in the liver and back.

**Rectum:** Diarrhea; bearing down in the abdomen and rectum.

**Urinary:** Constant urging to micturate. Green; frothy; contains bile, sugar (jaundice, diabetes).

**Modalities:** *Worse,* motion, lying on left side.

**Relationship:** Compare: *Tinospora cordifolia* (a Hindu medicine for chronic cases of fever with splenomegaly). *Polymnia uvedalia*—Bearsfoot (acute splenitis with tenderness over the left hypochondriac region; spleen enlarged, ague cake. Vascular atony, tissues sodden, flabby and non-elastic. Enlarged glands; influences all ductless glands). *Ceanothus thrysiflorus*—California lilac (pharyngitis, tonsillitis, nasal catarrh, diphtheria. Tincture internally and as a gargle).

Compare: *Berb., Myric., Cedr., Agar.* (spleen).

**Dose:** First attenuation. Locally as a hair tonic.

---

## CEDRON—SIMARUBA FERROGINEA

(Rattlesnake Bean) **Cedr.**

Periodicity is the most marked characteristic of this drug. It is particularly useful in tropical or in damp, warm, marshy countries. It has been, found curative in malarial affections, especially neuralgia. Adapted to people with a voluptuous disposition, excitable, nervous temperament. Has power to antidote snake bites and stings of insects. Tincture of pure bean is applied on wounds. Mania.

**Head:** Pain from temple to temple, across the eyes. Pain over the entire right side of the face, coming on at about 9 a.m. Crazy feeling from pain across the forehead; worse, working in blackness[1]. Roaring in ears as produced by *Chin.* The whole body seems numb with headache (meningitis).

**Eyes:** Shooting over the left eye. Severe *pain in the eyeball, radiating around the eye and* shooting into the nose. Scalding lachrymation. *Supra-orbital neuralgia, periodical.* Iritis, choroiditis.

**Extremities:** Lancinating pain in joints; worse, feet and hands. Sudden pain in the ball of right thumb (gout), extending up the arm, to the shoulder. Pain in the ball of right foot, extending to the knee. Shingles with radiating pains. Dropsy of the knee joint.

**Fever:** Chills towards evening; frontal headache extending to the parietal region. Eyes red. Heat, with itching in the eyes, tearing pain in limbs, *numbness of limbs.*

**Relationship:** Antidote: *Lach.*

Compare: *Ars., Chin.*

**Dose:** Tincture to third attenuation.

---

[1] On rising from bed, dizzy, cannot see to light a candle and could not tell when it was lighted (T. F. Allen, Handbook of Materia Medica).

# CENCHRIS CONTORTRIX—ANCISTRODON

(Copperhead Snake) **Cench.**

Like the other snake poisons, it affects the system profoundly. Like *Ars.*, it has dyspnea, mental and physical restlessness, thirst for small quantities of water; necessity for loose clothing like *Lach.* Marked alternation of moods; vivid dreams. Is a wonderful restorative and deep acting remedy. Increased sexual desire in both sexes. Ineffectual attempts to recline. Right ovarian region painful.

**Head:** Forgetful, absent-minded, alternating moods. Aching pain in the left frontal eminence and left side of teeth.

**Eyes**: Swelling around the eyes, aching and itching in the eyes.

**Heart:** Feels distended, fills the whole chest, as if it fell down in the abdomen; sharp stitches, fluttering under the left scapula.

**Sleep:** Dreams horrible and vivid; lascivious.

**Modalities:** *Worse,* pressure; lying down; afternoon and night.

**Relationship:** Compare: *Ars., Lach. Clotho arietans*—Puff adder: Should have a great sphere of usefulness in many conditions where excessive swelling is a leading feature (John H. Clarke, M. D.).

**Dose:** Sixth potency.

---

# CEREUS BONPLANDII

(A Night-blooming Cereus) **Cere-b.**

**Mind:** Great desire to work and to do something useful.

**Head:** Occipital headache and pain *through the globe of eyes* and orbits (*Cedr., Onos.*). Pain across the brain from left to right. Pain along the right malar bone extending to the temple.

**Chest:** Convulsive pain in the heart; feels as if transfixed. Pain in chest through the heart, pain extending towards the spleen. Pain in the left pectoral muscle and cartilages of left lower ribs. Sensation of a great weight on the heart and pricking pain. Hypertrophy of the heart. Difficult, sighing respiration, as if from some compression of the chest.

**Extremities:** Pain in the neck, back, shoulders, down the arms, hands and fingers. Pain in knees and joints of lower extremities.

**Skin:** Itching (*Dol., Sulph.*).

**Relationship:** Compare: *Cact., Spig., Kalm., Cereus serpentinus* (very irritable with a tendency to swear; wild anger and low morals. Disturbance in speech; while writing, leaves the last syllable. Paralyzed feeling. Pain in the heart, dwindling of sexual organs. Emissions, followed by pain in the testicles).

**Dose:** Third to sixth attenuation.

---

## CERIUM OXALICUM

(Oxalate of Cerium) **Cer-ox.**

Spasmodic reflex vomiting and spasmodic cough are within the sphere of this remedy. *Vomiting during pregnancy,* of half digested food. Whooping cough with vomiting and hemorrhage. Dysmenorrhea in fleshy, robust women. Better when flow is established.

**Relationship:** Compare: *Ingluvin* (made from gizzard of a fowl). Vomiting of pregnancy; gastric neurasthenia. Infantile vomiting and diarrhea. 3x trituration *Amygd., Lac-ac., Ip.*

**Dose:** First trituration.

---

## CHAMOMILLA

(German Chamomile) **Cham.**

The chief guiding symptoms belong to the mental and emotional group, which lead to this remedy in many forms of diseases. Especially for frequent employment in diseases of children where peevishness, restlessness and colic give the needful indications. A disposition that is mild, calm and gentle, sluggish and constipated bowels, contraindicate *Chamomilla.*

*Chamomilla* is *sensitive, irritable, thirsty, hot and numb.* Oversensitiveness from abuse of coffee and narcotics. *Pains unendurable* associated with numbness. Night sweats

**Mind:** *Whining restlessness.* Child wants many things which he refuses when given. Piteous moaning because he can not have what he wants. Child can only be quietened when carried about and petted constantly. *Impatient,* intolerant of being spoken to or interrupted; extremely sensitive to every pain; always complaining. Spiteful, *snappish.* Complaints from anger and vexation. Mental calmness contraindicates *Cham.*

**Head:** Throbbing headache in one-half of the brain (migraine). Inclined to bend head backward. Hot, clammy sweat on the forehead and scalp.

**Eyes**: Lids smart (blepharitis). Yellow sclera. Spasmodic closing of lids (blepherospasm).

**Ears:** Ringing in the ears. *Otalgia,* with soreness; *swelling and heat, driving the patient frantic.* Stitching pain. Ears feel obstructed.

**Nose**: Sensitive to all smells. Coryza, with inability to sleep.

**Face**: *One cheek red* and hot; the other pale and cold. Stitches in the jaw extending to the inner ear and teeth. Tooth ache *worse after a warm drink;* worse, coffee, at night. Drives to distraction[1]. Jerking of tongue and facial muscles (convulsions). Distress in teething children (*Calc-p., Ter.*).

**Mouth**: Toothache, if anything warm is taken, from coffee, during pregnancy. Nocturnal salivation.

**Throat**: Parotid and submaxillary glands swollen (mumps and parotiditis). Constriction and pain as if from a plug.

**Stomach**: Eructations, foul. Nausea after coffee. Sweats after eating or drinking. Aversion to warm drinks. Tongue yellow; taste bitter. Bilious vomiting (jaundice). Acid rising; regurgitation of food. Bitter, bilious vomiting. Pressive gastralgia, as if from a stone (*Bry., Abies-n.*).

**Abdomen**: Distended. Griping in the umbilical region, and pain in the lumbosacral region. Flatulent colic, after anger *with red cheeks and hot perspiration.* Hepatic colic. Acute duodenitis (*Kali-bi.* chronic).

**Stool:** Hot, *green,* watery, fetid, *slimy,* with colic. Chopped white and yellow mucus like chopped eggs and spinach. Soreness of the anus. Diarrhea during dentition. Hemorrhoids, with painful fissures.

**Female:** Uterine hemorrhages. Profuse discharge of clotted, *dark blood with labor-like pains* (dysmenorrhea). Labor pains spasmodic; press upward (*Gels.*). Patient intolerant of pain (*Caul., Caust., Gels., Hyos., Puls.*). Nipples inflamed; tender to touch. Infant's breasts tender (mastitis in infants). Yellow, acrid leucorrhea (*Ars., Sep., Sulph.*).

**Respiratory**: Hoarseness, hawking, *rawness of larynx. Irritable, dry, tickling cough;* suffocative tightness of the chest, with bitter expectoration during daytime. Rattling of mucus in the child's chest (asthma).

**Back:** Insupportable pain in loins and hips. Lumbago. Stiffness of neck muscles.

**Extremities**: Violent rheumatic pains drive him out of bed at night; compelled to walk around. Burning of soles at night (*Sulph.*). *Ankles give way* in *the afternoon.* Paralytic loss of power in the feet at night, unable to step on them.

**Sleep:** Drowsiness with moaning, weeping and wailing during sleep; anxious, frightened dreams with half open eyes.

**Modalities:** *Worse,* by *heat,* anger, open air, wind, *night. Better,* from being carried, warm wet weather.

---

[1] Driving the patient frantic (T. F. Allen, Handbook of Materia Medica).

**Relationship:** Compare: *Cypr., Anth., Acon., Puls., Coff., Bell., Staph., Ign.* Follows *Belladonna in* diseases of children and abuse of *Opium*. *Rubus villosus*—Blackberry (diarrhea of infancy; stools watery and clay colored).

Antidotes: *Camph., Nux-v., Puls.*

Complementary: *Bell., Mag-c.*

**Dose:** Third to thirtieth attenuation.

---

## CHAPARRO AMARGOSO

(Goat-bush) **Chap.**

Chronic diarrhea. Tenderness over the liver. Stools with little pain, but with profuse mucus. Dysentery. Acts as a tonic and antiperiodic.

**Relationship:** Compare: *Kali-c., Cupr-ar., Caps.*

**Dose:** Third attenuation.

---

## CHELIDONIUM MAJUS

(Celandine) **Chel.**

A prominent liver remedy, covering many of the direct reflex symptoms in the diseased conditions of this organ. The jaundiced skin and especially the *constant pain under the inferior angle of right scapula,* are certain indications. Paralytic drawing and lameness in single parts. Great general lethargy and an indisposition to make any effort, is also marked. Ailments brought on or renewed by change of weather. *Serous effusions. Hydrocele. Bilious complications during gestation.*

**Head:** Icy coldness of the occiput from the nape of the neck; *feels heavy as lead.* Heavy, lethargic; drowsiness, very marked, with general numbness; vertigo associated with hepatic disturbances. Inclination to fall forward. Right sided headache extending down, behind the ears and to the shoulder blade (migraine). *Neuralgia over the right eye,* right cheek bone and right ear, with excessive lachrymation, preceded by pain in the liver region.

**Eyes:** Dirty yellow color of the sclera. Sore sensation on looking up. Tears fairly gush out. Orbital neuralgia of the right eye, with profuse lachrymation; pupils contracted, relieved by pressure.

**Nose:** Flapping of alae nasi (*Lyc.*).

**Face:** *Yellow;* worse nose and cheeks. Wilted skin.

**Stomach:** Tongue yellow with imprint of teeth; large and flabby (*Merc., Hydr.*). Taste bitter, pasty. Halitosis. *Prefers hot food and drink.* Nausea, vomiting; *better, taking very hot water.* Pain through the stomach to the back and right shoulder blade. Gastralgia. *Eating relieves temporarily,* especially when accompanied with hepatic symptoms.

**Abdomen:** Jaundice due to hepatic and gall bladder obstruction. Gall colic (cholecystitis). Distention. Fermentation and sluggish bowels. Constriction across, as if by a string. Liver enlarged. Gallstones (*Berb.*).

**Stool:** Constipation; stools hard, round balls, like sheep's dung, bright yellow, pasty; clay colored, stools float in water; *alternation of diarrhea and constipation.* Burning and itching in the anus (*Rat., Sulph.*).

**Urinary:** Profuse urine, foaming, yellow urine, like beer (*Chen-a.*), dark, turbid.

**Female:** Menses too late and too profuse.

**Respiratory:** Very quick and short inspirations; pain on deep inspiration. Dyspnea. Short, exhausting cough; sensation of dust, not relieved by cough. Whooping cough; spasmodic cough; loose, rattling; expectoration difficult (pneumonia). Pain on the *right* side of the chest and shoulder with embarrased respiration. Small lumps of mucus fly from the mouth when coughing. Hoarse in the afternoon. Constriction of chest.

**Back:** Pain in the nape. Stiff neck, head drawn to the left. *Fixed pain under the inner and lower angle of right scapula.* Pain at the lower angle of left scapula.

**Extremities:** Pain in arms, shoulders, hands, finger tips. *Icy coldness of the finger tips;* wrists sore, tearing in metacarpal bones (rheumatism). Entire flesh sore to touch. Rheumatic pain in the hips and thighs; intolerable pain in the heels, as if pinched by a very narrow shoe; worse, right. Feels paralyzed. Paresis of the lower limbs with rigidity of muscles.

**Skin:** Dry heat of skin; itches, *yellow.* Painful red pimples and pustules. Old, spreading, offensive ulcers. Wilted skin. Sallow, cold, clammy.

**Modalities:** *Worse,* right side, motion, touch, change of weather, very early in the morning. *Better,* after dinner, from pressure.

**Relationship:** *Chelidoninum* (spasm of smooth muscles everywhere, intestinal colic, uterine colic, bronchial spasm, tachycardia, etc). *Boldo—Boldoa fragrans* (bladder atony; cholecystitis and biliary calculus. Bitter taste, no appetite; constipation, hypochondriasis, languor, congestion of liver; burning weight in liver and stomach. Painful liver diseases. Disturbed liver following malaria). *Elemuy gauteria* (stones in kidneys and bladder; grain doses of powdered bark in water or 5 drops of tincture. Pellagra).

*Sulph.* often completes its work.

Complementary: *Lyc., Bry.*

Antidote: *Cham.*

Compare: *Nux-v., Sulph., Bry., Lyc., Op., Podo., Sang., Ars.*

**Dose:** Tincture and lower attenuations.

## CHELONE GLABRA

(Snakehead) **Chelo.**

A remedy for liver affections with pain or soreness in the left lobe of liver extending downwards. Dumb ague[1]. Soreness of external parts, as if the skin was off; debility. Malaise, following intermittent fever. Dyspepsia with hepatic torpor. Jaundice. *Round and thread worms.* It is an enemy to every kind of worm infesting the human body.

**Dose:** Tincture, in one to five drop doses.

---

## CHENOPODIUM ANTHELMINTICUM

(Jerusalem Oak) **Chen-a.**

Characteristic pain in the scapula very marked. Symptoms of apoplexy, right hemiplegia (migraine), and aphasia. Stertorous breathing (*Opium*). Sudden *vertigo.* Meniere's disease. Affections of the auditory nerves (*Nat-sal.*). Oil of Chenopodium is useful for hookworms and roundworms.

**Ears:** Torpor of the auditory nerve. Hearing better for *high pitched* sounds. Comparative or progressive deafness to the human voice, but *great sensitiveness to the sound, as of passing vehicles,* and shrinks from low tones. Buzzing in the ears (tinnitus). Enlargement of tonsils. *Aural vertigo* (Menier's disease).

**Urinary:** Copious, yellow, foamy urine, with an acrid sensation in urethra. Yellowish sediment (*Chel.*).

**Back:** *Intense pain between the angle of the right shoulder blade near the spine* and the chest.

**Relationship:** Compare: *Op., Chin., Chel.*

**Dose:** Third potency. Oil of Chenopodium for hookworms, 10 minim doses every 2 hours for 3 doses; also *Carboneum tetrachloridum.*

---

## CHENOPODII GLAUCI APHIS

(Plant Lice from Chenopodium) **Aphis**

Properties similar to the plant on which the insect lives.

**Head:** Sad, aching worse motion. Brain feels loose in the cranial cavity.

**Eyes:** Right orbital neuralgia with profuse lachrymation.

---

[1] Ill defined paroxysm of aching and fever following severe malaria fevers. (Clarke — Dictionary of Practical Materia Medica).

**Ears:** Cannon-like noises in the ear.

**Nose:** Acrid coryza with burning or biting in the nostrils.

**Face:** Yellowish discoloration of the face.

**Mouth:** Toothache relieved by perspiration (*Cham.*), extends to the ears, temples and cheek bones (*Plan.*). Vesicles on the tip of the tongue.

**Stomach:** No appetite for meat and bread. Colic with rumbling and ineffectual urging to stool. Much mucus.

**Stool:** Hard and knotty. Diarrhea in the morning with painful urging and burning in the anus. Pressure in rectum and bladder.

**Urinary:** Voluptous feeling in the glans. Burning in the urethra. Frequent, copious frothy micturition.

**Back:** Severe pain in the region of *lower inner angle of left shoulder blade, radiating to the chest.*

**Fever:** Shuddering all over. Burning in the palms, hot sweat in bed.

**Relationship:** Compare: *Nat-s., Nux-v.*

**Dose:** Sixth to thirtieth potency.

---

## CHIMAPHILA UMBELLATA

(Pipsissewa) **Chim.**

Acts principally on the kidneys and genito-urinary tract; affects the lymphatic and mesenteric glands and the female mammae also. Plethoric young women with dysuria. Women with large breasts. Hepatic and renal dropsies; chronic alcoholics. Incipient and progressive cataracts.

One of the remedies whose symptoms point to its employment in bladder affections, notably catarrh, acute and chronic (cystitis). *Scanty urine loaded with ropy, muco-purulent sediment. Prostatic enlargement.*

**Head:** Pain in the left frontal protuberance. Halo around the light. Itching of the eyelids. Stabbing pain in the left eye with lachrymation.

**Mouth:** Toothache, worse after eating and exertion, better cool water. Pain as if the tooth was being gently pulled.

**Urinary:** Urging to micturate. Urine turbid, offensive, containing ropy or bloody mucus (hematuria) and depositing a copious sediment. Burning and scalding during micturition and straining afterwards. *Must strain* before flow comes. Scanty urine (nephritis). Acute prostatitis, retention, sensation *of a ball in the perineum* (*Cann-i.*). Fluttering in the region of kidney. *Sugar in urine* (diabetes). Unable to micturate without standing with feet wide apart and body inclined forward.

**Male:** Smarting in the urethra from the neck of the bladder to the meatus (urethritis). Gleet. Loss of prostatic fluid. Prostatic enlargement and irritation.

**Female:** Labia inflamed, swollen. Pain in the vagina. Hot flushes. Painful *tumor of mammae,* not ulcerated with undue secretion of milk (galactorrhea). Rapid atrophy of breasts. Women having *very large breasts* and tumor in the mammary gland with *sharp* pain through it.

**Extremities:** Sensation of a band above the left knee.

**Skin:** Scrofulous ulcers. Glandular enlargements.

**Modalities:** *Worse,* in damp weather; from sitting on cold stones or pavements: left side.

**Relationship:** Compare: *Chimaphila maculata* (intense gnawing hunger; burning fever; sensation of swelling in arm pits); *Uva, Led., Epig.*

**Dose:** Tincture to third attenuation.

---

## CHININUM ARSENICOSUM

(Arsenite of Quinine) **Chinin-ar.**

The symptoms of general *weariness and prostration* produced by the drug have been utilized in prescribing it homeopathically as a general tonic, often with very marked beneficial and prompt effects. In diphtheria with great prostration, especially cases that are prolonged and in malarial affections, neuralgia, etc., it has been found curative. Asthmatic attacks which recur periodically, with great prostration. Icy skin. Pressure in the solar plexus, with a tender spine.

**Head:** Tired feeling. Head feels too full. Throbbing. Great anxiety. Great irritability. Vertigo; worse looking up. Dull, heavy headache, frontal and occipital. Darting pains running up into the head.

**Eyes:** Intense photophobia and orbicular spasm; gushing hot tears. Flickering with pain and lachrymation.

**Mouth:** Tongue thickly furred; yellow, slimy coating. Bitter taste. No appetite.

**Stomach:** Alternation of hyperacidity and decrease of acid. Hyperchlorhydria (*Rob., Arg-n., Orexine tannate*). Thirst for water, yet it disturbs. *Anorexia. Eggs produce diarrhea.*

**Heart:** Palpitations. Sensation as if the heart had stopped (angina pectoris). Suffocative attacks, occurring in periodical paroxysms. Must have open air. Shortness of breath on ascending; cardiac dyspnea; circulatory weakness after acute infections; early myocardial degeneration.

**Extremities:** Weak limbs. *Cold hands and feet, knees and limbs.* Tearing pains.

**Sleep:** Sleeplessness due to nervous causes (single dose of 5th or 6th potency).

**Fever:** Continuous, with weakness. System depleted.

**Relationship:** Compare: *Chinin-s., also Ferrum citricum* (in nephritis with great anaemia; acid dyspepsia and chlorosis. Morbus maculosus Werlhoffii); *Chinin-m.* (in severe neuralgic pains around the eyes, with chills; exaggerated sensitiveness to alcohol and tobacco; prostration and restlessness). *Oenothera biennies* (effortless diarrhea with nervous exhaustion; incipient hydrocephalus). *Macrozamia spiralis* (extreme debility after illness; collapse).

**Dose:** Second and third trituration.

---

## CHININUM SULPHURICUM

(Sulphite of Quinine) **Chinin-s.**

A dose of *Chinin-s.* in high potency sometimes arouses suppressed malaria and brings back the paroxysm. Besides its undoubted influence over malaria, it is indicated homeopathically whenever there is marked periodicity and spinal sensitiveness. *Acute articular rheumatism.* Polyarticular gout. Pruritus and congested conditions of the rectum. Symptoms of *chronic interstitial nephritis.* Retro-bulbar neuritis with sudden loss of sight. Thready vessels. Hiccough.

**Head:** Pain in the forehead and temples, increasing gradually at noon, of malarial origin with vertigo and pulsation. Worse, left side. Falls in the street. Inability to remain standing. Amaurosis.

**Ears:** Violent ringing, buzzing, and *roaring in the ears, with deafness* (Meniere's disease).

**Face:** Neuralgia commences under the eye; extends into and around it. Pains return with great regularity; *relieved by pressure.*

**Urinary:** Bloody (hematuria). Turbid, slimy, clay colored, greasy sediment. Small amount of urea and phosphoric acid with excess of uric acid and abundance of chlorides accompanied by subnormal temperature. Excessive flow. Albuminuria.

**Circulatory System:** An immediate and rapid decrease in red blood cells and reduction in hemoglobin with increase in elimination of chlorides (hemoglobinuria). Tendency to polynucleated leucocytosis.

**Back:** *Great sensitiveness of the dorsal vertebrae;* pain on pressure. Last cervical sensitive. Pain extends to the head and neck.

**Fever:** Chills daily at 3 p. m. Painful swelling of various veins (phlebismus) during a chill. Shivering even in a warm room. Anguish. Subnormal temperature.

**Skin:** Itching; erythema, urticaria, icterus, vesication, pustules, purpura. Great sensitiveness. Shrivelled skin.

**Relationship:** Compare: *Chininum salicylicum* (deafness, tinnitus, and Meniere's disease). *Ars., Eup-per., Methylene blue. Camphora mono-bromata* is said to intensify the action of quinine and render it more permanent. *Baja,* an East Indian drug, said to be almost infallible in intermittent fever, quartan type; pulsating headache, injected eyes, flushed face. Liver and spleen enlarged. Eedema. Also *Pambotano,* Mexican remedy for intermittent and tropical fevers.

Antidotes: *Parthenium, Nat-m., Lach., Arn., Puls.*

**Dose:** First to third triturations; also thirtieth potency and higher.

---

# CHIONANTHUS VIRGINICA

(Fringe Tree) **Chion.**

This remedy is often of service in many types of headaches, neurasthenic, *periodical, sick,* menstrual and bilious. Taken for several weeks, drop doses, will often break up the sick headache habit. Pain in the forehead, chiefly over the eyes. Eyeballs very painful with pressure over the root of nose. Hepatic derangements. *Jaundice.* Enlarged spleen (*Cean.*). Jaundice, with arrest of menses. A prominent liver remedy. *Gallstones* (*Berb., Chol., Calc.*). *Diabetes mellitus.* Paroxysmal, abdominal pain.

**Head:** Listless, apathetic. Dull frontal headache over the root of nose, over the eyes and through the temples, worse stooping, motion, jar. *Yellow conjunctiva* (jaundiced).

**Mouth:** Dry sensation not relieved by water, also profuse saliva. Tongue broad with thick yellow fur.

**Abdomen:** Aching in the umbilical region, griping. Feels as if a string was tied in a "slip knot" around the intestines which was suddenly drawn tight and then gradually loosened. Sore; *enlarged, with jaundice* and constipation. Clay colored stool, also soft, yellow and pasty. Tongue heavily coated. No appetite. Bilious colic. Hepatic region tender. Pancreatic disease and other glandular disorders.

**Urinary:** High specific gravity; frequent micturition; bile and sugar in the urine. Urine very dark.

**Skin:** Yellow; marked moisture on the skin. Sallow, greenish, itching.

**Relationship:** Compare: *Chin., Cean., Chel., Card-m., Podo., Lept.*

**Dose:** Tincture and first attenuation.

# CHLORALUM HYDRATUM

(Chloral Hydrate) **Chlol.**

This drug, used in physiological doses, is a powerful hypnotic and cardiac depressant. It has a marked effect on the skin, producing erythema, ecchymosis, etc., is utilized homeopathically with much success, especially in the treatment of hives. Emotional excitability, hallucinations. Night terrors in children. Muscular prostration.

**Head:** Morning headache; worse in the forehead, also in the occiput, on motion; better in the open air. Passive cerebral hyperemia (use 30th). Sensation as if a hot band was drawn from temple to temple. Hears voices.

**Eyes:** Blood shot and watery. Circles of light, black spots. Illusions of sight when eyes are closed or at night. Dim vision. Conjunctivitis, burning in the eye and lids; eyeball feels too large; everything looks *white.*

**Respiratory:** Extreme dyspnea, with sensation of weight and constriction of chest (angina pectoris). Asthma with sleeplessness.

**Sleep:** Insomnia, hallucinations, horrid dreams. Somnolence.

**Skin:** Red blotches, like measles. *Urticaria, worse, spirituous liquors,* hot drinks. Erythema aggravated by alcoholic drinks with palpitations; causes pain in tendons and extensors. Intense itching. Surface of body *stone cold.* Wheals come on from a chill; better, warmth. Purpura (*Phos., Crot-h.*).

**Modalities:** *Worse,* after hot drinks, stimulants, eating, night.

**Relationship:** Antidotes: *Ammc., Atro., Dig., Mosch.*

Compare: *Bell., Op., Apis; Veronal* (a dangerous drug made by the action of alcohol upon urea, contains the same radical that alcohol does. Makes a man just as drunk as pure alcohol. Staggers, cannot stand up- Dr. Varney. Confluent, reddish spots; dermatitis, itching of glans and prepuce; circumscribed patch of dermatitis on the first metacarpo-phalangeal joint). *Luminal* (sleeplessness with skin symptoms in migraine; lethargy like epidemic encephalitis: Dr. Royal).

**Dose:** First trituration in hives, otherwise, higher potencies. Locally, in offensive foot sweat, bathe with one percent solution. For its physiological effects, five to twenty grains. Use cautiously.

---

# CHLOROFORMIUM

(Chloroform) **Chlf.**

General anesthetic, antispasmodic. Complete muscular relaxation. Weak and quick pulse, shallow or stertorous breathing. Convulsions, nephritic or biliary colic, gastralgia. Symptoms obtained by Dr. D. Macfarlan with the 6th potency.

Great weakness, especially on the right side. Limbs very tired from knees down. Increased perspiration all over the face and chest; drowsy and dizzy; dry lips and throat; dry tickling cough at night. Flatulence; food regurgitates; sore and bruised feeling in the stomach; catching pain around the heart. Sharp pain on the right side of chest when he takes a deep breath; shortness of breath on exertion.

**Head:** Delirium where excitement and violence predominate. Head drawn down upon the shoulders, eyes open and close rapidly, pupils contracted; rapid convulsive movements of the face, of muscles and extremities (delirium tremens, tetnus and convulsions).

**Relationship:** *Etherum:* Post-operative bronchitis (Prof. Bier). *Spiritus aetheris compositus*: Hoffman's Anodyne (flatulence; angina pectoris. Dose: 5m to 1 dram in water).

**Dose:** Higher attenuations, or sixth. *Phosphorus* is the remedy to give in narcosis of chloroform.

---

# CHLORUM

(Chlorine Gas in Water) **Chlor.**

Marked effect on the respiratory system producing spasm of the glottis, which is the chief symptom of this drug. Asthma with spasm of glottis. Useful externally and internally in gangrene.

**Mind:** Fear of becoming crazy. Marked loss of memory, *especially for names.*

**Nose:** Sooty, smoky nostrils Coryza with sudden gushes of sharp, corroding fluid, making nose sore inside and around the alae. *Constriction with suffocation.*

**Throat:** *Spasm of the glottis.* Irritation in the epiglottis, larynx, and bronchi. Aphonia from damp air. *Sudden dyspnea from spasm of vocal cords* with staring protruding eyes, blue face, cold sweat, pulse small (laryngismus).

**Respiration:** *Inspiration free with obstructed expiration* (asthma) (*Meph.*). Livid face. Prolonged, loud, whistling rales. Extreme dryness of the tongue.

**Dose:** Chlorine water, when required in full strength, must be freshly prepared. Fourth to sixth potency.

---

# CHOLESTERINUM

(Cholesterine—The Proximate Principle. Furnished by the Epithelium Lining of the Gall Bladder and the Larger Ducts)

**Chol.**

For cancer of the liver. *Obstinate hepatic engorgements.* Burning pain on the side; while walking holds his hand on the side, as it hurts him. Opacities of the vitreous. Jaundice; gallstones. Cholesterine is the physiological opponent of Lecithin. Both seem to play some unknown part in the growth of tumors. Gallstones and insomnia.

**Relationship:** Compare: *Taurocholate of soda* (*Natrium taurocholicum*) in homeopathy: Dr. I. P. Tessier, in an interesting study of the action of bile and its salts in hepatic affections, analyzes a number of experiments by leading authorities with the object of determining it's action, and concludes that in the *Taurocholate of Soda,* homeopathy has a useful remedy against certain forms of hypoglobular anemia. The claim that its pathogenesis and toxicology clearly indicate its value and that it should also serve us as a remedy in cases of hypertrophy of the spleen and ganglia. He calls our attention to the fact that it produces dyspnea, the Cheyne-Stokes rhythm, acute pulmonary edema and intense exaggeration of cardiac pulsations, offering a good field for clinical studies and experimentation of great interest which may give fruitful and important results.

**Dose:** Third trituration.

---

# CHROMICUM ACIDUM

(Chromic Acid)

**Chr-ac.**

Diphtheria, post-nasal tumors and epithelioma of the tongue have been benefited by this drug. Bloody, foul smelling lochia. Symptoms come and go *suddenly,* return periodically; offensive discharges.

**Nose:** Ulcers and scabs in the nose. Offensive smell. Corrosive pain. Ozena (*Aur.*).

**Throat:** Diphtheria; sore throat. Tough mucus with an inclination to swallow it; causing hawking. Post-nasal tumors (polyp).

**Stool:** Watery, frequent, copious, with nausea and vertigo. Hemorrhoids, internal and bleeding. Weakness in the lumbosacral region (lumbago).

**Extremities:** Uneasiness in the limbs. Pain in the shoulder blades and back of neck. Pain in the knees (arthritis) and balls of feet (gout). Drawing pains in the soles while walking.

**Relationship:** Compare: *Kali-bi., Rhus-t., Chromium sulphuricum* (in locomotor ataxia, goitre, *prostatic hypertrophy.* Herpes preputialis. Wry neck. Also in exophthalmic goitre, inhibits the vagus relieving tachycardia. Acts like a nerve tonic where there is lack of nervous tone. Fibroid tumors. Infantile paralysis. Dose for adults, 3 to 5 grains after meals and at bedtime).

**Dose:** Homeopathically, third to sixth trituration.

---

# CHRYSAROBINUM

(Goa Powder, Andira Araroba) **Chrysar.**

Acts as a powerful irritant of the skin and is used successfully in skin diseases, especially in *ringworm, psoriasis,* herpes and acne rosacea. Vesicular or squamous lesions, associated with a foul smelling discharge and crust formation with a tendency to become confluent giving the appearance of a single crust covering the entire area (Bernstein). *Violent itching in the* thighs legs and *ears.* Dry, scaly eruptions, especially around the eyes and ears, scabs with pus underneath (crusta lactea) (*Mez.*).

**Eyes:** Blepharitis, conjunctivitis, keratitis. Intense photophobia. Optical hyperesthesia.

**Ears:** Eczema behind the ears. Filthy, scabby condition with a tendency to form thick crusts. The whole ear and the surrounding tissue appears to be one scab.

**Relationship:** *Chrysarobinum* contains *Chrysophan,* which is rapidly oxydized into *Chrysophanic acid.* This is also contained in *Rhubarb* and *Senna.*

**Dose:** Locally, as a cerate, 4-8 grains to an ounce of vaseline. Internally, third to sixth potency. Used externally; should be used with caution on account of its ability to produce inflammation.

---

# CICUTA VIROSA

(Water Hemlock) **Cic.**

The action on the nervous system producing spasmodic affections, viz., hiccough, trismus, tetanus and convulsions, gives the pathological picture calling for this remedy, whenever this is further characterized by the more individual symptoms of the drug. Among these are the *bending of the head, neck and spine backwards* and the general action of the patient is *violent* with frightful distortions. Violent, strange desires. Sensation of an internal chill. Moaning and howling. Does absurd things. Marked action on the skin.

**Mind:** Delirium with singing, dancing and funny gestures. Everything appears strange and terrible. Confounds present with the past; feels like a child. Stupid feeling. Melancholy, with indifference. Mistrustful. *Epilepsy*; moaning and whining. Vivid dreams.

**Head:** *Head turned or twisted to one side. Cerebro-spinal meningitis. Cervical muscles contracted.* Vertigo with gastralgia and muscular spasms. Sudden, violent shocks through the head. Stares persistently at objects. *Convulsions* from concussion of the brain. Thick, yellow scabs on the head. Head symptoms relieved by emission of flatus.

**Eyes:** While reading, letters disappear. *Pupils dilated, insensible strabismus.* Objects recede, approach and seem double (diplopia). Eyes stare. Pupils go behind the upper lids as the head inclines. Effects of exposure to snow. Spasmodic affections of the eyes and its appendages. Strabismus; periodic, spasmodic after a fall or a blow.

**Ears:** Difficulty in hearing. Sudden detonations especially on swallowing. *Hemorrhage from the ears.*

**Face:** Pustules which run together forming thick, yellow scabs on the face and head, corners of mouth and chin, with a burning pain. *Red face.* Trismus; disposition to grind teeth.

**Throat:** Dry. Feels as if closed. Spasms of the esophagus; cannot swallow. Effects on esophagus from swallowing a sharp piece of bone.

**Stomach:** Thirst; burning pressure; *hiccough.* Throbbing in the pit of the stomach which is raised to the size of a fist. Desire for unnatural things, *like coal* (*Alum., Calc.*). Indigestion, with insensibility, frothing at mouth.

**Abdomen:** Flatulence with anxiety and crossness. Rumbling. Distended and painful. Colic with convulsions.

**Rectum:** Diarrhea in the morning with an irresistible desire to micturate. Itching in rectum.

**Respiratory:** Chest feels tight; can hardly breathe. Tonic spasm in the pectoral muscles. Heat in the chest.

**Back and Extremities:** Spasms and cramps in muscles of the nape of neck and spasmodic drawing of the head backward. Curved limbs cannot be straightened nor straight ones, bent. *Back bent backward like an arch* (opisthotonus). Jerking, tearing in coccyx, especially during menses.

**Skin:** Eczema; no itching, exudation forms into a *hard, lemon colored crust.* Suppressed eruption causes brain disease. Elevated eruptions, as large as peas. Chronic impetigo.

**Modalities:** *Worse,* from touch, draughts, concussion, tobacco smoke.

**Relationship:** Antidotes: *Op., Arn.*

Compare: *Cicuta maculata*—Water hemlock (effects very similar; the most prominent symptoms being: Falls unconscious, tetanic or clonic convulsions.

Body covered with sweat. Consider in epilepsy and tetanus. Tincture and lower potencies). *Hydr-ac., Con., Oean., Stry., Bell.*

**Dose:** Sixth to two hundredth attenuation.

---

## CIMEX LECTULARIS—ACANTHIA

(Bedbug) **Cimx.**

Of use in intermittent fever with weariness and an inclination to stretch. Hamstrings feel too short (*Am-m.*). Flexors mostly affected. Sensation of retraction of arm tendons. Stretching.

**Head:** Violent headache caused by drinking. Great rage; vehement at the beginning of chilly stage. Would like to tear everything to pieces. Pain under the right frontal bone.

**Rectum:** Constipation, feces dry, hard and in small balls (*Op., Plb., Thuj.*). Ulcer of rectum.

**Female:** Shooting pain from vagina, up towards the left ovary.

**Fever:** Chilliness of the whole body. Sensation as if wind blowing on the knees. *Pain in all joints, as if tendons were too short,* especially knee joints. Chills; worse lying down. Thirst during apyrexia, but little during the chilly stage; still less during the heat stage and none during sweating. Musty, offensive sweat.

**Dose:** Sixth to two hundredth attenuation.

---

## CIMICIFUGA RACEMOSA—ACTAEA RACEMOSA (MACROTYS)

(Black Snakeroot) **Cimic.**

Has a wide action on the cerebrospinal and muscular system, as well as on the uterus and ovaries. Especially useful in rheumatic, nervous subjects with ovarian irritation, uterine cramps and heavy limbs. Its muscular and crampy pains, primarily of neurotic origin, occurring in nearly every part of the body are characteristic. *Agitation and pain* indicate it. Pain like electric shocks here and there. Migraine. Symptoms referable to the pelvic organs prominent. "It lessens the frequency and force of the pulse, soothes pain and allays irritability."

**Mind:** Sensation of a cloud enveloping her. Great depression, with *dreams of impending evil.* Fears riding in a closed carriage, of being obliged to jump out. Incessant talking. Visions of rats, mice, etc. Delirium tremens; tries to injure himself. Mania following disappearance of neuralgia.

**Head:** Wild feeling in the brain. Shooting and throbbing pains in the head after mental worry, over study or as a reflex of uterine disease. Waving sensation or *sensation of opening and shutting in the brain.* Brain feels too large. *Pain, pressing outward* (meningitis).

**Eyes:** Asthenopia associated with pelvic problems. Deep seated throbbing and *shooting pains* in the eyes with photophobia from artificial light. *Intense aching in the eyeball. Pain from* eyes *radiating to the top of the head.*

**Ears:** Tinnitus. Ears sensitive to least noise.

**Stomach:** Nausea and vomiting caused by pressure on the spine and cervical region. Sinking in the epigastrium (*Sep., Sulph.*). *Gnawing pain.* Tongue pointed and trembling.

**Female:** Amenorrhea (use Macrotin preferably). Pain in the ovarian region; shoots upward and down the anterior surface of thighs. Pain immediately before menses. Menses profuse, dark, *coagulated,* offensive with backache (menorrhagia, dysmenorrhea), nervousness; always irregular. Ovarian neuralgia (ovaritis, cyst). *Pain across the pelvis, from hip to hip.* After-pains with great sensitiveness and *intolerance to pain.* Infra-mammary pains, worse left side. Facial blemishes in young women.

**Respiratory:** Tickling in the throat. Dry, short cough, *worse speaking* and at night. Cough when secretion is scanty, spasmodic, dry with muscular soreness and nervous irritation

**Heart**: Irregular, slow, trembling pulse. Tremulous action. Angina pectoris. Numbness of the left arm; feels as if bound to the side. Heart's action ceases suddenly, impending suffocation. Left sided infra-mammary pain.

**Back:** Spine very sensitive, especially the upper part (cervical spondylosis). *Stiffness and contraction in the neck and back* (cerebro-spinal meningitis). Intercostal rheumatism. Rheumatic pains in muscles of back and neck. Pain in the lumbar and sacral region, down the thighs, and through the hips. Crick in the back.

**Extremities:** Uneasy, restless feeling in the limbs. Aching in limbs and *muscular soreness*. Rheumatism affecting the belly of muscles, especially large muscles. Choreic movements accompanied by rheumatism. Jerking of limbs. Stiffness in tendo-Achilles. Heaviness in the lower extremities. Heavy, aching, tensive pain.

**Sleep:** Sleeplessness. Irritation of the brain in children during dentition.

**Skin:** Locally and internally for ivy poisoning.

**Modalities:** *Worse,* morning, cold (except headache), during menses; the more profuse the flow, the greater the suffering. *Better,* warmth, eating.

**Relationship:** Compare: *Rhamnus californica (muscular pains,* lumbago, pleurodynia, acute rheumatism). *Derris pinnata* (neuralgic headaches of rheumatic origin). *Aristolochia milhomens* (pain in tendo-Achilles; diabetes). *Caul., Puls., Lil-t., Agar., Macrotinum* (especially for lumbago).

**Dose:** First to thirtieth attenuation, third most frequently used.

---

# CINA MARITIMA

(Worm-seed) **Cina**

This is a children's remedy, big, fat, rosy, scrofulous, corresponding to many conditions that may be referred to intestinal irritation such as worms and accompanying complaints. An irritability of temper, variable appetite, grinding of teeth and even convulsions with screams and violent jerkings of the hands and feet are all within its range of action. The *Cina* patient is hungry, cross, ugly and wants to be rocked. *Pain in shocks.* Skin sensitive to touch.

**Mind:** Ill-humored. Child *very cross;* does not want to be touched, caressed or carried. Desires many things but rejects every thing offered. Abnormal consciousness, as if having committed some evil deed.

**Head:** Headache, alternating with pain in the abdomen. Relieved by stooping (*Mez.*). Headache on using the eyes.

**Eyes:** Dilated pupils; yellow vision. Weak sight from masturbation. Strabismus from abdominal irritation. Eyestrain, especially when presbyopia sets in. *Pulsations of the superciliary muscle.*

**Ears:** Digging and scratching in the ears.

**Nose:** Itching in the nose all the time. *Wants to rub it* and pick at it. *Bores the nose* till it bleeds.

**Face:** Intense, circumscribed redness of cheeks. *Pale,* hot, *with dark rings around the eyes.* Cold perspiration. *White and bluish discoloration around the mouth.* Grits teeth during sleep. *Choreic movements of face* and hands.

**Stomach:** Gets hungry soon after a meal. Hungry, digging, gnawing sensation. Epigastric pain; worse on waking in the morning and before meals. Vomiting and diarrhea immediately after eating or drinking. Vomiting with a clean tongue. Desires many and different things. Craving for sweets.

**Abdomen:** *Twisting pain around the navel* (*Spig.*). Bloated and hard abdomen.

**Stool:** White mucus, like small pieces of popped corn, preceded by pinching colic. *Itching in the anus* (*Teucr.*). Worms (*Sabad., Naphtin., Nat-p.*).

**Urinary:** Turbid, white urine; turns milky on standing (phosphaturia). Involuntary at night (nocturnal enuresis).

**Female:** Uterine hemorrhage before puberty.

**Respiratory:** Gagging cough in the morning. Whooping cough. Violent recurring paroxysms, down in the throat. Cough ends in a spasm. Cough violent enough to bring tears and sternal pain; feels as if something had been torn off (bronchitis). Periodic; returning in the spring and fall. Swallows after coughing. *Audible gurgling from the throat to the stomach after drinking.* Child is afraid to speak or move for the fear of bringing on a paroxysm of cough. After coughing, moans, anxious, gasps for air and turns pale.

**Extremities:** *Twitching* and jerking, distortion of limbs, trembling (epilepsy). Paralyzed shocks; patient will jump suddenly, as though in pain. Child throws arms from side to side. Nocturnal convulsions. *Sudden inward jerking of fingers of right hand. Child stretches out feet spasmodically.* Left foot in constant spasmodic motion.

**Sleep:** Child gets on hands and knees in sleep; on the abdomen. Night terrors in children; cries out, screams, wakes up frightened. *Problems while yawning.* Screams and talks in sleep. Grits teeth.

**Fever:** Light chill. High fever, associated with a clean tongue. Very hungry; colicky pains; chilliness with thirst. Cold sweat on the forehead, nose and hands. In *Cina* fever, face is cold and hands warm.

**Modalities:** *Worse,* looking fixedly at an object, from worms, at night, in the sun, in summer.

**Relationship:** Compare: *Santoninum* (often preferable in worm affections; same symptoms as *Cina*; corresponding to the "pain in shocks" produced by *Cina.* Visual illusions, *yellow* sight; violet light not recognized, colors not distinguishable. Urine, deep saffron in color. Spasms and twitchings, chronic gastric and intestinal problems, sometimes removed by a single dose (physiological) of *Santoninum.* Dahlke). *Helminthochortos*—Worm moss (acts very powerfully on intestinal worms, especially the lumbricoids). *Teucr., Ign., Cham., Spig.*

Antidote: *Camph., Caps.*

**Dose:** Third attenuation. In nervous irritable children, thirtieth and two hundredth preferable. *Santoninum* in first (with care) and third trituration.

---

## CINCHONA OFFICINALIS—CHINA

(Peruvian Bark) **Chin.**

*Debility* from exhausting discharges, from loss of vital fluids, together with a *nervous erethism* calls for this remedy. Periodicity is most marked. Sensitive to draughts. Seldom indicated in the earlier stages of acute diseases. Chronic gout. Chronic suppurative pyelitis. Post-operative gas pains, no relief from passing it.

**Mind:** Apathetic, indifferent, disobedient, taciturn, despondent. Ideas crowd in mind; prevent sleep. Disposition to hurt other people's feelings. Cries suddenly and tossing about.

**Head:** As if the skull would burst. Sensation as if the brain was balancing to and fro and striking against the skull, receiving great pain (*Sulph., Sul-ac.*). Intense *throbbing* in the head and carotids. Spasmodic headache in the vertex with subsequent pain, as if sides of head were bruised. Face flushed after hemorrhages, sexual excesses or loss of vital fluids. Relieved from pressure and warm room. Scalp sensitive; worse combing hair. Aches worse in open air, from temple to temple. Worse by contact, current of air, stepping. Dizzy when walking.

**Eyes:** Blue color around the eyes. Hollow eyes. Yellowish sclera. Black specks, bright dazzling illusions; night blindness (nyctalopia) in an anemic retina. Spots before the eyes. Photophobia. Distortion of eyeballs. Intermittent ciliary neuralgia. *Pressure in eyes.* Amaurosis; scalding lachrymation.

**Ears:** *Ringing* in ears, Meniere's disease. External ear sensitive to touch. Hearing sensitive to noise. Lobules red and swollen.

**Nose:** Checked catarrh. Epistaxis, especially on rising. Coryza, sneezing, watery discharge. Violent, *dry* sneezing. Cold sweat around the nose.

**Face:** Sallow complexion. Face bloated; red.

**Mouth:** Toothache; better pressing teeth firmly together, and by warmth. Tongue coated thick, dirty; tip burns, succeeded by ptyalism. Bitter taste. Food tastes too salty.

**Stomach:** Tender, cold. Vomiting of undigested food. Slow digestion. Weight after eating. Ill effects of tea. Hungry without appetite. Flat taste. Darting pain crosswise in the hypogastric region. Milk disagrees. Hungry, longing for food which lies undigested. *Flatulence; belching* of bitter fluid or regurgitation of food *gives no relief;* worse eating fruit. *Hiccough.* Bloatedness better by movement.

**Abdomen:** Severe flatulent colic; better bending double. *Tympanitic abdomen* (peritonitis). Pain in the right hypochondrium. *Gall stone colic* (*Triumfetta rhomboidea*). Liver and spleen swollen and enlarged. Jaundice. Internal coldness of stomach and abdomen. Gastro-duodenal catarrh.

**Stool:** Undigested (lienteria), frothy, yellow; *painless;* worse at night, after meals, during hot weather, from *fruit,* milk, beer. Very weakening with much flatulence. Difficult even when soft (*Alum., Plat.*).

**Male**: Excited, lascivious fancy. Frequent emissions (spermato- rrhea), followed by great weakness. Orchitis.

**Female**: Menses too early. *Dark clots and abdominal distention.* Profuse menses with pain (dysmenorrhea). Desire too strong. Bloody leucorrhea. Seems to take the place of the usual menstrual discharge. Painful heaviness in the pelvis.

**Respiratory**: Influenza with debility. Cannot breathe with head low. Labored, slow respiration; constant choking. *Suffocative catarrh;* rattling in the chest; violent, hacking cough *after every meal.* Hemorrhage from lungs. Dyspnea, sharp pain in the left lung (pleurisy). Asthma; worse damp weather.

**Heart**: Irregular with weak rapid beats followed by strong, hard beats. Suffocative attacks, syncope; anemia and dropsy.

**Back**: Sharp pain across the kidneys, worse movement and at night. Knife-like pains around the back (D. MacFarlan).

**Extremities**: *Pain in limbs and joints, as if sprained; worse, slight touch;* hard pressure relieves. Sensation of a string around the limb. Joints swollen; very sensitive, with dread of open air. Great debility, trembling, with a numb sensation. Averse to exercise; sensitive to touch. Weariness of joints; worse, mornings and when sitting (arthritis).

**Sleep**: Drowsiness. Unrefreshing sleep, constant stupor. Wakes up early. Protracted sleeplessness. Anxious, frightening dreams, confused consciousness on waking, cannot get rid of the dream and fear of dream remains. Snoring, especially in children.

**Fever**: Intermittent paroxysms return every week. All stages well marked. Chills, generally in the forenoon, commencing in the breast; thirst before chill, little and often. Debilitating night sweats. Free perspiration caused by every little exertion, especially on single parts. Hay fever, watery coryza, pain in the temples.

**Skin**: *Extreme sensitiveness to touch, but hard pressure relieves. Coldness;* increased sweat. One hand ice cold, the other warm. Anasarca (*Ars., Apis*). *Dermatitis;* erysipelas. Indurated glands; scrofulous ulcers and caries.

**Modalities**: *Worse, on slightest touch,* draught of air; every other day; loss of vital fluids; at night; *after eating;* bending over. *Better,* bending double; hard pressure; open air; warmth.

**Relationship:** Antidotes: *Arn., Ars., Nux-v., Ip.*

Compare: *Quinidinum* (paroxysmal tachycardia and *auricular fibrillation.* Heart is slowed, and the auriculo-ventricular conduction time is lengthened. Dose 1/2 grain t. i. d.). *Cephalanthus occidentalis*—Button bush (intermittent fever, sore throat, rheumatic symptoms, vivid dreams). *Ars., Cedr., Nat-s., Cydonia vulgaris*—Quince (supposed to be of use in strengthening the sexual organs and stomach).

Complementary: *Ferr., Calc-p.*

**Dose:** Tincture to thirtieth potency.

---

# CINERARIA MARITIMA

(Dusty Miller) **Cine.**

Has some reputation in the cure of cataract and corneal opacities. Is used externally by instilling into the eye, one drop four or five times a day. This must be kept up for several months. Most effective in traumatic cases. Compare in cataract, *Phos., Cann-s., Caust., Naphtin., Led., Nat-m., Sil., Platan.*

---

# CINNABARIS—MERCURIUS SULPHURATUS RUBER

(Mercuric Sulphide) **Cinnb.**

For certain forms of ciliary neuralgia and ulceration on a syphilitic base, this remedy is most effective. Sleepless at night.

**Head:** Congestion of the head.

**Eyes:** *Pain from the lachrymal duct radiates around the eye, to the temple, from the inner canthus, across the brow to the ear. Severe shooting pain in the bones of orbit, especially running from the inner to the outer canthus in the bone. Redness of the whole eye.* Lids granulated; canthi and lids red.

**Nose:** Pressive sensation, as if from heavy spectacles. Pain around the root, extending into the bones on each side (*Aur., Kali- i.*).

**Throat:** Stringy mucus passed through the posterior nares into the throat (post-nasal drip). Dryness of the mouth and throat; must rinse the mouth. Fiery looking ulcers in the mouth and throat (stomatitis).

**Male:** Prepuce swollen; *warts* on it, which bleed easily; testicles enlarged; buboes; angry looking chancres. Syphilides, squamous and vesicular.

**Female:** Leucorrhea. Sensation of pressure in the vagina.

**Extremities:** Pain in the forearm, from the elbow down, including hands. Pain in long bones when barometric level lowers; coldness in the joints.

**Skin:** *Very fiery red* looking ulcers. Nodes on shin bones. Buboes. Condyloma, easily bleeding.

**Modalities:** *Worse,* lying on the right side (feels as if the contents of the body were being dragged over to that side).

**Relationship:** Compare: *Hep., Nit-ac., Thuj., Sep.*

Antidotes: *Hep., Sulph.*

**Dose:** First to third trituration.

---

# CINNAMONUM CEYLANICUM

(Cinnamon) **Cinnm.**

Cancer where pain and fetor are present. Best when skin is intact. Its use in hemorrhages has abundant clinical verification. Epistaxis. Hemorrhages from the bowels, hemoptysis, etc. Strain in the loins or a false step brings on a profuse flow of bright blood. *Post-partum hemorrhage.* Flatulence and diarrhea. Feeble patients with languid circulation.

**Female:** Bearing down sensation. Menses *early, profuse, prolonged, bright red.* Sleepy. No desire for anything. Fingers seem swollen. Uterine hemorrhages caused by overlifting, during puerperal state; menorrhagia, metrorrhagia.

**Relationship:** Compare: *Ip., Sil., Tril-p.*

Antidote: *Acon.*

**Dose:** Tincture to third potency. For cancer, strong decoction, one-half pint in a day. *Oil of cinnamon* in aqueous solution, best local disinfectant. 3-4 drops in two quarts of water as a douche, wherever a germicide and disinfectant is needed. Three drops on sugar for hiccough.

---

# CISTUS CANADENSIS

(Rock Rose) **Cist.**

A deep acting, anti-psoric remedy, with a marked action on glandular affections, herpetic eruptions, chronic swellings when a patient is *extremely sensitive to cold. Sensation of coldness in various parts.* Scrofulous ophthalmia. Poisoned wounds, bites, phagedenic ulcers. *Carcinomatous diseases of glands in the neck. Cist.* has an affinity for the naso-pharynx; aborts colds, that center in the posterior nose. Sniffling. Hemicrania (migraine).

**Ears:** Watery discharge; also fetid pus (otorrhea). Tetter on and around the ears, extending to the external meatus.

**Face:** Itching, burning and crusts on the right zygoma. Lupus, caries; open, bleeding cancer. Tip of the nose, painful.

**Mouth:** Scorbutic swollen gums. *Mouth feels cold;* putrid, impure breath. *Pyorrhea* (*Merc-c., Caust., Staph., Kreos.*). *Hurts to protrude the tongue.*

**Throat:** Spongy feeling; *very dry* and *cold air passing over the parts causes pain.* Breath, tongue, and throat feel cold. Uvula and tonsils swollen. A small, dry spot in the throat; must sip water frequently. Hawking of mucus. Swelling and suppuration of glands in the throat (follicular tonsillitis). Head drawn to one side by swellings in neck (parotiditis). Sore throat from inhaling the least *cold air.* Heat and itching in the throat.

**Stomach:** *Cool feeling* in the stomach, before and after eating. *Cool feeling* in the entire abdomen. Desire for cheese.

**Stool:** Diarrhea from coffee and fruit, thin, yellow, urgent; worse in the morning.

**Female:** Induration and inflammation of mammae (mastitis). Sensitive to cold air. Bad smelling leucorrhea.

**Respiratory:** Asthmatic after lying down (trachea feels narrow), preceded by formication.

**Chest:** Coldness in the chest. The neck is studded with tumors. Induration of mammae. Hemorrhage from the lungs.

**Extremities:** Sprained pain in the wrist. Tips of fingers sensitive to cold. Tetter on hands. Cold feet. Syphilitic ulcers on the lower limbs, with a hard swelling around. White swelling.

**Sleep:** Cannot sleep from the coldness in the throat.

**Skin:** Itching all over. Small, painful pimples; lupus. *Glands inflamed and indurated.* Mercurio-syphilitic ulcers. Skin of hands hard, thick, dry, fissured; deep cracks. Itching in swollen hands and arms; general itching which prevents sleep.

**Modalities:** *Worse,* slightest exposure to cold air; mental exertion, excitement. *Better* after eating.

**Relationship**: Antidotes: *Rhus-t., Sep.*

Compare: *Con., Carb-v., Calc., Arg-n.*

**Dose**: First to thirtieth attenuation. Locally as a wash to arrest fetid discharges.

---

## CITRUS VULGARIS

(Bitter Orange) **Cit-v.**

Headache with nausea, vomiting and vertigo. Facial neuralgias mostly right sided. Thoracic oppression. Frequent and irresistible yawning. Disturbed sleep.

**Relationship**: *Citrus decumana*—Grape fruit (tinnitus, *noises in the head* and ringing in ears. Sensation of pressure in the temporal region). *Aurantium*—Orange (neuralgic and skin symptoms. Itching, redness and swelling of hands. Diseases of the aged with coldness and chilliness. Boiled, dried *orange peel* excites the intestines in a manner similar to other forms of cellulose or agar. There is an increased flow of bile which continues for hours. It unites both, a cholagogue action with a mechanical stimulus to peristalsis).

Compare: *Citrus limonum* (scorbutus, sore throat and cancer pains; checks excessive menstruation). *Citricum acidum* (useful in *scurvy,* chronic rheumatism and hemorrhages. All forms of *dropsy* are benefited with *Cit-ac.* and lemon juice, a tablespoonful every 3-4 hours. Pain from cancer of tongue. Used as a local application and mouth wash, one dram to 8 ozs. of water. For cancer pains generally, often effective).

---

## CLEMATIS ERECTA

(Virgin's Bower) **Clem.**

Scrofulous, rheumatic, gonorrheal and syphilitic patients. Acts especially on the skin, *glands* and genito-urinary organs, especially on the testicles. A remedy of marked importance in disturbances of sleep and neuralgic *pains* in various parts. Many of these pains are relieved by perspiration. Muscles, relaxed or twitching. Great emaciation. *Great sleepiness.* Distant pulsations in the entire body.

**Head**: Boring pains in the temples. *Feels confused; better in the open air.* Eruptions on the occiput, at the base of hair, moist, pustular, sensitive, itching.

**Eyes:** Heat in the eyes and *sensitive to air;* must close them. Chronic blepharitis with sore and swollen Meibomian glands (styes). Iritis, great *sensitiveness to cold.* Flickering before the eyes. Pustular conjunctivitis with tinea capitis; eyes inflamed and protruding (exopthalmos).

**Face:** White blisters on the face and nose, as if sun burnt. Swelling of the submaxillary glands with hard tubercles; throbbing, aggravated on being touched. Pain on the right side of the face radiating to the eye, ear and temple; better, holding cold water in the mouth.

**Mouth:** *Toothache; worse, at night and from tobacco.* Teeth feel too long.

**Stomach:** After eating, weakness in all the limbs and pulsation in arteries.

**Urinary:** Tingling in the urethra lasting some time after micturating. Frequent, scanty micturition; burning at the orifice. *Interrupted flow.* Urethra feels constricted. Urine emitted drop by drop. Inability to pass all the urine; dribbling after micturition. Pain worse at night, pain along the spermatic cord. Commencing stricture.

**Male:** Ilio-scrotal neuralgia. *Testicles indurated with a bruised feeling.* Swelling in the scrotum (orchitis), right half only. Problems from suppressed gonorrhea. Violent erections with stitches in the urethra. Testicles hang heavy or retracted, with pain along the spermatic cord; worse, right side.

**Skin:** Red, burning, vesicular, scaly, scabby. Itches terribly; worse, washing in cold water; worse face, hands and *scalp around the occiput. Glands* hot, painful, *swollen;* worse inguinal glands. Glandular indurations and tumors of breast. Varicose ulcers.

**Modalities:** *Better,* in open air. *Worse,* at night, and by warmth of bed, washing in cold water; new moon (monthly aggravation).

**Relationship:** Compare: *Clematis vitalba* (varicose and other ulcers). *Sil., Staph., Petr., Olean., Sars., Canth., Ph-ac., Puls.*

Antidotes: *Bry., Camph.*

**Dose:** Third to thirtieth potency.

---

## COBALTUM METALLICUM

(The Metal Cobalt) **Cob.**

Adapted to neurasthenic spinal states. Sexual disturbances. Fatigue, agitation and bone pains, worse in the morning.

**Mind:** All mental excitement increases suffering. Constant change in moods.

**Head:** Aches; worse, bending head *forward.* Itching of the hairy scalp and beard.

**Mouth:** Teeth feel too long. Toothache. Cracks across the tongue (fissures). Coated white (*Ant-c.*).

**Abdomen:** Shooting pains in the liver. Pain in the spleen.

**Rectum:** Constant dropping of blood from the anus, no blood with the stools.

**Male:** Pain in the right testicle; better, micturating. Emissions, without erection. Impotence. Backache in the lumbar region and weak legs. Lewd dreams. Pain at the end of urethra; greenish discharge (gonorrhea); brown spots on genitals and abdomen.

**Back:** *Pain in the back and sacrum; worse while sitting;* better, walking or lying. Weakness in legs and backache after emissions.

**Extremities:** Aching in wrist joints. Pain shooting into the thighs from the liver. *Weak knees.* Trembling in limbs. Tingling in feet. Foot-sweat, mostly between toes.

**Sleep:** Unrefreshing; *disturbed by lewd dreams.*

**Skin:** Dry and pimply. Pimples around the nates, chin, hairy scalp.

**Relationship:** Compare: *Cann-i., Sep., Zinc., Agn., Sel.*

**Dose:** Sixth to thirtieth potency.

---

# COCA—ERYTHROXYLON COCA

(The Divine Plant of the Incas—but the Spanish Priests Denounced it as "Un Delusio Del Demonio") **Coca**

A mountaineer's remedy. Useful in a variety of complaints incidental to mountain climbing, such as palpitations, dyspnea, anxiety and insomnia. Exhausted nervous system from physical and mental strain. Caries of teeth. *Loss of voice*: Give 5-6 drops, every half hour, two hours before expected demand on voice. Nocturnal enuresis. Emphysema (*Queb.*).

**Mind:** Melancholy; bashful, ill at ease in society, irritable, delights in solitude and obscurity. Sense of right and wrong abolished.

**Head:** Fainting fit from climbing mountains. Shocks coming from the occiput with vertigo. *Noises in the ear.* Headache with vertigo, preceded by flashes of light. Sensation of a band across the forehead. Diplopia. Tongue furred. *Headaches at high altitudes.* Tinnitus.

**Stomach:** Peppery sensation in the mouth. Longing for alcoholic liquors and tobacco. Great satiety for a long time. Incarcerated flatus; rises with noise and violence, as if it would split the esophagus. Tympanitic distention of the abdomen. No appetite but for sweets.

**Male:** Diabetes with impotency (*Ph-ac.*).

**Respiratory:** Hawking of small, transparent pieces of mucus. Weak vocal cords. *Hoarseness;* worse after talking. *Want of breath, short breath* especially in aged athletes and alcoholics. Hemoptysis. *Asthma,* spasmodic variety.

**Heart:** *Palpitations,* with a weak heart and dyspnea.

**Sleep:** Can find no rest anywhere, but sleepy. Nervousness and nocturnal restlessness during teething.

**Modalities:** *Better,* from wine; riding, fast motion in open air. *Worse,* ascending, high altitudes.

**Relationship:** Compare: *Ars., Paull., Cypr., Cham.*

Antidote: *Gels.*

**Dose:** Tincture to third attenuation.

---

# COCAINUM HYDROCHLORICUM

(An Alkaloid from Erythroxylon Coca) **Cocain.**

Besides the great usefulness of *Cocain.* as a local anesthetic, it has specific homeopathic uses, though the symptoms are mainly clinical.

Sensation *of small foreign bodies* or *worms under the skin.*

**Mind:** Talkative. Constant desire to do something great, *to undertake vast feats of strength.* Cerebral activity. Frightful persecutory hallucinations;

*sees and feels bugs and worms. Moral sense blunted.* Personal appearance neglected. Thinks he hears unpleasant remarks about himself. Hallucinations of hearing. Irrational *jealousy.* Insomnia.

**Head:** Throbbing and bursting sensation. Roaring and noises in the head.

**Eyes:** Glaucoma, increased tension, decreased corneal sensibility. Eyes staring, expressionless. *Pupils dilated.*

**Ears:** Acute hearing.

**Throat:** Dry, burning, tickling, constricted, paralysis of muscles of deglutition. Speech difficult.

**Stomach:** Loss of appetite for solid food. *Likes sweets. Hemorrhages* from bowels, stomach.

**Sleep:** Restless, cannot sleep for hours after retiring.

**Nervous System:** Chorea; paralysis agitans; alcoholic tremors and senile trembling. Local sensory paralysis. Formication and numbness in hands and forearms.

**Fever:** Coldness with intense pallor.

**Relationship:** Compare: *Stovaine* (an analgesic, a vasomotor dilator). Antidote to disagreeable effects occasionally resulting from injection of cocaine into the skin or gums, drop doses of nitro-glycerine 1% sol.

**Dose:** Lower potencies. As a local application to mucous membranes, 2-4%.

---

## COCCINELLA SEPTEMPUNCTATA

(Lady Bug) **Cocc-s.**

This remedy ought to be remembered in neuralgias, teeth, gums, mouth, etc. Is awakened by profuse accumulation of saliva. Uvula feels too long. Symptoms of hydrophobia; worse, by any bright object.

**Head:** Pain in the forehead over the right eye, sensitive to touch; from superior molars to the forehead (facial neuralgia). Aching in temples and occiput. Rush of blood to face. *Throbbing toothache. Cold sensation in the teeth* and mouth (*Cist.*). Periodical attacks of frontal neuralgia. Cannot open eyes during paroxysm. Pain, worse from any bright object; better, sleep.

**Stomach:** Hiccough and burning in the stomach.

**Back:** Pain in *the region of kidneys and loins.* Icy cold extremities.

**Relationship:** Compare: *Canth., Mag-c.*

**Dose:** Third potency.

---

# COCCULUS INDICUS

(Indian Cockle) **Cocc.**

Within the sphere of action of *Cocc.* are many spasmodic and paretic affections, notably those affecting one-half of the body. Affects the cerebrum, will not cure convulsive seizures proceeding from the spinal cord (A. E. Hinsdale). *Painful contracture* of limbs and trunk; tetanus. Many evil *effects of night watching* are relieved by it. It shows a special attraction *for light haired females,* especially during pregnancy, causing marked nausea and backache. Unmarried and childless women, sensitive and romantic girls, etc. All its symptoms are worse riding in a carriage or on shipboard; hence its used in seasickness. Sensation of *hollowness* or emptiness, as if parts had gone off to sleep. Feels too weak to talk loud.

**Mind:** Capricious. Heavy and stupid. *Time passes too quickly;* absorbed in reveries. Inclination to sing irresistible. Slow in comprehension. Mind benumbed. *Profound sadness.* Cannot bear contradiction. Speaks hastily. Very anxious about the health of others.

**Head:** Vertigo, nausea, *especially when riding* or sitting up. Sense of emptiness in the head. Headache in *the occiput* and nape (cerebro-spinal meningitis); worse, lying on the back of head. Sick headache from riding in a carriage, cannot lie on back part of head. Pupils contracted. Opening and shutting sensation, especially in the occiput. Trembling of head. Pain in eyes, as if torn out of the head.

**Face:** Paralysis of facial nerve. Cramp-like pain in masseter muscle; *worse, opening the mouth.* Prosopalgia in the afternoon with wide radiations of pain.

**Stomach:** Nausea from riding in cars, boat, etc., or looking at a boat in motion; worse on becoming cold or taking cold. Nausea, with faintness and vomiting. *Aversion to food,* drink, tobacco. *Metallic taste.* Paralysis of muscles preventing deglutition. Dryness in the esophagus. Seasickness (*Res.* lx). Cramps, in the stomach during and after a meal. Hiccough and spasmodic yawning. Loss of appetite. Desire for cold drinks, especially beer. Sensation in the stomach as if one had been without food for a long time until hunger had disappeared. Smell of food disgusts (*Colch.*).

**Abdomen:** Distended, with wind, and sensation as *if full of sharp stones when moving;* better, lying on one side or the other. *Pain in the abdominal ring,* as if something was forced through. *Abdominal muscles weak;* it seems as if hernia would occur.

**Female:** Dysmenorrhea, with profuse dark menses. Menses too early, clotted, with spasmodic colic. Painful pressing in the uterine region, followed by hemorrhoids. Purulent, gushing leucorrhea between menses; *very weakening,* can scarcely speak. So weak during menstruation, she is scarcely able to stand.

**Respiratory:** Sensation of emptiness and cramps in the chest. Dyspnea from constriction of trachea, as if irritated by smoke. Choking constriction in the upper part of the esophagus, oppressing respiration and inducing cough.

**Back:** Cracking of cervical vertebrae on moving the head. *Paralytic pain in the lumbosacral region.* Pain *in the shoulder and arms, as if bruised.* Pressure in the scapula and nape. Stiffness on moving the shoulders.

**Extremities:** Lameness; worse by bending. *Trembling* (chorea) and pain in limbs. Arms go to sleep. One sided paralysis; worse after sleep. Hands are alternately hot and cold; numbness and cold sweat now of one, now of the other hand. Numb and unsteady. *Knees crack on motion.* Lower limbs are very weak. Inflammatory swelling of knees (arthritis). Intensely painful, paralytic drawing. Limbs straightened out, painful when flexed.

**Sleep:** Spasmodic yawning. Coma vigil. Constant drowsiness. After loss of sleep, night watching, nursing.

**Fever:** Chills with flatulent colic, nausea, vertigo, coldness in the lower extremities and heat of head. Sweat general. Nervous form of low fever. *Chilliness, with perspiration and heat of skin.*

**Modalities:** *Worse,* eating, after loss of sleep, open air, smoking, riding, swimming, touch, noise, jar; afternoon, menstrual period, after emotional disturbance.

**Relationship:** Antidotes: *Coff., Nux-v.*

Compare: *Picrotoxinum*—alkaloid of Cocculus (epilepsy, attacks in the morning on leaving horizontal position, hernia, locomotor ataxia, night sweats); *Symphoricarpus racemosus* (morning sickness); *Petr., Puls., Ign.*

**Dose:** Third to thirtieth potency.

---

# COCCUS CACTI

(Cochineal) **Coc-c.**

The clinical application of the symptoms of this remedy place it among the medicines for spasmodic and whooping coughs and catarrhal conditions of the bladder; spasmodic pains in kidneys (nephritis), with visceral tenesmus (cystitis). Anuria, anasarca, ascites.

**Mind:** Sad, early in the morning or in the afternoon.

**Head:** Suboccipital soreness; worse after sleep and exertion. Headache, worse from lying on back, better with the head high.

**Eyes:** Dull pain over right eye in the morning. *Sensation of a foreign body between upper lid and eyeball.* Distress from cinders lodged in eye.

**Urinary:** Urging to micturate; *brick red sediment. Urinary calculi, hematuria, urates* and uric acid; lancinating pains from the kidney to the bladder. Deep colored, thick urine (gonorrhea). Dysuria.

**Female:** Menses too early, profuse, *black* and thick (menorrhagia); *dark clots* with dysuria. Intermittent menstruation (metrorrhagia); flow only in the evening and at night. *Large clots* escape when passing urine. *Labia* inflamed.

**Respiratory:** Constant hawking from an enlarged uvula; coryza, with inflamed fauces; *accumulation of thick viscid mucus,* which is expectorated with great difficulty. *Tickling in the larynx.* Sensation of a crumb behind the larynx, must swallow continuously; brushing teeth causes cough. Fauces very sensitive. Suffocative cough; worse, on waking with tough, white mucus, which strangles (asthma). Spasmodic morning cough. *Whooping cough attacks end with vomiting of tough mucus.* Chronic bronchitis complicated with gravel; large quantities of albuminous, tenacious mucus are expectorated. Walking against the wind takes the breath away.

**Heart:** Sensation as if everything was pressed towards the heart.

**Modalities:** *Worse,* left side, after sleep, touch, pressure of clothing, brushing teeth, slightest exertion. *Better,* walking.

**Relationship:** Compare: *Canth., Cact., Sars.*

**Dose:** Lower triturations.

---

## COCHLEARIA ARMORACIA—ARMORACIA SATIVA

(Horse-radish) **Coch.**

Frontal bone and sinus, antrum and salivary glands are specifically affected by this drug. Bloated sensation. Raises the vital force. Used as a gargle in scorbutic gums and sore throat. Hoarseness and in relaxed conditions of the fauces. Internally in gonorrhea. Useful as a condiment in enfeebled states of the stomach. An infusion of the root in cider for dropsy, causes copious diuresis. Locally, cures dandruff.

**Head:** Thinking is difficult. Anxiety, driven to despair by pain. Pressing, boring pain as if the frontal bone would fall out. Violent headache with vomiting (migraine). Impaired hearing.

**Eyes:** *Sore and scrofulous;* traumatic inflammation of the eyes, blearedness and cataract. Copious lachrymation from eyes (conjunctivitis).

**Stomach:** Pain towards the back; worse, pressure on dorsal vertebrae. Belching and cramps. Colic with backache. *Violent cramps radiating from the stomach through both the sides to the back.* Griping around the navel.

**Urinary:** Burning and cutting in the glans penis before, during and after micturition. Frequent micturition.

**Respiratory:** Dry, hacking, laryngeal cough, also post-influenzal cough, dry or loose, worse lying down. Chest is painful to touch. Coryza, with hoarseness. Mucoid asthma. Edema of lungs. Throat feels rough and hoarse.

**Back:** Pain in the back from incarcerated flatus, radiates *from the abdomen to the back and down into the sacrum.*

**Modalities:** *Worse* evening and at night.

**Relationship:** Compare: *Cann-s., Sin-n., Caps.*

**Dose:** First to third attenuation.

---

## CODEINUM

(An Alkaloid From Opium) **Cod.**

Trembling of the whole body. Involuntary twitching in the muscles of arms and lower limbs (chorea). *Itching,* with a sensation of warmth, numbness and prickling. Diabetes.

**Head:** Pain from the occiput to the back of neck. Skin of face and scalp sore after neuralgia.

**Eyes:** Involuntary twitching of lids (*Agar.*).

**Stomach:** Spasmodic pain in the pit of the stomach. Eructations. Great thirst, with desire for bitter substances.

**Respiratory:** Short and irritating cough; worse, at night. Copious, purulent expectoration. Nocturnal cough of phthisis.

**Relationship:** Compare: *Op., Agar., Hyos., Am-br.*

**Dose:** One-quarter of a grain doses to the third trituration.

---

## COFFEA CRUDA

(Unroasted Coffee) **Coff.**

Stimulates the functional activity of all organs, increasing the nervous and vascular activity. Drinking of coffee by aged, is likely to increase production of uric acid, causing irritation of kidneys; muscle and joint pains; with the increased susceptibility of old people to the stimulating action of coffee and tea, their use should be curtailed or carefully watched. Great nervous agitation and restlessness. Extreme sensitiveness characterizes this remedy. Neuralgia in various parts, always with great nervous excitability and *intolerance of pain,* driving to despair. *Unusual activity of mind and body.* Bad effects of sudden emotions, surprises, joys, etc. Nervous palpitations. *Coff.* is specially suited to tall, lean, stooping people with dark complexions, temperament choleric and sanguine. Skin hypersensitive.

**Mind:** Gaiety, easy comprehension, irritability, excited; senses acute. Impressionable, especially to pleasurable impressions. Full of ideas, quick to act. Tossing about in anguish (*Acon.*).

**Head:** Tight pain, worse from noise, smell, narcotics. Seems as if the brain was torn to pieces, *as if a nail was driven in the head.* Worse in open air. *Sensitive hearing.*

**Face:** Dry heat, with red cheeks. Prosopalgia extending to the molars, ears, forehead and scalp.

**Mouth:** Toothache; temporarily relieved by holding ice water in the mouth (*Mang-act.* opposite). Hasty eating and drinking. Delicate taste.

**Stomach:** Excessive hunger. Intolerance of tight clothing. After wine and liquor.

**Female:** Menses too early (menorrhagia) and long lasting. Dysmenorrhea, large clots of black blood. *Hypersensitive vulva and vagina.* Voluptuous itching (pruritus vulva).

**Respiratory:** Short, dry cough of measles in nervous, delicate children.

**Heart:** Violent irregular palpitations especially after excessive joy or surprise. Rapid high tension, pulse and urinary suppression.

**Extremities:** Crural neuralgia; worse, motion, afternoon and at night; better, by pressure.

**Sleep:** Wakeful; on a constant move. Sleeps till 3 a. m., after which only dozes. Wakes with a start, sleep disturbed by dreams. *Sleepless, on account of mental activity;* flow of ideas, with nervous excitability. Disturbed by itching in the anus.

**Modalities:** *Worse,* excessive emotions (joy), narcotics, strong odors, noise, open air, cold, night. *Better,* warmth, from lying down; holding ice in mouth.

**Relationship:** Incompatible: *Camph., Cocc.*

Complementary: *Acon.*

Compare: *Coffea tosta* (roasting develops certain vitamin-like substances (P. T. Mattei). Pigeons, who have developed "deficiency" neuritis and paralysis on a diet of polished rice lost their disabilities on the addition of 8cc to a 5% infusion of coffee to their food. Unroasted coffee was useless). *Caffeinum* (a crystalline alkaloid—is a direct heart stimulant and diuretic. Dropsy depending on cardiac insufficiency. Myocardial degeneration. Cardiac insufficiency in pneumonia and other infectious diseases. Raises the blood pressure, increases the pulse rate and stimulates the heart muscle; hence, supports in extreme weakness or threatened failure. Stimulates the respiratory centre, nerve centres and *increases diuresis.* One of the best stimulants of the vasomotor centres. Acute pulmonary edema. Brachialgia and other neuralgias characterized by nocturnal *exacerbations.* Jousset uses equal parts of caffein and sacchar. l. 3 grains taken in divided doses every other day. Hypodermically, 1/4 grain. Excruciating facial neuralgia from decaying teeth); *Acon., Cham., Nux-v., Cypr., Caffeinum* and plants containing it, like *Kola, Thea,* etc.

Strong black coffee, drunk as hot as possible, is indispensable as an antidote in a large number of poisons, especially narcotics. Hot coffee by rectum in cases of extreme collapse.

Antidotes: *Nux-v., Tab.*

**Dose:** Third to two hundredth potency.

---

# COLCHICUM AUTUMNALE

(Meadow Saffron) **Colch.**

Affects the muscular tissues, periosteum and synovial membranes of joints markedly. Has specific power in relieving the gouty paroxysms. It seems to be more beneficial in chronic affections of these parts. The parts are red, hot, swollen. Tearing pains; worse in the evening, at night and from touch; stubbing the toes hurts exceedingly. *There is always great prostration,* internal *coldness* and a tendency to collapse. Effects of night watching and hard study. Shocks as from electricity through one half of the body. Bad effects from suppressed sweat. Dreams of mice.

**Head**: Headache chiefly frontal and temporal, also occipital and in the nape of the neck, worse afternoon and evening.

**Eyes**: Pupils unequal; left pupil contracted. Variations in visual acuity (cataract). Lachrymation worse in open air; violent tearing pain in the eyes. Dim vision after reading (aesthenopia). Spots before the eyes.

**Ears**: Itching in the ears; sharp, shooting pains below the right tragus.

**Face**: Pain in facial muscles, worse moving about. Tingling and edematous swelling; cheeks red, hot, sweaty. Very irritable because of the pains (*Cham.*). Pain behind the angle of right lower jaw.

**Stomach**: Dry mouth, tongue burns, painful gums and teeth. *Thirst;* pain in the stomach with flatulence. The *smell of food causes nausea, even fainting,* especially fish. Profuse salivary secretion. Vomiting of mucus, bile and food; worse, any motion; *great coldness in the stomach. Craving for various things* but becomes averse to them on smelling, followed by nausea. Gouty gastralgia. Burning or icy coldness in the stomach and abdomen. Thirst for effervescent, alcoholic beverages. Pain in the transverse colon.

**Abdomen:** *Distention* of abdomen with gas and an inability to stretch out legs. Borborygmi. Pain over the liver region. Caecum and ascending colon very distended. Fullness and continuous rumbling. Ascites.

**Stool:** Painful, scanty, transparent, jelly-like mucus (intestinal catarrh); pain, as if anus was torn open (proctitis), with prolapse. Autumnal dysentery; stools contain *white shreddy particles* in large quantities. Ineffectual pressing; feels the faeces in the rectum, but cannot expel them.

**Urinary:** Dark, scanty or suppressed; bloody, brown, black, inky; contains clots of putrid, decomposed blood, albumin (nephritis) and sugar (diabetes).

**Female:** Pruritus of genitals. Cold sensation in the thighs after menses. Sensation of swelling in the vulva and clitoris.

**Heart:** Anxiety in the region of heart. Impulse not felt. Pericarditis with severe pain, oppression and dyspnea, pulse thread-like. Heart sounds become weaker with low tension pulse.

**Back:** Aching in the lumbar and lumbosacral region. Dull pain across the loins. Backache, better, rest and pressure.

**Extremities:** Sharp pain down the left arm. Tearing in the limbs during warm weather, stinging during cold. Pins and needles in hands and wrists, fingertips are numb. Pain in the front of thigh. Right plantar reflex abolished. Limbs, lame, weak, tingling. Pain worse in the evening and in warm weather. Joints stiff and feverish; shifting rheumatism; pains worse at night. Inflammation of the great toe, gout in the heel, *cannot bear to have it touched or moved.* Tingling in the finger nails. Knees strike together, can hardly walk (knock knees). Edematous swelling and coldness of legs and feet.

**Skin:** Blotchy, papular rash on face. Pink spots on the back, chest and abdomen. Urticaria.

**Modalities:** *Worse,* sunset to sunrise, motion, loss of sleep, smell of food, in the evening, mental exertion. *Better,* stooping.

**Relationship:** Antidotes: *Thuj., Camph., Cocc., Nux-v., Puls.*

Compare: *Colchicinum* (intestinal catarrh with shreddy membranes; convulsive jerkings of the right hand; rheumatic fever, gout, endo and pericarditis, pleurisy, arthritis deformans in the early stages; *intense pain of rheumatism,* 3x trituration). Also, *Carb-v., Arn., Lil-t., Ars., Verat.*

**Dose:** Third to thirtieth attenuation.

---

# COLLINSONIA CANADENSIS

(Stone Root) **Coll.**

Pelvic and portal congestion resulting in hemorrhoids and constipation, especially in females. Depressed arterial tension, general atony of muscular fibre. *Chronic nasal, gastric and pharyngeal catarrh* due to portal obstruction. Dropsy from cardiac disease. Pruritus in pregnancy, with piles. *Constipation in children from intestinal atony.* Said to be of special value when given before surgery for rectal diseases. Sense of weight and constriction. Venous engorgement.

**Head**: Dull frontal headache; from suppressed hemorrhoids. Chronic catarrh.

**Mouth:** Tongue coated yellow. Bitter taste (*Coloc., Bry.*).

**Rectum**: *Sensation of sharp sticks in the rectum. Sense of constriction.* Vascular engorgement of rectum. Dry feces. *Very obstinate constipation* with protruding hemorrhoids. Aching in the anus (proctitis) and hypogastrium. Constipation during pregnancy; with membranous dysmenorrhea, following labor (*Nux-v.*). Painful, bleeding piles. Dysentery with tenesmus. *Alternate constipation and diarrhea* and great flatulence (dyspepsia). *Itching in the anus* (*Teucr., Rat.*).

**Female**: Dysmenorrhea; *pruritus vulva;* uterine prolapse; swelling and dark redness (hyperemia) of genitals; pain on sitting down. Membranous dysmenorrhea with constipation. Cold feeling in the thighs after menstruation. Sensation of swelling in the labia and of the clitoris.

**Respiratory**: *Cough from excessive use of voice,* "minister's sore throat"; sharp pain in the larynx. Hoarseness. Harassing, dry cough.

**Heart**: Palpitations; rapid but weak. Dropsy. After heart symptoms relieved, piles or menses return (metastasis). Chest pains alternate with hemorrhoids. Oppression, faintness and dyspnea (*Acon-f.*). Murmurs.

**Modalities**: *Worse,* from the slightest mental emotion or excitement; cold. *Better,* heat.

**Relationship**: Antidote: *Nux-v.*

Compare: *Aesc., Aloe, Ham., Lycps-v., Neg., Sulph., Nux-v.*

**Dose**: Tincture to third attenuation. Higher potencies where there is an organic heart affection.

---

## COLOCYNTHIS

(Bitter Cucumber) **Coloc.**

Often indicated in the transition season when the air is cold, but the sun is still powerful enough to heat the blood.

Develops most of its symptoms in the abdomen and head, causing intense neuralgias. It is especially suitable for irritable people, easily angered and ill effects therefrom. Women with copious menses and sedentary habits. People with a tendency to corpulency. The neuralgic pains are nearly always relieved by pressure. Cramps, twitching and shortening of muscles. Constrictions and contractions. Cystospasm following surgery of orifices (*Hyper.*). Urinous odor of perspiration (*Berb., Nit-ac.*). *Agonizing pain in the abdomen,* causing the patient to bend double is most characteristic. Sensations; cutting, twisting, grinding, contracting and bruised; *as if clamped with iron bands.*

**Mind:** Extremely irritable. Becomes angry when questioned. Mortification caused by offense. Anger with indignation (*Cham., Bry., Nux-v.*).

**Head:** Vertigo on turning the head *to the left.* Lateral cutting headache with nausea, and vomiting (migraine). Pains (better pressure and heat), with soreness of *the scalp.* Burning pains, digging, grinding and tearing. Frontal headache; worse, stooping, lying on the back and moving eyelids.

**Eyes:** Pains sharp, boring, *better pressure.* Sensation, as if the eyes would fall out on stooping. Gouty affections of the eyes (cataract). Violent pain in the eyeballs which precede the development of glaucoma.

**Face:** Tearing and shooting pains with swelling of the face; especially the left side with great soreness. Gets relief from pressure (*Chin.*). Neuralgia, *with chilliness;* teeth seems too long. *Sounds re-echo in ears.* Pain in the stomach, always accompanied with pain in the teeth or head.

**Stomach:** Very *bitter* taste. Tongue rough, as if from sand and feels scalded. Canine hunger. Sensation in the stomach as if something would not yield; drawing pain.

**Abdomen:** Agonizing, cutting pain in the abdomen *causing the patient to bend double* and pressing the abdomen. Sensation as if stones were being ground together in the abdomen and it would burst. Intestines feel bruised. Colic with cramps in calves. Cutting in the abdomen, especially after anger. Each paroxysm is attended with general agitation and a chill over the cheeks, ascending from the hypogastrium. Pain in a small spot below the navel. *Dysenteric stool renewed each time by the least food or drink. Jelly-like* stools. Musty odor. Distention.

**Urinary:** Intense burning along the urethra during stool. Vesical catarrh, discharge like fresh white of egg. *Viscid* (*Ph-ac.*), fetid; small quantities with frequent urging. Itching at the orifice. Red, hard crystals, adhering firmly to the vessel. Tenesmus of the bladder (cystitis). *Dysuria, pain extends all over the abdomen.*

**Female:** *Boring pain in the ovary. Must bend double, with great restlessness.* Round, small cystic tumors in the ovaries or broad ligaments. Wants abdomen supported by pressure. Bearing down cramps, causing her to bend double (*Op.*).

**Extremities:** *Contraction of muscles.* All the limbs are drawn together. Pain in the right deltoid (*Guaco.*). *Cramp-like pains in the hip;* lies on the affected side; pain from the hip to the knee. Spontaneous luxation of the hip joints. Stiffness of joints and shortening of tendons. Sciatic pain, left side, drawing, tearing; better, *pressure and heat;* worse, gentle touch. Contraction of the muscles. Pain down the right thigh; muscles and tendons feel too short; numbness with pain (*Gnaph.*). Pain in the left knee joint.

**Modalities:** *Worse,* from anger and indignation. *Better,* doubling up, hard pressure, warmth, lying with head bent forward.

**Relationship:** Antidote: *Coff., Staph., Cham.*

*Coloc.* is the best antidote for lead poisoning (Royal).

Compare: *Lobelia erinus* (violent corkscrew-like pains in abdomen). *Dipodium punctatum* (*writhing.* Twisting like a dying snake. Intractable insomnia). *Dios., Cham., Cocc., Merc., Plb., Mag-p.*

**Dose:** Sixth to thirtieth potency.

---

## COMOCLADIA DENTATA

(Guao) **Com.**

Important eye and skin symptoms. Affections of the antrum. Sacro-iliac and abdominal pain. *Throbbing pains worse by heat.* Pain in the joints and ankles.

**Eyes:** Ciliary neuralgia with eyes feeling large and protruded (exophthalmos), especially *right. Worse, near a warm stove;* feels as if pressed outward. Sees only a glimmer of light with the left eye. Glaucoma, sense of fullness; *eyeball feels too large.* Motion of eyes aggravates.

**Face:** Swollen, with eyes projecting.

**Chest:** Acute pain in the left mammary gland. Pain from the right side of chest, radiates down the arm to fingers. Cough with pain under the left breast, extending to the left scapula.

**Skin:** Itchy, red with pimples. *Redness all over,* like scarlatina. Erysipelas. Deep ulcers with hard edges. Leprosy. Red stripes on the skin (*Euph.*). Eczema (papular), of the trunk and extremities; also of the pustular type.

**Modalities:** *Better,* open air, scratching; by motion. *Worse,* touch, warmth, rest; night.

**Relationship:** Compare: *Rhus-t., Anac., Euph.*

**Dose:** First to thirtieth potency.

---

# CONIUM MACULATUM

(Poison Hemlock) **Con.**

An old remedy, rendered classical by Plato's graphic description of its employment in the death of Socrates. The *ascending paralysis* it produces, ending in death by failure of respiration, shows the ultimate tendency of many symptoms produced in the provings for which *Con.* is an excellent remedy, such as a difficult gait (locomotor ataxia), trembling (chorea), sudden loss of strength while walking, painful stiffness of legs, etc. Such a condition is often found in old age, at a time of weakness, languor, local congestions and sluggishness. This is the special environment that *Con.* chooses to manifest its action. It corresponds to the debility, hypochondriasis, urinary problems, weak memory, sexual debility found here. Problems at menopause, in old maids and bachelors. Growth of tumors invite it also. General feeling as if bruised by blows. Great debility in the morning, in bed. *Weakness of body and mind, trembling* and palpitations. Cancerous diathesis. Arteriosclerosis. Caries in the sternum. Enlarged glands. Acts on the glandular system, engorging and indurating it, altering its structure like scrofulous and cancerous conditions. Tonic after gripe. Insomnia of multiple neuritis.

**Mind:** Excitement causes mental depression. Depressed, timid, averse to society and afraid of being alone. No inclination for business or study; takes no interest in anything. Memory weak; unable to sustain any mental effort.

**Head**: *Vertigo on lying down and when turning over in bed,* when turning head *sidewise* or turning the eyes; worse, shaking the head, slight noise or conversation of others[1], especially towards the left. Headache, stupefying, with nausea and vomiting of mucus (migraine), with the sensation of a foreign body under the skull. Scorched feeling on top. Tightness as if both temples were compressed; worse after a meal (*Gels., Atropinum*). Bruised, semilateral pains. Dull occipital pain on rising in the morning.

**Eyes**: *Photophobia and excessive lachrymation.* Corneal pustules. Dim sighted (cataract); worse, artificial light. On closing the eyes, he sweats. Paralysis of ocular muscles (ptosis) (*Caust.*). In superficial inflammations, as in phlyctenular conjunctivitis and keratitis. *The slightest ulceration or abrasion will cause the intensest photophobia.*

**Ears**: Defective hearing; discharge from ear blood colored (otorrhea).

**Nose**: Bleeds easily, becomes sore. Polypus.

**Stomach**: Soreness around the root of tongue. Terrible nausea, acrid *heartburn* and acid eructations; *worse on going in bed.* Painful spasms of the stomach. Amelioration from eating and aggravation a few hours after meals;

[1] To talking and any other noise (Clarke — Dictionary of Practical Materia Medica).

acidity and burning; painful spot at the level of the sternum (gastric ulcer).

**Abdomen**: Severe aching in and around the liver. Chronic jaundice and pain in the right hypochondrium (hepatomegaly). Sensitive, bruised, swollen, knife-like pains. Painful tightness (peritonitis).

**Stool**: Frequent urging; hard with tenesmus. *Tremulous weakness after every stool* (*Verat., Ars., Arg-n.*). Heat and burning in the rectum during stool.

**Urinary**: Difficulty in voiding urine. *It flows and stops again* (*Led.*). *Interrupted discharge* (*Clem.*). Dribbling in old men (*Cop.*).

**Male**: Desire increased; power decreased. Sexual nervousness, with feeble erection. *Effects of suppressed sexual appetite.* Testicles hard and enlarged (orchitis).

**Female**: Dysmenorrhea, with pain drawing down the thighs. Mammae lax and shrunken, *hard*, painful to touch (mastitis). *Stitches in the nipples.* Wants to press the breast hard with the hand. Menses delayed and scanty; parts sensitive. *Breasts enlarge and become painful* before and during menses (*Calc., Lac-c.*). Rash before menses. Itching around the pudenda. Unready conception (sterility). Induration of os and cervix. Ovaritis; ovary enlarged, indurated; lancinating pains. Ill effects of *repressed sexual desire* or suppressed menses or from excessive indulgence. Leucorrhea after micturition.

**Respiratory**: Dry cough, almost continuous, hacking; worse, evening and at night; *caused by a dry spot in the larynx* with *itching* in the chest and throat, *when lying down,* talking or laughing and during pregnancy. Expectoration only after prolonged coughing: Want of breath on the least exercise; oppressed breathing (asthma); constriction of chest; pain in the chest.

**Back**: Dorsal pain between shoulders. Ill effects of bruises and shocks to the spine. Coccygodynia. Dull aching in the lumbar and sacral region.

**Extremities**: Heavy, weary, paralyzed; trembling; hands unsteady; fingers and toes numb. *Muscular weakness,* especially of the lower extremities. *Perspiration of hands. Putting feet on chair relieves pain.*

**Skin**: *Axillary glands painful, with a numb feeling down the arm.* Induration after contusions. Yellow skin, with papular eruption; yellow finger nails (jaundiced). *Glands enlarged and indurated,* also mesenteric. Flying stitches through the glands. Tumors; piercing pains; worse, at night. Chronic ulcers with a fetid discharge. *Sweat as soon as one sleeps* or closes the eyes. Night and morning sweat, with an offensive odor and smarting of the skin.

**Modalities**: *Worse,* lying down, *turning* or rising in bed; *celibacy;* before and during menses, from taking cold, physical or mental exertion. Better, while fasting, in the dark, from letting the limbs hang down, motion and pressure.

**Relationship**: Compare: *Scirrhinum*—Cancer nosode (cancerous diathesis; enlarged glands; cancer of breast; worms); *Bar-c., Hydr., Iod., Kali-p., Hyos., Cur.*

**Dose**: Best in higher potencies given infrequently, especially for growths, paretic states, etc. Otherwise sixth to thirtieth.

---

# CONVALLARIA MAJALIS

(Lily of the Valley) **Conv.**

A heart remedy. Increases the energy of heart's action and renders it more regular. Of use when the ventricles are over distended and dilatation begins, when there is an absence of compensatory hypertrophy and when venous stasis is marked. Dyspnea, dropsy, and a tendency for aneurisms. *Anasarca.*

**Mind:** Dull intellect. Grieves easily. Hysterical manifestations.

**Head:** Dull headache; worse, ascending, hawking. Scalp sensitive. Irritability.

**Face**: Hydroa on the nose and lips; raw and sore. Epistaxis. Sees imaginary gray spot about three inches square.

**Mouth:** Grating of teeth in the morning. Coppery taste. Tongue feels sore and scalded; broad and thick with a heavy, dirty coating.

**Throat**: Raw feeling at the back of throat when inspiring.

**Abdomen**: Sensitive. Clothes feel too tight. Gurgling and pain on taking a deep breath. Movements in the abdomen like the fist of a child. Colicky pains.

**Urinary**: Aching in the bladder; feels distended. Frequent micturition; offensive; scanty urine.

**Female**: Great *soreness in the uterine region, with sympathetic palpitations of the heart.* Pain in the sacro-iliac joints, running down the leg. Itching at the urinary meatus and vaginal orifice.

**Respiratory**: Pulmonary congestion. Orthopnea. *Dyspnea* while walking. Sensation of heat in the throat.

**Heart**: Sensation as if the heart beats throughout the chest. Endocarditis, with extreme orthopnea. *Sensations as if the heart ceased to beat, then starts very suddenly.* Palpitations from the least exertion. Tobacco heart, especially when due to cigarettes. Angina pectoris. Extremely rapid and irregular pulse.

**Back and Extremities**: Pain and aching in lumbar region; aching in legs; in the big toe (gout). Trembling of hands. Aching in the wrists and ankles.

**Fever**: Chills beginning and extending down the back, followed by fever and a little sweat. Thirst and headache during chill. Dyspnea during fever.

**Modalities**: *Better,* in open air. *Worse,* in a warm room.

**Relationship**: Compare: *Dig., Crat., Lil-t., Adon.* (feeble heart action due to functional disturbance).

**Dose**: Third attenuation and for symptoms of heart failure, tincture, one to fifteen drops.

---

## COPAIVA OFFICINALIS

(Balsam of Copaiva) **Cop.**

Powerful action on the mucous membranes, especially that of the urinary tract, the respiratory system and the skin, here it produces a well-marked nettle rash. Colds and catarrhs.

**Head:** Excessive sensitiveness; pain in the occiput. Dull, frontal headache, extending to the occiput and back with throbbing, worse right side and motion. Scalp sensitive. Sensitive to sharp sounds.

**Nose**: Rawness and soreness of the nostrils with a stopped up feeling; dryness of the posterior nares. Profuse, thick, fetid discharge from the nasal passages, running down the throat at night. *Burning and dryness,* crusts on turbinate bones. Marked catarrhal conditions in the upper respiratory tract.

**Stomach**: Food seems too salty. Gastric problems during menstruation or following urticaria. Flatulence, urging to stool and difficult passage with pain.

**Rectum**: *Mucus colitis.* Stools covered with mucus accompanied, with colic and chills. Burning and itching in the anus, caused by piles.

**Urinary**: Burning pressure; painful micturition with dribbling. Retention, with pain in the bladder, anus and rectum. *Catarrh of the bladder* (cystitis); dysuria. Swelling of the orifice (urethritis). Constant desire to micturate. Urine smells of violets. Greenish, turbid color; peculiar pungent odor (gonorrhea).

**Male**: Testicles sensitive and swollen (orchitis).

**Female**: Itching in the vulva and anus with a bloody purulent discharge. Profuse, strong smelling menstrual discharge, with pains radiating to the hip bones and nausea.

**Respiratory**: Cough with profuse, gray, purulent expectoration. Tickling in the larynx, trachea and bronchi. Bronchial catarrh, with profuse greenish, offensive discharge (bronchitis).

**Skin**: Hives with fever and constipation. Roseola. Erysipelatous inflammation especially around the abdomen. Circumscribed, lenticular patches with itching; mottled appearance. Chronic urticaria in children. Bullous eruptions.

**Relationship**: Antidotes: *Bell., Merc.*

Compare: *Santalum* (aching in kidneys); *Cann-s., Canth., Baros., Cub., Apis, Vesp., Erig., Senec., Sep.*

**Dose**: First to third attenuation.

---

# CORALLIUM RUBRUM

(Red Coral) **Cor-r.**

The provings of coral develop much coryza, epistaxis, and even ulceration within the nostrils. It is to be thought of in whooping and spasmodic coughs especially when the attack comes on with a *very rapid* cough, and the attacks follow so closely that they almost run into each other. Often preceded by a sensation of smothering, followed by exhaustion. Congestion of the face after dinner. Purple face. *Violence of paroxysm,* may lead to hemoptysis. Sensation of cold air streaming through the skull and air passages. One is too cold when uncovered and too hot when covered; relieved by artificial heat.

**Head**: Feels very large; violent pain as if parietal bones were forced apart; worse stooping. Eyes hot and painful. Deep seated frontal headache with severe pain behind the eyeballs. Pain aggravated by breathing cold air through the nose.

**Nose**: Odors of smoke, onions, etc. Painful ulcer in the nostrils. *Post-nasal catarrh. Profuse secretion of mucus dropping through the posterior nares* (sinusitis); air feels cold. Dry coryza; nose stopped up and ulcerated. Epistaxis.

**Mouth**: Food tastes like sawdust. Bread tastes like straw. Beer tastes sweet. Pain during articulation on the left lower jaw. Craves salt.

**Male**: Ulcers on the glans and inner prepuce, with a yellow ichor (blenorrhea). Emissions and weakened sexual power. Profuse perspiration of genitals.

**Respiratory:** Hawking of profuse mucus. Throat very sensitive, *especially to air.* Profuse nasal catarrh. Inspired air feels cold (*Cist.*). *Profuse secretion of mucus dropping through the posterior nares* (post nasal drip). Dry, *spasmodic,* suffocative cough; very rapid cough, short, barking. Cough with great sensitiveness of air passages; *feels cold on deep inspiration.* Continuous hysterical cough. Feels suffocated and greatly exhausted after whooping cough.

**Skin**: Red, flat ulcers. Coral colored, then dark red spots, changing to copper colored spots[1]. Psoriasis of palms and soles.

**Modalities**: *Worse* in open air, changing from a warm to cold room.

**Relationship**: Complementary: *Sulph.*

Compare: *Bell., Dros., Meph., Caust.*

**Dose**: Third to thirtieth attenuation.

---

[1] Smooth spots on the palms and fingers, first of coral color, then dark red and finally copper colored (Clarke — Dictionary of Practical Materia Medica).

## CORALLORHIZA ODONTORHIZA

(Crawley Root) **Corh.**

Hectic fever, coming on between 9 to 10 a. m., lasting till mid-night. Intensely nervous and restless, burning of palms and soles; no thirst, chill or perspiration. Can bear only the slightest covering.

---

## CORNUS CIRCINATA

(Round-leaved Dogwood) **Corn.**

Chronic malaria, hepatitis, jaundice. Weakness in the morning. Pain in the pit of stomach, with a distended abdomen. Vesicular eruptions associated with chronic liver disease or aphthous stomatitis.

**Mouth**: Ulceration of the tongue, gums and mouth; aphthæ. Burning in the mouth, throat and stomach.

**Stool:** Loose, windy, dark stools, immediately after dinner. Burning in the anus. Dark, bilious, offensive diarrhea with a sallow complexion.

**Skin**: Vesicular eczema of the face in infants, with apthae.

**Relationship**: Compare: *Cornus alternifolia*—Swamp walnut (weak and tired; disturbed sleep, fever, restlessness, eczema; *skin cracked;* chest feels cold, as if full of ice); *Cornus florida* (chronic malaria; indigestion and distressing acid heart burn; general debility from loss of fluids and night sweats, neuralgic pain in the arms, chest and trunk, sensation as if broken in two; intermittent fever *with drowsiness;* great exhaustion at intervals; general clammy sweat. Chill is preceded by drowsiness, heat is associated with drowsiness. Headache after quinine).

**Dose**: Tincture to sixth attenuation.

---

## CORYDALIS FORMOSA—DICENTRA CANADENSIS

(Turkey-pea) **Cory.**

Syphilitic affections. Ulcers in the mouth and fauces (stomatitis). Cancer cachexia pronounced. Gummata and nocturnal pains. Chronic diseases with atony. Tongue clean, broad and full. Tissues flabby, doughy, cold. Gastric catarrh (*Hydr.*).

**Skin**: Dry, scaly scabs on the face of old people. Lymphatic glands swollen.

**Relationship**: *Nit-ac., Kali-i., Fl-ac.*

**Dose**: Tincture, twenty drops, three times a day.

# COTYLEDON UMBILICUS

(Pennywort) **Cot.**

Marked action on the heart; oppression of the chest; fullness in the throat. Epilepsy. Numb aching in the muscular and fibrous tissue. Sciatica. Well marked pains through the breast, to the scapula. Catarrh of larynx and trachea. Hysterical joint.

**Mind**: Lost, confused feeling. Difficult articulation for some time after awaking. Pressing pain in the vertex, headache. Ailments from suppressed emotions. *Sensation as if a part of the body was absent.*

**Chest**: Pain under the left nipple and aching in the right breast. Pain extends to the scapula from the left breast. Pain at the angles of scapulae. Full, bursting sensation, as if from an obstruction of the heart. Choking fullness of the throat. Breathing oppressed.

**Extremities**: Aching in the back and thighs. Aching in all joints. Skin sensitive, rubbing of trousers causes an acute sting. Legs and arms feel heavy and sore.

**Relationship**: Compare: *Ambr., Asaf., Hepat., Ign., Lach.*

**Dose**: Tincture to third potency.

---

# CRATAEGUS OXYACANTHA

(Hawthorn Berries) **Crat.**

Produces giddiness, lowered pulse, air hunger and reduction in blood pressure. Acts on the heart muscle and *is a cardiac tonic.* No influence on the endocardium.

Myocarditis. Failing compensation. *Irregularity of the heart.* Insomnia in aortic sufferers; anemia; edema; cutaneous chilliness. High arterial tension. Is a sedative in cross, irritable patients with cardiac symptoms.

Chronic heart disease, with extreme weakness. Very feeble and irregular heart action. General anasarca. Very nervous with pain at the back of head and neck. Collapse of typhoid. Hemorrhage from bowels. Cold extremities, pallor; irregular pulse and breathing. Painful sensation of pressure on the left side of chest, below the clavicle. Dyspepsia and nervous prostration with heart failure. In the beginning of heart disease, after rheumatism. *Arteriosclerosis. Said to have a solvent power on the crustaceous and calcareous deposits in the arteries.*

**Head**: Apprehensive, despondent. Very nervous and irritable, with pain at the back of head and neck. Mental dullness, conjunctival irritation and nasal discharges.

**Urinary**: *Diabetes,* especially in children.

**Heart**: *Cardiac dropsy.* Fatty degeneration. Aortic disease. *Extreme dyspnea on least exertion,* without a marked increase in pulse. Pain in the region of heart *and under the left clavicle.* Heart muscles seem flabby, worn out. Cough. *Heart dilated; first sound weak.* Pulse accelerated, *irregular, feeble, intermittent.* Valvular murmurs, angina pectoris. Cutaneous chilliness, cynosis of fingers and toes; aggravated by exertion or excitement. Sustains heart in infectious diseases.

**Sleep**: Insomnia in aortic patients.

**Skin**: Excessive perspiration. Skin eruptions.

**Modalities**: *Worse,* in a warm room. *Better,* fresh air, quiet and rest.

**Relationship**: *Stroph-h., Dig., Iber., Naja, Cact.*

**Dose**: Fluid extract or tincture, one to fifteen drops. Must be used for some time in order to obtain good results.

---

## CROCUS SATIVUS

(Saffron) **Croc.**

Is a remedy often useful in hemorrhages that are black and stringy. Tingling in various parts. Chorea and hysterical affections. Frequent and extreme changes in sensations and mental conditions. Anger with violence followed by repentance. *Laughing* mania. Drowsiness and *lassitude;* better by literary labor.

**Mind**: *Vacillating;* pleasant mania; sings and laughs. Happy and affectionate; then angry. Sudden changes from hilarity to melancholy. Vivid recollection from music heard[1] (*Lyc.*).

**Head**: Throbs, pulsates during climacteric; worse during menses.

**Eyes**: Appearance as of electric sparks. Must wipe the eyes sensation of mucus or water in them. *Sensation in eyes as after violent crying.* Sensation as if she had been looking through very sharp spectacles. *Eyes feel as if in smoke.* Pupils enlarged and react slowly. Lids heavy. Ciliary neuralgia, pain from the eyes extending to the top of the head. *Sensation as if cold air was rushing through the eye* (*Fl-ac., Syph.*). Asthenopia with extreme photophobia. Threatened glaucoma; embolism in central retinal artery.

**Nose**: Epistaxis. *Dark, stringy, clotted. Strings of dark blood* hanging down the nose.

**Abdomen**: *Obstinate constipation* due to portal stagnation. Constipation in infants. Crawling and stitches in the anus. *Sensation of something alive in*

---

[1] Sensitive to music, involuntarily joins in on hearing anyone sing (Clarke — Dictionary of Practical Materia Medica).

*the abdomen, stomach, etc.*, especially on the left side (*Calen.*). Abdomen swollen, feeling of something heavy.

**Female:** Threatened abortion, especially when hemorrhage is *dark and stringy.* Surging of blood to genitals. Menses dark, viscid, too frequent and copious, *black and slimy* (menorrhagia)· Uterine hemorrhage; *clots with long strings;* worse from least movement. Jerking pain in the interior of the left breast as if drawn towards the back by means of a thread (*Crot-t.*). A bounding feeling, as if something alive in the right breast.

**Respiratory**: Wheezy cough, with frothy expectoration, containing threads like fine twine; worse lying down. Breath has an offensive, sickly smell. Sensation as if the uvula is elongated in hysterical patients.

**Back**: Sudden feeling of coldness in the back, as if cold water was thrown over him; icy cold extremities.

**Extremities**: Spasmodic contractions and twitchings of a single set of muscles. Chorea and hysteria with great alterations in mood. The entire upper extremity falls asleep. Cracking in hip joint and *knees.* Weakness in the knees and legs. Pain in the ankles and soles.

**Modalities**: *Worse*, lying down, hot weather, warm room, in the morning, fasting, before breakfast, looking fixedly at an object. *Better,* in open air.

**Relationship**: Antidote: *Op., Bell.*

Compare: *Ip., Tril-p., Plat., Chin., Sabin.*

**Dose**: Tincture to thirtieth attenuation.

---

# CROTALUS HORRIDUS

(Rattlesnake) **Crot-h.**

Snake poisons are supposed to be chemically *cyanide hydrates of soda* and other salts. Alcohol is the natural solvent of these salts and is an antidote. Has a profound trophic action. Nutritional problems associated with old age.

Low septic states. General disorganization of blood, hemorrhages and jaundice. A crotalin injection decreases the rate of coagulation of blood. In epilepsy the average rate is far greater than in normal conditions. Decomposition of blood , *hemorrhages* (dark fluid that forms no clots), tendency to carbuncles, malignant scarlatina, *yellow fever,* plague, cholera, etc. give an opportunity to use this remedy. *Hemorrhagic diathesis.* Acts as a sedative. Sleeps into his symptoms. Affinity for the right side.

**Mind**: Lachrymose mood; clouded perception and memory; impatient. Loquacious, with a desire to escape. Sadness. Delusions of cerebral decay.

**Head**: Vertigo, with weakness and trembling. Dull heavy occipital pain, on the right side and right eye (meningitis). Headache with pain in the heart when lying on the left side. Headache; must walk on the tips of the toes to avoid jarring.

**Eyes**: Very sensitive to light (photophobia), especially *lamp light.* Yellow color of eyes. Illusions; blue colors. *Ciliary neuralgia;* tearing, boring pain, as if a cut had been made around the eye. *For absorption of intra-ocular hemorrhages* into the vitreous, but particularly for non-inflammatory retinal hemorrhages. Diplopia.

**Ears**: Auditory vertigo (Meniere's disease). Blood oozes from ears. Sensation of stoppage in the right ear.

**Nose**: Epistaxis, *blood black and stringy,* ozena, after exanthemata or syphilis.

**Face**: Acne. Lips swollen and numb. Lead colored and yellow face. Lockjaw.

**Mouth**: Tongue red and small, but feels swollen (glossitis). Tongue fiery red, dry in the center, smooth and polished. Mouldy smell of breath. Mouth fills up with saliva. Tongue on protruding, deviates to the right (paralysis). Spasmodic grinding of teeth at night. Cancer of the tongue with hemorrhage.

**Throat**: Dry, swollen, dark red. Spasms of the esophagus; cannot swallow any solid substance. Tight constriction. Gangrenous, with much swelling.

**Stomach**: Intolerance of clothing around stomach. Unable to retain anything; violent vomiting of food; bilious vomiting, vomiting of blood, hematemesis. Constant nausea and vomiting every month, after menstruation. Cannot lie on the right side, without vomiting a dark green matter (bilious vomiting). Black or coffee ground vomiting. Cancer of stomach with vomiting of bloody, slimy mucus. Trembling, fluttering feeling below the epigastrium. Intolerance of clothing around the epigastrium. Faintness and sinking in the stomach. Gastric ulcer. Atonic dyspepsia. Gastritis in chronic alcoholism. Hungry, craves stimulants, sugar; averse to meat.

**Abdomen**: Distended, hot, and tender. Pain in the region of liver (jaundice). Appendicitis.

**Rectum**: Black, thin, offensive like coffee grounds. Intestinal hemorrhage; blood dark, fluid, non-coagulable. Blood oozes from the rectum when standing or walking.

**Urinary**: Dark, bloody urine (hematuria). Casts. Inflamed kidney (nephritis). Albuminous, dark, scanty (*Merc-c.*).

**Female**: Prolonged menses. Dysmenorrhea; pain extends down the thighs, with aching in the heart region. Uterine hemorrhage (menorrhagia) with a sensation of faintness in the stomach. Puerperal fever; offensive lochia.

Phlegmasia alba dolens. Sensation as though uterus would drop out (prolapse). Painful, drawing pains in the uterine ligaments. Cannot keep legs still.

**Respiratory**: Cough, with bloody expectoration (hemoptysis). Tickling from a dry spot in the larynx.

**Heart:** Action feeble, pulse tremulous. Palpitations, especially at menstrual period. Trembling feeling in the heart (apoplexy).

**Extremities**: Hands tremble, swollen. Lower extremities go to sleep easily. *Right sided paralysis.*

**Sleep**: Dreams of the dead. Starting in sleep. Yawning. Smothering sensation on waking up.

**Fever**: Malignant fevers of a *hemorrhagic or putrescent character.* Low bilious remittents. Yellow fever. Bloody sweat. Cerebro-spinal meningitis (*Cic., Cupr-act.*). Cold sweats.

**Skin**: Swelling and discoloration, skin tense and shows every tint of color, with excruciating pain. Vesication. *Sallow.* Yellow color of the whole body (jaundice). Great sensitiveness of skin on *right half* of body. *Purpura hemorrhagica.* Hemorrhage from every part of body. Bloody sweat. Chilblains, felons. Dissecting wounds. Pustular eruptions. Insect stings. Post-vaccination eruptions. Bad effects of vaccination. Lymphangitis and septicemia. Boils, carbuncles, and eruptions are surrounded by purplish, mottled skin and edema. Anthrax. Sore sensation relieved by pressure.

**Modalities**: *Worse*, right side; open air; evening and in the morning; in spring, coming on in warm weather; yearly; on awaking; damp and wet; *jar.*

**Relationship**: Compare: *Both., Naja* (more nervous phenomena); *Lach.* (marked affinity for the left side); *Elaps corallinus* (preferable in otorrhea and affections of the right lung); *Crotalus cascavella* (thoughts and dreams of death. Paralysis of articulation, embarrassed stertorous breathing and semi-consciousness. A magnetic state is produced; cutting sensation all around the eyeball); *Bung.*—Krait (poliomyelitis).

Antidote: *Lach., Alcoholus.* Radiant heat; camphor.

**Dose**: Third to sixth potency.

---

## CROTON TIGLIUM

(Croton Oil Seed) **Crot-t.**

Is a valuable remedy in diarrhea, summer complaints and *skin affections.* These may alternate with each other. Feels tight all over. It is one of the antidotes to Rhus poisoning, as is evident from its wide and intense action upon the skin and mucous surface, causing both irritation and inflammation, with formation of vesicles and mucus discharges. Has an elective affinity for the skin of face and external genitals. *Burning in the esophagus.*

**Head**: Pressing pain in the forehead, especially orbits.

**Eyes**: Granular lids; pustules on the cornea (keratitis). Red and raw appearance (ophthalmia). *Feel drawn backwards.* Eruptions around the eyes. *Tensive pain above the right orbit.*

**Stool**: Copious watery stools with much urging; *always shoots out forcibly,* with gurgling in the intestines; worse, drinking the least quantity, or even while eating. Constant urging to pass stool, followed by sudden evacuation. Swashing sensation in the intestines.

**Urinary**: Urine at night foamy; dark orange colored; turbid on standing; greasy particles floating on top. Urine during the day is pale with a white sediment.

**Chest:** *Drawing pain through the left side of chest to the back. Asthma* with cough; cannot expand the chest. Nursing women; every time she suckles the child, it produces *pain from the nipple to the back.* Inflamed breasts (mastitis). Cough, as soon as he touches the pillow, must get up. Sensitive to deep breathing.

**Skin**: *Feels hide bound. Intense itching; but scratching is painful.* Pustular eruptions, especially on the face and genitals with fearful itching, followed by painful burning[1]. Vesicles; confluent oozing. Vesicular erysipelas, itching exceedingly. Herpes zoster; stinging, smarting pains in the eruption.

**Modalities**: *Worse,* least food or drink; during summer; touch, at night and in the morning, washing.

**Relationship**: Compare*: Momordica charantia*—Hairy mordica (has marked, drastic properties, producing colic, nausea, vomiting and cholera-like symptoms, abdomen seems full of fluid which is discharged explosively, thin, watery, yellow. Great thirst). *Rhus-t., Anag., Anac., Sep.*

Antidote*: Ant-t.*

**Dose**: Sixth to thirtieth potency.

---

## CUBEBA OFFICINALIS

(Cubebs) **Cub.**

Mucous membranes generally, but especially that of the urinary tract are chiefly affected by this remedy. Frequent micturition of a nervous origin. Leucorrhea in little girls.

---

[1] Patient can't bear to itch as it is followed by intense burning. (Clarke — Dictionary of Practical Materia Medica).

**Urinary**: Urethritis, with much mucus especially in women. Cutting pain after micturition with constriction. Hematuria. Prostatitis, with a thick yellow discharge (gonorrhea). Cystitis.

**Respiratory**: Catarrh of the nose and throat, with a fetid odor and expectoration. Mucus trickles from the posterior nares. Rawness of the throat with hoarseness.

**Relationship:** Compare: *Cuc-p., Cop., Pip-m., Santal.*

**Dose**: Second and third attenuation.

---

## CUCURBITA CITRULLUS

(Seeds of Watermelon) **Cuc-c.**

Infusion for painful micturition with a sense of constriction and backache.

---

## CUCURBITA PEPO

(Pumpkin Seed) **Cuc-p.**

Intense nausea immediately after eating. Vomiting of pregnancy. Seasickness. One of the most efficient and least harmful of tineafuges.

**Relationship**: Compare: *Filix mas; Cuprum oxydatum nigrum.*

**Dose**: Tincture. The seeds are a valuable remedy for tapeworm. Scald the seeds and peel off the outer skins when softened, the green inner pulp is the part to be used. Two ounces of seed, yield one of the pulp. May be mixed with cream and taken like porridge. Take in the morning after twelve hours fasting, and follow after two hours with castor oil.

---

## CUNDURANGO

(Condor Plant) **Cund.**

Stimulates the digestive functions and thus improves the general health. Allays the pain of gastralgia accompanying cancer of stomach. Modifies secretions of the digestive glands. Varicose ulcers. Lupus.

*Painful cracks at the corner of the mouth* is a guiding symptom of this drug. Chronic gastric catarrh, syphilis, and cancer. Tumors; stricture of the esophagus. The active principle (*Cunduranginus*) produces locomotor ataxia.

**Stomach:** Painful affections of the stomach; ulceration. Vomiting of food and indurations, constant burning pain. Stricture of the esophagus, with burning pain behind the sternum (heartburn), where food seems to stick. Vomiting of food, and indurations in the left hypochondrium with a constant burning pain.

**Skin**: Fissures around the muco-cutaneous outlets. Epithelioma of the lips or anus. Ulcerative stage of carcinoma cutis when fissures form.

**Relationship**: Compare: *Aster., Con., Hydr., Ars.*

**Dose**: Tincture or bark, 5 grain doses before meals, in water. Also the thirtieth potency, in tumors.

---

## CUPHEA VISCOSISSIMA

(Flux-weed) **Cuph.**

Vomiting of undigested food. *Cholera infantum,* severe acidity; frequent green, watery, acrid stools. Tenesmus with severe pain. High fever; restlessness and sleeplessness. Obstinate constipation.

**Relationship**: Compare: *Æth., Coto*—Para-coto bark (intestinal catarrh,; chronic, copious, exhausting diarrhea and dysentery; colliquitive sweats of phthisis and chronic diarrhea).

*Typha latifolia*—Cat-tail flag (diarrhea, dysentery, summer complaints in children. Tincture and first attenuation).

**Dose**: Tincture.

---

## CUPRUM ACETICUM

(Acetate of Copper) **Cupr-act.**

Hay fever, with burning excoriation, paroxysmal cough; tough, tenacious mucus and fear of suffocation. *Protracted labor.* Chronic psoriasis and leprosy.

**Head**: Violent throbbing and lancinating pains in the forehead. Left sided brow ague. Brain seems void. Inclined to gape and cry. Loses consciousness; *head reels when in a high ceiled room.* Constant protrusion and retraction of tongue (chorea) (*Lach.*). Neuralgia with heaviness in the head, burning, stinging and stitching in temples and forehead (cerebrospinal meningitis, hydrocephalus).

**Face**: Collapsed, hippocratic. Facial neuralgia in the cheek bone, upper jaw and behind the right ear. Better by chewing, pressure and external warmth.

**Stomach**: Violent spasmodic pains in the stomach and abdomen. Vomiting. Slimy, brown diarrhea. Violent tenesmus. Cholera.

**Respiratory**: Attacks of angina pectoris coming on when excited. Violent spasmodic cough (croup). Short, difficult respiration. Spasmodic constriction of the chest. Dyspnea.

**Skin**: Leprosy-like eruption, without itching, all over the body, in spots of various sizes.

**Modalities**: *Worse,* mental emotions, touch. *Better,* chewing, pressure, night, lying on the affected side and warmth.

**Relationship**: Action similarly to *Cupr.* but is more violent.

**Dose:** Third to sixth trituration.

---

# CUPRUM ARSENICOSUM

(Arsenite of Copper, Scheele's Green) **Cupr-ar.**

A remedy for symptoms depending on deficient renal action, various intestinal affections, cholera morbus and infantum; enterocolitis, diarrhea and dysentery. Gastrointestinal disturbances in influenza and typhoid. *Uremic convulsions,* headache, vertigo and unconscious conditions resulting from brain edema. Nephritis of pregnancy. Convulsions preceded by gastro-intestinal symptoms. Chlorosis. Bronchial asthma with emphysema. Purulent endocarditis (Royal). Painful neuroses, enteroptosis. Delirium and tremor cordis (chorea).

**Mouth**: Tongue thickly coated, dirty brown, white, metallic taste; thirst. Dry mouth.

**Abdomen:** Gastroenteritis. Violent abdominal pain. Diarrhea in phthisis. Cholera (*Ars., Verat., Camph.*). Rumbling and sharp cutting pain. Dark, liquidy stools.

**Urinary**: Renal inefficiency and uremia. *Garlicky odor.* Diabetes. Urine with a high specific gravity; increased acetones and diacetic acid.

**Male**: Perspiration on the scrotum; it is constantly damp and moist. Boils on the scrotum. Purulent white discharge from the urethra (gleet); tingling and burning in the urethra (urethritis); pain in the prostate and penis (syphilis).

**Heart**: Cardiac rhythm and force altered due to defective elimination.

**Back**: Persistent lameness. Pain in the lumbar region and in the lower part of left shoulder blade; chest feels tight.

**Extremities**: *Cramps in the calves,* worse after midnight, only relieved by getting out of bed and standing. Ulcers; gangrene.

**Skin**: Icy cold (hypothermia). Cold clammy perspiration of an intermittent nature. Acne, pustules on the face and in the cruro-genital region; ulcers look like chancre. Gangrene; carbuncles.

**Dose**: Third trituration.

# CUPRUM METALLICUM

(Copper) **Cupr.**

*Spasmodic affections, cramps,* convulsions, beginning in the fingers and toes, violent, contractive and intermitting pain, are some of the more marked expressions of the action of *Cupr.*, its curative range therefore includes tonic and clonic spasms, convulsions and epileptic attacks. Chorea brought on by fright. Nausea greater than in any other remedy. In epilepsy, aura begins in the knees, ascends to the hypogastrium; followed by unconsciousness, foaming and falling. Symptoms disposed to appear periodically and in groups. Complaints begin on the left side (*Lach.*). Tapeworm (colloidal *Cupr.* 3x).

Where eruptions strike in, as in scarlet fever, complaints such as excessive vomiting, stupor, convulsions, may result, which come within the sphere of this remedy. Pain is aggravated by movement and touch.

**Head:** Fixed ideas, malicious and morose. Uses words not intended. Fearful. Empty feeling. Purple, red swelling on the head with convulsions. Bruised pain in the brain and eyes on turning them. Meningitis. Sensation as if water was poured over the head. Giddiness accompanies many ailments, head falls forward on the chest.

**Eyes:** Aching over the eyes. Fixed, stary, sunken, glistening, turned upward. Crossed. Quick rolling of the eyeballs, with closed eyes.

**Nose:** Violent congestion of the nose (*Meli.*).

**Face:** Distorted, pale, *bluish,* with blue lips (cyanosed). *Contraction of jaws,* with foam in the mouth (epilepsy).

**Mouth:** *Strong metallic, slimy taste,* with flow of saliva. Constant protrusion and retraction of the tongue, like a snake (*Lach.*). Paralysis of the tongue. Stammering speech.

**Stomach:** Hiccough preceding the spasms. *Nausea.* Vomiting, relieved by drinking cold water; with colic, diarrhea, spasms. Strong metallic taste (*Rhus-t.*). *While drinking, the fluid descends with a gurgling sound* (*Laur.*). Craves cool drinks.

**Abdomen:** Tense, hot and tender to touch; *contracted.* Neuralgia of abdominal viscera. *Colic,* violent and intermittent. Intussusception.

**Stool:** Black, painful, bloody, with tenesmus and weakness (dysentery). Cholera; with cramps in abdomen and calves.

**Female:** Menses too late, protracted. Cramps, extending into chest, before, during or after suppression of menses. Also, from suppressed foot sweats (*Sil.*). Ebullition of blood; palpitations. Chlorosis. *After-pains.*

**Respiratory:** Cough has a gurgling sound, better by drinking cold water. Suffocative attacks, worse 3 a. m. (*Am-c.*). *Spasm and constriction* in the chest;

spasmodic asthma, alternating with spasmodic vomiting. Whooping cough, better, swallowing cold water, with vomiting, spasms and a purple face. Spasm of the glottis. Dyspnea with epigastric uneasiness. Spasmodic dyspnea before menstruation. Angina with asthmatic symptoms and cramps (Clarke).

**Heart:** Angina pectoris. Slow pulse; or hard, full and quick. Palpitations, precordial anxiety and pain. Fatty degeneration (*Phyt.*).

**Extremities:** Jerking, twitching of muscles. Coldness of the hands. Cramps in the palms. Great weariness of limbs. *Cramps in calves and soles.* Epilepsy; aura begins in the knees. Clenched thumb. Clonic spasms, beginning in the fingers and toes.

**Sleep:** Profound, with shocks in the body. Constant rumbling in the abdomen during sleep.

**Skin:** *Bluish* (cyanosed), marbled. Ulcers, itching spots, and pimples in the folds of joints. Chronic psoriasis and leprosy (Hughes).

**Modalities:** *Worse,* before menses, from vomiting, contact. *Better,* during perspiration, drinking cold water.

**Relationship:** Antidotes: *Bell., Hep., Camph.* Copper is found in *Dulc., Staph., Con.* and some other plants. Also in King-crab *(Limulus cyclops).*

Complementary: *Calc.*

Compare: *Cuprum sulphuricum* (*burning at the vertex;* incessant, spasmodic cough; worse at night; tongue and lips bluish; locally, *Cupr- s.* in 1-3 percent solution in inoperable sarcoma). *Cuprum cyanatum* (meningitis basilaris); *Cholas terrapina* (cramps in calves and feet; rheumatism, with cramp like pains); *Plumb., Nux-v., Verat. Cuprum oxydatum nigrum* lx (all kinds of worms, including tapeworms and trichinosis according to Zopfy's 60 years' experience).

**Dose:** Sixth to thirtieth potency.

---

## CURARE—WOORARI

(Arrow Poison) **Cur.**

Muscular paralysis without impairing sensation and consciousness. Paralysis of respiratory muscles. *Reflex action diminished.* Debility in the aged (*Baryta*) and from loss of fluid. Catalepsy. Nervous debility. Trismus. Glycosuria with motor paralysis. *Cur.* decreases the output of adrenalin. Vomiting of bile in cirrhosis of liver. Diabetes mellitus, 4th dilution (Dr. Barkhard).

**Mind:** Indecision; no longer wishes to think, or act for herself.

**Head:** Lancinating pains all over the head. Head drawn backward (tetnus). Falling out of hair. Brain feels full of fluid.

**Eyes:** Sharp, stitching pains over the right eye. Black spots before vision. Ptosis on the right side.

**Ears:** Noises; unbearable otalgia. Lancinating pains start from the ears (otitis); extending down, to the legs. Swelling of the ear lobes.

**Nose:** Ozena. Tubercles on the nose; fetid lumps of pus.

**Face:** Facial and buccal paralysis. Tongue and mouth drawn. Red face. Tongue and mouth drawn to the right.

**Female:** Dysmenorrhea. Menses too early, during menses, colic, headache, renal pain. Leucorrhea, thick, purulent, offensive (vaginitis).

**Respiratory:** Threatened *paralysis of respiration* on falling asleep. Short breath (emphysema). Short dry cough; provokes vomiting, followed by fainting. *Chest sore to pressure. Very distressing dyspnea.*

**Extremities:** Tired, pain up and down the spine. *Arms weak, heavy.* Cannot lift the fingers. Weakness of hands and fingers in pianists. Legs tremble; give way when walking. Debility; paralysis. Catalepsy. Favors development of corns. Reflexes lessened or abolished. Locomotor ataxia.

**Skin:** Leprosy. Dirty looking skin. Boils. Tubercles on the nose. Liver spots. Blood oozes through. Itching.

**Modalities:** Worse, dampness, cold weather, cold wind; 2 a. m., right side.

**Relationship:** Compare: *Cytisinum* (motor paralysis); *Con., Caust., Crot-h., Nux-v., Curare* antidotes *Strych.*

**Dose:** Sixth to thirtieth potency.

---

# CYCLAMEN EUROPAEUM

(Sow-bread) **Cycl.**

Large doses produce violent purging and vomiting; disturbed digestion with very salty saliva. Anemic and chlorotic conditions. Affections of the uterus. Gastro-intestinal and genito-urinary tracts affected, inducing secondary anemia and various reflexes. *Sleepiness, moroseness and lassitude.* Cough at night while asleep without waking, especially in children (*Cham., Nit-ac.*).

**Mind:** Terrors of conscience. Grieves over neglected duty. Depression, with sobbing, desire to be alone.

**Head:** Aching in the morning, with *flickering before the eyes.* Vertigo; things turn in a circle; better in room; worse, open air. One sided headache (migraine).

**Eyes:** Dim vision (amaurosis), worse on waking up, with spots before the eyes. *Flickering of various colors.* Convergent strabismus. *Sees countless stars.* Diplopia. Disturbance of vision, associated with gastric disturbances.

**Nose:** Frequent sneezing with itching in the ears.

**Stomach:** *Salty taste;* hiccough-like eructations worse, after fatty food. Diarrhea after every cup of coffee; hiccough. Satiety after a few mouthfuls only. Disgust for meat, especially pork. Desire for lemonade. No thirst all day.

**Rectum:** *Pain around the anus and perineum,* as if a spot was suppurating, when walking or sitting[1].

**Female:** Menses *profuse, black,* membranous, *clotted, too early with labor-like pains* from back to pubes (dysmenorrhea). Flow less when moving around. Menstrual irregularities (metrorrhagia) with migraine and blindness, or fiery spots before the eyes. *Hiccough during pregnancy.* Post-partum hemorrhage with colicky bearing down pains, relief after gush of blood. After menses, swelling of breasts with milky secretion.

**Extremities:** Pains in parts where bones lie near the surface. Burning, *sore pain in the heels.* Cramp-like contractions in the right thumb and index finger. Pains in the periosteum. Chilblains.

**Skin:** Acne in young women, pruritus better scratching and by appearance of menses.

**Modalities:** *Worse,* open air, evenings, sitting, standing, and cold water. *Better,* during menstrual flow, by moving around, rubbing parts; in warm room, lemonade.

**Relationship:** Compare: *Ambr., Puls., Chin., Ferr-cit-et-chin.*

**Dose:** Third attenuation.

---

## CYPRIPEDIUM PUBESCENS

(Yellow Lady's Slipper) **Cypr.**

The skin symptoms correspond to those of poisoning by Rhus, for which it has been found an efficent antidote. Nervousness in children; from teething and intestinal problems. Debility after gout. *Hydrocephaloid* symptoms, result of long, exhausting diarrhea. *Sleeplessness.* Cerebral hyperesthesia in young children, often the result of over stimulation of the brain.

**Head:** Child cries out at night; is awake and begins to laugh and play. Headaches in elderly people and during climacteric.

**Relationship:** Compare: *Ambr., Kali-br., Scut., Valer., Ign.* Skin relatives: *Grin., Anac.*

**Dose:** Tincture to sixth attenuation. For Poison oak, 5 drops of tincture per dose, also locally.

---

[1] Drawing pressure in the anus and perineum, as from a subcutaneous ulceration, when walking or sitting (Clarke — Dictionary of Practical Materia Medica).

## CYTISUS LABURNUM

(Laburnum) **Cyt-l.**

All parts of this shrub are poisonous, producing an inflammation of the stomach and intestines, with vomiting, diarrhea, headache, pale face and cold skin. Wide spread anesthesia, and convulsions are some of the chief effects of this drug. Cerebrospinal meningitis. Great prostration, sense of constriction in the throat, stiffness of the nape, tearing pains from the nape to the occiput, lustreless eyes.

**Head:** Stupefaction; indifference (*Ph-ac.*). Unequally dilated pupils; *giddiness;* twitching of facial muscles (*Agar.*). Hydrocephalus. Constant vertigo, intense sleepiness.

**Stomach:** Excessive thirst. Constant nausea, vomiting; burning pain in the epigastrium.

**Urinary:** Tenesmus and erections. Grass green urine.

**Extremities:** Numbness and pain in the hands. Difficulty in moving them.

**Relationship:** Compare: *Nux-v., Gels. Cystinum* (produces motor paralysis resembling that of *Curare* and death through respiratory paralysis).

**Dose:** Third potency.

---

## DAMIANA

(Turnera) **Dam.**

Said to be of use in sexual neurasthenia; impotency. Sexual debility from nervous prostration. Incontinence in old people. Chronic prostatic discharge. Renal and cystic catarrh; frigidity in females. Aids the establishment of normal menstrual flow in young girls.

**Dose:** Tincture and fluid extract, ten to forty drop doses.

---

## DAPHNE INDICA

(Spurge Laurel) **Daph.**

Acts on the lower tissues, muscles, bones and skin. Sudden, lightening jerks in different parts of the body. *Craving for tobacco.* Burning in the stomach. Parts of the body feel separated (*Bapt.*). *Fetid* breath, urine, sweat.

**Head:** Feels as if the skull would burst; *as if the head was separated from the body.* Heat in the head, especially vertex.

**Mouth:** Tongue *coated on one side only* (*Rhus-t.*). Foul smelling, saliva hot.

**Urinary:** Thick, turbid, yellowish, like rotten eggs.

**Extremities:** Right toe swollen, painful (gout). Pain shoots upward to the abdomen and heart. Rheumatic pains in the thighs and knees. Buttocks feel cold. Shooting pains, shift rapidly; worse, cold air.

**Sleep:** Complete inability to sleep; sometimes caused by aching in bones. Dreams, with nightmare. Dreams of cats, black cats. Starting on falling to sleep with chilliness and claminess.

**Relationship:** Antidotes: *Bry., Rhus-t.*

Compare: *Fl-ac., Aur., Mez., Staph.*

**Dose:** First to sixth attenuation.

---

## DIGITALIS PURPUREA

(Foxglove) **Dig.**

Comes into play in all diseases where the heart is primarily involved, where the pulse is *weak, irregular, intermittent, abnormally slow* and dropsy of external and internal parts. *Weakness and dilatation of the myocardium.* Its greatest indication is failure of compensation, especially when *auricular fibrillation has set in.* Slow pulse in a recumbent posture, but irregular and dicrotic on sitting up. Auricular flutter and fibrillation especially when subsequent to rheumatic fever. Heart block, very slow pulse. Other symptoms of organic heart disease, such as great weakness and sinking of strength, faintness, coldness of skin and irregular respiration; cardiac irritability and ocular problems after tobacco; jaundice from induration and *hypertrophy of the liver,* frequently call for *Dig.* Jaundice with heart disease. Faint, as if dying. *Bluish* (cyanosed) appearance of the face. *Cardiac muscular failure,* when asystole is present. Stimulates the heart muscles, increases the force of systole, and the length. Prostration from slight exertion. Collapse.

**Mind:** Despondency; fearful; anxious about the future. Dullness of senses. Every shock strikes in the epigastrium[1]. Melancholia, dull lethargic, with *a slow* pulse.

**Head:** Vertigo, when walking and on rising, in cardiac and hepatic affections. Sharp, shooting frontal pain, extending into the nose, after drinking cold water or eating ice-cream. Heaviness of the head, with sensation as if it would fall backward. Face bluish. Confusion, fullness and noises in the head. Cracking sounds during a nap. Blue tongue and lips (cyanosis).

---

1 Stomach, sensitiveness, sinking on bad news (1001 Small Remedies, Edited by Dr. F. Schroyens).

**Eyes:** Blueness of eyelids. Dark bodies, like flies, before the eyes. *Change in the acuteness for the perception of different shades of green.* Objects appear green and yellow. Mydriasis; lid margins red, swollen, agglutinated in the morning (blepharitis). Detachment of retina. Dim vision (amaurosis), irregular pupils, diplopia.

**Stomach:** Sweet taste with constant ptyalism. *Excessive nausea,* not relieved by vomiting. Faintness, *great weakness in the stomach.* Burning in the stomach extending to the esophagus. After taking cold water or ice-cream, sharp pain in the forehead, extending to the nose. *Faintness* and vomiting from motion. Discomfort, even after eating a small quantity of food or from the mere sight or smell. *Tenderness in the epigastrium.* Copious salivation. *Neuralgic pain in the stomach not related to the ingestion of food.*

**Abdomen:** Pain on the left side, apparently in the descending colon and under the false ribs. Severe abdominal pain, pulsations in the abdominal aorta, epigastric constriction. *Enlarged, sore, painful liver* (jaundice).

**Stool:** *White, chalk-like, ashy, pasty stools.* Diarrhea during jaundice.

**Urinary:** Continuous urging, in drops, dark, hot, burning, with sharp cutting or *throbbing* pain at the neck of the bladder, *as if a straw was being thrust back and forth;* worse at night. Suppressed. Ammoniacal and turbid. *Urethritis,* phimosis, strangury. Sensation of fullness after micturition. Constriction and burning, as if the urethra was too small. Brick-dust sediment.

**Male:** Nocturnal emission (*Digitalinum*), with great weakness of genitals after coitus. Hydrocele; scrotum enlarged like a bladder. Gonorrhea, balanitis (*Merc.*), with edema of the prepuce. Dropsical swelling of genitals (*Sulph.*). Enlarged prostate.

**Female:** Labor-like pains in the abdomen and back before menses. Uterine hemorrhage.

**Respiratory:** Desire to take a deep breath. Breathing irregular, difficult; deep sighing. Cough, with raw, sore feeling in the chest. Expectoration sweetish. Senile pneumonia. Great weakness in the chest. *Dyspnea,* constant desire to breathe deeply, lungs feel compressed (asthma). Chronic bronchitis; passive congestion of the lungs, with bloody sputum due to a failing myocardium. *Cannot bear to talk.* Hemoptysis with a weak heart.

**Heart:** The least movement causes violent palpitations, sensation as if it would cease beating, if he moves (opposite, *Gels.*). Frequent stitches in the heart. *Irregular heart especially due to mitral disease. Very slow pulse. Intermits; weak.* Cyanosis. Inequality of pulse; it varies. *Sudden sensation as if the heart stood still. Pulse weak, and quickened by the least movement.* Pericarditis, copious serous exudation. Dilated heart, tired, irregular, with a slow, feeble pulse. Hypertrophy with dilatation. Cardiac failure following fevers. Cardiac dropsy.

**Extremities:** Swelling of the feet. Fingers go to sleep easily. Coldness of the hands and feet. Rheumatic pain in the joints. Shining, white swelling of joints. Muscular debility. Nocturnal swelling in fingers. Sensation as *if a red hot wire* suddenly darted through the legs (Dudgeon).

**Sleep:** *Starts from sleep in alarm* that he is falling from a height. Continuous sleepiness.

**Fever:** Sudden flushes of heat, followed by great nervous weakness.

**Skin:** Erythema, deep red, worse on the back, like measles. Blue distended veins on lids, ears, lips and tongue. *Dropsical.* Itching and jaundiced.

**Modalities:** *Worse,* when sitting erect, after meals and music. *Better*, when stomach is empty; in open air.

**Relationship:** Antidotes: *Camph., Serpentaria aristolochia.*

Incompatible: *Chin.*

Compare: *Nerium odorum* (resembles *Dig.* in heart symptoms, also has an action like strychnia on the spinal cord. Spasms appear more in the upper part of the body. Palpitations; weak heart will be strengthened by it. Lock jaw). *Adon., Crat.* (a true heart tonic); *Kalm., Spig., Liatris spicata.*

Compare also: *Digitoxinum* (*Dig.* dissolved in chloroform; which has yellow vision very marked, and distressing nausea, *aggravated* by *champagne and aerated waters). Nitri spiritus dulcis* increases action of *Dig. Ichthyotoxinum; Eel serum* (experiments show great analogy between the serum and the venom of vipera. Indicated whenever the systole of the heart is insufficient, decompensated valvular disease, irregular pulse due to auricular fibrillation. Asystole, feeble, frequent, irregular pulse, dyspnea and scanty urine. Liver enlarged, dyspnea, albuminuria. No edema). *Convallaria majalis* (heart disease with vertigo and digestive disturbances). *Quinidinum*—Isomeric methoxyl compound (restores normal rhythm in auricular fibrillation, often supplements the action of *Dig.* Two doses of 3 grains each, three hours apart if no symptoms of cinhonism develop, 4 doses 6 grs. each daily (C. Harlan Wells.). Paroxysmal tachycardia. Establishes, normal heart rhythm at least temporarily, less in valvular lesions).

**Dose:** The third to thirtieth attenuation will bring about a reaction when the drug is homeopathically indicated; but for palliative purposes, the physiological dosage is required. For this purpose, the tincture made from the *fresh* plant, in doses of five to twenty drops, when cardiac stimulation is desired, or the infusion of 1½ per cent. Dose, one-half to one ounce if the diuretic action is desired. The tincture may be given on sugar or bread, and no liquid should be taken for twenty minutes before and after its administration. Powdered leaves, ½ to 2 grains in capsules. *Digitoxinum* 1-250 grain. No matter what form of *Dig.* is given, the dose should be reduced as soon as the pulse rate reaches 80 beats a minute and the normal rhythm is partially or completely restored. Under such conditions a good rule is to cut the dose in half and still more if there be a sudden fall in the urinary output.

---

# DIOSCOREA VILLOSA

(Wild Yam) **Dios.**

As a remedy for many kinds of *pain,* especially colic, and in severe, painful affections of the abdominal and pelvic viscera; it ranks with the polychrests of the materia medica. People with feeble digestive powers; tea drinkers, with much flatulence. *Gall stone colic.*

**Mind:** Calls things by the wrong name.

**Head:** Dull pain in both the temples; better pressure, but worse afterwards. Buzzing in the head.

**Stomach:** Mouth dry and bitter in the morning, tongue coated, no thirst. Belching of large quantities of offensive gas. Neuralgia of the stomach. *Sinking in the pit of the* stomach, pyrosis. *Pain along the sternum, extending to the arms.* Eructations of sour, bitter wind, with *hiccough.* Sharp pain in the epigastrium, relieved by standing erect.

**Abdomen:** Pains suddenly shift to different parts; *appear in remote localities, as fingers and toes.* Rumbling, with emission of much flatus. Griping, cutting in the hypogastric region, with intermittent cutting in the stomach and small intestines. Colic; better walking around; pains radiate from the abdomen to the back, chest, arms; worse, bending forward and while lying. *Sharp pains from the liver, shooting upward to the right nipple.* Pain from the gall bladder radiates to the chest, back, and arms. Renal colic, pain in the extremities. Hurried desire for stool.

**Rectum:** Hemorrhoids with darting pains extending to the liver; looks like a bunch of grapes or red cherries; protrude after stool, with pain in the anus. Diarrhea worse in the morning, yellowish, followed by exhaustion, as if flatus and feces were hot.

**Male:** *Relaxation and coldness of the organs.* Pains shoot into the testicles from the region of kidneys. *Strong smelling sweat* on the scrotum and pubes. *Emissions* in sleep or from sexual atony *with weak knees.*

**Female:** Uterine colic; pains radiate from the uterus. Vivid dreams.

**Respiratory:** Tight feeling all along the sternum. Chest does not seem to expand on breathing. Short winded.

**Heart:** Angina pectoris; pain behind the sternum radiates to the arms, labored breathing; *feeble action of the heart,* especially with flatulence pain through the chest and tightness across.

**Extremities:** Lameness of the back; worse, stooping. Aching and stiffness in joints. Sciatica; pains shoot down the thigh; worse, right side; better, when perfectly still. *Felons* in the beginning, when pricking is first felt. Nails brittle. Cramps in flexors of fingers and toes.

**Modalities:** *Worse,* evening and night, *lying down,* and *doubling up. Better,* standing erect, motion in open air; pressure.

**Relationship:** Antidotes: *Cham., Camph.*

Compare: *Coloc.* (differs in modalities); *Nux-v., Cham., Bry.*

**Dose:** Tincture to third potency.

---

## DIOSMA LINCARIS

(Buku—from Cape of Good Hope) **Diosm.**

Pathogenically it produces: Somnolence; nervous insomnia; night sweats. Erratic pains with bad humor, desire to weep or fear of sickness. Violent vertigo. Cephalagia, chiefly frontal, radiating to the occiput. Eyes brilliant with lachrymation or itching, the conditions are accompanied with an expression of stupefaction, hardness of hearing or noises from aural pressure. Earthy face with disseminated rosaceous eruptions. Nausea, fetid breath with sensation of emptiness. *Sensation of meteorism with stinging pains in the spleen.* Painful sensation in the abdomen, with pubic pressure, the pressure of clothes becomes insupportable with emission of highly colored, bloody urine. Frequent yellow diarrhea, worse at night. Catamenia abundant, anticipating, sometimes metrorrhagic in type; crampy pains on ingesting food. Sensation of heat or of cold in the hands, with convulsive movements of the fingers. Weakness of the legs, aggravated by sitting down.

Clinically, this pathogeny should be useful in cerebral affections with dullness or stupefaction; in convulsive or epileptiform attacks; in *hysteria;* in *hepatitis* (cirrhosis or atrophy); in hematuria with ovarian or uterine lesions.

In splenitis, where it surpasses *Cean.* Mental disorders in nervous or ascetic individuals, particularly where there is constant fear of death, erotic or maniacal attacks. *Gastralgia. Gastroenteritis.* Sudden fright with trembling and weakness of the legs (Dr. C. Leal La Rota).

---

## DIPHTHERINUM

(Potentized Diphtheritic Virus) **Diph.**

Adapted to patients prone to catarrhal affections of the respiratory organs, scrofulous individuals. Diphtheria, laryngeal diphtheria, *post-diphtheritic paralysis.* Malignancy from the start. Glands swollen; tongue red, swollen;

breath and discharge very offensive. Diphtheritic membrane thick, dark. Epistaxis; profound prostration. Swallows without pain, but fluids are vomited or returned by the nose.

**Relationship:** Compare: *Diphtherotoxinum* (Cahis) (chronic bronchitis with rales. Cartier suggests it in the vago-paralytic forms of bronchitis in the aged or in toxic bronchitis after influenza).

**Dose:** Thirtieth, two hundredth or C. M. potency. Must not be repeated too frequently.

---

## DOLICHOS PURIENS—MUCUNA

(Cowhage) **Dol.**

A right sided medicine, with pronounced liver and skin sypmtoms. A general, *intense itching* without eruptions. Exalted nervous sensibility. Senile pruritus. Hemorrhoidal diathesis.

**Throat:** *Pain in the throat, worse swallowing, below the right angle of jaw, as if a splinter was imbedded vertically.* Pain in the gums prevents sleep.

**Abdomen:** Colic from getting feet wet. *Constipation, with intense itching; bloated abdomen.* White stools. Swelling of the liver (hepatomegaly-jaundice). *Hemorrhoids,* with a burning sensation.

**Skin:** *Intense, itching,* with no swelling or rash; worse across the shoulders, also around the elbows, knees and hairy parts. Jaundice. Yellow in spots; itching excessively at night. Herpes zoster (*Ars.*).

**Modalities:** *Worse,* at night, scratching, right side.

**Relationship:** Compare: *Rhus-t., Bell., Hep., Nit-ac., Fago.*

**Dose:** Sixth potency. Tincture, drop doses, in hemorrhoids.

---

## DORYPHORA DECEMLINEATA

(Colorado Potato Bug) **Dor.**

The center of this drug's action seems to be in the urinary organs, hence its employment in gonorrhea and gleet. Urethritis in children from local irritation and gleet. Severe trembling in the extremities. Prostration. Swelling of the body. *Burning sensation.*

**Urinary:** Difficult micturition. Urethra inflamed (urethritis), with excruciating pain on micturition (dysuria). Pain in the back and loins. Severe trembling in limbs.

**Relationship:** Antidote: *Stram.*

Compare: *Agar., Apis, Canth., Lach., Cocc-s.*

**Dose:** Sixth to thirtieth potency.

## DROSERA ROTUNDIFOLIA

(Sundew) **Dros.**

Affects markedly the respiratory organs and was pointed out by Hahnemann as the principal remedy for whooping cough. *Dros.* can break down resistance to tubercles and should therefore be capable of raising it (Dr. Tyler). Laryngeal phthisis is benefited by it. Phthisis pulmonaris; vomiting of food due to coughing with gastric irritation and profuse expectoration. Pain around the hip joint. Tubercular glands.

**Head:** Vertigo when walking in the open air, with an inclination to fall on the *left side.* Coldness of the left half of face, with stinging pains and dry heat in the *right half.*

**Stomach:** Nausea. Aversion to and bad effects from acids.

**Respiratory:** Spasmodic, dry irritating cough, like whooping cough, the *paroxysms follow each other very rapidly;* can scarcely breathe; chokes. Cough very deep and hoarse; worse, after midnight; yellow expectoration, *with bleeding from the nose* and mouth; *retching. Deep, hoarse voice; hoarseness;* laryngitis. Rough, scraping sensation deep in the fauces and soft palate. Sensation of crumbs in the throat, of a feather in the larynx. Laryngeal phthisis with rapid emaciation. Harassing and titillating cough in children, not at all through out the day, but commences as soon as the head touches the pillow, at night. Clergyman's sore throat, with rough, scraping, dry sensation deep in the fauces; voice hoarse, deep, toneless, cracked, requires exertion to speak. *Asthma when talking,* with contractions of the throat at every word uttered.

**Extremities:** Paralytic pains in the coccy-femoral joint and thighs. Stiffness in the joints of feet. All limbs feel lame. Bed feels too hard.

**Fever:** Internal chilliness; shivering, with a hot face, cold hands, no thirst. Is always too cold, even in bed.

**Modalities:** Worse, after midnight, lying down, on getting warm in bed, drinking, singing, laughing.

**Relationship:** Antidote: *Camph.*

Compare: *Fluoroformium* (2 percent watery solution, 2-4 drops, after paroxysms, considered specific for whooping cough). *Ouabain* from leaves of Carissa schimperi—Arrow poison (respiratory spasm-whooping cough is cut short in the first stage, reduced frequency of attacks and hastens convalescence). *Chel., Cor-r., Cupr., Cast., Arg-met., Meny.*

**Dose:** First to twelfth attenuation.

# DUBOISINUM

(Corkwood Elm) **Dub.**

Acts chiefly on the nervous system, eyes, upper respiratory tract. Recommended in pharyngitis sicca with black, stringy mucus. It dilates the pupil, dries the mouth, checks perspiration, causes headache and drowsiness. On the eye it acts more promptly than Atropia, much stronger as a mydriatic. *Red spots float in the field of vision.* Sensation as if stepping in an empty space. *Vertigo with a pale face* (anemia); not gastric in origin. Scarlet fever; locomotor ataxia. Palliative in exophthalmic goitre.

**Mind**: Absent-minded, incoherent, *silly and nonsensical,* memory impaired.

**Head**: Impossible to stand with eyes shut, tendency to fall backwards.

**Eyes**: *Conjunctivitis,* acute and chronic. Mydriasis. Paralysis of accommodation. Hyperemia of the retina with weakness of accommodation, fundus red, blood vessels full and tortuous; pupils dilated, with dim vision. *Pain over the eyes,* between them and the brow.

**Respiratory**: Larynx dry, voice hoarse, phonation difficult. Dry cough with oppressed breathing.

**Extremities**: Loss of power in limbs, staggers; feels as if he has stepped in an empty space. Trembling, numbness and weakness.

**Relationship:** It antagonises *Muscarinum. Duboisin sulphate* 1-100 gr. *sedative in mania.* 2-4 milligrams a day. Hystero-epilepsy. Motor restlessness in insane. *Has been used as a substitute for Atropia* in doses of 1-20 of a grain hypodermically.

Antidotes: *Morph., Pilo.*

Compare: *Bell., Stram., Hyos.*

**Dose**: Third to twelfth potency.

---

# DULCAMARA

(Bitter-sweet) **Dulc.**

Hot days and cold nights towards the close of summer are especially favorable for the action of *Dulcamara,* is one of the remedies whose symptoms corresponds to the conditions found in effects of damp weather, colds after exposure to wet, especially diarrhea. It has a specific relation to the *skin, glands* and digestive organs; *mucous membranes* secrete more profusely while the skin is inactive. The rheumatic *problems* induced by damp cold are aggravated by every cold change and are somewhat relieved by moving about. Results from sitting on a cold, damp ground. Icy coldness. One sided spasms with speechlessness. Paralysis of single parts. Congestive headache with neuralgia and a dry nose. Patients living or working in damp, cold basements (*Nat-s.*). Eruptions on the hands, arms or face around the menstrual period.

**Head:** Mental confusion. Occipital pain ascending from the nape of the neck (meningitis). Headache relieved by conversation. Rejects things asked for. Back part of head chilly, heavy, aching, during cold weather. Tinea capitis. *Scald head, thick brown crusts,* bleeding when scratched. Buzzing in the head.

**Eyes:** Every time he takes a cold, it settles in the eyes. Thick, yellow discharge; granular lids (blepharitis, ophthalmia). Hay fever; profuse, watery discharge, worse in the open air.

**Ears:** Otalgia, buzzing, stitches and swelling of parotids (mumps, parotiditis). Middle ear catarrh (otitis media, otorrhea) (*Merc-d., Kali-m.*).

**Nose:** Dry coryza. Complete stoppage of the nose. *Stuffs up when there is a cold rain.* Thick, yellow mucus, bloody crusts. Profuse coryza. Wants to keep the nose warm, least cold air obstructs the nose. Coryza in the new born.

**Face:** Tearing in the cheek extending to the ear, orbit, and jaw, *preceded by coldness of parts, and attended by canine hunger.* Humid eruptions on the cheeks and face generally; facial neuralgia; worse, *slightest exposure to cold.*.

**Mouth:** Saliva tenacious, soapy. Dry, rough tongue, rough scraping in the throat, after taking cold in damp weather. Cold sores on the lips.

**Stomach:** Vomiting of white, tenacious mucus. *Aversion to food. Burning thirst for cold drinks.* Heartburn. Nausea accompanies the desire for stool. Chills during vomiting.

**Abdomen**: Colic from cold. Acts prominently on the umbilical region. *Cutting pain around the navel.* Swelling of the inguinal glands (*Merc.*).

**Rectum:** Green, watery, slimy, bloody *mucus,* especially in summers, when the weather suddenly becomes cold; *from damp, cold weather* and suppressed eruptions.

**Urinary:** Must micturate *on getting chilled.* Strangury, painful micturition. Catarrh of the bladder (cystitis) from taking cold. Urine has thick, *mucoid,* purulent sediment (pyuria). Ischuria from wading. with bare feet in cold water.

**Female:** Suppression of menses from cold or dampness. Before appearance of menses, *a rash appears on the skin* or sexual excitement. Dysmenorrhea with blotches all over; mammae engorged and sore, delicate, sensitive to cold.

**Respiratory:** Cough worse cold, wet weather, with free expectoration, tickling in the larynx. Cough, hoarse, spasmodic. Whooping cough, with excessive secretion of mucus. Winter coughs, dry, teasing. Asthma with dyspnea. Loose, rattling cough; worse wet weather. Must cough for a long time to the expel phlegm. Cough *after physical exertion. Adenitis.*

**Back:** Stiff neck. *Pain in the small of back* (lumbosacral region), as after stooping for a long time. Stiffness and lameness across the neck and shoulders, after getting cold and wet (cervical spondylosis).

**Extremities:** Paralysis; paralyzed limbs, *feet icy cold.* Warts on hands. Perspiration on the palms. Pain in the shin bones. Rheumatism alternates with diarrhea. Rheumatic symptoms after acute skin eruptions.

**Fever:** Dry, burning heat all over. Chills towards the evening, mostly in the back. Icy coldness, with pains. Dry heat with burning of skin. Chills with thirst.

**Skin:** *Pruritus, always worse in cold, wet weather.* Herpes zoster, pemphigus. Swelling and indurated glands from exposure to cold. Vesicular eruptions. Sensitive, bleeding ulcers. Little boils. Red spots, *urticaria,* brought on by exposure, or sour stomach. Humid eruptions on the face, genitals, hands, etc. *Warts,* large, smooth, on the face and palmar surface of hands. Anasarca. Thick, brown-yellow crusts, bleeding when scratched.

**Modalities:** *Worse,* at night; from *cold* in general, *damp, rainy weather. Better,* from moving about, external warmth.

**Relationship:** Antidotes: *Camph., Cupr.*

Complementary: *Bar-c.*

Incompatible: *Bell., Lach.*

Compare: *Pimpinella saxifraga*—Bibernell: Respiratory mucous membrane sensitive to draughts, pain and coldness in the occiput and nape. Whole body weak; heavy head and drowsiness; lumbago and stiff neck; pain from the nape to the shoulder; chilliness. *Rhus-t., Cimic., Calc., Puls., Bry., Nat-s.*

**Dose:** Second to thirtieth potency.

---

## ECHINACEA ANGUSTIFOLIA—RUDBECKIA

(Purple Cone Flower) **Echi.**

We are indebted to the eclectic school for this remarkable medicine as a "corrector of blood dyscrasia." Acute autoinfection. Symptoms of *blood poisoning, septic conditions generally.* Diarrhea during typhoid. Gonorrhea. Boils. *Erysipelas* and foul ulcers. *Gangrene.* Goitre with exophthalmic symptoms; full doses, can also inject 5-10 drops into the thyroid gland. Tendency to malignancy in acute and subacute disorders. Last stages of cancer, to ease pain. *Venom infection.* Cerebro-spinal meningitis. Puerperal infections. *Tired feeling.* Piles. Pustules. Acts on the vermiform appendix, thus has been used for appendicitis, but remember it promotes suppuration and a neglected appendicitis with pus formation would probably rupture sooner under its use. Lymphatic inflammation; crushing injuries. *Snake bites,* bites and stings in general. Foul discharges with emaciation and great debility.

**Head:** Confused, depressed. Aches with a peculiar periodical flushing of the face, even to the neck; dizziness and profound prostration.

**Nose:** Foul smelling discharge, membranous formations protruding (diphtheria). Post-nasal catarrh with ulceration and fetor (ozena). Nose feels stuffed up. Right nostril raw, bleeding.

**Mouth:** Canker; gums recede and bleed easily (scorbutic); corners of mouth and lips crack; tongue dry and swollen; sores; dirty brownish. Tongue, lips, and fauces *tingle* with a sense of fear around the heart (*Acon.*). White coating of tongue, with red edges. Promotes the flow of saliva.

**Throat:** Tonsils purple or black, gray exudation extending to posterior nares and air passages. Ulcerated sore throat.

**Stomach:** Sour belching and heartburn. Nausea; better lying down.

**Urinary:** Albuminous, scanty, frequent and involuntary.

**Female:** *Puerperal septicemia;* discharges suppressed; abdomen sensitive and tympanitic; offensive, excoriating leucorrhea.

**Chest:** Pain as if a lump in the chest, under the sternum. Pain in the pectoral muscles (*Arist-m.*).

**Extremities:** *Aching in limbs* and general lassitude.

**Fever:** *Chilliness with nausea.* Cold flashes all over the back. *Malarial fever.*

**Skin:** Recurring boils. Carbuncles. Irritations from insect bites and poisonous plants. Lymphatics enlarged (lymphangitis). Old tibial ulcers. Gangrene.

**Relationship:** Compare: *Cench., Both., Ars., Lach., Bapt., Rhus-t., Cist., Hep., Calen.*

**Dose:** Tincture, one to ten drops, every two hours and larger doses.

*Locally,* as a cleansing and antiseptic wash.

---

# ELAPS CORALLINUS

(Coral Snake) **Elaps**

Similar to snake poisons generally. Has very marked *black discharges. Cold things disagree.* Desire for sweetened buttermilk. Nausea and vomiting. Prostrating diarrhea of consumption. Acidity of the stomach with a faint feeling. Sudden pain in the stomach. Spasms of the esophagus; pharynx constricted; food and liquids suddenly arrested, and then fall heavily into the stomach.

Spasms followed by paresis. *Cold feeling in the stomach.* Fruits and ice water lie very cold. *Right sided paralysis.* Must have oscillatory motion. Rheumatic constitutions. Ear, nose and throat symptoms important.

**Mind:** Depressed; imagines that he hears someone talking; dreads to be left alone. *Fear of rain.* Can speak, but cannot understand speech. Fears apoplexy.

**Head:** Violent headache, extending from the forehead *to the occiput;* first one eye, then the other. Otalgia. Vertigo with a tendency to fall forward. Weight and pain in the forehead. Fullness of the head.

**Eyes:** Aversion to light (photophobia); letters run together when reading. Veil before the eyes (amaurosis). Burning in lids. Edema around the eyes in the morning. Large, red, fiery spots before the eyes.

**Ears:** Cerumen *black* and hard with difficulty in hearing; a serous, *greenish* discharge, offensive; buzzing, and auditory illusions. Sudden attack of nocturnal deafness with roaring and crackling in the ears, crackling in ears on swallowing. Intolerable itching in the ear.

**Nose:** *Chronic nasal catarrh with fetid odor and greenish crusts.* Ozena; yellowish-green discharge. Mucous membrane wrinkled; nostrils plugged up with dry mucus. Pains from the nose to the ears on swallowing. *Nostrils stopped up.* Epistaxis. Pain at the root of nose. Eruptions around the nose.

**Throat:** Thick, very offensive, dry, greenish-yellow crusts on the posterior pharyngeal wall and extremely foul breath. Spasmodic contractions of the *esophagus;* passage of fluids arrested.

**Stomach:** *Feels cold.* Sensation as if the food turns like a corkscrew on swallowing; desire for sweetened buttermilk. Acidity after every mouthful.

**Female:** Dysmenorrhea with black blood. Discharge of black blood between menses (metrorrhagia). Itching of vulva and vagina.

**Chest:** *Coldness in the chest after drinking.* Hemorrhage from the lungs, black like ink and watery; stitches *in the apex of right lung* (phthisis). Fainting caused by stooping. Oppression on going upstairs. Peeling off of skin from palms and fingers. *Cough,* with terrible pain through the lungs. Worse right side and expectoration of black blood (hemoptysis). Sensation of a sponge in the esophagus.

**Extremities:** Icy cold feet. Vesicular eruptions on feet. Arms and hands swollen, bluish. Knee joints feel sprained. Pricking under the nails.

**Sleep:** Dreams about dead people.

**Fever:** Cold perspiration all over. Typhoid when ulcers have eaten into the tissues, and black blood is discharged.

**Skin:** Glands and skin of axillae affected; itching with tetter. Tips of fingers peel off. Itching eruptions in the axillae.

**Modalities:** *Worse* eating fruit; cold drinks; *wet weather.*

**Relationship:** Compare: *Kino*—from *Pterocarpus erinaceus* (hemoptysis and hemorrhage from intestines). *Eucalyptus rostrata* (offensive dark discharge from the right ear). *Crot-h., Alumn., Carb-v., Ars., Lach.*

**Dose:** Sixth to thirtieth potency.

---

## ELATERIUM—ECBALIUM

(Squirting Cucumber) **Elat.**

This is an invaluable remedy in violent vomiting and purging, especially if the evacuations are copious and watery. It is a very efficient remedy in certain forms of dropsy. Marked yawning and stretching. *Beriberi;* choleraic conditions; urticaria and mental disorders coming on as a consequence of suppressed malaria. An irresistible desire to wander away from home at night. Effects of damp weather.

**Stomach:** Nausea and vomiting with great weakness. Griping pain in the bowels.

**Rectum:** *Watery, copious, forceful. Squirting diarrhea;* frothy, olive green, with cutting in the abdomen.

**Extremities:** Sharp pain in fingers, thumbs, knees, toes, and instep. Gouty pain in both the great toes. Pain extends down the extremities; pain in the hip joints with diarrhea. Arthritic nodules.

**Fever:** Chill comes on with marked *yawning and stretching,* lasting all through the chill. Pain in extremities, darting to the fingers and toes. Chills and fever, with spurting diarrhea.

**Skin:** Smarts, stings, and burns. Dropsical. Urticaria from suppressed intermittent fever. Skin, orange colour.

**Modalities:** *Worse,* from exposure on a damp ground.

**Relationship:** Compare: *Bry., Crot-t., Gamb.*

**Dose:** Third to thirtieth potency. As a hydragogue cathartic to produce free discharge in dropsies, *Elat.* 1-20 of a grain. Palliative only.

---

## EOSINUM

**Eos.**

A remedy for cancer, polyarthritis. Proved in potencies by Dr. B. C. Woodbury.

**Mind:** Peculiar sensation of being very tall with a tendency for vertigo.

**Mouth:** Redness, burning and *numbness* of the tongue (glossitis).

**Extremities:** *Burning* under finger nails and toe nails, in soles. *Itching* and redness of knee caps. *Redness* of palms.

**Skin:** Burning in various parts on skin. Shifting location after scratching which relieves.

**Dose:** Second decimal (1% solution).

## EPIGEA REPENS

(Trailing Arbutus) **Epig.**

Chronic cystitis with *dysuria;* tenesmus after micturition; *muco-pus and uric acid deposit,* gravel, renal calculi. Fine sand in the urine of a *brown color.* Burning in the neck of the bladder whilst micturating and tenesmus afterwards. Pyelitis, incontinence of urine. Croaking noise and rumbling in bowels.

**Relationship:** Compare: *Uva, Chim., Lyc., Pareir. Epig.* contains arbutin and formic acid.

**Dose:** Tincture in 5 drop doses every three hours.

## EPIPHEGUS VIRGINIANA—OROBANCHE

(Beechdrop) **Epiph.**

A remedy for sick, neurasthenic and nervous headaches, especially in women, brought on or aggravated by exertion, shopping, etc. Tongue coated yellow; bitter taste. Drowsy after meals. Loose stools. *Subinvolution* with dysmenorrhea and congestion.

**Head:** Pressing pain in the temples, *pressing inwards; worse, left side. Viscid salivation;* constant inclination to spit. Sick headache, coming on when deviating from ordinary pursuits. Headaches from nerve tire caused by mental or physical exhaustion, *preceded by hunger.*

**Modalities:** *Worse,* from working in open air. *Better,* from sleep.

**Relationship:** Compare: *Iris, Meli., Sang., Fagu*—Beech nuts (headache and salivation; swelling in the mouth; dread of water).

**Dose:** First to thirtieth potency.

## EQUISETUM HYEMALE

(Scouring Rush) **Equis-h.**

Principal action is on the bladder. A remedy for enuresis and dysuria.

**Urinary:** Severe, dull pain with a feeling of fullness in the bladder, not relieved by micturating. Frequent urging with severe pain *at the close of micturition.* Urine flows only drop by drop. Sharp, *burning,* cutting pains in the urethra while micturating.

Incontinence in children, with dreams or nightmares when passing urine. Incontinence in old women, with involuntary stools. Retention and dysuria during pregnancy and after delivery. Much mucus in urine. Albuminuria. Involuntary micturition (enuresis).

Deep pain in the region of right kidney, extending to the lower abdomen with an urgent desire to micturate. Right lumbar region painful.

**Modalities:** *Worse,* right side, movement, pressure, touch, sitting down; *better,* in the afternoon from lying down.

**Relationship:** Compare: *Hydrang., Ferr-p., Apis, Canth., Lina., Chim. Equis-h.* contains silica in an appreciable quantity.

**Dose:** Tincture to sixth potency. A decoction, teaspoonful doses or the tincture in hot water is found useful to allay irritability of the urinary tract, calculus, dysuria, etc., also for pleuritic effusion and dropsy.

---

## ERECHTHITES HIERACIFOLIA

(Fire-weed) **Erech.**

A hemorrhagic remedy. Epistaxis of bright red blood. Hemorrhage from any part, especially lungs; always attended by excitement of circulation. Flashes of heat and coldness. Scanty urine, edema of the extremities.

**Skin:** *Symptoms like Rhus poisoning.*

**Relationship:** Compare: *Erig., Mill., Ham., Rhus-t.*

**Dose:** Tincture. Locally for Poison oak.

---

## ERIGERON CANADENSE—LEPTILON CANADENSE

(Fleabane) **Erig.**

Hemorrhages are caused and cured by this remedy. Persistent hemorrhage from the bladder. Hemorrhage from the uterus with dysuria. *Profuse bright red blood.* Pain in the left ovary and hip. Chronic gonorrhea with burning micturition; continuous dribbling. *Dysentery* with soreness and burning in the bladder. *Tympanites.*

**Female:** Metrorrhagia with violent irritation of the rectum and bladder, prolapsus uteri. Bright red flow. Menorrhagia; profuse leucorrhea; *bloody lochia returns after least motion,* comes in gushes; between periods, *leucorrhea with urinary irritation;* pregnant women with a "weak uterus"; a bloody discharge on the slightest exertion. Bleeding hemorrhoids; epistaxis instead of menses (*Bry.*).

**Modalities:** *Worse,* left side.

**Relationship:** *Terebinthiniae oleum* similar.

**Dose:** Tincture to third potency. Oil of Erig. 1x internally *for tympanites.* An enema of one dram of the oil with the yolk of an egg and a pint of milk will reduce the most enormous tympanites.

---

## ERIODYCTION CALIFORNICUM

(Yerba Santa) **Erio.**

A remedy for asthmatic and bronchial affections. Bronchial phthisis with night sweats and emaciation. Asthma relieved by expectoration. *Cough after influenza.* Stimulates absorption of pleural effusion. Poor appetite with an impaired digestion. Whooping cough.

**Head:** Dizzy, feels intoxicated. Pressure outwards; worse, occiput.

**Ears:** Otalgia.

**Nose:** Coryza with burning in the throat. Coryza with dizziness and sneezing.

**Mouth:** Foul taste in the morning.

**Male:** Sore, dragging in the testicle, cannot bear any pressure; better gentle support.

**Respiratory:** Wheezing; asthma, with coryza and *mucus secretions.* Dull pain in the right lung. Burning in the fauces. Chronic bronchitis, bronchial tuberculosis, with profuse, easily raised bronchial secretion, giving relief.

**Relationship:** Compare: *Grin., Aral., Eucal., Ip.*

**Dose:** Tincture in doses of 2 to 20 drops and attenuations.

---

## ERYNGIUM AQUATICUM

(Button Snakeroot) **Ery-a.**

A remedy for urinary disorders. Strangury, etc., with nervous erethism. *Thick, yellow mucoid discharges.* Influenza. Uridrosis, sweat with a urinous odor in the evening.

**Urinary:** Tenesmus of the bladder (cystitis) and urethra (urethritis). Difficult and frequent micturition. Pain behind the pubes. Spasmodic stricture. *Renal colic* (*Pareir., Calc.*). Congestion of kidneys (nephritis) with a dull pain in the back, running down to the ureters and limbs. Irritable bladder from an enlarged prostate or from pressure of the uterus.

**Male:** Discharge of prostatic fluid on the slightest cause (prostatorrhea). Seminal emissions without erections, with lassitude (spermatorrhea) (*Dios., Ph-ac.*).

**Respiratory:** Cough with a sense of constriction. Smarting in the throat and larynx.

**Relationship:** Compare: *Con., Cann-s., Dios., Oci., Clem.*

**Dose:** Tincture to third potency.

---

## ESCHSCHOLTZIA CALIFORNICA

(California Poppy) **Esch.**

Experiments on animals shows that it acts more powerfully than morphine which is contained in the plant. It causes general weakness, torpor, accelerated respiration and complete paralysis of the limbs. Slowing of circulation.

A soporic remedy which is harmless. Use the tincture.

---

## EUCALYPTUS GLOBULUS

(Blue Gum Tree) **Eucal.**

*Eucal.* is a powerful antiseptic and is destructive to the lower forms of life, a stimulating expectorant and an efficient diaphoretic. Atonic dyspepsia, gastric and intestinal catarrh. A remedy with marked effects on catarrhal processes, malaria and intestinal disturbances. *Influenza.* Fevers of a *relapsing* character. Produces diuresis and a great increase of urea. Hemorrhages, internally and locally (*Ham.*). *Typhoid.* Symptoms of exhaustion and toxemia. Disorders of the mucous membranes of the air passages, genito-urinary organs and gastro-intestinal tract. A gastro-intestinal irritant with pain in the stomach and upper intestines, several hours after eating.

**Head:** Exhilaration. Desire for exercise. Dull, congestive headache. *Coryza;* sore throat.

**Eyes:** Eye smart and burn.

**Nose:** *Stuffed up sensation;* thin, watery coryza; nose does not stop running; tightness across the bridge. *Chronic catarrhal, purulent and fetid discharge.*

Ethmoid and frontal sinus involved (sinusitis).

**Throat:** Relaxed, aphthous condition of the mouth and throat. Excessive secretion of saliva. Burns, feels full. Constant sensation of phlegm in the throat. Enlarged, ulcerated tonsils and an inflamed throat (use tincture locally).

**Stomach:** *Slow digestion.* Marked flatulence, fetid. All gone sensation with pulsations in the epigastrium. Spleen hard and contracted. Pain in the epigastrium and upper abdomen, ameliorated by food. Malignant disease of the stomach with vomiting of blood (hematemesis) and sour fluid.

**Rectum:** *Acute diarrhea.* Aching pains in the bowels with a feeling of impending diarrhea. *Dysentery* with rectal heat; tenesmus; hemorrhage. Diarrhea; stools thin, watery, preceded by sharp pains. Diarrhea of typhoid.

**Urinary:** *Acute nephritis complicating influenza.* Hematuria. Suppurative inflammation of the kidneys (pyelonephritis). Urine contains pus (pyuria) and is deficient in urea. Sensation of loss of expulsive force in the bladder. Burning and tenesmus; *catarrh of the bladder* (cystitis); diuresis; *urethral caruncle* (nodule). Spasmodic stricture; gonorrhea.

**Female**: Leucorrhea, acrid, fetid. Ulcer around the urethral orifice.

**Respiratory:** *Asthma* with great dyspnea and palpitations. Moist asthma. Expectoration of white, thick mucus. Bronchitis in the aged. Bronchorrhea (*Bals., Peru.*). Profuse expectoration of offensive muco-pus. Irritating cough. Whooping cough in rachitic children. Fetid form of bronchitis, bronchial dilatation and emphysema.

**Extremities:** Rheumatic pains; worse at night, walking or carrying anything. Stiff, weary sensation. *Prickling sensation, followed by painful aching.* Nodular swellings over the metacarpal and metatarsal joints.

**Fever:** Elevation of temperature. Continuous and typhoid fevers. Scarlet fever (protective and curative). Discharges show a tendency to foulness, high temperature, accelerated but not a strong pulse. Use the tincture.

**Skin:** Glandular enlargements and nodular swelling over joints. Foul and indolent ulcers. Herpetic eruptions.

**Relationship:** Compare: *Oleum eucalyptus* (produces a remarkable physical exhaustion, no desire for any motion, unable to do any real mental work, study, etc. The volatile oil possesses, in common with other terpenes, the property of converting water, in the presence of air and sunlight, into hydrogen peroxide, or to convert oxygen into ozone which is the explanation usually given for its deodorizing and antiseptic properties (Merrel). Locally, in catarrhal affections, especially when of a suppurating or putrid nature). *Eucalyptus tereticoris* (menstrual cough and *prostration). Eucalyptolum* (depresses the temperature of the healthy body more than quinine; acts on the kidneys like *Ter.*); *Anac., Hydr., Kali-s. Eucal.* neutralizes ill effects of

*Strychninum. Angophora lanceolatum*—Red gum (dysentery, pains, tenesmus; better lying flat on the face; obstinate constipation). *Eucalyptus rostrata; Kino.*

**Dose:** Tincture in one to 20 drop doses and lower potencies. Also *Oleum eucalyptolum* in five drop doses.

---

# EUGENIA JAMBOS—JAMBOSA VULGARIS

(Rose-apple) **Eug.**

*Eug.* produces a state of intoxication like alcohol. Everything appears beautiful and larger; excitement soon changes to depression. Acne, simple and indurated. The pimples and some area around it is painful. Acne rosacea. Nausea, *better smoking. Comedones.*

**Head:** Headache as if a board was lying on the right side. Talkative. *Hot lachrymation.*

**Extremities:** *Nocturnal cramps in soles of feet* (*Cupr., Zing.*). Skin cracks around the toes. Fissures between toes (tinea pedis). Skin recedes from the nails, forming pus (paronychia, onychia, panatrium).

**Relationship:** Compare: *Eugenia cheken—Myrtus chekan* (chronic bronchitis); *Ant., Berb-a.*

---

# EUONYMUS ATROPURPUREA

(Wahoo. Burning Bush) **Euon-a.**

Brunettes more easily affected, producing headache, mental disturbances and distress in the hepatic and renal region; albuminuria. Migraine. Passive congestion and torpor of the liver; chronic catarrhal affections of the stomach and intestines. Weak heart. Chronic rheumatism and gout.

**Mind:** Mental confusion, despondent, irritable; loss of memory, unable to recall familiar names.

**Head:** Heavy frontal headache. Sore, tired feeling; bruised feeling of the scalp. Pain over the right eye extending back through the head. Bilious headache; coated tongue, bad taste, constipation. Vertigo, obscure vision and gastric derangement associated with albuminuria. Headache over the eyebrows.

**Stomach:** Mouth dry, pasty taste; thirsty, stomach full and uncomfortable.

**Abdomen:** Flatulance and pain. Anus very sore and burning. Constipation with hemorrhoids and severe backache. Diarrhea; stools variable and profuse, bloody. Pain around umbilical region.

**Urinary:** Urine scanty, high colored; acidity increased.

**Back:** Dull pain between the shoulders and around the renal and splenic region; pain in the lumbar region better lying down.

**Extremities:** Aching in all joints, especially ankles. Feet feel swollen and tired.

**Modalities:** *Better* cool draught, pressure. *Worse* evening.

**Relationship:** *Euonymus europaea*—Spindle tree (liver disorders, biliousness, lumbago, gastric derangements with albuminuria. Cutting pains in malar bones, tongue, penis up to the bladder); *Podo., Am-pic., Chel., Euonin.* lx trituration (albuminuria).

**Dose:** Tincture and lower attenuations.

---

# EUPATORIUM AROMATICUM

(Pool-root) **Eup-a.**

Nervous erethism; restlessness and morbid watchfulness[1]. Hysteria and chorea. Low fevers, with extreme restlessness.

Aphthous disease. *Sore nipples.* Sore mouth in infants (stomatitis). Vomiting of bile, pain in the stomach, headache, and fever.

**Relationship**: *Lapsana communis*—Nipple wort: Useful in sore nipples and piles. *Hyos., Passi., Hydraz-m.*

**Dose**: Tincture, locally, on the sore mouth and sore nipples. Internally, tincture to third attenuation.

---

# EUPATORIUM PERFOLIATUM

(Thoroughwort) **Eup-per.**

Known as "Bone-set," from the prompt manner in which it relieves pain in limbs and muscles which accompanies some forms of febrile disease, like malaria and influenza. *Eup-per.* acts principally upon the gastro-hepatic organs and bronchial mucous membrane. It is a boon in miasmatic districts, along the rivers, marshes, etc., and in all conditions where there is a great deal of *bone pain.* Cachexia from old, chronic, bilious intermittents. Worn out constitutions from inebriety. Sluggishness of all organs and functions. Bone pains, general and severe. Soreness. Marked periodicity (*Ars., Chin., Cedr.*).

---

[1] Morbid irritation of the nerveous system (Clarke — Dictionary of Practical Materia Medica).

**Head**: Throbbing pain. Pressure as if a cap of lead was pressed over the whole skull. Vertigo; sensation of falling to *the left.* Vomiting of bile. Pain on top and back of head with pain *and soreness of the eyeballs.* Periodical headache, every third and seventh day. *Occipital pain after lying down, with a sense of weight.*

**Mouth**: Cracks at the corners of the mouth, yellow coated tongue, thirst.

**Stomach**: Tongue yellow. Taste bitter. Hepatic region sore (jaundice). Great thirst. Vomiting and purging of bile, several quarts at a time. Vomiting preceded by thirst. *Hiccough (Sul-ac., Hydr- ac.).* Avoids tight clothing.

**Rectum**: Stools frequent, green, watery. Cramps. Constipated with a sore liver.

**Respiratory:** Coryza with sneezing. *Hoarseness and cough with soreness in the chest;* must support it. *Influenza* with great soreness of the muscles and bones. *Chronic,* loose cough, chest sore; *worse at night.* Cough relieved by getting on hands and knees.

**Extremities:** *Aching pain in the back. Aching in the bones of the extremities with soreness of flesh. Aching in arms and wrists.* Swelling of the left great toe. Gouty soreness and inflamed nodosities of joints, associated with headache. Dropsical swelling (arthritis).

**Fever:** Perspiration relieves all symptoms except headache. Chill between 7 and 9 a. m., *preceded by thirst, great soreness and aching in bones.* Nausea, vomiting of bile at the end of chills or hot stage; throbbing headache. Knows chill is coming on because he cannot drink enough.

**Modalities:** *Worse,* periodically. *Better,* by conversation, by getting on hands and knees.

**Relationship:** Compare: *Bry., Sep., Nat-m., Chel. Nyctanthes arbor tristis* (bilious fever; insatiable thirst; bitter vomiting at the end of chill; also constipation in children).

**Dose:** Tincture to third attenuation.

---

## EUPATORIUM PURPUREUM

(Queen of the Meadow) **Eup-pur.**

Albuminuria, diabetes, strangury, *irritable bladder,* enlarged prostate are the special fields of action for this remedy. Excellent in renal dropsy. Chills and pains run upwards. Impotency and sterility. Homesickness.

**Head:** *Left sided headache with vertigo.* Pain from the left shoulder to the occiput. Sick headache beginning in the morning, worse afternoon and evening, worse in cold air.

**Urinary:** Deep, dull pain in the kidneys (nephritis). Burning in the bladder and urethra (urethritis) on micturating. Insufficient flow; milky (albuminuria). Strangury. Hematuria. Constant desire; bladder feels dull. Dysuria. *Vesical irritability* in women (cystitis). *Diabetes insipidus.*

**Female:** Pain around the left ovary. Threatened abortion. External genitals feel as though wet.

**Back:** Weight and heaviness in the loins and back.

**Fever:** *No thirst* during chill, but severe frontal ache. *Chill commences in the back.* Violent shaking with comparatively little coldness. Bone pains.

**Relationship:** Compare: *Senec., Cann-s., Helon., Ph-ac., Tritic., Epig.*

**Dose:** First potency.

---

## EUPHORBIA LATHYRIS

(Gopher Plant, Caper Spurge) **Euph-l.**

The fresh milky juice is exceedingly acrid when applied to the skin and the fruit is highly purgative and poisonous. The juice causes redness, itching, pimples and sometimes gangrene. The symptoms point to its use in erysipelas, Poison oak, etc. Rheumatic pains during rest. Paralytic, weakness of joints.

**Mind:** Delirium and hallucinations. Stupor, coma.

**Eyes:** Almost closed from *edema of lids.*

**Nose:** End of nose very inflamed externally. Very *sensitive and edematous* mucous membranes with ulceration.

**Face:** At first, a ruddy glow on the cheeks, afterwards, a death- like pallor. Cold perspiration in beads on the forehead. Red, puffed and suppurating in spots. Erythema, beginning on the face, gradually extending into the hairy parts, and then spreading over the whole body, taking eight days to do so; eruptions glossy, rough, edematous, with burning and smarting; aggravated by touch and cold air; ameliorated in a closed room and by sweet oil applications. Fine bran-like desquamation. Sensation of cobwebs. Stinging, smarting and burning of the face when touched.

**Mouth:** Tongue coated, slimy; acrid taste. Breath cold, musty odor.

**Stomach:** Nausea and vomiting of copious, clear water, intermingled with white, gelatinous lumps.

**Rectum:** Drastic purgation from large doses; mild laxative condition from smaller doses; followed several weeks later by obstinate constipation. Stools of white, transparent, gelatinous mucus; later mingled with blood.

**Urinary:** Copious flow of urine.

**Male:** Inflammation of the scrotum, resulting in deep acrid ulcers, with intense itching and burning; worse, touching the parts, from washing.

**Respiratory:** Labored breathing. Breath, cold with a musty odor. Cough; first, hacking, as from inhalation of sulphur; later on, paroxysmal, like whooping cough, in regular paroxysms, ending in diarrhea and vomiting with sleepiness between each paroxysm.

**Heart:** Weak and fluttering heart action. Pulse 120, full, bounding, somewhat irregular.

**Sleep:** Restlessness at night. Sleep disturbed, anxious dreams.

**Fever:** Temperature increased. Body bathed in profuse perspiration, standing out like beads on the forehead; later, cold, clammy perspiration on the forehead.

**Skin:** Erythema, beginning on uncovered parts, on face, and spreading all over the body; glossy, rough, edematous, with burning and smarting. Fine bran-like desquamation following erythema. Eruptions rough, scaly, smarting and burning; when scratched, forms deep, ragged ulcers; skin where ulcers remains red.

**Modalities:** *Worse,* touch and cold air; *better,* closed room and sweet oil application.

**Relationship:** Antidoted by *Rhus-t.* (skin symptoms); *Verat.* (vomiting, purging, cough and coma).

**Dose:** Third to thirtieth potency.

---

## EUPHORBIA POLYCARPA

(Golondrina) **Euph-po.**

An antidote to snake poison. Its use also renders the body immune to the influence of the snake venom, and is thus used as a prophylactic (*Indg.*).

**Relationship:** Compare: *The Euphorbias. Euphorbia prostata* (used by Indians as an infallible remedy against bites of poisonous insects and snakes, especially the rattle snake). *Plumeria cellinus-* Tincture internally and locally every 15 minutes for snake poisoning (Dr. Correa). *Cedron. Mikania guaco,* a Brazilian snake cure. *Selaginella apus:* Macerate in milk, locally and internally for bites of snakes and spiders. *Iodium,* tincture for rattle snake bites externally and one drop dose every 10 minutes. *Gymnema sylvestre* (will abolish the taste of bitter things; *sense of taste altered;* powdered root for snake bite); *Sisyrinchium galaxoides*—Blue eyed grass: Ten to fifteen drop doses of tincture (rattlesnake bites).

# EUPHORBIUM OFFICINARUM

(Spurge—The Resinous Juice of Euphorbia Resinifera) **Euph.**

An irritant to the skin and mucous membranes. Burning pain in bones. Pain in limbs and paralytic weakness in the joints. Important respiratory and skin symptoms. Terrible burning pains. *Pains of cancer.* Everything appears larger than it really is.

**Head:** Acute mania. Violent, pressive headache.

**Eyes:** Inflamed and agglutinated in the morning (conjunctivitis).

**Nose:** Nasal pruritus with mucus secretions from the nasopharynx.

**Face:** Erysipelas; yellow blisters. Burning in cheeks; worse, left. Red swelling of cheeks.

**Stomach:** Great hunger. Sialorrhea (profuse salty saliva). Waterbrash. Thirst for cold drinks.

**Abdomen:** Sunken; spasmodic, flatulent colic. Stools fermented, profuse, clayey. Feels hollow.

**Respiratory:** Breathing oppressed, as if the chest was not wide enough. Spasmodic, dry cough, day and night with asthma. Violent, fluent coryza, with burning and cough. Constant cough, with stitches radiating from the pit of the stomach to the sides of the chest. Croup, dry, hollow, cough. A warm feeling in the chest, as if hot food had been swallowed.

**Extremities:** Paralytic pains. Pain in the hip joint and coccyx.

**Skin:** Erysipelatous inflammation, especially of the cheek. Biting and stinging, red, swollen. Vesicular erysipelas. Carbuncle; old, torpid, indolent ulcers with biting, lancinating pain. Old torpid ulcer, pustules; *gangrene* (*Echi., Sec.*). Ulcerating carcinoma and epithelioma of the skin.

**Relationship:** Compare: *Euphorbia amygdaloides*—Wood spurge (pain in the antrum, illusion of smell, *odor of mice.* Sense of taste blunted. Diarrhea; stools difficult, with painful anal spasm).

*Euphorbia corollata*—Large flowering spurge (a diaphoretic expectorant and cathartic of the old school in gastro-enteric disturbances, with deathly nausea. Vomiting of food, water, and mucus, copious evacuations. Attacks recur after short intermissions. Sensation of clawing in the stomach; cold sweat) (*Verat.*).

*Euphorbia marginata*—Snow on the mountain (honey from the flowers is poisonous, detected by the hot, acrid taste. The milky juice produces skin symptoms like *Rhus-t.*).

*Euphorbia pilulifera*—Pillbearing spurge (humid asthma, cardiac dyspnea, hay fever and bronchitis. Urethritis with intense dysuria and much urging. Acrid leucorrhea; worse least movement. Hemorrhages from sunstroke and traumatism).

Compare, also: *Psoralea*—A Columbian plant (pain of cancer, ulcers. Leucorrhea fetid. Pruritus. Uterine tumors). *Crot-t., Jatr-c., Colch.*

Antidotes: *Camph., Op.*

**Dose:** Third to sixth potency.

---

## EUPHRASIA OFFICINALIS

(Eyebright) **Euphr.**

Manifests itself in inflaming the conjunctival membrane especially, producing profuse lachrymation. Patient is better in the open air. Catarrhal affections of the mucous membranes especially of the eyes and nose. Profuse *acrid* lachrymation and bland coryza; worse, evening. Hawking up of offensive mucus.

**Head:** Bursting headache with dazzling of the eyes. *Catarrhal headache* with profuse discharge from the eyes and nose.

**Eyes:** *Catarrhal* conjunctivitis; discharge of an acrid matter. *The eyes water all the time.* Acrid lachrymation; bland coryza (opposite: *All-c.*). Discharge thick and excoriating (*Merc.* thin and acrid). Burning and swelling of the lids (blepharitis). Frequent inclination to blink. Free discharge of acrid matter. Sticky mucus on the cornea; must wink to remove it (phlyctenulae). Pressure in the eyes (glaucoma). Little blisters on the cornea. Opacities (cataract). Rheumatic iritis. Ptosis (*Gels., Caust.*).

**Nose:** *Profuse, fluent coryza,* with violent cough and abundant expectoration.

**Face:** Redness and heat of cheeks. Stiffness of the upper lip.

**Stomach:** Vomiting from hawking mucus. Nausea and bitterness after smoking.

**Rectum:** Dysentery. Prolapse ani. Pressure down in the anus, while sitting. *Constipation.*

**Male:** Spasmodic retraction of genitals, with pressure above the pubic bone. Condyloma and sycotic excrescences. *Prostatitis.* Nocturnal irritability of the bladder; dribbling urine.

**Female:** Menses *painful; flow lasts only an hour or day;* late, scanty, short. *Amenorrhea with ophthalmia.*

**Respiratory:** Frequent yawning when walking in the open air. Profuse, fluent coryza in the morning, with cough and expectoration. Influenza. Gags, on clearing the throat in the morning. Whooping cough, only during day time, with profuse lachrymation.

**Sleep:** Yawning when walking in the open air. Sleepy during the day.

**Fever:** Chilly and cold. Sweat mostly on the chest, at night during sleep.

**Skin:** First stage of measles; eye symptoms marked. Consequence of external injuries.

**Modalities:** *Worse,* in the evening, indoors, warmth, south winds, from light. *Better,* from coffee, in the dark.

**Relationship:** Antidotes: *Camph., Puls.* Compare: *Hydrophyllum virginicum*—Burr flower (catarrhal inflammation of the eyes; hot lachrymation with itching, swollen lids, dull headache; also for effects of Poison oak); *All-c., Ars., Gels., Kali-i., Sabad.*

**Dose:** Third to sixth potency.

---

## EUPIONUM

(Wood Tar Distillation) **Eupi.**

Marked female symptoms and backache. A remedy for *uterine displacements*. Pain in the back, followed by a bland leucorrhea. Menses too early and copious; flow thin. *Intense sweat from the slightest exertion.* Disgusting dreams. Sensation as if the whole body was made of jelly.

**Head:** Vertigo; everything turns around on sitting up in bed. Heat at the vertex; stitches radiating from the vertex down the limbs and into the abdomen and genitals. Sore, painful spots on the head. Painful pulsations in the forehead.

**Female:** *Burning in the right ovary. Gushing leucorrhea.* Chronic tubal disease. Uterine flexions. Menses too early and copious (menorrhagia). During menses, irritable and disinclined to talk; burning and stitches in the chest and heart. After menses, yellow *leucorrhea with severe backache.* When backache ceases, the discharge gushes out. Sore pain between the labia during micturition. Pruritus pudendi; labia swollen.

**Back:** Sacrum painful, as if broken. Severe backache; must lean against something for support. Pains extend into the pelvis.

**Extremities:** *Cramps in the calves;* worse at night.

**Relationship:** *Kreos., Graph., Lach.*

**Dose:** Third potency.

---

## FABIANA IMBRICATA

(Pichi) **Fab.**

A South American shrub cultivated in Southern California. It is a terebinthine diuretic. It has also tonic and chologogue properties, used in the treatment of nasal catarrh, jaundice, dyspepsia and to increase the secretion of bile (Albert Schneider). Useful in uric acid diathesis, cystitis, gonorrhea, *prostatitis,* dysuria, cystitis with suppurative *prostatic* conditions; post-gonorrheal urinary conditions; cholelithiasis and liver affections. Cystitis and burning after micturition. Excoriiting urine and calculi.

**Dose:** Ten to twenty drops of the tincture.

---

## FAGOPYRUM ESCULENTUM

(Buckwheat) **Fago.**

Its action on the skin, producing pruritus, is very marked. Visible pulsations of the arteries. Fluent coryza. Offensive excretions. Itching erythema. *Pruritus senilis.* Post-nasal catarrh; dry crusts, granular appearance of the posterior nares with itching.

**Head:** Inability to study or remember. Depressed and irritable. Pain, deep in the head, *with an upward pressure.* Itching in and around the eyes and ears. Head hot, better bending backward, with a tired neck. Occipital headache. Bursting pain. Cerebral hyperemia.

**Eyes:** *Itching* and smarting, swelling, heat and soreness.

**Nose:** Sore, red, inflamed. Fluent coryza, with sneezing, followed by dryness and crust formation.

**Throat:** Soreness and feeling of excoriation, deep down in the pharynx. Uvula elongated, tonsils swollen (tonsillitis).

**Stomach:** Eructations of *scalding, hot,* acid, watery substance; better, coffee. Bad taste in the morning. Persistent, morning nausea. Drooling.

**Female:** *Pruritus vulvae, with yellow leucorrhea* worse, rest. Burning in the right ovary.

**Heart:** Pain around the heart, better lying on the back, extending to the left shoulder and arm (angina pectoris). *Throbbing in all the arteries* after retiring. Palpitations with oppression. Pulse irregular, intermittent, rapid. Light feeling in the chest.

**Extremities:** Stiffness with a bruised sensation in the muscles of the neck, sensation as if the neck cannot support the head (cervical spondylosis). Pain in the shoulder, with pain along the fingers. *Vehement itching in arms and legs;* worse towards the evening. Feet numb and prickling. Streaking pains in the arms and legs.

**Skin:** *Itching;* better by bathing in cold water; worse scratching, touch and retiring. Sore, red blotches. Blind boils. Itching in knees elbows and hairy portions. *Itching deep in the hands.* Vesicular, pustular, phlegmonous dermatitis. Skin hot, swollen.

**Modalities:** *Better,* cold water, coffee; *worse,* in the afternoon; from sunlight, scratching.

**Relationship:** Compare: *Dol., Bov., Urt-u.*

**Dose:** Third potency and 12x.

---

## FEL TAURI

(Ox Gall) **Fel.**

Increases the duodenal secretion, emulsifies fats and increases the peristaltic action of the intestines. Liquifies bile and acts as a purgative and cholegogue. Disordered digestion, diarrhea and pain in the nape of the neck are among its chief symptoms. Obstruction of the gall ducts. Biliary calculi. Jaundice.

**Stomach:** Eructations, gurgling in the stomach and epigastric region. Violent peristaltic movements. *Tendency to sleep after eating.*

**Relationship:** Compare: *Merc-d., Chol.* In biliary lithiasis, *Chin. Calculus biliari*-Triturated gall stones—10-12x (gall stones).

**Dose:** Lower triturations. Purified oxgall 1 to 10 gr.

---

## FERRUM IODATUM

(Iodide of Iron) **Ferr-i.**

Scrofulous affections, glandular enlargements and tumors call for this remedy. Crops of boils. Acute nephritis following eruptive diseases. Uterine displacements. Body emaciated. Anemia. Exophthalmic goitre following suppression of menses. Debility following a drain upon the vital forces. Impetigo of the cheek.

**Throat:** Sore, as if a splinter in the throat, shooting in different directions. Hoarseness.

**Stomach:** Food seems to push up, into the throat, as if it had not been swallowed.

**Abdomen:** Fullness, even after eating a little food; stuffed feeling, as if she could not lean forward.

**Urinary:** Urine dark. Sweet smelling (diabetes). *Crawling sensation in the urethra and rectum.* Sensation as if urine was stopped at fossa navicularis. Difficulty in retaining urine. Incontinence in anemic children.

**Female:** On sitting, *sensation as if something was pressed upwards in the vagina.* Severe bearing down. Retroversion and prolapse of uterus. Leucorrhea like boiled starch. Menses suppressed or scanty. Itching and soreness of the vulva and vagina.

**Respiratory:** Coryza; discharge of mucus from the nose, trachea and larynx (bronchorrhea). Pressure beneath the sternum. Scrofulous swelling of the nose. Chest feels oppressed. Hemoptysis (phthisis).

**Dose:** Third trituration. Does not keep long.

---

# FERRUM MAGNETICUM

(Loadstone) **Ferr-ma.**

Marked symptoms in the intestinal tract. Pain in the nape of neck. Paralytic weakness. Small warts on the hands.

**Stomach:** During a meal, flatulence; afterwards lassitude, taciturn, heat, pain in the epigastrium, especially on breathing.

**Abdomen:** Movements and grumbling in the abdomen. Loose evacuations with much flatulence, especially on the left side with a pulling pain in the legs. Abundant and frequent emission of fetid flatus.

**Dose:** Third potency.

---

# FERRUM METALLICUM

(Iron) **Ferr.**

Best adapted to young weak people, anemic and chlorotic, with pseudo-plethora, who flush easily; cold extremities; *oversensitiveness;* worse after any active effort. *Weakness* merely from speaking or walking, though *looks* strong. *Pallor* of skin, mucous membranes, face alternating with flushes. Orgasms of blood to the face, chest, head, lungs, etc. Irregular distribution of blood. Pseudo-plethora. Muscles flabby and relaxed.

**Mind:** Irritability. *Even slight noises are unbearable.* Excited from the slightest opposition. Sanguine temperament.

**Head:** Vertigo on seeing flowing water. Stinging headache. Ringing in the ears before menses. Hammering, pulsating, congestive headache; pain extends to the teeth, with cold extremities. Pain in *the back of head,* with roaring (throbbing) in the neck. Scalp painful. Must take down the hair.

**Eyes:** Watery, dull red; photophobia; letters run together.

**Nose:** Mucous membrane relaxed, boggy, anemic, pale.

**Face:** Fiery red and *flushed from the least pain, emotion, or exertion. Red parts become white,* bloodless and puffy.

**Mouth:** *Pain in the teeth; relieved by icy cold water.* Earthy, pasty taste, like rotten eggs.

**Stomach:** *Voracious* appetite or absolute loss of appetite. Loathing for sour things. Attempts to eat bring on diarrhea. *Spits up food by the mouthful* (*Phos.*). Eructations of food after eating, without nausea. Nausea and vomiting after eating. *Vomiting immediately after eating. Vomiting after midnight. Intolerance of eggs.* Distention and pressure in the stomach after eating. Heat and burning in the stomach. Soreness of the abdominal walls. Flatulent dyspepsia.

**Rectum:** Undigested (lienteria) stools, at night, while eating or drinking, painless. Ineffectual urging; stools hard, followed by backache or cramping pain in the rectum; prolapsus recti; itching in the anus, especially in young children.

**Urinary:** Involuntary; worse daytime. Tickling in the urethra extending to the bladder.

**Female:** Menses remit a day or two and then return. Discharge of long pieces from the uterus. Women who are weak, delicate, chlorotic, yet have a fiery red face. Menses too early, too profuse, last too long; pale, watery (menorrhagia). Sensitive vagina. Tendency to abortion. Prolapse of vagina.

**Respiratory:** Chest *oppressed;* breathing difficult (asthma). Surging of blood to the chest. Hoarseness. Cough dry, spasmodic. Hemoptysis (*Mill.*). With cough, pain in occiput.

**Heart:** Palpitations; worse movement. Sense of oppression. Anemic murmur. *Pulse full, but soft and yielding; also, small and weak. Heart contracts suddenly, filling the blood vessels and then suddenly draws a reflux resulting in pallor.*

**Extremities:** Rheumatism of the shoulder. Dropsy after loss of vital fluids. Lumbago; better, walking slowly. Pain in the hip joint, tibia, soles and heel.

**Fever:** General coldness of extremities; head and face hot. *Chill at 4 a. m.* Heat in palms and soles. Profuse, debilitating sweat.

**Skin:** Pale; flushes readily, pits on pressure.

**Modalities:** *Better,* walking slowly. Better after rising. *Worse,* while sweating; sitting still. After cold washing and overheating. *Midnight aggravation.*

**Relationship:** Antidotes: *Ars., Hep.*

Complementary: *Chin., Alum., Ham.*

Compare: *Rumx.* (similar symptoms in the respiratory and digestive sphere, contains organic iron).

*Ferrum aceticum* (alkaline urine in acute diseases. Pain in the right deltoid. Epistaxis; especially adapted to thin, pale, weak children who grow rapidly and are easily exhausted; *varices of the feet;* copious expectoration of greenish pus; asthma; worse, sitting still and lying; phthisis, constant cough, vomiting of food after eating, hemoptysis).

*Ferrum arsenicosum* (enlarged liver and spleen with fever; lienteria; albuminuria. Simple and pernicious anemia, chlorosis. Skin dry. Eczema, psoriasis, impetigo. Use 3x trituration).

*Ferrum bromatum* (sticky, excoriating leucorrhea; uterus heavy and prolapsed, scalp feels numb).

*Ferrum cyanatum* (neuroses with irritable weakness and hyper-sensitiveness, especially of a periodical character; *epilepsy;* cardialgia with nausea, flatulence, constipation, alternating with diarrhea; chorea).

*Ferrum magneticum* (small warts on the hands).

*Ferrum muriaticum* (arrested menstruation; tendency to seminal emissions or copious micturition at puberty; very dark, watery stools; diphtheria; phlegmonous erysipelas; pyelitis; hemoptysis of dark, clotted blood; dysparunia; pain in *right shoulder,* right elbow, and a marked tendency to cramps and round red spots on the cheeks; bright crystals in urine. Anemia, 3x, after meals. Tincture 1-5 drops, 3 times daily in chronic interstitial nephritis).

*Ferrum sulphuricum* (watery and painless stools; menorrhagia, pressing, throbbing between periods with rush of blood to the head. Basedow's disease. Erethism. Pain in the gall bladder; toothache; acidity; eructation of food in mouthfuls).

*Ferrum pernitricum* (cough, with florid complexion).

*Ferrum tartaricum* (cardialgia; heat at the cardiac orifice of stomach).

*Ferrum protoxalatum* (anemia). Use 1x trituration. Compare also: *Graph., Mang-act., Cupr.*

**Dose:** States of debility where blood is poor in hematin; requires material doses; plethoric, hemorrhagic conditions call for small doses, from the second to the sixth potency.

---

# FERRUM PHOSPHORICUM

(Phosphate of Iron) **Ferr-p.**

In the early stages of febrile conditions, it stands midway between asthenic activity of *Acon.* and *Bell.,* with the asthenic sluggishness and torpidity of *Gels.* The typical *Ferr-p.* subject is not full blooded and robust, but nervous, sensitive, anemic with the false plethora and easy flushing of *Ferr.* Prostration is marked; face more active than *Gels.* The superficial redness never assumes the dusky hue of *Gels.* Pulse soft and flowing; no anxious restlessness of *Acon.* Susceptibility to chest problems . Bronchitis in young children. In acute exacerbation of tuberculosis, a fine palliative with a wonderful power. Corresponds to Grauvogl's oxygenoid constitution, the inflammatory, febrile, emaciating, wasting consumptive.

Remedy for the first stage of all febrile disturbances and inflammations before exudation sets in; especially for catarrhal affections of the respiratory tract. *Ferr-p.* 3x increases hemoglobin. In pale, anemic subjects, with violent local congestions. Hemorrhages, bright from any orifice.

**Head:** Soreness to touch, cold, noise, jar. Rush of blood to the head. Ill effects of sun (sun stroke). Throbbing sensation. Vertigo. Headache *better cold applications.*

**Eyes:** Red, inflamed with a burning sensation (conjunctivitis). sensation of sand under the lids. Hyperemia of the optic disc and retina with blurred vision.

**Ears:** Noises. Throbbing. First stage of otitis. Membrana tympani red and bulging. Acute otitis; when *Bell.* fails, prevents suppuration.

**Nose:** First stage of cold in the head. Predisposition to colds. *Epistaxis;* bright red blood.

**Face:** Flushed; cheeks sore and hot. Florid complexion. Facial neuralgia; worse, shaking the head and on stooping.

**Throat:** Mouth hot; fauces red, inflamed (stomatitis). Ulcerated sore throat. Tonsils red and swollen (tonsillitis). Eustachian tubes inflamed. Sore throat of singers. Subacute laryngitis with fauces inflamed and red (2x). After surgery of throat and nose to control bleeding and to relieve soreness. First stage of diphtheria. Ranula in vascular, sanguine constitutions.

**Stomach:** Aversion to meat and milk. Desire for stimulants. *Vomiting of undigested food.* Vomiting of bright red blood (hematemesis). *Sour eructations.*

**Abdomen:** First stage of peritonitis. Hemorrhoids. Stools watery, bloody, undigested. First stage of dysentery with blood in the discharges.

**Urinary:** Urine spurts with every cough. Incontinence. Irritation at the neck of the bladder. Polyuria. *Diurnal enuresis.*

**Female:** Menses every three weeks (metrorrhagia and dysmenorrhea) with bearing down sensation and pain on top of the head. Vaginismus. Vagina dry and hot.

**Respiratory:** *First stage of all inflammatory affections.* Congestion of the lungs. Hemoptysis. Short, painful, tickling cough. Croup. Hard, dry cough, with sore chest. Hoarseness. *Expectoration of pure blood in pneumonia (Mill.).* Cough better at night.

**Heart:** Palpitations; pulse rapid. First stage of cardiac diseases. *Short, quick, soft pulse.*

**Extremities:** Stiff neck. Articular rheumatism. Crick in back. Rheumatic pain in the shoulder; pain extends to the chest and wrist. Whitlow. Palms hot. Hands swollen and painful.

**Sleep:** Restless and sleepless. Anxious dreams. Night sweats of anemia.

**Fever:** Chill daily at 1 p. m. All catarrhal and inflammatory fevers; first stage.

**Modalities:** *Worse,* at night and 4 to 6 a. m., touch, jar, motion, right side. *Better,* cold applications.

**Relationship:** Compare: (Oxygenoid constitution: *Acon., Chin., Ars., Graph., Petr.). Ferrum pyrophosphoricum* (congestion of brain and headache following great loss of blood; tarsal cysts); *Acon., Gels., Chin.*

**Dose:** Third to twelfth potency.

---

## FERRUM PICRICUM

(Picrate of Iron) **Ferr-pic.**

Is considered as a great remedy to complete the action of other medicines. The symptom that specially calls for it is failure of the function of an organ under exertion; e. g., the voice fails after public speaking. Acts best in dark haired patients, plethoric, with sensitive livers. Warts and epithelial growths; corns with yellowish discoloration. *Senile hypertrophy of the prostate. Epistaxis.* Chronic deafness and tinnitus due to gout. Meatus dry. Pseudo-leukemia.

**Ears:** Deafness before menses. Crackling in the ears and low pitched voice. Vascular deafness. Dental neuralgia, radiating towards the ears and eyes. Humming in the ears as if from telegraph wires. Tinnitus.

**Stomach:** Indigestion, furred tongue, headache after meals, especially in bilious, dark haired people.

**Urinary:** Pain along the entire length of urethra (urethritis). *Frequent micturition at night, with a full feeling and pressure in the rectum. Smarting at the neck of the bladder* and penis (*Barosma crenulatum*). Retention of urine.

**Extremities:** Pain on the right side of neck, radiates down the right arm. Locomotor ataxia, ocular stage. Hands covered with warts.

**Dose:** Second and third trituration.

---

## FICUS RELIGIOSA

(Sacred Fig, Ashwathwa) **Fic-r.**

This East Indian drug causes and cures hemorrhage of many kinds, hematemesis, menorrhagia, hemoptysis, hematuria, etc. Bloody urine.

**Head**: Melancholic, quiet. Burning at vertex. Vertigo and slight headache.

**Eyes:** Dim sight.

**Stomach:** Nausea; vomiting of bright red blood (hematemesis); pain and sick feeling in the stomach.

**Respiratory:** Difficult breathing; cough with vomiting of blood; pulse very weak.

**Relationship:** Compare: *Acal., Ip., Mill., Thlas.*

**Dose**: First potency.

---

## FILIX MAS—ASPIDIUM

(Male Fern) **Fil.**

A remedy for worm symptoms, especially with constipation. Tapeworm. Soporific conditions. *Torpid inflammation of the lymphatic glands* (maceration of fresh root). Pulmonary tuberculosis in young patients, no fever with limited, ulcerated lesions, formerly classified as scrofula.

**Eyes:** Blindness, monocular amblyopia.

**Abdomen**: Bloated. Gnawing pain; worse eating sweets. Diarrhea and vomiting. Worm colic with itching in the nose, pale face, blue rings around the eyes. Painless hiccough.

**Relationship**: Compare: *Aspidium panna, Panna*—3 doses, 2 grammes each, in half hour, fasting, in a glass of milk. Tasteless and will remove tapeworm. *Cina, Gran., Kousso.*

**Dose**: First to third potency. For the expulsion of tapeworm, a full dose of 1/2 to 1 dram of the Oleoresin, fasting.

---

## FLUORICUM ACIDUM

(Hydrofluoric Acid) **Fl-ac.**

Especially adapted to chronic diseases with syphilitic and mercurial history. *Glabella region bloated.* Acts especially on the lower tissues and is indicated in deep, destructive processes, bed sores, ulcerations, varicose veins and ulcers. Patient is compelled to move around energetically. Complaints of old age or the prematurely aged, with weak, distended blood vessels. Hob-nailed liver of alcoholics. *Goitre* (Dr. Woakes) (*Kalium fluoratum* produced bronchocele in dogs). Early decay of teeth (caries). Old cases of nocturnal fever, coming on periodically.

**Mind**: Indifference towards those loved most; inability to realize responsibility; buoyancy. Mentally elated and gay.

**Head:** Alopecia. Caries of the skin. Pressure on the sides of head, from within outward. Caries in the ossicles and mastoid, with copious discharge; worse warmth (*Silicea;* worse cold.). Exostosis.

**Eyes:** *Sensation as if wind is blowing through the eyes.* Lachrymal fistula. Violent itching of the inner canthus.

**Nose:** Chronic nasal catarrh with ulceration of the septum; nose obstructed and dull heavy pain in the forehead.

**Mouth:** Dental fistula with persistent bloody, salty discharge. Syphilitic ulcerations of the throat, which is very sensitive to cold. Teeth feel warm. Affects teeth and bones of the upper jaw.

**Stomach:** Heaviness and weight in the stomach. Heat in the stomach before meals. Sour eructations (gastric ulcer). Averse to coffee, wants fancy dishes. Stomach symptoms relieved by tight clothes. Desire for highly seasoned food. Craves cold water, hungry. Warm drinks produce diarrhea.

**Abdomen:** Soreness over the liver. Flatus and eructations.

**Stool**: Bilious diarrhea, with an aversion to coffee.

**Urinary:** Scanty, dark urine. In dropsy, produces frequent and free discharge, with great relief.

**Male:** Burning in the urethra (urethritis). Sexual passion and desire increased with erections at night, during sleep. *Swollen scrotum* (hydrocele).

**Female:** Menses copious, frequent, too long (metrorrhagia, menorrhagia). Ulcerations of the uterus and os. Copious and excoriating leucorrhea. Nymphomania.

**Respiratory:** Oppression of the chest, difficult breathing, great dyspnea (asthma). Hydrothorax.

**Extremities:** Inflammation of the finger joints (rheumatism). Sensation of a splinter under the nail. Nails crumble. Caries and necrosis, especially of long bones. Coccygodynia. Ulcer over the tibia.

**Skin:** *Varicose veins.* Nevi. Ulcers; red edges and vesicles. Decubitus; worse, warmth. Syphilitic rupia. Itching in cicatrices. Feels as if burning vapors were emitted from the pores. *Itching especially in the orifices* and in spots, worse warmth. Nails grow rapidly. Periosteal abscess (osteomyelitis). Profuse, sour, offensive perspiration. Syphilitic tubercles. *Dropsy of limbs* in old, feeble constitutions. Atony of capillary and venous system. Tissues bloated (edema).

**Modalities:** *Worse,* warmth, morning, warm drinks. *Better,* cold, while walking.

**Relationship:** Compare: *Thiosinaminum* (action on cicatricial tissues; adhesions, strictures, tumors); *Calc-f., Sil.*

Complementary: *Sil.*

**Dose:** Sixth to thirtieth potency.

# FORMALINUM

(Aqueous Solution (35 percent) of Formaldehyde Gas)

**Formal.**

Is a powerful disinfectant and deodorant; a potent poison. Prevents growth and kills almost any pathogenic micro-organism. It seems to have the peculiar property of eating into malignant tumors, leaving the surrounding healthy tissue uncharred and unchanged. A plug of cotton wool soaked in a 20 percent solution of formaldehyde, and applied for a few hours, will produce a necrotic slough, which must be scraped away before the next application, otherwise it hardens.

*Formal. in hot water, as vapors is a valuable therapeutic agent in pertussis,* phthisis and in catarrhal affections of the upper air passages.

**Mind:** *Forgetfulness.* Anxiety. Unconscious.

**Head:** Coryza; eyes water; *vertigo.*

**Mouth:** Ptyalism, thick saliva; loss of taste.

**Stomach:** Food feels like a ball in the stomach. Burning in the mouth and stomach.

**Abdomen:** Intense urging for stool, watery stools.

**Urinary:** Anuria; albuminuria.

**Respiratory:** Dyspnea. *Laryngismus stridulus. Whooping cough.*

**Fever:** Chills in the forenoon, followed by long fever. Bones ache during the entire paroxysm. During fever, forgets where he was.

**Skin:** Puckered skin like leather; wrinkles; scales off. Eczema in the neighborhood of a wound. Damp sweat, most marked on the right upper extremity.

**Relationship:** Antidote: *Ammonia water.*

Compare: *Ammonium formaldehydum,* known commercially as *Cystogen* (dose, five to seven grains, two to four times daily, dissolved in hot water, after meals. Prevents the decomposition of urine in the bladder, kidneys and ureters. Turbid urine rendered clear and non-irritating; phosphatic deposits dissolved and growth of pyogenic bacteria arrested). Also, *Urotropinum* (a diuretic and solvent of uric acid concretions; relieves cystitis associated with putrefaction. Three to five grains well diluted. When administered invariably appears in the cerebro-spinal fluid and is therefore advised in threatened meningeal infection).

**Dose:** As vapor in hot water for respiratory affections; 1 percent spray, otherwise 3x potency.

---

# FORMICA RUFA—MYRMEXINE

(Crushed Live Ants) **Form.**

An *arthritic* medicine. Gout and articular rheumatism; pains worse, motion; better, pressure. Right side most affected. Chronic gout and stiffness in joints. Acute outbursts of gouty poisons, especially when assuming the neuralgic form. Tuberculosis, carcinoma and lupus; chronic nephritis. Complaints from overlifting. Apoplectic diseases. *Has a marked deterrent influence on the formation of polypi.*

**Head:** Vertigo. Headache with cracking in the left ear. Brain feels too heavy and large. Sensation as if a bubble burst in the forehead. Forgetful in the evening. *Exhilarated.*

**Eyes:** Rheumatic iritis.

**Ears:** Ringing and buzzing (tinnitus). Cracking in the left ear with headache. Parts around the ear feel swollen. Polypi.

**Nose:** *Nasal polypi. Coryza* with a *stopped up* feeling in the nose.

**Stomach:** Constant pressure at the cardiac end of the stomach with a burning pain. Nausea with headache (sick headache) and vomiting of yellowish bitter mucus. Pain shifts from the stomach to the vertex. Gas cannot be passed.

**Abdomen:** Pain in the bowels before stool, with shuddering chilliness. Drawing pain *around the navel,* before stool.

**Rectum:** In the morning, difficult passages of small quantities of flatus; afterwards diarrhea like urging in the rectum.

**Urinary:** Bloody, albuminous with much urging; quantities of urates (nephritis).

**Male:** Seminal emissions; weakness. "Slothful to venery."

**Respiratory:** Hoarseness, with a dry, sore throat; cough worse at night, with aching in the forehead and constrictive pain in the chest; pleuritic pain.

**Extremities:** Rheumatic pains; stiff and contracted joints. Muscles feel strained and torn from their attachment. *Weakness of the lower extremities.* Paraplegia. Pain in the hips. *Rheumatism comes on suddenly and with restlessness. Sweat does not relieve.* Relief after midnight and from rubbing.

**Skin:** *Red, itching and burning.* Nettle rash. Nodes around the joints (*Am-p.*). Profuse sweat without relief.

**Modalities:** *Worse,* cold and cold washing, dampness before a snowstorm. *Better,* warmth, *pressure,* rubbing. Combing hair.

**Relationship:** Compare: *Formicicum acidum* (chronic myalgia. Muscular pain and soreness. Gout and articular rheumatism, which appear suddenly. Pains usually worse on the right side, motion and better from pressure. *Failing vision.* Increases muscular strength and resistance to fatigue. Feels stronger and more "fit". Marked diuretic effect, greater elimination of products of disassimilation, particularly urea. *Tremor.* Tuberculosis, chronic nephritis and carcinoma, lupus, etc., have been treated successfully with injections of *Form-ac.* in a dilution corresponding to the 3rd and 4th centesimal. For prescribing it for varicose veins, polypi, catarrh, Dr. J. H. Clarke orders an ounce or two of a solution of *Form-ac.* in the proportion of one part of the acid to eleven parts of distilled water. Of this, one teaspoonful is taken in a tablespoonful of water after food, once or twice daily. Pain in aponeurosis and muscles of head, neck and shoulders before a snowstorm). *Rhus-t., (Dulc., Urtica* and *Juniperus* contain *Form-ac.*), *Wood alcohol,* when taken as a constituent of a beverage so common in these prohibition days is not eliminated easily and is slowly converted into *Formic acid,* attacking the brain and causes death or blindness.

Dr. Sylwestrowicz of the Hering Research Laboratory in the Hahnemann College, Philadelphia contributes his experience with *Form- ac.,* as follows:

"The best field for *Form-ac.* treatment are cases of a typical gout. Also worthy of mention are disturbances in the muscles such as myositis; periostitic processes of the bones in form of doughy swellings, changes in the fascias such as Dupyutren's contraction, skin problems such as chronic eczema, psoriasis and loss of hair, kidney disturbances such as subacute and chronic nephritis. In these cases *Form-ac.* in 12x and 30x, hypodermically 1 c.c. is indicated at intervals of 2-4 weeks. Eight to twelve days after the first injection an aggravation is often noticed.

In acute rheumatic fever and acute gonorrhric arthritis *Form-ac.* 6x, every six days 1 c.c., sometimes 12x in sensitive patients shows splendid results in abolishing the pains and preventing recurrence.

Chronic arthritis needs a special discussion. Clinical experiments in the Hering Research Laboratory of the Hahnemann Medical College of Philadelphia in a great number of arthritis cases with *Form-ac.* showed, that it acts preferably on the ligaments, capsula and bursa of the joints. Such kind of cases respond very readily to treatment.

The prognosis depends to a large extent upon the etiology of the case. The most satisfactory cases are chronic arthritis in connection with gouty diathesis. Chronic arthritis following an attack of acute rheumatic fever also shows remarkable results although often, pains of a neuralgic character persist in certain spots stubbornly. Finally, chronic arthritis of a traumatic nature can be cured by *Form-ac.* In the latter case, *Form-ac.* 6x showed quicker and better results than 12x or 30x which are indicated in the previous cases. In general the disappearance, of stiffness in the joints is the first sign of improvement. Then the pain and swelling cease gradually in 1-6 months time.

The prognosis of *Form-ac.* treatment is not so favorable in chronic arthritis in which deformans processes have already taken place on the articular surfaces.

Such processes in the beginning can be checked completely, advanced cases frequently show an improvement. But there is always the possibility that this improvement is only temporary. This is particularly to be expected in the cases of the so called arthritis deformans in which even the inflammations on the ligaments and capsula are of a very progressive character."

**Dose:** Sixth to thirtieth attenuation.

## FRAGARIA VESCA

(Wood Strawberry) **Frag.**

Acts on digestion and mesenteric glands. Prevents formation of calculi, removes tartar from teeth and prevents attacks of gout. The fruit has refrigerant properties. Strawberries produce symptoms of poisoning in certain susceptible individuals, such as urticarial rashes (strawberry anaphylaxis). Here, give *Frag.* in a high potency.

Chilblains; worse during hot weather. Lack of mammary secretion. *Psilosis* (Spruce).

**Mouth:** Tongue *swollen; strawberry* tongue (glossitis).

**Skin:** *Urticaria;* petechial and erysipelatous eruptions. Swelling of the whole body (anasarca).

**Relationship:** Compare: *Apis, Calc.*

## FRANCISCEA UNIFLORA

(Manaca) **Franc.**

Chronic stiffnes of the muscles. Gonorrheal rheumatism. Syphilis and rheumatism, great heat over the body, much aching, better sweat. Pain at the back of the head and spine; band-like feeling around the head. Pericarditis with rheumatism. Rheumatic pains in the feet and lower part of legs. Urine contains uric acid.

**Dose:** Tincture or fluid extract, 10 to 60 minims.

## FRAXINUS AMERICANA

(White Ash) **Frax.**

Enlargement of the uterus. Fibrous growths, subinvolution, and prolapse. Uterine tumors with bearing down sensations. Fever sores on lips. Cramps in feet. Cold creeping and hot flashes. Infantile eczema.

**Head:** Throbbing pain at the back of head. Depression, with nervous restlessness, anxiety. *Hot spot on* top of the head.

**Abdomen**: Tenderness in the left inguinal region; bearing down pain, extending down the thigh.

**Female:** *Uterus enlarged* and patulous. Watery, non-irritating leucorrhea. Fibroids with a bearing down sensation, cramps in feet, worse in the afternoon and night. Dysmenorrhea.

**Relationship**: Compare: *Fraxinus excelsior*—European ash (*gout*; rheumatism. infusion of ash leaves. Rademacher). *Galega officinalis*—Goat's rue: Backache; debility; anemia and impaired nutrition. Increases the quantity and quality of the milk in nursing women, also the appetite. *Epiph., Sep., Lil-t.*

**Dose**: Ten to fifteen drops of the tincture, three times a day.

---

## FUCHSINUM—MAGENTA

(A Coloring Substance Used in Adulteration of Wine) **Fuch.**

Produces redness (hyperemia) of the ears, deep red discoloration of the mouth, swollen gums, with burning and a tendency to salivation (stomatitis); deep red urine, albuminous and light red, profuse diarrhea with abdominal pains. Cortical substance of kidneys degenerated. Useful in cortical nephritis with albuminuria.

**Dose:** 6x to 30th potency.

---

## FUCUS VESICULOSUS

(Sea Kelp) **Fuc.**

A remedy for obesity and *non-toxic goitre;* also exophthalmic goitre. Digestion is furthered and flatulence diminished. Obstinate constipation; forehead feels as if compressed by an iron ring. Thyroid enlargement in obese subjects.

**Relationship**: Compare: *Phyt., Thyr., Bad., Iod.*

**Dose:** Tincture, five to sixty drops, three times a day, before meals.

---

## FULIGO LIGNI

(Soot) **Fuli.**

Acts on the glandular system, mucous membranes and obstinate ulcers, epidermis, tetters and eczema. Chronic irritation of the mucous membranes of the mouth; pruritus vulvae; uterine hemorrhage; cancer, especially of the scrotum, chimney sweeper's cancer; epithelial cancers; cancer of the womb with metorrhagia; sadness; thoughts of suicide.

**Relationship**: Compare: *Kreos.*

**Dose**: Sixth trituration.

---

## GALANTHUS NIVALIS

(Snow-drop) **Gala.**

Proving by Dr. A. Whiting, Vancouver.

Faintness, sinking sensations. Sore dry throat with a dull headache. Semiconscious with a worried feeling during sleep. Heart weak with a sensation of collapse, as if she must fall. Pulse very irregular, rapid and uneven, violent palpitations. Systolic murmur at the apex. Therapeutically, of decided benefit in cases of mitral regurgitation with broken down compensation. *Myocarditis* with some degree of mitral insufficiency.

**Dose:** First potency to the fifth.

---

## GALIUM APARINE

(Goose Grass) **Gali.**

*Gali.* acts on the urinary organs, is a diuretic and is of use in dropsies, gravel and calculi. Dysuria and cystitis. Has power of suspending or modifying cancerous action. Has clinical confirmation of its use in cancerous ulcers and nodulated tumors of the tongue. Inveterate skin affections and scurvy. Favors healthy granulations on ulcerated surfaces.

**Dose:** Fluid extract; half-dram doses, in a cup of water or milk, three times a day.

---

# GALLICUM ACIDUM

(Gallic Acid) **Gal-ac.**

Should be remembered as a remedy in *phthisis.* It checks the morbid secretions, gives tone to the stomach and increases the appetite. Passive hemorrhages when pulse is feeble and capillaries relaxed, cold skin. Hematuria. Hemophilia. Itching of skin. *Pyrosis.*

**Mind:** Wild delirium at night; very restless, jumps out of bed; sweats; is afraid to be alone; is rude and abuses every one.

**Head:** Pain in the back of the head and neck.

**Eyes:** Photophobia with burning of lids.

**Nose:** Thick, stringy discharge from the nose. Epistaxis.

**Rectum:** Copious stool; anus feels constricted. Faint feeling after stool. Chronic mucoid discharges.

**Urinary:** Kidneys painful, distress along the ureters upto the bladder. Dull heavy pain in the bladder, directly over the pubis (cystitis). Urine loaded with thick, cream colored mucus.

**Respiratory:** Pain in lungs; *pulmonary hemorrhage;* excessive expectoration (phthisis). Accumulation of mucus in the throat, in the morning. Dry at night.

**Relationship:** Compare: *Ars., Iod., Phos.*

**Dose:** First trituration and pure acid, 2 to 5 grain doses.

---

# GAMBOGIA—GARCINIA MORELLA

(Gummi Gutti) **Gamb.**

The use of this drug in homeopathy has been confined to its action on the alimentary tract. It produces a diarrhea very similar to *Crot-t.* From its pathogenesis, it is very evident that it has a very intense and definite action on the gastroenteric tract.

**Head:** Heavy with inertia and drowsiness.

**Nose:** Itching and burning in eyes; lids stick together (conjunctivitis), with *sneezing.*

**Mouth:** Sensation of coldness at the edge of teeth. Burning, smarting and dryness of the tongue and throat.

**Stomach:** Great irritability of the stomach. Pain after food (gastritis).

**Abdomen:** Pain and distention, flatulence after stool. *Rumbling* and *rolling.*

**Rectum:** Dysentery, with retained scybala, and pain in the sacral region.

Diarrhea with *sudden and forcible ejection of* bilious stools. *Tenesmus after, with burning in anus* (proctitis). Ileo-caecal region sensitive to pressure. Profuse, watery diarrhea in hot weather, particularly old people. Pain in coccyx.

**Modalities:** *Worse,* towards evening and at night.

**Relationship:** Compare: *Crot-t., Aloe, Podo.*

**Dose:** Third to thirtieth potency. *Gamb.* painted on the chest in pulmonary tuberculosis is considered by Abrams specific, and incipient cases are symptomatically cured in several weeks.

---

## GAULTHERIA PROCUMBENS

(Wintergreen) **Gaul.**

Inflammatory rheumatism, pleurodynia, sciatica and other neuralgias, come within the sphere of this remedy. Cystic and prostatic irritation, undue sexual excitement and renal inflammation (nephritis).

**Head**: Neuralgia of the head and face.

**Stomach**: Acute gastritis, severe pain in the epigastrium; *prolonged vomiting*. Uncontrollable appetite, not withstanding an irritable stomach. Gastralgia from nervous depression (give five drops of 1x of oil).

**Skin**: Smarting and burning. Intense erythema, worse cold bathing; better, olive oil and cool air blowing on part.

**Relationship**: Compare: *Spiraea ulmaria. Gaul.* contains Arbutin. *Sal-ac., Methylium salicylicum* (an artificial Gaultheria oil for rheumatism, espccially when the salicylates cannot be used. Pruritus and epididymitis, locally). After *Canth.* in burns.

**Dose**: Tincture and and lower potencies.

---

## GELSEMIUM SEMPERVIRENS

(Yellow Jasmine) **Gels.**

Centers its action upon the nervous system, causing various *degrees of motor paralysis.* General prostration. *Dizziness, drowsiness, dullness and trembling.* Slow pulse, tired feeling, mental apathy. *Paralysis* of various groups of muscles around the eyes, throat, chest, larynx, sphincter, extremities, etc. Post-diphtheritic paralysis. *Muscular weakness.* Complete relaxation and prostration. Lack of muscular co-ordination. General depression from heat of sun (sunstroke). Sensitive to a falling barometer; cold and dampness brings on many complaints. Children fear falling, grab the nurse or crib. Sluggish circulation. Nervous affection of cigarmakers. *Influenza*. Measles. Pellagra.

**Mind:** Desire to be quiet, to be left alone. *Dullness, languor, listless.* "Discernings are lethargic." *Apathy regarding his illness.* Absolute lack of fear. Delirious on falling asleep. Emotional excitement, fear, etc., lead to physical ailments. Bad effects from fright, fear, exciting news. Stage fright. Child starts, grasps the nurse and screams as if afraid of falling (*Borx.*).

**Head**: *Vertigo,* spreading from the occiput. Heaviness of head; *band-like sensation* around *the head* and *occipital* headache (cerebrospinal meningitis). *Dull,* heavy ache, with heaviness of the eyelids; bruised sensation; better, compression and lying with the head high. *Pain in the temples, extending to the ear, alae* of nose and chin. Headache with muscular soreness of the neck and shoulders (cervical spondylosis). Headache preceded by blindness; better, profuse micturition. Scalp sore to touch. Delirious on falling asleep. Wants to raise the head on the pillow.

**Eyes:** Ptosis; *eyelids* heavy; patient can hardly open them.

Diplopia. Disturbed muscular apparatus. Corrects blurring and discomfort in the eyes even after accurately adjusted glasses. Vision blurred, smoky (*Cycl., Phos.*). *Dim sighted;* pupils dilated and insensible to light. *Orbital neuralgia with contraction and twitching of muscles.* Bruised pain behind the orbits. One pupil dilated, the other contracted. Deep inflammations, with haziness of the vitreous fluid. Serous inflammations. Albuminuric retinitis. Detached retina, glaucoma and descemetitis. *Hysterical amblyopia*

**Nose:** Sneezing; fullness at the root of nose. Dryness of nasal fossae. Swelling of turbinates. Watery, excoriating discharge. Acute coryza, with dull headache and fever.

**Face:** *Hot, heavy, flushed, besotted looking* (*Bapt., Op.*). Facial neuralgia. Dusky hue of the face, with vertigo and dim vision. Facial muscles contracted, especially around the mouth. Chin quivers. Lower jaw dropped (tetnus, epilepsy).

**Mouth:** Putrid taste and breath. Tongue numb, thick, coated, yellowish, *trembles,* paralyzed.

**Throat:** Difficulty in swallowing, especially warm food. Itching and tickling in the soft palate and naso-pharynx. Pain in sternocleidomastoid, behind the parotid. Pain radiates to the ear. Throat feels rough, burns. *Post-diphtheritic paralysis.* Tonsillitis; shooting pain, extending into ears. *Sensation of a lump in the throat* that cannot be swallowed. Aphonia. Swallowing causes pain in the ear (*Hep., Nux-v.*). *Pain from the throat to the ear.*

**Stomach:** As a rule, the *Gels.* patient has no thirst. Hiccough; worse in the evening. Sensation of emptiness and weakness in the pit of the stomach, or of an oppression, like a heavy load.

**Stool:** Diarrhea *from emotional excitement*, fright, bad news (*Ph-ac.*). Stools painless or involuntary. Cream colored (*Calc.*), *tea-green.* Partial paralysis of the rectum and sphincter.

**Urinary**: *Profuse, clear, watery,* with chilliness and tremulousness. Dysuria. Partial paralysis of the bladder; flow intermittent (*Clem*). *Retention.*

**Male:** Spermatorrhea *without erections.* Genitals cold and relaxed (*Ph-ac.*). Scrotum continuously covered with sweat. Gonorrhea, first stage; discharge scanty; tendency to corrode; little pain, but much heat; smarting at the meatus.

**Female:** Rigid os (*Bell.*). Vaginismus. False labor pains; pains pass up the back. *Dysmenorrhea* with scanty flow; menses retarded. Pain extends to the back and hips. Aphonia and sore throat during menses. Sensation as if the uterus was squeezed (*Clem., Nux-v., Ust.*).

**Respiratory:** Slow breathing with great prostration. Oppression of the chest. Dry cough, with a sore chest and fluent coryza. *Spasm of the glottis.* Aphonia; acute bronchitis, respiration quickened, spasmodic affections of the lungs and diaphragm.

**Heart**: *Sensation as if it is necessary to keep in motion or else the heart's action would cease.* Slow pulse (*Dig., Kalm., Apoc.*). Palpitations; pulse soft, weak, full and flowing. Pulse slow when quiet, but greatly accelerated on motion. *Weak, slow pulse of old age.*

**Back:** Dull, heavy pain. Complete relaxation of the entire muscular system. Languor; muscles feel bruised. Every little exertion causes fatigue. Pain in the neck, especially in the sternocleidomastoid muscles. Dull aching in the lumbosacral region, extending upward. Pain in the muscles of the back, hips and lower extremities, mostly deep seated (myalgia).

**Extremities:** Loss of power of muscular control. Cramps in muscles of the forearm. Professional neuroses. Writer's cramp. Excessive *trembling* and weakness of all limbs. Hysterical convulsions. Fatigue after slight exercise.

**Sleep:** Cannot get enough sleep. Delirious on falling asleep. Insomnia from exhaustion, from uncontrollable thinking; tobacco. Yawning. Sleepless from nervous irritation (*Coff.*).

**Fever**: *Wants to be held, because he shakes so much.* Pulse slow, full, soft, compressible. Chills up and down the back. Heat and sweat stages, long and exhausting. Dumb ague with marked muscular soreness, great prostration and violent headache. *Nervous chills.* Bilious remittent fever with stupor, dizziness, faintness; thirstless, prostrated. Chill, without thirst, along the spine; wave-like, extending upward, from the sacrum to the occiput.

**Skin:** Hot, dry, itching, measle like eruptions. Erysipelas. *Measles, catarrhal symptoms; aids in bringing out eruptions.* Retrocedent, with livid spots. Scarlet fever with stupor and a flushed face.

**Modalities:** *Worse,* damp weather, fog, before a thunderstorm, emotion, or excitement, *bad news,* tobacco smoking, thinking of his ailments; at 10 a. m. *Better,* bending forward, profuse micturition, open air, continuous motion, stimulants.

**Relationship:** Compare: *Ign.* (gastric affections of cigarmakers); *Bapt., Ip., Acon., Bell., Cimic., Mag-p.,* (*Gels.* contains some *Mag-p.*). *Culx.* (vertigo on blowing the nose with fullness in the ears).

Antidotes: *Chin., Coff., Dig.* Alcoholic stimulants relieve all complaints where *Gels.* is useful.

**Dose:** Tincture to thirtieth attenuation; first to third most often used.

---

## GENTIANA LUTEA

(Yellow Gentian) **Gent-l.**

Stomach symptoms predominate. Acts as a tonic, increasing the appetite.

**Head:** Vertigo, worse, rising or motion; better open air. Frontal headache, better eating and in the open air. Brain feels loose, head tender. Aching in the eyes.

**Throat:** Dry. Thick saliva.

**Stomach:** Acid risings, ravenous hunger, nausea, weight and aching in the stomach. Inflation and tension of the stomach and abdomen (*Ictod.*). Colic, umbilical region sensitive to touch. Flatulence.

**Relationship:** Compare: *Gentiana quinqueflora* (intermittent fever; dyspepsia, cholera infantum, weakness); *Gentiana cruciata* (throat symptoms in addition to similar stomach symptoms; dysphagia; vertigo with headache; sensation as if eyes pressing inwards, constricted throat, head and abdomen. Distention, fullness and tightness of the abdomen. Creeping sensation all over body, as if from fleas). *Hydr., Nux-v.*

**Dose:** First to third attenuation.

---

## GERANIUM MACULATUM

(Crane's Bill) **Ger.**

Habitual sick headaches. *Profuse hemorrhages,* pulmonary and from different organs. Hematemesis. *Ulceration of the stomach. Atonic and foul ulcers.* Summer complaints.

**Head:** Giddiness with diplopia; better, closing the eyes. Ptosis and dilated pupils. Sick headache.

**Mouth:** Dry; tip of tongue burning. Pharyngitis

**Stomach:** Catarrhal gastritis with profuse secretion, tendency to ulceration and passive hemorrhage. *Decreases the vomiting* in *gastric ulcer.*

**Rectum:** Constant desire for stool with an inability to pass anything for some time. Chronic diarrhea with offensive mucus. Constipation.

**Female:** Menses too profuse (menorrhagia). Post-partum hemorrhage. Sore nipples (*Eup-a.*).

**Relationship:** Compare. *Gerin.* 1x. Constant hawking and spitting in elderly people. *Erodium cicutarium*—Hemlock—Stork's bill (a popular hemostatic in Russia, especially used in metrorrhagia and menorrhagia); *Hydrastininum, Chin., Sabin.*

**Dose:** Tincture, half-dram doses in gastric ulcer. Tincture to third attenuation, as a general rule. Locally on ulcers, it will destroy the pyogenic membrane.

---

## GETTYSBURG WATER

**Get.**

*Stringy mucus* from throat and posterior nares. *Rawness.* Neck muscles rigid. Joints weak. Cannot lift things. *Ligaments rigid.* Subacute gouty state. Evaporated and residue triturated to 6x. Of use in sub-acute and chronic rheumatism. White coated tongue. Highly colored urine with a red sandy sediment. Sensation of rigidity, *worse movement,* especially in the lumbar region and joints of hips, shoulders and wrists. *Not perceived when quiet.* More in the morning. Cannot remain long in one position. Stiffness of muscles on moving. Pain in the ligaments relieved by rest.

**Modalities:** *Worse,* stiffness of muscles on moving. *Better,* rest (ligaments and stiffness of muscles).

**Relationship:** *Lyc., Phos., Rhus-t., Puls.,* but modalities differ.

**Dose:** Lower triturations. Also thirtieth potency.

---

## GINSENG QUINQUEFOLIUM

(Aralia Quinquefolia, Wild Ginseng, Panax) **Gins.**

Said to be a stimulant to the secretory glands, especially salivary. Acts on the lower part of the spinal cord. *Lumbago, sciatica, and rheumatism.* Paralytic weakness. *Hiccough.* Skin symptoms, itching pimples on the neck and chest.

**Head:** Vertigo, with gray spots before the eyes; semi-lateral headache (migraine); occipital.

**Eyes:** Difficulty in opening the eyelids; diplopia.

**Throat:** Tonsillitis, just like *Bell.*, but in dark complexioned people.

**Abdomen:** Tense, painful, rumbling. Pain on the right side. Loud gurgling in the ileo-caecal region. Perityphlitis.

**Male:** Rheumatic pains after frequent emissions. Weakness of genital organs. Voluptuous tickling at the end of the urethra. Sexual excitement. Pressure in testicles.

**Extremities:** Hands feel swollen. Skin feels tight. Contraction. Coldness of the back and spine. Bruised pain in the lumbosacral region and thighs; nocturnal digging pains in the right lower limb extending to the toes. Burning heat in fingertips. Eruption, on upper inner thighs. *Stiff, contracted joints,* heaviness of lower limbs. Crackling in joints. Stiffness of the back.

**Relationship:** Compare: *Aral., Coca. Hed.*—Ivy (mental depression and skin irritation antidoted by *Gunpowder).*

**Dose:** Tincture to third potency.

---

## GLONOINUM = GL = Glycerine<br>O = Oxygen<br>N = Nitrogen

(Nitro-glycerine, Spirits Glycerinus Nitrate) **Glon.**

Recent German provings of *Glonoinum* confirm the original American provings and clinical indications, and bring out very marked nervous disturbances. Great lassitude, no inclination to work; extreme irritability, easily excited by the slightest opposition, ending in congestive head symptoms. The sixth potency alone produced itching all over the body followed by acne and furuncle formation, also bulimia.

A great remedy for congestive headaches, hyperemia of the brain from excess of heat or cold. Excellent for intracranial, climacteric disturbances, or problems due to menstrual suppression. Children get sick on sitting before an open fire. *Surging of blood to the head and heart.* Tendency to sudden and violent irregularities in circulation. Violent convulsions associated with cerebral congestion (meningitis). *Sensation of pulsations throughout the body. Pulsating pain.* Cannot recognize localities. Sciatica in atheromatous subjects, with cold shriveled limbs; seasickness.

**Head:** *Confusion,* with dizziness. Effects of sunstroke; heat on head, as in type-setters and people who work under gas and electric light. *Head heavy, but cannot lay it on a pillow. Cannot bear any heat around the head.* Better from uncovering the head. *Throbbing* headache. Angio-spastic neuralgia of the head and face. Very irritable. Vertigo on assuming an upright position. Cerebral congestion. Head feels enormously large, as if the skull was too small for the brain. Sun headaches; increases and decreases with the sun (sunstroke). Shocks in the head, synchronous with the pulse. Headache in place of menses. Rush of blood to the head in pregnant women. Threatened apoplexy. Meningitis.

**Eyes:** Sees everything half light, half dark. Letters appear smaller. Sparks before the eyes.

**Ears:** Throbbing; each heart beat is heard in the ears; full feeling.

**Face:** Flushed, hot, livid, pale; sweaty; pain in the root of the nose; faceache. Dusky face.

**Mouth:** Pulsating toothache.

**Throat:** Neck feels full (goitre). Collar must be opened. Chokes and swelling under the ears.

**Stomach:** Gastrlagia in anaemic patients with feeble circulation. Nausea and vomiting. Faint, gnawing, and empty feeling in the pit of the stomach. Abnormal hunger.

**Abdomen:** Constipation, with itching, painful hemorrhoids, with pinching in the abdomen, before and after stool. Diarrhea; copious blackish, lumpy stools.

**Female:** Menses delayed, or sudden cessation with congestion of the head. Climacteric flushing.

**Heart:** Laborious action. Fluttering. Palpitations with dyspnea (angina pectoris). Cannot go uphill. Any exertion brings on rush of blood to the heart with fainting spells. Throbbing in the whole body including finger tips.

**Extremities:** Itching all over, worse extremities. Pain in the left biceps. Drawing pain in all limbs. Backache.

**Modalities:** *Better*, brandy. *Worse,* in the sun; exposure to sun-rays, gas, open fire; jar, stooping, having a hair cut; peaches, stimulants; lying down; from 6 a. m. to noon; left side.

**Relationship:** Antidote: *Acon.*

Compare: *Aml-ns., Bell., Op., Stram., Verat-v.*

**Dose:** Sixth to thirtieth potency

**Non-homeopathic Uses:** For palliative (non-homeopathic) purposes, in angina pectoris, asthma, heart failure, etc., physiological doses—i. e., 1-100 of drop—must be given. Here it is the great emergency remedy. The conditions calling for it are small, wiry pulse, pallor, arterial spasm, anaemia of the brain, *collapse,* feeble heart, syncope, dicrotic pulse, vertigo—the opposite of those indicating a homeopathic dosage. Thus often used to lower the arterial tension in chronic interstitial nephritis.

# GLYCERINUM

(Glycerine) **Glyc.**

Used homeopathically, dynamized glycerine seems to be a long, deep acting remedy, building up tissues, hence it is of great use in marasmus, mental and physical debility, diabetes, etc. It disturbs the nutrition in its primary action, and in the secondary action, seems to improve the general state of nutrition (Dr. Wm. B. Griggs).

**Head:** Feels full, throbs; mentally confused. Severe headache two days before menses. Occiput feels full.

**Nose:** Stopped up, sneezing, irritating coryza. Sensation of crawling on the mucous membrane. Post-nasal dripping.

**Stomach:** Fermentation, burning in the stomach and esophagus.

**Urinary:** Profuse and frequent micturition. Increased specific gravity and sugar. Diabetes.

**Female:** Profuse, long lasting flow with a bearing down heaviness in the uterus (dysmenorrhea). General sense of exhaustion.

**Chest:** Hacking cough with a sense of weakness. Chest seems full. Influenzal pneumonia.

**Extremities:** Rheumatic pains of a remittent type. Feet painful and hot, feel enlarged.

**Relationship:** Compare: *Lac-ac., Gels., Calc.*

**Dose:** Thirtieth and higher potencies. Pure glycerine in teaspoonful doses, t. i. d., with lemon juice for pernicious anemia.

---

# GNAPHALIUM POLYCEPHALUM

(Cud-weed, Old Balsam) **Gnaph.**

A remedy of unquestioned benefit in sciatica, when pain is associated with *numbness* of the part affected. Rheumatism and morning diarrhea. Polyuria.

**Face:** Intermittent pains of the superior maxillary nerve on both sides.

**Abdomen:** Borborygmus. Colic; pain in various parts of the abdomen. Irritated prostate. First stage of cholera infantum; vomiting and purging.

**Female:** Weight and fullness in the pelvis. *Dysmenorrhea,* with scanty and painful menses.

**Back:** Chronic backache in the lumbar region; better resting on the back. Lumbago with numbness of the lower part of back and weight in pelvis.

**Extremities:** Cramps in the calves of legs and feet when in bed. Rheumatic pains in the ankle joints and legs. *Intense pain along the sciatic nerve; numbness* *alternates with pain.* Frequent pain in calves and feet. Gouty pain in the big toes. Better, drawing, limbs up, flexing the thigh on the abdomen. Gouty concretions (*Am-be.*). Anterior crural neuralgia (*Staph.*). Pain in the joints, as if they lacked oil. Chronic muscular rheumatism of the back and neck.

**Relationship:** Compare: *Xan., Cham., Puls.*

**Dose:** Third to thirtieth potency.

---

# GOSSYPIUM HERBACEUM

(Cotton Plant) **Goss.**

A powerful emmenagogue, used in physiological doses. Homeopathically, it corresponds to many reflex conditions, depending on disturbed uterine functions and pregnancy. *Goss.* will relieve tardy menses, especially with the sensation that the flow is about to start but does not do so. Tall, bloodless patients (anemic), with nervous chills.

**Head:** Pain in the cervical region with a tendency of the head to draw backward with nervousness (cervical spondylosis).

**Stomach:** Nausea, with an inclination to vomit before breakfast. Anorexia with an uneasy feeling at the scrobiculum at the time of menses.

**Female:** Labia swollen and itchy. *Intermittent pain in the ovaries.* Retained placenta. Tumor of the breast with swelling of the axillary glands. Morning sickness, with a sensitive uterine region. Suppressed menstruation. Menses too watery. Backache, weight and dragging in the pelvis. Uterine subinvolution and fibroids, with gastric pain and debility.

**Relationship:** Compare: Action similar to ergot when made from fresh green root. *Lil-t., Cimic., Sabin.*

**Dose:** Tincture to sixth attenuation.

---

# GRANATUM

(Pomegranate) **Gran.**

As a vermifuge for the expulsion of tapeworm and homeopathically for the following symptomatic indications; *salivation* with nausea and vertigo. Spasm of the glottis.

**Head:** Feels empty. Sunken eyes; pupils dilated; weak sight. *Vertigo very persistent.*

**Stomach:** *Constant hunger.* Poor digestion. Losses flesh. Vomiting at night.

**Abdomen:** Pain in the stomach and abdomen; worse *around the umbilicus* (*Cocc., Nux-m., Plb.*); ineffectual urging. Itching in the anus. Dragging in the vaginal region, as if hernia would protrude. Swelling resembling umbilical hernia.

**Chest:** Oppressed, with sighing. Pain between the shoulders; even clothing is oppressive.

**Extremities:** Pain around the shoulders, as if a heavy load had been carried. Pain in all the finger joints (rheumatic arthritis). Tearing in the knee joint (osteoarthritis). Convulsive movements.

**Skin:** *Itching in the palms.* Sensation as if pimples would break out. Jaundiced complexion.

**Relationship:** Compare: *Pelletierinum* (one of its constituents—an anthelmintic, especially for tapeworm); *Cina; Kousso.*

**Dose:** First to third potency.

---

## GRAPHITES

(Black Lead, Plumbago) **Graph.**

Like all the carbons, this remedy is an anti-psoric of great power, especially active in patients who are rather stout, of fair complexion, with a tendency to skin affections and constipation, *fat, chilly and costive* (constipated), with delayed menstrual history, takes cold easily. Children impudent, teasing, laugh at reprimands. Has a particular tendency to develop the skin phase of internal disorders. *Eradicates tendency to erysipelas.* Anemia with redness of the face. Tendency to obesity. Swollen genitals. Gushing leucorrhea. Aids absorption of cicatricial tissue. Induration of tissue. Cancer of pylorus. Duodenal ulcer.

**Mind:** Great tendency to start. Timid. Unable to decide. Want of disposition to work. Fidgety while sitting at work. *Music makes her weep.* Apprehensive, despondency, indecision.

**Head:** Rush of blood to the head with a flushed face and epistaxis, distention and flatulence. Headache in the morning on waking, mostly on one side, with an inclination to vomit (migraine). Sensation of a cobweb on the forehead. Feels numb and pithy. Rheumatic pains on one side of head, extending to the teeth and neck. *Burning on the vertex.* Humid, itchy eruptions on the hairy scalp, emitting a fetid odor. Cataleptic condition.

**Eyes:** Ophthalmia with intolerance of artificial light. Eyelids *red and swollen.* Blepharitis. Dryness of the lids. *Eczema of lids; fissured.*

**Ears:** *Dryness of the inner ear.* Cracking in ears when eating. *Moisture and eruptions behind the ears. Hears better in noise.* Hardness of hearing.

Hissing in the ears. Detonation in the ear like the retort of a gun. A thin, white, scaly membrane covering membrana tympani, like exfoliated epithelium. Fissures in and behind the ear.

**Nose:** Sore on blowing it; is painful internally. Smell abnormally acute; cannot tolerate flowers. Scabs and fissures in nostrils.

**Face:** Feels as if cobwebs were on it. Eczema of the nose. Itching pimples. Moist eczema around the mouth and chin. Erysipelas, burning and stinging.

**Mouth:** Rotten odor from the mouth. Breath smells like urine. Burning blisters on the tongue, salivation (aphthae). Sour eructations.

**Stomach:** Aversion to meat. Sweets nauseate. *Hot drinks disagree.* Nausea and vomiting after each meal. Morning sickness during menstruation. Pressure in the stomach. Burning in the stomach, causing *hunger.* Eructations difficult. *Constrictive, pain in the stomach.* Recurrent gastralgia. Flatulence. Stomach pain is temporarily relieved by eating, hot drinks especially milk and lying down.

**Abdomen:** Nauseous feeling in the abdomen. Fullness and hardness of the abdomen, as from incarcerated flatulence; *must loosen clothing;* presses painfully at the abdominal ring. Croaking in the abdomen. Inguinal region sensitive, swollen (inguinal hernia). Flatulent colic, opposite the side on which he lies. Chronic diarrhea, stools brownish, liquid, undigested, *offensive.* Very fetid gas is passed preceded by colic.

**Rectum:** Constipation; large, difficult, knotty stools united by mucus threads. Burning hemorrhoids. Prolapse, diarrhea; stools, brownish, fluid, mixed with undigested substance (lienteric), *very fetid,* sour odor. Smarting, sore anus, itching. Lumpy stool, conjoined with threads of mucus. Varices of the rectum. Fissure in the anus (*Rat., Paeon.*).

**Urinary:** Turbid, with a sediment. Sour smelling.

**Male:** Sexual debility with increased desire; aversion to coition; too early or no ejaculation; herpetic eruption on organs.

**Female:** Menses *too late,* with constipation; pale and scanty, with tearing pains in the epigastrium, and itching *before.* Hoarseness, coryza, cough, sweats and morning sickness, during menstruation. Leucorrhea, *pale,* thin, *profuse, white, excoriating,* with great weakness of the back. Mammae swollen and hard. Induration of the ovaries, uterus and mammae (cancerous affectious). Nipples sore, cracked, and blistered. Decided aversion to coitus.

**Respiratory:** Constriction of the chest; spasmodic asthma, suffocative attacks, wakes up from sleep; must eat something. Pain in the middle of the chest, with cough, scraping and soreness. Chronic hoarseness with skin affections. Inability to control the vocal cords, hoarseness on beginning to sing and for breaking voice.

**Extremities:** Pain in the nape of neck, shoulders, back and limbs. Spinal pains. Pain in the lumbosacral region with great weakness. Excoriation between the thighs. Left hand numb; arms fall asleep; finger nails *thick,* black and rough; matrix inflamed (*Psor., Fl-ac.*). Edema of the lower limbs. Toe nails crippled. Stiffness and contraction of toes. Nails brittle and crumbling. Nails deformed, painful, sore, thick, and crippled. Cracks or fissures in the fingertips. Offensive foot sweat.

**Skin:** Rough, hard, persistent dryness in portions of skin unaffected by eczema. Early stage of keloid and fibroma. Pimples and acne. *Eruptions, oozing out a sticky exudation.* Rawness in the bends of limbs, groins, neck, behind ears. *Unhealthy skin; every little injury suppurates.* Ulcers discharging a *glutinous* fluid, thin and sticky. Swelling and induration of glands. Gouty nodosities. Cracks in nipples, mouth, between toes, anus. Phlegmonous erysipelas of the face; burning and stinging pain. Swelling of feet. *Wens.* Chronic Poison oak.

**Modalities:** *Worse,* warmth, at night, during and after menstruation. *Better,* in the dark, from wrapping up.

**Relationship:** Complementary: *Arg-n.* (follows well in gastric derangements); *Caust., Hep., Lyc., Ars., Tub.*

Compare: *Petr., Sep., Sulph., Fl*-ac. Associated constipation with mucus covered stools and flatulence should be taken into consideration to differentiate it from remedies such as *Petr.* and *Lyc.* (Raue).

Antidote: *Nux-v., Acon., Ars.*

**Dose:** Sixth to thirtieth potency. Locally as cerate, in sore nipples.

---

# GRATIOLA OFFICINALIS

(Hedge Hyssop) **Grat.**

Acts especially on the gastro-intestinal tract. Chronic catarrhal conditions, leucorrhea and gonorrhea. Obstinate ulcers. Useful in mental problems from overweening pride. Especially useful in females. *Nux-v.* symptoms in females often met by *Grat.*

**Head:** Sick headaches. *Rush of blood to the head* with loss of vision (blindness). Sensation as if the brain was contracting and head was becoming smaller. Tightness in the forehead, with wrinkles on the skin.

**Eyes:** Loss of vision with rush of blood to the head. Eyes dry, burn. Myopia.

**Stomach:** Vertigo during and after meals; hunger and sensation of emptiness after meals. Dyspepsia with distention of the stomach. Cramps and colic after supper and at night, with swelling of the abdomen and constipation. Dysphagia for liquids.

**Rectum:** Diarrhea; *green, frothy water,* followed by burning in the anus, *forcibly evacuated without pain. Constipation,* with gouty acidity. Hemorrhoids with hypochondriasis. Rectum constricted.

**Female:** *Nymphomania.* Menses too profuse, premature, and too long (metrorrhagia). Leucorrhea.

**Sleep:** Insomnia.

**Modalities:** *Worse,* drinking too much water.

**Relationship:** Compare: *Dig., Euph., Tab., Cham., Am-pic., Nux-v.*

**Dose:** Second to third potency.

---

# GRINDELIA ROBUSTA

(Rosin-wood) **Grin.**

Both *Grindelia robusta* and *Grindelia squarrosa* have been used for the symptoms recorded here. There is no practical difference in their action, although the *Grindelia squarrosa* is credited with more *splenic* symptoms, dull pains and fullness in the left hypochondrium; chronic malaria; gastric pains associated with splenic congestion. Induces paralysis, beginning in the extremities. Its action is shown on the heart, first quickening if, then retarding it.

Acts on the cardio-pulmonary distribution of the pneumo-gastric nerve in dry catarrh (*Ant-t.* in muco-purulent). Produces paresis of the pneumo-gastric nerve, interfering with respiration. *Smothering after falling asleep.* Asthmatic conditions, chronic bronchitis. Bronchorrhea with tough mucus, difficult to detach. Raises the blood pressure. Nausea and retching of gastric ulcer. Diabetes. An effective antidote to Rhus poisoning, locally and internally; also for burns, blisters, vaginal catarrh and herpes zoster. Hyperchlorhydria when attended with asthmatic and other neurotic symptoms. Hyperemia of the gastric mucosa with difficult respiration.

**Head:** Feels full, as from quinine.

**Eyes:** *Pain in the eyeballs,* running back to the brain; worse, moving the eyes. Pupils dilated. Purulent ophthalmia and iritis.

**Abdomen:** Cutting pains in the region of spleen, extending to the hips. Splenomegaly (*Cean., Card-m.*).

**Respiratory:** An efficacious remedy for wheezing and oppression in bronchitic patients. The sibilant rales are disseminated with foamy mucus, very difficult to detach. Acts on the pulmonary circulation. Asthma, with profuse tenacious expectoration, which relieves. *Stops breathing on falling asleep;* wakes *up with a start,* and gasps for breath. Must sit up to breathe. *Cannot* *breathe when lying down.* Pertussis with profuse mucous secretion (*Coc-c.*). Bronchorrhea with tough, whitish, mucous expectoration. Sibilant rales. Weak heart and respiration. Cannot breathe while lying down. Cheyne-Stokes respiration.

**Skin:** Rash-like roseola, with severe burning and itching. Vesicular and papular eruptions. Herpes zoster. Itching and burning. *Poison oak* (locally as a wash). Ulcers with swollen, purplish skin.

**Relationship:** Compare: *Ant-t., Erio., Lach., Sang.*

**Dose:** Tincture in 1 to 15 drop doses, also lower potencies.

---

# GUACO

(Mikania, Climbing Hemp Weed) **Gua.**

Acts on the nervous system and female organs. An antidote to bites of scorpions and serpents (*Euph-po.*). Cholera. *Bulbar paralysis. Syphilis.* Cancer. Deafness; tongue heavy and difficult to move (paralysed). *Spinal irritation.* Spinal symptoms very marked and verified. Beer drinkers threatened with apoplexy. *Diarrhea and dysentery with aching in the sacrum and loins.*

Headache, red face. Heaviness and difficulty in moving the tongue (apoplexy).

**Throat:** Larynx and trachea constricted; dysphagia. Tongue feels heavy, difficult to move.

**Urinary:** Increased, cloudy, phosphatic. Pain over the region of bladder (cystitis).

**Female:** Leucorrhea copious, corroding, putrid, debilitating. Itching and smarting at night, as if fire was running out of the parts.

**Back:** Pain between scapulae, extending to the forearm. Burning in the nape of shoulders. *Pain along the spine; worse,* bending. Weariness through the hips and lumbar region.

**Extremities:** Pain in the deltoid, shoulders, elbows, arms, and fingers. Pain around the hip joint. Legs heavy. Pain in the ankle joints and soles. *Paralysis of the lower extremities.*

**Modalities:** *Worse,* from motion.

**Relationship:** Compare: *Ox-ac., Lath., Caust.*

**Dose:** Third to sixth potency.

---

# GUAIACUM OFFICINALE—GUAJACUM OFFICINALE

(Resin of Lignum Vitae) **Guaj.**

Chief action on fibrous tissue and is especially adapted to the arthritic diathesis, rheumatism and tonsillitis. Secondary syphilis. Very valuable in acute rheumatism. *Frees foul secretions. Unclean odor from the whole body.* Promotes suppuration of abscesses. Sensitiveness and aggravation from local heat. Contraction of limbs, stiffness and immobility. Feeling that he must stretch.

**Mind:** Forgetful; thoughtless; staring. Slow to comprehend.

**Head:** *Gouty and rheumatic pain in the head* and face, *extending to the neck.* Tearing pain in the skull; worse, cold, wet weather. Feels swollen and blood vessels are distended. Aching in the left ear. *Pains often end in a stitch,* especially in the head.

**Eyes:** Pupils dilated. Eyelids appear too short[1]. Pimples, around the eyes.

**Throat:** Rheumatic sore throat with weak throat muscles. Throat dry, burns, swollen, stitches towards the ear. *Acute tonsillitis.* Syphilitic sore throat.

**Stomach:** Tongue furred. *Desire for apples* and other fruits. Aversion to milk. Burning in the stomach. Constricted epigastric region (hyperchlorhydria).

**Abdomen:** Intestinal fermentation. Excessive flatus in bowels. Diarrhea, cholera infantum.

**Urinary:** Sharp stitches after micturating. Constant desire.

**Female:** Ovaritis in rheumatic patients with irregular menses and dysmenorrhea, irritable bladder (cystitis).

**Respiratory:** *Feels suffocated* (asthma). Dry, tight cough. Halitosis after coughing. *Pleuritic stitches.* Pain in the articulations of the ribs, with shortness of breath till expectoration sets in.

**Back:** Pain from the head to neck. *Aching in the nape. Stiff neck and sore shoulders* (cervical spondylosis). Stitches between the scapulae and occiput. Contractive pain between scapulae.

**Extremities:** Rheumatic pain in the shoulders, arms and hands. *Growing pains* (*Ph-ac.*). Pricking in the nates. Sciatica and lumbago. Gouty tearing with contractions. Immovable stiffness. Pain in the ankles, extending up the leg, causing lameness. Joints swollen, painful and intolerant to pressure; can not bear heat. Stinging pain in the limbs. Arthritic lancinations followed by contraction of limbs. *Sensation of heat* in the affected limbs.

**Modalities:** *Worse,* from motion, heat, cold wet weather; pressure, touch, from 6 p. m. to 4 a. m. *Better,* external pressure.

---

1 Protrusion of the eyeballs (exophthalmos) (1001 Small Remedies, Edited by Dr. F. Schroyens).

**Relationship:** *Guajacolum* (in the treatment of gonorrheal epididymitis, 2 parts to 30 vaseline, locally).

Antidote: *Nux-v.*

Follows: *Sep.*

Compare: *Merc., Caust., Rhus-t., Mez., Rhod.*

**Dose:** Tincture to sixth attenuation.

---

# GUARANA

(Paullinia Sorbilis) **Guar.**

Contains a large percentage of caffein, which may explain its use as a remedy for certain forms of sick headache.

**Head:** Intellectual excitement. Sick headaches in people who have used tea and coffee in excess. Throbbing headache after liquor.

**Rectum:** Stools profuse, bloody, bright green; flakes intermixed; odorless. Cholera infantum.

**Sleep:** Uncontrollable sleepiness and heaviness of the head, with a flushed face after eating.

**Skin:** Chloasma on temples and arms. Urticaria (*Dulc., Apis, Chlol.*).

**Dose:** Must be given in material doses, fifteen to sixty grains of the powder.

---

# GUAREA TRICHILOIDES

(Ballwood) **Guare.**

Eye symptoms have been verified. Chemosis and pterygium have been cured with it. Lupus of an ochre-red color.

**Head:** Sensation as if the brain was falling forwards; as if from a blow on the head.

**Eyes:** Conjunctiva inflamed, swollen (conjunctivitis). Tearing pain in the eyeballs; tension, forced out feeling (glaucoma). Objects appear gray, upside down. Eye symptoms alternate with diminished hearing. Epiphora.

**Respiratory:** Cough with sweat, pain and tightness of the chest; larynx irritated.

**Dose:** Tincture.

---

## GYMNOCLADUS CANADENSIS

(American Coffee Tree) **Gymno.**

Sore throat, dark, livid redness (hyperemia) of the fauces and erysipelatous swelling of the face are most marked. Hives. Desire for heat and quiet. Headache, throbbing in the forehead temples and over the eyes, with *a bluish-white coating of tongue.* Burning in the eyes.

**Face:** Sensation of flies crawling over the face. Erysipelas.

**Mouth:** Great sensitivity of teeth.

**Throat:** Sore; dark livid redness of fauces and tonsils. Sticking pain. Mucus in the throat with hawking. Tickling, with dry cough.

**Relationship:** Compare: *Lachn., Lach., Ail., Rhus-t.*

**Dose:** Lower attenuations.

---

## HAEMATOXYLON CAMPECHIANUM

(Logwood) **Hem.**

Sense of constriction is characteristic. *Sensation as if a bar lay across the chest.* Angina pectoris.

**Head:** Feels constricted; heavy, hot. Eyelids heavy.

**Stomach:** Painful digging from the abdomen to the throat, causing pain in the region of heart with oppression. Colic, tympanites. Borborygmi and diarrhea. Swollen (distention), painful.

**Female:** Pain in the hypogastrium attended with slimy, whitish leucorrhea. *Weak feeling with painful bearing down sensation during the menstrual period* (dysmenorrhea).

**Chest:** Constriction, extending to the epigastrium. Sensation of a bar across the chest. Convulsive pain in the heart region with oppression. Great soreness in the region of heart. Palpitations.

**Relationship:** Compare: *Cact., Coloc., Naja.*

**Dose:** Third potency.

---

## HAMAMELIS VIRGINIANA

(Witch-hazel) **Ham.**

Venous congestion, hemorrhages, varicose veins and hemorrhoids, with *bruised soreness of the affected parts* seems to be the special sphere of this remedy. Acts upon the coats of the veins causing relaxation with consequent engorgement. Passive venous hemorrhages from any part, of great value in open, painful wounds with weakness from loss of blood. After surgery, supercedes the use of morphia (Helmuth).

**Head:** Wants "the respect due to me" shown. Sensation of a bolt, from temple to temple. Fullness, followed by epistaxis. Numbness over the frontal bone (forehead).

**Eyes:** Painful weakness; *sore pain* in the eyes; bloodshot appearance; inflamed vessels greatly injected. Hastens absorption of intraocular hemorrhage. Eyes feel forced out.

**Nose:** Profuse epistaxis, flow passive, non-coagulable with tightness in the bridge of nose. Bad odor from the nose.

**Mouth:** Tongue feels burnt. Thirst. Blisters on the sides.

**Throat:** Mucous membrane distended and bluish; varicosis of the throat (pharynx).

**Stomach:** Hematemesis of black blood. Throbbing and pain in the stomach.

**Rectum:** Anus feels sore and raw. *Hemorrhoids, bleeding profusely with soreness.* Dysentery. Pulsations in the rectum.

**Urinary:** Hematuria with increased desire.

**Male:** Pain in the spermatic cord, radiating to the testies. Varicocele. Pain in the testicles. Orchitis. Testicles enlarged, hot, and painful. Epididymitis.

**Female:** Ovarian congestion and neuralgia; feels very sore. Vicarious menstruation. Uterine hemorrhage, bearing down pain in the back. Menses *dark, profuse, with soreness in the abdomen* (dysmenorrhea). *Metrorrhagia, occurring midway between menstrual periods.* Intermenstrual pain (Jas. W. Ward). Vagina very tender (vaginitis). Profuse leucorrhea. Pruritus vulva. Milk leg, hemorrhoids, and sore nipples, after confinement. Metrorrhagia; passive flow. Vaginismus, ovaritis, soreness over the entire abdomen. Phlegmasia alba.

**Respiratory:** Hemoptysis; tickling cough. Chest feels sore and constricted.

**Back:** Sore pain down the cervical vertebrae. Severe pain in lumbar and hypogastric region, extending down the legs.

**Extremities:** Tired feeling in the arms and legs. Very sore muscles and joints. Varicose veins. Chills in the back and hips, extending down the legs. Neuralgia of the internal saphenous nerve.

**Skin:** Bluish chilblains. Phlebitis. Purpura. Varicose veins and ulcers; very sore. Burns. Ecchymosis. Traumatic inflammations (*Arn.*).

**Modalities:** *Worse,* warm, moist air.

**Relationship:** Compare in hemorrhoids: *Calc-f., Aloe, Mur-ac.* in varicose veins. *Mangifera indica.*

Compare: *Arn., Calen., Tril-p., Bell., Sul-ac., Puls.*

Antidote: *Arn.*

Complementary: *Ferr.*

**Dose:** Tincture to sixth attenuation. Distilled extract locally.

## HEDEOMA PULEGIOIDES

(Pennyroyal) **Hedeo.**

Female symptoms are very marked; usually associated with nervous disturbances. Red sand in urine. *Pain along the ureter.* Flatulent colic. Antidotes effects of Poison oak (*Grin.*).

**Head:** Dull, heavy feeling in the morning. Sore pain, as if from a cut. Weak, faint; better, lying down.

**Stomach:** Gastritis. *Everything taken into the stomach causes pain.* Tongue coated thin white. Nausea.

**Abdomen:** Distended, sore, and sensitive.

**Urinary:** Frequent urging, cutting pains. Pain along the left ureter. Dragging pain from the kidney to the bladder. Dull burning pain over the left kidney. Burning irritation at the neck of the bladder causing frequent intense desire to micturate and an inability to retain urine for more than a few minutes, better micturating.

**Female:** Bearing down pains with severe backache; worse, least movement. Leucorrhea with itching and burning. Ovaries congested and painful; bearing down spasmodic contractions.

**Extremities:** *Pain in the thumb joint.* Pain, coldness, and paretic condition. Twitchings, jerkings, soreness. Tendo-Achilles painful, as if sprained and swollen; walking painful.

**Relationship:** Compare: *Mentha; Sep., Lil-t., Oci.* (uric acid diathesis, pain in ureters). *Hedera helix*—Common ivy (delirium and chronic convulsions. Chronic hydrocephalus. Rhinorrhea, cerebro-spinalis. Cataract. Acts on the blood vessels, menorrhagia). *Glechoma hederacea*—Ground ivy (hemorrhoids with *rectal irritation* and bleeding. Diarrhea. Anus feels raw and sore. Cough with laryngeal and tracheal irritation. Glandula sub-mentalis inflamed).

**Dose:** First potency.

---

## HECLA LAVA—HEKLA LAVA

(Lava Scoriae From Mt. Hecla) **Hecla**

Marked action upon *the jaws.* Of great use in exostosis, gum abscess, difficult teething. Nodosities, caries of bone, etc. Osteitis, periostitis, osteosarcoma; rachitis. *Tumors* in general. Bone necrosis. Necrosis and sinus after mastoid operation.

**Face:** Ulceration of nasal bones. *Facial neuralgia from carious teeth* and after extraction. Toothache with swelling around the jaws. Abscess of gums.

*Enlargement of the maxillary bone*[1]. Cervical glands enlarged and indurated.

**Relationship:** Compare: *Sil., Merc., Phos., Conchiolinum*—Mother of pearl (diaphysis of bone affected; parts extremely sensitive to touch).

*Amphisbaena vermicularis*—Snail-like lizard (great affinity for the jaw bones, worse by air and dampness).

*Slag* (Great itching of parts).

**Dose:** Lower triturations.

---

## HELIANTHUS ANNUUS

(Sunflower) **Helia.**

Old cases of intermittent fever. Coryza, catarrh, nasal hemorrhage and thick scabs in the nose. Rheumatic pain in the left knee. Vomiting, black stools, congestion and dryness of the mouth and pharynx, redness and heat of skin. Symptoms aggravated by heat and relieved by vomiting. Spleen remedy. Marked effects on the stomach, with nausea and vomiting. Stools black (*Lept.*). Dry mouth. Externally, as a vulnerary like *Arn.* and *Calen.*

---

## HELLEBORUS NIGER

(Snow-rose) **Hell.**

Produces a condition of *sensorial depression.* Sees, hears, tastes imperfectly and general *muscular weakness,* which may go on to complete paralysis accompanied with dropsical effusions. Hence, a remedy in low states of vitality and serious diseases. Characteristic aggravation from 4 to 8 p.m. (*Lyc.*). *Sinking sensation.* State of effusion in hydrocephalus. Mania of a melancholic type.

**Mind:** Slow in answering. Thoughtless; staring. *Involuntary sighing. Complete unconsciousness. Picks lips and clothes.*

**Head:** Forehead wrinkled in folds. Cold sweat. Stupefying headache. *Rolls head* day and night; moaning, sudden screams. *Bores head into the pillow;* beats it with hands (meningitis). Dull pain in the occiput with sensation of water swashing inside (hydrocephalus). Headache culminates in vomiting (migraine).

**Eyes:** Eyeballs turn upwards; squinting, vacant look (epilepsy). Pupils dilated. Eyes wide open, sunken. Night blindness.

---

[1] Exostosis, lower jaw (1001 Small Remedies, Edited by Dr F. Schroyens).

**Nose:** Dirty, dry nostrils. Rubs nose. Smell diminished. Nose pointed.

**Face:** Pale, sunken. Cold sweat. Wrinkled. Neuralgia of the left side; parts so tender, he cannot chew.

**Mouth:** *Horrible smell from the mouth.* Lips dry and cracked. Tongue red and dry. *Falling of lower jaw* (tetnus). Meaningless picking of lips. Grinding of teeth. *Chewing motion.* Greedily swallows cold water, though unconscious. Child nurses greedily with disgust for food. Ptyalism, with sore corners of the mouth.

**Abdomen:** Gurgling, as if bowels were full of water. Swollen, painful to touch.

**Rectum:** Jelly-like, white mucus; involuntary.

**Urinary:** Suppressed; scanty, dark; coffee ground sediment. Frequent urging. Child cannot micturate. Bladder overdistended (cystitis).

**Respiratory:** Frequent sighing. Respiration irregular. Chest constricted; gasps for breath. Hydrothorax (*Merc-sul.*).

**Extremities:** *Automatic motion of one arm and leg.* Limbs heavy and painful. Stretching of limbs. Thumb drawn into the palm (*Cupr.*). Vesicular eruption between fingers and toes.

**Sleep:** Screams suddenly in sleep. Soporous sleep. *Cri encephalique.* Cannot be fully aroused.

**Skin:** *Pale, dropsical,* itchy. Livid spots on the skin. Sudden, watery, swelling of the skin. Falling off of hair and nails. Angio-neurotic edema.

**Modalities:** *Worse,* from evening till morning, from uncovering.

**Relationship:** *Helleborus foetidus* or, *Polymnia uvedalia*—Bear's foot: Acts especially on the spleen (*Cean.*); also rectum and sciatic nerve. Splenic pain extends to the scapula, neck and head, worse left side and evening; chronic ague cake; hypertrophied uterus; glandular enlargements; hair and nails fall off; skin peels. *Helleborus orientalis* (salivation).

Antidote: *Camph., Chin.*

Compare: Threatening effusion; *Tub., Apis, Zinc., Op., Chin., Cic; Iodof.*

**Dose:** Tincture to third potency.

---

## HELODERMA

(Gila Monster) **Helo.**

The result of the bite is a benumbing paralysis like paralysis agitans or locomotor ataxia. There is no tetanic phase—a condition almost reverse in objective symptoms to *Hydr-ac. or Stry*. The most unusual action of this drug is noted upon the eye of a mouse. *The eyeball becomes more prominent* and the cornea shows opacities. The exophthalmus is due to the pressure of the blood behind the eyeball (Boyd). Homeopathically, it is indicated in many forms of diseases characterized by great coldness, "arctic" coldness. Cold waves from the occiput to the feet or ascending.

**Head:** Very depressed. Sensation of falling to the right side. *Cold* band around the head; cold pressure within the skull. Eyelids heavy. Pain beginning in the right ear, extending around the back of head to the left ear.

**Face:** Cold crawling feeling, as if facial muscles were tight.

**Mouth:** Tongue cold, tender and dry. Very thirsty. Dysphagia. Breath cold.

**Chest:** Cold feeling in the lungs and heart. Slow labored thumping of the heart (oppressed action of the heart).

**Back:** Coldness across the scapulae. Burning along the spine.

**Extremities:** Numbness and trembling (paralysis agitans). Cyanosis of the hands. Coldness. Sensation as if walking on a sponge, and as if feet were swollen. Staggering gait. Cock's gait. When walking, lifts feet higher than usual, and the heel comes down hard (locomotor ataxia). Feet cold as ice or burn. Stretching relieves pain in the muscles and limbs.

**Fever:** *Internal coldness,* as if frozen to death. Cold rings around the body. Cold waves (*Abies-c., Acon.*). *Cold spots.* Arctic coldness. Temperature subnormal—96 degree (*Camph.*).

**Relationship:** Compare: *Lacerta agilis*—Green lizard (skin eruptions. Vesicles under the tongue. Increased mental acumen. Dysphagia. Constant accumulation of saliva in the mouth. Nausea; violent pressure in the stomach). *Camph., Lach.*

**Dose:** Thirtieth potency.

---

## HELONIAS DIOICA—CHAMAELIRIUM

(Unicorn Root) **Helon.**

Sensation of weakness, dragging and weight in the sacrum and pelvis with great languor and prostration are excellent indications for this remedy. There is a sensitiveness expressed as consciousness of the womb. Tired, women with tendancy to backaches. The weakness shows itself as a tendency to prolapse and as other malpositions of the womb. Menses are often suppressed and the kidneys congested. It seems as if the monthly congestion (menses), instead of venting itself as it should, through the uterine vessels, vents itself via the kidneys. With all these symptoms, there is a profound melancholia. Patient must do something to engage his mind. Remember it in women with prolapse from atony, enervated by indolence and luxury (better when attention is engaged, hence when the doctor comes), or for those worn out with hard work; tired, strained muscles burn and ache; sleepless. Diabetes mellitus and insipidus. Constant aching and tenderness over the kidney region.

**Mind:** Profound melancholy. *Patient is better when kept busy,* when mind is engaged, when doing something. Irritable; cannot endure the least contradiction.

**Head:** Burning sensation on top of the held. Headache, better mentai exertion.

**Urinary:** *Albuminous,* phosphatic; profuse and clear, saccharine. Diabetes.

**Female:** Dragging in the sacral region, with prolapse, especially after a miscarriage. *Pruritus vulvae.* Backache after miscarriage (*Kali-c.*). Weight and soreness in the womb; *conscious of the womb. Menses too frequent, too profuse* (menorrhagia). Leucorrhea. Breasts swollen, nipples painful and tender (mastitis). Parts hot, red, swollen; burn and itch terribly. Albuminuria during pregnancy. Debility attending menopause.

**Back:** *Pain and weight in the back;* tired and weak. Aching and burning across the lumbar region; *can trace the outlines of the kidneys by constant burning.* Boring pain in the lumbar region, extending down the legs. Great languor, better exercising.

**Extremities:** Sensation as if cool wind streamed up the calves of legs. Feet feel numb when sitting.

**Modalities:** *Better,* when doing something (mental diversion). *Worse,* motion, touch.

**Relationship:** Compare: *Agrimonia eupatoria*—Cockleburr (painful kidneys, impaired digestion and menstrual problems; bronchorrhea and dysuria. Cough with profuse expectoration attended with expulsion of urine. Tincture 1-10 gtt). *Alet., Lil-t., Puls., Senec., Stann.*

**Dose:** Tincture to sixth attenuation.

---

## HEPAR SULPHURIS CALCAREUM

(Hahnemann's Calcium Sulphide) **Hep.**

Suits especially the scrofulous and lymphatic constitutions who are inclined to eruptions and glandular swellings. Unhealthy skin. Blondes with a sluggish character and weak muscles. *Great sensitiveness to all impressions.* Sweating patient pulls a blanket around himself. Locally, it has a special affinity for the respiratory mucous membrane, producing croupous, catarrhal inflammation, profuse secretion; also easy perspiration. After abuse of mercury. Infected sinus with pus formation. *The tendency to suppuration* is most marked, and has been a strong guiding symptom in practice. The lesions spread by the formation of small papules around the side of the old lesion. Chilliness, hypersensitiveness, splinter-like pains, craving for sour and strong things are very characteristic. *Sensation as if wind was blowing on some part.* The side of the body on which he lies at night becomes gradually, insufferably painful; he must turn. *Pellagra* (material doses required). Syphilis after antispecific gross medication.

**Mind:** Anguish in the evening and night with thoughts of suicide. *The slightest cause irritates him.* Dejected and sad. Ferocious. Hasty speech.

**Head:** Vertigo and headache on shaking the head or riding. Boring pains in the right temple and in the root of the nose every morning. Scalp sensitive and sore. Humid scald head, itching and burning.[1] Cold sweat on the head.

**Eyes:** *Ulcers on the cornea.* Iritis, with pus in the anterior chamber; purulent conjunctivitis with marked chemosis, profuse discharge, great sensitiveness to touch and air. Eyes and lids red and inflamed (blepharitis). Pain in the eyes, as if pulled back into the head. Boring pain in the upper bones of the orbits. Eyeballs sore to touch. Objects appear red and too large. Vision obscured by reading; field reduced in one half. Bright circles before the eyes. *Hypopion.*

**Ears:** Scurfs on and behind the ears. Discharge of fetid pus from the ears (otorrhea). Whizzing and throbbing in ears, with hardness of hearing (tinnitus). Deafness after scarlet fever. Pustules in the auditory canal and auricle. Mastoiditis.

**Nose:** Sore, ulcerated. Soreness of the nostrils with catarrh. Sneezes every time he is exposed to cold, dry wind, with a running nose, later, thick, offensive discharge. Stopped up every time he goes out into cold air. *Smell, like old cheese. Hay fever* (*Hep.* 1x will often start secretions and profuse drainage in stuffy colds).

**Face:** Yellowish complexion. Middle of the lower lip cracked. Vesicular erysipelas with pricking in parts. Neuralgia of the right side, extending in a streak to the temple, ear, alae and lip (facial neuralgia). Pain in the facial bones, especially when touched. Ulcers at the corners of mouth. Shooting in the jaw on opening the mouth.

**Mouth:** Ptyalism. Gums and mouth painful to touch (stomatitis) and bleed readily (scorbutic).

**Throat:** On swallowing, sensation of a plug and *of a splinter in the throat.* Quinsy *with impending suppuration.* Stitches in throat extending to the ear on swallowing. Hawking up of mucus.

**Stomach:** Longing for acids, wine and strong tasting food. Aversion to fatty food. Frequent eructations without taste or smell. Distention of the stomach,

---

1 Humid scabs on the head, feeling sore on scratching, of fetid smell, itching violenty on rising in the morning (Clarke — Dictionary of Practical Materia Medica).

compelling him to loosen the clothing. Burning in the stomach. Heaviness and pressure in the stomach after a slight meal.

**Abdomen:** Stitching in the region of liver when walking, coughing, breathing, or when touching it (*Bry., Merc.*). Hepatitis, hepatic abscess; abdomen distended, tense; chronic abdominal affections.

**Rectum:** Clay colored and soft. *Sour,* white, lienteric, *fetid.* Loss of power to expel even soft stool.

**Urinary:** Voided slowly, without force, drops vertically, bladder weak. Seems as if some urine always remained. Greasy pellicle on the urine. Diseases of the bladder in old men (*Phos., Sulph., Cop.*).

**Male:** Herpes, sensitive, bleed easily. Ulcers externally on the prepuce similar to a chancre (*Nit-ac.*). Excitement and emission without amorous fancies. Itching of the glans, frenum and scrotum. Suppurating inguinal glands. Figwarts with an offensive odor. Humid soreness of the genitals and between the scrotum and thigh. Obstinate gonorrhea "does not get well."

**Female:** Discharge of blood from the uterus. Itching of pudenda and nipples, worse during menses. Menses late and scanty. *Abscesses of labia with great sensitiveness.* Extremely offensive leucorrhea. Smells like old cheese (*Sanic.*). Profuse perspiration at climacteric (*Til., Jab.*).

**Respiratory:** Aphonia and cough (bronchitis) when exposed to dry, cold wind. Hoarseness with aphonia. Cough troublesome when walking. Dry, hoarse cough. Cough excited *whenever any part of the body gets cold or uncovered,* or from eating anything cold. Croup with loose, rattling cough; worse in the morning (pneumonia). *Choking cough.* Rattling, croaking cough; suffocative attacks; has to rise up and bend the head backwards. Anxious, wheezing, moist breathing, asthma worse in dry cold air; better in damp. Palpitations of the heart.

**Extremities:** Finger joints swollen (rheumatoid arthritis); tendency to easy dislocation. Nail of the great toe painful on slight pressure.

**Fever:** Chilly in the open air or from *the slightest draught.* Dry heat at night. *Profuse sweat;* sour, sticky, offensive.

**Skin:** Abscesses; suppurating glands are very sensitive. *Papules* prone to suppurate and extend. Acne in the youth. Suppurate with prickly pain. Bleed easily. Angio-neurotic edema. *Unhealthy skin; every little injury supputrates.* Chapped skin, with *deep cracks on the hands and feet* (rhagades). Ulcers, with bloody suppuration, smelling like old cheese (carbuncles). *Ulcers very sensitive* to contact, burning, stinging, easily bleeding. Sweats day and night without relief. *"Cold-sores" very sensitive.* Cannot bear to be uncovered; *wants to be wrapped up warmly.* Sticking or pricking in afflicted parts. Putrid ulcers, *surrounded by little pimples.* Great sensitiveness to the slightest touch. *Chronic* *and recurring urticaria.* Small pox. Herpes circinatus, wens and whitlows. Constant offensive exhalations from the body.

**Modalities:** *Worse,* from dry cold winds; cool air; slightest draught; from mercury, touch; lying on the painful side. *Better,* in damp weather, from wrapping up the head, from warmth, after eating.

**Relationship:** Antidotes: *Bell., Cham., Sil.*

Compare: *Acon., Spong., Staph., Sil., Sulph., Calc-s., Myris. Hep.* antidotes bad effects from *Mercury, Iodine, Potash, Cod liver oil.* Removes the weakening effects of ether.

**Dose:** First to 200th. The higher potencies may abort suppuration, the lower promote it. If it is necessary to hasten it, give 2x.

---

## HEPATICA TRILOBA

(Liver-wort) **Hepat.**

Pharyngeal catarrh with profuse, serous sputa and hoarseness. Tickling and irritation of the throat. *Scraping and rough sensation.* Induces free and easy expectoration. Viscid, thick, tenacious phlegm causes continuous hawking. Soreness of the nostrils. Sensation *as if particles of food remained in the epiglottis.* Sputa sweet, profuse, creamy.

**Dose:** Second potency.

---

## HERACLEUM SPHONDYLIUM—BRANCA URSINA

(Hogweed) **Hera.**

Recommended as a spinal stimulant; in epilepsy with flatulence, gout and skin symptoms.

**Head:** Aches with drowsiness, worse moving in open air, better tying the head up with cloth. *Marked fatty* (oily) *perspiration on the head* with violent itching. Seborrhea capitis. Sick headache.

**Stomach:** Pain with an inclination to vomit. Bitter risings and taste. Hungry but unable to eat. Abdominal and splenic pain.

**Dose:** Third potency.

---

## HIPPOMANES

(A Meconium Deposit Out of the Amniotic Fluid Taken From the Colt) **Hipp.**

The old famous aphrodisiac of the Greek authors.

**Stomach**: *Icy coldness* in stomach.

**Male:** Sexual desire increased. Prostatitis. Drawing pain in the testicles.

**Extremities:** Violent pain in the wrist (rheumatism). Paralysis of wrists. *Sprained sensation in wrist.* Great weakness of hands and fingers. Weakness in joints of feet, knee, and soles. *Chorea.* Marked weakness after growing too fast.

**Relationship:** Compare: *Caust.*

**Dose:** Sixth to thirtieth potency.

---

## HIPPOZAENINUM

(Gladerine Mallein, Farcine) **Hippoz.**

This powerful nosode introduced by Dr. J. J. Garth Wilkinson, covers symptoms which suggest integral parts of consumption, cancer, syphilis, etc., and promises useful service in the treatment of ozena, scrofulous swellings, pyemia, erysipelas. Chronic rhinitis; saneous secretion.

**Nose:** Red, swollen. *Catarrh, ozena,* ulceration. Discharge acrid, corroding, bloody, offensive. Tubercles on alae nasi. Papules and ulceration in the frontal sinus and pharynx.

**Face:** All glands swollen (parotitis); painful; form abscesses.

**Respiratory:** Hoarseness. Bronchial asthma. Noisy breathing; short, irregular. Cough, with dyspepsia. Excessive secretion. Suffocation imminent. *Bronchitis in the aged,* where suffocation from excessive secretion is imminent. Tuberculosis.

**Skin:** Lymphatic swellings. Articular non-fluctuating swellings. Nodules in the arm. Malignant erysipelas. Pustules and abscesses. Ulcers. Rupia. Eczema.

**Relationship:** Compare: *Mucotoxinum* (Cahis' preparation with the *Micrococcus catarrhalis.* Friedlander's Bacillus of pneumonia and the *Micrococcus tetragenius* for acute and chronic mucus catarrhs in children and old people); *Aur., Kali-bi., Psor., Bac.*

**Dose:** Thirtieth potency.

---

## HIPPURICUM ACIDUM

(Proved by Dr. Wm. B. Griggs) **Hip-ac.**

Its chief action is on the external tissues of the eyes and nasal pharynx, joint surfaces, liver and mucous membranes. Right side especially affected, general muscular soreness.

**Eyes:** Pain over the right eye, dull, constant, worse in a warm room. Eyelids inflamed and swollen (blepharitis).

**Throat:** Sore, raw, dry, with dysphagia, halitosis; gummy exudate; thickness and infiltration of all tissues around the throat.

**Stomach:** Acid rising. Lump in the pit of the stomach. Soreness and pressure over the liver.

**Female:** Menstrual flow for three weeks with complete relief of muscular and joint pains.

**Extremities:** Backache extending down the hips. Pain in the shoulders and extremities, sore, swollen joints. Pain in the middle of the thigh, posteriorly shooting down the right leg. Tired, grating sensation in the joints (arthritis).

**Skin:** Itching, burning. Papules looking like goose flesh on the chest.

**Relationship:** *Benz-ac.* seems to be an analogue.

**Dose:** Lower potencies.

---

## HOANG NAN—STRYCHNOS GAULTHERIANA

(Tropical Bind Weed) **Strych-g.**

Exhaustion with vertigo. Numbness with tingling in hands and feet; involuntary action of lower jaw. Pustules and boils; tertiary syphilis and paralysis, eczema prurigo, old ulcers, leprosy, cancer of glandular structures and bites of serpents. Removes fetor and hemorrhage in cancer, revives the healing process. Follows *Ars*.

**Dose:** Five drops of the tincture. May be increased to twenty.

---

## HOMARUS

(Digestive Fluid of a Live Lobster) **Hom.**

Dyspepsia, sore throat and headache seems to be a combination that may be controlled by this remedy. Frontal and temporal pain chiefly, with soreness in the eyes. Throat sore, *raw,* burns with tough mucus. Pain in the stomach and abdomen, better after eating. Belching. Chilliness and pain all over. Itching of skin.

**Modalities:** *Worse,* from milk, after sleep. *Better,* from motion, after eating.

**Relationship:** Compare: *Sep., Aster., Astac., Aeth.*

**Dose:** Sixth potency.

---

## HURA BRAZILIENSIS

(Assacu) **Hura**

Used in leprosy, when skin feels as if it was hide bound. Tense vesicles; sensation of splinters under the thumb nails. Skin of the forehead feels drawn tight. Stiff neck, pain in the back. Throbbing in the finger tips. Itching, pimples on all projecting portions of the bone, malar bones, etc.

**Relationship:** Compare: *Calotropis* or *Madura album* (leprosy; livid and gangrenous tubercles; thickening of the skin).

**Dose:** Sixth potency.

---

## HYDRANGEA ARBORESCENS

(Seven-barks) **Hydrang.**

A remedy for gravel, profuse deposit of white amorphous salts in urine. Calculus, renal colic, hematuria. Acts on the ureter. Pain in the lumbar region. Dizziness. Oppression of the chest.

**Urinary:** Burning in the urethra and frequent desire (urethritis). Urine hard to start. Heavy deposit of mucus. *Sharp pain in the loins,* especially left. Great thirst with abdominal symptoms and an *enlarged prostate* (*Ferr-pic., Sabal*). Gravelly deposits. Spasmodic stricture. Profuse deposit of white amorphous salts.

**Relationship:** Compare: *Lyc., Chim., Berb., Pareir., Uva, Sabal, Oxyd., Geum*—Water avens (severe jerking pains, from deep in the abdomen to the end of urethra; affections of the bladder, with pain in the penis; worse, eating; relaxed mucous membranes, with excessive and depraved secretions; imperfect digestion and assimilation). *Polytrichum juniperinum*—Haircap moss (according to Dr. A. M. Cushing in mother tincture or infusion for an enlarged prostate—prostatitis).

**Dose:** Tincture.

# HYDRASTIS CANADENSIS

(Golden Seal) **Hydr.**

Acts especially on the mucous membranes, relaxing them and producing a *thick, yellowish, ropy* secretion. The catarrh may be anywhere, throat, stomach, uterus, urethra, it is always characterized by a peculiar mucoid discharge. *Hydr.* is especially active in old, easily tired people, cachectic individuals with great debility. Cerebral effects prominent, feels his wits sharpened, head cleared, facile expression. Weak muscular power, poor digestion and obstinate constipation. Lumbago. Emaciation and prostration. Its action on the liver is marked. Cancer and cancerous state, before ulceration, when pain is the principal symptom. *Goitre* of puberty and pregnancy. *Small pox* internally and locally. *Hydr.* abolishes the distressing symptoms of small pox, shortens its course, making it less dangerous and greatly mitigates its consequences (J. J. Garth Wilkinson).

**Mind:** Depressed; sure of death, and desires it.

**Head:** Dull, pressing frontal pain, especially associated with constipation. Myalgic pain in the scalp and muscles of the neck (*Cimic.*). Eczema of the forehead along the line of hair. *Sinusitis,* after coryza.

**Ears:** Roaring. Muco-purulent discharge. Deafness. *Eustachian catarrh* with a high pitched voice.

**Nose:** *Thick, tenacious secretion from the posterior nares to* the throat (post-nasal drip). Watery, *excoriating* discharge. Ozena, with ulceration of septum. Tends to blow the nose all the time.

**Mouth:** Peppery taste. Tongue white, swollen, large, flabby, slimy; *shows imprint of teeth* (*Merc.*); as if scalded; stomatitis. Ulceration of the tongue, fissures toward the edges (glossitis).

**Throat:** Follicular pharyngitis. Raw, smarting, excoriating sensation. Hawking of yellow, tenacious mucus (*Kali-bi.*). Child is aroused suddenly from sleep by this tenacious post-nasal dropping. Goitre of puberty and pregnancy.

**Stomach:** Sore feeling in the stomach more or less constant. Weak digestion. *Bitter taste.* Pain as if from a hard cornered substance. All gone sensation. Pulsation, in the epigastrium. Cannot eat bread or vegetables. Atonic dyspepsia. Ulcers and cancer. Gastritis.

**Abdomen:** Gastro-duodenal catarrh. Liver torpid, tender. Jaundice. Gallstones. Dull dragging in the right groin with a cutting sensation in the right testicle.

**Rectum:** Prolapsed; anus fissured. *Constipation*, with a sinking feeling in the stomach, dull headache. During stool, smarting pain in the rectum. After stool, long lasting pain (*Nit-ac.*). Hemorrhaids; even a light flow exhausts. Contraction and spasm.

**Urinary:** *Gleety discharge.* Urine smells decomposed.

**Male:** Gonorrhea, second stage; discharge thick and yellow.

**Female:** Erosion and excoriation of the cervix. Leucorrhea, worse after menses (*Bov., Calc.*); acrid and corroding, shreddy, tenacious. Menorrhagia. Pruritus vulvae with profuse leucorrhea (*Calc., Kreos., Sep.*). Sexual excitement. Tumor of the breast; nipple retracted.

**Respiratory:** Chest raw, sore, burning. Dry, harsh cough. Bronchial catarrh, later stages. Bronchitis in old, exhausted people, *with thick, yellow, tenacious expectoration.* Frequent fainting spells, with cold sweat all over. Feels suffocated on lying on the left side (asthma). Pain from the chest to the left shoulder.

**Back:** Dull, heavy, dragging pain and stiffness, particularly *across the lumbar region, must use arms to raise himself from the seat.*

**Skin:** Eruptions like variola. Lupus; *ulcers*, cancerous formations. General tendency to profuse perspiration and unhealthy skin (*Hep.*).

**Relationship:** Antidote: *Sulph.*

Useful after too much Chlorate of Potash for sore throat.

Compare: *Xanthorrhiza apifolia, Kali-bi., Con., Ars-i., Phyt., Galium aparine* (cancer—nodulated tumor of the tongue); *Aster., Stann., Puls.* Also *Manzanita* (diarrhea, gonorrhea, gleet, leucorrhea, catarrhal conditions). *Hydrastininum muriaticum*—Muriate of hydrastia (locally, in an aphthous sore mouth, ulcers, ulcerated sore throat, ozena, etc. Internally, third decimal trituration. Is a uterine hemostatic and vasoconstrictor; metrorrhagia, especially from fibroids; hemorrhages; *in dilatation of the stomach,* and chronic digestive disorders). *Hydrastinin sulphuricum* lx (hemorrhage from the bowels in typhoid).

*Marrubium album*—Hoarhound (a stimulant to mucous membranes, especially laryngeal and bronchial; chronic bronchitis, dyspepsia and hepatic disorders; colds and coughs).

**Dose:** Tincture to thirtieth attenuation. Locally colorless *Hydr.*, mother tincture or fluid extract.

---

# HYDROCOTYLE ASIATICA

(Indian Pennywort) **Hydrc.**

Curative in disorders that exhibit interstitial inflammation and cellular proliferation in any part. Hypertrophy and induration of connective tissue. Has considerable reputation in *leprosy* and *lupus* when there is no ulceration. The skin symptoms are very important. Of great use in ulceration of the womb. Difficulty in maintaining the upright position. Very copious perspiration. Pains of cervical cancer.

**Face:** Pain in left cheek bone.

**Female:** Pruritus of vagina. Inflammation of the bladder neck. *Heat within the vagina. Granular ulceration of womb.* Profuse leucorrhea. Dull pain in the ovarian region. Cervical redness. Severe labor-like pain in uterus and appendages.

**Skin:** Dry eruptions. *Great thickening of epidermoid layer and exfoliation of scales* (ichthyosis). *Psoriasis gyrata,* on trunk and extremities, palms and soles. Pustules on chest. Circular spots with scaly edges. *Intolerable itching, especially of soles.* Profuse sweat. Syphilitic affections. *Acne.* Leprosy. *Elephantiasis* (*Ars.*). Lupus non-exedens.

**Relationship:** Compare: *Elaeis guineensis*—South American palm (scleroderma, elephantiasis, leprosy, skin thickened, itching and hardened. Anesthesia). *Hura; Strychnos gaultheriana* (bites of serpents, ulcers and cutaneous affections generally). *Chaulmoogra oil* from seeds of *Tarakiogenos; Hydr., Ars., Aur., Sep.*

**Dose:** First to sixth potency.

---

# HYDROCYANICUM ACIDUM

(Prussic Acid) **Hydr-ac.**

One of the most toxic agents known. Convulsions and paralysis (hemiplegia) express the action of this remedy. Spasmodic constriction in the larynx, feeling of suffocation, pain and tightness in the chest, palpitations; pulse weak, irregular. Sinking *sensation in the epigastrium.* Hysterical and epileptic convulsions. Cyanosis. Collapse, due to pulmonary disease, not a cardiac collapse. Catalepsy. Cholera. Stage of collapse (*Ars., Verat.*). Coldness. Tetanus narcolepsy.

**Mind:** Unconscious. Wild delirium. Fear of imaginary problems. *Fears* everything—horses, wagons, houses falling, etc.

**Head:** Violent, stupefying headache. Brain feels on fire. Pupils motionless or dilated. Supra-orbital neuralgia, with flushing on the same side of face.

**Face:** Jaws clenched in rigid spasm (tetnus). Froth in the mouth (epilepsy). Pale, bluish lips.

**Stomach:** Tongue cold. *Drink rumbles through the throat and stomach.* Gastralgia; worse when stomach is empty. *Great sinking in the pit of the stomach.* Pulsating pain in the precordial region.

**Respiratory:** Noisy and agitated breathing. Dry, spasmodic, suffocative cough. Asthma, with contraction of the throat. Whooping cough. Paralysis of the lungs (*Aspidosperma*). Marked cyanosis; venously congested lung.

**Heart:** Violent palpitations. Pulse, *weak, irregular.* Cold extremities. Torturing pain in chest. Angina pectoris (*Spig., Ox-ac.*).

**Sleep:** Yawning, with shivering. Irresistible drowsiness. Vivid, incoherent dreams.

**Relationship:** Antidotes: *Ammc., Camph., Op.*

Compare: *Cic., Oena., Camph., Laur.*

**Dose:** Sixth and higher potencies.

---

# HYOSCYAMUS NIGER

(Henbane) **Hyos.**

Disturbs the nervous system profoundly. As if some diabolical force took possession of the brain and prevented its functions. It produces a perfect picture of *mania in a quarrelsome and obscene character.* Inclined to be unseemly and immodest in acts, gestures and expressions. Very talkative and persists in stripping herself, or uncovering genitals. Is jealous, afraid of being poisoned, etc. Its symptoms also point to weakness and *nervous agitation;* hence typhoid and other infections with *coma vigil. Tremulous weakness and twitching of tendons.* Subsultus tendinum. Muscular twitchings, spasmodic affections, generally with delirium (delirium tremens). Non-inflammatory cerebral activity. *Toxic gastritis.*

**Mind:** *Very suspicious.* Talkative, obscene, lascivious mania, uncovers the body; jealous, *foolish.* Great hilarity; *inclined to laugh at everything.* Delirium, with an attempt to run away. Low, muttering speech; *constant carpholagia, deep stupor.*

**Head:** Feels light and confused. Vertigo as if intoxicated. Brain feels loose, fluctuating. Inflammation of the brain, with unconsciousness (meningitis); head shakes to and fro.

**Eyes:** Pupils dilated, sparkling, fixed. Eyes open, but does not pay attention; downcast and dull, fixed (tetanus). Strabismus. Spasmodic closing of lids. Diplopia. Objects have colored borders.

**Mouth:** Tongue dry, red, cracked, stiff and immovable, protruded with difficulty; speech impaired. Foam in the mouth (epilepsy). Teeth covered with sordes. Lower jaw drops.

**Throat:** Stinging dryness. Constriction. Cannot swallow liquids. *Uvula elongated.*

**Stomach:** Hiccough, eructations empty, bitter. Nausea, with vertigo. Vomiting, with convulsions; hematemesis; violent cramps, relieved by vomiting; burning in the stomach; epigastrium tender. *After irritating food.*

**Abdomen:** Colic, as if the abdomen would burst. Distention. Colic with vomiting, belching, hiccough, screaming. Tympanites. Red spots on the abdomen.

**Stool:** Diarrhea, colicky pains; *involuntary,* aggravated by mental excitement or during sleep. Diarrhea during the lying-in period. Involuntary defecation.

**Urinary:** *Involuntary* micturition (enuresis). Bladder paralyzed. Has no will to micturate (*Caust.*).

**Male:** Impotence. Lascivious; exposes his person; plays with genitals during fever.

**Female:** Before menses, hysterical spasms. Excited sexual desire (nymphomania). During menses, convulsive movements, urinary flux and sweat. Lochia suppressed. Spasms in pregnant women. Puerperal mania.

**Chest:** Suffocating fits. Spasm, forcing to bend forward. *Dry, spasmodic cough at night, worse lying* down; better sitting up, from itching in the throat, as if the uvula was too long. Hemoptysis.

**Extremities:** *Picking at bed clothes;* plays with hand; reaches out for things. Epileptic attacks ending in deep sleep, Spasms and convulsions. Cramps in calves and toes. Child sobs and cries without waking.

**Sleep:** Intense sleeplessness. Sopor with convulsions. *Starts up frightened.* Coma vigil.

**Nervous System:** Great restlessnes; *every muscle twitches* (paralysis agitans, chorea). Will not be covered.

**Modalities:** *Worse,* at night, during menses, after eating, when lying down. *Better,* stooping.

**Relationship:** Antidotes: *Bell., Camph.*

Compare: *Bell., Stram., Agar., Gels.*

*Hyoscyaminum hydrobromatum—Scopolaminum bromhydricum.* (paralysis agitans; *tremors of disseminated sclerosis.* Sleeplessness and nervous agitation. Dry cough in phthisis. Similar in its effects to alcohol, both recent and remote. Corresponds to the effects of strong poisons introduced into or generated within the body. Symptoms of uremia and acute nervous exhaustion. A remedy for shock. Third and fourth decimal trituration. In physiological dosage (1-200 gr.) mania and chorea; insomnia). *Scopola* (Japanese Belladonna)—chemically identical with Hyoscine (joyous delirium, licking of lips and smacking of mouth; sleepless; tries to get out of bed; sees cats, picks imaginary hairs, warms hands before an imaginary fire, etc).

**Dose:** Sixth to 200th potency.

# HYPERICUM PERFORATUM

(St. John's Wort) **Hyper.**

The great remedy for injuries to nerves, especially of fingers, toes and nails. Crushed fingers, especially tips. Excessive painfulness is a guiding symptom for its use. Prevents lock jaw. *Punctured* wounds. Relieves pain after operations. Supersedes the use of morphia after an operation (Helmuth).

Spasms after every injury. Has an important action on the rectum; hemorrhoids. *Coccygodynia.* Spasmodic asthmatic attacks with changes of weather or before storms, better by copious expectoration. Injured nerves from bites of animals. Tetanus. Neuritis, tingling, burning and numbness. Constant drowsiness.

**Mind:** Feels as if lifted high in the air, or anxiety, lest he falls from a height. Mistakes in writing. Effects of shock. Melancholy.

**Head:** Heavy; feels as if touched by *an icy cold hand. Throbbing in the vertex;* worse in a close room. Brain seems compressed. Right side of face aches. Brain fag and neurasthenia. Facial neuralgia and toothache of a pulling, tearing character with sadness. *Head feels longer*—elongated to a point. In a fractured skull, bone splinters. Brain feels alive. Pain in the eyes and ears. Falling out of hair.

**Stomach:** Craving for wine. Thirst; *nausea.* Tongue coated white at the base, tip clean. Sensation of a lump in the stomach (*Abies-n., Bry.*).

**Rectum:** Urging, dry, dull, pressing pain. *Hemorrhoids* with pain, bleeding and tenderness.

**Respiratory:** Asthma *worse* foggy weather and relieved by profuse perspiration.

**Back:** Pain in the nape of neck. *Pressure over the sacrum.* Spinal, concussion. Coccyx injury from a fall, with pain radiating up the spine and down the limbs. Jerking and twitching of muscles.

**Extremities:** Darting pain in the shoulders. Pressure along the ulnar side of arm. Cramps in the calves. Pain in toes and fingers, especially in the tips. *Crawling in the hands and feet.* Lancinating pain in upper and lower limbs (sciatica). *Neuritis* with tingling, burning pain, numbness and flossy skin. Joints feel bruised. Hysterical joints. Tetanus (*Phys., Kali-br.*). Traumatic neuralgia and neuritis.

**Skin:** Hyperidrosis, sweating on the scalp, worse in the morning after sleep; falling of hair from injury; eczema on hands and face, intense itching, eruptions seems to be under the skin. Herpes zoster. Old ulcers or sores in the mouth, very sensitive. Lacerated wounds with marked prostration from loss of blood.

**Modalities:** *Worse*, in cold; dampness, in a *fog*; in a closed room; least exposure; touch. *Better*, bending head backward.

**Relationship:** Compare; *Led.* (punched wounds and bites of animals); *Arn., Staph., Calen., Ruta, Coff.*

Antidotes: *Ars., Cham.*

**Dose:** Tincture to third potency.

---

# IBERIS AMARA

(Bitter Candytuft) **Iber.**

State of nervous excitement. Has a marked action upon the heart. Possesses great efficacy in cardiac diseases. Controls vascular excitement in hypertrophy with thickening of the cardiac walls. Cardiac debility after influenza. Liver region full and painful (hepatomegaly). White stools (jaundice).

**Mind:** Sad and sighing; fearful and trembling. Irritable.

**Head:** Vertigo and pain around the heart. Constant hawking of thick, stringy mucus until after a meal. Hot, flushed face. Vertigo, *as if the occiput was turning around;* eyes feel forced outwards.

**Heart:** Conscious of the heart's action. On turning to the left side, stitching pain, sensation of needles through the ventricles is felt at each systole. Palpitations, *with vertigo and choking in the throat.* Stitching pains in the cardiac region (angina pectoris). *Pulse full, irregular, intermittent.* Worse, least motion and in a warm room. Sensation of weight and pressure, with occasional sharp, stinging pains. Dropsy with an enlarged heart. Violent palpitations *induced by slightest exertion, or by laughing or coughing. Darting pains through the heart. Cardiac dyspnea.* Dilation of the heart. Wakes up with palpitations around about 2 a.m. Throat and trachea fill up with mucus. Cough causes redness of the face. *Tachycardia.*

**Extremities:** Numbness and tingling in the left hand and arm. Whole body sore, lame and trembling.

**Modalities:** Worse, lying down; on the left side; motion, exertion; warm room.

**Relationship:** Compare: *Cact., Dig., Aml-ns., Bell.*

**Dose:** Tincture and first potency.

---

# ICHTHYOLUM

(A Combination of Sulphonated Hydrocarbons; a Fossil Product of Complex Structures found in Tyrol, Supposed to be Fish Deposits, Contains 10% Sulphur.) **Ichth.**

Its action on skin, mucous membranes and kidneys is prompt and useful. It is strongly antiparasitic; redness, pain and inflammation; decreases tension. Excellent in winter coughs of old people. Polyarthritis. Chronic rheumatism. *Uric acid diathesis.* Hay fever. *Chronic hives. Tuberculosis, aids nutrition.* Bad effects of alcoholism, when nothing will stay in the stomach.

**Mind:** Irritable and depressed. Forgetful, lack of concentration.

**Head:** Dull, aching; better cold, pressure. Dull frontal and supra-orbital headache; worse moving the eyes, cold air; better, warmth.

**Eyes:** Burn, red; worse, change of temperature.

**Nose:** Bland coryza; stuffed feeling; feels sore inside. Irresistible desire to sneeze.

**Face:** Skin feels dry and itches. Acne on the chin.

**Throat:** Irritated; pain radiates to the ears; sore, dry, with hawking and expectoration.

**Stomach:** Disagreeable taste, burning sensation, very thirsty. *Nausea. Increased appetite.*

**Abdomen:** Disposition to soft, shapeless stools. Griping in the umbilical and left hypogastric region. Early morning diarrhea.

**Urinary:** Increased in quantity and frequency. Burning pain in the meatus. Uric acid deposits.

**Female:** Fullness in the lower abdomen. Nausea at the time of menses.

**Respiratory:** Coryza: *dry, teasing cough.* Bronchiectasis and phthisis. Bronchitis, especially in the aged.

**Extremities:** Lameness in the right shoulder and right lower extremity.

**Skin:** Heat and irritation; *itching.* Scaly and itching eczema. *Crops of boils.* Pruritus of pregnancy. Psorisis, acne rosacea, erysipelas.

**Relationship:** Compare: *Hep., Calc., Sil., Sulph., Ars., Petr.*

**Dose:** Lower potencies.

Externally, it is used as an ointment, with lanoline 20 to 50 per cent; for chronic eczema and psoriasis, also acne rosacea and gouty joints. Chilblains, scabies. Rectal suppositories for senile prostate.

# ICTODES FOETIDA

(Pothos foetidus, Skunk Cabbage) **Ictod.**

For asthmatic complaints; worse from inhaling any dust. *Hysteria.* Erratic spasmodic pains. "Will-o'-the-wisp" like character of its subjective symptoms and its physiometric property are special features (Samuel Jones). *Inflation and tension in the abdomen.* Millar's asthma.

**Head:** Absent-minded, irritable. Headache in *single spots,* with *violent pulsations of the temporal arteries.* Outward, drawing pain from the glabella. Better in the open air (*Puls.*). Hyperemic swelling across the nose bridge.

**Abdomen:** *Inflation and tension* in the abdomen (flatulence).

**Respiratory:** Spasmodic croup. Troublesome respiration, with sudden feeling of anguish and sweat. Sneezing, with pain in the throat. Pain in the chest, with difficulty in breathing. Tongue feels numb. *Asthma; relieved by stool.*

**Dose:** Tincture and lower potencies.

---

# IGNATIA AMARA

(St. Ignatius Bean) **Ign.**

Produces a marked hyperesthesia of all the senses and a tendency to clonic spasms. Mentally, *the emotional element is upper most and co-ordination of function is interfered with.* Hence, it is one of the chief remedies for hysteria. It is especially adapted to the nervous temperament, women of sensitive, easily excitable nature, dark, mild disposition, quick to perceive, rapid in execution. Rapid change of mental and physical condition, opposite to each other. Great contradictions. Alert, nervous, apprehensive, rigid, trembling patients who suffer acutely mentally or physically, at the same time, made worse by drinking coffee. The *superficial* and *erratic character* of its symptoms is most characteristic. *Effects of grief* and worry. Cannot bear tobacco. Pain in small, circumscribed spots (*Ox-ac.*). *Plague.* Hiccough and hysterical vomiting.

**Mind:** Changeable mood; introspective; silently brooding. Melancholic, sad, tearful. Not communicative. *Sighing and sobbing.* After shocks, grief, disappointment.

**Head:** Feels hollow, heavy; *worse, stooping.* Headache as if a nail was driven out through the side. Cramp-like pains over the root of nose. Congestive headaches following anger or grief; *worse, smoking or smelling tobacco,* inclines head forward.

**Eyes:** *Asthenopia,* with spasms of the lids (blepharospasm) and neuralgic pain around the eyes (*Nat-m.*). Flickering zigzags.

**Face:** *Twitching of muscles* of the face and lips (chorea). Changes color when at rest.

**Mouth:** *Sour taste.* Easily bites the inside of cheeks. Constantly full of saliva. Toothache; worse after drinking coffee and smoking.

**Throat:** Sensation of a lump in the throat that cannot be swallowed. Tendency to choke, globus hystericus. Sore throat; stitches, when not swallowing; better, eating something solid. Stitches between acts of swallowing. Stitches extend to the ear (*Hep.*). Tonsils inflamed, swollen, *with small ulcers. Follicular tonsillitis.*

**Stomach:** Sour eructation. All gone feeling in the stomach; *much flatulence;* hiccough. Cramps in the stomach; worse slightest contact. Averse to an ordinary diet; longs for a great variety of indigestible articles. Craving for acid things. *Sinking in the stomach, relieved by taking* a *deep breath.*

**Abdomen:** Rumbling in the bowels. Weak feeling in the upper abdomen. Throbbing in the abdomen (*Aloe, Sang.*). Colicky, griping pain in one or both sides of the abdomen.

**Rectum:** Itching and stitching pains up the rectum. *Prolapse.* Stools pass with difficulty; *painful constriction of the anus after stool.* Stitches in hemorrhoids during cough. Diarrhea from fright. Stitches from anus deep into the rectum. Hemorrhage and pain; worse when stool is loose. *Pressure as of a sharp instrument from within outward.*

**Urinary:** Profuse, watery urine (*Ph-ac.*).

**Female:** Menses, *black,* too early, too profuse or scanty. During menses great languor, with spasmodic pain in the stomach and abdomen. Feminine sexual frigidity. Suppression from grief.

**Respiratory:** Dry, spasmodic cough in quick successive shocks. Spasm of the glottis (*Calc.*). Reflex cough. Coughing increases the desire to cough. *Much sighing.* Hollow spasmodic cough, worse in the evening, little expectoration, leaving pain in trachea.

**Extremities:** Jerking of limbs (convulsions, epilepsy). Pain in tendo-Achilles and calf. Ulcerative pain in soles.

**Sleep:** Very light. Jerking of limbs on going to sleep. Insomnia from grief, cares, with itching of arms and violent yawning. Dreams continuing a long time; troubling him.

**Fever:** Chill, with thirst; not relieved by external heat. During fever, itching; nettle rash all over the body.

**Skin:** Itching, nettle rash. Very sensitive to draught of air. Excoriation, especially around the vagina and mouth.

**Modalities:** *Worse,* in the morning, open air, after meals, *coffee,* smoking, liquids, external warmth. *Better,* while eating, change of position.

**Relationship:** Compare: *Zinc., Kali-p., Sep., Cimic. Panacea arvensis*•—Poor man's mercury (sensitiveness over the gastric region with hunger but an aversion to food).

Complementary: *Nat-m.*

Incompatible: *Coff., Nux-v., Tab.*

Antidotes: *Puls., Cham., Cocc.*

**Dose:** Sixth to 200th potency.

---

# ILLICIUM ANISATUM

(Anise) **Anis.**

Should be remembered in the treatment of flatulent conditions. So called three months colic, especially if it recures at regular hours; rumbling in the abdomen. One symptom is worthy of a special mention: *pain in the region of the third rib,* about an inch or two from the sternum, generally on the right side and occasionally on the left. Cough, frequent with this pain. Purulent tracheal and gastric catarrh in old drunkards. Old asthmatics. Vomiting, epileptiform convulsions with biting of the tongue.

**Nose:** Sharp stitches beneath the lips. Acute catarrh.

**Mouth:** Burning and numbness of the inner lower lip.

**Respiratory:** Dyspnea. Pain near the third intercostal cartilage. Cough with pus like phlegm. Palpitations with apthae. Hemoptysis.

**Dose:** Third potency.

---

# ILEX AQUIFOLIUM

(American Holly) **Ilx-a.**

Intermittent fever. Marked eye symptoms, spleen, pain in. All symptoms better in winter.

**Eyes:** Infiltrations of the cornea; staphyloma; nocturnal burning in the orbits, rheumatic inflammation of the eye; psilosis.

**Relationship:** *Ilex paraguariensis*—Yerba mate (persistent epigastric pain; sense of dryness in the mouth and pharynx, anorexia, pyrosis, nervous depression, neurasthenia. Somnolence; incapacity for work, diminution of urinary secretion, headache and pruritus. Migraine. Renal colic. Is said to be of use as a prophylactic against sunstroke, being a safe stimulant for circulation, diaphoresis and diuresis). *Ilex vomitoria*—Yaupon (emetic properties—possesses tonic and digestive qualities, free from sleepless effects. Has an active principle said to act as a powerful diuretic—employed in nephritis and gout). *Ilex cassine*—Christmas berry tea (excellent diuretic and substitute for tea).

---

## INDIGO TINCTORIA

(Indigo—Dye Stuff) **Indg.**

Marked action on the nervous system, and of an undoubted benefit in the treatment of epilepsy with great sadness. Excited mood and desire to be busy. Neurasthenia and hysteria. Pure powdered indigo placed on the wound cures snake and spider poison (*Kali-perm., Euph-po., Cedr.*). Stricture of the esophagus; blue color (*Cupr.*).

**Head:** Vertigo with nausea. Convulsions. Sensation of a band around the forehead. Undulating sensation throughout the head. Sensation as if the brain was frozen. Gloomy; cries at night. Hair feels pulled from the vertex. Head feels frozen.

**Ears:** Pressure and roaring (tinnitus).

**Nose:** Excessive sneezing and epistaxis.

**Stomach:** Metallic taste. *Eructations.* Bloating. Anorexia. Flushes of heat rising from the stomach to the head.

**Rectum:** Prolapse of rectum. Aroused at night with horrible itching in the anus (pin worms).

**Urinary:** Constant desire to micturate. Urine turbid. Catarrh of bladder (cystitis).

**Extremities:** *Sciatica.* Pain from the middle of the thigh to the knee. Boring pain in the knee joint; better, walking. *Pain in the limbs worse after every meal.*

**Nervous System:** Hysterical symptoms where pain predominates. Excessive nervous irritation. Epilepsy; flashes of heat from the abdomen to the head; fit begins with dizziness. Aura from a painful spot between the shoulders (epilepsy). Reflex spasms from worms.

**Modalities:** *Worse*, during rest and sitting. *Better,* pressure, rubbing, motion.

**Relationship:** Compare: *Cupr., Oestrus cameli,* an Indian medicine for epilepsy.

**Dose:** Third to thirtieth potency.

# INDIUM METALLICUM

(The Metal Indium) **Ind.**

Headaches and migraine. Seminal emissions. *Backache.*

**Head:** Pain in the *head when straining at stool.* Bursting in the head during stool. Dull pain in the temples and forehead *with nausea,* weakness, *sleepiness.* All gone sensation in the stomach around 11 a. m. Violent attack of sneezing. Sexual psychopathy.

**Face:** Painful suppurating pimples. Corners of mouth cracked and sore (*Cund.*).

**Throat:** Uvula enlarged, ulcerated; thick, tough mucus in the posterior part of pharynx. Worse evening.

**Male:** Horribly offensive smell of urine after standing for a short time. Emissions too frequent. Diminished power. Testicles tender (orchitis); drawing pains along the spermatic cord.

**Extremities:** Stiffness in the neck and shoulders. Pain, especially in the left arm. Legs restless and weary. Toes itch (*Agar.*).

**Relationship:** Compare: *Sel., Titan.* (male sexual organs).

---

# INDOLUM

(A Crystalline Compound Derivable from Indigo, but also a Product of Putrefaction of Proteids) **Indol.**

Primary action is to increase the elimination of Indican. Auto-intoxication. Compare: *Skatol.*

Persistent desire to sleep, dull, discontented mental state, hideous. Delusions and nervousness, constant motion of fingers and feet (chorea). Intestinal putrefaction.

**Head:** Dull occipital and frontal headache in the afternoon. Dull sensation over the eyes. Eyeballs hot and hurt when moved. Pupils dilated with headache.

**Stomach:** Bloated feeling. Hungry sensation after a full meal. Great thirst. Constipation.

**Extremities:** Very tired and sore lower limbs. Feet burn. Knee joints sore.

**Sleep:** *Sleepiness.* Continuous dreaming.

**Dose:** Sixth attenuation.

---

# INSULINUM

(An Active Principle from the Pancreas Which Affects Sugar Metabolism) **Ins.**

Besides the use of *Ins.* in the treatment of diabetes, restoring the lost ability to oxidize carbohydrate and storing glycogen in the liver, some use of it homoeopathically has been made by Dr. Wm. F. Baker, showing its applicability in acne, carbuncles, erythema with itching eczema. In the gouty, transitory glycosuria when skin manifestations are persistent, give three times daily after eating. In a persistent case of skin irritation, boils or varicose ulceration with polyuria, it is indicated.

**Dose:** 3x to 30x.

---

# INULA HELENIUM

(Scabwort) **Inul.**

A medicine for mucous membranes. Bearing down sensations in the pelvic organs and bronchial symptoms are most marked. Substernal pain. Diabetes.

**Head:** Vertigo on stooping; throbbing after eating, pressure in the temples and forehead.

**Rectum:** Pressing towards the rectum as if something was extruding (prolapse).

**Urinary:** Frequent urging to micturate; passes only drops. Violet odor (*Ter.*).

**Female:** Menses too early and painful (dysmenorrhea). Labor-like pains; urging to stool; dragging in the genitals with violent backache. Itching in the legs during menses, chattering of teeth from cold during menstruation. Sensation as if something moving about in the abdomen, stitches in the genitals. Chronic metritis.

**Respiratory:** Dry cough; worse at night and lying down; larynx painful. Chronic bronchitis; cough with thick expectoration, languor and weak digestion. Stitches behind the sternum. Teasing cough with marked, free expectoration. Palliative in tubercular laryngitis.

**Extremities:** Pain in the right shoulder and wrist; tearing in the left palm, unable to double fingers; pain in the lower limbs, feet and ankles.

**Relationship:** Compare: *Croc., Ign., Arum-d.* (loose cough worse at night, on lying down).

**Dose:** First to third potency.

# IODOFORMIUM

(Iodoform) **Iodof.**

Should not be forgotten in the treatment of tubercular meningitis, both as a local application to the head and internally (*Bac.*). *Tuberculous conditions.* Subacute and chronic diarrhea in children.

**Head:** Sharp, neuralgic pain. Head feels heavy, as if it cannot be lifted from the pillow. Itching in the occiput. *Meningitis.* Sleep interrupted by sighing and cries. Very drowsy.

**Eyes:** Pupils, *dilated;* contract unequally, react poorly. Diplopia. Failing sight due to retro-bulbar neuritis, central scotoma, partial atrophy of the optic disc.

**Abdomen:** Scaphoid abdomen. Chronic diarrhea with suspected tuberculosis. Abdomen distended; mesenteric glands enlarged. *Cholera infantum. Chronic diarrhea; stools greenish, watery, undigested, with an irritable temper.*

**Chest:** Sore pain in the apex of the right lung. Sensation of a weight on the chest, as if smothering. Cough and wheezing on going to bed. Pain in left breast, like a hand grasping at the base of the heart. Hemoptysis (phthisis). Asthmatic breathing.

**Extremities:** Legs weak; cannot stand and walk with eyes closed (locomotor ataxia). Weakness of the knees when going upstairs.

**Dose:** Second trituration. Three grains on the back of the tongue will relieve an attack of asthmatic breathing.

---

# IODIUM

(Iodine) **Iod.**

Rapid metabolism: *Loss of flesh* with great appetite. Hungry with much thirst. Better after eating. *Great debility, the slightest effort induces perspiration. Iod.* individual is exceedingly thin, dark complexioned, with enlarged lymphatic glands, has a voracious appetite but loose flesh. Tubercular type.

All glandular structures, respiratory organs, circulatory system are especially affected; they atrophy. *Iod.* arouses the defensive apparatus of the system by assembling the mononuclear leucocytes whose phagocytic action is marked, at a given point. Lead poisoning. Tremor. *Iod.* craves cold air.

*Acute exacerbation of chronic inflammation.* Arthritis deformans. *Acts prominently on the connective tissue. Plague. Goitre.* Abnormal vaso-constriction; capillary congestion followed by oedema, ecchymosis, hemorrhages and nutritive disturbances are the pathological conditions at the base of its symptomatology. Sluggish vital reaction, hence chronicity in many of its aspects. Acute catarrh of all mucous membranes, rapid emaciation, not withstanding a good appetite and glandular atrophy call for this remedy, in numerous wasting diseases and in scrofulous patients. Acute affections of the respiratory organs. *Pneumonia,* rapid extension. *Iod.* is warm, and wants cool surroundings. Weakness and loss of breath on going upstairs. *Adenoid vegetations.* Tincture internally and locally for swollen glands and rattle snake bites.

**Mind:** Anxiety *when quiet. Present* anxiety and depression, no reference to the future. Sudden impulse to run and get violent. Forgetful. Must be busy. Fear of people, shuns every one. Melancholy. Suicidal tendency.

**Head:** Throbbing; *rush of blood,* and sensation of a tight band. Vertigo; worse from stooping, worse in a warm room. Chronic, congestive headache in old people (*Phos.*).

**Eyes:** Violent lachrymation. Pain in the eyes. Pupils dilated. Constant motion of the eyeballs (nystagmus). *Acute dacryocystitis.*

**Nose:** Sneezing. Sudden, violent influenza. Dry coryza becomes fluent in the open air, also a *fluent hot coryza* with general heat of the skin. Pain at the root of nose and frontal sinus. Nose stopped up. Tendency to ulceration (ozena). Anosmia. *Acute nasal engorgement* associated with high blood pressure

**Mouth:** Gums loose and bleed easily (scorbutic). Foul ulcers and salivation. Profuse, fetid saliva. Tongue thickly coated. Halitosis.

**Throat:** Larynx feels constricted. *Eustachian deafness.* Thyroid enlarged. Goitre, with a sensation of constriction. Swollen submaxillary glands. Uvula swollen.

**Stomach:** Throbbing in the pit of the stomach. *Ravenous hunger* and marked thirst. Empty eructations, as if every particle of food was turned into gas. Anxious and worried if he does not eat (*Cina, Sulph.*). Looses flesh, yet hungry and eating well (*Abrot.*).

**Abdomen:** Liver and spleen sore and enlarged (hepato-splenomegaly). Jaundice. Mesenteric glands enlarged (Hodgkin's disease). Pancreatic disease. Cutting pain in abdomen.

**Rectum:** Hemorrhage with every stool. Diarrhea, whitish, frothy, fatty. Constipation with ineffectual urging; better by drinking cold milk. Constipation alternating with diarrhea (*Ant-c.*).

**Urinary:** Frequent and copious, *dark yellow-green (Bov.),* thick, acrid with a cuticle on the surface.

**Male:** Testicles swollen and indurated. Hydrocele. Loss of sexual power with atrophied testes.

**Female:** Great weakness during menses (*Alum., Carb-an., Cocc., Hem.*). Menses irregular. Uterine hemorrhage. *Ovaritis* (*Apis, Bell., Lach.*). *Wedge-like pain from* the ovary to the uterus. *Dwindling of mammary glands.* Nodosities on the skin of mammae. Acrid leucorrhea, thick, slimy, corroding the linen. *Wedge-like pain* in *the right ovarian region.*

**Respiratory:** Hoarse. *Raw* and tickling feeling, provoking a dry cough. *Pain in the larynx.* Laryngitis, with painful roughness; worse during cough. Child grasps throat when coughing. Right sided pneumonia with high temperature. Difficult expansion of the chest, blood streaked sputum; internal dry heat, external coldness. Violent heart action. Pneumonia. Hepatization spreads rapidly with persistent high temperature; absence of pain in spite of great involvement, worse warmth; craves cool air. Croup in scrofulous children with dark hair and eyes (*Brom.* opposite). Difficult inspiration. Dry, morning cough, from tickling in the larynx. Croupy cough with difficult respiration; wheezy. *Cold extends downwards* from the head to the throat and bronchi. Great weakness in the chest. Palpitations from least exertion. Pleuritic effusion. Tickling all over the chest. *Iod.* cough is worse indoors, in warm, wet weather and when lying on the back.

**Heart:** Heart feels squeezed. Myocarditis, painful compression around the heart (angina pectoris). Feels as if squeezed by an iron hand (*Cact.*) followed by great weakness and faintness. Palpitations from least exertion. Tachycardia.

**Extremities:** Joints inflamed and painful. Pain in the bones at night. White swelling. Gonorrheal rheumatism. Rheumatism of the nape and upper extremities. Cold hands and feet. Acrid sweat of feet. Pulsations in large arterial trunks. Rheumatic pains, nocturnal pain in joints; constrictive sensations.

**Fever:** Flushes of heat all over the body. Marked fever, restlessness, red cheeks, apathetic. Profuse sweat.

**Skin:** Hot, dry, yellow and withered. Glands enlarged. Nodosities. Anasarca from cardiac disease.

**Modalities:** *Worse,* when quiet, in warm room, right side. *Better,* walking in open air.

**Relationship:** Pathogenesis is similar to that of *Carb-ac.*

Antidotes: *Hep., Sulph., Grat.*

Complementary: *Lyc., Bad.*

Compare: *Brom., Hep., Merc., Phos., Abrot., Nat-m., Sanic., Tub.*

**Dose:** The crude drug in a saturated solution may be required. Third to thirtieth potency. Ioduretted solution of Potass. iod. (35 grains Potass and 4 grains Iodine to 1 oz. of water, 10 drops, three times a day) expels dead tapeworms.

Locally, the most powerful, least harmful and easily managable microbicide. Ideal agent to keep wounds clean and disinfected. Bites of insects, reptiles, etc. In gunshot wounds and compound fractures, it is excellent. Great skin disinfectant.

---

# IPECACUANHA

(Ipecac Root) **Ip.**

The chief action is on the ramifications of the pneumogastric nerve, producing spasmodic irritation in the chest and stomach. Morphia habit. The principal feature of *Ipecacuanha* is its *persistent nausea* and vomiting, which form the chief guiding symptoms. Indicated after indigestible food, raisins, cakes, etc. Especially indicated in fat children and adults, who are feeble and catch cold in a relaxing atmosphere; warm, moist weather. Spasmodic affections. Hemorrhages *bright red* and *profuse.*

**Mind:** Irritable; holds everything in contempt. Full of desires, for what they do not know.

**Head:** Bones of skull feel crushed or bruised. Pain extends to the teeth and root of tongue.

**Eyes:** Inflamed, red (conjunctivitis). Pain through the eyeballs. Profuse lachrymation. Cornea dim (keratitis). Eyes tire from near vision (hypermetropia). State of vision constantly changing. Spasms of accommodation from irritable weakness of ciliary muscle. Nausea from looking at moving objects.

**Nose:** Coryza, with obstruction of the nose and nausea. Epistaxis.

**Face:** Blue rings around the eyes. Periodical orbital neuralgia, with lachrymation, photophobia and smarting eyelids.

**Stomach:** *Tongue usually clean.* Mouth, moist; *increased saliva. Constant nausea* and vomiting, with a pale face, twitching of face. Vomits food, bile, blood, mucus (gastric ulcer). Stomach feels relaxed, as if hanging down. Hiccough.

**Abdomen:** Amoebic dysentery with tenesmus; while straining pain so great that it nauseates; little thirst. Cutting, clutching; *worse, around the navel.* Body rigid; stretched out stiff.

**Stool:** Pitch like, green as grass, *like frothy molasses,* with griping at the navel. Dysenteric, slimy.

**Female:** Uterine hemorrhage, *profuse, bright, gushing, with nausea.* Vomiting during pregnancy. *Pain from the navel to the uterus.* Menses too early and too profuse (menorrhagia).

**Respiratory:** Dyspnea; constant *constriction in the chest.* Asthma. Annual attacks of asthma. Continuous sneezing; coryza; wheezing cough. *Cough incessant and violent, with every breath* (bronchitis). Chest seems full of phlegm, but does not yield to coughing. Bubbling rales. Suffocative cough; child becomes stiff, and blue in the face (cyanosed). Whooping cough with epistaxis and bleeding from the mouth. Bleeding from the lungs *with nausea;* sensation of constriction; rattling cough. Croup. Hemoptysis from the slightest exertion (phthisis) (*Mill.*). *Hoarseness,* especially at the end of a cold. Complete aphonia.

**Extremities:** Body stretched stiff, followed by spasmodic jerking in the arms towards each other (tetnus).

**Sleep:** With eyes half open. Shocks in all the limbs on going to sleep (*Ign.*).

**Fever:** Intermittent fever, irregular cases after quinine. *Slightest chill* with *much* heat, *nausea,* vomiting and dyspnea. Relapses from an improper diet.

**Skin:** Pale, lax. Blue around the eyes. Miliary rash.

**Modalities:** *Worse,* periodically; from veal, moist warm wind, lying down.

**Relationship:** Compare: *Emetinum*—principal alkaloid of *Ip.* (a powerful amoebicide, but is not a bactericide. Specific for amoebiasis; of remarkable value in the treatment of amoebic dysentery; also as a remedy in pyorrhea, 1/2 gr. daily for three days, then less). *Emetinum,* 1/2 gr. hypodermically in psoriasis. Emetin hydrocin. 2x, diarrhea with colicky, abdominal pains and nausea. Emetin for entamoebic dysentery. In physiological doses must be carefully watched. May produce hepatization of the lungs, rapid heart action, tendency for the head to fall forward and lobar pneumonia. In hematemesis and other hemorrhages, compare: *Gelatin* (which has a marked effect on the coagulability of the blood. Hypodermically or orally, a 10 per cent jelly, about 4 oz., three times a day). *Ars., Cham., Puls., Ant-t., Squil. Convolvulus* (colic and diarrhea). *Typha latifolia*—Cat tail flag (dysentery, diarrhea and summer complaints). *Euphorbia hypericifolia*—Garden spurge (very similar to *Ip.* irritation of the respiratory and gastrointestinal tracts and female organs). *Lippia mexicana* (persistent dry, hard, bronchial cough asthma and chronic bronchitis).

In asthma, compare: *Blatta-o.*

Antidotes: *Ars., Chin., Tab.*

Complementary: *Cupr., Arn.*

**Dose:** Third to 200th potency.

# IRIDIUM METALLICUM

(The Metal) **Irid-met.**

Intestinal putrefaction and septicemia. Anemia, increases red blood corpuscles. Epilepsy; lupus. Rheumatism and gout. Uterine tumors. Spinal paresis. *Exhaustion after disease.* Children who are puny, weak limbed and grow too fast. Nephritis of pregnancy.

**Head:** Difficulty in concentration of thought. Sensation as if the mind was void, though confused. "Woody" feeling on the right side of the head. Right side of the scalp sensitive. Profuse, watery coryza, better indoors. Ozena.

**Respiratory:** Hoarse cough, worse talking; posterior nares feel raw, inflamed, profuse, thick, yellowish discharge. Chronic laryngeal catarrh.

**Back and Extremities:** Weakness in the kidney region. Spinal paresis, especially in the aged and after a disease. Pressing in the groin and left thigh. Tension in both the thighs, especially left. Left hip joint feels dislocated with dull pain towards the left gluteal region.

**Relationship:** Compare: *Iridium muriaticum* (produces salivation and stiffness of the jaws followed by head and nervous symptoms. Congestion of the nares and bronchi. Dragging pain in the lower back. Headache worse right side, heavy feeling as of liquid lead).

Compare: *Plat., Pall., Osm.*

**Dose:** Sixth and higher.

---

# IRIS VERSICOLOR

(Blue Flag) **Iris**

Thyroid, *pancreas,* salivary, intestinal glands and gastrointestinal mucous membrane are especially affected. Increases the flow of bile. Sick headaches and cholera morbus provide the special therapeutic field for its action.

**Head:** Frontal headache with nausea (migraine). Scalp feels constricted. Right temples especially affected. Sick headache, worse rest; begins with a blur before the eyes, after relaxing from a mental strain. Pustular eruptions on the scalp.

**Ears:** Roaring, buzzing, *ringing* in ears with deafness. Aural vertigo, with intense noises in the ears (Meniere's disease).

**Face:** Neuralgia after breakfast, beginning in the infra-orbital nerve and involving the whole face.

**Throat:** Mouth and tongue feel scalded. Heat and smarting in the throat. *Burning.* Profuse flow of saliva; ropy. *Goitre.*

**Stomach:** *Burning in the entire alimentary canal. Vomiting,* sour, bloody, bilious. Nausea. Profuse flow of saliva (*Merc., Ip., Kali-i.*). *Deficient appetite.*

**Abdomen:** Liver sore. Cutting pain. Flatulent colic. Diarrhea; stools watery, with *burning in the anus* and throughout the intestinal canal. Periodical, nocturnal diarrhea with pain and green discharges (dysentery). *Constipation* (give 30th).

**Extremities:** Shifting pains. Sciatica, as if the left nip joint was wrenched. Pain extends to the popliteal space. Gonorrheal rheumatism (use *Irisinum*).

**Skin:** Herpes zoster, associated with gastric derangements. Pustular eruptions. Psoriasis; irregular patches with shining scales. Eczema, with nocturnal itching.

**Modalities:** *Worse,* in the evening and at night, from rest. *Better,* from continuous motion.

**Relationship:** Antidote: *Nux-v.*

Compare: *Iris florentina*—Orris-root (delirium, convulsions, and paralysis); *Iris factissima* (headache and hernia); *Iris germanica*—Blue garden iris (dropsy and freckles); *Iris tenax*—*Iris minor* (dry mouth; deathly sensation at a point in the stomach, *pain in the ileo-ceacal region;* appendicitis. Pain from adhesions after). *Pancreatinum*—a combination of several enzymes (indicated in intestinal indigestion; pain an hour or more after eating. Lienteric diarrhea. Dose: 3-5 grains, better not given during the active period of gastric digestion). *Pepsinum* (imperfect digestion with pain in the gastric region. Marasmus in children who are fed on artificial foods. Diarrhea due to indigestion. Dose: 3-4 grains. Diseases of pancreas, gout, diabetes); *Ip., Podo., Sang., Ars., Ant-c.*

**Dose:** Tincture to thirtieth potency. Favorable reports from the very highest potencies.

---

## JABORANDI

(Pilocarpus Microphyllus) **Jab.**

*Jaborandi* is a powerful glandular stimulant and a very efficient diaphoretic. Its most important effects are diaphoresis, salivation and myosis. Hot flushes, nausea, salivation and profuse perspiration. The face, ears and neck with in a few minutes of taking a dose become deeply flushed, and drops of perspiration break out all over the body whilst at the same time the mouth waters and saliva pours out in an almost continuous stream. Other secretions like lachrymal, nasal, bronchial and intestinal are also affected, but in a lesser degree. The sweat and saliva produced by a single dose is often enormous in quantity, can be almost half a pint.

It is homoeopathic to *abnormal sweats* and has achieved great success in *night sweats* of phthisis. Acts upon the thyroid and its sudorific action may possibly be due to it. *Exophthalmic goitre* with increased action of the heart and pulsations in the arteries; tremors and nervousness; heat and sweating; bronchial irritation A valuable remedy in limiting the duration of mumps.

**Eyes:** *Eye strain* from whatever cause. Irritability of the ciliary muscle (ciliary spasm). Eyes easily tire from the slightest use (aesthenopia). Heat and burning in the eyes on use. Headache; smarting and pain in the globe on use. Glaucoma. Everything at a distance appears hazy; vision becomes indistinct every few moments. Retinal images retained long after using the eyes. Irritation from electric or other artificial light. *Pupils contracted;* do not react to light. Staring eyes. *Near sighted* (myopia). Vertigo and nausea after using eyes. *White spots before the eyes. Smarting* pain in the eyes. Lids twitch. Atrophic choroiditis. Spasm of the accommodation while reading.

**Ears:** Serous exudation into the tympaniticum cavities. Tinnitus (*Pilocarpinum* 2x).

**Mouth:** Saliva viscid, like white of egg. Dryness. Free salivation (mumps), *with profuse sweating.*

**Stomach:** Nausea on looking at moving objects; vomiting; pressure and pain in the stomach.

**Abdomen:** Diarrhea, painless; during the day with a flushed face and profuse sweat.

**Urinary:** Scanty; pain over the pubes with much urging.

**Respiratory:** Bronchial mucous membrane inflamed (bronchitis). Inclination to cough with difficult respiration. Edema of the lungs (hydrothorax). Foamy sputa. Profuse, thin, serous expectoration. Slow, sighing respiration.

**Heart:** Pulse irregular, dicrotic. Oppression of the chest. Cyanosis; collapse. Nervous cardiac affections.

**Skin:** *Excessive perspiration on all parts of the body.* Persistent dryness of the skin. Dry eczema. Semi-lateral sweats. Chilliness with sweat.

**Relationship:** Compare: *Aml-ns., Atrop., Phys., Lyc., Ruta, Pilocarpinum muriaticum* (Meniere's disease, rapidly progressive phthisis, with free hemorrhages, profuse sweating, 2x trituration). *Atropinum* is the antagonist to *Pilocarpinum*, in dose of one one-hundredth grain for one-sixth of *Pilocarpinum.*

**Non-homeopathic Uses:** Chiefly used as a powerful and rapid diaphoretic. It is of efficient service in renal disease, especially with uremia, eliminating both water and urea. Scarlatinal dropsy. Contra-indicated in *heart failure, post-puerperal uremia* and in senile cases. Dose: One-eighth to one-fourth grain hypodermically.

**Dose:** Third trituration.

---

## JACARANDA CAROBA

(Brazilian Caroba Tree) **Jac-c.**

Has reputation as a remedy for venereal diseases and rheumatism. Morning sickness. Urinary and sexual symptoms are important. Rheumatic symptoms.

**Head:** Vertigo on rising, with a heavy forehead.

**Eyes:** Painful; are inflamed and watery.

**Nose:** Coryza with a heavy head.

**Throat:** Sore, dry, constricted. Vesicles in the pharynx.

**Urinary:** Urethra inflamed (urethritis); discharge of yellow matter (gonorrhea).

**Male:** Heat and pain in the penis (balanitis); painful erections; phimosis. Prepuce painful and swollen. Chancroid (syphilis). Chordee. Itching pimples on the glans and prepuce.

**Extremities:** Rheumatic pain in the right knee. Weakness of the lumbar region. Morning soreness and stiffness of muscles. Gonorrheal rheumatism. Itching pimples on the hands. Gonorrheal and syphilitic arthritis.

**Relationship:** Compare: *Thuj., Cor-r., Jac-g.* (in syphilitic symptoms, especially of the eye and throat. Chancroids; *atonic ulcers.* Dark, painless diarrhea).

**Dose:** Tincture to third potency.

---

## JALAPA—EXOGONIUM PURGA

(Jalap) **Jal.**

Causes and cures colic and diarrhea. The child is good all day, but screams and is restless and troublesome at night.

**Mouth:** Tongue, smooth, glazed, dry, smarting (glossitis).

**Abdomen:** Pain in the right hypochondrium. Flatulence and nausea. Pinching and griping (colitis). Abdomen distended. Face cold and blue.

**Stool:** Watery diarrhea; thin, muddy stools. Anus sore.

**Extremities:** Aching in the arms and legs. Pain in the large joint of the great toe (gout). Smarting at the root of the nail. Burning in the soles.

**Relationship:** Antidotes: *Elat., Cann-s.*

Compare: *Camph., Coloc.*

**Dose:** Third to twelfth potency.

---

# JATROPHA CURCAS

(Purging Nut) **Jatr-c.**

Of value in cholera and diarrhea. The abdominal symptoms are most important. Suppressed measles (H. Farrington).

**Stomach:** Hiccough, followed by copious vomiting. Nausea and vomiting brought on by drinking, with an acrid feeling in the throat. Great thirst. *Very easy vomiting.* Heat and burning in the stomach, with crampy, constrictive pains in the epigastrium (gastritis).

**Abdomen:** Distended, with gurgling noises. Pain in the hypochondria. Pain in the region of liver and under the right scapula extending to the shoulder. Violent urge to micturate.

**Stool:** Sudden, profuse, watery, like rice water. *Diarrhea; forced discharge; loud noise in the abdomen like gurgling of water coming out of a bung hole,* associated with coldness, cramps, nausea, and vomiting (cholera).

**Extremities:** Cramps in the muscles, especially calves, legs, and feet. *Coldness* of the whole body. Pain in the ankles, feet and toes. Heels sensitive.

**Modalities:** *Better,* by placing hands in cold water.

**Relationship:** Compare: *Camph., Verat., Gamb., Crot-t., Jatropha urens*—Sponge nettle (edema and cardiac paresis).

**Dose:** Third to thirtieth potency.

---

# JONOSIA ASOCA—SARACA INDICA

(The Asoka Tree) **Joan.**

Has an extensive sphere of action on female organs. Amenorrhea and metrorrhagia.

**Head:** Unilateral headache (migraine); reflex uterine, congestive headache better open air and by free flow.

**Eyes:** Pain in the eyeballs; supraorbital pain, photophobia.

**Nose:** Nasal catarrh; profuse; watery discharge. Anosmia.

**Stomach:** Desire for sweets, acid things. Thirsty, excessive nausea.

**Rectum:** Obstinate constipation, hemorrhoids.

**Female:** Delayed and irregular menses. Menstrual colic; amenorrhea. Pain in the ovaries before flow; menorrhagia, irritable bladder; leucorrhea.

**Back:** Pain along the spine, radiating to the abdomen and thighs.

**Sleep:** Disturbed. Dreams of travelling.

**Dose:** Tincture.

---

## JUGLANS CINEREA

(Butternut) **Jug-c.**

A faulty elimination that produces jaundice and various skin eruptions is pictured by this drug. The sharp, *occipital headache,* usually associated with liver disturbances, is very characteristic. Pain in the chest, axilla and scapula, with a sensation of suffocation (angina pectoris). Sensation as if all the internal organs were too large, especially those of the left side. Cholelithiasis.

**Head:** Dull, full head. Eruptions on the scalp. *Sharp, occipital headache* (migraine). Head feels enlarged. Pustules on the lids and around the eyes.

**Nose:** Tingling in the nose; sneezing. Coryza, preceded by *pain under the sternum,* with threatening suffocation. Later, copious, bland, thick mucus discharge.

**Mouth:** Acrid feeling in the mouth and throat. Soreness in the region of tonsils externally. Dryness of the root of the tongue and fauces.

**Stomach:** Atonic dyspepsia with marked eructations and flatulent distention. Soreness in the region of liver.

**Rectum:** Yellowish-green, with tenesmus and burning in the anus. Camp diarrhea.

**Back:** Muscles of the neck rigid, lame. Pain between the scapula and under the right scapula. Pain in the lumbar vertebrae.

**Skin:** Red, like flush of scarlatina. Jaundice, with pain around the liver and right scapula. *Itching* and pricking when heated. *Pustules.* Eczema, especially on the lower extremities, sacrum and hands. Erythema and erysipelatous redness.

**Modalities:** Better, on getting heated, exercise, scratching, on rising in the morning. worse, walking.

**Relationship:** Compare: *Juglandin* (duodenal catarrh; bilious diarrhea); *Chel., Bry., Iris.*

**Dose:** Tincture to third potency.

# JUGLANS REGIA

(Walnut) **Jug-r.**

Skin eruptions are prominent.

**Head:** Confused; feels as if the head was floating in air. *Sharp pain in the occiput. Styes.*

**Female:** Menses early, black, pitch like coagula. Abdomen distended.

**Skin:** Comedones and acne on the face. Crusta lactea, with soreness around the ears. Itching and eruptions of small red pustules (acne rosacea). Scalp red and itches violently at night. Chancre-like ulcer (syphilis). Axillary glands suppurate.

**Relationship:** Compare: *Jug-c.*

**Dose:** Tincture and lower potencies.

---

# JUNCUS EFFUSUS

(Common Rush) **Junc-e.**

A diuretic. Urinary affections. Dysuria, strangury and ischuria. *Asthmatic symptoms in hemorrhoidal subjects.* Bubbling sensations. Abdominal flatulence. Arthritis and lithiasis.

**Dose:** Tincture and first potency.

---

# JUNIPERUS COMMUNIS

(Juniper Berries) **Juni-c.**

Catarrhal inflammation of the kidneys. Dropsy, with suppression of urine. Old people, with poor digestion and scanty secretion of urine. Chronic pyelitis.

**Urinary:** Strangury; bloody, scanty urine, violet odor (*Ter.*). Weight in the kidney region. Prostatic discharge. Renal hyperemia (*Eucalyptolum*).

**Respiratory:** Cough with scanty, loaded urine.

**Relationship:** Compare: *Sabin; Juniperus virginianus*—Red cedar (violent cystitis. Persistent dragging in the back; hyperemia of the kidneys; pyelitis and cystitis, dropsy in the aged with suppressed urine. Dysuria, burning cutting pain in the urethra which micturating. Constant urging apoplexy, convulsions, strangury, uterine hemorrhage). *Ter.*

**Dose:** Best form is the infusion. One ounce to a pint of boiling water. Dose, one-half to two ounces, or tincture, one to ten drops.

# JUSTICIA ADHATODA

(Vasaka, An Indian Shrub) **Just.**

Highly efficacious medicine for acute catarrhal conditions of the respiratory tract (used in the beginning).

**Head:** Irritable, remitive to external impressions; hot, full and heavy head.

**Nose:** Lachrymation with *coryza, profuse,* fluent with constant sneezing; loss of smell and taste; *coryza with cough.*

**Throat:** Dry, pain during empty swallowing; tenacious mucus, mouth dry.

**Respiratory:** Dry cough from the sternal region extending all over the chest (bronchitis). Hoarseness, larynx painful. *Paroxysmal cough* with suffocative obstruction of respiration. *Cough with sneezing.* Severe dyspnea with cough. *Tightness across the chest.* Asthmatic attacks, cannot endure a close, warm room. *Whooping cough.*

**Relationship:** Seems to come between *All-c.* and *Euphr.,* which compare.

**Dose:** Third potency and higher. Severe aggravation has been noticed from lower potencies.

---

# KALIUM ARSENICOSUM

(Fowler's Solution) **Kali-ar.**

The *Kali-ar.* patient tends towards malignancy and inveterate skin diseases. He is restless, nervous and anemic.

**Female:** Cauliflower-like excrescences on os uteri, with flying pains, foul smelling discharge and pressure below the pubis.

**Skin:** Intolerable itching, worse undressing. *Dry,* scaly, wilted. Acne; pustules worse during menses. Chronic eczema; itching worse *from warmth,* walking, undressing. *Psoriasis,* lichen. Phagedenic ulcers. Fissures in the bends of arms and knees. Gouty nodosities; worse, change of weather. Skin cancer, where suddenly an alarming malignancy without any external signs sets in. Numerous small nodules under the skin.

**Relationship:** *Rad-br.*

**Dose:** Third to thirtieth potency.

---

# KALIUM BICHROMICUM

(Bichromate of Potash) **Kali-bi.**

The special affinities of this drug are the mucous membranes of the stomach, bowels and air passages; bones and fibrous tissues. Kidneys, heart and liver are also affected. Incipient parenchymatous nephritis. Nephritis with gastric disturbances. Cirrhosis of the liver. Anemia and absence of fever are characteristic. General weakness bordering on paralysis. It is especially indicated in fleshy, fat, light complexioned people subject to catarrhs or with a syphilitic or scrofulous history. Symptoms are worse in the morning; *pain migrates quickly,* rheumatic and gastric symptoms alternate. More adapted to the subacute stage rather than the violent acute stage. Mucous membranes affected everywhere. Catarrh of the pharynx, larynx, bronchi and nose with a *tough, stringy, viscid secretion*, which is a very strong guiding symptom for this drug. *Perforation of the septum.* Chronic atonic catarrh. Polypus. Dilatation of the stomach and heart.

**Head:** Vertigo with nausea when rising from a seat. Headache over *the eyebrows,* preceded by a blurred vision. *Aching and fullness in the glabella.* Semilateral headache in small spots (migraine), and from suppressed catarrh. Frontal pain; usually over one eye. *Bones and scalp feel sore.*

**Eyes:** Supra-orbital neuralgia, right side. Eyelids burn, swollen, edematous (blepharitis). Discharge *ropy* and yellow. Corneal ulcers (keratitis), no pain or photophobia. *Descemetitis,* with only moderate irritation of the eye. Croupous conjunctivitis; granular lids with pannus. Iritis, with punctate deposits on the inner surface of the cornea. Slight pain with severe ulceration or inflammation (*Con.* opposite).

**Ears:** Swollen, with tearing pains (otitis). Thick, yellow, stringy, fetid discharge (otorrhea). Sharp stitches in the left ear.

**Nose:** Snuffles in children, *especially fat, chubby babies. Pressure and pain at the root of the nose,* sticking pain in the nose. *Septum ulcerated;* round ulcer. *Fetid smell. Discharge thick, ropy, greenish-yellow. Tough, elastic plugs* from the nose; leave a raw surface (ozena). Inflammation extends to the frontal sinuses, with distress and fullness at the root of the nose. Dropping from the posterior nares (*Hydr.*). *Loss of smell* (anosmia). Marked hawking. Inability to breathe through the nose. Dryness. *Coryza with obstruction* of the nose. *Violent sneezing.* Profuse, watery nasal discharge. Chronic inflammation of the frontal sinus with a stopped up sensation (sinusitis).

**Face:** Florid complexion. Blotchy, red appearance. Acne (*Jug-r., Kali-ar.*). Bones sensitive, especially beneath the orbits.

**Mouth:** Dry; viscid saliva. Tongue mapped, *red, shiny, smooth* (glossitis), *and dry,* with dysentery; broad, flat, indented, thickly coated. Sensation of a hair on the tongue.

**Throat:** Fauces red and inflamed. Dry and rough. Parotid glands swollen (mumps). Uvula relaxed, *edematous, bladder-like.* Pseudo-membranous deposit on the tonsils and soft palate. Burning, extending to the stomach. Aphthae. Diphtheria, with profound prostration and soft pulse. Discharge from the mouth and throat, tough and stringy.

**Stomach:** Nausea and vomiting after beer. Load immediately after eating. Feels as if digestion has stopped. Dilatation of the stomach. Gastritis. *Round ulcer of the stomach* (gastric ulcer). Stitches in the region of liver and spleen, which radiate to the spine. Dislikes water. Cannot digest meat. Desire for beer and acids. Gastric symptoms are relieved after eating and the rheumatic symptoms reappear. Vomiting of bright yellow water.

**Abdomen:** Cutting pain in the abdomen, soon after eating. Chronic intestinal ulceration (ulcerative colitis). Soreness in the right hypochondrium, fatty infiltration of the liver and increase in soft fibrous tissue. Painful retraction, soreness and burning.

**Stool:** Jelly-like, gelatinous; *worse, mornings.* Dysentery; tenesmus, stools brown, frothy. Sensation of a plug in the anus. Periodic constipation with pain across the loins, brown urine.

**Urinary:** Burning in the urethra (urethritis). *After micturition, a drop seems to remain which cannot be expelled.* Ropy mucus in the urine. Urethra becomes clogged up. Congestion of the kidneys; nephritis with scanty, albuminous urine and casts. Pyelitis; urine mixed with epithelial cells, mucus, pus, or blood. *Hematochyluria.*

**Male:** Itching and pain in the penis, with pustules. Ulcers, with paroxysmal stitches; aggravated at night. Constriction at the root of the penis, at night on awakening. Syphilitic ulcers, with cheesy, tenacious exudation. Erections (*Pic-ac.*).

**Female:** Yellow, tenacious leucorrhea. Pruritus vulva, with great burning and excitement. Prolapsus uteri; *worse in hot weather.*

**Respiratory:** Voice hoarse; worse, evening. Metallic, hacking cough. *Profuse, yellow expectoration, very glutinous and sticky,* coming out as a long, stringy, and very tenacious mass. Tickling in the larynx. Catarrhal laryngitis, cough has a brassy sound. True membranous croup, extending to the larynx and nares. Cough, with pain in the sternum, extending to shoulders; worse when undressing. Pain at the bifurcation of the trachea on coughing; from mid-sternum to the back (bronchitis).

**Heart:** Dilatation, especially from a co-existing renal lesion. Cold feeling around the heart (*Kali-n.*).

**Back:** *Cutting through the loins;* cannot walk; extends to the groins. Pain in the coccyx and sacrum extending up and down (coccygodynia).

**Extremities:** Pains fly rapidly from one place to another (*Kali-s., Puls.*). Wandering pains, along the bones; worse cold. Left sided sciatica; better, motion. Bones feel sore and bruised. *Very weak.* Tearing pains in the tibia; syphilitic rheumatism (*Mez.*). Pain, swelling, stiffness and crackling of all the joints. Soreness in the heels when walking. Tendo-Achilles swollen and painful. Pains in small spots (*Ox-ac.*).

**Skin:** Acne. Papular eruptions. *Ulcer with punched out edges,* with tendency to penetrate and tenacious exudation. Pustular eruptions, resembling smallpox, with burning pains. Itching with vesicular eruption.

**Modalities:** *Better,* from heat. *Worse,* beer, morning, hot weather, undressing.

**Relationship:** Compare: *Ant-t., Brom., Hep., Ind., Calc., Ant-c.* In the production of false membranes compare: *Brom., Am-caust., Sul-ac., Ip.*

Antidotes: *Ars., Lach.*

**Dose:** Third trituration, also thirtieth attenuation and higher.

The lower preparations of this salt should not be kept for too long.

---

## KALIUM BROMATUM

(Bromide of Potash) **Kali-br.**

Like all Potash salts, this weakens the heart and lowers the temperature. Brominism (bromium poisoning) is caused by it. General failure of mental power, loss of memory, melancholia, anesthesia of the mucous membranes, especially of the eyes, throat and skin; acne; loss of sexual desire, paralysis. Leading remedy in psoriasis. Nodular form of chronic gout. *Symptoms of apoplectic attacks,* uremic or otherwise; somnolence and stertor, convulsions, aphasia, albuminuria. Epilepsy (with a salt free diet).

**Mind:** Profound, melancholic delusion; feeling of moral deficiency; religious depression; delusions of conspiracies against him. Imagines he is singled out as an object of divine wrath. Loss of memory. Must do something, moves about; gets fidgety (*Tarent.*). Fear of being poisoned (*Hyos.*). Amnesic aphasia; can pronounce any word told, but cannot speak otherwise. *Night terrors.* Horrid illusions. Active delirium.

**Head:** Suicidal mania with tremulousness. Face flushed. *Numb feeling in the head.* Brain fag. Coryza extends to the throat.

**Throat:** Congestion of the uvula and fauces. *Anesthesia* of the fauces, pharynx, and larynx. Dysphagia, especially of liquids (*Hyos.*).

**Stomach:** Vomiting with *intense thirst,* after each meal. *Persistent hiccough* (*Sul-ac.*).

**Abdomen:** Sensation as if the bowels were falling out. *Cholera infantum,* with reflex cerebral irritation, jerking and twitching of muscles. Green, watery stools with intense thirst, vomiting, eyes sunken. Prostration. *Internal coldness* of the abdomen. Dysentery. Green, watery stools. *Retraction* of the abdomen.

**Urinary:** Sensitivity of the urethra diminished. Urine profuse, with thirst. Diabetes (*Ph-ac.*).

**Male:** Debility and impotence. Effects of sexual excesses, especially loss of memory, impaired co-ordination, numbness and tingling in the limbs. Sexual excitement during partial slumber.

**Female:** Pruritus. Ovarian neuralgia with great nervous uneasiness. *Exaggerated sexual* desire. Ovarian cysts.

**Respiratory:** Spasmodic croup. Reflex cough during pregnancy. Dry, fatiguing, hacking cough at night.

**Extremities:** *Fidgety hands;* busy twitching of fingers. Jerking and twitching of muscles.

**Sleep:** Restless sleep. Extreme drowsiness. Sleeplessness due to worry, grief and sexual excess. Night terrors. Grinds teeth in sleep. Horrible dreams. Somnambulism.

**Skin:** *Acne* of face, pustules. Itching; worse on the chest, shoulders, and face. Anesthesia of the skin. *Psoriasis.*

**Modalities:** *Better,* when occupied mentally or physically.

**Dose:** A few grains of the crude salt to the third trituration. Remember the unstable character of this salt. Said to be much more active, if salt is eliminated from the diet.

---

## KALIUM CARBONICUM

(Carbonate of Potassium) **Kali-c.**

The weakness characteristic of all Potassium salts is seen especially in this, with a soft pulse, coldness, general depression and characteristic *stitches,* which may be felt in any part of the body, or in connection with any affection. All Kali pains are *sharp and cutting;* nearly all are better by motion. Never use any salts of Potash when there is fever (T. F. Allen). Sensitive to every atmospheric change and *intolerance of cold weather.* One of the best remedies following labor. Miscarriage, for consequent debilitated states. Early morning aggravation is very characteristic. Fleshy, aged people with dropsical and paretic tendencies. *Sweat, backache, and weakness.* Throbbing pains. Tendency to dropsy. Tubercular diathesis. Pain from within out, and of a stinging character. "Giving-out" sensation. Fatty degenerations. Stinging pain in the muscles and internal parts. Twitching of muscles. Pain in a small spot on the left side. Hypothyroidism. Coxitis.

**Mind:** Despondent. Alternating moods. *Very irritable.* Full of fear and imaginations. Anxiety felt in the stomach. Sensation as if the bed was sinking. Never wants to be left alone. Never quiet or contented. Obstinate and *hypersensitive* to pain, noise, touch.

**Head:** Vertigo on turning. Headache *from riding in the cold wind.* Headache comes on with yawning. Stitches in the temples; aching in the occiput, one sided, with nausea (migraine), on riding in a carriage. Loose feeling in the head. Great *dryness of hair*; falls out (*Fl-ac.*).

**Eyes:** Stitches in the eyes. Spots, gauze and black points before the eyes. Lids stick together in the morning. Swelling *over the upper lid, like little bags.* Swelling of glabella between the brows. Asthenopia. Weak sight from excessive sexual indulgence. On shutting eyes, painful sensation as if light penetrating the brain.

**Ears:** Stitches in the ears. Itching, cracking, ringing and roaring.

**Nose:** Nose *stuffs up in a warm room.* Thick, fluent, yellow discharge. Post-nasal dropping (*Spig.*). Sore, scurfy nostrils; bloody nasal mucus. Crusty nasal openings. Epistaxis on washing the face in the morning. *Ulcerated nostrils.*

**Mouth:** Gums separate from teeth; pus oozes out. Pyorrhea. Aphthae. Tongue white. Profuse saliva, constantly in the mouth. Bad, slimy taste.

**Throat:** Dry, parched, rough. Sticking pain, as from a fish bone. Dysphagia; food goes down the esophagus slowly. Mucus accumulates in the morning.

**Stomach:** Flatulence. Desire for sweets. Sensation of a lump in the pit of the stomach. Gagging. Dyspepsia in old people; burning acidity, bloating. Gastric disorders from ice water. *Sour eructations. Nausea;* better lying down. Constant feeling, *as if the stomach was full of water.* Sour vomiting; throbbing and cutting pain in the stomach. Disgust for food. *Anxiety felt in the stomach.* Epigastrium, sensitive externally. Easy choking when eating. Epigastric pain radiates to the back.

**Abdomen:** Stitches in the region of liver. Old chronic liver problems, with soreness. Jaundice and dropsy. Distention and coldness of the abdomen. Pain from the left hypochondrium through the abdomen; must turn on the right side before he can rise.

**Rectum:** *Large,* difficult stools with stitching pain an hour before.

Hemorrhoids, large, swollen, painful. Itching, ulcerated pimples around the anus. Large quantity of blood discharged with natural stool. Pain in the hemorrhoids when coughing. Burning in the rectum and anus. Easy prolapse (*Graph., Podo.*). Itching (*Ign.*).

**Urinary:** Obliged to rise several times at night to micturate. Pressure in the bladder long before urine comes. Involuntary micturition when coughing, sneezing, etc.

**Male:** Complaints from coition. Deficient sexual instinct. Excessive emissions, *followed by weakness.*

**Female:** Menses early, profuse (*Calc.*), or *too late, pale and scanty,* with soreness around the genitals; pain from the back passes down, through the gluteal muscles, with cutting in the abdomen. Pain through the left labium, extending through the abdomen to the chest. Delayed menses in young girls with chest symptoms (hydrothorax) or ascites. Difficult, first menses. *Complaints after parturition.* Uterine hemorrhage; constant oozing after copious flow, with violent backache (dysmenorrhea), relieved by sitting and pressure.

**Respiratory:** Cutting pain in the chest; worse lying on the right side. Hoarseness and aphonia. Dry, hard cough around 3 a. m., with *stitching pains* and dryness of the pharynx. Bronchitis, *the entire chest is very sensitive.* Expectoration scanty and tenacious, but *increasing* in the morning and after eating; aggravated in the right lower chest and by lying on the painful side. *Hydrothorax.* Leaning forward relieves chest symptoms. Expectoration must be swallowed; cheesy taste; copious, offensive, lump. *Coldness of the chest. Wheezing* (asthma). Cough *with a relaxed uvula.* Tendency to tuberculosis; and to take cold; *better in a warm climate.*

**Heart:** Sensation as if the heart was suspended. Palpitations and *burning in the heart region. Weak, rapid pulse; intermits* due to digestive disturbance. Threatened heart failure.

**Back:** Great exhaustion. Stitches in region of kidneys and right scapula. *Lumbosacral region feels weak.* Stiffness and paralytic feeling in the back. Burning in the spine (*Guaj.*). Severe backache during pregnancy, and after miscarriage. Hip disease. Pain in the nates, thighs and hip joint. Lumbago with sudden sharp pains extending up and down the back and extending to the thighs.

**Extremities:** *Back and legs give out.* Uneasiness, heaviness, and tearing in the limbs and jerking. Tearing pain in the limbs with swelling (sciatica). Limbs sensitive to pressure. White swelling of knee. Tearing in arms from the shoulder to the wrist. Lacerating pain in the wrist joint. Paralysis in old people, and dropsical affections. Limbs go to sleep easily. Tips of toes and fingers painful. *Soles very sensitive.* Itching in the great toe, with pain (gout). *Pain from the hip to the knee. Pain in the knees* (arthritis).

**Sleep:** Drowsy after eating. Wakes up around 2 o' clock and cannot sleep again.

**Skin:** Burning as from a mustard plaster.

**Modalities:** *Worse,* after coition; in cold weather; from soup and coffee; in the morning around three o'clock; lying on the left and painful side. *Better,* in warm weather, though moist; during the day, while moving around.

**Relationship:** Complementary: *Carb-v.* (lowness of vitality may suggest a preliminary course of *Carb-v.* to nurse up recuperation to the point that *Kali-c.* would come in helpfully). Follows *Nux-v.* often in stomach and bladder problems.

Compare: *Kalium salicylicum* (vomiting, especially of pregnancy; arteriosclerosis, with chronic rheumatism); *Kalium silicicum* (gouty nodosities); *Kalium aceticum* (diabetes, diarrhea, dropsy, alkaline urine, very much increased in quantity); *Kalium citricum* (Bright's disease—1 gr. to a wine glass of water); *Kalium ferrocyanatum*—Prussian blue (physical and mental prostration following infection. Inability to sustaine routine work. Neuralgic affections depending on impoverished blood supply and exhausted nerve centers, especially spinal. Fatty and functional heart problems. Pulse weak, small, irregular. Uterine symptoms, like *Sep.* bearing down sensation and gastric sinking; profuse, pus-like leucorrhea and passive hemorrhage; use 6x); *Kalium oxalicum* (lumbago, convulsions); *Kalium picro-nitricum* and *Kalium picricum* (jaundice, violent eructations); *Kalium tartaricum* (paraplegia); *Kalium telluricum* (garlicky odor of breath, salivation, swollen tongue). Also compare: *Calc., Am-p., Phos., Lyc., Bry., Nat-m., Stann., Sep.*

Antidotes: *Camph., Coff.*

**Dose:** Thirtieth and higher. Sixth trituration. Do not repeat too often. Use cautiously in old gouty cases, advanced Bright's disease and tuberculosis.

---

# KALIUM CHLORICUM

(Chlorate of Potassium—$KClO_3$) **Kali-chl.**

Acts very destructively upon the kidneys, producing croupous nephritis, hemoglobinuria, etc. Parenchymatous nephritis with stomatitis. Produces acute ulcerative and follicular stomatitis. *Noma. Toxemic conditions of pregnancy* (urinary symptoms). *Chronic nephritis;* hepatitis. Septicemia. Anemia.

**Mouth:** Profuse secretion of acrid saliva. Entire mucous membrane red, tumid, with gray based ulcers. Tongue swollen (glossitis). *Stomatitis*—aphthous and *gangrenous.* Fetor. Mercurial stomatitis (as a mouth wash).

**Stomach:** Sensation of weight in the epigastric and umbilical region. Flatulence. Vomiting of greenish-black matter (hematemesis).

**Rectum:** Diarrhea; profuse with greenish mucus.

**Urinary:** Albuminous, scanty, suppressed. Hematuria; diuresis. Nucleo-albumin and bile, high phosphoric acid, with low total solids.

**Skin:** Jaundice. Itching miliary or papular eruptions. Discolored; chocolate tint.

**Dose:** Second to sixth potency. Use cautiously, locally as it is poisonous.

---

# KALIUM CYANATUM

(Potassium Cyanide) **Kali-cy.**

Sudden sinking sensation. Cancer of the tongue and agonizing neuralgias have been benefitted by this drug. Sick headache; sciatica; epilepsy.

**Mouth:** Ulcer of the tongue, with indurated edges. Speech difficult. Power of speech lost but intelligence intact.

**Face:** Severe neuralgia in the temporal region, recurring daily at the same hour. Pain in the orbital and supra-maxillary region, with screaming and loss of consciousness.

**Respiratory:** Cough prevents sleep; respiration weak; cannot take a deep breath.

**Modalities:** *Worse,* from 4 a. m. to 4 p. m.

**Relationship:** Compare: *Plat., Stann., Cedr., Mez., Mur-ac.*

**Dose:** Sixth potency and 200th.

---

# KALIUM HYDRIODICUM

(Iodide of Potassium) **Kali-i.**

The profuse, watery, acrid coryza that the drug produces, serves as a sure guiding symptom, especially when associated with pain in the frontal sinus. It acts predominantly on the fibrous and connective tissues, producing infiltration. Edema, etc. *Glandular swellings.* Purpura and hemorrhagic diathesis. *Syphilis* may be indicated in all stages:

1. In acute form with evening remitting fever, going off with nocturnal perspiration.
2. Second stage, mucous membranes and skin ulcerates.
3. Tertiary symptoms; nodes. Give material doses.

*Diffused sensitiveness* (glands, scalp, etc.). Rheumatism of the *neck, back,* feet, especially heels and soles; worse, cold and wet. *Kali-i.* in material doses acts in different forms of fungal diseases (thrush, ringworm, etc.), often simulating syphilis and bacterial diseases like tuberculosis. Symptoms like loss of weight, hemoptysis, etc. Tea taster's cough after inhaling the fungus; often brings about a favorable reaction in many chronic ailments even when not clearly, symptomatically indicated.

**Mind:** Sad, anxious; harsh temper. Irritable; congestion of the head, heat and throbbing.

**Head:** Pain through *the sides* of head. Violent headache. Cranium swells up in a hard lump. Pain intense over the eyes and at *the root of nose.* Brain feels enlarged. Hard nodes, with severe pain; *pneumococcic meningitis.*

**Eyes:** Conjunctiva red, injected; profuse lachrymation (conjunctivitis). *Syphilitic iritis.* Pustular keratitis and chemosis. Bony tumors of the orbit.

**Ears:** Noises in the ear (tinnitus). Boring pain in the ears (otalgia).

**Nose:** Red, swollen. Tip of the nose red; *profuse, acrid, hot, watery, thin discharge. Ozena, with a perforated septum.* Sneezing. Nasal catarrh, involving the frontal sinus. Stuffiness and dryness in the nose, without discharge. Profuse, *cool,* greenish, non-irritating discharges.

**Stomach:** Saliva increased. Faintness in the epigastrium. Cold food and drink, especially milk, aggravate. Marked thirst. Throbbing, painful, burning. Flatulence.

**Female:** Menses late, profuse. During menses uterus feels as if squeezed. Corrosive leucorrhea, with subacute inflammatory conditions of the womb in young married women. Fibroid tumors, metritis, sub-involution, hypertrophy, 1x or 1 gr. crude, 3 times a day.

**Respiratory:** Violent cough; worse in the morning. Pulmonary edema. *Larynx feels raw.* Laryngeal edema. Wakes up due to choking. *Expectoration like soap suds, greenish.* Pneumonia, when hepatization commences. Stitching pains through the lungs extending to the back. Asthma. Dyspnea on ascending, with pain in the heart. Hydrothorax (*Merc-sul.*). *Pleuritic effusion. Cold travels downwards to the chest.*

**Extremities:** Severe bone pains. Periosteum thickened, especially the tibia; sensitive to touch (*Kali-bi., Asaf.*). Rheumatism; pain at night and in damp weather. Contraction of joints. *Rheumatism of the knees with effusion.* Pain in the lumbosacral region and coccyx. Pain in the hip, forcing him to limp. *Sciatica;* cannot stay in bed; worse at night and lying on the affected side. Formication in the lower extremities when sitting, better lying down.

**Skin:** Purple spots (petechae); worse on the legs (erythema nodosum). Acne, hydroa. Small boils. Glands enlarged, indurated. Hives. *Rough nodules* all over, worse covering; heat of body intense. Fissured anus in infants. Tendency to edematous swellings, eyelids, mouth, uvula, etc. *Acne rosacea.*

**Modalities:** *Worse,* warm clothing, warm room, at night, damp weather. *Better,* motion, open air.

**Relationship:** Antidote: *Hep.*

Compare: *Iod., Merc., Sulph., Mez. Chopheenee,* a Hindu remedy for syphilitic eruptions, ulcerations and bone pains. Used in tincture.

**Dose:** Crude drug in material officinal dosage, but remember Dr. Meyhoffer's statements in his chronic diseases of organs of respiration: "From the moment the drug produces pathogenetic symptoms, it exaggerates the function of the tissue, exhausts the already diminished vitality and thence, instead of stimulating the organic cell in the direction of life, impairs or abolishes its power of contraction. We use, as a rule, the first dilution, 6 to 20 drops a day; if after a week no decided progress is visible, one drop of the tincture of *Iod.* is added to each hundred of the first dilution. In this way, the mucus tubercles, gummy deposits and ulcerations resulting therefrom in the larynx undergo a favorable termination in laryngeal syphilis." When strictly homoeopathically indicated, as in acute respiratory affections the third potency is indicated.

---

## KALIUM MURIATICUM

(Chloride of Potassium—KCl) **Kali-m.**

Although not proven, this remedy has a wide clinical use, through its introduction by Schussler. It is certainly of a great value in catarrhal affections, in sub-acute inflammatory states, fibrinous exudations and glandular swellings (Hodgkin's diseases). *White or gray coating at the base of the tongue* and expectoration of thick, white phlegm, seem to be the special guiding symptoms. Bursitis prepatellaris.

**Head:** Imagines he must starve. Headache with vomiting. Crusta lactea. Dandruff.

**Eyes:** White mucus, purulent scabs. Superficial ulcer. Trachoma. Corneal opacities.

**Ears:** *Chronic, catarrhal conditions of the middle ear* (otitis media). Glands around the ear swollen. *Snapping and noises in the ear.* Threatened mastoiditis. Great effusion around the auricle.

**Nose:** Catarrh; phlegm white, thick. Vault of pharynx covered with adherent crusts. Stuffy cold. Epistaxis (*Arn., Bry.*).

**Face:** Cheek swollen and painful.

**Mouth:** Aphthae; thrush; white ulcers in the mouth. Swollen glands around the jaw and neck. Coating on the tongue *grayish-white,* dryish, or slimy.

**Throat:** *Follicular tonsillitis.* Tonsils inflamed; enlarged so much, can hardly breathe. Grayish patches or spots in the throat and tonsils (diphtheria). Adherent crusts in the pharyngial vault. "Hospital" sore throat. Eustachian catarrh.

**Stomach:** *Fatty* or *rich food causes indigestion.* Vomiting of white, opaque mucus; water gathers in the mouth (waterbrash). Pain in the stomach, with constipation. Bulimia; hunger disappears by drinking water.

**Abdomen:** Abdominal tenderness and swelling. Flatulence. Thread worms, causing itching in the anus.

**Rectum:** Constipation; light colored stools. Diarrhea after fatty food; clay colored, white, or slimy stools (jaundice). Dysentery; purging, with slimy stools. *Hemorrhoids;* bleeding; blood dark and thick; fibrinous, clotted.

**Female:** Menses, too late or suppressed, checked or too early; excessive discharge; *dark clotted,* or tough, black blood, like tar (*Plat.*). Leucorrhea; discharge of milky white mucus, thick, non-irritating, bland. Morning sickness, with vomiting of white phlegm. Bunches in the breast, feel quite soft and are *tender.*

**Respiratory:** Aphonia; hoarseness. Asthma, with gastric derangements; mucus white and hard to cough up. Loud, gastric cough; cough short, acute and spasmodic, like whooping cough; expectoration thick and white. Rattling sounds of air passing through thick, tenacious mucus in the bronchi; difficult to cough up.

**Back and Extremities:** Rheumatic fever; exudation and *swelling around the joints.* Rheumatic pains felt only during motion, or increased by it. Nocturnal rheumatic pains; worse by warmth of bed; lightening-like pain extending from the lumbosacral region to the feet (sciatica); must get out of bed and sit up. Hands get stiff while writing.

**Skin:** Acne, erythema and eczema, with *vesicles* containing a thick, white matter. Dry, flour-like scales on the skin (*Ars.*). Bursitis.

**Modalities:** *Worse,* rich food, fats, motion.

**Relationship:** Compare: *Bell.* which *Kali-m.* follows well in catarrhal and hypertrophic conditions. *Kino* (otorrhea, with stitches in the right ear); *Bry., Merc., Puls., Sulph.*

**Dose:** Third to twelfth potency.

External use in skin affections with a burning sensation.

# KALIUM NITRICUM—NITRUM

(Nitrate of Potassium, Saltpeter) **Kali-n.**

Often indicated in asthma, also valuable in cardiac asthma; of great value in *sudden dropsical swellings over the whole body* (anasarca). Gastro-intestinal inflammation, with marked debility and relapse in phthisis, call for this remedy. Suppurative nephritis.

**Head:** Scalp very sensitive. Headache with vertigo, as if falling to the right side and backwards; worse, stooping. Ennui.

**Eyes:** Vision becomes clouded (cataract). Turbid corpus vitreum (*Arn., Ham., Sol-n., Phos.*). Variegated colored rings before eyes. Burning and lachrymation.

**Nose:** Sneezing. Swollen sensation; *worse, right nostril.* Point red and itchy. Polypus (*Sangin-n.*).

**Mouth:** Tongue red (glossitis), with burning pimples; burns at tip. Throat constricted and sore.

**Stool:** Thin, watery, bloody (dysentery). Membranous shreds with tenesmus. *Diarrhea from eating veal.*

**Female:** Menses too early, profuse, *black;* preceded and with violent backache (dysmenorrhea) Leucorrhea. Burning pain in the ovarian region only during menses (*Zinc.* after).

**Respiratory:** Hoarseness. Dry, morning cough, with pain in chest and hemoptysis. Bronchitis with sharp, short, dry, hacking cough. *Asthma,* with excessive dyspnea, nausea, dull stitches and burning in the chest. Dyspnea so great that breath cannot be held long enough to drink, though thirsty. Chest feels constricted. Oppression worse in morning. Sour smelling expectoration. Expectoration of clotted blood, after hawking mucus. Acute exacerbations in phthisis; congestion of the lungs. *Spasmodic croup;* paroxysm of crowing respiration. Laryngeal diphtheria.

**Heart:** Pulse weak, *small,* thready. Violent stitch in precordia, and palpitations (angina pectoris).

**Extremities:** Stitches between the shoulder blades. Tearing and sticking in the shoulders and joints. Hands and fingers seem swollen (rheumatism).

**Modalities:** *Worse,* eating veal; towards morning and in the afternoon. *Better,* drinking sips of water.

**Relationship:** Antidotes: *Op., Nit-s-d.*

Antidote to opium and morphine poisoning, 8-10 grains to glass of water.

Compare: *Gunpowder* (Nitre with sulphur and charcoal 2x trituration "Blood poisoning." Septic suppuration. Protective against wound infection.

Antidote to Ivy and Primula rash (Clarke). *Herpes facialis;* crops of boils. Carbuncles. Osteomyelitis. *Cann-s.* (which contains a large amount of *Kali-n.). Lyc., Sang., All-s., Ant-i.*

**Dose:** Third to thirtieth potency.

---

# KALIUM PERMANGANICUM

(Permanganate of Potassium) **Kali-perm.**

Intense irritation in the nose, throat and larynx. Diphtheria. Dysmenorrhea. Bites of serpents and of other animal poisons. Septic conditions; tissues infiltrated with a tendency to sloughing.

**Nose:** Epistaxis. Nasal discharge. Smarts and irritates. Constrictive, smarting sensation in the throat. Larynx feels raw. Short, hacking cough.

**Throat:** Swollen and painful. Everything hawked up is streaked with blood. Posterior nares painful. Muscles of the neck feel sore. Swollen uvula. Kalitosis.

**Respiratory:** Constrictive, smarting sensation in the throat. Larynx feels raw. Short hacking cough.

**Dose:** Locally, 1 dram in a quart of water, to correct fetor in cancer, ulcer, ozena and other foul odors. Also as an injection in leucorrhea and gonorrhea. Internally, 2x dilution in water. Saturated solution locally in eruption of smallpox.

Potassium permanganate for morphine poisoning: Potassium permanganate is recognized as being the most effective chemical antidote in cases of morphine or opium poisoning, acting directly on the morphine and oxidizing it to less toxic substances. To be effective, the permanganate must come in direct contact with the opium or morphine in the stomach; hypodermic or intravenous injections are absolutely useless, as the salt will be decomposed by the blood serum at once. The approved treatment is administration of two to five grains of potassium permanganate in dilute aqueous solution as soon as possible after the poison is taken, this amount is to be increased if very large doses of the poison have been taken. Washing out the stomach with a quantity of 1 to 500 solution of permanganate is also recommended, using at least a pint of this solution either by a stomach pump or by enforced vomiting. *Permanganate of Potash* counteracts the effects of alkaloids of many poisonous plants. Owing to its oxidizing powers, if given before the alkaloid has been absorbed (Dr. Chestnut in Dept. of Agriculture).

---

# KALIUM PHOSPHORICUM

(Phosphate of Potassium) **Kali-p.**

One of the greatest nerve remedies. *Prostration.* Weak and tired. Especially adapted to the young. Marked disturbance of the sympathetic nervous system. Conditions arising from *want of nerve power,* neurasthenia, mental and physical depression, are wonderfully improved by this remedy. The causes are usually excitement, overwork and worry. Besides, *it corresponds to states of adynamia and decay,* gangrenous conditions. In these two directions it has won many clinical laurels. Remember it in the treatment of suspected malignant tumors. After removal of cancer, when the skin is drawn *tight* over the wound during the healing process. Delayed labor.

**Mind:** Anxiety, *nervous dread,* lethargy. Indisposition to meet people. Extreme lassitude and depression. Very nervous, starts easily, *irritable.* Brain fag; hysteria; *night terrors.* Somnambulance. Loss of memory. *Slightest labor seems* like a *heavy task.* Great despondency about business. Shyness; disinclined to converse.

**Head:** Occipital headache; better, after rising. Vertigo, from lying or standing up from sitting and when looking upward (*Gran.*). *Cerebral Anemia.* Headache in students, and those worn out by fatigue. Headaches are relieved by gentle motion. Headache, with a weary, empty, all gone feeling is the stomach (*Ign., Sep.*).

**Eyes:** Sight weak loss of perceptive power; after diphtheria; from exhaustion. Ptosis (*Caust.*).

**Ears:** *Humming and buzzing in the ears* (tinnitus).

**Nose:** Nasal diseases, with offensive odor; fetid discharge.

**Face:** Livid and sunken, with hollow eyes. Right sided neuralgia, relieved by cold applications.

**Mouth:** *Breath offensive, fetid* (halitosis). Tongue coated brownish, like mustard. *Excessively dry,* in the morning. Toothache with easily bleeding gums; they have a bright red seam on them. Gums spongy and receding (scurvy) (*Caps., Ham., Lach.*).

**Throat:** Gangrenous sore throat. Paralysis of the vocal cords.

**Stomach:** A nervous "gone" sensation in the pit of the stomach (*Ign., Sep., Sulph.*). Feels seasick without nausea.

**Rectum:** Diarrhea; foul, *putrid odor;* after fright, with depression and exhaustion. Diarrhea while eating. Dysentery; stools consist of pure blood; patient becomes delirious; abdomen swells. Cholera; stools have the appearance of rice water (*Verat., Ars., Jatr-c.*). Prolapsus recti (*Ign., Podo.*).

**Urinary:** Enuresis. Incontinence of urine. Bleeding from the urethra. *Very yellow urine.*

**Male:** Nocturnal emissions; sexual power diminished; utter prostration after coitus (*Kali-c.*).

**Female:** Menstruation *too late or too scanty* in pale, irritable, sensitive, lachrymose females. Very profuse discharge, deep red or blackish-red, thin and non-coagulating; sometimes with an offensive odor. Feeble and ineffectual labor pains.

**Respiratory:** Asthma; least food aggravates. Short breath on going upstairs. Cough; yellow expectoration.

**Extremities:** Paralytic lameness of the back and extremities. Exertion aggravates. Pains, with depression and subsequent exhaustion.

**Fever:** Subnormal temperature.

**Modalities:** *Worse,* excitement, worry, mental and physical exertion; eating, cold, early morning. *Better,* warmth, rest, nourishment.

**Relationship:** Compare: *Kalium hypophosphoricum (debility with wasting of muscular tissue.* Phosphaturia with general anemia or leucocythemia. Effects of excessive tea drinking. Chronic bronchitis where the expectoration is *thick and fetid,* sometimes *scanty and tough.* Dose: 5 grains of crude to 3x). *Genista tinctoria* —Dyer's weed (contains scopolamine; frontal headache and vertigo, worse motion, better open air and eating. Dry throat, wakes up with waterbrash. Itching eruptions on the elbows, knees and ankles. Promotes diuresis in dropsical conditions). *Macroziama spiralis* (extreme debility after severe illness; collapse. Weariness from no assignable cause, no pains. Boring pain in the vertex; vomiting and retching all night; impossible to open eyes, giddiness and cold). *Zinc., Gels., Cimic., Lach., Mur-ac.*

**Dose:** Third to twelfth trituration. The highest potencies seem to be indicated in certain cases.

---

# KALIUM SILICICUM

(Silicate of Potash) **Kali-sil.**

A deep acting remedy. Lassitude is very marked. Desire to lie down all the time. Emaciation.

**Head:** Absent-minded, anxious, indolent, timid. Feeble will power. Head congested, blood surges from the body to the head. Vertigo, coldness of the head; photophobia.

**Nose:** Nasal catarrh, discharge *bloody*, excoriating, offensive nose, swollen, ulcerated (ozena).

**Stomach:** Weight in the stomach after eating, nausea, pain, flatulence. Pain in liver region.

**Rectum:** Constipation. Constriction of anus during stool.

**Extremities:** Stiffness all over the body and limbs. Creeping sensation over limbs. Twitching of muscles (chorea). Weak and weary.

**Modalities:** *Worse,* open air, drafts, cold, exertion, motion uncovering, bathing.

**Dose:** Higher potencies.

---

# KALIUM SULPHURICUM

(Potassium Sulphate) **Kali-s.**

Ailments accompanied by profuse desquamation. Applicable to the later stages of inflammation. *Yellow,* mucus and serous discharges, profuse and intermittent. Has been found of much use in oxaluria.

**Head:** Rheumatic headache, beginning in the evening. Bald spots. Dandruff and scaldhead (crusty eruptions).

**Ears:** Eustachian deafness. Discharge of *yellow* matter (otorrhea) (*Hydr.*).

**Nose:** Colds, *with yellow,* slimy expectoration. Nose obstructed. Anosmia (*Nat-m.*). *Engorgement of the naso-pharyngeal mucous membrane,* breathing through the mouth, snoring, etc., remaining after removal of adenoids.

**Face:** Aches in a heated room. Epithelioma.

**Stomach:** Tongue coated yellow and slimy. Insipid, pappy taste. Gums painful. Burning thirst, nausea and vomiting. Sensation of a load. Dread of hot drinks.

**Abdomen:** Colicky pains; abdomen feels cold to touch; tympanitic, tense. Yellow, slimy diarrhea. Constipation with hemorrhoids (*Sulph.*).

**Male:** Gonorrhea; discharge slimy, yellowish-green. Orchitis. Gleet.

**Female:** Menses too late, scanty, with sensation of a weight in the abdomen. Metrorrhagia.

**Respiratory:** Coarse rales. *Rattling of mucus* in the *chest* (*Ant-t.*). Post-influenzal cough, especially in children. Bronchial asthma, with yellow expectoration. Cough; worse in the evening and in hot atsmosphere. Croupy hoarseness (*Hep., Spong.*).

**Extremities:** Pain in the nape, back and limbs, worse in a warm room. *Shifting, wandering pains.*

**Fever:** Rise of temperature at night. Intermittent fever, with a yellow, slimy tongue.

**Skin:** Psoriasis (*Ars., Thyr.*). Eczema; burning, itching, papular eruption. Nettle rash. Polypi. Epithelioma. Seborrhea. Favus. Ringworm of scalp or beard with abundant scales.

**Modalities:** *Worse,* in the evening, heated room. *Better,* cool, open air.

**Relationship:** Compare: *Kalium sulphuricum chromicum*—Alum of chrome—3x (produces in the nasal passages, very fine threads from the septum to the external wall; affections of the nasal fosse and hay-fever. Chronic colds. Sneezing, red, watery eyes, irritation of the mucous membrane). *Puls., Kali-bi., Nat-m.*

**Dose:** Third to twelfth potency.

---

## KALMIA LATIFOLIA

(Mountain Laurel) **Kalm.**

A rheumatic remedy. Pains shift rapidly. Nausea and slow pulse frequently accompanying. Also has a prominent action on the heart. In small doses, it accelerates the heart's action; in larger, it moderates it greatly. Neuralgia; *pains shoot downward, with numbness. Fulgurating pains of locomotor ataxia.* Protracted and continuous *fevers,* with tympanites. Paralytic sensations; pain and aching in the limbs accompany nearly every group of symptoms. *Albuminuria.*

**Head:** *Vertigo;* worse stooping. Confusion of brain. Pain in front and temporal region from the head to the nape and to the teeth; from cardiac origin.

**Eyes:** Vision impaired. *Stiff, drawing sensation on moving the eyes.* Rheumatic iritis. Scleritis, *pain increased by moving the eye.*

**Face:** Neuralgia; worse *right side.* Stitches in the tongue. Stitches and tearing in the bones of jaw and face.

**Stomach:** Warm, glowing sensation in the epigastrium. Nausea; vomiting. *Pain in the pit of the stomach; worse bending forward; relieved by sitting erect.* Bilious attacks with nausea, vertigo and headache. Sensation of something being pressed under the epigastrium.

**Urinary:** Frequent, with sharp pains in the lumbar region. Post-scarlatinal nephritis.

**Female:** Menses too early, or suppressed, with pain in the limbs, back and inside of thighs. Leucorrhea follows menses.

**Heart:** Weak, *slow* pulse (*Dig., Apoc.*). Fluttering of heart with anxiety. *Palpitations; worse leaning forward.* Gouty and rheumatic metastasis of the heart. Tachycardia, with pain (angina pectoris) (*Thyr.*). Tobacco heart. Dyspnea and pressure from the epigastrium towards the heart. *Sharp pains take away* *the breath.* Shooting through the chest, above the heart, into the shoulder blades. Frequent pulse. Heart's action tumultuous, rapid and visible. Paroxysms of anguish around the heart.

**Back:** Pain from the neck radiates down the arm (cervical spondylosis); in the upper three dorsal vertebrae extending to the shoulder blade. Pain down the back, as if it would break (lumbago); in localized regions of the spine; through the shoulders. *Lumbar pain, of nervous origin.*

**Extremities:** Deltoid rheumatism especially right. Pain from the hips to the knees and feet. *Pains affect a large part of a limb,* or several joints, and pass through quickly. Weakness, numbness, pricking, and a sense of coldness in the limbs. *Pains along the ulnar nerve*, index finger. Joints red, hot, swollen. Tingling and numbness of the left arm.

**Sleep:** Sleepless, *wakes up very early in the morning.*

**Modalities:** *Worse,* leaning forward (opposite, *Kali-c.*); looking down; motion, open air.

**Relationship:** Compare: *Kalm.* contains Arbutin g. *v. Derris pinnata* (of great service in neuralgic headaches of rheumatic origin).

Compare: *Spig., Puls.*

Complementary: *Benz-ac.*

**Dose:** Tincture to sixth potency.

---

# KOLA

(Sterculia) **Kola**

Neurasthenia. Regulates the circulation, is a tonic and antidiarrheic, regulates cardiac rhythm and acts diuretically. Weak heart.

A remedy for the drinking habit. It promotes appetite and digestion, and decreases the craving for liquor. *Asthma.* Gives power to endure prolonged physical exertion without taking food and without feeling fatigued.

**Relationship:** *Coca.*

**Dose:** Three to ten drops, even one dram doses, three times a day.

---

# KAOLINUM

(Bolus Alba, China Clay, Alumina Silicata) **Alum-sil.**

Refer *Alumina silicata* on page 36.

---

# KOUSSO—BRAYERA

(Hagenia Abyssinica) **Kou.**

A *Vermifuge*—nausea and vomiting, vertigo, precordial anxiety slowing and irregular pulse, subdelirium and collapse. Rapid and extreme prostration. To expel tapeworm's.

**Relationship:** Compare: *Mallotus philippinensis*—Kamala: An efficient remedy for tapeworm in 30-60 minims of tincture taken in cinnamon water.

**Dose:** ½ oz. Mix with warm water and let it stand for 15 minutes; stir well and administer. May be preceded with a little lemon juice (Merrell).

---

# KREOSOTUM

(Beechwood Kreosote) **Kreos.**

*Kreosotum* is a mixture of phenols obtained from its distillation.

Pulsations all over the body and profuse bleeding from small wounds. Very severe, old, neuralgic affections; pain aggravated by rest. *Excoriating,* burning and offensive discharges. Hemorrhages, ulcerations, cancerous affections. Rapid decomposition of fluids and secretions; burning pains. Overgrown, poorly developed children. Post-climacteric diseases. Tumefaction, puffiness, gangrene. Aliments in teething children.

**Mind:** Music causes weeping and palpitations. Vanishing of thoughts; stupid, forgetful, peevish, irritable. Child wants everything but throws it away when given.

**Head:** Dull pain, as if a board was pressing against the forehead. Menstrual headache. Occipital pain (*Gels., Zinc-pic.*).

**Eyes:** Salty lachrymation. Lids red and swollen (blepharitis).

**Ears:** Eruption around and pimples within. Difficult hearing and buzzing (tinnitus).

**Nose:** Offensive smell and discharge (ozena). Chronic catarrh in old people. Acrid rawness. Lupus (*Ars.*).

**Face:** Sick, suffering expression; cheeks red, hot.

**Mouth:** Lips red, bleeding. Very painful dentition; child will not sleep. *Very rapid decay of teeth* (caries), *with spongy, bleeding gums* (scorbutic); teeth dark and crumbly (*Staph., Ant-c.*). Putrid odor and bitter taste.

**Throat:** Burning, choking sensation. *Putrid odor.*

**Stomach:** Nausea; vomiting of food several hours after eating; of sweetish water in the morning. Sensation of coldness, as if ice water is in the stomach.

Soreness; better eating. Painful hard spot. Hematemesis. Bitter taste after a mouthful of water.

**Abdomen:** Distended. Burning hemorrhoids. Diarrhea; very offensive; dark brown. Bloody, fetid stools. *Cholera infantum* in connection with painful dentition, green stools, nausea, dry skin, exhaustion, etc.

**Urinary:** *Offensive.* Violent itching in vulva and vagina, worse when micturating. Can micturate only when lying; cannot get out of bed fast enough during first sleep. Dreams of micturating. Enuresis in the first part of night. *Must hurry when desire comes to micturate.*

**Female:** Corrosive pruritus vulva, burning and swelling of the labia; violent itching between labia and thighs. During menses, *difficult hearing;* buzzing and roaring; eruptions afterwards. Burning and soreness in the external and internal parts. Leucorrhea, yellow, acrid; odor of green corn; worse between periods. Hemorrhage after coition. Menses too early, prolonged (metrorrhagia). Vomiting of pregnancy, with ptyalism. *Menstrual flow intermits* (*Puls.*); ceases on sitting or walking; reappears on lying down. Pain worse after menses. Lochia offensive; *intermits.*

**Respiratory:** *Hoarse, with pain in the larynx.* Cough; worse evening with retching and pain in the chest. Raw burning in the chest; pain and oppression. Cough after influenza (*Erio.*). Winter coughs in old people, *with heavy pressure on the sternum.* Gangrene of the lungs. After every cough, *copious, purulent expectoration.* Hemoptysis; periodic attacks (phthisis). Sternum feels pressed in.

**Back:** Dragging backache, extending to the genitals and down the thighs. Great debility.

**Extremities:** Pain in joints, hip and knee. Boring pain in the hip joints. Scapulae sore.

**Sleep:** Disturbed with tossing. Paralytic sensation in the limbs on waking. Anxious dreams of pursuit, fire, erections, etc.

**Skin:** Itching, worse towards the evening. Burning in the soles. Senile gangrene. Small wounds bleed freely (*Crot-h., Lach., Phos.*). Pustules and herpes. Ecchymosis (purpura); dorsal surface of fingers and hands eczematous.

**Modalities:** *Worse,* in open air, cold, rest, when lying; after menstruation. *Better,* from warmth, motion, warm diet.

**Relationship:** Antidote: *Nux-v.*

Inimical: *Carb-v.*

Complementary: In malignant diseases: *Ars., Phos., Sulph.*

*Guaiacolum* (is the principal constituent of *Kreos.*, and similar in action. Used in pulmonary tuberculosis. Dose 1 to 5 m.).

*Matico—Artanthe elongata or Piper augustifolia* (gonorrhea, hemorrhage from the lungs; catarrhal conditions of genito-urinary organs and gastro-intestinal tract. Topically a hemostatic. Difficult, dry, deep, winter cough. Use tincture).

Compare also: *Fuli., Carb-ac., Iod., Lach.*

**Dose:** Third to thirtieth potency. The 200th in sensitive patients.

---

# LAC CANINUM

(Dog's Milk) **Lac-c.**

This remedy is of undoubted value in certain forms of sore throat, diphtheria and rheumatism. Corresponds to a low vitiated, non-feverish type of sickness. The keynote symptom is, *erratic pains, alternating sides.* Feels as if walking on air, or of not touching the bed when lying down. Great lassitude. Ozena. Decided effect in drying up milk in women who cannot nurse the baby. *Great weakness and prostration.* Sinking spells every morning. Mastitis.

**Mind:** Very forgetful while writing, makes mistakes. *Despondent;* thinks her disease is incurable. Attacks of rage. *Visions of snakes.* Thinks himself to be of little consequence.

**Head:** Sensation of walking or floating in air (*Stict.*). Pain first on one side, then on the other. Blurred vision, nausea and vomiting at the height of an attack of headache (migraine). Shooting pain in the occiput extending to the forehead. Sensation as if the brain was alternately contracted and relaxed.

**Ears:** Reverberation of voice. Noises in ears.

**Nose:** Coryza; one nostril is stuffed up, the other free; alternate. Alae nasi and corners of the mouth cracked. Bones of the nose sore to pressure. Bloody pus discharged (ozena).

**Mouth:** Tongue coated white with bright red edges; profuse salivation. Drooling in diphtheria. *Cracking of jaw while eating* (*Nit-ac., Rhus-t.*). Putrid taste increased by sweets.

**Throat:** Sensitive to touch. Painful swallowing; pain extends to the ears. Sore throat and cough with menstruation. *Tonsillitis and diphtheria symptoms change repeatedly from side to side. Shining glazed* appearance of deposits, *pearly white or* like pure white porcelain. *Stiffness of the neck* and tongue. Throat feels burned, raw. Tickling sensation causes constant cough. Sore throat beginning and ending with menses.

**Female:** Menses too early, profuse, *flow in gushes. Breasts swollen; painful before* (*Calc., Con., Puls.*) and better on appearance of menses. Mastitis; *worse, least jar. Helps to dry up milk.* Sinking in the epigastrium. Sexual organs easily excited. Backache; spine very sensitive to touch or pressure. *Galactorrhea.*

**Extremities:** Sciatica, right side. Legs feel numb and stiff, cramps in feet. Rheumatic pains in the extremities and back, from one side to the other. Pain in the arms extending to the finger. Burning in palms and soles.

**Sleep:** Dreams of snakes.

**Modalities:** *Worse,* morning of one day and in the evening of next. *Better,* cold, cold drinks.

**Relationship:** Compare: *Lach., Con., Lac felinum*—Cat's milk (ciliary neuralgia; eye symptoms, photophobia; asthenopia; dysmenorrhea); *Lac vaccinum*—Cows' milk (headache, rheumatic pains, constipation); *Lac vaccinum coagulatum*—Curds (nausea of pregnancy); *Lactis vaccini flos*—Cream (diphtheria, leucorrhea, menorrhagia, dysphagia); *Lac-ac.*

**Dose:** Thirtieth and the highest potencies.

---

# LAC DEFLORATUM

(Skimmed Milk) **Lac-d.**

A remedy for diseases with faulty nutrition; sick headaches, with profuse flow of urine during pain. *Car sickness.*

**Head:** Despondent. Pain begins in the forehead and radiates to the occiput, in the morning, on rising. *Intense throbbing,* with nausea, vomiting, blindness and obstinate constipation; worse, noise, light, motion, during menses, with great prostration and better by pressure and bandaging the head tightly (migraine).

**Stool:** *Constipation.* Stools hard, large, after great straining; painful, lacerating anus.

**Relationship:** Compare: *Colostrum* (diarrhea in infants. The whole body smells sour. Colic). *Nat-m.*

**Dose:** Sixth to thiritieth potency and higher.

---

# LACHESIS MUTUS

(Bushmaster or Surucucu) **Lach.**

Like all snake poisons, *Lach.* decomposes the blood, rendering it more fluid; hence a hemorrhagic tendency is marked. Purpura, septic states, diphtheria and other low forms of disease, when the system is thoroughly poisoned and the prostration is profound. The modalities are most important in guiding to the remedy. Delirium tremens with marked trembling and confusion. Very important during climacteric and for patients with a melancholic disposition. Ill effects of suppressed discharges. Diphtheritic paralysis (*Botul.*). Diphtheria carriers. Sensation of tension in various parts. Cannot bear anything tight anywhere.

**Mind:** Great *loquacity.* Amative. Sad in the morning; no desire to mix with the world. Restless and uneasy; does not wish to attend to business; wants to be off somewhere all the time. Jealous (*Hyos.*). Mental labor best performed at night. Euthanasia. Suspicious; nocturnal delusion of fire. Religious insanity (*Verat., Stram.*). Derangement of *time sense.*

**Head:** Pain through the head on awaking. Pain at the root of the nose. Pressure and burning in the vertex. Waves of pain; worse after moving. Sun headaches, with headache, flickerings, dim vision, very pale face (apoplexy). Vertigo (Meniere's disease). Relieved by the onset of a discharge (menses or nasal catarrh).

**Eyes:** Defective vision after diphtheria, extrinsic muscles too weak to maintain focus. Sensation as if the eyes were drawn together by cords which were tied in a knot at the root of the nose.

**Ears:** Tearing pains from the zygoma into the ear; with a sore throat. Cerumen hard, dry.

**Nose:** Epistaxis, nostrils sensitive. Coryza, preceded by headache. Hay asthma; paroxysms of sneezing (*Sil., Sabad.*).

**Face:** Pale. Trigeminal neuralgia, left side, heat running up to the head (*Phos.*). Tearing pains in the jaw bones (*Amph., Phos.*). Purple, mottled, puffed; looks swollen, bloated, jaundiced, chlorotic.

**Mouth:** Gums swollen, spongy, bleed (scorbutic). Tongue swollen, burns, trembles, red, dry and cracked at the tip, catches in between teeth (glossitis). *Aphthous and denuded spots* with burning and rawness. Nauseous taste. *Toothache, pain extends to the ears.* Pain in the facial bones.

**Throat:** Sore, *worse left side, swallowing liquids. Quinsy.* Septic parotiditis. Dry, intensely swollen, externally and internally. Diphtheria; membrane dusky, blackish; pain *aggravated by hot drinks;* chronic sore throat, with much hawking; mucus sticks, *and cannot be forced up or down. Very painful; worse slightest pressure, touch is even more annoying.* In diphtheria, etc., the trouble *begins on the left side.* Tonsils purplish. Purple, livid color of the throat. Sensation as if something was swollen which must be swallowed; *worse, swallowing saliva or liquids. Pain radiates to the ear. Collar and neck band must be very loose.* Empty swallowing more painful than swallowing solids.

**Stomach:** Craving for alcohol, oysters. Any food causes distress. Pit of the stomach painful to touch. Hungry, cannot wait for food. Gnawing pressure, *better by eating* (gastric ulcers), but returning in a few hours. Perceptible trembling movement in the epigastric region.

**Abdomen:** Liver region sensitive, *cannot bear anything around the waist* (jaundice). Especially suitable to drunkards. Abdomen tympanitic, sensitive, painful (*Bell.*).

**Rectum:** Constipated, *offensive stool.* Anus *feels tight,* as if nothing could go through it. Pain darting up the rectum every time he sneezes or coughs. Hemorrhage from the bowels like charred straw, *black particles.* Hemorrhoids protrude, become *constricted, purplish.* Stitches in them on sneezing or coughing. Constant urging in the rectum, not for stool.

**Male:** Intense excitement of sexual organs.

**Female:** Climacteric problems, palpitations, flashes of heat, hemorrhages, headache in the vertex, fainting spells; worse, pressure of clothes. Menses too short, too feeble; *pains, all relieved* by *the flow* (*Eupi.*). Left ovary very painful and swollen, indurated. Mammae inflamed, bluish (mastitis). Coccyx and sacrum painful, especially on *rising* from a sitting posture. Acts especially well at the beginning and close of menstruation.

**Respiratory:** Upper part of the trachea is very susceptible to touch. Sensation of suffocation and strangulation on lying down edema of the lungs, particularly *when anything is around the throat;* compels the patient to spring from the bed and rush for an open window. Spasms of the glottis (laryngismus); feels as if something ran down, from the neck to the larynx. Feels *he must take a deep breath.* Cramp-like distress in the precordial region. Cough; dry, suffocative fits, tickling (asthma). Little secretion and much sensitiveness; worse, pressure on the larynx, *after sleep,* open air. *Breathing almost stops on falling asleep* (*Grin.*). Larynx painful to touch. Sensation of a plug (*Anac.*) which moves up and down, with a short cough.

**Heart:** Palpitations, with fainting spells, especially during climacteric. Constricted feeling causing palpitations with anxiety. Cyanosis. Irregular beats.

**Back:** Neuralgia of the coccyx *worse rising from a sitting posture;* must sit perfectly still. Pain in the neck, worse cervical region (cervical spondylitis). Sensation of threads stretched from the back to the arms, legs, eyes, etc.

**Extremities:** Sciatica, right side, better lying down. *Pain in the tibia* (may follow sore throat). Shortening of tendons.

**Sleep:** Patient *sleeps into an aggravation.* Sudden starting on falling asleep. Sleepiness, yet cannot sleep (*Bell., Op.*). Wide awake in the evening.

**Fever:** Chills in the back; feet icy cold; hot flushes and hot perspiration. Paroxysm returns after acids. Intermittent fever every spring.

**Skin:** Hot perspiration, *bluish, purplish appearance.* Boils, carbuncles, ulcers, with bluish-purple surroundings. Dark blisters. Bed-sores with black edges. Blue-black swellings (ecchymosis). Pyemia; dissecting wounds. Purpura with intense prostration. *Senile erysipelas.* Wens. Cellulitis. Varicose ulcers.

**Modalities:** *Worse,* after sleep (*Kali-bi.*). *Lach.* sleeps into aggravation; ailments that come on during sleep (*Calc.*); left side, in the spring, warm bath, pressure or constriction, hot drinks. Closing eyes. *Better,* appearance of discharges, warm applications.

**Relationship:** Antidotes: *Ars., Merc., Heat, Alcoholus, Salt.*

Complementary: *Crotalus cascavella* often completes curative work of *Lach.*, (*Murx.*) *Lyc., Hep., Salam.*

Incompatible: *Acet-ac., Carb-ac.*

Compare: *Cotyledon umblicus* (climacteric problems); *Nat-m., Nit-ac., Crot-h., Amphisbaena vermicularis*—Snake lizard (right jaw swollen and painful, lancinating pains; headaches. Eruption of vesicles and pimples); *Naja, Lepi.*

**Dose:** Eighth to 200th potency. Doses ought not be repeated too frequently. If well indicated, a single dose should be allowed to exhaust its action.

---

# LACHNANTES TINCTORIA

(Spirit Weed) **Lachn.**

Head, chest and circulation are affected. Bridge of nose seems as if pinched. A remedy for torticollis, rheumatic symptoms of the neck. *Tuberculosis* in light complexioned people. Early stages and established chest cases, with severe coldness. Produces a desire to talk, a flow of language and the courage to make a speech.

**Head:** Right sided pain, extending down to the jaw; *head feels enlarged;* worse, least noise. Scalp painful. Sleepless. Circumscribed, red cheeks; scalp feels sore, as if hair was standing on ends; burning in palms and soles. Bridge of nose feels as if pinched.

**Chest:** Sensation of heat, bubbling and boiling around the heart region rising to the head.

**Back:** *Chilliness between the shoulder blades;* pain and stiffness in the back. Neck *drawn over to one side* during a sore throat. Rheumatism (spondylosis) of the neck. Stiffness of the neck. Pain in the nape, as if dislocated.

**Skin:** Body icy cold; face yellow, tendency to sweat.

**Relationship:** Compare: *Dulc., Bry., Puls.,* also *Fel.* (pain in the nape of the neck, and great tension there).

**Dose:** Third potency. Tincture in phthisis, unit doses, once or twice a week, or three drops every four hours.

---

## LACTICUM ACIDUM

(Lactic Acid) **Lac-ac.**

Morning sickness, *diabetes* and rheumatism offer a field for this remedy. *Problems in the breasts.* Locally, in the tuberculous ulceration of vocal cords.

**Throat:** Fullness or lump like a puff ball. Keeps swallowing. Constricted low down.

**Stomach:** Tongue dry, parched. Thirst; voracious hunger. Canker, *copious salivation and waterbrash. Nausea;* morning sickness, especially *in pale, anemic* women. Hot, acrid eructation. *Nausea;* better, *eating.* Burning, hot gas from the stomach to the throat, causing profuse secretion of tenacious mucus, worse *smoking.*

**Urinary:** Large quantities passed, frequently. Saccharine (diabetes).

**Chest:** Pain in the breasts, with enlargement of *axillary glands, and pain extends into hand.*

**Extremities:** Rheumatic pains in the joints, shoulders, wrists, *knees* with much weakness. Trembling of the whole body while walking. Limbs feel chilly.

**Relationship:** Compare: *Sarcol-ac.q.v., Lith-c., Ph-ac.*

**Dose:** Third to thirtieth potency. Six to ten drops in a small glass of water in acute gastroenteritis (Cartier).

---

## LACTUCA VIROSA

(Acrid Lettuce) **Lact.**

This remedy acts principally upon the brain and circulatory system. Delirium tremens with sleeplessness, coldness, and tremor. Hydrothorax and ascites. Impotence. Sensation of lightness and *tightness* affecting the whole body, especially the chest. Seems to be a *true galactogogue.* Marked action on the extremities.

**Mind:** Stupefaction of sense. Great restlessness.

**Head:** Dull, heavy, confused, dizzy. Heat of face and headache, with general coldness. Headache, with affections of the respiratory system.

**Abdomen:** Sensation of weight, fullness; borborygmi; abundant emissions of wind. Colic, early morning, abdomen tense, relieved somewhat by evacuation and passing of wind.

**Female:** Promotes catamenia. *Increase of* milk in breasts (*Asaf.*).

**Chest:** Difficult breathing (asthma). Suffocative breathing from dropsy of the chest (hydrothorax). Constant tickling cough. Incessant, spasmodic cough, as if the chest would fly to pieces (bronchitis). Squeezing sensation in lower chest (angina pectoris).

**Extremities:** Lame hip, down left side; worse walking. Coldness and numbness of feet and legs. Tremor in the hands and arms. Cramps in the shin bones, extending to the toes and side of leg involving the calves.

**Sleep:** Restless; impossible to get sleep. Deep, comatose sleep.

**Relationship:** Antidotes: *Acet-ac., Coff.*

Compare: *Nabalus serpentarius—Prenanthes serpentaria*—Rattlesnake root—White lettuce, similar to Lactuca (chronic diarrhea, worse after eating, at nights and towards the morning. Pain in the abdomen and rectum; emaciation. Constipation and somnolence; susceptible to the aura of others. Dyspepsia with acid burning eructation. *Craving for acid food.* Leucorrhea with throbbing in the uterus); *Lach., Kali-c., Spira.* (galactagogue).

**Dose:** Tincture.

---

## LAMIUM ALBUM

(White Nettle) **Lam.**

Has a special affinity for the female and urinary organs.

Headache *with backward and forward motion of the head.* Leucorrhea and menses too early and scanty. Hemorrhoids; hard stools, with blood. Sensation in the urethra, as though a drop of water was passing through it. Tearing in the extremities. Hemoptysis. Blisters on heel from slight rubbing. Ulcers on the heel (*All-c.*).

**Dose:** Third potency.

---

## LAPIS ALBUS

(Silico-fluoride of Calcium) **Lap-a.**

Affections of the glands, *goitre,* pre-ulcerative stage of carcinoma. Burning, stinging pain in the breast, stomach and uterus (carcinogenic stage). Connective tissue around the glands specially affected. Fatty anemic babies with an appetite like *Iod.* Ravenous appetite. Remarkably successful in scrofulous affections, except in malarial cases. *Uterine carcinoma.* Fibroid tumors with *intense burning* pains through the part with *profuse hemorrhage.* Glands have a certain elasticity and pliability about them rather than the stony hardness of *Calc-f.* and *Cist.*

**Ears:** Otitis media suppurativa. Where *Sil.* is indicated, progress is hastened by *Lap-a.* (Bellows).

**Chest:** Persistent pains in the mammary region. Glandular hardening.

**Skin:** Scrofulous abscesses and sores. Enlargement and induration of the glands, *especially cervical.* Lipoma, sarcoma, carcinoma. Pruritus.

**Relationship:** Compare: *Sil., Bad., Ars-i., Calc-i., Con., Kali-i., Aster.*

**Dose:** First to sixth potency.

---

## LAPPA ARCTIUM

(Burdock) **Lappa**

Very important in skin therapeutics. Eruptions on the head, face, and neck; pimples; acne. Styes and ulcerations on the edge of the eyelids. Profuse and frequent micturition. Crops of boils and styes (*Anthraci.*).

**Female:** Uterine displacements. An exceedingly sore, bruised feeling in the uterus, with great relaxation of the vaginal tissues; apparently complete lack of tonicity of pelvic contents. These symptoms are all aggravated by standing, walking, taking a misstep or sudden jar.

**Dose:** Tincture to third potency.

---

## LATHYRUS SATIVUS

(Chick-pea) **Lath.**

Affects the lateral and anterior columns of the cord. Does not produce pain. *Reflexes always increased.* Paralytic affections of lower extremities; spastic paralysis; lateral sclerosis; Beri-beri. Athetosis. Locomotor ataxia. Infantile paralysis. After influenza and wasting, exhaustive diseases where there is much weakness and heaviness, slow recovery of nerve power. Sleepy, constant yawning.

**Mind:** Depressed; hypochrondriacal. Vertigo when standing with eyes closed.

**Mouth:** Burning pain on the *tip of the tongue;* with tingling and numbness of the tongue and lips, as if scalded.

**Urinary:** Increased bladder reflex. Frequent, must hurry, else voided involuntarily.

**Extremities:** Tips of fingers numb. Tremulous, tottering gait. Excessive rigidity of legs; spastic gait. Knees knock against each other when walking. Cramps in legs worse cold, and cold feet. Cannot extend or cross legs when sitting. Myelitis with marked spastic symptoms. Rheumatic paralysis. Gluteal muscles and lower limbs emaciated (paraplegia). Legs blue; swollen, if hanging down. Stiffness and lameness of ankles and knees, toes do not leave the floor, heels do not touch the floor. Muscles of calves very tense. Patient sits bent forward, straightens up with difficulty.

**Relationship:** Compare: *Oxyt., Sec., Petiveria tetandra,* a South American plant (paralysis; paraplegia with numbness. Sensation of internal coldness). *Agrostema githago*—Corncockle (burning sensation, in the stomach, through the esophagus extends into the throat, in lower abdomen and anus; nausea, bitter vomiting, impaired locomotion; difficulty in remaining erect; vertigo and *headache, burning from the lower jaw to the vertex).*

**Dose:** Third potency.

---

# LATRODECTUS MACTANS

(Spider) **Lat-m.**

The bite produces tetanic effects that last several days. A picture of *angina pectoris* is presented by the action of the drug. The precordial region seems to be the center of attack. Constriction of chest muscles, with radiation to the shoulders and back. Lowered coagulability.

**Head:** Anxiety. Screams with pain. Pain in the neck extends to the back of head. Occipital pain.

**Respiratory:** Extreme apnea. Gasping respiration. Fears losing breath.

**Chest:** Violent, precordial pain extending to the axilla and down the arm and forearm to the fingers, with numbness of the extremity. Pulse feeble and rapid. Sinking sensation in the epigastrium. Cramping pains from the chest to the abdomen.

**Extremities:** Pain in the left arm, feels paralyzed. Weakness of legs followed by cramps in the abdominal muscles. Paraesthesia of lower limbs.

**Skin:** Coldness of the entire surface. Skin cold as marble.

**Relationship:** Compare: *Latrodectus hasselti*—New South Wales Black spider (long lasting effects seem to indicate it in *"chronic"* blood poisoning. Arrests intense pain in pyemia. Great edema in the neighbourhood of a wound;

paralysis of limbs, with great wasting of muscles. Violent, darting, burning pains preceding paralysis; vertigo, tendency to fall forward; septicemic conditions; constant delusion of *flying.* Loss of memory. Roaring noises). *Aran., Mygal., Ther., Latrodectus katipo*—New Zealand spider (lymphangitis and nervous twitchings, scarlet burning eruption). *Triatema*—Kissing bug (swelling with violent itching in fingers and toes. Smothering sensation and difficult respiration succeeded by fainting and a rapid pulse).

**Dose:** Sixth potency.

---

# LAUROCERASUS

(Cherry Laurel) **Laur.**

Spasmodic tickling cough, especially in cardiac patients, is often magically influenced by this drug. *Lack of reaction,* especially in chest and heart affections. *Drink rolls audibly through the esophagus and intestines.* General coldness, not ameliorated by warmth. Violent pain in the stomach with loss of speech. Spasm of facial muscles and esophagus. Asphyxia neonatorum.

**Respiratory:** Cyanosis and dyspnea; worse, sitting up. Patient puts hands on the heart. Cough with valvular disease. Exercise causes pain around the heart. Tickling, *dry cough.* Dyspnea (asthma). Constriction of the chest. Cough, with copious, jelly like or bloody expectoration. Small and feeble pulse. Threatening paralysis of the lungs. *Gasping for breath;* clutches the heart.

**Heart:** Mitral regurgitation. Clutching the heart and palpitations. Cyanosis neonatorum.

**Extremities:** Toe and finger nails become knotty. Skin blue (cyanosed). Sprained pains in hips, thighs and heels. Cold, clammy feet and legs. Clubbing of fingers. Veins of hands distended.

**Sleep:** Spells of deep sleep, with snoring and stertorous breathing.

**Fever:** Coldness; chills and heat alternate. Thirst, with a dry mouth in the afternoon.

**Relationship:** Compare: *Hydr-ac., Camph., Sec., Am-c., Ambr.*

**Dose:** Tincture to third potency. Cherry laurel water, two to five drop doses.

---

# LECITHINUM

(A Phosphorus Containing Complex Organic Body Prepared From the Yolk of an Egg and Animal Brains) **Lec.**

*Lecithinum* is important in the vital processes of plant and animal organisms. *Lec.* has a favorable influence upon the nutritive condition and especially upon the blood, hence it is used in anemia, convalescence, neurasthenia and insomnia. Increases the number of red blood corpuscles and amount of hemoglobin. Excellent galactagogue, renders milk more nourishing and increases quantity.

Causes an immediate decrease in the excretion of phosphates. Mental exhaustion and impotency. Tuberculosis, causing marked improvement in nutrition and general improvement. Tired, weak, short breath, loss of flesh; symptoms of a general breakdown. Sexually weak.

**Mind:** Forgetful, dull, confused.

**Head:** Aching, especially in the occiput, pulsating and ringing in the ears (tinnitus).

**Face:** Pain in zygoma; face pale.

**Stomach:** Loss of appetite, thirsty, craves wine and coffee, bloated, sore pain in the stomach rising towards the throat.

**Urinary:** Scanty with phosphates (phosphaturia), sugar (diabetes) or albumen (albuminuria).

**Male:** Male power lost or enfeebled. Impotence.

**Female:** An aphrodisic and ovarian insufficiency.

**Extremities:** Soreness, aching, lack of energy. Tired and weak.

**Relationship:** Compare: *Phos.*

**Dose:** One-half to 2 grains of crude and potencies. Twelfth potency.

---

# LEDUM PALUSTRE

(Marsh Tea) **Led.**

Especially affects the rheumatic diathesis, going through all the changes, from functional pain to altered secretions and deposits of solid, earthy matter in the tissues. The *Led.* rheumatism begins in the feet, and travels upward. It also affects the skin, producing an eruption like Poison oak, and is antidotal thereto, as well as to stings of insects. *There is a general lack of animal heat,* and yet heat of bed is intolerable. For punctured wounds, produced by sharp pointed instruments or bites, particularly if the *wounded parts are cold,* this is the remedy. Tetanus with twitching of muscles near the wound.

**Head:** Vertigo when walking, with a tendency to fall on one side. Distress when the head is covered. Epistaxis (*Meli., Bry.*).

**Eyes:** Aching in eyes. Extravasation of blood in the lids (black eye), conjunctiva, aqueous or vitreous. Contused wounds. Cataract with gout.

**Face:** *Red pimples on the forehead and cheeks;* stinging when touched. Crusty eruptions around the nose and mouth.

**Mouth:** Dry, retching with eructations. Musty taste with catarrhal affection.

**Rectum:** *Anal fissures.* Hemorrhoidal pain.

**Respiratory:** Burning in the nose. Cough with hemoptysis. Dyspnea; chest feels constricted (asthma). Suffocative, arrest of breathing. Pain along the trachea. Bronchitis with emphysema in the aged. Oppressive constriction of the chest. Tickling in the larynx; spasmodic cough. Hemoptysis, alternating with rheumatism. Chest hurts when touched. Whooping cough; spasmodic, *double inspiration* with sobbing.

**Extremities:** Gouty pains shoot through the foot, limb and joints, but especially in the small joints. Swollen, hot, pale. Throbbing in the right shoulder. Pressure in the shoulder, worse motion. Cracking in joints; worse, warmth of bed. Gouty nodosities. Ball of great toe swollen (*Both.*). Rheumatism begins in the lower limbs and ascends (*Kalm.* opposite). Ankles swollen. *Soles painful,* can hardly step on them (*Ant-c., Lyc.*). Easy spraining of ankles.

**Fever:** Coldness, want of animal heat. Sensation as if cold water over the parts; general coldness with heat of face.

**Skin:** Acne on the forehead, sticking pain therein. Eczema (facial). Itching in the feet and ankles; worse, scratching and warmth of bed. Ecchymosis. Long discoloration after injuries. *Carbuncles* (*Anthraci., Tarent-c.*). *Antidotes Rhus poisoning* (*Grin., Cypr., Anac.*).

**Modalities:** *Better,* from cold, putting feet in cold water. *Worse,* at night and from heat of bed.

**Relationship:** Compare: *Led.* antidotes spider poisons. *Ruta, Ham., Bell-p., Arn.*

**Dose:** Third to thirtieth potency.

---

## LEMNA MINOR

(Duckweed) **Lem-m.**

A catarrhal remedy. Acts especially on the nostrils. *Nasal polypi; swollen turbinates. Atrophic rhinitis.* Asthma from nasal obstruction; worse in wet weather.

**Nose:** *Putrid smell;* anosmia. Crusts and mucopurulent discharge very abundant (ozena). Post-nasal dripping. Pain like a string from the nostrils to the ear. Reduces nasal obstruction in an edematous condition. Dryness of the naso-pharynx.

**Mouth:** *Putrid taste* on rising in the morning. Dry pharynx and larynx.

**Abdomen:** Disposition to noisy diarrhea.

**Modalities:** *Worse,* in damp, rainy weather, especially *heavy rains.*

**Relationship:** Compare: *Dulc.* (damp surroundings and foggy weather). *Calc., Teucr., Calen., Nat-s.*

**Dose:** Third to thirtieth potency.

---

## LEPIDIUM BONARIENSE

(Cress, Brazilian Cress) **Lepi.**

Affections of the breast (mastitis) and heart with lancinating pains.

With heart symptoms, numbness and pain in the left arm, sensation of sinking in the pit of the stomach.

Left side of the head, face, chest, hip to knee, all have lancinating pain.

A streak of pain from the temple to the chin, as if the face was cut with a razor (facial neuralgia). Burning in the throat, roaring in ears (tinnitus). Sensation of a tight girdle around the chest, as if a knife piercing the heart (angina pectoris). Pain in the neck, back and extremities.

**Relationship:** Compare: *Arn., Lach.*

---

## LEPTANDRA VIRGINICA

(Culver's Root) **Lept.**

A liver remedy with jaundice and *black, tarry stools.* Bilious states. Enfeebled portal circulation. Malarial conditions.

**Head:** Dull frontal pain; vertigo, drowsiness and depression. Smarting and aching in the eyes.

**Stomach:** Tongue coated *yellow.* Great distress in the stomach and intestines, with a desire for stool. Aching in the liver region extending to the spine, which feels chilly.

**Stool:** Profuse *black, fetid stools* with pain in the umbilicus. Bleeding piles. Typhoid stools turn black and look like tar. Clay colored stools with jaundice. Prolapse of rectum with hemorrhage.

**Relationship:** Compare: *Podo., Iris, Bry., Merc., Ptel., Myric.*
**Dose:** Tincture to third potency.

---

## LIATRIS SPICATA—SERRATULA TINCTORIA

(Colic Root) **Liat.**

A vascular stimulant. Increases the functional activity of the skin, mucous membranes.

Of use in dropsy due to liver and spleen diseases, also renal dropsy. Here suppressed micturition is most favorably influenced. *General anasarca* due to cardiac and renal disease. *Diarrhea,* with violent urging and pain in the lower part of the back. Colic. Locally, applied on ulcers and unhealthy wounds. A prompt diuretic.

**Dose:** 1 to 4 drams of tincture or infusion.

---

## LILIUM TIGRINUM

(Tiger Lily) **Lil-t.**

Manifests powerful influence over the pelvic organs and is adapted to many reflex states dependent on some pathological condition of uterus and ovaries. More often indicated in unmarried women. Action on the heart is very marked. Pain in small spots (*Ox-ac.*). Rheumatic arthritis.

**Mind:** Tormented about her salvation. Consolation aggravates. *Profound depression of spirits.* Constant inclination to weep. Anxious; *fears some organic and incurable disease.* Disposed to curse, strike, thinks obscene things. *Aimless, hurried manner;* must keep busy.

**Head:** Hot, dull, heavy. Faints in a warm room. Wild feeling in the head.

**Eyes:** Hyperesthesia of the retina. Pain, extending back into the head; lachrymation; and impaired vision. *Myopic astigmia.* Useful in restoring power to the weakened ciliary muscle (*Arg-n.*).

**Stomach:** Flatulent; nausea with sensation of a lump in the stomach. Hungry; longs for meat. Thirsty, drinks often and much, and before severe symptoms.

**Abdomen:** Abdomen sore, distended; trembling sensation in the abdomen. Pressure downwards and backwards against the rectum and anus; worse, standing; better, walking in the open air. Bearing down sensation in the lower part of the abdomen.

**Rectum:** Constant desire to defecate, *from pressure in the rectum,* worse standing. Pressure down the anus. Early morning urgent stool. Dysentery; mucus and blood, with tenesmus, especially in plethoric and nervous women at the change of life (menopause).

**Urinary:** Frequent urging. Urine milky, scanty, *hot.*

**Female:** Menses early, scanty, *dark, clotted, offensive; flow only when moving about. Bearing down sensation with an urgent desire for stool, as though all the organs would escape. Ceases when resting (Sep., Lac-c., Bell.). Congestion of the uterus,* prolapse and anteversion. Constant desire to support parts externally. Pain in the ovaries and down the thighs. Acrid, brown leucorrhea; smarting in the labia. Sexual instinct awakened. Bloated feeling in the uterine region. Sub-involution. Pruritus pudendi.

**Heart:** Sensation as if the heart was grasped in a vise (*Cact.*). Feels full to bursting. Pulsations all over the body. Palpitations; irregular pulse; very rapid. Pain in the cardiac region, with sensation of a load on the chest. Cold feeling around the heart. Suffocative feeling in a crowded and warm room. Angina pectoris with pain in the right arm.

**Extremities:** Cannot walk on the uneven ground. Pain in the back and spine, with trembling, but often in the front, of a pressing down character[1]. Pricking in fingers. Pain in the right arm and hip. Legs ache; cannot keep them still. Pain in the ankle joint. Burning in palms and soles.

**Sleep:** Unrefreshing, with disagreeable dreams. Unable to sleep, with a wild feeling in the head.

**Fever:** Great heat and lassitude in the afternoon, with throbbing throughout the body.

**Modalities:** *Worse*, consolation, warm room. *Better,* fresh air.

**Relationship:** Compare: *Cact., Helon., Murx., Sep., Plat., Pall.*

Antidote: *Helon.*

**Dose:** The middle and higher potencies seem to have done best. Its curative action sometimes is slow in developing itself.

---

## LIMULUS CYCLOPS (XIPHOSURA)

(Horse Foot, King Crab) **Lim.**

*Lim.* was introduced by C. Hering and was partially proved by him and Lippe. Hering was surprised to see that the blood of the King crab that he dissected, was blue, which on investigation, was found to contain copper as he

---

1 Stitching pain from ilium to ilium or from the pubes to the sacrum (Clarke — Dictionary of Practical Materia Medica).

had surmised and which he thought would prove to be another medicine for cholera. Further provings are necessary to establish this, though symptoms so far observed make this probable. Hering's fertile mind always lead him to pioneer paths into practical therapeutics.

Physical and mental exhaustion; drowsiness *after sea bathing.* Gastro-enteric symptoms. Painful fullness of the entire right side of the body.

**Head:** Mental depression. Difficulty in remembering names, confused with heat of the face, rush of blood to the face (apoplexy), worse when meditating. Pain behind the left eyeball.

**Nose:** Fluent coryza. Sneezing, worse drinking water. Constant nasal dropping. Pressure above the nose and behind the eyes.

**Abdomen:** Colic with heat. Cramp-like pain with watery stools. Abdomen hot and constricted. Piles, constriction of the anus.

**Respiratory:** Husky voice. Dyspnea after drinking water. Oppression of the chest.

**Extremities:** Crural neuralgia. Soles of feet ache, feel numb. Pain in the right hip joint. Heels sore.

**Skin:** *Itching spots and vesicles* on the face and *hands.* Burning in palms.

**Relationship:** Compare: *Aster., Hom., Cupr.*

**Dose:** Sixth potency.

---

## LINARIA VULGARIS

(Toad-flax, Snap Dragon) **Lina.**

Acts prominently within the domain of the pneumogastrics. Eructations, nausea, salivation, pressure in the stomach. Jaundice, hepato-splenomegaly. Enteric symptoms and *great drowsiness* very marked. Cardiac *fainting.* Enuresis. Rectal symptoms. Tongue rough, dry; throat constricted. Coldness. Confusion in the head. Irresistible sleepiness. Symptoms worse walking in open air.

**Dose:** Third potency.

---

## LINUM USITATISSIMUM

(Common Flax) **Linu-u.**

The application of Linseed poultice has produced in sensitive subjects, severe respiratory disturbances, such as asthma, hives, etc. Its action in such cases is marked by *intense irritation.* It has been found to contain a small quantity of Hydrocyanic acid, which may account for this intensity. The decoction is of service in inflammation of the urinary passages, cystitis, strangury, etc. Also in diseases of the intestinal tract. It has a place in the treatment of asthma, hay fever and urticaria. Trismus and paralysis of the tongue.

**Relationship:** Compare: *Linum catharticum*—Purging flax (similar respiratory symptoms, but also colic and diarrhea).

**Dose:** Lower potencies.

---

# LITHIUM CARBONICUM

(Carbonate of Lithium) **Lith-c.**

Chronic *rheumatism connected with heart lesions* and asthenopia offer a field for this remedy. Rheumatic nodes. Uric acid diathesis. The whole body is *sore.* Gout and tophi.

**Head:** Tension, as if bound; better, sitting and going out. Externally sensitive. *Headache ceases while eating.* Trembling and throbbing. Pain in the heart; extends to the head. Dizzy states with ringing in the ears (Meniere's disease). Both cheeks covered with dry, bran-like scales.

**Eyes:** Half vision (hemiopia); invisible right half. Photophobia. Pain over the eyes. Dry lids. Eyes pain after reading (aesthenopia).

**Stomach:** Acidity, nausea, *gnawing, relieved by eating* (*Anac.*). Cannot endure the slightest pressure, even of clothes (*Lach.*).

**Urinary:** Tenesmus. Turbid urine with mucus and red deposits. Pain in the region of the right kidney and ureter. Free and colorless. While micturating, pressure in the heart. Cystitis, subacute and chronic. Soreness of the bladder. Urine scanty and dark, acrid; sandy deposit (albuminuria).

**Respiratory:** Constriction of the chest. Violent cough when lying down. Air feels cold when inspired. Pain in the mammary glands, *which extends into the arms and fingers.*

**Heart:** Rheumatic soreness in the cardiac region. Sudden shocks in the heart (angina pectoris). Throbbing, dull stitch in the cardiac region. Pain in the heart before menses, associated with pain in the bladder, before micturition; better, after. Trembling and fluttering in the heart, extending to the back.

**Extremities:** Paralytic stiffness all over. Itching around the joints. Rheumatic pains throughout, the small joints are generally affected. Pain in the hollow of the foot, extending to the knee. Swelling and tenderness of finger and toe joints; better, hot water. Nodular swellings in joints. Ankles pain when walking.

**Skin:** Scabby, tettery eruption on the hands, head and cheeks, preceded by a red, raw skin. Dull stitch, ending in itching. *Barber's itch* (use high). Rough rash all over the body, loose epithelium, tough, dry, itchy skin.

**Modalities:** *Worse,* in the morning, right side. *Better,* rising and moving about.

**Relationship:** Compare: *Lyc., Am-p., Benz-ac., Calc., Lithium muriaticum* (symptoms of cinchonism, viz., *dizzy* head, full, *blurring of vision.* Ringing in the ears; marked tremors; *general weakness;* marked muscular and general prostration; no gastro-intestinal effects. Nose sore, heartburn, pain in teeth). *Lithium lacticum* (rheumatism of shoulder, and small joints relieved by moving about; worse, resting). *Lithium benzoicum* (deep seated pains in the loins; in lumbosacral region; uneasiness in the bladder. Cystitis. Gallstones. Frequent desire. Diminishing uric acid deposit) *Lithium bromatum* (cerebral congestion, threatened apoplexy, insomnia and epilepsy).

**Dose:** First to third trituration.

---

# LOBELIA INFLATA

(Indian Tobacco) **Lob.**

Is a vasomotor stimulant; increases the activity of all the vegetative processes; spends its force mainly upon the pneumogastric nerve, producing a depressed, relaxed condition with oppression of the chest and epigastrium, impeded respiration, nausea and vomiting.

Languor, relaxation of muscles, *nausea, vomiting and dyspepsia* are the general indications that point to the use of this remedy, in asthma and gastric affections. Best adapted to light complexioned, fleshy people. Bad effects of drunkeness. *Suppressed discharges* (*Sulph.*). Diphtheria. *Catarrhal jaundice* (*Chion.*).

**Head:** Vertigo and fear of death. Gastric headache with nausea. vomiting and great prostration; worse, afternoon till midnight; tobacco. Dull, heavy pain.

**Ears:** *Deafness due to suppressed discharges* or eczema. Shooting pain from the throat.

**Face:** Bathed in cold sweat. Sudden pallor.

**Mouth:** Profuse flow of saliva; acrid burning taste; *mercurial taste;* tenacious mucus, tongue coated white.

**Stomach:** Acidity, flatulence, shortness of breath after eating. Heartburn with profuse flow of saliva. *Extreme nausea and vomiting.* Morning sickness.

*Faintness and weakness in the epigastrium. Profuse salivation, with a good appetite.* Profuse sweat and prostration. Cannot bear the smell or taste of tobacco. Acrid, burning taste; acidity, with a contractive feeling in the pit of the stomach. Flatulence, shortness of breath after eating. Heartburn.

**Urinary:** Deep red color and copious red sediment.

**Respiratory:** *Dyspnea from constriction of the chest;* worse, any exertion. Sensation of pressure or weight on the chest; *better by walking rapidly.* Feels as if the heart would stop. Asthma; attacks, with weakness, felt in the pit of the stomach and preceded by *prickling* all over. Cramps, ringing cough, short breath, catch in the throat. Senile emphysema.

**Back:** Pain in the sacrum; cannot bear the slightest touch. Sits leaning forward.

**Skin:** Prickling, itching with intense nausea.

**Modalities:** *Worse*, tobacco, afternoon, slightest motion, cold, especially cold washing. *Better,* by rapid walking (chest pain), towards the evening and from warmth.

**Relationship:** Antidote: *Ip.*

Compare: *Tab., Ars., Ant-t., Verat., Rosa.*

*Lobelia syphilitica or coerulea* (gives a perfect picture of sneezing, influenza, involving the posterior nares, palate, and fauces. Very depressed. Pain in the forehead, over the eyes; pain and gas in the bowels, followed by copious watery stools with tenesmus and soreness of the anus. Pain in the knees. Prickling in soles. *Great oppression in the lower part of chest,* as if air could not reach there. *Pain in chest under the short ribs of left side.* Dry, hacking cough. Breathing difficult. Dull, aching pain over the root of nose. Eustachian catarrh. Pain in the posterior part of spleen).

*Lobelia erinus* (*malignant growths,* extremely rapid development; colloid cancer of the omentum; cork screw like pains in the abdomen; great dryness of the skin, nasal and buccal mucous membranes; distaste for brandy; dry, eczematous patches which can be covered by the finger tips. Malignant disease of the face. Epithelioma).

**Dose:** Tincture to thirtieth potency. Locally the tincture is antidotal to Poison oak. Often *Lobelia acetum* acts better than any other preparation. *Lob.* hypodermically acts clinically almost as precisely as the antitoxin of diphtheria does upon the infection and renders the system stronger to resist future infections (F. Ellingwood).

---

# LOBELIA PURPURASCENS

(Purple Lobelia) **Lob-p.**

Profound prostration of all the vital forces and of the nervous system; *respiratory paralysis. Nervous prostration of influenza.* Coma. Tongue white and paralyzed.

**Head:** Confused and depressed. Headache with nausea, vertigo; especially between the eyebrows. Cannot keep eyes open; spasmodic closure of lids (blepharospasm).

**Eyes:** Impossible to keep open. Drowsy.

**Chest:** Superficial respiration; heart and lungs feel paralyzed; respiration slow. Heart beats sound like booms of a drum to the patient.

**Relationship:** Compare: *Bapt., Lobelia cardinalis* (debility, especially of lower extremities; oppressed breathing, pleurisy, *sticking* pain in the chest on taking a long breath. Pain in the *left* lung, intermitting, pricking during the day).

**Dose:** Third potency.

---

# LOLEUM TEMULENTUM

(Darnel) **Lol.**

Has been used in cephalalgia, sciatica, paralysis. Prostration and restlessness.

**Head:** Anxious and depressed, confused. Vertigo; must close the eyes. Head heavy. Noises in the ears (tinnitus).

**Stomach:** Nausea, vomiting. Pain in the pit of the stomach and abdomen. Severe purging.

**Extremities:** Gait unsteady. *Trembling of all limbs* (chorea). Loss of power in extremities. *Violent pain in calves, as if bound with cords.* Cold extremities. Spasmodic motions of arms and legs. Cannot write; cannot hold a glass of water (Writer's cramp). Trembling of hands in paralysis.

**Relationship:** Compare: *Sec., Lath., Oxyt.*

**Dose:** Sixth potency.

---

# LONICERA XYLOSTEUM

(Fly-woodbine) **Lon-x.**

Convulsive symptoms. Uremic convulsions. Albuminuria. Syphilis.

**Head:** Congestion of the head and chest; coma. Contraction of one pupil and dilatation of the other. Sopor, eyes half open, red face.

**Extremities:** Jerking of limbs. Trembling of the whole body. Violent convulsions. Limbs and head fall over as if paralyzed. Extremities cold. Cold perspiration.

**Relationship:** Compare: *Lonicera periclymenum*—Honey suckle (irritability of temper, with violent outbursts). *Croc.*

**Dose:** Third to sixth potency.

---

# LUPULUS HUMULUS

(Hops) **Lup.**

Is a good remedy in unstrung conditions of the nervous system attended with nausea, dizziness, headache following a night's debauch. *Infantile jaundice.* Urethral burning. Drawing and twitching in almost every muscle. Nervous tremors; wakefulness and delirium of drunkards. *Giddiness* and *stupefaction. Slow* pulse. Perspiration profuse, clammy, greasy.

**Head:** Morbid vigilance. Highly excited. Dull, heavy headache with dizziness. Drawing and twitching in every muscle.

**Male:** Painful erections. Emissions, *depending on sexual weakness and after onanism.* Spermatorrhea.

**Sleep:** *Drowsy* during the day, Sopor.

**Skin:** Scarlatina-like eruption on the face. Sensation of insects crawling under the skin; feels chapped, skin peels.

**Relationship:** Antidotes: *Coff., Vinegar.*

Compare: *Nux-v., Urt-u., Cann-i.*

**Dose:** Tincture to third potency. *Lupulinum* lx trituration (best in seminal emissions. Locally in painful cancers).

---

# LYCOPERSICUM ESCULENTUM

(Solanum Lycopersicum, Tomato) **Lycpr.**

Marked symptoms of rheumatism and influenza. Severe aching pains all over the body. *Pains after influenza.* Head always shows signs of acute congestion. Hay fever with marked aggravation from breathing the least dust. Frequent micturition and profuse watery diarrhea.

**Head:** Bursting pain, beginning in the occiput and spreading all over. The entire head and scalp feels sore, bruised, after the pain has ceased.

**Eyes:** Dull, heavy; pupils contracted; eyeballs feel contracted; aching in and around the eyes. Eyes suffused.

**Nose:** Profuse, watery coryza; drops down the throat. Itching in the anterior chamber; worse, breathing any dust; better, indoors.

**Urinary:** Constant dribbling *in open air.* Must get up at night to micturate.

**Respiratory:** Voice husky. Pain in the chest, extending to the head. Hoarseness; constant desire to clear the throat. Expulsive cough, deep and harsh. Chest oppressed; dry, hacking cough coming on at night and keeping one awake.

**Heart:** Decided decrease in pulse rate with anxiety and apprehensiveness.

**Extremities:** Aching throughout the back. Dull pain in the lumbar region. *Sharp pain in the right deltoid and pectoral muscles.* Pain deep in the middle of the right arm. Rheumatic pains in the right elbow and wrist, and both the hands. Intense aching in the lower limbs. Right crural neuralgia. Tingling along the right ulnar nerve.

**Modalities:** *Worse,* right side, open air, continuous motion, jars, noises. *Better,* warm room, tobacco.

**Relationship:** Compare: *Bell.* (follows well); *Eup-per., Rhus-t., Sang., Caps.*

**Dose:** Third to thirtieth potency.

---

# LYCOPODIUM CLAVATUM

(Club Moss) **Lyc.**

This drug is inert until the spores are crushed. Its wonderful medicinal properties are only disclosed by trituration and succussion.

In nearly all the cases where *Lyc.* is indicated, evidence of urinary or digestive disturbance will be found. It corresponds to Grauvogl's carbo-nitrogenoid constitution, the non-eliminative lithemic. *Lyc.* is especially adapted to ailments developing gradually, functional power weakens, failure of the digestive powers, when the liver function is seriously disturbed. *Atony. Malnutrition.* Mild temperaments of lymphatic constitution with catarrhal tendencies; older people, with an earthy complexion, uric acid diathesis, skin shows yellowish spots, etc., also precocious, weak children. Symptoms characteristically run from *right to left,* acts especially on *the right* side of the body and are worse from about 4 to 8 p. m. In kidney affections, *red sand in urine,* backache in the renal region; worse before micturition. Intolerant of cold drinks; *craves everything warm.* Best adapted to intellectually keen people, but of weak, muscular power. Deep seated, progressive, chronic diseases. Carcinoma. *Emaciation.* Debility in the morning. Marked regulating influence upon the glandular (sebaceous) secretions. *Pre-senility.* Ascites in liver disease. *Lyc.* patient is thin, withered, full of gas and dry. Lacks vital heat; has poor circulation, cold extremities. Pains come and go suddenly. Sensitive to noise and odors.

**Mind:** *Melancholy; afraid to be alone.* Little things annoy. Extremely sensitive. Averse to undertaking new things. Headstrong and haughty when sick. Loss of self confidence. Hurried when eating. Constant fear of breaking down under stress. *Apprehensive.* Weak memory, confused thoughts; *spells or writes wrong words* and syllables. Failing brain power (*Anac., Phos., Bar-c.*). Cannot bear to see anything new. Cannot read what he writes. Sadness in the morning on awaking.

**Head:** Shakes head without any apparent cause. Twists face and mouth. Pressing headache on the vertex; worse from 4 to 8 p. m. and from lying down or stooping, if not eating regularly (*Cact.*). Throbbing headache after every paroxysm of cough. Headaches over the eyes in severe colds; *better, uncovering* (*Sulph.*). Vertigo in the morning on rising. Pain in the temples, as if they were screwed together. Tearing pain in the occiput; better, fresh air. Severe hairfall. Eczema; moist oozing behind the ears. Deep furrows on the forehead. Premature baldness and gray hair.

**Eyes:** Styes on the lids near the inner canthus. Day blindness (hemeralopia) (*Both.*). Night blindness (nyctalopia) more characteristic. Sees only one-half of an object (hemiopia). Ulceration and redness of the lids (blepharitis). Eyes half open during sleep.

**Ears:** Thick, yellow, offensive discharge. Eczema around and behind the ears. Otorrhea and deafness with or without tinnitus; after scarlatina. *Humming and roaring with hardness of hearing;* every noise causes a peculiar echo in the ear.

**Nose:** Sense of smell very acute. Sensation of dryness posteriorly. Scanty, excoriating discharge anteriorly. Ulcerated nostrils. Crusts and elastic plugs (*Kali-bi., Teucr.*). Fluent coryza. *Nose stopped up.* Snuffles; child starts from sleep rubbing nose. *Fan-like motion of alae nasi* (*Kali-br., Phos.*).

**Face:** Grayish-yellow discoloration of the face, with blue circles around the eyes. Withered, shrivelled and emaciated; copper colored eruption. *Dropping of lower jaw,* in typhoid fever (*Lach., Op.*). Itching; scaly herpes on the face and corner of mouth.

**Mouth:** Teeth excessively painful to touch. Toothache, with swelling of cheeks; relieved by warm application. Dryness of mouth and tongue, without thirst. Tongue dry, black, cracked, swollen; oscillates to and fro. Mouth waters. *Blisters on the tongue.* Halitosis.

**Throat:** Dryness of the throat, without thirst. Food and drink regurgitates through the nose. Inflammation of the throat, with stitches on swallowing; *better, warm drinks.* Swelling and suppuration of tonsils. Ulceration of tonsils, *beginning on the right side.* Diphtheria; *deposits spread from right to left; worse, cold drinks.* Ulceration of vocal bands. Tubercular laryngitis, especially when ulceration commences.

**Stomach:** Dyspepsia due to farinaceous and fermentable food, cabbage, beans, etc. Excessive hunger. Aversion to bread, etc. Desire for sweet things. *Food tastes sour.* Sour eructations. Great weakness of digestion. Bulimia, with much bloating. After eating, pressure in the stomach, with bitter taste in mouth. *Eating ever so little creates fullness.* Cannot eat oysters. Rolling of flatulence (*Chin., Carb-v.*). Wakes up at night feeling hungry. Hiccough. *Incomplete, burning eructations rise only up to the pharynx, where they burn for hours.* Likes to take the hot food and drink. Sinking sensation; worse night.

**Abdomen:** Immediately after a light meal, abdomen is *bloated, full.* Constant sense of fermentation in the abdomen, like yeast; upper left side. Hernia, right side. Liver sensitive. Brown spots on the abdomen. Dropsy, due to hepatic disease. Hepatitis, atrophic form of nutmeg liver. Pain shooting across the lower abdomen, from right to left.

**Rectum:** Diarrhea. Inactive intestinal canal. Ineffectual urging. Stool *hard, difficult, small,* incomplete. *Hemorrhoids; very painful to touch, aching* (*Mur-ac.*).

**Urinary:** Pain in the back before micturating; ceases after flow; *slow in coming, must strain.* Retention. *Polyuria at night. Heavy red sediment.* Child cries before micturating (*Borx.*).

**Male:** No erectile power; *impotence.* Premature emission (*Calad., Sel., Agn.*). Enlarged prostate. Condylomata.

**Female:** Menses too late; last too long, too profuse. Vagina dry. Coition painful. Pain in the right ovarian region. Varicose veins of pudenda. Leucorrhea, acrid, with burning in the vagina. Discharge of blood from genitals during stool.

**Respiratory:** Tickling cough. Dyspnea. Tensive, constrictive, burning pain in the chest. Cough worse going down hill. Cough deep, hollow (whooping cough). Expectoration gray, thick, bloody, purulent, *salty* (*Ars., Phos., Puls.*). Nocturnal cough, tickling as from sulphur fumes. Catarrh of the chest in infants, seems full of mucus, rattling. Neglected pneumonia with great dyspnea, flaying of alae nasi and presence of mucus rales.

**Heart:** *Aneurism* (*Bar-c.*). Aortic disease. Palpitations at night. Cannot lie on the left side.

**Back:** *Burning* between scapulae as if from hot coals. Pain in the small of back (lumbosacral region).

**Extremities:** Numbness, also drawing and tearing in limbs (sciatica), especially when at rest or at night. Heaviness of arms. Tearing in the shoulder and elbow joints. Chronic gout, with chalky deposits in the joints. Profuse foot sweat. Pain in the heels on treading, as if from a pebble. Painful callosities (corns) on the soles; toes and fingers contracted. *Sciatica, worse right side. Cannot lie on the painful side.* Hands and feet numb. Right foot hot, left cold. Cramps in calves and toes at night in bed. Limbs go to sleep. Twitching and jerking (locomotor ataxia).

**Sleep:** Drowsy during the day. Starting in sleep. Dreams of accidents.

**Fever:** Chill between 3 and 4 p. m., followed by sweat. Icy coldness. Feels as if lying on ice. One chill is followed by another (*Calc., Sil., Hep.*).

**Skin:** Ulcerates. Abscesses beneath the skin; worse warm applications. Hives; worse, warmth. Violent itching; fissured eruptions (rhagades). *Acne.* Chronic eczema associated with urinary, gastric and hepatic disorders; bleeds easily. Skin becomes thick and indurated. Varicose veins, nevi, erectile tumors. Brown spots, freckles worse on left side of face and nose. *Dry* shrunken, especially palms; hair becomes prematurely gray. Dropsies. Offensive secretions; *viscid and offensive perspiration,* especially of feet and axilla. Psoriasis.

**Modalities:** *Worse,* right side, from right to left, from above downward, 4 to 8 p. m., from heat or in a warm room, hot air, bed. Warm applications, except throat and stomach which are better from warm drinks. *Better,* by *motion,* after midnight, from warm food and drink, on getting cold, from being uncovered.

**Relationship:** Complementary: *Lyc.* acts with special benefit *after Calc.* and *Sulph. Iod., Graph., Lach., Chel.*

Antidotes: *Camph., Puls., Caust.*

Compare: Carbo-nitrogenoid constitution: *Sulph., Rhus-t., Urt-u., Merc., Hep. Alum.* (*Lyc.* is the only vegetable that takes up aluminum. T. F. Allen). *Ant-c., Nat-m., Bry., Nux-v., Both.* (day blindness; can scarcely see after sunrise;

pain in the right great toe (gout). *Plumbago littoralis*—A Brazilian plant (costive with red urine, pain in kidneys, joints and the body generally; milky saliva, ulcerated mouth). *Hydr.* follows *Lyc.* in indigestion.

**Dose:** Both the lower and the highest potencies are credited with excellent results. For purposes of aiding elimination, the second and third attenuation of the tincture, a few drops, 3 times a day, have proved efficacious, otherwise the 6th to 200th potency and higher, in not too frequent doses.

---

## LYCOPUS VIRGINICUS

(Bugle-weed) **Lycps-v.**

Lowers the blood pressure, reduces the heart rate and increases the length of systole to a great degree. Passive hemorrhages (*Adren.* 6x).

A heart remedy and of use in exophthalmic goitre and hemorrhoidal bleeding. Indicated in diseases with tumultuous action of the heart and more or less pain. *Hemoptysis due to valvular heart disease.* Beneficial in toxic goitre used in the pre-operative stage. Dose, 5 drops of tincture (Beebe).

**Head:** Frontal headache; worse, frontal eminences; often succeeded by a labored heart. Epistaxis (due to high blood pressure).

**Eyes:** Protrusion, pressing, outward, with tumultuous action of heart (exophthalmos). Supraorbital pain, with aching in the testicles.

**Mouth:** Toothache in the lower molars.

**Rectum:** Bleeding from the rectum. Hemorrhoids.

**Urinary:** Profuse flow of limpid, watery urine, especially when the heart is very irritable; also scanty urine (Bright's disease). Bladder feels distended when empty. Diabetes. *Pain in the testicles.*

**Respiratory:** Wheezing. Cough with *hemoptysis* (phthisis), bleeding small but frequent.

**Heart:** Rapid heart action in smokers. Precordial pain; constriction, tenderness, pulse, weak, irregular, intermittent, tremulous, rapid. Cyanosis. Heart's action tumultuous and forcible. Palpitations from nervous irritation, with oppression around the heart. Rheumatoid, flying pains, associated with heart disease. Cardiac asthma (*Sumb.*).

**Sleep:** Wakefulness and morbid vigilance with inordinately active, but weak circulation.

**Relationship:** Compare: *Ephedra vulgaris*—Teamster's tea (in exophthalmic goitre; eyes feel pushed out with *tumultuous* action of heart); *Fuc., Spartin-s., Crat., Adren.* 6x.

**Dose:** First to thirtieth potency.

# LYSSINUM

(Hydrophobinum—Saliva of a Rabid Dog) **Lyss.**

Affects principally on the nervous system; aching in bones. Complaints from abnormal sexual desire. Convulsions brought on by dazzling light or sight of running water (hydrophobia).

**Head:** Lyssophobia; fear of becoming mad. Emotion and bad news aggravates; also, thinking of fluids. *Hypersensitiveness of all senses.* Chronic headache. Boring pain in forehead.

**Mouth:** Constant spitting; saliva tough, viscid. Sore throat; constant desire to swallow, which is difficult; gagging when swallowing water. Froth in the mouth.

**Rectum:** Desire for stool on hearing or seeing running water. Profuse, watery stools, with pain in the bowels; worse, evening.

**Urinary:** Constant desire to micturate on seeing running water.

**Male:** Lascivious; priapism with frequent emissions. No emission during coition. Atrophy of testicles. Complaints from abnormal sexual desire.

**Female:** Uterine sensitiveness; conscious of womb (*Helon.*). Feels prolapsed. Vagina sensitive, rendering coition painful (dysparunia). (*Berb.*). Uterine displacements.

**Respiratory:** Voice altered in tone. Breathing held for some time. Spasmodic contraction of respiratory muscles.

**Modalities:** *Worse*, sight or sound of running water or pouring water, or even thinking of fluids; dazzling or reflected light; heat of sun; stooping.

**Relationship:** Compare: *Xanthium spinosum*—Cockle (said to be specific for hydrophobia and is recommended for chronic cystitis in women). *Canth.*, *Bell.*, *Stram.*, *Lach.*, *Nat-m.*

**Dose:** Thirtieth potency

---

# MAGNESIUM CARBONICUM

(Carbonate of Magnesia) **Mag-c.**

Gastro-intestinal catarrh with marked acidity. Often used with advantage for complaints arising in people who have been taking this drug to sweeten the stomach. Is frequently indicated in children; whole body smells sour, and is disposed to boils. Broken down, "worn out" women, with uterine and climacteric disorders. With numbness and distention in various parts and nervous prostration. Sensitive to the least start, noise, touch, etc. Affections of the antrum of Highmore. Effects of shock, blows, mental distress. Sensation of numbness; nerve prostration; tendency to constipation after nervous strain; *sensitive to least touch,* it causes starting. Sensitive to cold winds or weather or from excess of care and worry with constipation and heaviness. Intense neuralgic pains.

**Head:** Sticking pain in the side of the head on which he lies, as if the hair was pulled; worse, mental exertion. Itching of scalp worse in damp weather. Pain above the margin of right orbit. Black motes before the eyes.

**Ears:** Diminished hearing. Deafness; comes suddenly and varies. Numbness of the outer ear. Feeling of distention in the middle ear. Subdued tinnitus.

**Face:** Tearing pain on one side; worse, quiet; must move about. Toothache, especially during pregnancy; worse at night; worse, cold and quiet. Teeth feel too long. Ailments from cutting wisdom teeth (*Cheir.*). Pain in the malar bone, worse during rest, night. Swelling of the malar bone with pulsating pain, worse exposure to cold wind.

**Mouth:** Dry at night. Sour taste. Vesicular eruption; bloody saliva. Sticking pain in the throat; hawking up of fetid, pea colored particles.

**Stomach:** Desire for fruit, acids and vegetables. Eructations *sour, and vomiting of bitter water.* Craving for meat.

**Abdomen:** Rumbling, gurgling. Dragging towards the pelvis. *Very heavy;* contractive, pinching pains in the right iliac region.

**Stool:** Preceded by griping, colicky pain. *Green, watery, frothy, like a frog pond's scum.* Bloody mucus with stools (dysentery). *Milk passes undigested in nursing children. Sour,* with tenesmus (*Rheum*). Constipation after mental shock or severe nervous strain.

**Female:** *Sore throat before menses appear.* Before menses, coryza and nasal obstruction. Menses too *late and scanty,* thick, dark, like pitch; mucoid leucorrhea. Menstrual flow only during sleep; more profuse at night (*Am-m.*), or when lying down; ceases when walking.

**Respiratory:** Tickling cough, with *salty,* bloody expectoration (hemoptysis). Constrictive pains in the chest with dyspnea. Soreness in the chest during motion.

**Extremities:** Tearing in shoulders as if dislocated. Right shoulder painful, cannot raise it (*Sang.*). The entire body feels tired and painful, especially legs and feet. Swelling in the bend of knee.

**Sleep:** Unrefreshing; more tired on rising than on retiring.

**Fever:** Chilly in the evening. Fever at night. Sour, greasy perspiration.

**Skin:** Earthy, sallow and parchment-like; emaciation. Itching vesicles on hands and fingers. Nodosities under the skin. Sore; sensitive to cold.

**Modalities:** Worse, warmth of bed; change of temperature; cold wind or weather; every *three weeks;* rest. *Better,* warm air; walking in open air.

**Relationship:** Antidotes: *Ars., Merc.*

Complementary: *Cham.*

Compare: *Rheum, Kreos., Aloe, Cheiranthus cheiri*—Wall flower (deafness, otorrhea, nose stopped up at night *from irritation of cutting wisdom teeth*).

**Dose:** Third to thirtieth potency.

---

# MAGNESIUM MURIATICUM

(Muriate of Magnesia) **Mag-m.**

A liver remedy with pronounced characteristic constipation. Chronic liver affections with tenderness and pain, extending to the spine and epigastrium, worse after food. Especially adapted in diseases of women, with a long history of indigestion and uterine disease; children who cannot digest milk. Evil effects of sea bathing.

**Head:** Sensitive to noise; bursting headache; worse, motion, open air; better, pressure, and wrapping up warmly (*Sil., Stront-c.*). Profuse perspiration on the head (*Calc., Sil.*).

**Nose:** Nostrils ulcerated (ozena). Coryza. Nose stopped and fluent. *Loss of smell and taste,* following catarrh. Cannot lie down. Must breathe through the mouth.

**Face:** Neuralgic pains, dull, aching, worse damp weather, slightest draft, better pressure, heat.

**Mouth:** Blisters on lips. Gums swollen, bleed easily (scorbutic). Tongue feels burnt and scalded. Throat dry, with hoarseness.

**Stomach:** Appetite poor, bad taste in the mouth. Eructations like rotten eggs. Continuous rising of a white froth in the mouth. *Cannot digest milk.* Urine can be passed only by pressing the abdominal muscles.

**Abdomen:** Pressing pain in the liver; worse lying on the right side. *Liver enlarged* (hepatomegaly) *with bloating of the abdomen;* yellow tongue. Congenital scrotal hernia. Must use abdominal muscles to enable him to micturate.

**Stool:** Constipation in infants during dentition; only passing a small quantity; *stools knotty,* like sheep's dung, *crumbling at the verge of anus.* Painful, smarting hemorrhoids.

**Urinary:** Urine difficult to void. Bladder can only be emptied by straining and pressure.

**Female:** Menses black, clotted. Pain in the back and thighs. Metrorrhagia; worse at night. Great excitement at every period. Leucorrhea with every stool and after exercise. Tinea ciliaris, eruptions on the face and forehead worse before menses.

**Respiratory:** Spasmodic dry cough; worse in the first part of night, with burning and a sore chest.

**Heart:** Palpitations and cardiac pain *while sitting* (angina pectoris)*; better by moving around* (*Gels.*). Functional cardiac affections *with hepatomegaly.*

**Extremities:** Pain in the back and hips; in arms and legs. Arms "go to sleep" when waking in the morning.

**Sleep:** Sleep during day; restless at night on account of heat and shock; anxious dreams.

**Modalities:** *Worse,* immediately after eating, lying on the right side; *from sea bathing. Better,* from pressure, motion; open air, except headache.

**Relationship:** Antidotes: *Camph., Cham.*

Compare: *Nat-m., Puls., Sep., Am-m., Nasturtium aquaticum*—Water-cress (useful in scorbutic affections and constipation, related to strictures of the urinary apparatus; supposed to be aphrodisiacal in its action. Is also antidotal to tobacco narcosis and is a sedative in neurotic affections, neurasthenia, hysteria. Cirrhosis of liver and dropsy).

**Dose:** 5 drops of tincture. Third to 200th potency.

---

## MAGNESIUM PHOSPHORICUM

(Phosphate of Magnesia) **Mag-p.**

The great anti-spasmodic remedy. Cramping of muscles with radiating pains. Neuralgic pains *relieved by warmth.* Especially suited to tired, languid, exhausted subjects. Indisposition for mental exertion. Goitre.

**Mind:** Laments all the time about pain. Inability to think clearly. Sleepless on account of indigestion.

**Head:** Vertigo on moving, falls forward on closing the eyes, better walking in open air. Aches after mental labor, with chilliness; always better by warmth (*Sil.*). Sensation as if the contents of the skull were liquid, as if the parts of brain were changing places or as of a cap was on the head.

**Eyes:** Supraorbital pains; worse, right side; relieved by warmth applied externally. Increased lachrymation. Twitching of lids. Nystagmus, strabismus, ptosis. Eyes hot, tired, vision blurred, colored lights before eyes.

**Ears:** *Severe neuralgic pain;* worse behind the right ear; worse, by going into cold air, and *washing face and neck with cold water.*

**Mouth:** *Toothache; better by heat and hot liquids.* Ulceration of teeth (caries), with swelling of the glands on the face, throat and neck, *and swelling* of tongue (glossitis). *Complaints in teething children.* Spasms without febrile symptoms.

**Throat:** Soreness and stiffness, especially on the right side; parts seem puffy, *with chilliness,* and aching all over.

**Stomach:** Hiccough, with retching day and night. Thirst for very cold drinks.

**Abdomen:** *Enteralgia,* relieved by pressure. *Flatulent colic, forcing the patient to bend double; relieved by rubbing, warmth, pressure; accompanied with belching of gas, which gives no relief. Bloated, full sensation in the abdomen; must loosen the clothing, walk about, and constantly pass flatus.* Constipation in rheumatic subjects due to flatulence and indigestion.

**Female:** *Menstrual colic. Membranous dysmenorrhea.* Menses too early, dark, stringy. Swelling of external parts. Ovarian neuralgia. Vaginismus.

**Respiratory:** Asthmatic oppression of the chest. Dry, tickling cough. *Spasmodic cough,* with difficulty in lying down. *Whooping cough* (*Cor-r.*). Voice hoarse, larynx sore and raw. Intercostal neuralgia.

**Heart:** *Angina pectoris.* Nervous spasmodic palpitation. Constricting pains around the heart.

**Extremities:** Involuntary shaking of hands. Paralysis agitans. Cramps in calves. Sciatica; feet very tender. Darting pains. Twitchings. *Chorea.* Writer's and player's cramp. Tetanic spasms. Weakness in arms and hands, finger tips stiff and numb. General muscular weakness.

**Fever:** *Chilliness* after dinner, in the evening. *Chills run up and down the back, with shivering,* followed by a suffocating sensation.

**Modalities:** *Worse,* right side, cold, touch, night. *Better,* warmth, bending double, pressure, friction.

**Relationship:** Compare: *Kali-p., Coloc., Sil., Zinc., Dios.*

Antidotes: *Bell., Gels., Lach.*

**Dose:** First to twelfth potency. Sometimes the highest potencies are preferable. Acts especially well, when given in hot water.

---

## MAGNESIUM SULPHURICUM

(Epsom Salt) **Mag-s.**

The skin, *urinary* and female symptoms are most marked. The purgative action of the Sulphate of Magnesia is not a quality of the drug, but a quality of its physical state, which renders its absorption impossible. The properties inherent in the substance itself can only be discovered by attenuation (Percy Wilde).

**Head:** Apprehensive; vertigo; head heavy during menses. Eyes burn, noises in ears (tinnitus).

**Stomach:** Frequent eructations, tasting like bad eggs. Rising of water in the mouth (waterbrash).

**Urinary:** Stitches and burning in the orifice of the urethra after micturating (urethritis). Stream intermits and dribbles. Urine passed in the morning is copious, bright yellow, it soon becomes turbid, and deposits a copious red sediment. Urine is greenish when passed; is of a clear color, and in a large quantity. Diabetes (*Ph-ac., Lac-ac., Ars-br.*).

**Female:** Thick leucorrhea, as profuse as menses, with weary pain in the lumbosacral region and thighs, on moving about. Bleeding between menses (metrorrhagia). Menses return after fourteen days; the discharge is thick, black, and profuse. Menses too early, intermits.

**Back:** Bruised and ulcerative pain between the shoulders, with the sensation of a lump, as large as the fist, on account of which she cannot lie upon her back or side; relieved by rubbing. Violent pain in the lumbosacral region, as if bruised, and as before menstruation.

**Extremities:** The left arm and foot fall asleep in bed, in the morning after waking.

**Fever:** Chills from 9 to 10 a. m. Shuddering in the back; heat in one part and chill in another.

**Skin:** Small pimples over the whole body, that itch violently. Suppressed itch (*Sulph.*). Crawling in the tips of the fingers of the left hand; better on rubbing. *Warts.* Eyrsipelas (applied locally as a saturated solution). Dropsy (physiological doses).

**Relationship:** It is claimed that the addition of a small amount of *Mag-s.* to the usual hypodermic of morphine increases the value of the hypodermic from 50 to 100%.

**Physiologic Dosage:** *Mag-s.* is of diagnostic and therapeutic value in gallstone colic. From 2 to 4 teaspoonfuls in a glass of hot water taken at the onset of a colicky attack may abort or stop the colic.

Epsom salt is one of the most active saline cathartics, operating with little pain or nausea, especially if pure. It has but little, if any effect on intestinal peristalsis, its action causes a rush of fluid into the intestines, which by producing a distention of the bowel produces evacuation. It causes little or no irritation in the intestine. In common with the other salines, it is the classical evacuant to be employed in connection with mercurials and antihelmintics and in cases of poisoning. Epsom salt usually acts within one or two hours, acts faster if taken in hot water and in the morning before breakfast. The ordinary dose as a mild laxative is a heaping teaspoonful; as a cathartic, two to four teaspoonfuls. The taste may be improved, if necessary, by the addition of a little lemon juice and sugar.

Besides its chief use as a saline cathartic, magnesium sulphate is used to a considerable extent externally in saturated solution as an antiphlogistic and antipruritic in erysipelas, ivy poisoning, cellulitis and other local inflammations. Use as a compress saturated with the solution.

**Dose:** The pure salt to the third potency. Locally 1:4 in water in septic conditions, erysipelas, orchitis, boils, etc.

---

## MAGNOLIA GRANDIFLORA

(Magnolia) **Magn-gr.**

Rheumatism and cardiac lesions are prominent features in the symptomatology of this drug. *Stiffness* and soreness. Alternating pains between spleen and heart. Patient is tired and stiff. Soreness when quiet. Erratic, shifting of pains.

**Heart:** Oppression of the chest with an inability to expand the lungs. Sensation of a large bolus of food which distresses the stomach. Sensation of suffocation when walking fast or when lying on the left side. Dyspnea. Crampy pains in the heart. Angina pectoris. Endocarditis and pericarditis. Tendency to faint. *Sensation as if the heart had stopped beating.* Pain around the heart accompanied by itching in the feet.

**Extremities:** Stiffness and sharp erratic pains; worse in joints. *Feet itch.* Numbness in the left arm. Rheumatic pain in clavicles. Shooting in all limbs.

**Modalities:** *Worse,* damp air, lying on the left side; in the morning, on first rising. *Better,* dry weather, motion; intermenstrual flow (*Ham., Bov., Bell., Elaps*).

**Relationship:** Compare: *Rhus-t., Dulc., Aur.*

**Dose:** Third potency.

---

## MALANDRINUM

(Grease in Horses) **Maland.**

A very effectual protection against smallpox. Ill effects of vaccination (*Thuj., Sil.*). Efficacious in clearing of the remnants of cancerous deposits (Cooper).

**Skin:** Scab on the upper lip, with stinging pain when torn off. Aching in the forehead. *Dry, scaly; itching; rhagades of hands and feet in cold weather and from washing.* Toes feel scalded and itch terribly. Bone like protuberances (exostosis).

**Dose:** Thirtieth potency and highest.

---

## MANCINELLA

(Hippomane—Manganeel Apple) **Manc.**

Skin symptoms are most marked. Dermatitis with excessive vesiculation, oozing of a sticky serum and formation of crusts. To be remembered in mentally depressed states at puberty and at climacteric, with exalted sexuality (Hering). *Loss of vision.* Pain in the thumb.

**Mind:** Silent mood, sadness. Wandering thoughts. *Sudden vanishing of thoughts.* Bashful. *Fear of becoming insane.*

**Head:** Vertigo; head feels light, empty. Scalp itches. Hair falls out after an acute sickness.

**Nose:** Illusions of smell, of gunpowder, dung, etc. Pressure at the root of the nose.

**Mouth:** Feels peppery. Copious, offensive saliva. Taste of blood. Burning of fauces. Dysphagia from constriction of the throat and esophagus.

**Stomach:** Continuous choking sensation rising from the stomach. Vomiting of ingesta, followed by griping and copious stools. Burning pains and black vomit (hematemesis).

**Extremities:** Icy cold hands and feet. Pain in the thumb.

**Skin:** Intense erythema. *Vesicles.* Fungoid growths. Erysipelas. *Large blisters, as from scalds.* Heavy, brown crusts and scabs. *Pemphigus.*

**Relationship:** Compare: *Crot-t., Jatr-c., Canth., Anac.*

**Dose:** Sixth to thirtieth potency.

---

## MANGANUM ACETICUM

(Manganese Acetate) **Mang-act.**

*Mang-act.* causes anemia with destruction of the red corpuscles. Jaundice, nephritis with albuminuria. Fatty degeneration of the liver. Paralysis agitans. *Cellulitis,* subacute stage, promotes suppuration and hastens regeneration.

Symptoms of chronic poisoning, according to Professor von Jaksch, were involuntary laughter, involuntary weeping and walking backwards. Strongly exaggerated reflexes and physical disturbances, evidenced by men making fun of each other's gait. Paraplegia progressive; wasting, feeble and staggering gait.

Inflammation of bones (osteomyelitis) or joints (arthritis), with nocturnal digging pains. Asthmatic people who cannot lie on a feather pillow. Syphilitic and chlorotic patients with general anemia and paralytic symptoms are often benefitted by this drug. Gout. Chronic arthritis. For speakers and singers. Great accumulation of mucus. Growing pains and weak ankles. General soreness and aching; every part of the body feels sore when touched; early stage of tuberculosis.

**Head:** Anxiety and fear; *better lying down.* Feels large and heavy, with rush of blood; pain from above downward. Field of vision contracted. Stolidy, mask-like face.

**Ears:** Feel stopped; cracking on blowing the nose. *Pain from other parts extends to the ears.*Deafness in *damp weather.* Whistling tinnitus.

**Nose:** Dry, obstructed. Chronic catarrh, with epistaxis, dryness; *worse in cold damp weather.*

**Mouth:** Nodes on palate. Toothache; *worse,* anything cold (*Coff.* opposite). Hemming all the time. Low, monotonous voice. Tongue sore and irritable with ulcers (apthae) or warts.

**Abdomen:** Flatulence; chronic hepatomegaly (jaundice).

**Female:** Derangements of menstruation, amenorrhea; menses too early and scanty, in anemic subjects. *Flushes of heat at climacteric.*

**Respiratory:** *Chronic hoarseness.* Larynx dry, rough, constricted. Tuberculosis of the larynx. Cough; worse evening, and *better lying down* and worse in damp weather. Mucus difficult to loosen. Stitches in the larynx extending to the ear. Heat in the chest. Hemoptysis. *Every cold rouses up a bronchitis* (*Dulc.*).

**Extremities:** Muscular twitching. Cramps in calves. Stiffness in muscles of legs. Inflammation of bones and joints with insupportable nocturnal digging pains. *Every part of body feels sore when touched.* Cannot walk backwards without falling. *Tendancy to fall forward. Walks stooping forward.* Legs feel numb. Wilson's disease. Paralysis agitans. Peculiar slapping gait, walks on the metatarso-phalangeal joint (locomotor ataxia); walks backwards. Ankles painful. Bones very sensitive. Shiny red swelling of joints. *Knees pain* and itch. Rheumatism of feet. Intolerable pain in the skin of the lower limbs. Burning spots around the joints. Periosteal inflammation (periostitis). Suppuration of skin around the joints.

**Sleep:** Languor and sleepiness. Vivid dreams. Sleepy very early in the evening.

**Skin:** Suppuration of skin around joints. Red, elevated spots. *Itching;* better, scratching. Deep cracks in bends of elbows, etc. Psoriasis and pityriasis. Burning around ulcers. *Chronic eczema* associated with amenorrhea, worse at menstrual period or at menopause.

**Modalities:** *Worse,* cold wet weather, change of weather. *Better,* lying down (cough).

**Relationship:** Compare: *Colloidal Manganese* (boils and other staphylococcal infections); *Manganum muriaticum* (painful ankles, bone-pains); *Manganum oxydatum* (pain in the tibia, dysmenorrhea, colic and diarrhea. Easily fatigued and heated; sleepy. Stolid, mask like face; low monotonous voice, "economical speech." Muscular twitching (chorea), cramps in calves; stiff leg muscles; occasional uncontrollable laughter. Peculiar slapping gait. Symptoms similar to paraylsis agitans, progressive lenticular degenerations and pseudo-sclerosis. Workers in *Manganum binoxide* are frequently affected with bulbar paralysis. Use 3x homoeopathically). *Manganum sulphuricum* (liver affections, excess of bile; a powerful intestinal stimulant); *Arg-met., Rhus-t., Sulph.*

Antidotes: *Coff., Merc.*

**Dose:** Third to thirtieth potency.

---

# MANGIFERA INDICA

(Mango Tree) **Mangi.**

One of the best general remedies for passive hemorrhages, uterine, renal, gastric, pulmonary and intestinal. Rhinitis, sneezing, pharyngitis, and other acute throat problems, suffocative sensation, as if the throat would close. Relaxation of the mucous membranes of the alimentary canal. Catarrhal and serous discharges, chronic intestinal irritation. Varicose veins. Drowsiness. Atonic conditions, poor circulation, relaxed muscles.

**Skin:** Itching of palms. Skin as if sunburnt, swollen. White spots, intense itching. Lobes of ears and lips swollen.

**Relationship**: Compare: *Erig., Epil.*

**Dose:** Tincture.

---

# MEDORRHINUM

(The Gonorrheal Virus) **Med.**

A powerful and deep acting medicine, often indicated for chronic ailments due to suppressed gonorrhea. For women with chronic pelvic disorders. Chronic *rheumatism*. Great disturbance and irritability of nervous system. Pain intolerable, tensive; nerves quiver and tingle. Children dwarfed and stunted. Chronic catarrhal conditions in children. Nose dirty, tonsils enlarged, thick yellow mucus from the nostrils; lips thickened due to breathing from the mouth. State of collapse and *trembling all over.* History of sycosis. Often restores a gonorrheal discharge. Intensity of all sensations. Edema of limbs; dropsy of serous sacs. Disseminated sclerosis.

**Mind:** Weak memory. Looses the thread of conversation. Cannot speak without weeping. *Time passes too slowly* (*Cann-i., Arg-n.*). Is in a great hurry. Hopeless of recovery. Difficult concentration. Fears of going insane (*Manc.*). Sensibility exalted. Nervous, restless. Fear in the dark, sensation as if some one behind her. Melancholy with suicidal thoughts.

**Head:** Burning pain in the brain; worse, occiput. Head heavy and drawn backward (epilepsy). Headache from jarring of cars, exhaustion, or hard work. Weight and pressure in the vertex. Hair dry, crisp. Itching of scalp; dandruff.

**Eyes:** Feels *as if she stared* at everything. Eyeballs ache. Sensation of sticks in the eyes. Lids irritated (blepharitis).

**Ears:** Partial deafness, pulsations in the ears. Quick, darting pains in the right ear.

**Nose:** Intense itching. Coldness of the tip. Posterior nares obstructed. Chronic nasal and pharyngeal catarrh.

**Face:** Pallor, acne, blotches of a reddish color. *Small boils* break out during menses.

**Mouth:** Tongue coated brown and thick, blistered; canker sores. Blisters on the inner surface of lips and cheeks.

**Stomach:** Coppery taste and eructations of sulphuretted hydrogen. Ravenous hunger soon after eating. *Very thirsty.* Craving for liquor, salt, sweets, etc., warm drinks. Pernicious vomiting of pregnancy.

**Abdomen:** Violent pain in the liver and spleen. Rests more when comfortably lying on the abdomen.

**Rectum:** Can pass stool only by leaning very far back. Painful sensation of a lump on the posterior surface of the sphincter. Oozing of fetid moisture. *Intense itching in the anus.*

**Urinary:** Painful tenesmus when micturating. *Nocturnal enuresis.* Renal colic (*Berb., Oci., Pareir.*). Urine flows very slowly.

**Male:** Nocturnal emissions, followed by great weakness. *Impotence.* Gleet; the entire urethra feels sore. Urethritis. Enlarged and painful prostate with frequent urging and painful micturition (gonorrhea).

**Female:** Intense pruritus. Menses *offensive,* profuse, dark, clotted; stains difficult to wash out, micturates frequently at that time. *Sensitive spot near os uteri.* Leucorrhea thin, acrid, excoriating, fishy odor. Sycotic warts on the genitals. Ovarian pain, worse left side, or from ovary to ovary. *Sterility.* Metrorrhagia. Intense menstrual colic. Breasts *cold,* sore, and sensitive.

**Respiratory:** Oppressed respiration. Hoarse while reading. Pain and soreness through the chest and mammae. Incessant, dry, nocturnal cough. Asthma. Incipient phthisis. Larynx feels sore. Dyspnea; cannot exhale (*Samb.*). Cough; better lying on the stomach.

**Extremities:** Pain in the back, with burning heat. Legs heavy; ache all night; *cannot keep them still* (*Zinc.*). Ankles turn easily when walking. Burning of hands and feet. Finger joints enlarged, puffy. Gouty concretions. *Heels and balls of feet tender* (*Thuj.*). *Soreness of soles.* Restless; better, clutching hands.

**Sleep:** Dreams she is drinking (*Ars., Phos.*). Sleeps in the knee-chest position.

**Fever:** Wants to be fanned all the time. Chills up and down the back; coldness of the legs, hands, and forearms. Flashes of heat in the face and neck. Night sweat and hectic sweat.

**Skin:** Yellow. Intense and incessant *itching;* worse at night and when thinking of it. Fiery red rash around the anus in babies. Copper colored spots. Favus. Tumors and abnormal growths.

**Modalities:** *Worse,* when thinking of the ailment, *from daylight to sunset,* heat, inland. *Better,* at the seashore, lying on the stomach, damp weather (*Caust.*).

**Relationship:** Compare: (Lactation: *Galega officinalis; Lactuca virosa). Sulph., Syph., Zinc.*

**Dose:** The very highest potencies are only of service. Must not be repeated often.

---

## MEDUSA

(Jelly-fish) **Medus.**

Whole face puffed and edematous, eyes, nose, ears, lips.

**Female:** Marked action on the *lacteal glands.* The secretion of milk was established after lack of it in all previous confinements.

**Skin:** Numbness; burning, pricking heat. Vesicular eruption, especially on the face, arms, shoulders, and breasts. *Nettle rash* (*Apis, Chlol., Dulc.*).

**Relationship:** Compare: *Pyrar., Physal.* (urticaria); *Urt-u., Hom., Sep.*

# MEL CUM SALE

(Honey with Salt) **Mel-c-s.**

Prolapsus uteri and chronic metritis, especially when associated with subinvolution and inflammation of the cervix. The special symptom leading to its selection is sensation *of soreness across the hypogastrium from ileum to ileum.* Uterine displacements, at the commencement of metritis. Sensation as if the bladder was too full. Pain from sacrum towards the pubes. Pain as if in the ureters.

**Dose:** Third to sixth potency. Honey for itching of anus (threadworms) and worms.

---

# MELILOTUS OFFICINALIS

(Yellow Melilot, Sweet Clover) **Meli.**

Congestions and hemorrhages seem to be the special manifestations of this drug. Violent congestive and nervous headaches. Infantile spasms. Epilepsy from a blow on the head. *Pain* and *debility* point to it. Coldness but also an increase in temperature; tenderness, and pain. Muscular system depressed. Dreams and emissions.

**Mind:** Unable to fix the mind. Memory treacherous. Stupor. Wants to run away and hide. Delusions; thinks every one is looking at her, fears to talk loud, etc.

**Head:** Headache with retching, vomiting, sense of pressure over the orbits, pallor, cold hands and feet, black spots before the eyes. Heavy, oppressed; *frontal, throbbing,* undulating sensation in the brain. *Sick headache;* relieved by epistaxis or menstrual flow. *Fullness all over the head.* Eyes heavy; blurred sight; wants to close them tightly for relief. *Neuralgia* around and over right side of head and neck. Scalp sore and tender to touch.

**Nose:** Stopped up, dry, must breathe through the mouth; dry, hard clinkers in the nose; *profuse epistaxis.*

**Face:** Intensely red and flushed with throbbing carotids (*Bell.*).

**Rectum:** Difficult, painful, constipated. Anus feels constricted, full, *throbs.* No desire until there is a large accumulation (*Bry., Alum.*).

**Female:** Menses *scanty, intermits,* with nausea and bearing down pain. Sticking pain in external parts. Dysmenorrhea. Ovarian neuralgia.

**Respiratory:** Feels as if smothered, especially from rapid walking. Hemoptysis. Weight on the chest. Tickling in the throat with cough.

**Extremities:** Pain in the knee; wants to stretch the leg, but does not relieve. Joints sore. Skin and extremities cold. Numbness and aching in knee joints.

**Modalities:** *Worse*, rainy, changeable weather, approach of storm, motion; 4 p. m.

**Relationship:** Compare: *Melilotus alba*—White clover: Practically the same action (hemorrhages, congestive headaches, engorged blood vessels, spasms). *Aml-ns., Bell., Glon.*

**Dose:** Tincture, for inhaling; lower potencies.

---

## MENISPERMUM CANADENSE

(Moon Seed) **Menis.**

A remedy for migraine, associated with restlessness and dreams. Pain in the spine. Dryness, itching all over. Dry mouth and throat. Also useful in uterine hemorrhage.

**Head:** Pressure *from within outward, with stretching and yawning* and pain down the back. Sick headache; pain in the forehead and temples, shifting to the occiput. Tongue swollen and increased saliva.

**Extremities:** Pain in the back, thighs, elbows, shoulders. Legs sore, as if bruised.

**Relationship:** Compare: *Cocc., Bry.*

**Dose:** Third potency.

---

## MENTHA PIPERITA

(Peppermint) **Menth.**

Stimulates the temperature receptors so that just after taking it, a current of air at the ordinary temperature seems cold. Marked action on the respiratory organs and skin. Useful in gastrodynia, flatulent colic.

**Abdomen:** Bloated, disturbing sleep. Infantile colic. Bilious colic with great accumulation of gas.

**Respiratory:** Voice husky. Tip of nose sore, to touch. Throat dry and sore, as if a pin was placed crosswise in it. *Dry cough, worse from cold air in the larynx, tobacco smoke, fog,* talking; *with irritation in the suprasternal fossa* (*Rumx.*). *Trachea painful to touch.*

**Skin:** Every scratch becomes a sore. Itching in the arm and hand when writing. Vaginal pruritus. Herpes zoster (*Ars., Ran-b.*).

**Relationship:** Compare: *Rumx., Lach., Mentha pulegium*—European pennyroyal (pain in the bones of the forehead and extremities). *Mentha viridis*—Spearmint (scanty urine with frequent desire).

**Dose:** Tincture, 1 to 20 drops, to thirtieth potency. Locally, in pruritus vaginae.

---

## MENTHOLUM

**Mentho.**

The stearopten from the essential oil of Mentha. Mucous membranes of the naso-pharynx and spinal nerve plexus affected, producing neuritic pains and paresthesias. *Mentho.* has proved curative in acute nasal catarrh; in acute eustachian catarrh; pharyngitis; laryngitis; neuralgias, etc. (Wm. B. Griggs, M. D.). Itching, especially *pruritus vulvae.*

**Head:** Frontal headache, pain over the frontal sinus, descends to the eyeballs. Mental confusion. Supra-orbital pain over the left eye. Pain in the face above zygoma with numbness. Pain in eyeballs.

**Ears:** Eustachian tubes feel blocked and some deafness.

**Nose:** Coryza with post nasal dripping (sinusitis). Cold sensation in the nose.

**Respiratory:** Tickling in the fauces. Stabbing pains in the precordia, radiating over the entire chest. Short, dry cough, worse smoking. Asthmatic breathing with congestive headache.

**Extremities:** Muscular pain in the cervical region. Soreness of lumbar muscles.

**Relationship:** Compare: *Kali-bi., Spig.*

**Dose:** Sixth potency. Externally for itching, use 1 percent solution or ointment.

---

## MENYANTHES TRIFOLIATA

(Buck-bean) **Meny.**

A remedy for certain headaches, intermittent fever. Coldness of the abdomen. Twitchings. Sensation of tension and compression. Fidgets and urinary problems in women. Diabetes.

**Head:** Pressing in the vertex; *better, hard pressure with the hand.* Pain pressing together. Weight pressing on the brain with every step on ascending.

Pain from the nape extending over the whole brain; better, stooping, sitting; worse, going upstairs. Cracking in the jaw and twitching of facial muscles (tetanus, epilepsy).

**Stomach:** No thirst at any time. Ravenous hunger; passing away after eating a little. Desire for meat. Sensation of coldness extending up to the oesophagus.

**Abdomen:** Distended and full; increased by smoking tobacco. Coldness of the abdomen.

**Extremities:** *Icy coldness of hands and feet.* Cramp-like pain. As soon as patient lies down, *legs jerk and twitch* (convulsions).

**Fever:** Coldness predominates; felt most acutely in the abdomen, legs and tip of the nose.

**Modalities:** *Worse,* during rest, ascending. *Better,* pressure on the affected part, stooping, motion.

**Relationship:** Compare: *Caps., Puls., Calc., Ph-ac., Sang.*

Antidote: *Camph.*

**Dose:** Third to thirtieth potency.

---

# MEPHITIS PUTORIUS

(Skunk) **Meph.**

A great medicine for *whooping cough.* In order to insure its full success, it should be given in the lower dilutions from lx to 3x. Suffocative feeling, asthmatic paroxysms, spasmodic cough; cough so violent, seems as if each spell would terminate life. Child must be raised up, gets blue in the face (cyanosed), cannot exhale. Mucus rales through the upper part of chest. Patient wants to bathe in ice cold water.

**Mind:** Excited, full of fancies. Can neither sleep nor work.

**Eyes:** Pain from over exertion; blur; unable to distinguish letters; conjunctiva red; eyes hot and painful (conjunctivitis).

**Mouth:** Painful jerks in the root of the teeth. Bloated face. Coppery taste, as after eating onions.

**Respiratory:** Sudden contraction of the glottis (laryngismus), when drinking or talking. *Food goes down the wrong way.* False croup; cannot *exhale. Spasmodic and whooping cough. Few paroxysms during daytime, but many at night,* with vomiting after eating. Asthma, as if inhaling sulphur; cough from talking; hollow, deep, with rawness, hoarseness, and pain through the chest. *Violent spasmodic cough; worse* at night.

**Sleep:** Wakes up at night with rush of blood to the lower part of legs. Vivid dreams of water, fire, etc.

**Relationship:** Compare: *Dros., Cor-r., Stict.*

**Dose:** First to third potency. Has a very short action.

---

## MERCURIALIS PERENNIS

(Dog's Mercury) **Merl.**

Great exhaustion and drowsiness. Tumor at the ensiform appendix, very sensitive. Affections of the muscular fibres of stomach, intestines, bladder.

**Head:** Vertigo on going down stairs. Head confused. Pain as from a band, tightly across the forehead. Nostrils sore, conscious of the nose, feels as if she has two noses.

**Mouth:** Great dryness of the mouth and throat, tongue feels heavy, dry and numb. Burning blisters on the tongue, lips and cheeks. Ulcers on the palate, tonsils and the posterior part of pharynx. Dryness of the throat.

**Female:** *Amenorrhea,* scanty menses, accompanied with orgasms. Pains and swelling of the breasts. Dysmenorrhea.

**Relationship**: Compare: *Borx., Crot-t., Euph.*

**Dose:** Third potency.

---

## MERCURIUS SOLUBILIS—HYDRARGYRUM

(Quicksilver) **Merc.**

Every organ and tissue of the body is more or less affected by this powerful drug; it transforms healthy cells into decrepit, inflamed and necrotic wrecks, decomposes the blood, producing profound anemia. This malignant medicinal force is converted into a useful life saving and life preserving service if employed homoeopathically, guided by its clear cut symptoms. The lymphatic system is especially affected with all the membranes, *glands,* internal organs, bones, etc. Lesions produced by mercury are very similar to those of syphilis. Very often indicated in the *secondary* stage of syphilis where there is febrile chloro-anemia, rheumatoid pains behind the sternum, around the joints, etc., ulceration of the mouth and throat, falling of hair, etc. These are the special conditions and stages to which *Merc.* is homoeopathic and where the 2x trituration will do surprising work. Again, hereditary syphilitic manifestations, are within its range; bullae, abscesses, snuffles, marasmus, stomatitis or destructive inflammations. *Tremors* everywhere. Weakness with ebullitions and tremblings from least exertion. All *Merc.* symptoms are *worse at night,* from warmth of bed, from damp, cold, rainy weather, *worse during perspiration.* Complaints increase with sweat and rest; all symptoms are associated with a great deal of weariness, prostration and trembling. A human "thermometer." Sensitive to heat and cold. Parts are very swollen, with a raw, sore feeling; the profuse, oily perspiration does not relieve. *Breath,* excretions and body smell foul. Tendency to formation of pus, which is thin, greenish, putrid; streaked with thin blood.

**Mind:** Slow in answering questions. Memory weakened and loss of will power. Weary of life. Mistrustful. Thinks he is losing his reason.

**Head:** Vertigo, when *lying on the back.* Sensation of a band around the head. One sided, tearing pains (migraine). *Tension around the scalp, as if bandaged.* Catarrhal headaches; much heat in the head (meningitis). Stinging, burning, fetid eruptions on the scalp. Loss of hair. Exostosis, with a feeling of soreness. Scalp tense; oily sweat on the head.

**Eyes:** Lids red, thick, swollen (blepharitis). *Profuse, burning, acrid discharge* (purulent conjunctivitis). Floating black spots. *After exposure to a glare of fire; it foundry men. Parenchymatous keratitis* of syphilitic origin with burning pain. Iritis, with hypopyon.

**Ears:** Thick, *yellow discharge;* fetid and bloody (otorrhea). *Otalgia, worse warmth of bed;* at night. sticking pains. Boils in the external canal (*Calc-pic.*).

**Nose:** Marked sneezing. Sneezing *in sunshine. Nostrils raw, ulcerated;* nasal bones swollen. Yellow-green, fetid, pus-like discharge (ozena). Coryza; acrid discharge, but too thick to run down the lip; worse, warm room. Pain and *swelling of the nasal bones and caries, with greenish, fetid ulceration.* Epistaxis at night. Copious discharge of corroding mucus. Coryza with sneezing; sore, raw, smarting sensation; worse, damp weather; *profuse, fluent.*

**Face:** Pale, *earthy,* dirty looking, puffy. Aching in the facial bones. Syphilitic pustules on the face.

**Mouth:** Sweetish metallic taste. *Salivary secretions greatly increased;* bloody and viscid. Saliva fetid, coppery. Speech difficult on account of the trembling tongue. *Gums spongy,* recede, bleed easily (scorbutic, scurvy). Sore pain on touch and from *chewing.* Whole mouth *moist.* Crown of teeth decay. Teeth loose, feel tender and elongated. *Furrow on the upper surface of the tongue lengthwise.* Tongue heavy, *thick; moist coating; yellow, flabby, teeth indented;* feels as if burnt, with ulcers (apthae). *Fetid odor* from mouth (halitosis); can smell it all over the room. Alveolar abscess, worse at night. *Great thirst, with a moist mouth.*

**Throat:** Bluish-red swelling. Constant desire to swallow. Putrid sore throat; worse right side. *Ulcers* and inflammation appearing at every change in weather. Stitches extend to the ear on swallowing; fluids return through the nose. Quinsy, with dysphagia, *after pus has formed.* Sore, raw, smarting, burning throat. Complete aphonia. Burning in the throat, as if from ascending hot vapor.

**Stomach:** Putrid eructations. *Intense thirst for cold drinks.* Weak digestion, with *continuous hunger.* Stomach sensitive to touch. Hiccough and regurgitation. Feels replete and constricted.

**Abdomen:** Stabbing pain, with chilliness. Boring pain in the right groin. Flatulent distention, with pain. Liver enlarged (hepatomegaly); sore to touch, indurated. Jaundice (obstructive). Bile secreted deficiently.

**Rectum:** Greenish, *bloody and slimy, worse at night; with pain and tenesmus. Never-get-done feeling.* Discharge accompanied by chilliness, sick stomach, cutting colic, and tenesmus. Whitish-gray stools.

**Urinary:** Frequent urging. Greenish discharge from the urethra; burning in the urethra when beginning to micturate. Urine dark, scanty, bloody, albuminous.

**Male:** Vesicles and ulcers; soft chancre. Cold genitals. Prepuce irritated; itches. Nocturnal emissions, stained with blood.

**Female:** Menses profuse, with abdominal pain (dysmenorrhea). Leucorrhea excoriating, greenish and bloody; *sensation of rawness* in parts. *Stinging pain* in the ovaries (*Apis*). Itching and burning; worse, after micturating; better, washing with cold water. Morning sickness, with profuse salivation. Mammae painful and full of milk during menses.

**Respiratory:** Soreness from the fauces to sternum. *Cannot lie* on *the right side* (left side, *Lyc.*). Cough, with yellow, mucopurulent expectoration. Paroxysms of two; worse, night, and from warmth of bed. Catarrh, with chilliness; dread of air. Stitches from the lower lobe of the right lung to the back. Whooping cough with epistaxis (*Arn.*). Cough worse, tobacco smoke.

**Back:** Bruised pain in the lumbosacral region, especially when sitting. Tearing pain in the coccyx; better, pressing on the abdomen.

**Extremities:** Weakness of limbs. Bone pains, pain in the limbs; worse, night. Patient is very sensitive to cold. Oily perspiration. *Trembling extremities, especially hands; paralysis agitans.* Lacerating pain in joints. Cold, clammy sweat on legs at night. Dropsical swelling of feet and legs.

**Fever:** Generally gastric or bilious, with profuse nocturnal perspiration; debility, slow and lingering. Heat and shuddering alternately. Yellow perspiration. *Profuse perspiration without relief. Creeping chilliness;* worse in the evening and into night. Alternate flashes of heat in single parts.

**Skin:** Almost *constantly moist.* Persistent dryness of the skin contraindicates *Merc.* Excessive, odorous, viscid perspiration; worse, night. *General tendency to free perspiration, but patient is not relieved thereby.* Vesicular and pustular eruptions. Ulcers, irregular in shape, edges undefined. Pimples around the main eruption. *Itching;* worse from warmth of bed. Crusta lactea; yellowish-brown crusts, considerable suppuration. Glands swell every time patient takes cold. Buboes. Orchitis (*Clem., Ham., Puls.*).

**Modalities:** *Worse,* at night, wet, damp weather, lying on the right side, perspiring; warm room and warm bed.

**Relationship:** Compare: *Capparis coriaccea* (polyuria, glandular affections, mucus diarrhea; influenza); *Epilobium palustre*—Willow herb (chronic diarrhea with tenesmus and mucus discharges; ptyalism, dysphagia; wasting of the body and marked debility; cholera infantum); *Kali-i.* (in hard chancre); *Mercurius aceticus* (congestion with stiffness, dryness and heat of parts affected. Eyes inflamed, burn and itch. Lack of moisture. Throat dry, talking difficult. Pressure in lower part of sternum; chancre in urethra; Tinea capitis favosa, margin of ulcers painful); *Mercurius auratus* (psoriasis and syphilitic catarrh; brain tumors; lues of nose and bones; ozena; swelling of testicles); *Mercurius bromatus* (secondary syphilitic skin affection); *Mercurius nitrosus*—Nitrate of mercury (especially in pustular conjunctivitis and keratitis; gonorrhea and mucous patches, with *sticking pains;* syphilides); *Mercurius phosphoricus* (nervous diseases from syphilis; exostoses); *Mercurius precipitatus ruber* (suffocative attacks at night on lying down when *on the point of falling asleep,* obliged to jump up suddenly which relieves; gonorrhea; *urethra feels like a hard string;* chancroid; phagedenic ulcer and bubo; pemphigus, mucus patches, eczema with rhagades and fissures, barber's itch; blepharitis, internally and externally; leaden heaviness in occiput, with otorrhea); *Mercurius tannicus* (syphilides in patients with gastro-intestinal diseases, or, if very sensitive, to ordinary mercurial preparations); *Erythrinus*—South American Red Mullet fish (in pityriasis rubra and syphilis; red rash on chest; pityriasis); *Lolium temulentum* (in *trembling* of hands and legs); *Mercurius cum kali* (inveterate colds, acute facial paralysis). *Heuchera americana*—Alum root (gastroenteritis, nausea, vomiting of bile and frothy mucus; stools watery, profuse, slimy, tenesmus, never get done feeling. Dose, 2 to 10 drops of tincture).

Compare: *Mez., Phos., Syph., Kali-m., Aeth-a.*

Antidote: *Hep., Aur., Mez.*

Complementary: *Bad.*

**Dose:** Second to thirtieth potency.

---

# MERCURIUS CORROSIVUS

(Corrosive Sublimate) **Merc-c.**

This salt leads all other remedies in tenesmus of the rectum, which is incessant and is not relieved by stool. The tenesmus often involves the bladder as well. Bright's disease. Gonorrhea; second stage, with continuous tenesmus. Destroys the secreting portions of the kidneys. This process is slow, but sure. Albuminuria in early pregnancy (*Phos.* later and at full term).

**Head:** Delirium, stupor. Frontal pain, congestion of the head, with burning in the cheeks. Drawing pain in the periosteum of skull.

**Eyes:** Pain behind the eyeballs, as if forced out. Phlyctenulae; deep ulcers on the cornea. Excessive photophobia and *acrid lachrymation. Iritis,* ordinary or syphilitic (give in association with atropin locally for prevention of adhesions). Pain severe at night; burning, shooting, tearing. Little tendency to pus formation. *Iris muddy in color, thick, neither contracts nor dilates.* Retinitis albuminuric, ophthalmia neonatorum. *Lids edematous,* red, excoriated (blepharitis). *Severe burning. Soreness of the eyes.*

**Ears:** Violent pulsations. Fetid pus (otorrhea).

**Nose:** Excessive coryza. Ozena with perforation of septum nasi (*Kali-bi.*). Rawness and smarting in nostrils. Post-nasal swelling, mucous membrane dry, red, and covered with bloody mucus.

**Face:** Swollen. Red, puffy. Lips black, swollen. Sordes. Facial neuralgia within the bones.

**Mouth:** Teeth loose. Gums purple, swollen, and spongy (scorbutic). Tongue swollen and inflamed (glossitis). Salivation. Pyorrhea. Ptyalism. Taste salty and bitter.

**Throat:** *Red, swollen, painful, intensely inflamed. Uvula swollen. Swallowing painful.* Severe pain is *the post-nasal area with sharp pains radiating to the ears. Burning pain with great swelling; worse, slight external pressure.* All glands around thorax swollen.

**Stomach:** Incessant, green, bilious vomiting. Epigastrium very sensitive.

**Abdomen:** Bruised sensation; caecal region and transverse colon painful (intussusception, ulcerative colitis). Bloated; very painful to least touch.

**Rectum:** Dysentery; tenesmus, not relieved by stool; incessant. Stool hot, bloody, slimy. offensive, with cutting pains and shreds of mucous membrane.

**Urinary:** Intense burning in the urethra (urethritis). Urine hot, burning, scanty or *suppressed;* bloody, *greenish discharge.* Albuminous. *Tenesmus of bladder.* Stabbing pain extending up the urethra into the bladder (cystitis). Perspiration after micturition.

**Male:** Penis and testies enormously swollen (balanitis and orchitis). Chancres assume a phagedenic appearance (syphilis). *Gonorrhea;* urethral orifice red, swollen; glans sore and hot. Discharge greenish, thick.

**Respiratory:** Pain in the larynx as if cut with a knife. Aphonia. Cough with hemoptysis. Pulse rapid and intermittent. Stitches through the side of chest.

**Fever:** Chilly from slightest exposure. Profuse perspiration; surfaces cold.

**Modalities:** *Worse,* evening, night, acids. *Better,* while at rest.

**Relationship:** Compare: *Ars., Lach., Leonurus cardiaca*—Mother-wort influences pelvic organs, allays spasm and nervous irritability, promotes secretion and reduces febrile excitement. Valuable in suppressed menses and *lochia;* dysentery; vomiting, severe pains in the abdomen, violent thirst. Tongue dry and cracked). *Monsonia ovata*—An African plant belonging to Geraniaceae used for dysentery in material doses).

Antidote: *Calcium sulphide* is antidotal to Bichloride poisoning. Use intravenous injection of 71/2 grains in 71/2 ozs. boiled water.

**Dose:** Sixth potency. In solution 1 : 1000, hypodermically injected under the conjunctiva in choroditis with progressive myopia. Stops immediately the severe aching pain behind eyeballs (Dr. G. D. Hallet).

---

# MERCURIUS CYANATUS

(Cyanide of Mercury) **Merc-cy.**

Acute infections, pneumonia, nephritis. Its action is similar to that of the toxins of infectious diseases. Great and rapid prostration, tendency towards hemorrhages, from different orifices, of dark fluid blood, cyanosis, rapid respiration and heart action, albuminuria, twitching and jerking of muscles. Typhoidal pneumonia.

Livid states from great struggling, where suffocation is imminent and paralysis of, lung threatening; profuse sweat.

Affects the buccal cavity most prominently. This, together with marked prostration, gives it a place in the treatment of *diphtheria,* where it has achieved unquestionably great results. Malignant types, with prostration. Coldness and nausea. Syphilitic ulcers when perforation threatens.

**Head:** Great excitement, fits of passion; fury; talkativeness. Atrocious headache. Eyes sunken; face pale.

**Mouth:** Covered with ulcerations (stomatitis). Tongue pale. Free salivation. Halitosis. Pain and swelling of the salivary glands. Astringent taste. *Ulcerations* of the mouth have a gray membrane.

**Throat:** Feels raw and sore. Mucous membranes broken down, ulcerated. Looks raw in spots, especially in public speakers. Hoarseness, and talking is painful. *Necrotic destruction of soft parts of the palate and fauces.* Intense hyperemia of the fauces. Swallowing is very difficult. Dark blood from the nose. Diphtheria of the larynx and nose (*Kali-bi.*).

**Stomach:** Nausea, vomiting, bilious, bloody; hiccough; abdomen painful, tender on pressure.

**Rectum:** Intolerable pain. Redness around the anus. Frequent hemorrhage; stools with tenesmus (dysentery). Discharge of a fetid liquid with a gangrenous odor. Black stools.

**Urinary:** Amber color, dysuria, albuminous, scanty. Nephritis with great debility and chilliness. Suppression of urine.

**Skin:** Moisture, with icy coldness.

**Dose:** Sixth to thirtieth potency. Aggravation is apt to occur from potencies below the sixth.

---

## MERCURIUS DULCIS

(Calomel) **Merc-d.**

Has a marked effect on the catarrhal inflammation of the ear and is useful in eustachian catarrh and deafness. Diarrhea with soreness of the anus. *Prostatitis.* Remittent bilious attacks. *Pallor, flabby, bloatedness,* and turgid flaccidity. Inflammation with plastic exudate. Especially indicated in systems disposed to remittent bilious fevers; in peritonitis and meningitis *with plastic exudation.* Dropsies due to combined renal and cardiac diseases, especially with jaundice (Hale). Cirrhosis of the liver, especially in the hypertrophic form. Use 1x (Jousset).

**Ears:** Otitis media; closure of the eustachian tube; ear problems in scrofulous children; membrana tympani retracted, thickened and immovable.

**Mouth:** Halitosis; salivation; sore gums. Ulcers. Tongue black. Constant flow of dark, putrid saliva; very offensive. Ulceration of the throat with dysphagia. Granular pharyngitis.

**Stomach:** Nausea and vomiting. Cyclic vomiting in infants (*Cupr-ar., Iris*).

**Rectum:** Scanty, bloody mucus, with bile and *constant desire*, without tenesmus. Dark green, watery with griping. *Anus sore* and burning. Dysentery; small stools of *mucus and blood, covered with bile.*

**Skin:** *Flabby and ill nourished.* Swollen glands. Phagedenic ulcers. Copper colored eruptions.

**Relationship:** Compare: *Kali-m.*

**Dose:** Third to sixth trituration. For palliative (non-homoeopathic) purposes, to secure evacuation of bowels, two or three grain doses of first decimal trituration, repeated several times every hour.

---

## MERCURIUS IODATUS FLAVUS

(Proto-iodide of Mercury) **Merc-i-f.**

Throat affections with greatly swollen glands and characteristic coating of the tongue. Worse, right side. Chancre; induration remains for a long time. Swollen inguinal glands, large and hard. *Mammary tumors* with a tendency to profuse, warm perspiration and gastric disturbances.

**Mouth:** *Tongue coated thickly, yellow at the base.* Tip and edges may be red (glossitis) and take imprint of teeth.

**Throat:** Lacunar tonsillitis. When only the superficial part of the tonsil is involved. Cheesy exudates with halitosis. Swelling begins on the right side. Small ulcers on the posterior pharyngeal wall. Easily detached patches on the inflamed pharynx and fauces (diphtheria); *worse on the right tonsil;* profuse tenacious mucus. Sensation of a lump. *Constant inclination to swallow.*

**Relationship:** Compare: *Plb-i.* (in mammary tumors).

**Dose:** Second trituration.

---

## MERCURIUS IODATUS RUBER

(Bin-iodide of Mercury) **Merc-i-r.**

Diphtheria and ulcerated sore throats, especially on the left side, with marked glandular swelling. Chronic suppurating buboes. Hard chancres. Old cases of syphilis in scrofulous patients. Early stages of cold, especially in children.

**Nose:** Coryza and dull hearing; right side of nose, hot. Hawks mucus from the posterior nares. Turbinated bones swollen. Polyp. Boggy mucous membrane in the nose and throat; closure of the eustachian tube, opening with a pop.

**Mouth:** Gums swollen; toothache; glands swollen. Scalded feeling on the tongue. Aphthae. Profuse saliva. Tongue feels stiff at the base, and pains on moving.

**Throat:** Diphtheria; submaxillary glands painfully engorged, fauces dark red; *worse, left tonsil.* Parenchymatous tonsillitis. Will often abort peritonsillitis if given frequently. Cough from an elongated uvula, with a sore throat. Laryngeal disease with aphonia. *Fauces dark red;* swallowing painful. Phlegm in nose and throat. Disposition to hawk, with sensation of a lump in throat (goitre). *Stiffness in the muscles of the throat and neck.*

**Skin:** Small fissures and cracks; hard papules; *Huntarian chancre;* syphilitic ulcers. Bubo. Sarcocele.

**Dose:** Third trituration. Iodide salts of mercury is far more active as a bactericide than the other mercurials, including the chloride.

---

# MERCURIUS SULPHURICUS—HYDRARG. OXYD. SUB-SULPH.

(Turpethum Minerale, Yellow Sulphate of Mercury)

**Merc-sul.**

Watery stools, burning in the anus. Sore tip of tongue. Edema of the legs. Sneezing from direct rays of the sun. Diarrhea, early in the morning; stool bursts out in a hot stream of yellow matter. Intense evacuations, like rice water. Scanty, clear, scalding urine. *Intense dyspnea;* must sit up. Respiration rapid, short; burning in the chest. *Hydrothorax* (*Ars.*). Cardiac pain and weakness.

**Relationship:** Compare: *Merc-act.* (cutting in the urethra when last drop is flowing out).

---

# METHYLENE BLUE

(One of the Aniline Dyes) **Methyl.**

A remedy for neuralgia, neurasthenia, malaria; *typhoid,* here it diminishes the tympanites, delirium and fever; pus infection. Tendency to tremor, chorea and epilepsy. Nephritis (acute parenchymatous), scarlatinal nephritis. Urine acquires a green color. Bladder irritation from its use antidoted by a little nutmeg. Surgical condition of kidney with a large amount of pus in the urine (pyuria). Gonorrheal rheumatism and cystitis. Backache, sciatica. Later states of apoplexy (Gisevius).

**Dose:** 3x attenuation. A 2 percent solution locally, in chronic otitis with a foul smelling discharge.

A 1 percent aqueous solution for ulcers and abscesses of cornea.

# MEZEREUM

(Spurge Olive) **Mez.**

Skin symptoms, affections of the bones and neuralgias most important, especially around the teeth and face. Bruised, weary feeling in joints, with drawing and stiffness. *Pain of various kinds, with chilliness and sensitiveness to cold air.* Bone pains. Eruptions after vaccination. Burning, darting sensation in the muscles; subsultus tendinum. Pain shoots upward and seems to draw the patient out of bed. Semi-lateral complaints. *Patient is very sensitive to cold air.*

**Head:** Hard work to talk[1]. Headache; worse from talking. Stupefying headache on the right side. Affections of the external head; scaly eruptions, white scabs. Head covered with *thick, leathery crusts, under which pus collects* (crusta lactea). Violent neuralgia around the face and teeth, extending to the ear, at night; *worse, eating;* better nearhot stove. Roots of teeth decay. Teeth feel elongated.

**Eyes:** *Ciliary neuralgia after surgery* especially after removal of eyeball. Pain radiates and shoots downward, *with a cold feeling and stiffness of the bone.*

**Ears:** Feel too open, *as if the tympanum was exposed to cold air and it blew into the ear.* Desire to bore fingers in.

**Nose:** Sneezing, coryza; interior of nose, excoriated. Post nasal adenoids.

**Face:** Red. Eruptions around the mouth, with coryza.

**Stomach:** Desire for ham-fat. Burning in the tongue, extending to the stomach. *Mouth waters.* Nausea felt in the throat; better, eating. Chronic gastritis; burning, corroding pain; nausea, vomiting, chocolate color. *Gastric ulcer* with severe burning.

**Abdomen:** Swelling of glands with a large abdomen in children. Pressure in the inguinal ring (hernia). Flatulent colic with shivering and difficult respiration.

**Rectum:** Constipation after confinement. Prolapse of rectum. Diarrhea with small, white particles. *Green discharges.* Constipation, with hepatic and uterine inertia. Constriction of the anus; stitches and prolapse of rectum.

**Urinary:** Red flakes float on top of urine. Hot, bloody. Biting, burning in the forepart of the urethra at the close of micturating (urethritis). Hematuria preceded by crampy pain in the bladder. After micturating, a few drops of blood are passed.

---

1 Aversion to talking, seems like hard work to even utter a word (Clarke — Dictionary of Practical Materia Medica).

**Male:** *Enlargement of testicles* (orchitis). Violent sexual desire. Gonorrhea with hematuria.

**Female:** Menses too frequent, soon, profuse (menorrhagia). Leucorrhea like albumen; very corroding.

**Respiratory:** Soreness and burning in the bones of thorax. Constriction across the chest. Cough; worse, eating, irritation lower than can be reached, on taking a warm drink.

**Back and Extremities:** Pain in the neck and back; worse, motion and at night; intolerant of all touch. *Pain* and burning in the tibia and long bones. Legs and feet go to sleep. Pain in hip and knee.

**Skin:** Eczema; *intolerable itching;* chilliness with pruritus. Worse in bed. Ulcers itch and burn, surrounded by vesicles and shining, fiery red areola. Herpes zoster, with burning pain. *Bones,* especially long bones, inflamed and swollen; caries, exostosis; pain worse night, touch, damp weather (*Merc., Syph.*). *Eruptions ulcerate and form thick scabs under which purulent matter exudes* (*Chrys-ac.*).

**Modalities:** *Worse*, cold air; night, evening until midnight, warm food, touch, motion. *Better,* open air.

**Relationship:** Compare: *Dirca palustris*—Leather wood (a gastro-intestinal irritant inducing salivation, emesis and purgation; cerebral hyperemia, neuralgic pains, with depression, palpitation and dyspnea); *Merc., Phyt., Rhus-t., Guaj., Syph.*

Antidotes: *Kali-i., Merc.*

**Dose:** Sixth to thirtieth potency.

---

# MICROMERIA DOUGLASII

(Yerba Buena) **Micr.**

A California mint-like plant acting on the stomach and bowels. Used as a tea to cure colic and relieve flatulence. Is a pleasant beverage and febrifuge, blood purifier and tonic.

**Stomach:** Nausea; pain in the stomach and bowels; flatulence.

**Dose:** Tincture.

---

## MILLEFOLIUM

(Yarrow) **Mill.**

An invaluable remedy for various types of hemorrhages; blood, bright red. Incarcerated hernia; small-pox, with great pain in the pit of the stomach. After surgery for calculi. Bad effects of falling from a height; overlifting. *Continuous high temperature.* Hemoptysis.

**Head:** Vertigo when moving slowly. Sensation as if he had forgotten something. The head seems full of blood. Convulsions and epilepsy from suppressed menses. *Piercing thrusts* of pain.

**Nose:** *Epistaxis* (*Erech.*). Piercing pain from the eyes to the root of the nose.

**Stool:** Hemorrhage from the bowels. Bleeding hemorrhoids.

**Urinary:** Hematuria (*Senec.*).

**Female:** Menses early, profuse, protracted (menorrhagia). Hemorrhage from the uterus; bright red, fluid. *Painful varices during pregnancy.*

**Respiratory:** Hemoptysis in incipient phthisis. Cough, with bloody expectoration, in suppressed menses or hemorrhoids. Violent palpitations.

**Relationship:** Compare: *Ficus venosa*—Pakur (hemorrhage from bowels and lungs). *Acal.* and *Helx.*—Snail (in hemoptysis, diseases of the chest, consumption); also, *Sec.*, *Ip.*, *Erech.*, *Ger.*, *Ham.*

**Dose:** Tincture to third potency.

---

## MITCHELLA REPENS

(Partridge Berry) **Mit.**

Bladder symptoms accompany complaints, especially uterine congestion.

**Urinary:** Irritation at the neck of the bladder, with urging to micturate (*Eup-pur.*, *Apis*). Dysuria. Catarrh of the bladder (cystitis).

**Female:** Cervix dark red, swollen (cervicitis). Dysmenorrhea and uterine hemorrhage; blood bright red.

**Relationship:** Compare: *Chim.*, *Senec.*, *Uva*, *Ger.*, *Goss.*

**Dose:** Tincture.

---

# MOMORDICA BALSAMINA

(Balsam Apple) **Mom-b.**

Griping, colic, pain in the back and hypogastrium with dysmenorrhea. Accumulation of flatus in the splenic flexure of colon. Dropsy.

**Head:** Dizzy, contents of the head feel lighter; mist before the eyes.

**Abdomen:** Rumbling, griping, colicky pains, starting from the back, spreading over the entire abdomen.

**Female:** Painful and profuse menses; labor-like pains, followed by gushes of blood; pain at the lumbosacral region extending towards the front of the pelvis.

**Relationship:** *Momordica charantia*—Indian variety (more severe symptoms—intestines full of yellow watery fluid, discharged *explosively*, cramps, thirst, prostration. Cholera-like symptoms. Similar to *Crot-t., Elat.* Use 3x.).

**Dose:** Tincture. Also used externally as a liniment and poultice for burns, chapped hands, etc.

---

# MORPHINUM

(An Alkaloid of Opium) **Morph.**

Morphine bears the same relation to *Opium* as Atropine to *Belladonna* i. e., represents its nervous side. It is less stimulating, less convulsant and more decidedly hypnotic. Constipates less and affects the contractility of the bladder more. It is less diaphoretic and more pruritic.

**Mind:** *Profound depression.* Irritable, fault finding, hysterical. *Shock induced by terror. Dream-like state.*

**Head:** *Vertigo from the least movement of the head.* Headache, with a sensation of being "wound up." Bursting pain; head drawn back (tetanus, convulsions).

**Eyes:** Bluish, drooping lids. *Itching in the eyes.* Delusions of vision on closing the eyes. Staring, injected; diverging strabismus. Pupils unequally contracted. *Look unsteady.* Ptosis. *Paresis of rectus interni.*

**Ears:** Left ear throbs painfully; better, heat. *Seems to hear the circulation all over the body.*

**Nose:** Sneezing in paroxysms. *Itching* and tingling on the tip of the nose.

**Face:** *Dusky red or pallid lividity of the face, lips, tongue, mouth or throat.*

**Mouth:** *Very dry.* Tongue dry, brown violet in the middle. *Thirst.* Loss of appetite *with an aversion to meat.*

**Throat:** Dry and constricted. Pharynx paralyzed, swallowing is almost impossible; better hot drinks, worse solids.

**Stomach:** Nausea *incessant and deathly,* faintness, constant retching. Vomiting of green fluid (bile). *Nausea and vomiting on rising up.*

**Abdomen:** Distended. Acute pain in the abdomen and along the spinal cord. *Tympanites.*

**Stool:** Diarrhea watery; brown, or black with horrible tenesmus. Constipation; stools large, dry, knotty, with a tendency to bruise and fissure.

**Urinary:** Paresis of the bladder. *Strangury; slow and difficult micturition.* Retention of urine from prostatic hypertrophy. *Uremia,* acute and chronic.

**Male:** Impotency. Pain in the right spermatic cord (*Ox-ac.*).

**Respiratory:** Faint and struggling for breath; diaphragmatic paralysis; hiccough; dyspnea, paroxysmal, on first falling asleep (*Lach., Grin.*). Cheyne-Stokes respiration. Chest tight. Pain in the middle of the sternum. Dry, hard, *teasing,* exhausting cough, worse at night. Strangling cough with viscid mucoid sputum; thin, scanty, but sounds loose and abundant.

**Heart:** *Alternation of tachycardia and bradycardia.* Cardiac muscular tissue is intact, even if severely exhausted. Pulse small, weak, dicrotic.

**Back:** Pain along the spine. Weakness in the loins. Aching across the lumbosacral region; cannot walk erect (*Cimic.*).

**Extremities:** Staggering gait (locomotor ataxia). *Numbness.*

**Sleep:** Yawning, *drowsy;* prolonged, deep sleep. Sleepless; restless sleep, with frequent startings. Sleepy, but cannot sleep.

**Nervous System:** Restlessness and hyperesthesia; trembling, twitching, jerking, convulsions. *Extremely susceptible to pain.* Pain causes twitching and jerking of limbs (chorea). Violent, *sudden* neuralgic pains and sudden fainting. *Delirium, melancholic in character.* Neuralgias *intensely painful;* left supraorbital; right intercostal, better from heat; *multiple neuritis.* Sore feeling all over. *Bed feels too hard.* Aggravation after sleep (*Lach.*). Neuralgia after zoster (*Mez.*).

**Fever:** Chills. Icy coldness. Burning heat; profuse sweat.

**Skin:** *Livid;* purple spots; zoster-like herpes. *Itching.* Skin looses its elasticity. Urticaria appearing at climaxis.

**Dose:** Third to sixth trituration.

# MOSCHUS

(Musk) **Mosch.**

A remedy for hysteria and nervous paroxysms, *fainting fits* and convulsions, catalepsy, etc. The characteristic condition being aggravation by cold; there is great sensitiveness to air. Marked nervous trembling and frequent fainting. Great flatulence. Diseases do not follow a normal course. Coldness. Tension in the muscles, skin and mind.

**Mind:** *Uncontrollable laughter*. Scolding. Anxiety with palpitations; starting as if frightened. Sexual hypochondriasis.

**Head:** Compressive pain over the root of nose. Pressure on top of the head. Vertigo on least motion; sensation as if falling from a great height. Scalp sensitive. Sounds in the ears as if from the retort of a cannon.

**Stomach:** Desire for black coffee, stimulants. Aversion to food. Everything tastes flat. With stomach symptoms, anxiety in the chest. Distended. Faints when eating. Abdomen greatly distended. *Spasmodic, nervous hiccough* (*Hydr-ac., Sul-ac., Ign., Caj.*).

**Urinary:** Profuse micturition. *Diabetes.*

**Male:** *Violent desire;* involuntary emissions. Impotence, associated with diabetes (*Coca*). Premature senility. Nausea and vomiting after coition.

**Female:** Menses too early, too profuse (menorrhagia), with a disposition to faint (*Nux-m., Verat.*). Sexual desire, with intolerable titillation in parts (nymphomania). Drawing and pushing in the direction of the genitals; sensation as if menses would appear.

**Respiratory:** Tightness of the chest, is obliged to take a deeper breath. Sudden constriction of larynx (laryngismus) and trachea. *Difficult respiration; chest oppressed;* hysterical spasm of chest; asthma. Spasms of the glottis. Impending paralysis of lungs. Asthma with intense anxiety, fear and smothering sensation. *Cough ceases, mucus cannot be expectorated.* Globus hystericus.

**Heart:** Hyterical palpitations (angina pectoris). Trembling around the heart. Weak pulse and fainting.

**Modalities:** *Better,* in the open air, rubbing. *Worse*, cold. Open air feels very, very cold.

**Relationship:** Compare: *Nux-m., Asaf., Valer., Sumb., Ign., Castm.*

Compatible: *Ambr.*

Antidotes: *Camph., Coff.*

**Dose:** First to third potency.

# MUREX PURPUREA

(Purple Fish) **Murx.**

Symptoms of the female sexual organs are most prominent, and have been clinically verified. Especially adapted to nervous, lively, affectionate women. Patient weak and run down.

**Mind:** Great sadness, anxiety and dread.

**Stomach:** Sinking, all gone sensation in the stomach (*Sep.*). Hungry, must eat.

**Urinary:** Urine frequent at night; smells like Valerian; constant urging (*Kreos.*).

**Female:** Conscious of the womb. Pulsations in the neck of the uterus. *Sensation* as if something was pressing on a sore spot in the pelvis; worse sitting. *Pain from the right side of womb to the right or left breast.* Sore pain in the uterus. *Desire, easily excited, nymphomania.* Least contact of parts causes *violent sexual excitement.* Menses irregular, profuse, frequent, large clots (menorrhagia, metrorrhagia). Sensation of protrusion. Prolapse; enlargement of the uterus (cancer of uterus), with pelvic tenesmus and sharp pains, extending towards the breasts; aggravated by lying down. Dysmenorrhea and chronic endometritis with displacement. *Must keep legs tightly crossed.* Leucorrhea green or bloody, alternates with mental symptoms and aching in the sacrum. Benign tumors of the breasts. Pain in the breasts during menstrual period.

**Modalities:** *Worse,* least touch.

**Relationship:** Compare: *Plat., Lil-t., Sep.* (the latter lacks sexual erethism of *Murx.*).

**Dose:** Third to thirtieth potency.

---

# MURIATICUM ACIDUM

(Muriatic Acid) **Mur-ac.**

This acid has an elective affinity for the blood, producing a septic condition similar to that found in low fevers with high temperature and great prostration. Patient becomes so weak that she slides down the bed. Decomposition of fluids. Involuntary stools while passing urine. Hemorrhages. Mouth and anus chiefly affected.

**Mind:** Irritable and peevish; fretful. *Loud moaning.* Great restlessness. Sad, taciturn; *suffers in silence.*

**Head:** Vertigo; *worse lying on the right side;* occiput heavy as if filled with lead. Sound of voice is intolerable. Pain as if the brain was crushed.

**Nose:** *Hemorrhage;* intense sneezing.

**Face:** Lower jaw falls; pimples and freckles; lips raw, dry, cracked.

**Mouth:** Tongue, pale, swollen, dry, leathery, paralyzed. Deep ulcers on the tongue. Hard lumps on the tongue. Epithelioma; edges bluish-red (*Carb-ac.*). Aphthous mouth. Gums and glands swollen. Fetid breath. *Sordes on teeth.*

**Throat:** Uvula swollen. Ulcers and false membrane (diphtheria). Edematous, dark, raw. An attempt to swallow produces spasms and choking.

**Stomach:** Cannot bear sight or thought of meat. At times, ravenous appetite and constant desire to drink. Achlorhydria and fermentation of food.

**Rectum:** Tendency to involuntary evacuations while micturating. *Hemorrhoids, extremely sensitive to any touch;* even a sheet of toilet paper is painful. Anal itching and prolapsus ani while micturating. *Hemorrhoids during pregnancy; bluish, hot, with violent stitches.*

**Urinary:** Cannot micturate without having bowel movement at the same time.

**Female:** Menses appear too soon. Leucorrhea. During menses, soreness in the anus. Ulcers on the genitals.

**Heart:** Pulse rapid, *feeble and small. Intermits every third beat.*

**Extremities:** Heavy, painful, and weak. Tottering gait. Pain in tendo-Achilles.

**Fever:** Cold extremities. Heat without thirst. Typhoid type, stupid. Hemorrhages. Restlessness. Involuntary discharges. Bed sores. Pulse rapid and feeble. Excessive prostration.

**Skin:** Papular and vesicular eruptions with great itching (*Rhus-t.*). Carbuncles; foul smelling ulcers on the lower extremities. Scarlet fever, livid, with petechiae; scanty eruption. Eczema on the back of hands.

**Modalities:** *Worse*, in damp weather, before midnight. *Better*, lying on the left side.

**Relationship:** Compare: *Ph-ac., Ars., Bapt.*

Follows well after *Bry.* and *Rhus-t.*

Antidote: *Bry.*

**Dose:** First to third potency.

---

## MYGALE LASIODORA

(Black Cuban Spider) **Mygal.**

Weakness, palpitations, nervousness, fear, like other spider preparations. Chorea is the principal therapeutic field of this. Sexual symptoms are important.

**Mind:** Delirious, restless, sad; fears death; despondent.

**Face:** *Twitching of facial muscles.* Mouth and eyes open in rapid succession. Hot and *flushed.* Tongue dry and parched; protruded with difficulty. Head jerks to one side. Grating of teeth at night.

**Stomach:** Nausea, with weak sight. Aversion to food. Excessive thirst.

**Male:** Violent erections. Chordee (*Kali-br., Camph.*).

**Extremities:** Unsteady gait (locomotor ataxia). *Constant motion of the whole body.* Tremulous. Intense redness in streaks, following course of lymphatics (lymphangitis). Twitching of limbs. Restless hands. Convulsive, uncontrollable movements of arms and legs. Limbs drag while walking.

**Modalities:** *Better*, during sleep. *Worse*, in the morning.

**Relationship:** Compare: *Agar., Tarent., Cupr., Ziz.*

**Dose:** Third to thirtieth potency.

---

## MYOSOTIS SYMPHYTIFOLIA

(Forget-me-not) **Myos-s.**

Chronic bronchitis and phthisis. Night sweats.

**Respiratory:** Cough with profuse muco purulent expectoration (bronchitis), gagging and vomiting during cough; worse while or after eating. Bronchorrhea. Pain in the left lung (lower); painful while coughing and sensitive to percussion.

**Dose:** Tincture to second potency.

---

## MYRICA CERIFERA

(Bayberry) **Myric.**

Marked action on the liver and mucous membranes. Persistent sleeplessness. *Jaundice.*

**Mind:** *Despondent, irritable,* indifferent. *Gloomy.*

**Head:** Scalp feels tight. Headache with drowsiness; yellow sclera; aching in the eyeballs. Pressure in the vertex and forehead. *Dull, heavy aching in temples and forehead on waking up in the morning.* Pain and stiffness in the nape of neck (cervical spondylosis).

**Face:** Yellow. Itching and stinging. Creeping sensation.

**Mouth:** Tongue furred with a bad taste in the mouth and nausea. *Tenacious, thick, nauseous secretion.* Tender, spongy and bleeding gums (scorbutic) (*Merc.*).

**Throat:** Constricted with a rough feeling and a constant desire to swallow. Stringy mucus; detached with difficulty.

**Stomach:** Taste bitter and nauseous, with halitosis. Complete loss of appetite, with a feeling of fullness in the stomach after a hearty meal. Strong desire for acids. Weak, sinking feeling in the epigastrium, approaching nausea; increased after eating; relieved by rapid walking.

**Abdomen:** Dull pain in the liver region. Complete jaundice with bronze-yellow skin; loss of appetite. Fullness in the stomach and abdomen. Scanty, yellow, frothy urine.

**Rectum:** Constant discharge of flatus when walking. Urging to stool, with no results other than the expulsion of a great amount of flatus. Loose, light colored stool; ash colored, destitute of bile.

**Urinary:** Dark, frothy, scanty, high colored, biliary.

**Extremities:** Staggering gait. Pain under the shoulder blades and back of neck, in all the muscles and in the hollow of the right foot.

**Sleep:** Disturbed, bad dreams and frequent waking; insomnia.

**Skin:** Yellow and itching. *Jaundice. Creeping sensation, as if from insects.*

**Relationship:** Compare: *Ptel., Corn., Chel., Lept., Fago.*

Antidote: *Dig.* (jaundice).

**Dose:** Tincture to third potency.

---

## MYRISTICA SEBIFERA

(Brazilian Ucuba) **Myris.**

A remedy of great antiseptic powers. Inflammation of the skin, cellular tissue (cellulitis), and periosteum (periostitis). Traumatic infections. Parotiditis. Fistulas. Carbuncles. *Specific action in panaritium.* Pain in the finger nails with swelling of the phalanges. Hands are stiff, as if from squeezing something for a long time. Coppery taste and burning in the throat. Tongue white and cracked. Phlegmonous inflammations. Hastens suppuration and shortens its duration. Often prevents the use of a knife. Otitis media, suppurative stage. Fistula in ano. Often acts more powerfully than *Hep.* or *Sil.*

---

## MYRTUS COMMUNIS

(Myrtle) **Myrt-c.**

The leaves contain Myrtol, an active antiseptic. Chest pains, as often found in phthisis call for this remedy. Incipient phthisis. Nerve sedative and stimulant to mucous membranes, bronchitis, cystitis and pyelitis.

**Chest:** Stitching pain *in the left breast, radiating to the shoulder blade* (*Anis., Ther., Pix*). Dry, hollow cough, with tickling in the chest. *Worse* in the morning. Sensation of burning in the left chest.

**Relationship:** Compare: *Myrtus chekan* (chronic bronchitis with dense, yellowish sputum, difficult to detach. Copious expectoration, distressing the patient and cough).

**Dose:** Third potency.

---

## NAJA TRIPUDIANS

(Virus of the Cobra) **Naja**

*Naja* produces a typical bulbar paralysis (L. J. Boyd). Causes no hemorrhage but only edema, hence the victims of this reptile frequently bear very little sign of external injury, a small scratch or puncture being the only indication where the fangs have worked their havoc. The tissue lying beneath the wound is dark purple and a large quantity of viscid blood-like fluid collects in the vicinity of the wound. An intense burning pain at the spot bitten is the first symptom. In man there follows an interval before fresh symptoms occur. The average is about an hour. Once developed, the symptoms follow a rapid course. A feeling of intoxication is produced, followed by a loss of power over the limbs. The patient is bereft of speech, swallowing, and looses control over the movement of lips. The saliva is ejected in large quantities, respiration gradually becomes slower and slower, and at length ceases. Conscious all the time. Is not a hemorrhagic or septic medicine like *Lach.* and *Crot-h.* Its action settles around the heart; valvular problems. Marked surging of blood upwards, marked dyspnea, inability to lie on the left side. Hypertrophy, and valvular lesions. *Organs seem to be drawn together.* Very susceptible to cold. With heart symptoms, pain in the forehead and temples. Diseases primarily depending upon the degeneration of motor cells. Control of sphincters lost.

**Mind:** Broods constantly over imaginary problems. Suicidal insanity (*Aur.*). Depressed. Aversion to talking. Blurred speech. Melancholy. Dread of being left alone. Fear of rain.

**Head:** *Pain in the left temple and left orbit, extending to the occiput with nausea and vomiting* (migraine). Hay fever, with dry larynx. Suffocative spells after sleeping (*Lach.*).

**Eyes:** Staring. Ptosis of both lids.

**Ears:** Illusions of hearing; otalgia; chronic otorrhea, black discharges; smells like herring brine.

**Female:** Neuralgia in the left ovary; often serviceable in obscure pains of left groin, especially in post-operative cases; *seems; to be drawn to the heart.*

**Respiratory:** Grasping at the throat, with sense of choking. *Irritating, dry cough, dependent on cardiac lesions* (*Spong., Laur.*). Sticky mucus and saliva. Asthmatic constriction in the evening. Asthma beginning with coryza.

**Heart:** Dragging and anxiety in the precordia. Sensation of weight on the heart. Angina pains extending to the nape of neck, left shoulder and arm with anxiety and fear of death. Pain in the forehead and temples with heart symptoms. Pulse *irregular in force.* Threatened paralysis of the heart, body cold, pulse slow, weak, irregular, tremulous. *Acute and chronic endocarditis.* Palpitations. Stitching pain in the region of heart. *Damaged heart after infectious diseases.* Marked symptoms of *low* tension (*Elaps, Vip.*).

**Sleep:** Profound; like a log with stertorous breathing, a typical reptilian state.

**Modalities:** *Worse*, from use of stimulants; *better*, from walking or riding in open air.

**Relationship:** Compare: Serpent poisons generally. *Bungarus fasciatus* (Banded krait). This venom produces a condition like acute polioencephalitis and myelitis, both symptomatically and histologically. *Lach., Crot-h., Spig., Spong.*

**Dose:** Sixth to thirtieth potency.

---

# NAPHTHALINUM

(A Chemical Compound From Coal-tar, Tar Camphor)

**Naphtin.**

Coryza, hay fever, phthisis pulmonalis, also gonorrhea have been influenced favorably by this drug. Pyelonephritis. Irritation of the periphery of the urinary apparatus. Whooping cough.

**Head:** Lying as if stupefied by a narcotic. Restless. Face pale. Yellowish hue.

**Eyes:** Marked affinity for the eye. It produces detachment of the retina; papillo-retinal infiltration; deposits in patches on the retina; amblyopia and consecutive amaurosis; sparkling synchisis; soft cataract. Exudation in the retina, choroid and ciliary body. Cataract. *Opacity of the cornea* (leucoma).

**Urinary:** Irresistible desire. Meatus red, swollen and edema of prepuce (balanitis). Black urine. Cutting pain down the penis. Pain in the bladder (cystitis). Terribly offensive odor of decomposing ammoniacal urine.

**Respiratory:** Sneezing; eyes inflamed; painful; head hot. *Hay fever. Spasmodic asthma*; better in open air. Soreness in the chest and stomach; must loosen the clothing. *Dyspnea* and sighing inspiration. Emphysema in the aged with asthma. *Whooping cough,* long and continued paroxysms of coughing, unable to take a breath. Acute laryngo-tracheitis. Bronchitis when the spasmodic element is associated with tenacious expectoration and oppression (Cartier).

**Skin:** Dermatitis; itching infiltration. Eruptions at corners of mouth and pigmentation around the nails.

**Relationship:** Compare: *Dros., Cor-r., Coc-c. Terpin-hydras.* (whooping cough, hay asthma and bronchial affections. 1-2 grain doses).

**Non-homoeopathic Uses:** For worms, especially pinworms, one-gram dose. Externally in skin diseases, five percent ointment.

**Dose:** Third trituration.

---

# NARCISSUS POETICIUS

(Daffodil) **Narc-po.**

Symptoms of nausea followed by violent vomiting and diarrhea.

Daffodil bulbs contain an alkaloid, the action of which, according to authorities, varies as to whether the alkaloid is extracted from the flowering bulb or from the bulb after flowering. In the former case the alkaloid *produces dryness of the mouth, checks cutaneous secretions, dilates the pupil, quickens the pulse and slows and weakens the heart contractions.* On the other hand, the alkaloid from the bulbs after flowering, *produces copious salivation, increases cutaneous secretion, contracts the pupil of the eye, produces a slight relaxation of the pulse, and slight faintness and nausea—The Lancet.*

A remedy for cough and bronchitis. Continuous cough. Coryza; frontal headache. Convulsive stage of whooping cough.

**Skin:** Erythema of a papular, vesicular and pustular type, aggravation in wet weather.

**Dose:** First attenuation.

# NATRIUM ARSENICOSUM

(Arseniate of Sodium) **Nat-ar.**

A remedy for nasal catarrh with headache, pain at the root of the nose, dry and painful eyes. Psoriasis (*Ars., Chry-ac., Thyr.*). Bronchitis in children over seven years. Facilitates the termination of cold and conserves strength and appetite (Cartier.).

**Head:** Floating sensation on turning the head quickly; aching in the frontal region and root of the nose, over the orbits. Headache; worse, pressure and tobacco smoke.

**Eyes:** Catarrhal conjunctivitis and blepharitis marginalis. Eyes feel weak, stiffness of the balls and tendency of the lids to close. Feel heavy and droop (ptosis). Lachrymation on exposure to wind. Agglutination in the morning. Dry, painful, burning; tire soon. Edema in the orbital region. Supraorbital pain.

**Nose:** Watery discharge; drops into the throat. *Feels obstructed; pain at the root.* Dry crusts, on removal, leave mucous membrane raw. Post-nasal dropping of thick, bland, yellowish mucus. *Crusts in nose.*

**Throat:** Dark, *purplish, swollen, edematous;* red and glassy (diphtheria).

**Respiratory:** Racking cough with profuse greenish expectoration. *Oppression of the chest and around the heart,* also in the larynx. Miner's asthma. Lungs feel as though smoke had been inhaled.

**Extremities:** Aching in the arms; worse in the shoulder. Pain in anterior crural nerves. Joints stiff. Feels tired all over. Knee joints crack (arthritis).

**Relationship:** Compare: *Ars., Kali-c., Apis.*

**Dose:** Third to thirtieth potency.

---

# NATRIUM CARBONICUM

(Carbonate of Sodium) **Nat-c.**

All the *Natriums* stimulate cellular activity and increase oxidation and metabolism. Great debility *caused by summer heat;* chronic effects of sunstroke; exhaustion; anemic; milky, watery skin; very weak ankles, are all peculiar *Natrium carbonicum* conditions.

**Mind:** Unable to think; difficult, slow comprehension. Mental weakness and depression; worries; very sensitive to noise; colds, change of weather. Anxious and restless during thunderstorm; worse from music (*Ambr.*). Marked gaiety. Sensitive to the presence of certain individuals.

**Head:** Aches from the *slightest mental exertion,* worse from *sun or working under gas light* (*Glon.*). Feels too large. Oversensitive to hearing. Headaches with the return of hot weather. Vertigo from exposure to sun.

**Nose:** All the problems of the external nose which may attain a morbid size, pimples and puffiness. Constant coryza; obstruction of the nose. *Catarrh; bad smell of nasal secretions.* Several problems of the external nose (*Caust.*). *Posterior nasal catarrh. Hawking profuse mucus from the throat; worse, slightest draught.*

**Face:** Freckles, *yellow spots, pimples.* Swelling of the upper lip. Pale, with blue rings around the eyes and swollen lids.

**Stomach:** Feels swollen and sensitive. Ill effects of drinking cold water when overheated. Waterbrash. Hungry at 5 a.m. *Very weak digestion,* caused by the slightest error in the diet. Averse to milk. Depressed after eating. Bitter taste. Old dyspeptics, always belching, have a sour stomach and rheumatism. Dyspepsia relieved by soda biscuits.

**Stool:** Sudden call for stool. Escapes with haste and noise. *Yellow substance, like pulp of orange in discharge.* Diarrhea from milk.

**Female:** Induration of the cervix. Pudenda sore. Bearing down sensation (prolapse) (*Sep., Murx.*). Heaviness; worse, sitting; better, by moving. Menses late, scanty, like meat washings (*Nit-ac.*). Leucorrheal discharge, offensive, irritating, preceded by colic.

**Respiratory:** Dry cough, when coming into a warm room from out doors. Cough with coldness of the left breast or chest.

**Extremities:** Old sprains. Great weakness of limbs, especially in the morning. *Easy dislocation and spraining of ankles.* Foot bends under (*Caust.*). Soreness between toes and fingers. Heel and tendo-Achilles affected. Chapped hands. The hollow of the knee is painful on motion. Icy cold up to knees.

**Sleep:** Wakes up very early in the morning. Amorous dreams. Drowsy during the day.

**Skin:** Inclination to perspire easily, or dry, rough, cracked skin. Eruptions on the finger tips, knuckles and toes. Vesicular eruption in patches and circles. Veins full. Soles of feet raw and sore.

**Modalities:** *Worse*, sitting, from music, summer *heat,* mental exertion, *thunderstorm.* Least draught, changes in weather, sun. *Better,* by moving, by boring in ears and nose..

**Relationship:** Compare: *Sodii bicarbonas* (in vomiting of pregnancy with acetonuria, 30 grains in water spread over twenty-four hours); *Nat-s., Caust., Natrium cacodylicum* (foul breath and mouth with bad odor. Dry dermatitis of the abdominal skin. Malignant growths. In phthisis, 5 centigrams hypodermically, daily. Increase number of red blood corpuscles to double.

Also in *malignant disease*). *Arsynal*—Disodium methylarsenate. Introduced by M. A. Gautier, for phthisis in the second stage 4 to 6 centigrammes per day for one week followed by a week's intermission. But much smaller doses, i. e., lx to 3x are followed by improvement, lower fever, night sweat and hemoptysis ceasing.

Antidote: *Ars., Camph.*

**Dose:** Sixth potency.

---

# NATRIUM HYPOCHLOROSUM

(Chlorate of Sodium, Labarraque's Solution)

**Nat-hchls.**

In congested and atonic states of the uterus and its ligaments, with hepatic disorders. Chronic catarrhal diseases of the middle ear. *Flabby, debilitated constitution.* Both hands swollen in the morning. Phlegmatic. Depressed, faint.

**Head:** Vertigo, with aching across the forehead. Sensation of swimming, as if the top of the head would float off. Epistaxis in the form of clots.

**Mouth:** Sore irritable spots along the sides of tongue and throat, gums sore, tongue swollen; aphthous ulceration. Putrid taste. Furred tongue, large, flabby, indented. Cough with aphonia.

**Stomach:** *Drowsy after meals.*

**Urinary:** Dark with albumen and casts. Diffuse nephritis. Severe pain across the lumbosacral region.

**Female:** Sensation as if the uterus was pushed up on sitting down (*Ferr-i.*). Feels as if it opened and shut. Severe metrorrhagia. Leucorrhea with backache. Passive, bearing down sensation due to a heavy uterus. Womb is heavy, sodden with a tendency to prolapse. Subinvolution.

**Extremities:** Hands swollen every morning. Extreme weakness in ankles and knees.

**Relationship:** Compare: *Aur-m-n., Calc., Sep., Heliotropium peruvianum* (uterine displacement, with active bearing down sensation and aphonia; membranous dysmenorrhea).

Antidotes: *Puls., Guaj.*

**Dose:** Fifteen to twenty drops of Labarraque's solution in water. Third attenuation made with dilute alcohol, lower with water.

---

# NATRIUM MURIATICUM

(Chloride of Sodium) **Nat-m.**

Prolonged intake of excessive salt causes profound nutritive changes in the system, resulting in salt retention, evidenced by dropsies, edemas and alteration in the blood causing a condition of anemia and leucocytosis. There also seems to be a retention of effete materials in the tissues giving rise to symptoms loosely described as gouty or rheumatic gout. The provings are full of such symptoms (Dr. Stonham.). A great remedy for certain forms of intermittent fever, anemia, chlorosis, several disturbances of the alimentary tract and skin. Great debility; maximum weakness is felt in the morning, in bed. *Coldness.* Emaciation most notable in the neck. Great liability to take cold. *Dry mucous membranes.* Constrictive sensation throughout the body. *Great weakness and weariness*. Oversensitive to all sorts of influences. Hyperthyroidism. Goitre. Addison's disease. Diabetes.

**Mind:** Psychic causes of disease; ill effects of grief, fright, anger, etc. Depressed, particularly in chronic diseases. *Consolation aggravates.* Irritable; gets into a passion about trifies. Awkward, hasty. Wants to be alone to cry. Tears with laughter.

**Head:** Throbs. *Blinding* headache. Aches as if a thousand little hammers were knocking on the brain in the morning on awakening, *after menstruation*, from *sunrise to sunset.* Feels too large; cold. Anemic headache in school girls; nervous, discouraged, broken down. Chronic headache, semi-lateral, congestive, from sunrise to sunset, with a pale face, nausea, vomiting; periodical; from eye strain; menstrual. Before attack, numbness and tingling in the lips, tongue and nose, relieved by sleep. Frontal sinus inflamed (sinusitis).

**Eyes:** Feel bruised, *with headache in school children* (eye strain). Eyelids heavy. *Muscles weak and stiff.* Letters run together. Sees sparks. Fiery, zigzag appearance around all objects. Burning in eyes. Give out on reading or writing. Stricture of the lachrymal duct with suppuration. Escape of muco-pus when pressing on the sac. Lachrymation, burning and acrid. Lids swollen (blepharitis). Eyes appear wet with tears. *Tears stream down the face on coughing* (*Euphr.*). *Asthenopia* due to insufficiency of *internal recti muscles* (*Gels.* and *Cupr-act.*, when due to *external* muscles). *Pain in the eyes when looking down.* Cataract, *incipient* (*Sec.*).

**Ears:** Noises; roaring and ringing (tinnitus).

**Nose:** *Violent, fluent coryza,* lasting for one to three days, followed by obstruction of the nose, making breathing difficult. Discharge thin and watery, *like raw white of egg.* Violent sneezing, coryza. *Infallible for stopping a cold commencing with sneezing.* Use thirtieth potency. *Loss of smell and taste.* Internal soreness of the nose. Dryness.

**Face:** Oily, shiny, as if greased. Earthy complexion. *Fever blisters.*

**Mouth:** Frothy coating on the tongue, with bubbles on the side. Sense of dryness. Scorbutic gums. *Numbness, tingling in the tongue,* lips, and nose. Vesicles and burning in the tongue, as if there was a hair on it. Eruptions around the mouth and *vesicles like pearls on lips* (herpes labialis). Lips and corners of mouth dry, ulcerated and cracked. Deep crack in the middle of lower lip. *Tongue mapped* (*Ars., Rhus-t., Tarax.*). Loss of taste. Large vesicle on lower lip, which is swollen and burns. Immoderate thirst.

**Stomach:** Hungry, yet looses flesh (*Iod.*). Heartburn with palpitations. Unquenchable thirst. *Sweats while eating*. Craving for salt. Aversion to bread, to anything slimy, like oysters, fats. Throbbing in the pit. Sticking sensation in the cardiac orifice.

**Abdomen:** Cutting pain in the abdomen. Distended. Pain in the abdominal ring on coughing.

**Rectum:** Burning pains and stitching after stool. Anus contracted, *torn, bleeding.* Constipation; stool dry, crumbling (*Am-m., Mag-m.*). Painless and copious diarrhea, preceded by pinching pain in the abdomen.

**Urinary:** Pain just *after* micturating (*Sars.*). Increased, involuntary when walking, coughing, etc. Has to wait for a long time for it to pass *if others are present* (*Hep., Mur-ac.*).

**Male:** Emission, even after coitus. Impotence with retarded emission.

**Female:** Menses irregular; usually profuse. Vagina dry. Leucorrhea acrid, watery. Bearing down pains; worse in the morning (*Sep.*). Prolapsus uteri, with cutting in the urethra. Ineffectual labor pains. Suppressed menses (follow with *Kali-c.*). Hot during menses.

**Respiratory:** Cough from a tickling in the pit of the stomach, accompanied by stitches in the liver and spurting of urine (*Caust., Squil.*). Stitches all over the chest. Cough with bursting pain in the head. Shortness of breath, especially on going upstairs (*Calc.*). Whooping cough with *lachrymation.*

**Heart:** Tachycardia. Sensation of coldness in the heart. Heart and chest feel constricted. Fluttering, palpitating; intermittent pulse. Pulsations of the heart shake the body. *Intermits on lying down.*

**Extremities:** Pain in the back, *with a desire for some firm support* (*Rhus-t., Sep.*). Every movement accelerates the circulation. *Palms hot and perspiring.* Arms, legs, especially knees, feel weak. *Hangnails.* Dryness and cracking around the finger nails. *Numbness and tingling* in the fingers and lower extremities. Ankles weak and turn easily. Painful contraction of hamstrings (*Caust.*). Cracking in joints on motion. *Coldness of legs* with congestion of the head, chest and stomach.

**Sleep:** Sleepy in the forenoon. Nervous jerking during sleep. Dreams of robbers. Sleepless from grief.

**Fever:** Chill between 9 and 11 a. m. Heat; violent thirst, increases with fever. Fever blisters. *Coldness of the body* and *continuous chilliness* very marked. Hydremia in chronic malarial states with weakness, constipation, loss of appetite, etc. Sweats on every exertion.

**Skin:** Greasy, oily, especially on hairy parts. Dry eruptions, especially on the margin of the hairy scalp and bends of joints. Fever blisters. Urticaria; itch and burn. Crusty eruptions in the *bends of limbs, margin of scalp,* behind ears (intertrigo) (*Caust.*). Warts on palms. Eczema; raw, red, and inflamed; worse, eating salt, at seashore. Affects hair follicles. Alopecia. Hives, itching after exertion. *Greasy* skin.

**Modalities:** *Worse,* noise, music, warm room, lying down; around 10 a. m., at the sea shore, mental exertion, consolation, *heat,* talking. *Better,* open air, cold bathing, going without regular meals, lying on the right side; pressure against the back, tight clothing.

**Relationship:** Complementary to *Apis, Sep., Ign.*

Compare: *Aqua marina*—Isotonic plasma (marine plasma is sea water taken some miles away from the shore and at some depth, below surface, filtered and diluted with twice as much pure fresh water. It acts primarily on the blood, as in intoxications, scrofulous conditions, enteritis. It disintoxicates in cancer, administered subcutaneously in the treatment of skin, renal and intestinal diseases, *gastroenteritis and tuberculosis. Scrofulous affection of children.* Lymphadenitis. Lupus, eczema, varicose ulcers. A great "blood purifier and vitalizer." Potentized sea water is indicated in weakness, lack of reaction; symptoms worse seaside. Goitre). *Sal marinum,* sea salt, (indicated in chronic enlargements of glands, especially cervical. Suppurating glands. It is useful as an auxiliary remedy, if not as a principal, in the treatment of diseases in patients of a strumous diathesis. Also useful in constipation). *Natrium selenicum* (laryngeal phthisis with expectoration of small lumps of bloody mucus and slight hoarseness). *Natrium silicicum* (hemophilia; scrofulous bone affections; given intravenously every 3 days for *senile pruritus* (*Dol., Fago.*). *Ign., Sep., Thuj., Graph., Alum.*

Antidotes: *Ars., Phos., Spir-n-d.*

**Dose:** Twelfth to thirtieth and higher. The very highest potencies often yield the most brilliant results. In infrequent dosage.

---

# NATRIUM NITRICUM

(Nitrate of Sodium) **Nat-n.**

A Rademacherian remedy for *inflammations.* Hemoptysis. Hematuria. Purpura hemorrhagica. Hemorrhagic variola. Drowsiness. Pains of tabes. *Influenza.* Hemorrhages from mucous membranes, particularly nasal. Hemoglobinuria. Uric acid diathesis. Asthma with urine supersaturated with solids. Anemia and hydremia. Exhaustion, must rest frequently when walking.

**Head:** Dull. Indisposed to mental and physical exertion. Pain pressing inwards. Inward pressing in malar bones.

**Ears:** Otalgia. *Epistaxis.*

**Stomach:** Sour eructations. Aversions to coffee. Flatulence, with pressure in the pit of the stomach and pain in the chest; worse motion, better eructation.

**Abdomen:** Abdominal muscles contract painfully towards the spine. Distended. Difficult stool (constipation); feels as if more remained to pass (unsatisfactory stools).

**Heart:** Pain in the region of heart (angina pectoris). Pulse slower and softer.

**Dose:** Second trituration, also watery solution; 1 dram of salt to 8 oz. water. Dram doses.

---

# NATRIUM PHOSPHORICUM

(Phosphate of Sodium) **Nat-p.**

*Natrium phosphoricum* is the remedy for conditions arising from excess of lactic acid, often resulting from too much sugar. Ailments, *with excess of acidity.* Sour eructations and taste. Sour vomiting. *Yellow, creamy coating of the tongue and posterior portion of the roof of mouth.* Inflammation of any part of the throat, with sensation of a lump in the throat. Flatulence, with sour risings. Colic, with symptoms of worms. Cracking of joints. *Jaundice* (lx trituration). Oxaluria.

**Mind:** Imagines, on waking at night, that pieces of furniture are people; that he hears footsteps in the next room. *Fear.*

**Head:** Feels dull in the morning, feels full and throbbing.

**Eyes:** Discharge of *a golden-yellow, creamy matter* from the eyes. Dilation of one pupil. Scelera, dirty yellow (jaundice).

**Ears:** One ear red, hot, frequently itchy, accompanied by gastric derangements and acidity.

**Nose:** Offensive odor. Itching in the nose. Naso-pharyngeal catarrh, with thick, yellow, offensive mucus (ozena).

**Face:** Paleness or a bluish, florid appearance of the face.

**Mouth:** Canker sores of lips and cheeks. *Blisters on the tip of the tongue,* with stinging in the evening. *Thin, moist coating on the tongue. Yellow, creamy coating on the posterior part of the roof of mouth. Dysphagia.* Thick, creamy membrane over the tonsils and soft palate.

**Stomach:** *Sour eructations, sour vomiting, greenish diarrhea.* Spits mouthful of food.

**Male:** Emissions without dreams, with *weakness in the back and trembling in limbs.* Desire without erection. Gonorrhea.

**Female:** Menses too early; pale, thin, watery. Sterility with acid secretions from the vagina. Leucorrhea; discharge creamy or honey colored, or acid and watery. Sour smelling discharges from the uterus. Morning sickness, with sour vomiting.

**Back:** Weariness; aching in the wrists and finger joints. Hamstrings sore. *Synovial crepitation.* Rheumatic arthritis.

**Extremities:** Rheumatism of the knee joint (osteoarthritis).

**Skin:** Yellow. Itching in various parts, *especially ankles. Hives.* Smooth, red, shining. Erysipelas. Feet icy cold during day time, burn at night. Swelling of lymphatic glands.

**Relationship:** Compare: *Natrium lacticum* (rheumatism and gout; gouty concretions; rheumatism with diabetes); *Natrium nitrosum* (angina pectoris. Cyanosis, fainting, copious liquid stools at night; throbbing and fullness; faintness, nervous pains in the head, nausea, eructations, blue lips). *Natrium silicofluoricum*—Salufer (a cancer remedy; tumors, bone affection, caries, lupus, ethmoiditis. Must be used carefully); *Natrium selenicum* (chronic laryngitis and laryngeal phthisis; hoarseness of singers, expectorate small lumps of mucus with frequent clearing of throat); *Natrium sulphurosum* (diarrhea with yeasty stools); *Natrium sulphocarbolicum* (pyemia; purulent pleurisy, 3 to 5 grains every three hours); *Natrium telluricum* (breath has an odor of garlic; night sweats of phthisis). *Calc., Rob., Phos.* In oxaluria 1x four times daily prevents formation of calculi; keeps the oxalate of lime in solution (Schwartz).

**Dose:** Third to twelfth trituration. In jaundice lx.

**Non-homeopathic Uses:** Phosphate soda is used hypodermically for morphine habit, by Dr. M. J. Luys. Phosphate soda, 75 gr. daily, for constitutional iodism, thyroidism and Grave's disease.

---

# NATRIUM SALICYLICUM

(Salicylate of Sodium) **Nat-sal.**

Has an extensive range of action affecting the head, ear, throat, kidneys, liver and on metabolism. Hemorrhages, especially epistaxis. Produces marked effects upon the internal ear with vertigo, deafness, noises in the ears and loss of bone conduction, hence, its useful in Meniere's disease. *One of the best remedies for the prostrating after effects of influenza.* Lassitude, drowsiness, listlessness, tremors. Incipient dementia. Increases the quantity of bile. Follicular tonsillitis.

**Head:** Perfectly rational periods alternate with manifestations of insanity of a sombre character. *Vertigo; worse,* raising head. All objects seem to move to the right. Dull headache and confusion. Fibrositis of the scalp.

**Eyes:** Retinal hemorrhage, albuminuric retinitis with hemorrhage. Iridocyclitis due to traumatism with infection, and in sympathetic disease, secondary to it (Dr. Gradel).

**Ears:** *Tinnitus* of a low tone. Deafness. Auditory vertigo.

**Chest:** Dyspnea; breathing noisy, shallow, panting; pulse irregular. Complete aphonia.

**Skin:** Edema, urticaria, red in circumscribed patches. Tingling and itching. Pemphigoid eruption.

**Relationship:** Compare: *Lobelia purpurascens* (drowsiness; dizzy headache between eyebrows; cannot keep eyes open; tongue white—feels paralyzed, as also the heart and lungs; intense prostration of all vital forces; deadly chill, without shivering; useful for the low, nervous prostration of influenza); *Gaul., Chin. Pyrus malus*—Crab apple tree (labyrinthine vertigo, Dr. Cooper).

**Non-homeopathic Uses:** In acute articular rheumatism, lumbago, sciatica, etc. Usual doses, ten to twenty grains every three hours. Must be used carefully, as it is often destructive of kidney tissue. Ordinary allopathic doses allay the pain of dysmenorrhea and promote menstrual flow.

**Dose:** Third potency.

---

# NATRIUM SULPHURICUM

(Sulphate of Sodium, Glauber's Salt) **Nat-s.**

A liver remedy, especially indicated for the so called hydrogenoid constitution, where the complaints are as such due to living in damp houses, basements, cellars. They are worse in rainy weather, from water in any form.

*Feels every change from dry to wet;* cannot even eat plants growing near water nor fish. Always feels best in warm, dry air. Clinically, it has been found to be a valuable remedy for *spinal meningitis,* head symptoms *from injuries to the head,* mental problems therefrom. Every spring, the skin affections return. Tendency to warts. Fingers and toes affected. Chronic gout (*Lyc.*).

**Mind:** Lively music saddens. Melancholy with periodical attacks of mania. Suicidal tendency; *must exercise restraint.* Inability to think. Dislikes speaking, or to be spoken to.

**Head:** Occipital pain. Piercing stitches in the ears. Vertigo; relieved by sweat on the head. Sensation of bursting on coughing. Hot feeling on top of the head. Boring in the right temple, preceded by burning in stomach. Ill effects of falls and injuries to the head, mental problems arising therefrom. Dreams of running water.

**Eyes:** Conjunctiva yellow (jaundice). Granular lids. *Photophobia* (*Graph.*).

**Ears:** Sticking pain, otalgia, lightening-like stitches in damp weather.

**Nose:** Nasal catarrh, with thick, yellow discharge and salty mucus. Coryza. Epistaxis. Ethmoiditis.

**Mouth:** Slimy, thick, tenacious, white mucus. *Bitter taste,* blisters on the palate.

**Throat:** Thick, yellow mucus, drops from the posterior nares.

**Stomach:** Sour vomit. *Brown, bitter coating on the tongue.* Yellow complexion. Thirst for something cold. Bilious vomiting, *acid* dyspepsia, with heartburn and flatulence.

**Abdomen:** Duodenal catarrh; hepatitis; icterus and vomiting of bile; liver sore to touch, with sharp, stitching pains; cannot bear tight clothing around the waist, worse, lying on left side. *Flatulence;* wind colic in the ascending colon; worse, before breakfast. Burning in the abdomen and anus. Bruised pain and urging to stool.

**Stool:** Diarrhea yellow, watery. *Loose morning stools;* worse, after a spell of wet weather. Stools involuntary, when passing flatus. *Great size of the fecal mass.*

**Urinary:** Loaded with bile. Brick-dust sediment. Excessive secretion. Diabetes.

**Male:** Condylomata; soft, fleshy excrescenses; greenish discharges. Gonorrhea; discharge thick, greenish; little pain.

**Female:** Epistaxis during menses, which is acrid and profuse. Burning in pharynx during menstruation. Herpetic vulvitis. *Leucorrhea* yellowish-green, *following gonorrhea in female.* Leucorrhea with hoarseness.

**Respiratory:** Dyspnea during damp weather. *Must hold the chest when coughing.* Humid asthma; rattling in the chest between 4 and 5 a. m. *Cough* with thick ropy, greenish expectoration; all gone sensation in the chest. Constant desire to take deep, long breaths. *Asthma in children,* as a constitutional remedy. Delayed resolution in pneumonia. Springs up in bed as cough hurts; holds the painful side (*Bry.*). Pain through *the lower left chest.* Every fresh cold brings on an attack of asthma.

**Back:** Itching when undressing. Violent pains at the back of the neck *and at the base of the brain.* Piercing pain between scapulae. Spinal meningitis; opisthotonus.

**Extremities:** Swelling of axillary glands (lymphadenopathy). Inflammation around root of nails (paronychia). Burning in the soles; edema of feet (phlagmesia alba dolens); itching between the toes (tinea pedis). Gout. Pain in limbs (sciatica), compels frequent change in position. Run around[1]. Pain in the hip joints, worse left side, worse, stooping. Stiffness of knees, cracking of joints. Rheumatism, worse in damp cold weather.

**Skin:** Itching while undressing. Jaundiced, watery blisters. Sycotic excrescences; wart-like red lumps all over the body.

**Modalities:** *Worse,* music (makes her sad); lying on the left side; dampness of basements, damp weather. *Better,* dry weather, pressure, changing position.

**Relationship:** Compare: *Natrium succinicum* (5 gr. every 3 hours. Catarrhal jaundice). *Malaria officinalis*—decomposed vegetable matter (has power to cause the disappearance of the plasmodium of malaria. Malarial cachexia. General sense of weariness. Splenic affections. Malaria and rheumatism. Functional hepatic diseases. Sixth potency and higher). *Natrium choleinicum*—Fel tauri depuratum (constipation; chronic gastric and intestinal catarrh; cirrhosis of the liver; diabetes; *pain in the nape* of *neck; tendency to sleep after eating;* flatus; ascites); *Momordica balsamina*—Balsam apple (colic, dysmenorrhea with gushes of blood). *Pulmo vulpis*—Wolf's lung (persistent shortness of breath causing a paroxysm of asthma on the slightest motion. Strong, sonorous bubbling rales. lx trituration). *Peumus boldus—Boldo* (atonic states of stomach and intestinal canal; liver states following malaria. Burning weight in the region of liver and stomach, bitter taste, languor; abscess of liver; asthma, bronchitis, catarrh, edema of the lungs); *Natrium iodatum* (incipient rheumatic endocarditis; chronic bronchitis, rheumatism and tertiary syphilis. Chronic catarrhal affections, arteriosclerosis. Here various symptoms, such as *angina pectoris,* vertigo, dyspnea become less marked after it continuous use of 6-10 grs., 3 times a day). *Natrium hyposulphurosum* (liver spots, locally and internally); *Sulph., Thuj., Merc., Still.*

Complementary: *Ars., Thuj.*

**Dose:** First to twelfth trituration.

[1] Compels one to move again after a short time (Clarke — Dictionary of Practical Materia Medica).

# NICCOLUM METALLICUM

(Metallic Nickel) **Nicc-met.**

Periodical nervous sick headaches with asthenopia, weak digestion, constipation. Catarrh. Suits debilitated, nervous, literary patients, with frequent headaches, dyspepsia and constipation.

**Head:** Cracking in cervical vertebrae when moving the head. Pain on top as if from a nail. Pressure on the vertex, in the morning; worse till noon and in a warm room. Stitches. Objects appear too large. Migraine; first on the left side. Twitching of the upper lip.

**Nose:** Violent sneezing; stopped up. Nasal catarrh, with redness and swelling of the tip of the nose. Acute pain at the root of the nose, extending to the vertex and through the temples.

**Mouth:** Sour, fetid secretions ooze from the molar teeth (decayed).

**Throat:** Sore; right side with great tenderness; *soreness* to *touch externally.* Strangulated feeling.

**Stomach:** All gone, empty feeling in the epigastrium, *without a desire for food.* Acute gastralgia with pains extending to the shoulder. Thirst and *intense hiccough.*

**Stool:** Diarrhea and tenesmus after milk.

**Female:** Menses late, scanty, with great debility and burning in the eyes. Profuse leucorrhea; worse, after micturition (*Mag-m., Plat.*); also worse after menses.

**Respiratory:** Hoarseness. Dry, hacking cough, with stitches in the chest. *Obliged to sit up and hold the head. Must put the arms on the thighs when coughing.*

**Skin:** Itching all over, worse on the neck, not relieved by scratching.

**Modalities:** *Worse,* periodically, every two weeks; yearly, forenoon. *Better,* in the evening.

**Dose:** Third trituration.

---

# NICCOLUM SULPHURICUM

(Sulphate of Nickel) **Nicc-s.**

Useful in climacteric disturbances. Periodic neuralgias of malarial origin. Urine and saliva increased. Coppery taste. Weak, asthenopic, literary people with weak digestion and constipation, are worse in the morning and suffer from periodic headaches and hoarseness.

**Head:** Nervous, uneasy, desire to recline, tired, cannot settle down to any occupation. Periodic headaches, occipital pain, extending down the spine, worse lying on the back; sore pain in the eyes.

**Female:** Dull aching in the ovaries with a sensation as if menses would appear. *Hot flushes,* followed by perspiration on parts touching each other, when they are separated they become dry.

**Back:** Stiff, numb sensation, worse in the neck (cervical spondylosis). Spine sore. Wakes up in the morning with burning soles. Spinal pains, legs and arms heavy and weak, cannot lie on the back.

**Dose:** Second trituration.

---

# NITRICUM ACIDUM

(Nitric Acid) **Nit-ac.**

Selects for its special seat of action the outlets of the body where the mucous membrane and skin meet; pain *as from splinters. Sticking* pains. Marked improvement in all symptoms while riding in a carriage. Acts best on dark complexioned people past their middle life. Syphilis, after abuse of mercury. Pains appear and disappear quickly (*Bell.*). Hydrogenoid constitution. Sycotic remedy.

Blisters and ulcers in the mouth, tongue, genitals; bleed easily. Fissures, with pain during stool, as if the rectum was torn. All discharges are very offensive, especially urine, feces and perspiration. People who have chronic diseases, take cold easily and are disposed to diarrhea. Excessive physical irritability. Cachexia, due to syphilis, scrofula, intermittent fever with liver involvement, anemia, etc. Gravel; arthritis. Capilary bleeding after currettage.

**Mind:** *Irritable,* hateful, vindictive, headstrong. Hopeless despair. Sensitive to noise, pain, touch, jar. Fear of death.

**Head:** Sensation of a *band around the head.* Headache from pressure of a hat; full feeling; worse from street noises. Hair falls out. Scalp sensitive.

**Eyes:** Diplopia; *sharp, sticking pains.* Ulceration of the cornea. Gonorrheal ophthalmia, photophobia, constant lachrymation. Syphilitic iritis.

**Ears:** Difficult hearing; better by riding in a carriage or train. *Very sensitive to noise,* like the rattle of wagons over pavements (*Coff., Nux-v.*). Cracking in ears when chewing.

**Nose:** Ozena. Green casts from the nose every morning. Coryza, with sore and bleeding nostrils. Tip red. Stitches, sensation of a splinter in the nose. *Caries of mastoid. Epistaxis* with chest affections. Chronic nasal catarrh with yellow, offensive, *corrosive* discharge. Nasal diphtheria, with watery and exceedingly excoriating discharge.

**Mouth:** Putrid breath. Salivation. Bleeding from gums. Painful pimples on the sides of the tongue. *Tongue clean, red and wet with a central furrow* (glossitis). Teeth become loose; gums soft and spongy (scorbutic). *Ulcers on the soft palate, with sharp, splinter-like pains* (stomatitis). Salivation and fetor oris. *Bloody saliva.*

**Throat:** Dry. Pain extends to the ears. Hawks mucus constantly. White patches and *sharp points, as if from splinters* on swallowing.

**Stomach:** Great hunger, with a sweetish taste. Longing for indigestible things, chalk, earth, etc. Pain in the cardiac orifice (gastric ulcer). Dyspepsia with excess of oxalic acid, uric acid and phosphates in urine, great mental depression. *Loves fat and salt* (*Sulph.*).

**Abdomen:** Great straining, but little passes. Rectum feels torn. Bowels constipated, with fissures in the rectum. Tearing pains during stools. Violent cutting pains *after stools, lasting for hours* (*Rat.*). Hemorrhages from the bowels, profuse, bright. Prolapsus ani. Hemorrhoids bleed easily. Diarrhea, slimy and offensive. After stools, irritable and exhausted. Colic relieved from tightening clothes. Jaundice, aching in the liver region.

**Urinary:** Scanty, dark, *offensive.* Smells like horse's urine. *Cold on passing.* Burning and stinging. Hematuria and albuminuria (Bright's disease). Alternation of cloudy, phosphatic urine with profuse urinary secretion in old prostatic cases.

**Male:** Soreness and burning in the glans and beneath the prepuce. Ulcers; burn and sting; exude an, offensive matter (syphilis).

**Female:** External parts sore, with ulcers (*Hep., Merc., Thuj.*). Leucorrhea brown, flesh colored, watery, or stringy, offensive. Hair on genitals fall out (*Nat-m., Zinc.*). Uterine hemorrhages. Menses early, profuse, like muddy water, with pain in the back, hips and thighs. Stitches through vagina. Metrorrhagia after parturition.

**Respiratory:** Hoarseness. Aphonia, with dry hacking cough, from tickling in the larynx and pit of stomach (bronchitis). Soreness at the lower end of sternum. *Short breath on going upstairs* (*Ars., Calc.*). Cough during sleep (*Cham.*).

**Extremities:** Fetid foot sweat, causing soreness of toes, with sticking pain; chilblains. Sweating of palms, hands; cold, blue nails. Offensive sweat in axillae at night.

**Skin:** Warts, large jagged; bleeds on washing. Ulcers bleed easily, sensitive; splinter-like pains; zigzag, irregular edges; base looks like raw flesh. Exuberant granulations. Black pores on the face (comedones, freckles), papules worse on the forehead.

**Modalities:** *Worse,* evening and night, cold climate, and also hot weather. *Better,* while riding in a carriage (reverse: *Cocc.*).

**Relationship:** Complementary: Ars., *Calad., Lac-c., Sep.*

Inimical: *Lach.*

Compare: *Merc., Kali-c., Thuj., Hep., Calc.*

**Dose:** Sixth potency. As the *Nit-ac.* patient begins to improve, skin symptoms may appear for a time, a favorable indication.

---

## NITRI SPIRITUS DULCIS

(Sweet Spirits of Nitre) **Nit-s-d.**

*Sensorial apathy* in low fevers when there is stupor, difficulty in arousing the patient, is met by this remedy. Dry skin, nausea, flatulence. Salty taste. *Ill effects of salt* (halophagia) (*Ars., Phos.*). Catching cold in stormy weather. Acute nephritis following scarlet fever. Dropsy, is an excellent diuretic.

**Face:** Prosopalgia with photophobia. Burning in cheeks and vomiting, *followed by lassitude.* Boring in facial bones; in angles of lower jaw. Very sensitive to cold.

**Respiratory:** Very rapid breathing after a short walk. Painful constriction beneath the sternum.

**Modalities:** *Worse,* from mental disturbance, during winter and spring.

**Relationship:** Increases the action of *Dig.*

Compare: *Ph-ac., Lyc.*

**Dose:** A few drops of the pure spirits in water every two or three hours.

---

## NITROSO-MURIATICUM ACIDUM

(Aqua Regia) **Nit-m-ac.**

Almost a specific in oxaluria. Removes the distressing skin symptoms resembling psoriasis. Three to five drops, three times a day. So called bilious conditions; torpid liver, hepatitis and early cirrhosis of liver. More adapted to hepatic torpor and gastric catarrh, common in hot and damp climates and aggravated by eating meat and alcohol (Hale). Constricted anus. Gravel.

**Mouth:** Gums bleed easily (scurvy). Ptyalism. *Constant drooling at night* (*Merc.*). Cankers; small, superficial ulceration inside the mouth and on the tongue (cancrum oris). Metallic taste (*Cupr.*).

**Stomach:** Sour eructations, with an empty, hungry feeling in the stomach; not relieved by eating. *Salivation; worse at night.*

**Rectum:** Constipated, with ineffectual urging. Sphincter constricted. Anus moist and sore.

**Urinary:** Cloudy. Burning in the urethra (urethritis). Oxaluria.

**Dose:** Five to ten drops, well diluted.

---

## NUPHAR LUTEUM

(Yellow Pond Lily) **Nuph.**

Produces nervous weakness, with marked symptoms in the sexual sphere.

**Stool:** Enterocolitis. Yellow diarrhea; worse in the morning. Diarrhea during typhoid.

**Male:** Complete absence of sexual desire; parts relaxed; penis retracted. Impotency, with involuntary emissions during stool, micturition. Spermatorrhea. Pain in the testicles and penis.

**Relationship:** Compare, in sexual weakness; *Agn., Kali-br., Lyc., Sel., Yohim.* In diarrhea: *Chel., Gam., Sulph., Nymphaea odorata*—Sweet water lily (early morning diarrhea, backache; acrid leucorrhea, offensive ulcers; bronchorrhea; ulcerative sore throat).

**Dose:** Tincture to sixth potency.

---

## NUX MOSCHATA

(Nutmeg) **Nux-m.**

Marked tendency to *fainting fits* with heart failure. Cold extremities, *extreme dryness of the mucous membranes* and skin. Strange feeling, with irresistible *drowsiness.* Indicanuria. General inclination to become unconscious during acute attacks. Lypothymia (mental prostration after grief (*Ign.*). Staggers, when trying to walk (locomotor ataxia).

**Mind:** Changeable; laughing and crying. Confused, impaired memory. Bewildered sense, as in a dream. Thinks she has two heads.

**Head:** Vertigo when walking in open air; aches from eating a little too much. Sensation of expansion, *with sleepiness.* Pulsations in the head. Cracking sensation in the head. Sensitive to the slightest touch, even a draught of air. Bursting headache; *better hard pressure.*

**Eyes:** Objects look larger, very distant or vanish. Motes before the eyes. Mydriasis.

**Nose:** Oversensitive to smell; epistaxis, dark blood; dry, stopped up.

**Mouth:** Very dry. Tongue adheres to the roof of the mouth; but no desire for water. Saliva like cotton (*Berb.*). Toothache in pregnancy. Tongue numb, paralyzed. *Dryness* in the throat.

**Stomach:** *Excessively bloated. Flatulent dyspepsia.* Hiccough and craving for highly seasoned food. Retrocession gout to stomach.

**Abdomen:** Paralytic weakness of intestines. *Enormously distended.* Stool is soft, and yet is *unable to expel it,* even after long straining (*Alum.*). *Fainting during or after stool.* Protruding piles.

**Female:** Uterine hemorrhage. Menses too long, dark, thick. Leucorrhea muddy and bloody. Suppression, with persistent fainting attacks and sleepiness (*Kali-c.*). *Variableness of menstruation, irregularity of time and quantity.*

**Respiratory:** Aphonia from walking against the wind (*Hep.*). Cough when getting warm in bed.

**Heart:** Trembling, fluttering. Sensation as if something grasped the heart. Palpitations; pulse intermits.

**Extremities:** Pain in the right hip, radiating to the knee; worse, motion, especially going upstairs. Rheumatism from getting feet wet, from exposure to draughts. Rheumatism relieved by dry, warm clothes. Fatigue on the slightest exertion.

**Fever:** Chill begins in the left hand (*Carb-v.*). Chilliness and heat without thirst; *want of perspiration. Dryness of the skin* and of the inner parts, also of eyes, nose, lips, mouth, tongue, throat, etc.

**Sleep:** Great drowsiness (*Indol.*). *Complaints cause sleepiness.* Coma.

**Modalities:** *Worse,* cold moist wind, cold food, cold washing, lying on the painful side, motion, jar. *Better,* warmth, dry weather.

**Relationship**: *Oleum myristicae*—Oil of Nutmeg (as a remedy for boils, felons, poisonous ulcers, it has been used in the 2x potency); *Ornithogalum (flatulence,* swollen feeling across the lower chest; whenever she turns in bed, *feels as if a bag of water* also turned; gastric ulcer and cancer). *Myristica sebifera* (phlegmonous inflammations, hastens suppuration; powerful antiseptic. Ulcerative tendency in all tissues. Said to act more powerfully than *Hep.* and *Sil.*).

Compare: *Nux-v., Puls., Rhus-t., Ign., Asaf.*

Antidotes: *Camph., Gels., Valer.*

**Dose:** First to sixth potency.

# NUX VOMICA

(Poison Nut) **Nux-v.**

Is the greatest of polychrests, because the bulk of its symptoms correspond in similarity with those of the commonest and most frequent of diseases. It is frequently the first remedy indicated after over dosing, establishing a sort of equilibrium of forces and counteracting chronic effects.

*Nux-v.* is pre-eminently the remedy for many of the conditions incident to modern life. The typical *Nux-v.* patient is rather thin, spare, quick, active, nervous and irritable. He does a good deal of mental work; has mental strains and leads a sedentary life, found in prolonged office work, overstudy and close application to business, with its cares and anxieties. This indoor life and mental strain seeks stimulants, coffee, wine, possibly in excess; or, again, he hopes to quieten his excitement, by indulging in the sedative effects of tobacco, if not really a victim, to the seductive drugs, like opium, etc. These things are associated with other indulgences; at table, he takes preferably rich and stimulating food; wine and women play their part to make him forget the close application of the day. Late hours are a consequence; a thick head, dyspepsia and an irritable temper are the next day's inheritance. Now he takes some cathartic, liver pills or mineral water and soon gets into the habit of taking these things, which still further complicate matters. Since these frailties are more yielded to by men than women, *Nux-v.* is pre-eminently a male remedy. These conditions produce an *irritable,* nervous system, hypersensitive and over impressionable, which *Nux-v.* will do much to soothe and calm. Especially adapted to digestive disturbances, portal congestion, and hypochondriacal states depending thereon. Convulsions, with consciousness; worse, touch, moving. *Zealous fiery temperament. Nux-v.* patients are easily chilled, avoid open air, etc. *Nux-v.* always seems to be out of tune; inharmonious spasmodic action.

**Mind:** Very *irritable;* sensitive to all impressions. Ugly, malicious. *Cannot bear noises, odors, light,* etc. Does not want to be touched. Time passes too slowly. Even the least ailment affects him greatly. Disposed to reproach others. *Sullen, fault finding.*

**Head:** Headache in the occiput or over the eyes, with *vertigo;* brain feels as if turning in a circle. Oversensitiveness. *Vertigo with momentary loss of consciousness.* Intoxicated feeling; worse morning, mental exertion, tobacco, alcohol, coffee, open air. Pressing pain in the vertex, as if a nail was driven in. Vertigo in the morning and after dinner. Scalp sensitive. Frontal headache, with a desire to press the head against something. Congestive headache, associated with hemorrhoids. *Headache in the sunshine* (sunstroke) (*Glon., Nat-c.*). Feels distended and sore within, after a debauch.

**Eyes:** Photophobia; worse in the morning. Smarting dry sensation in the inner canthi. Infra-orbital neuralgia, with watering of eyes. Optic nerve atrophy from the habitual use of intoxicants (amblyopia, amaurosis). Paresis of ocular muscles; worse, tobacco and stimulants. Orbital twitching radiating towards the occiput. Optic neuritis.

**Ears:** Itching in the ear through out the eustachian tube. Auditory canal dry and sensitive. Otalgia; worse in bed. Hyperesthesia of the auditory nerves; loud sounds are painful, and anger him.

**Nose:** Stuffed up, especially at night. *Stuffy colds, snuffles,* after exposure to dry, cold atmosphere; worse, in a warm room. Odors tend to produce fainting. Coryza; fluent at daytime; *stuffed up at night and outdoors;* or alternates between nostrils. Epistaxis in the morning (*Bry.*). Arid discharge, but *with a stuffed up feeling.*

**Mouth:** Jaws contracted. Small aphthous ulcers with *bloody saliva* (stomatitis). First half of tongue clean; posterior covered with a deep fur; white, yellow, cracked edges. Toothache; worse cold things. Gums swollen, white, and bleeding (scorbutic).

**Throat:** *Rough, scraped feeling. Tickling* after waking up in the morning. Sensation of *roughness,* tightness and tension. Pharynx constricted. Uvula swollen. *Stitches extend to the ear.*

**Stomach:** Sour taste and *nausea in the morning, after eating. Weight and pain in the stomach; worse, eating, some time after.* Flatulence and pyrosis. Sour, bitter eructations. *Nausea and vomiting,* with much retching. Ravenous hunger, especially, about a day before an attack of dyspepsia. *Region of stomach very sensitive to pressure* (*Bry., Ars.*). Epigastrium bloated, with pressure, as of a stone, *several hours after eating.* Desire for stimulants. Loves *fats* and tolerates them well (*Puls.* opposite). Dyspepsia from drinking strong coffee. Difficult belching of gas. Wants to vomit, but cannot.

**Abdomen:** *Bruised soreness of abdominal walls* (*Apis, Sulph.*). Flatulent distention with spasmodic colic. Colic from uncovering. Liver engorged, with stitches and soreness. Colic with upward pressure, causing short breath, and desire for stool. *Weakness in the region of abdominal ring.* Strangulated hernia (*Op.*). Forcing in of lower abdomen towards the genitals. Umbilical hernia in infants.

**Rectum:** Constipation *with frequent ineffectual urging,* incomplete and unsatisfactory; *feeling as if a part remained unexpelled.* Constriction of the rectum. Irregular, peristaltic action; hence *frequent ineffectual desire or passing but small quantities at each attempt. Absence of all desire for defecation is a contraindication.* Alternate constipation and diarrhea, after abuse of purgatives. Urge for stool if felt throughout the abdomen. *Itching, blind hemorrhoids,* with ineffectual urging to stool; very painful; after drastic drugs. Diarrhea after a debauch; worse, morning. Frequent small evacuations. Scanty stool, with marked urging. Dysentery; stools *relieve pains for some time. Constant uneasiness in the rectum.* Diarrhea with jaundice (*Dig.*).

**Urinary:** Irritable bladder; from spasmodic sphincter. Frequent calls; little and often. Hematuria (*Ip., Ter.*). Ineffectual urging, spasmodic and strangury. Renal colic extending to genitals (renal calculi) with dribbling urine. While micturating, itching in the urethra and pain in the neck of the bladder.

**Male:** Easily excited desire. Emissions from high living. Bad effects of sexual excesses. Constrictive pain in the testicles. Orchitis (*Ham., Puls.*). Spermatorrhea with dreams, backache, burning in the spine, weakness and irritability. Hydrocele.

**Female:** Menses *too early,* last too long; *always irregular,* blood *black* (*Cycl., Lach., Puls.*) with fainting spells. *Prolapsus uteri. Dysmenorrhea* with pain in the sacrum, and constant urging to stool. Inefficient labor pains; extend to the rectum, with desire for stool and frequent micturition (*Lil-t.*). Desire too strong. Metrorrhagia with *sensation as if the bowels wanted to move.*

**Respiratory:** Catarrhal hoarseness with scraping in throat. Spasmodic constriction. *Asthma, with fullness in the stomach, in the morning or after eating.* Cough, with sensation as if something had been torn loose in the chest. *Shallow respiration. Oppressed breathing.* Tight, dry, hacking cough; at times with hemoptysis. *Cough brings on a bursting headache* and bruised pain in the epigastric region.

**Back:** Backache in the lumbar region. Burning in the spine (myelitis); worse 3 to 4 a.m. Cervico-brachial neuralgia; worse, touch. *Must sit up in order to turn in bed.* Bruised pain below scapulae. Sitting is painful.

**Extremities**: Arms and hands go to sleep. Paresis of arms, with shocks. Legs numb; feel paralyzed; cramps in calves and soles. Partial paralysis, from over exertion or getting soaked (*Rhus-t.*). Cracking in knee joints during motion. Drags his feet when walking (locomotor ataxia). Sensation of sudden loss in power of arms and legs, in the morning.

**Sleep**: *Cannot sleep after 3 a.m. till, towards the morning; wakes up feeling wretched.* Drowsy after meals, and in early evening. Dreams full of bustle and hurry. *Better after a short sleep,* unless aroused.

**Fever**: Cold stage predominates. Paroxysms anticipated in the morning. Excessive rigor, with *blueness of finger nails.* Aching in limbs and back, and gastric symptoms. Chilly; must *be covered* in every stage of fever. Perspiration sour; only one side of the body. *Chilliness on being uncovered, yet he does not allow being covered.* Dry heat of the body.

**Skin**: *Body burning hot, especially the face; yet cannot move or uncover* *without feeling chilly.* Urticaria with gastric derangement. Acne, skin red and blotchy.

**Modalities**: *Worse,* morning, mental exertion, after eating, touch, spices, stimulants, narcotics, dry weather, cold. *Better,* from a nap, if allowed to finish it; in the evening, while resting in damp, wet weather (*Caust.*), hard strong pressure.

**Relationship**: *Nux-v.* seeds contain copper, notice the cramp causing proclivities of both.

Complementary: *Sulph., Sep.*

Inimical: *Zinc.*

Compare: *Stry.* and *Kali-c., Hydr., Bry., Lyc., Graph.*

Antidotes: *Coff., Ign., Cocc.*

**Dose**: First to thirtieth potency and higher. *Nux-v.* is said to act best when given in the evening.

---

## NYCTANTHES ARBORTRISTIS

(Paghala Malli, Sad Tree) **Nyct.**

Bilious and obstinate remittent fever; sciatica; rheumatism. Constipation in children.

**Mind:** Anxious and restless.

**Head:** Dull headache.

**Mouth:** Tongue coated.

**Stomach:** Burning sensation, better cold applications. Bilious vomiting. Thirst. Nausea.

**Abdomen:** Tenderness of liver.

**Stool:** Constipation. Profuse, bilious stool (jaundice).

**Fever:** Thirst, before and during chill and heat; better by vomiting at end of chill; sweat not marked.

**Dose:** Tincture, drop doses.

---

## OCIMUM CANUM

(Brazilian Alfavaca) **Oci.**

Is to be remembered in diseases of the kidneys, bladder and urethra (nephritis, cystitis and urethritis). Uric acid diathesis. Red sand in the urine is its chief characteristic and frequently verified. Swelling of glands, inguinal and mammary. Renal colic, especially right side. Symptoms of renal calculus are pronounced.

**Urinary:** High acidity, formation of spike crystals of uric acid. Turbid, thick, purulent (pyuria), bloody (hematuria); *brick-dust red* or yellow *sediment. Odor of musk.* Pain in ureters. Cramps in kidneys (calculus).

**Male:** Heat and swelling of left testicle (orchitis).

**Female:** Vulva swollen; darting pains in labia. Nipples painful to least contact. Breasts feel full and tense; itching. Prolapsus vaginae.

**Relationship:** Compare: *Berb., Hedeo., Lyc., Pareir., Urt-u.*

**Dose:** Sixth to thirtieth potency.

---

## OENANTHE CROCATA

(Water Dropwart) **Oena.**

Epileptiform convulsions; worse, during menstruation and pregnancy. Puerperal eclampsia; convulsions. Burning in the throat and stomach, nausea and vomiting. Red spots on the face. Convulsive, facial twitching. Skin affections, especially leprosy and ichthyosis.

**Head:** Pain all over the head, dizzy. Sudden and complete unconsciousness. Furious delirium, giddiness. Countenance livid, eyes fixed, pupils dilated, *convulsive twitching of facial muscles,* trismus, foaming at mouth, locked jaws (epilepsy, hystero-epilepsy). Much yawning. Tendency to cry over little things.

**Respiratory:** Tickling cough, with rattling in the lower part of chest, thick, frothy expectoration. Heavy, spasmodic, stertorous breathing.

**Extremities:** Convulsions; opisthotonos (tetanus). Pain along the crural and sciatic nerves (sciatica), commencing in the back. Cold hands and feet. Numbness of a hand and foot.

**Relationship:** Compare: *Cic., Kali-br.*

**Dose:** First to sixth potency.

---

## OLEANDER—NERIUM ODORUM

(Rose-laurel) **Olnd.**

Has a marked action on the skin, heart and nervous system, producing and curing paralytic conditions with cramp-like contractions of upper extremities. Hemiplegia. Difficult articulation.

**Mind:** Memory weak; slow perception. Melancholy, with obstinate constipation.

**Head:** Vertigo and diplopia, when looking down. Vertigo when looking fixedly at an object and on rising from bed. Pain in the brain, as if the head would burst (meningitis). Numb feeling. Dull, unable to think. Indolence. *Eruptions on the scalp.* Humid, fetid spots *behind the ears* (*Graph., Petr.*) and occiput, with red, rough herpetic spots in front. *Corrosive itching on the forehead and margine of hair;* worse, heat.

**Eyes:** Can see objects only when looking at them sideways (strabismus). Eyes water on reading. Diplopia. *Sensation as if the eyes were drawn back into the head.*

**Face:** Pale, sunken, with blue rings around the eyes (*Ph-ac.*).

**Stomach:** *Canine hunger, with hurried eating,* without appetite. Thirst. Empty belching. Vomiting of food; bile. Throbbing in the pit.

**Abdomen:** Borborygmus, with profuse, fetid flatus. Gnawing around the navel. Ineffectual urging. *Undigested feces* (lienteria). *Stool passes when emitting flatus.* Burning pain in the anus.

**Chest:** Oppression as if from a weight; asthmatic when lying down. *Palpitations,* with weakness and empty feeling in the chest. Dyspnea. Obtuse stitches in the chest.

**Extremities:** *Weakness of the lower limbs.* Paralysis of legs and feet. Want of animal heat in limbs. Painless paralysis. Constant cold feet. Swelling, burning stiffness of fingers (rheumatic arthritis). Veins of hands swollen. Edema. Stiffness of joints.

**Skin:** Itching, scurfy pimples; herpes; sensitive and numb. Nocturnal burning. *Very sensitive skin* (hyperesthesia); slightest friction causes soreness and chapping. *Violent itching eruption, bleeding, oozing* (eczema); want of perspiration. Pruritus, especially of scalp, which is sensitive.

**Modalities:** *Worse,* undressing, rest, friction of clothes.

**Relationship:** Compare: *Con., Nat-m., Rhus-t., Caust., Lath.* Oleander contains Oleandrin and also Nerein of which the latter is said to be closely related if not identical with Digitalin. The pulse becomes slower, more regular, more powerful. *Diuresis;* palpitations, edema and dyspnea of valvular disease, disappear.

Antidotes: *Camph., Sulph.*

**Dose:** Third to thirtieth potency.

---

# OLEUM ANIMALE AETHEREUM

(Dippel's Animal Oil) **Ol-an.**

Acts on the nervous system, especially in the pneumo-gastric region. Useful in migraine and neuralgia of spermatic cord. Burning pains and stitches. *"Pulled upward"* and *"from behind, forward" pains.*

**Head:** Tearing pain, with sadness and irritability; worse after dinner; relieved by rubbing. Itching, burning vesicles; better, friction. Malar bones feel pulled forcibly upward. Migraine with polyuria.

**Eyes:** Smarting in the eyes; misty vision (amblyopia, cataract). Glistening bodies before eyes. Lachrymation when eating. Short sighted (myopia). Twitching of lids (*Agar.*).

**Nose:** Watery, excoriating discharge; worse in the open air.

**Face:** Feels drawn. Cramp-like pains. *Twitching of lips.* Malar bone feels pulled upward. Toothache, *better pressing teeth together.*

**Mouth:** Bites cheek while eating (*Caust.*). Tongue feels sore. Greasy feeling in the mouth.

**Throat:** Sore, dry, constricted. Air feels cold.

**Stomach:** Sensation *of water in the stomach;* of coldness, of constriction, and of burning; better, eructations.

**Abdomen:** Flatulence and rumbling. Ineffectual urging for stool, with burning in the anus. After stool, bruised pain in the abdomen.

**Urinary:** *Polyuria.* Greenish urine, frequent and urgent need to micturate, with tenesmus and scanty emission. Itching in urethra.

**Male:** Desire increased; ejaculation too soon. Pain along the spermatic cord to the testicles. *Testicles feel seized and pulled forcibly upward* (retracted); worse, right. *Pressure in the perineum.* Prostatic hypertrophy.

**Female:** *Early and scant menstruation;* flow black.

**Respiratory:** Chest feels constricted. Asthma from suppressed foot sweat. Oppression. *Stitches in the breast from behind forward.*

**Extremities:** Sprained feeling in the lumbosacral region. Cracking of vertebrae on raising the head (*Aloe; Nat-c., Thuj.*). Restlessness. Rheumatic pain in shoulders. Sweat of heels has a fish brine odor.

**Modalities:** Worse, after eating, from 2 to 9 p. m. *Better* by rubbing, eructation, open air.

**Relationship:** *Puls., Ars., Sil., Sep.*

Antidotes: *Camph., Op.*

**Dose**: Third to thirtieth potency and higher.

## OLEUM JECORIS ASELLI

(Cod Liver Oil) **Ol-j.**

Internally, a nutrient, hepatic and pancreatic remedy (Burnett). Emaciation, lassitude, scrofulous diseases, rheumatic affections. *Atrophy in infants; emaciati*on with hot hands and head; restless and feverish at night. *Pain in the liver region. Tuberculosis* in the beginning stage.

**Chest**: Hoarseness. Sharp stitching pains. Burning spots. *Dry, hacking, tickling cough, especially* at night. Whooping cough in miserable, scrofulous children. Here give drop doses, increasing daily one drop up to twelve, then descend in the same way (Dahlke). *Soreness through the chest. Hemopty*sis (phthisis) (*Acal., Mill.*). *Palpitations, accompany* other symptoms. *Yellowness.* Children who cannot take milk.

**Extremities:** Aching in elbows, knees and *sacrum.* Chronic rheumatism, with rigid muscles and tendons. *Burning in palms.*

**Fever**: Constantly chilly towards the evening. *Hectic fever.* Night sweats.

**Relationship:** Compare: *Cholesterinum, Tub., Phos., Iod.* One litre of *Ol-j.* contains 0.4 gram Iod. *Gadus morrhua*—Cod (frequent breathing, with flapping of alae nasi; rush of blood to chest; pain in the lungs and cough; dry heat in palms).

**Dose**: First to third trituration. Locally in *ringworm,* and nocturnal rubbing, in dwarfish, emaciated babies.

---

## OLEUM SANTALI

(Oil of Sandalwood) **Ol-sant.**

The action in the urinary and sexual spheres is most marked, especially in gonorrhea. It is also a stimulating, disinfectant expectorant. Two or three drops on sugar will frequently relieve hacking cough, when little sputum is expectorated.

**Urinary**: Frequent, burning, smarting, swelling and redness of meatus. Stream small and slow. *Acute aching in the kidney region.* Sensation of a ball pressing against the urethra; worse standing. Gleet, with profuse, thick discharge; chronic cystitis.

**Male**: Painful erections; swelling of the prepuce. Thick, yellowish, muco-purulent discharge. Deep pain in the perineum.

**Dose**: Two to 10M in capsules.

---

## ONISCUS ASELLUS—MILLEPEDES

(Wood Louse) **Onis.**

Has distinct diuretic properties; hence useful in dropsies. Asthmatic conditions with bronchial catarrh.

**Head**: Boring pain behind the right ear in the mastoid process (*Caps.*). Violent pulsation of arteries (*Ictod., Glon.). Painful* pressure above the root of nose.

**Stomach**: Persistent pressure at the cardiac orifice. Vomiting.

**Abdomen**: Distended; *meteorism; very severe colic.*

**Urinary**: Cutting, burning in urethra (urethritis). *Tenesmus of the bladder* (cystitis) *and rectum,* with absence of stool and urine.

**Relationship**: Compare: *Ictod., Canth.*

**Dose**: Sixth potency.

---

## ONOSMODIUM VIRGINIANUM

(False Gromwell) **Onos.**

Want of power of concentration and co-ordination. Vertigo, numbness and muscular prostration. Marked association of head and eye symptoms, with muscular fatigue and weariness.

A remedy for *migraine.* Headaches from eyestrain and sexual weakness. It produces diminution of sexual desire in both sexes; hence its homoeopathicity, in *sexual neurasthenia.* Depressed or lost sexual life in women. Neuralgic pains. General prostration. Acts as if born tired.

**Head:** Loss of memory. Nose feels dry. Confused. Dull, heavy, dizzy, pain pressing upward in the occiput. Occipito-frontal pain in the morning on waking, *chiefly left sided.* Pain in the temples and mastoid (*Caps.*).

**Eyes:** Vision blurred (amblyopia); optic disc hyperemic and retinal vessels enlarged. Strained feeling in the eyes; worse, using eyes. Eyes heavy and dull, muscular asthenopia; *ocular muscles tense.* Internal eye muscles paretic. *Pain in the eyeballs* between orbit and the ball, extending to the left temple.

**Throat:** Severe dryness. Discharge from posterior nares. Raw, scraping. Stuffed feeling in posterior nares. Symptoms worse by cold drinks.

**Abdomen:** Craving for ice water and cold drinks; wants to drink often. Abdomen feels bloated.

**Male:** Constant sexual excitement. *Psychical impotence.* Loss of desire. Speedy emissions. Deficient erections.

**Female:** Severe pain in the uterus; bearing down pains; old pains return. *Sexual desire completely destroyed.* Feels as if menses would appear. Aching in the breasts. Nipples itch. Menses too early and too prolonged (menorrhagia). Soreness in the uterine region. Leucorrhea, yellow, acrid, profuse.

**Chest:** Sore, aching in breasts; feels swollen and sore (mastitis). Pain in the heart; pulse, rapid, irregular, weak (angina pectoris).

**Back:** Pain in dorsal and lumbar regions. Numbness and tingling in legs and feet.

**Extremities:** Pain in the back. *Tired and numb* feeling in the legs, popliteal spaces, and below the knees. *Staggering gait* (locomotor ataxia). Sidewalk seems too high. Pain in left scapular region. Great muscular weakness and weariness.

**Modalities:** *Worse,* from motion, jar, and tight clothing. *Better,* when undressed, lying down on the back, from cold drinks, and eating.

**Relationship:** Compare: *Nat-m., Lil-t., Gels., Ruta.*

**Dose:** Thirtieth attenuation.

---

# OOPHORINUM

(Ovarian Extract) **Ov.**

Suffering following ovariotomy. *Climacteric disturbances* generally. Ovarian cysts. Cutaneous disorders and acne rosacea. Prurigo.

**Relationship:** Compare: *Orchitinum*: Testicular extract (after ovariotomy, sexual weakness, senile decay).

**Dose:** Low triturations.

---

# OPERCULINA TURPETHUM

(Nishope) **Oper.**

A remedy for plague, fever and diarrhea.

**Mind:** Delirium associated with restlessness, loquacity, Tendency to escape from bed; ravings, pains causes fainting.

**Rectum:** Watery diarrhea, profuse with a sinking sensation. Cholera morbus. Hemorrhoids.

**Skin:** Lymphatic glands enlarged and indurated. Boils and slowly suppurating abscesses.

# OPIUM—PAPAVER SOMNIFERUM

(Dried Latex of the Poppy) **Op.**

Hahnemann says that it is much more difficult to estimate the action of *Opium,* than of almost any other drug. The effects of *Opium* as shown in the insensibility of the nervous system, depressive drowsy stupor, painlessness, torpor, general sluggishness and lack of vital reaction, constitute the main indications for the drug when used homoeopathically. All complaints are characterized by *sopor.* They are *painless* and are accompanied by *heavy, stupid sleep, stertorous breathing. Sweaty skin.* Dark, mahogany-brown face. Serous apoplexy, venous, passive congestion. Want of sensitiveness to the action of medicines. Reappearance and aggravation from becoming heated. *Opium* lessens voluntary movements, contracts pupils, depresses higher intellectual powers, reduces self control and power of concentration, judgement; stimulates the imagination and checks all secretions except that of the skin. Want of susceptibility to remedies even though indicated. Diseases that originate from fright.

**Mind:** Patient wants nothing. Complete *loss of consciousness; apoplectic state.* Frightful fancies, daring, gay, bright. Unable to understand or appreciate his sufferings. Thinks he is not at home. Delirious talking, with wide open eyes.

**Head:** Vertigo; *head feels light in old people.* Dull, heavy stupid. Delirium. Vertigo after fright. Pain at the back of head; sensation of great weight (*Gels.*). Bursting feeling. Complete insensibility; no mental grasp for anything. Paralysis of brain.

**Eyes:** Half closed, dilated; pupils insensible, contracted (epilepsy). Ptosis (*Gels., Caust.*). Staring, glassy.

**Face:** Red, bloated, *swollen, dark, suffused, hot.* Looks intoxicated, besotted (*Bapt., Lach.*). Spasmodic facial twitching especially at the corners of mouth. Veins of face distended. *Hanging down of lower jaw.* Distorted.

**Mouth:** Dry. Tongue black, *paralyzed.* Bloody froth. Intense thirst. Blubbering of lips. Difficult articulation and swallowing.

**Stomach:** Vomiting, with colic and convulsions. Fecal vomiting (intestinal obstruction). Incarcerated hernia. Hungry; no desire to eat.

**Abdomen:** Hard, bloated, tympanitic. Lead colic. During colic, urging to stool and discharge of hard feces.

**Stool:** Obstinate constipation; no desire to go to stool. *Round, hard, black balls.* Feces protrude and recede (*Thuj., Sil.*). Spasmodic retention of feces in small intestines. Stool involuntary, black, offensive, frothy. Violent pains in the rectum, as if pressed asunder.

**Urinary:** Slow to start; feeble stream. *Retained* or involuntary, after fright. Loss of power or sensibility of bladder.

**Female:** Suppressed menses from fright. Cessation of labor pains with coma and twitching. Puerperal convulsions; drowsiness or coma between paroxysms. Threatened abortion and suppression of lochia, from fright, with sopor. Horrible labor-like pains in the uterus, with urging to stool.

**Respiratory:** Breathing stops on going to sleep; must be shaken to start it again (*Grin.*). Hoarse. *Deep snoring; rattling, stertorous breathing.* Difficult, intermittent, deep, unequal respiration. Heat in chest; burning around heart. Cough, with dyspnea and blue face (cynosis); with hemoptysis.

**Back and Extremities:** Opisthotonos. Swollen veins of neck. Painless paralysis (*Olnd.*). *Twitching of limbs* (chorea). Numbness. Jerks as if flexors were overacting. Convulsions; worse from glare of light; coldness of limbs.

**Sleep:** Great drowsiness (*Gels., Nux-m.*). Falls into a heavy, stupid sleep. Profound coma. Loss of breath on falling asleep (*Grin.*). Coma vigil. Picking at bedclothes. Very sleepy, but cannot go to sleep. Distant noises, cocks crowing, etc., keep him awake. Child dreams of cats, dogs, black forms. Bed feels very hot, cannot lie on it. Pleasant, fantastic, amorous dreams. Shaking chill; then heat, with sleep and sweat. Thirst only during heat.

**Fever:** Pulse *full* and *slow.* Heat extending all over the body. *Hot* perspiration. Fever characterized by stupor, snoring respiration, twitching of limbs, intense thirst and sleepiness. General low temperature with inclination to stupor.

**Skin:** Hot, damp, sweating. Constant desire to uncover. *Hot perspiration all over the body except lower limbs.*

**Modalities:** *Worse,* heat, during and after sleep (*Apis, Lach.*). *Better.* cold things, constant walking.

**Relationship:** Compare: *Apis, Bell., Gels., Nux-m., Morph.* (extreme susceptibility to pain; twitching; tympanites; severe itching); *Codeinum* (dry, teasing, incessant cough; twitching of muscles, especially of the eyelids); *Eschscholtzia californica*—California poppy (a harmless soporific).

Antidote: Acute *Opium* poisoning: *Atropinum* and Black coffee. Chronic *Opium* poisoning: *Ip., Nux-v., Passi., Berb.* is useful to counteract the opium habit.

**Non-homeopathic Preparations and Uses:** *Palliative only* in great pain, sleeplessness, peritonitis, and to check excessive secretion in diarrhea, diabetes, etc.

*Opium* (crude): Official dose, 1 grain.

Laudanum (tincture): Dose, 5 to 20 drops. Extract of Opium ¼ to 1 grain.

*Paregoric:* Tinctura Camphora Composita. Contains in each dram ¼ grain of Opium equal to 1/30 grain of Morphine. Dose ½ to 1 fluid dram for adults. For an infant 3 to 5 drops.

*Dover's Powder* consists of Opium, Ipecac and Sulphate of Potash. It contains 10% each of Opium and Ipecac. Dose 5 to 15 grains.

Morphine: 1/8 to ¼ grain.

Magendie's solution: 16 grains to 1 oz. or 5 drops equal to 1/6 grain.

Codein: ½ to 1 grain.

Apomorphia: 1/20 to 1/10 grain hypodermically

**Dose:** Third to thirtieth and 200th potency.

---

# OPUNTIA FICUS

(Ficus Indica, Bengalensis, Prickly Pear) **Opun-f.**

Diarrhea, with nausea. *Feels as if bowels had settled down in the lower abdomen.* Sick feeling in lower third of abdomen. Enteroptosis with loose and frequent evacuations.

It stops bleeding from the throat or mouth, blood, pure red. In dysentery and piles, it exerts a powerful influence to arrest the progress of bleeding. In bloody dysentery with great urging, colic and tenesmus it is an excellent remedy (*Merc-c.*).

**Relationship:** Compare: *Chaparro amargoso* (which Mexican physicians laud as a specific in chronic diarrhea). *Ricinus communis* (diarrhea, dysentery, obstinate chronic diarrhea).

**Dose:** Second attenuation.

---

# OREODAPHNE CALIFORNICA

(California Laurel) **Oreo.**

Neuralgic headache, cervico-occipital pain, cerebro-spinal meningitis, atonic diarrhea and intestinal colic.

**Head:** Dizziness; worse on stooping or moving. Head heavy, eyelids heavy, twitching. Intense aching, *with pressure at the inner angle of either orbit,* generally left, extending through the brain, across the scalp to the base of occiput; worse, light, noise; better, closing the eyes and in perfect silence. Constant, dull ache in the *cervical and occipital region* (cervical spondylosis), extending to the scapula and down the spine, into the head; pain extends into the ears. Great heaviness of the head, with a constant desire to move the head, which does not relieve. Drooping eyelids (ptosis). Twitching. Atonic diarrhea.

**Stomach:** Eructations, with nausea and shuddering.

**Dose:** First to third potency. Olfaction of the tincture.

---

# ORIGANUM MAJORANA

(Sweet Marjoram) **Orig.**

Acts on the nervous system generally, and is effective in masturbation and excessively aroused sexual impulses. Affections of the breasts (*Bufo*). Desire for active exercise *impelling her to run.*

**Female:** *Erotomania;* powerful lascivious impulses; leucorrhea; hysteria. Lascivious ideas and dreams.

**Relationship:** Compare: *Ferula glauca* (in violent sexual excitement in women; icy coldness in the occiput); *Plat., Valer., Canth., Hyos.*

**Dose:** Third potency.

---

# ORNITHOGALUM UMBELLATUM

(Star of Bethlehem) **Orni.**

To be considered in chronic gastric and other abdominal indurations, possibly cancer of the intestinal tract, especially of the stomach and caecum. Center of action is the pylorus, causing painful contraction with duodenal distension.

Depression of spirits. Complete prostration. Feeling of sickness keeps the patient awake at night.

**Stomach:** Tongue coated. Agonizing feeling in the chest and stomach, starting from the pylorus with flatus that rolls in balls from one side to the other, loss of appetite, phlegmy retchings and loss of flesh. Gastric ulceration with hemorrhage. *Pain increases when food passes the pyloric outlet. Vomiting of coffee ground* looking matter (hematemesis). Distension of the stomach. Frequent belching of offensive flatus. Painful sinking across the epigastrium.

**Dose:** Single doses of mother tincture and await action.

---

## OSMIUM METALLICUM

(The Element) **Osm.**

Irritation and catarrh of respiratory organs. Eczema. Albuminuria. *Pain in the trachea.* Increases and gives odor to local perspiration. Causes *adhesion of the nail fold.*

**Head:** Sensation of a band around the head. Falling of hair (*Kali-c., Fl-ac.*).

**Eyes:** *Glaucoma;* with iridescent vision. Violent supra and infra-orbital neuralgia; violent pains and lachrymation. *Green color surrounds candle light.* Conjunctivitis. Increase in intraocular tension, dim sight, photophobia.

**Nose:** Coryza, with full feeling in the nose. Nose and larynx sensitive to air. Small lumps of phlegm from posterior nares.

**Respiratory:** Acute laryngitis; cough and expectoration of tough, stringy mucus. Convulsive cough; feels as though the laryngeal membrane was torn. Noisy, *dry, hard, cough,* in violent, short outbursts, coming from low down, shaking the whole body. Talking causes pain in the larynx. Hoarse; *pain in the larynx;* sore sternum. Twitching of fingers with spasmodic cough.

**Skin:** Eczema, with pruritus. Irritated skin. Itchy pimples. Bromidrosis, sweat in axilla smelling of garlic, worse evening and night. Fold remains attached to the growing nail.

**Relationship:** Compare: *Arg-met., Irid., Sel., Mang.*

**Dose:** Sixth potency.

---

## OSTRYA VIRGINICA

(Ironwood) **Ost.**

Of great value in anemia from malaria. Bilious conditions and intermittent fever.

**Stomach:** *Tongue coated yellow at the root.* Loss of appetite. *Frequent nausea,* with dull, frontal headache (sick headache). Sickening pains.

**Dose:** First to third potency.

---

## OVI GALLINAE PELLICULA

(Membrane of Egg Shell) **Ovi-p.**

Sudden pains. Bearing down sensation. Intolerance of bands on wrists, arms, waist, etc. Backache and pain in the left hip. Debility. Pain in the heart and left ovary.

**Relationship:** Compare: *Calc., Naja, Ova tosta—Tosta praeparata*—Roasted egg shells. *Calcarea ovorum* (leucorrhea and backache. Sensation as if the spine was broken and wired, or tied together with a string. Pain of cancer. Warts). Also *egg vaccine for asthma.* A lot of interest is shown in Dr. Fritz Talbot's method of curing asthma in children by the use of an egg vaccine. Asthma due to susceptibility of the protein substance in eggs can be cured by immunizing against egg poisons by repeated doses of egg white. After the skin has been cleansed with soap and alcohol, the egg white is rubbed into a slight scratch.

---

# OXALICUM ACIDUM

(Sorrel Acid) **Ox-ac.**

Although certain oxalates are constant constituents of vegetable food and of the human body, the acid itself is a violent poison when taken internally, producing gastroenteritis, motor paralysis, collapse, stupor and death.

Influences the spinal cord, and produces motor paralysis. Pain very violent, *in spots* (*Kali-bi.*), *worse,* motion, and *thinking of it. Periodical remissions.* Spasmodic symptoms of throat and chest. *Rheumatism of the left side. Neurasthenia.* Tuberculosis.

**Head:** Sense of heat. Meningitis. Confusion and vertigo. Headache, before and during stool.

**Eyes:** Severe pain in the eyes; feel expanded. *Hyperesthesia of retina.*

**Stomach:** Violent pain in the epigastrium, discharge of flatus relieves. Gastralgia, pyrosis, sensation of coldness below the epigastrium. Burning pain, extending upwards; slightest touch causes excruciating pain. Bitter and sour eructation, worse at night. Cannot eat strawberries.

**Abdomen:** Pain in the upper part and region of naval two hours after eating, with much flatulence. Stitches in the liver. Colic. Burning in small spots in the abdomen. Diarrhea from coffee.

**Urinary:** Frequent and copious. Burning in the urethra (urethritis) and pain in the glans when micturating. Must micturate when thinking of it. Urine contains oxalates (oxaluria).

**Male:** *Terrible neuralgic pains in the spermatic cord.* Testicles feel contused and heavy (indurated). Seminal vesiculitis.

**Respiratory:** Nervous aphonia with cardiac derangement (*Coca, Hydr-ac.*). Burning sensation from throat down. Breathing spasmodic, with constriction of the larynx and chest. *Hoarseness. Left lung painful. Aphonia.*

Paralysis of the tensors of vocal cord. *Dyspnea; short, jerking inspirations.* Sharp pain through the lower region of left lung, extending down to the epigastrium.

**Heart:** Palpitations and dyspnea in organic heart disease; worse, when thinking of it. Pulse feeble. Heart symptoms alternate with aphonia, *angina pectoris; sharp, lancinating pain in the left lung coming on suddenly, depriving breath.* Precordial pains which dart to the left shoulder. Aortic insufficiency.

**Extremities:** Numb, weak, tingling sensation. Pains start from the spine and extend through the extremities. Drawing and *lancinating pains* shooting down the extremities. *Backache;* numb, weak. Myelitis. Muscular prostration. Wrist painful, as if sprained (*Ulm.*). Lower extremities blue, cold, insensible (cyanosed). Sensation of numbness. Multiple cerebral and posterior spinal sclerosis. Lancinating pains in various parts; jerking pains (convulsions, tetnus).

**Skin:** Sensitive, smarting and soreness, worse shaving; mottled, marbled in circular patches. Perspires easily.

**Modalities:** *Worse, left* side; slightest touch; light; shaving. Aroused around, 3 a. m. with gastric and abdominal pain. *All conditions worse by thinking of self.*

**Relationship:** Compare: *Ars., Colch., Arg-met., Pic-ac., Cicer arietinum*—Chick-pea (lithiasis, jaundice, liver affections; diuretic). *Scolopendra morsitans*—Centipede (terrible pains in the back and loins, extending down the limbs; return periodically, commencing in the head, extending to the toes. Angina pectoris. Inflammation, pain and gangrene. pustules and abscesses). *Caesium metallicum* (pain in the lumbar region and testicle. Headache, darting through the temples. Diarrhea and colic. Languor).

*Lime Water:* Antidote to *Ox-ac.* poisoning

**Dose:** Sixth to thirtieth potency.

---

# OXYDENDRON ARBOREUM— ANDROMEDA ARBOREA

(Sorrel Tree) **Oxyd.**

A remedy for dropsy—ascites and anasarca. Urine suppressed. Deranged portal circulation. Prostatic enlargement. Vesical calculi. Irritation of the bladder neck. Great difficulty in breathing. Tincture.

**Relationship:** Compare: *Cerefolium sativum* (dropsy, Bright's disease, cystitis).

---

# OXYTROPIS LAMBERTI

(Loco-weed) **Oxyt.**

Marked action on the nervous system. Trembling, emptiness. Walks backwards. Congestion of the spine and paralysis. Pains come and go quickly. Sphincters relaxed. Staggering gait. Reflexes lost.

**Mind:** Desire to be alone. Disinclined to work or talk. Worse, thinking of symptoms (*Ox-ac.*). *Mental depression.* Vertigo (*Gran.*).

**Head:** Vertigo. Full, warm feeling around the head. Feeling of intoxication with loss of vision. Pain in the maxillary bones and masseter muscles. Mouth and nose dry.

**Eyes:** Sight obscured (amblyopia); pupils contracted; do not respond to light. Paralysis of nerves and muscles of eyes.

**Stomach:** Eructations with colicky pains. Epigastrium tender.

**Rectum:** Sphincter seems relaxed (paralysis of the rectum). Stools slip from the anus, like *lumps of jelly,* mushy.

**Urinary:** Urging to micturate when thinking of it. *Profuse flow.* Pain in kidneys (*Berb.*).

**Male:** No desire or ability. Pain in the testicles (orchitis) and along the spermatic cord, down the thighs.

**Extremities:** Pain along the ulnar nerve. Numb feeling around spine. *Staggering gait.* Loss of co-ordination (locomotor ataxia). Patellar tendon reflex lost. Pains come and go quickly, but muscles remain sore and stiff.

**Sleep:** Restless, dreams of a quarrel.

**Modalities:** *Worse,* thinking of symptoms (maniacal tendency). *Worse,* every other day. *Better,* after sleep.

**Relationship:** Compare: *Astra-m., Lath., Ox-ac., Bar-c.* (Loco plant is rich in *Bar-c.*). *Lol.*

**Dose:** Third potency and higher.

---

# PAEONIA OFFICINALIS

(Peony) **Paeon.**

The rectal and anal symptoms are most important. Chronic ulcers on the lower parts of the body, leg, foot, toe, breast and rectum.

**Head:** Rush of blood to the head and face. Nervous. Vertigo when moving. Burning in the eyes and ringing in the ears.

**Rectum:** Biting, *itching in anus* (threadworms); orifice swollen (proctitis). Burning in the anus after stool; followed by internal chilliness. Fistula ani, diarrhea, with burning in the anus and internal chilliness. Painful ulcer, oozing offensive moisture on the perineum. *Hemorrhoids, fissures, ulceration of the anus and perineum, purple, covered with crusts.* Atrocious pains with and after each stool. Sudden, pasty diarrhea, with faintness in the abdomen.

**Chest:** Sticking pains in the left chest. Heat in the chest. Dull shooting from front to back through the heart.

**Extremities:** Pain in the wrist and fingers; knees and toes. Weakness of legs, inhibiting walking.

**Sleep:** Terrifying dreams, nightmares.

**Skin:** Sensitive, painful. Ulcers below the coccyx, around the sacrum: varicose veins. Ulcers in general, from pressure, bedsores, etc. Itching, burning, as from nettles.

**Relationship:** Compare: *Glechoma hederacia*—Ground ivy (rectal symptom). *Ham., Sil., Aesc., Rat. (great constriction* of the anus; stools forced out with a great effort).

Antidotes: *Rat., Aloe.*

**Dose:** Third potency.

---

# PALLADIUM METALLICUM

(The Metal) **Pall.**

An ovarian remedy; produces the symptom complex of chronic oophoritis. Useful where the parenchyma of the gland is not totally destroyed. Acts also on the mind and skin. Motor weakness, averse to exercise.

**Mind:** Lachrymose mood. *Love of approbation.* Pride; *easily offended.* Inclined to use violent language. *Keeps up brightly when in company,* very exhausted afterwards, with aggravation of pain.

**Head:** Feels as if swung backward and forwards. Temporo-parietal neuralgia with pain in the shoulder. *Pain across the top of head, from ear to ear;* worse after an evening's entertainment, with irritability and sour eructations. Sallow complexion.

**Abdomen:** Shooting pain from the navel to the pelvis. Sensation as if intestines were bitten off. Intestines feel strangulated. Soreness of the abdomen, swelling in the right groin (hernia). Flatulence.

**Female:** Uterine prolapse and retroversion. Subacute pelvic peritonitis with right sided pain and backache; menorrhagia. Cutting pain in the uterus;

relieved after stool. Pain and *swelling in the region of right ovary.* Shooting or burning pains in the pelvis, bearing down; relieved by rubbing. Soreness and shooting pain from the navel to the breast. Glairy leucorrhea. Menstrual discharge while nursing. Stitches in right breast near the nipple. It is indicated in gynecological conditions where the disease had its inception in the right ovary, uterine prolapse and retroversion, subacute pelvic peritonitis and concomitant symptoms being secondary (F. Aguilar, M. D.).

**Extremities:** Pruritus. Tired feeling in the lumbosacral region. Fleeting, neuralgic pains in the extremities. Heavy and tired feeling in limbs. Darting pains from toes to hips. Rheumatic pain in the right shoulder; right hip. Sciatica.

**Relationship:** Complementary: *Plat.*

Compare: *Arg-met., Helon., Lil-t., Apis.*

**Dose:** Sixth to thirtieth potency.

---

# PARAFFINUM

(Purified Paraffin) **Paraf.**

Valuable in uterine affections. Particularly serviceable, in constipation. Knife-like pains. Pain extends from one part to another, and alternate. Pain in the stomach alternates with pain in the throat and spine.

**Head:** Left side of the head and face suffer most; pains stinging and twisting (migraine, facial neuralgia). Pain as if a nail was driven into the left side of vertex. Twisting in the left ear.

**Eyes:** Vision dim (amblyopia); black specks before the eyes. Lids red (blepharitis). Sensation as if there was fat in the eyes.

**Mouth:** Tearing, twisting pain in the teeth extending down to the lower jaw. Full of saliva; feels sticky; bitter taste.

**Stomach:** Hungry all the time. Pain across the stomach. Pain in the stomach alternates with pain in the throat and spine, extends to the chest with belching. Fixed pain in the left hypochondrium, as if parts were being twisted. Palpitations with stomach pains.

**Abdomen:** Pain in the lower abdomen, extending to the genitals, rectum and coccyx; better, sitting.

**Rectum:** Frequent desire for stool. *Obstinate constipation in children* (*Alum., Nyct.*). Chronic constipation with hemorrhoids and continuous urging to stool, without result.

**Female:** Menses too late, black, abundant. Milky leucorrhea. Nipples pain when touched, as if sore inside. Stabbing pain in mons veneris. Very hot urine with burning pain in the vulva.

**Extremities:** Pain in the spine extending to the inguinal region and in both loins, when ascending the stairs. Sensation of electric shocks in all joints. Wrenching pain in calves, extending into the toes, in joints. Feet swollen with tearing in ankles and soles.

**Skin:** Burns, even of third degree, with sloughing and sepsis. Wash with sterile water and dry, spray with paraffine, and, cover with a thin layer of cotton. Also useful also in frost bites.

**Relationship:** Compare: *Naphtin., Petr., Kreos., Eupi.*

**Dose:** Lower triturations and thirieth potency.

---

## PAREIRA BRAVA—CHONDODENDRON TORMENTOSUM

(Virgin-vine) **Pareir.**

The urinary symptoms are most important. Useful in renal colic, prostatic affections and catarrh of the bladder. Sensation as if the bladder was distended, with pain. *Pain going down the thigh.*

**Urinary**: Black, bloody, thick mucoid urine. *Constant urging; great straining; pain down thighs while making efforts to micturate.* Can emit urine only when he goes on his knees, pressing the head firmly against the floor. Bladder feels distended; neuralgic pain in the anterior crural region (*Staph.*). Dribbling after micturition (*Sel.*). *Violent pain in glans penis.* Itching along the urethra; urethritis with prostatic problems (hypertrophy). Inflammation of urethra; becomes almost cartilaginous (gonorrhea).

**Relationship:** Compare: *Parietaria officinalis* (renal calculi; nightmares, patient dreams of being buried alive); *Chim.* (chronic catarrhal congestion following cystitis; acute prostatitis; sensation of a ball in the perineum when sitting); *Fab.*, see *Pichi* (dysuria; post-gonorrheal complications; gravel; vesical catarrh); *Uva, Hydrang., Berb., Oci., Hedeo.*

**Dose:** Tincture to third potency.

---

## PARIS QUADRIFOLIA

(One-berry) **Par.**

Head symptoms marked and verified. Sensation of expansion and consequent tension. Coldness of the right side of body, left hot. Catarrhal complaints, stuffed feeling in the root of nose. Disorder of sense of touch.

**Mind:** Imaginary foul smells. Feels too large. *Garrulous,* prattling, vivacious.

**Head:** Sensation as if the scalp was contracted and bones scraped. Soreness on top of the head; cannot brush hair. Aches, as if *pulling a string from the eyes to the occiput.* Occipital headache, with a sensation of weight. Head feels very large, expanded. Scalp sensitive. Numb feeling on the left side of head.

**Eyes:** Affections of the eyebrows. Eyes feel heavy, as if they were projected; *sensation of a string through the eyeballs.* Expanded, as though lids cannot cover (exophthalmos).

**Face:** Neuralgia; hot stitches in the left malar bone, which is very sore. Has relieved inflammation of the antrum, where eye symptoms coexisted.

**Mouth:** *Tongue dry on waking up.* Coated white, *without thirst,* with bitter or diminished taste.

**Respiratory:** Stuffed condition and fullness at the root of nose. Periodical, painless *hoarseness.* Cough as if from vapors of sulphur in the trachea. Constant hawking, on account of viscid, green mucus in the larynx and trachea.

**Extremities:** Sense of *weight and weariness in the nape of neck* and across the shoulders. Neuralgia, beginining in the left intercostal region and extending into the left arm (brachial neuralgia). Arm becomes stiff, fingers clenched. Neuralgia of coccyx; pulsating, sticking, when sitting. *Fingers often feel numb.* Numbness of the upper limbs. Everything feels rough.

**Relationship:** Compare: *Pastinaca sativa*—Parsnip (loquacity; delirium tremens; illusions of vision; intolerance of milk; roots used dietetically, cooked in water or as a broth or as a salad for consumptives and "kidney stones"). *Sil., Calc., Nux-v., Rhus-t.*

Incompatible: *Ferr-p.*

Antidote: *Coff.*

**Dose:** Third potency.

---

## PARTHENIUM HYSTEROPHORUS—ESCOBA AMARGO

(Bitter-broom) **Parth.**

A Cuban remedy for fevers, especially malarial. Increased flow of milk. Amenorrhea and general debility. Cheyne-Stokes breathing. After quinine.

**Head:** Aches, extending to the nose; feels swollen; pain in the frontal eminence. Aching in teeth. *Teeth feel on edge;* too long.

**Eyes:** Heavy; eyeballs ache.. Disordered vision.

**Ears:** Ringing in ears. Tinnitus and otalgia.

**Nose:** Pain at the root; feels swollen.

**Mouth:** Aching in teeth. *Teeth feel on edge;* too long.

**Abdomen:** Pain in the left hypochondrium. Splenic affections (hypertrophy).

**Modalities**: *Worse,* after sleep, sudden motion. *Better,* after rising, and walking about.

**Relationship:** Compare: *Chin., Cean., Helia.*

---

## PASSIFLORA INCARNATA

(Passion Flower) **Passi.**

An efficent anti-spasmodic. Whooping cough. Morphine habit. Delirium tremens. Convulsions in children; neuralgia. Has a quieting effect on the nervous system. Insomnia, produces normal sleep, no disturbance of cerebral functions, neuroses in children, worm fever, teething, spasms. *Tetanus.* Hysteria; puerperal convulsions. Painful diarrhea. Acute mania. *Atonic condition* generally present. *Asthma,* 10-30 gtt. every ten minutes for a few doses. Locally, in erysipelas.

**Head:** Violent ache as if the top of head would come off.

**Eyes**: Felt as if pushed out.

**Stomach:** Leaden, dead feeling after or between meals; flatulence and sour eructations.

**Sleep:** Restless and wakeful, resulting from exhaustion. Especially in the feeble, infants and the aged. Insomnia in infants, aged and the mentally worried and overworked people with a tendency to convulsions. Nocturnal cough.

**Dose:** Large doses of mother tincture are required, thirty to sixty drops, repeated several times.

---

## PENTHORUM SEDOIDES

(Virginia Stonecrop) **Pen.**

A remedy for coryza, with rawness and wet feeling in the nose. Throat feels raw. Chronic disorders of the mucous membranes, with irritability. Chronic post-nasal catarrh; chronic pharyngitis, mucous membrane purple and relaxed. Posterior nares feel moist and raw; nose and ears feel full. Aphonia, hoarseness, relaxed vocal cords. Hypersecretion of mucous membranes. Itching in the anus and burning in the rectum. Diseases of the pharyngeal vault and eustachian tube.

**Nose:** *Constant wet feeling in the nose,* which no amount of blowing will relieve. Discharge thick, pus like, streaked with blood. *Post-nasal catarrh* of puberty.

**Relationship:** Compare: *Pen.* often follows *Puls., Sang., Hydr.*

**Dose:** Not very active, and better adapted to chronic affections; it should be used for some time. Lower potencies.

---

# PERTUSSINUM

(Coqueluchin) **Pert.**

Taken from the glairy and stringy mucus containing the virus of whooping cough. Introduced by John H. Clarke for the treatment of whooping cough and other spasmodic coughs.

**Relationship:** Compare: *Dros., Cor-r., Cupr., Naphtin., Meph., Passi., Coc-c., Mag-p.*

**Dose:** The thirtieth potency.

---

# PETROLEUM

(Crude Rock Oil) **Petr.**

Strumous diathesis, especially the dark type, who suffer from catarrhal conditions of the mucous membranes, gastric acidity and cutaneous eruptions.

Very marked skin symptoms, acts on sweat and oil glands. Ailments are worse during the winter season. Ailments from riding in cars, carriages, or ships; lingering gastric and lung problems; chronic diarrhea. *Long lasting complaints* follow mental states—fright, vexation, etc. Chlorosis in young girls with or without gastric ulceration.

**Mind:** Marked aggravation from mental emotions. Loses his way in streets. Thinks he is double, or someone else is lying alongside. *Feels that death is near, must hurry to settle affairs.* Irritable, easily offended, vexed at everything. *Low spirited, with dimness of vision.*

**Head:** Sensitive, *as if a cold breeze was blowing on it.* Feels numb, as if made of wood; *occiput heavy, as if made of lead* (*Op.*). *Vertigo on rising,* felt in the occiput, as if intoxicated or like seasickness. *Moist eruptions on the scalp;* worse, back and ears (crusta lactea). Scalp sore to touch, followed by numbness. Headache, must hold the temples to relieve pain; provoked by shaking, while coughing. Use thirtieth.

**Eyes:** Loss of eyelashes. Dim sight; far sighted; cannot read fine print without glasses (hypermetropia); blenorrhea of the lachrymal sac; *marginal blepharitis.* Canthi fissured. Skin around eyes dry and scurfy.

**Ears:** Noise unbearable, especially when several people talking together. Eczema, intertrigo, etc. in and behind the ears with intense itching. Parts sore to touch. Fissures in the meatus. dry catarrh, with deafness and noises. Ringing and cracking in ears. Chronic eustachian catarrh. Diminished hearing.

**Nose:** *Nostrils ulcerated, cracked, burn;* tip of nose itches. Epistaxis. Ozena, with scabs and muco-purulent discharge.

**Face:** Dry; feels constricted, as if covered with albumin.

**Stomach:** Heartburn; hot, sharp, sour eructation. Distention. Marked sensation of emptiness. Strong aversion to fatty food, meat; worse, eating cabbage. *Hunger,* immediately after stool. *Nausea,* with accumulation of water in the mouth. Gastralgia when stomach is empty; relieved by constant eating (*Anac., Sep.*). Ravenous hunger. Must rise at night and eat (*Psor.*). Odor of garlic.

**Stool:** *Diarrhea only during daytime;* watery, gushing and *itching in the anus.* Diarrhea after cabbage; with an empty feeling in the stomach.

**Male:** Herpetic eruptions on the perineum. Prostate inflamed and swollen (prostatitis). Itching in the urethra.

**Female**: Before menses, throbbing, in the head (*Kreos.*). Leucorrhea, profuse, albuminous (*Alum., Borx., Bov., Calc-p.*). Genitals sore and moist. Sensation of moisture (*Eup-pur.*). Itching and mealy (bran-like) coating of nipple.

**Respiratory:** Hoarseness (*Carb-v., Caust., Phos.*). Dry cough with oppression of chest at night. Cough produces headache. Oppression of chest; worse, cold air. Dry cough at night, coming deep from the chest. Croup and laryngeal diphtheria.

**Heart:** Sensation of coldness (*Carb-an., Nat-m.*). Fainting, with ebullitions, of heat, and palpitations.

**Back:** Pain in the nape of neck, stiff and painful. Weakness in the lumbosacral region. Coccyx painful.

**Extremities:** Chronic sprains. Fetid sweat in axillae. Knees stiff. *Tips of fingers rough, cracked, fissured every winter.* Scalding sensation in knee. Cracking in joints.

**Fever:** Chilliness, followed by sweat. Flushes of heat, particularly on the face and head; worse at night. Perspiration on feet and axillae.

**Skin:** Itching at night. Chilblains, moist, itch and burn. Bed sores. *Skin dry, constricted, very sensitive, rough and cracked, leathery.* Herpes. Slightest scratch makes skin suppurate (*Hep.*). Intertrigo; psoriasis of hands. *Thick, greenish crusts, burning and itching; redness, raw; cracks bleed easily.* Eczema. Rhagades *worse in winter.*

**Modalities:** *Worse, dampness,* before and during a thunderstorm, from riding in cars, *passive motion; in winter,* eating, from mental states. *Better,* warm air; lying with head high; dry weather.

**Relationship:** Compare: *Carb-v., Graph., Sulph., Phos.*

Complementary: *Sep.*

Antidotes: *Nux-v., Cocc.*

**Dose:** Third to thirtieth and higher potencies. Material doses often better.

---

## PETROSELINUM SATIVUM

(Parsley) **Petros.**

The urinary symptoms give the keynotes for this remedy. *Piles with severe itching.*

**Stomach**: Thirsty and hungry, but desire fails on beginning to eat or drink.

**Urinary**: Burning, tingling, from perineum, extending throughout the urethra; *sudden urging to micturate;* frequent, voluptuous tickling in fossa navicularis. Gonorrhea; *sudden, irresistible desire to micturate; intense biting, itching, deep in the urethra;* milky discharge.

**Relationship**: Compare: *Apiolum*—the active principle of parsley (in dysmenorrhea); *Canth., Sars., Cann-s., Merc.*

**Dose**: First to third potency.

---

## PHASEOLUS NANUS

(Dwarf Bean) **Phase.**

Heart symptoms are quite pronounced. Diabetes.

**Head**: Aches chiefly in the forehead or orbits from fullness of brain; worse any movement or mental exertion.

**Eyes**: Pupils dilated, insensible to light. Eyeballs painful to touch.

**Urinary**: Diabetic urine.

**Heart**: Fearful, palpitations and sensation that death is approaching.

**Chest**: Breathing slow and sighing. Pulse rapid. *Palpitations.* Sick feeling around the heart, with a weak pulse. Right ribs sore. Dropsical effusion into pleura or pericardium (pleurisy, pericarditis, hydrothorax).

**Relationship**: Compare: *Crat., Lach.*

**Dose**: Sixth and higher. A decoction of the shells as a drink for diabetes, but look out for severe headache.

---

## PHELLANDRIUM AQUATICUM

(Water Dropwort) **Phel.**

The respiratory symptom is most important, and has been frequently verified clinically. A very good remedy for the *offensive expectoration and cough in phthisis,* bronchitis and emphysema. Tuberculosis generally affecting the middle lobes. *Everything tastes sweet.* Hemoptysis, hectic and colliquative diarrhea.

**Head**: *Weight on the vertex; aching and burning in temples and above the eyes.* Crushing sensation in the vertex. Vertigo, dizzy when lying down.

**Eyes**: Ciliary neuralgia; worse on any attempt to use the eyes; burning in eyes. Lachrymation. Cannot bear light (photophobia). Headache; involving nerves going to the eyes.

**Female**: *Pain in milk ducts;* intolerable between nursing. Pain in nipples (mastitis).

**Chest**: *Sticking pain in the right breast near the sternum, extending to the back, near shoulders.* Dyspnea and continuous cough, early in the morning. Cough, with profuse and fetid expectoration; compels him to sit up. Hoarseness.

**Extremities**: Tired feeling when walking.

**Fever**: Hectic; profuse and debilitating perspiration; intermittent, with pain in arms. Desire for acids.

**Relationship**: Compare: *Con., Phyt., Sil., Ant-i., Myos-a.*

**Dose**: Tincture to sixth potency. In phthisis not below the sixth.

---

## PHOSPHORICUM ACIDUM

(Phosphoric Acid) **Ph-ac.**

The common acid "debility" is very marked in this remedy, producing a nervous exhaustion. *Mental debility* first; later physical. A congenial soil for the action of *Ph-ac.* is found in young people who grow rapidly and who are over taxed, mentally or physically. Whenever the system has been exposed to the ravages of acute disease, excesses, grief, loss of vital fluids, we obtain conditions calling for it. Pyrosis, flatulence, diarrhea, diabetes, rhachitis and periosteal inflammation. Neurosis in the stump, after amputation. Hemorrhages in typhoid. Useful in relieving pain of cancer.

**Mind:** Listless. Impaired memory (*Anac.*). *Apathetic, indifferent.* Cannot collect his thoughts or find the right word. Difficult comprehension. Effects of grief and mental shock. Delirium with great stupefaction. Settled despair.

**Head:** Heavy; *confused.* Pain with sensation as if temples were crushed together. Worse, *shaking or noise. Crushing headache. Pressure on top.* Hair gray early in life; falls out. Dull headache after coition; from eye strain (*Nat-m.*). *Vertigo towards the evening, when standing or walking.* Hair thins out, turns gray early.

**Eyes:** *Blue rings around.* Lids inflamed (blepharitis) and cold. Pupils dilated. Glassy appearance. Averse to sunlight (photophobia); sees colors as of a rainbow. Feel too large. Ambylopia in masturbators. Optic nerves seem torpid. Pain *as if the eyeballs were frocibly pressed together and into the head.*

**Ears:** Roaring, with difficulty in hearing. Intolerance of noises.

**Nose:** Epistaxis. Bores fingers into the nose. *Itching.*

**Face:** Pale, earthy; feeling of tension as from dried albumen. Sensation of coldness on one side of face.

**Mouth:** Lips dry, cracked. Bleeding gums; retract from teeth (scurvy). Tongue swollen, dry, with viscid, frothy mucus. Teeth feel cold. At night, bites tongue involuntarily (epilepsy).

**Stomach:** Craves juicy things. Sour risings. Nausea. *Symptoms following sour food and drink.* Pressure as if from a weight, with sleepiness after eating (*Fel*). *Thirst for cold milk.*

**Abdomen:** Distention and fermentation in bowels. Splenomegaly (*Cean.*). *Aching in the umbilical region.* Loud rumbling.

**Stool:** Diarrhea, *white,* watery, involuntary, *painless,* with much flatus; not very exhausting. Diarrhea in weak, delicate, rachitic children.

**Urinary:** Frequent, profuse, watery, *milky. Diabetes.* Micturition, preceded by anxiety and followed by burning. *Frequent micturition at night.* Phosphaturia.

**Male:** Emissions at night and at stool. Seminal vesiculitis (*Ox-ac.*). Sexual power deficient (impotence); testicles tender and swollen (orchitis). Parts relax during embrace (*Nux-v.*). Prostatorrhea even when passing soft stool. Eczema of the scrotum. Edema of prepuce, and swollen glans penis (balanitis). Herpes preputialis. Sycotic excrescences (*Thuj.*).

**Female:** Menses too early and profuse, with pain in the liver region. Itching; yellow leucorrhea after menses. Milk scanty; health deteriorated from nursing.

**Respiratory:** Chest problems develop after brainfag. Hoarseness. Dry cough from tickling in the chest. Salty expectoration. Difficult respiration. *Weak feeling in the chest from talking* (*Stann.*). *Pressure behind the sternum,* rendering breathing difficult (asthma).

**Heart:** Palpitations in children who grow too fast; after grief, self abuse. Pulse irregular, intermittent.

**Back:** Boring pain between scapulae. Pain in the back and limbs, as if beaten.

**Extremities:** Weak. Tearing pains in joints, bones and periosteum (osteomyelitis). Cramps in upper arms and wrists. *Great debility.* Pains at night, *as if bones were scraped.* Stumbles easily and makes misteps. Itching, between fingers or in folds of joints.

**Sleep:** *Somnolence.* Lascivious dreams with emissions.

**Fever:** Chills. *Profuse sweat* at night and in the morning. Low types of fever, with dull comprehension and stupor.

**Skin:** Pimples, acne, blood boils. Ulcers with very offensive pus. Burning red rash (erysipelas). Formication in various parts. *Falling out of hair* (*Nat-m., Sel.*). Tendency to abscess after fever.

**Modalities:** *Better*, from keeping warm. *Worse,* exertion, from being talked to; loss of vital fluids; sexual excesses. Everything impeding circulation causes aggravation of symptoms.

**Relationship:** Compare: *Oenothera biennis*—Evening primrose (effortless diarrhea with nervous exhaustion. Incipient hydrocephalus. Whooping cough and spasmodic asthma). *Nectranada amara* (watery diarrhea, dry tongue, colic, bluish ring around sunken eyes, restless sleep). *Chin., Nux-v., Pic-ac., Lac-ac., Phos.*

Antidotes: *Coff.*

**Dose**: First potency.

---

# PHOSPHORUS

(Phosphorus) **Phos.**

*Phosphorus* irritates, inflames and degenerates mucous membranes, irritates and inflames serous membranes, inflames spinal cord and nerves, causing paralysis, destroys bone, especially the lower jaw and tibia; and disorganises blood. Causes fatty degeneration of blood vessels and every tissue and organ of the body, thus giving rise to hemorrhages, and hematogenous jaundice.

Produces a picture of destructive metabolism. Causes yellow atrophy of the liver and sub-acute hepatitis. Tall, slender people, narrow chested, with thin, transparent skin, weakened by loss of animal fluids, with great nervous debility, emaciation, amative tendencies, seem to be under the special influence of *Phosphorus.* Great susceptibility to external impressions, to light, sound, odors, touch, electrical changes and thunderstorms. *Suddenness* of symptoms, sudden prostration, faints, sweats, shooting pains, etc. Polycythemia. Bloody extravasations; *fatty degenerations,* cirrhosis, caries, are pathological states often calling for *Phosphorus.* Muscular pseudo-hypertrophy, neuritis. Inflammation of the respiratory tract. Paralytic symptoms. Ill effects of iodine and excessive use of salt; worse, *lying on the left side.* Tertiary syphilis, skin lesions, and nervous debility. *Scurvy. Pseudo-hypertrophic paralysis.* Ataxia and adynamia. Osteomyelitis. Bone fragility.

**Mind:** Great depression of spirits. Easily vexed. Fearfulness, as if something was creeping out of every corner. Clairvoyant state. Great tendency to start. Over sensitive to external impressions. Loss of memory. Paralysis in the insane. Ecstasy. Dread of death when alone. Brain feels tired. Insanity, with an exaggerated idea of one's own importance. Excitable, produces heat all over. Restless, fidgety. Hyposensitive, indifferent.

**Head:** Vertigo in the aged, *after rising* (*Bry.*). *Heat comes from the spine.* Neuralgia; parts must be kept warm. Burning pains. Chronic congestion of head. Brain fag, with *sensation of coldness in the occiput.* Vertigo, with faintness (pernicious anemia). Skin of forehead feels too tight. Itching of scalp, dandruff, falling out of hair in large bunches (alopecia areata).

**Eyes:** Cataract. Sensation as if everything was covered with a mist, veil, dust, or as it something was pulled tightly over the eyes. Black points seem to float before the eyes. Patient sees better by shading eyes with hand. Fatigue of eyes and head even without much use of eyes. *Green halo around the candle light* (*Osm.*). *Letters appear red. Atrophy* of optic nerve. Edema of lids and around eyes. Pearly white conjunctiva and long curved lashes. Partial loss of vision from abuse of tobacco (*Nux-v.*). Pain in orbital bones. Paresis of extrinsic muscles. Diplopia, due to deviation of the visual axis. Amaurosis from sexual excess. Glaucoma. Thrombosis of retinal vessels and degenerative changes in retinal cells. Degenerative changes where soreness and curved lines are seen in old people. Retinal problems with perception of light and hallucination of vision (retinitis).

**Ears:** *Hearing difficult,* especially to human voice. Re-echoing of sounds (*Caust.*). Dullness of hearing after typhoid.

**Nose:** Fan-like motion of nostrils (*Lyc.*). Bleeding; *epistaxis instead of menses* (vicarious menses). Over sensitive to smell (*Carb-ac., Nux-v.*). Periostitis of nasal bones. Foul imaginary odors (*Aur.*). Chronic catarrh, *with small hemorrhages* (ozena); handkerchief is always bloody. *Polypi; bleeding easily* (*Calc., Sang.*).

**Face:** Pale, sickly complexion; blue rings under the eyes. Hippocratic countenance. Tearing pain in facial bones; circumscribed redness in one or both the cheeks. *Swelling and necrosis of lower jaw* (*Amph., Hecla*).

**Mouth:** Swollen and easily *bleeding gums,* ulcerated (scurvy). Toothache after washing clothes. Tongue dry, *smooth, red* or white (glossitis), not thickly coated. Persistent bleeding after tooth extraction. Nursing sore mouth. Burning in the esophagus. Dryness in the pharynx and fauces. *Thirst for very cold water.* Stricture of esophagus.

**Stomach:** Hungry soon after eating. Sour taste and sour eructations after every meal. Belching large quantities of wind, after eating (dyspepsia, achlorhydria). *Throws up ingesta by the mouthfuls.* Vomiting; *water is thrown up as soon as it gets warm in the stomach. Post-operative vomiting.* Cardiac opening seems contracted, too narrow; the food scarcely swallowed, comes up again (*Bry., Alum.*). Pain in stomach; relieved by cold food, ices. Region of stomach painful to touch, or on walking. Inflammation of stomach (gastritis), with burning extending to the throat and bowels. *Bad effects of eating too much salt.*

**Abdomen:** Feels cold (*Caps.*). Sharp, cutting pains. *A very weak, empty, all gone sensation* felt in the whole abdominal cavity. Liver congested. Acute hepatitis. Fatty degeneration (*Carbn-tm., Ars., Chlf.*). Jaundice. Pancreatic disease. Large, yellow spots on the abdomen.

**Stool:** *Extremely fetid stools and flatus.* Long, narrow, hard, like a dog's. Difficult to expel. Desire for stool on lying on left side. *Painless,* copious *debilitating* diarrhea. Green mucus with sago like particles. Involuntary; seems as if the anus remained open. *Great weakness after stool.* Discharge of blood from rectum, during stool. *White,* hard stools. Bleeding hemorrhoids.

**Urinary:** Hematuria, especially in acute Bright's disease (*Canth.*). Turbid, brown, with red sediment.

**Male:** Lack of power (impotence). *Irresistible desire;* involuntary emissions, with lascivious dreams.

**Female:** Metritis. Chlorosis. Phlebitis. Fistulous tracks after mammary abscess. Slight hemorrhage from uterus between periods (metrorrhagia). Menses too early and scanty, not profuse, *but last too long.* Weeps before menses. Stitching pain in mammae. Leucorrhea profuse, smarting, corrosive, instead of menses. Amenorrhea, with vicarious menstruation (*Bry.*).

*Suppuration of mammae* burning, watery, offensive discharge. Nymphomania. Uterine polyps.

**Respiratory:** Hoarseness; worse evenings. *Larynx very painful* (laryngitis). Clergyman's sore throat; violent tickling in the larynx while speaking. Aphonia, worse evenings, with rawness. *Cannot talk on account of pain in the larynx.* Cough from tickling in throat; *worse, cold air,* reading, laughing, *talking,* on going from a warm room into cold air. Sweetish taste while coughing. Hard, dry, tight, racking cough (bronchitis). Congestion of lungs. Burning pains, heat and oppression of chest. *Tightness across chest; great weight on chest.* Sharp stitches in chest; respiration *quickened, oppressed. Marked heat in chest.* Pneumonia, with oppression; *Worse, lying on the left side.* The whole body *trembles,* with cough. Sputa rusty, blood colored or purulent. Tuberculosis in tall, rapidly growing young people. Do not give it too low or too frequently here, it may but hasten the destructive degeneration of tubercular masses. Repeated hemoptysis (*Acal.*). Pain in throat on coughing. Nervous cough provoked by strong odors, entrance of stranger; worse in the presence of strangers; worse lying on the left side; in a cold room.

**Heart:** Violent palpitations with anxiety, while lying on the left side. Pulse rapid, small, and *soft.* Heart dilated, especially right. Sensation of warmth in heart.

**Back:** Burning in the back; pain as if broken. *Heat between the shoulder blades.* Weak spine.

**Extremities:** Ascending sensory and motor paralysis from ends of fingers and toes. Stitches in elbow and shoulder joints. Burning in feet. Weakness and trembling, from every exertion. Can scarcely hold anything with his hands. Tibia inflamed and becomes necrosed. *Arms and hands become numb.* Can lie only on the right side. Post-diphtheritic paralysis, with formication of hands and feet. *Joints suddenly give way.*

**Sleep:** Great drowsiness, especially after meals. Coma vigil. Sleeplessness in old people. Vivid dreams of fire; of hemorrhage. Lascivious dreams. Goes to sleep late and awakens weak. *Short naps and frequent wakings.*

**Fever:** Chilly every evening. Cold knees at night. *Adynamic with lack of thirst, but unnatural hunger.* Hectic, with a small, quick pulse; viscid night sweats. Stupid delirium. Profuse perspiration.

**Skin**: *Wounds bleed profusely, even if small;* they heal and break out again. Jaundice. Little ulcers on the outside of larger ones. Petechiae. Ecchymosis. *Purpura hemorrhagia. Scurvy.* Fungus hematodes and excrescences.

**Modalities:** *Worse,* touch; physical or mental exertion; twilight; warm food or drink; change of weather, from getting wet in hot weather; evening; lying on the left or painful side; during a thunderstorm; ascending stairs. *Better,* in dark, lying on the right side, cold food; cold; open air; washing with cold water; sleep.

**Relationship:** Complementary: *Ars., All-c., Lyc., Sil. Sanguisuga officinalis* 30—Leech (*persistent hemorrhages;* effects of use of leeches). *Phosphorus pentachloratus* (great soreness of the mucous membrane of eyes and nose, throat and chest sore).

Incompatible: *Caust.*

Compare: *Tub.* follows *Phos.* well and compliments its action. *Phosphorus hydrogenatus* (crumbling teeth; hyperesthesia; locomotor ataxia); *Amph.* (right jaw swollen and painful). *Thymolum* (typical sexual neurasthenia; irritable stomach; aching throughout the lumbar region; worse, mental and physical exertion); *Calc., Chin., Ant-c., Sep., Lyc., Sulph.* In pneumonia, *Pneumococcinum* 200 and *Pneumotoxinum* (Cahis) taken from the Diplococcus lanceolatus of Fraenkel. Pneumonia and paralytic phenomena; pleuritic pain and pain in the ilio-ceacal region (Cartier).

Antidote: Antidote of *Phos.* poisoning: Turpentine with which it forms an insoluble mass. Also *Potassium permang., Nux-v.*

*Phos.* antidotes the nausea and vomiting of chloroform and ether.

**Dose:** Third to thirtieth potency. Should not be given too low or in too continuous doses, especially in tuberculous cases. It may act as euthanasia here.

---

# PHYSALIS ALKEKENGI — SOLANUM VESICARIUM

(Alkekengi, Winter Cherry) **Physal-al.**

Marked urinary symptoms confirming its ancient uses in gravel, etc. Lithiasis; marked diuretic action. Languor and muscular weakness.

**Head:** Vertigo, hazy feeling; memory weakened; desire to talk constantly. Throbbing pain, heaviness over the eyes. Facial paralysis. Dryness of the mouth.

**Urinary:** Acrid, foul, retained, abundant. Polyuria. Sudden inability to hold it in women. Nocturnal incontinence. *Enuresis.*

**Respiratory:** Cough. Hoarse voice; throat irritated; chest oppressed, causing insomnia. Stabbing pains in the chest.

**Extremities:** Stiff limbs; tonic cramps. Paralysis. When walking, every jar seems to repeat in the head.

**Fever:** Chilly in open air. Feverish in the evening. Sweat during stool, with a creeping sensation, and abundant urine. Pain in the liver region during fever.

**Skin:** Excoriation between fingers and toes; pustules on thighs; nodes on forehead.

**Modalities:** *Worse,* cold damp evening, after getting heated.

**Dose:** Tincture to third attenuation. The juice of the berries is used in dropsical conditions and irritable bladder.

---

# PHYSOSTIGMA VENENOSUM

(Calabar Bean) **Phys.**

This remedy and its active principle, *Eserine,* form a valuable addition to materia medica. Stimulates the heart, raises blood pressure and increases peristalsis. Causes contraction of the pupil and ciliary muscles. Induces a condition of short sightedness (myopia) *Spinal irritation,* loss of motility, prostration, with very sensitive vertebrae. Fibrillary tremors (chorea). Rigidity of muscles; paralysis. Depresses the motor and reflex activity of the cord and causes loss of sensibility to pain, muscular weakness, followed by complete paralysis, although muscular contractility is not impaired. Paralysis and tremors, chorea. Meningeal irritation, with rigidity of muscles. *Tetanus* and trismus. Poliomyelitis anterior. Eserine is used locally to produce contraction of pupil.

**Head:** Constant pain on top; vertigo, with a constrictive feeling in the head. Pain over the orbits; *cannot bear to raise eyelids.* Cerebro-spinal meningitis; general tetanic rigidity. Spastic conditions of the facial muscles.

**Eyes:** Night blindness (opposite, *Both.*); photophobia; *contraction of pupils; twitching of ocular muscles.* Lagophthalmus. Muscae volitantes; flashes of light; partial blindness. *Glaucoma;* paresis of accommodation; astigmatism. Profuse lachrymation. *Spasm of ciliary muscles, with irritability after using eyes. Increasing myopia.* Post-diphtheritic paralysis of the eye and accomodation muscles.

**Nose:** Fluent coryza; burning and tingling of nostrils; nose stuffed and hot. Fever blisters around nostrils.

**Mouth:** *Tip of tongue feels sore.* Sensation of a ball in the throat (globus hystericus).

**Throat:** Strong heart pulsations felt in the throat.

**Stomach:** Great pain immediately after eating. Sensitive to pressure in the epigastric region. Pain extends to the chest and down the arms. Gastralgia; chronic constipation.

**Female:** Irregular menstruation with palpitations. Congestion of eyes. Rigid muscles.

**Heart:** Feeble pulse; palpitations; spasmodic action, with feeling of pulsations throughout the body. Heart beats distinctly perceptible in chest and head. *Fluttering of heart felt in the throat.* Fatty degeneration (*Cupr-act.*).

**Extremities:** *Pain in the right popliteal space.* Burning and tingling in spine. Hands and feet numb. Sudden jerking of limbs on going to sleep. Tetanic convulsions. Locomotor ataxia. Numbness in paralyzed parts, crampy pains in limbs.

**Relationship:** Compare: *Eserinum*—the alkaloid of *Phys.* (slows action of heart and increases arterial tension; in ciliary spasm and spasmodic *astigmatism* due to irregular action of ciliary muscles; blepharo-spasms; *pupils contracted.* Twitching of lids, soreness of eyeballs, blurring of vision *after using the eyes,* pain around eyes and head). Used locally to contract the pupil. *Eserinum* contracts the pupils dilated by *Atropinum,* but not those dilated by *Gelsemium.* Internally 6x).

*Eserinum salicylicum* (post-operative intestinal paralysis; meteorism. Hypodermically 1/60-1/40 gr.).

Compare also: *Muscin., Con., Cur., Gels., Thebin.* (tetanus); *Piperazinum* (uric acid conditions. Pruritus. Gout and urinary calculi. *Constant backache.* Skin dry, urine scanty. Rheumatic arthritis. Give one grain daily in carbonated water. First and second decimal trituration three times a day).

Antidote: Atropia. In full medicinal doses will relieve most of the effects of Physostigmine.

**Dose:** Third potency. The neutral sulphate of *Eserinum* is instilled into the eye, from one-half to four grains to one ounce distilled water, to induce *contraction of pupil,* in mydriasis, injuries to the eye, iritis, corneal ulcers, etc.

---

# PHYTOLACCA DECANDRA

(Poke-root) **Phyt.**

Aching, soreness, restlessness, prostration, are general symptoms guiding to *Phyt.* Pre-eminently a glandular remedy. Glandular swellings with heat and inflammation. Has a powerful effect on fibrous and osseous tissues; fasciae and muscle sheaths; acts on scar tissue. Syphilitic bone pains; chronic rheumatism. Sore throat, quinsy and diphtheria. Tetanus and opisthotonos. Decrease of weight. Retarded dentition.

**Mind:** Loss of personal delicacy,[1] disregard of surrounding objects. Indifferent to life.

**Head:** Vertigo on rising. Brain feels sore. Pain from the frontal region backward. Pressure in temples and over the eyes. Rheumatism of scalp; pains come on every time it rains. Scaly eruptions on the scalp.

**Eyes:** *Smarting.* Sensation of sand under the lids (trachoma). Tarsal edges feel hot. Fistula lachrymalis (*Fl-ac.*). *Abundant lachrymation, hot.*

**Nose:** Coryza; flow of mucus from *one nostril and from the posterior nares.*

**Mouth:** Teething children with an irresistible desire *to bite the teeth together.* Teeth clenched; lower lip drawn down; lips everted; jaws firmly set; chin drawn down on the sternum, tongue *red,* feels rough and scalded (glossitis); bleeding from the mouth; blisters on the side. Mapped, indented, fissured, with a yellow patch down the center. Profuse stringy saliva.

**Throat:** *Dark red or bluish-red.* Pain at the root of tongue; soft palate and tonsils swollen. Sensation of a lump in the throat (*Bell., Lach.*). *Throat feels rough, narrow, hot. Tonsils swollen,* especially right; dark red appearance. *Shooting pain extending to the ears on swallowing.* Pseudo-membranous exudation, grayish-white; thick, tenacious yellowish mucus, difficult to dislodge. *Cannot swallow anything hot* (*Lach.*). Tension and pressure in the parotid gland. Ulcerated sore throat and diphtheria; *throat feels very hot; pain at the root of tongue extending to the ear.* Uvula large, dropsical. *Quinsy; tonsils and fauces swollen,* with burning pain; cannot swallow even water. *Mumps. Follicular pharyngitis.*

**Abdomen:** Sore spot in right hypochondrium. Rheumatism of abdominal muscles. Colic at the navel. Burning, griping pains. Bruised feeling in the epigastrium and abdomen. Constipation in the aged and those with weak heart. Bleeding from the rectum.

**Urinary:** Scanty, suppressed, *with pain in the kidney region.* Nephritis.

**Male:** Painful induration of testicles (orchitis). *Shooting along the perineum to the penis.*

**Female:** Mastitis; *mammae hard and very sensitive.* Tumors of the breasts with enlarged axillary glands. Cancer of breast. Breast is hard, painful and of a purple hue. Mammary abscess. When child nurses, *pain radiates from the nipple, all over the body.* Cracks and small ulcers around nipples. Irritable breasts, before and during menses. Galactorrhea (*Calc.*). Menses too copious and frequent. Ovarian neuralgia of right side.

---

[1] complete shamelessness and indifference to exposure of her person (Clarke — Dictionary of Practical Materia Medica).

**Respiratory:** Aphonia. Dyspnea (asthma); dry hacking, tickling cough; worse at night (*Menth., Bell.*). Aching pains in the chest, through mid-sternum; with cough. Rheumatism of lower intercostals.

**Heart:** Sensation as if the heart leaped into the throat (*Podo.*). Shock of pain in the cardiac region alternating with pain in the right arm (angina pectoris).

**Back:** Aching pain in the lumbar region; pains streaking up and down the spine. Weakness and dull pain in the region of kidneys. Back stiff, especially in the morning on rising and during damp weather.

**Extremities:** Shooting pain in right shoulder with stiffness and an inability to raise the arm (see Heart). Rheumatic pains; worse in the morning. *Pains fly like electric shocks,* shooting, lancinating, shifting rapidly (*Puls., Kali-bi.*). Pain on the under side of thighs. Syphilitic sciatica. *Aching in heels;* relieved by elevating feet. Pain, like shocks. Pain in legs, patient dreads to get up. Feet puffed; pain in ankles and feet. Neuralgia in toes (gout).

**Fever:** High fever, alternating with chilliness and great prostration.

**Skin:** Itches, becomes dry, shrunken, pale. Papular and pustular lesions. Very useful in early stages of cutaneous diseases. *Disposition to boils,* when sloughing occurs. Squamous eruptions. Syphilitic eruptions. Swelling and induration of glands (adenitis). *Venereal buboes.* Scarlatina-like rash. Warts and moles.

**Modalities:** *Worse,* sensitive to electric changes. Effects of getting wet, when it *rains,* exposure to *damp,* cold weather, night, exposure, motion, right side. *Better,* warmth, dry weather, rest.

**Relationship:** Compare: Tincture of *Phytolacca berry* (sore throats and in the treatment of obesity); *Bry., Rhus-t., Kali-i., Merc., Sang., Arum-t.*

Inimical: *Merc.*

Antidotes: Milk and salt; *Bell., Mez.*

**Dose:** Tincture to third potency. Externally for mastitis

---

# PICRICUM ACIDUM

(Picric Acid, Trinitrophenol) **Pic-ac.**

Causes degeneration of the spinal cord with paralysis. Brain fag and sexual excitement. Acts upon the generative organs probably through the lumbar centers of the spinal cord; prostration, weakness, pain in the back and pins and needle sensation in the extremities. *Neurasthenia* (*Ox-ac.*). Muscular debility. Heavy, tired feeling. Myelitis with spasms and prostration. Writer's palsy. Progressive, pernicious anemia. *Uremia* with complete anuria. A one percent solution applied on lint, is the best application for burns till granulations begin to form. Sallow complexion.

**Mind:** Lack of will power; disinclined to work. Cerebral softening. Dementia with prostration, sits still and listless.

**Head:** Head pains; *relieved by bandaging tightly. Occipital pain;* worse, slightest mental exertion. Vertigo and noises in the ear(tinnitus). Boils *within* ears and back of neck. After prolonged mental strain, with anxiety and dread of failure during examination. Brain fag.

**Eyes:** Chronic catarrhal conjunctivitis with copious, thick yellow discharge.

**Stomach:** Bitter taste. Aversion to food.

**Urinary:** *Scanty;* complete anuria. Dribbling micturition. Urine contains much indican, granular cylinders and fatty, degenerated epithelium. Inflammation of kidneys (nephritis) with profound weakness, dark, bloody, scanty urine (hematuria). Nocturnal urging.

**Male:** Emissions profuse, followed by great exhaustion, without sensual dreams. *Priapism;* satyriasis. Hard erections, with pain in the testicles radiating up the cord (orchitis). Prostatic hypertrophy, especially in cases which have not advanced too far.

**Female:** Pain in the left ovary and leucorrhea before menstruation. Pruritus vulvae.

**Extremities:** Burning along the spine. *Great weakness. Tired, heavy feeling all over the body, especially limbs; worse, exertion.* Feet cold. Cannot get warm. Acute ascending paralysis (hemiplegia).

**Modalities:** *Worse,* least exertion, especially mental, after sleep, wet weather. A summer or hot weather remedy; patient is worse then. *Better,* from cold air, cold water, tight pressure.

**Relationship:** Compare: *Ox-ac., Gels., Phos., Sil., Arg-n.* Compare: *Zinc-pic.* (facial palsy and paralysis agitans); *Ferr-pic.* (buzzing in ears, deafness; chronic gout; epistaxis; prostatic troubles); *Calc-pic.* (boils in and around ears).

**Dose:** Sixth potency.

---

# PINUS SYLVESTRIS

(Scotch Pine) **Pin-s.**

Has been found to be of real use in the treatment of *weak ankles* with tardiness in walking, in scrofulous and rachitic children. Emaciation of lower extremities. *Pinus sylvestris* combines rheumatic, bronchial and urticarious symptoms; the chest is thin and seems to give way.

**Extremities:** Stiffness; gouty pain in all joints, especially finger joints (rheumatism). Cramps in calves.

**Skin:** Nettle rash. Itching all over, especially around the joints and on the abdomen. Nose itches.

**Relationship:** Compare: *Pinus lambertiana*—Sugar pine (constipation, amenorrhea, abortions. *Pinus lambertiana* sap is a decided carthartic. Delayed and painful menstruation).

Also, *Abies-c., Abies-n.*

**Dose:** Tincture to third potency.

---

## PIPER METHYSTICUM

(Kava-kava) **Pip-m.**

The intoxication produced by Kava is of a silent and drowsy character with incoherent dreams; loss of muscular power.

Urinary and skin symptoms have been verified. Marked modality. *Arthritis deformans.* Colic with flatulence.

**Mind:** Very sensitive. Exaltation of mind. *Amelioration of pain for some time by diverting attention.* Restless, desire to change position.

**Urinary:** Increased. Burning during micturition, gonorrhea and gleet. Cystitis. *Chordee.*

**Extremities:** Pain in the right arm. Hands feel paralyzed. Pain in the thumb joint.

**Skin:** Scaly. Fall of scales leaves *white spots,* which often ulcerate (eczema). Leprosy. Ichthyosis.

**Modalities:** *Better,* by thinking of another topic; changing position.

**Relationship:** Compare: *Chaulmoogra*—Taraktogenos (the oil and its derivatives are to a certain extent effective in the treatment of *leprosy,* especially in early cases).

*Bixa orellana,* a South American plant related to Chaulmoogra, recommended for leprosy, eczema and elephantiasis.

**Dose:** Tincture and lower potencies.

---

## PIPER NIGRUM

(Black Pepper) **Pip-n.**

Sensation of burning and pressure everywhere.

**Mind:** Sad, apprehensive, unable to concentrate; starts at any noise.

**Head:** Heavy headache, as if the temples were pressed in.

**Eyes:** Inflamed and burning. Bursting pain in eyeballs.

**Nose:** Itchy, epistaxis, sneezing.

**Face:** Pressure in the nasal and facial bones. Hyperemic burning. Lips dry and cracked.

**Throat:** Sore, feels raw, burns. Burning pain in tonsils.

**Stomach:** Gastric discomfort. Sensation of fullness. Great thirst. Flatulence. Tympanites. Colic and cramps.

**Urinary:** Burning in the bladder and urethra. Difficult micturition. Bladder feels full, swollen; frequent inclination without success. Priapism.

**Chest:** Dyspnea, cough with pain in chest in spots, feels as if spitting blood. Palpitations, cardiac pain, slow intermittent pulse. Profuse flow of milk.

**Dose:** Low attenuations.

---

# PITUITARIA GLANDULA

(Pituitary Gland) **Pitu-gl.**

*Pitu-gl.* exercises a superior control over the growth and development of the sexual organs, stimulates muscular activity and overcomes uterine inertia. Its influence over unstriped muscular fibre is marked. Cerebral hemorrhage. Checks hemorrhages and aids in the absorption of clots. Uterine inertia in the second stage of labor where the os is fully dilated. High blood pressure, chronic nephritis, prostatitis. Ten drops after meals (Dr. Geo Fuller). Vertigo, difficult mental concentration, confusion and fullness, deep in the frontal region. Use the 30th potency

**Relationship:** *Pituitrinum* (is a vaso-constrictor and parturient. Used chiefly for its action on the uterus either to aid in childbirth or to check bleeding after delivery. In doses of 1 c.c.m. intravenously to stimulate labor pains, expulsive period only. Contraindicated in myocarditis, nephritis and arteriosclerosis. A watery solution made from the posterior portion of the gland is put up in ampules containing about 15 minims each and is considered as the hypodermic dose. No effect per os).

---

## PIX LIQUIDA

(Pine Tar) **Pix.**

Tar and its constituents act on various mucous membranes.

Its skin symptoms are most important. A great medicine for cough. Bronchial irritation after influenza (*Kreos., Kali-bi.*). Scaly eruptions. Severe itching. *Constant vomiting of a blackish fluid, with pain in the stomach* (hematemesis). Alopecia (*Fl-ac.*).

**Chest:** *Pain at a spot, around the third left costal cartilage where it joins the rib.* Rales through the lungs, and muco-purulent sputum; offensive odor and taste. Chronic bronchitis.

**Skin:** Cracked; *itches intolerably;* bleeds on scratching. Eruptions on the *back of hands.*

**Relationship:** Compare its constituents: *Kreos., Petr., Pin-s., Eupi., Ter., Carb-ac.*

**Dose:** First to sixth potency.

---

## PLANTAGO MAJOR

(Plantain) **Plan.**

Has considerable clinical reputation in the treatment of otalgia, toothache and enuresis. Sharp pain in the eyes, a reflex from decayed teeth or inflammation of the middle ear. Eyeball, very tender to touch. Pain plays between teeth and ears. Pyorrhea alveolaris. Depression and insomnia of chronic nicotinism. Causes an aversion to tobacco.

**Head:** Periodical prosopalgia, worse 7 a. m. to 2 p. m., accompanied with flow of tears, photophobia; pain radiates to temples and lower face.

**Ears:** Hearing acute; noise painful. Sticking pain in the ears. Neuralgic otalgia; *pain goes from one ear to the other through the head.* Otalgia with toothache. Loud noises go through one.

**Nose:** Sudden, yellowish, watery discharge.

**Mouth:** Teeth ache and are sensitive and sore to touch. Swelling of cheeks. Salivation; teeth feel too long; worse, cold air and contact. Toothache, better while eating. Profuse flow of saliva. Toothache with reflex neuralgia in eyelids.

**Rectum:** Wants to defecate; goes often, but cannot. Piles so bad, can hardly stand. Diarrhea, with brown watery stools.

**Urinary:** Profuse flow; *nocturnal enuresis* (*Rhus-a., Caust., Bell.*).

**Skin:** Itching and burning; papulae. Urticaria, chilblains *(Agar., Tam.)*.

**Relationship:** Compare: *Kalm., Cham., Puls.*

**Dose:** Tincture and lower potencies. Local use in toothache, in hollow teeth, otorrhea, pruritus, and Poison oak. Incised wounds.

---

# PLATANUS OCCIDENTALIS

(Sycamore Buttonwood) **Platan-oc.**

*Tarsal tumors.* Apply the tincture. Both acute and old neglected cases, where destruction of tissues occurred and cicatricial contraction caused marked deformity of the lid, has been restored to practically normal conditions. Acts best in children. Must be used for some time. Ichthyosis.

---

# PLATINUM METALLICUM

(The Metal) **Plat.**

Is pre-eminently a woman's remedy. Strong tendency to paralysis, anesthesia, localized *numbness and coldness* are shown. Hysterical spasms; pains increase and decrease gradually (*Stann.*). Tremulousness.

**Mind:** Irresistible impulse to kill. Self exaltation; *contempt for others.* Arrogant, proud. Weary of everything. Everything seems changed. Mental problems, associated with suppressed menses. Physical symptoms disappear as mental symptoms develop.

**Head:** Tense, pressing pain, confined to a small spot. *Cramp-like, squeezing pain.* Constriction around the forehead and right temples. *Numbness, with headache.*

**Eyes:** *Objects look smaller than they are.* Twitching of lids (*Agar.*). Eyes feel cold. Cramp-like pain in orbits.

**Ears:** Feels numb. Cramp-like twinges. Roaring and rumbling.

**Face:** Prosopalgia, with a numb feeling in the malar bones, as if the parts were between screws. Pain at the root of nose, as if squeezed in a vise. *Coldness, creeping, and numbness,* on the right side of face. Pains increase and decrease gradually (*Stann.*).

**Stomach:** Fermentation, much flatulence; *constriction; ravenous* hunger; persistent nausea with anxiety and weakness.

**Abdomen:** Painter's colic. Pain in the umbilical region; extending to the back. Pressing and bearing down in the abdomen, extending into the pelvis.

**Stool:** Retarded; faeces scanty; evacuated with difficulty. Adheres to the rectum, like soft clay. *Sticky stool.* Constipation in travellers, who are constantly changing food and water. Stool as if burnt.

**Female:** Parts hypersensitive. Tingling internally and externally (*Kali-br., Orig.*). Ovaries sensitive and burn. Menses too early, too profuse (menorrhagia), dark clotted with spasms and painful bearing down sensation (dysmenorrhea), chilliness, and sensitiveness of parts. Vaginismus. Nymphomania. Excessive sexual development; vaginismus. Pruritus vulvae. Ovaritis with sterility. Abnormal sexual appetite and melancholia.

**Extremities:** Tightness of thighs, as if too tightly wrapped. Numb and weary sensation. Feel paralyzed.

**Sleep:** Sleeps with legs far apart (*Cham.*).

**Modalities:** *Worse,* sitting and standing; evening. *Better,* walking.

**Relationship:** Compare: *Rhod., Stann., Valer., Sep.* Compare, also: *Platinum muriaticum* (this remedy has achieved beneficial results after Iodide of Potash failed to cure in syphilitic affection; violent occipital headaches, dysphagia, and syphilitic throat and bone affections; caries in bones of feet); *Platinum muriaticum natronatum* (polyuria and salivation); *Sedum acre* (sexual irritability, relieves irritation of nerve centers and gives rest).

Antidote: *Puls. Plat.* antidotes the bad effects of lead.

**Dose:** Sixth trituration to thirtieth potency.

---

# PLUMBUM METALLICUM

(Lead) **Plb.**

A great drug for general sclerotic conditions. Lead paralysis is chiefly of extensors, forearm or upper limb, from center to periphery with partial anesthesia or excessive hyperesthesia preceded by pain. Localized neuralgic pains, neuritis. Blood, alimentary and nervous systems are the special seats of action of *Plb.* Hematosis is interfered with, rapid reduction in the number of red blood corpuscles; hence pallor, icterus, anemia. Constrictive sensation in internal organs.

Delirium, coma and convulsions. Hypertension and arteriosclerosis. *Progressive muscular atrophy.* Infantile paralysis. Locomotor ataxia. Excessive and rapid emaciation. Bulbar paralysis. Important in peripheral affections. The points of attack for *Plb.* are the neuroaxons and the anterior horns. Symptoms of multiple sclerosis, posterior spinal sclerosis. Contractions and boring pain. All the symptoms of acute nephritis with amaurosis and cerebral symptoms. Chronic gout.

**Mind:** *Mental depression. Fear of being assassinated.* Quiet melancholy. Slow perception; loss of memory; amnesic aphasia. Hallucinations and delusions. Intellectual apathy. Memory impaired (*Anac., Bar-c.*). Paretic dementia.

**Head:** Delirium alternating with colic. Pain as if a ball rose from the throat to the brain. Hair very dry. Tinnitus (*Chin., Nat-sal., Carbn- s.*).

**Eyes:** Pupils contracted. Yellow (jaundiced). Optic nerve inflamed. Intraocular, suppurative inflammation. *Glaucoma,* especially if secondary to a spinal lesion. Optic neuritis, central scotoma. Sudden loss of sight after fainting (amaurosis).

**Face:** *Pale and cachetic.* Yellow, corpse-like; cheeks sunken. Skin of face greasy, shiny. Tremors of naso-labial muscles (epilepsy).

**Mouth:** Gums swollen, pale; *distinct blue lines along margines of gums.* Tongue tremulous, red on the margin. Cannot put it out, seems paralyzed.

**Stomach:** Contraction in esophagus and stomach; pressure and tightness. *Gastralgia.* Constant vomiting. Solids cannot be swallowed.

**Abdomen:** Excessive colic, *radiating to all parts of the body. Abdominal wall feels drawn by a string to the spine.* Pain causes a desire to stretch. Intussusception; strangulated hernia. *Abdomen retracted.* Obstructed flatus, with intense colic. Colic alternates with delirium and pain in atrophied limbs.

**Rectum:** Constipation; *stools hard, lumpy, black, with urging and spasms in the anus.* Obstructed evacuation from impaction of feces (*Plat.*). Neuralgia of the rectum (proctalgia). *Anus drawn up with constriction.*

**Urinary:** Frequent, ineffectual tenesmus. Albuminous; low specific gravity. *Chronic interstitial nephritis,* with severe pain in the abdomen. Urine scanty. Tenesmus of the bladder. Emission drop by drop.

**Male:** *Loss of sexual power.* Testicles drawn up, feel constricted.

**Female:** *Vaginismus,* with emaciation and constipation. *Induration of mammary glands.* Vulva and vagina hypersensitive. Stitches and burning pain in the breasts (*Apis, Con., Carb-an., Sil.*). Tendency to abortion. Menorrhagia with sensation of a string pulling from the abdomen to the back. Disposition to yawn and stretch.

**Heart:** Cardiac weakness. Pulse soft and small, dichrotic. Wiry pulse, cramp-like constriction in peripheral arteries.

**Back:** Spinal cord sclerosed. Lightening-like pains; temporarily better by pressure. Paralysis of lower extremities (paraplegia).

**Extremities:** Paralysis of single muscles. Cannot raise or lift anything with the hand. Extension is difficult. Paralysis from overexertion of the extensor muscles in piano players (*Cur.*). Pain in muscles of thighs; *come in paroxysms* (sciatica). *Wrist drop.* Cramps in calves. Stinging and tearing in limbs, also twitching and tingling, numbness, pain or tremor. Paralysis. Feet swollen. Pain in the atrophied limbs alternates with colic. Loss of patellar reflex. Hands and feet cold. Pain in the *right big toe* at night, very sensitive to touch (gout).

**Skin:** Yellow, dark brown liver spots. Jaundice. Dry. Dilated veins of forearms and legs (varices).

**Modalities:** *Worse,* at night, motion. *Better,* rubbing, hard pressure, physical exertion (*Alumn.*).

**Relationship:** Compare: *Plumbum aceticum* (painful cramps in paralyzed limbs; severe pain and muscular cramps in gastric ulcer; locally, as an application (non-homoeopathic) in moist eczema, and to dry up secretions from mucous surfaces. Care must be used, as sufficient lead can be absorbed to produce lead poisoning, one to two drams of the *liquor plumbi subacetatis* to an ounce of water; also in pruritus pudendi, equal parts of the *liquor plumbi and glycerin). Plumbum iodatum* (has been used empirically in various forms of paralysis, sclerotic degenerations, especially of spinal cord, atrophies, arteriosclerosis, pellagra. *Indurations of mammary glands, especially when a tendency to become inflamed appears; sore and painful.* Indurations of great hardness and associated with a very dry skin. Lancinating pain of *tabes*).

Compare: *Alum., Plat., Op., Podo., Merc., Thal. Plectranthus fruticosus* (paralysis, spastic, spinal form); *Plumbum chromicum* (convulsions, with terrible pain; pupils greatly dilated; retracted abdomen); *Plumbum phosphoricum* (loss of sexual power; *locomotor ataxia*).

Antidotes: *Plat., Alum., Petr.*

**Dose**: Third to thirtieth potency.

---

# PODOPHYLLUM PELTATUM

(May-apple) **Podo.**

Is especially adapted to people with a bilious temperament. It chiefly affects the *duodenum,* small intestines, liver and *rectum.* The *Podo.* disease is gastroenteritis with colicky pain and bilious vomiting. Stool is watery with jelly like mucus, painless, *profuse.* Gushing and offensive. Problems during pregnancy; pendulous abdomen after confinement; prolapsus uteri; painless cholera morbus. Torpidity of the liver; portal engorgement with a tendency to hemorrhoids, hypogastric pain, fullness of superficial veins, jaundice.

**Mind:** Loquacity and delirium from eating acid fruits. Depression of spirits.

**Head:** Vertigo, with a tendency to fall forward. Headache, dull pressure, worse morning, with a heated face and bitter taste; *alternating with diarrhea.*

*Rolling of head from side to side,* with moaning and vomiting (hydrocephalus). Eyelids half closed. Perspiration on the head during sleep in children.

**Mouth:** Grinding teeth at night; *intense desire to press gums together* (*Phyt.*). Difficult dentition. *Tongue broad, large, moist.* Foul, putrid taste. *Burning sensation on the tongue.*

**Stomach:** Hot, sour belching; nausea and vomiting. Thirst for large quantities of cold water (*Bry.*). Vomiting of hot, frothy mucus. Heartburn; gagging or empty retching. Vomiting of milk.

**Abdomen:** Distended; heat and emptiness. *Sensation of weakness or sinking.* Can lie comfortably only on the stomach. Liver region painful, *better rubbing the part.* Rumbling and shifting of flatus in ascending colon.

**Stool:** Cholera infantum and morbus. Long standing; *early in the morning; during dentition, with hot, glowing cheeks* while being bathed or washed; in hot weather after acid fruits. Morning, painless diarrhea which is not due to venous stasis or intestinal ulceration. Green, watery, *fetid, profuse,* gushing. *Prolapse of rectum* before or with stool. Constipation; clay colored, hard, dry, difficult. Constipation alternating with diarrhea (*Ant-c.*). Internal and external piles.

**Female:** Pain in the uterus, and *right ovary, with shifting noises along the ascending colon.* Suppressed menses with pelvic tenesmus. *Prolapsed uteri,* especially after parturition. Hemorrhoids with prolapsus ani during pregnancy. Prolapse from overlifting or straining; during pregnancy.

**Extremities:** Pain between the shoulders, under the right scapula, in loins and lumbar region. Pain in the right inguinal region; shoots down to the inner thigh and knees. Paralytic weakness on the left side.

**Fever:** Chill at 7 a.m., with pain in hypochondria, knees, ankles and wrists. *Great loquacity* during fever. Profuse sweat.

**Modalities:** *Worse,* early in the morning, in hot weather, during dentition.

**Relationship:** Compare: *Mandragora officinarum*—also called Mandrake (must not be confounded with *Podo.* Great desire for sleep; exaggeration of sounds and enlarged vision. Bowels inactive; stools large, white and hard). *Aloe, Chel., Merc., Nux-v., Sulph. Prunella vulgaris*—Self-heal (colitis).

**Dose:** Tincture to sixth potency. The 200th and 1000th seem to do good work in cholera infantum, when indicated.

---

# POLYGONUM PUNCTATUM (HYDROPIPER)

(Smartweed) **Poly-h.**

Metrorrhagia, also amenorrhea in young girls. *Varicosis;* hemorrhoids and rectal pockets. Burning in the stomach followed by sensation of coldness in the pit of stomach.

**Abdomen:** Griping pain, with great rumbling, nausea and liquid faeces. *Flatulent colic.*

**Rectum:** Interior of anus studded with itching eminences. *Hemorrhoids.* Liquid feces.

**Urinary:** Painful constriction at the neck of the bladder.

**Female**: Aching pain in hips and loins. *Sensation as if the hips were being drawn together.* Sensation of weight and tension in the pelvis. Shooting pain through the breasts. Amenorrhea.

**Skin:** *Superficial ulcers and sores on lower extremities,* especially in females at climacteric.

**Relationship:** Compare: *Card-m.* (ulcers); *Ham., Senec., Polygonum persicaria* (renal colic and calculi; *gangrene); Polygonum sagittatum*—Arrow-leaved tear-thumb (2x for *nephritic colic;* suppurative nephritis; lancinating pains along spine; itching in the hard palate; burning inner side of right foot and ankle. C.M. Boger); *Polyganum aviculare*—Knot grass (in material doses of tincture, found useful in phthisis pulmonalis and intermittent fever, especially in *arteriosclerosis.* Erythema).

**Dose:** Tincture.

---

# POLYPORUS PINICOLA

(Pine Agaric) **Polyp-p.**

Useful in intermittent, remittent and bilious fevers with headache, yellow coated tongue, constant nausea, faintness in the epigastrium and constipation. Similar to its botanical relative, *Polyporus officinalis,* or *Boletus laricis, q.v.* Deep dull, severe pain in shin bones, preventing sleep.

**Fever:** Great lassitude and congestion of head with vertigo. Face hot and flushed, prickling sensation all over; restless at night from pain in wrists and knee; rheumatic pains; profuse perspiration. Headache about 10 a. m. with pain in the back, ankles and legs, increasing till 3 p. m., then gradually decreasing.

---

# POPULUS CANDICANS

(Balm of Gilead) **Pop-c.**

Seems to have a remarkable power over acute colds, especially when accompanied by a deep, hoarse voice, or even aphonia. General insensibility of the surface[1] (worse, back and abdomen); rubbing and pounding borne without pain, and is grateful on account of warmth produced. Finger ends thickened, horny; insensible to pinching and pricking. Instantaneous voice producer (*Coca*).

**Head:** Discusses her symptoms with every one. Hot head with cold extremities. Cold sores on lips (*Nat-m.*). Tongue feels thick and numb. Burning irritation of eyes, nose, mouth, throat, and air passages.

**Respiratory:** *Acute hoarseness.* Throat and nostrils burn. Sits bent forward with dry cough. Pharynx and larynx feel dry, the voice is weak and toneless. Rawness and soreness of the chest and throat. Cough in children caused by naso-pharyngeal catarrh; mucus drops from posterior nares.

**Dose:** Tincture.

---

# POPULUS TREMULOIDES

(American Aspen) **Pop.**

The gastric and urinary symptoms point to its usefulness in dyspepsia and catarrh of the bladder, especially in old people. A good remedy for vesical problems of the bladder after surgery and in pregnancy. Cystitis. Fullness of head and sensation of heat on the surface of the body. *Night sweats. Ague.*

**Stomach:** *Indigestion, with flatulence and acidity.* Nausea and vomiting.

**Urinary:** Severe tenesmus; dysuria scalding. Urine contains mucus and pus (pyuria). Prostate enlarged. Pain behind the pubis, at end of micturition.

**Relationship:** Compare: *Nux-v., Chin., Corn-f., Cann-s., Canth.*

**Dose:** Tincture or *Pop.* trituration 1x.

---

# PRIMULA OBCONICA

(Primrose) **Prim-o.**

The poison of Primrose is fozund in its *glandular hairs,* which break easily and discharge an irritating fluid which is absorbed into the skin.

---

[1] Surface anesthesia with or without numbness (Clarke — Dictionary of Practical Materia Medica).

But the skin symptoms of poisoning appear in sensitive patients even without coming in direct contact with the plant, mere nearness is sufficient, just like Poison ivy. Intermittency of symptoms; worse right side. Pain in the liver and spleen. Deep infiltration and tension of tissues; blisters. *Paralyzed sensation. Weakness.* Pharyngeal soreness alternates with diminished facial irritation.

**Face:** Moist eczema. Papular eruption on the chin. Burns at night. Urticaria-like eruption. Eyelids swollen.

**Extremities:** Eczema on arms, wrists, forearms, hands, papular and excoriated. Rheumatic pain around the shoulder. Palms dry and hot. Cracking over joints and fingers. Eruptions between fingers. Purple blotches on the back of hands, palmar surface stiff. Blisters on fingers.

**Skin:** *Great itching,* worse at night, red and swollen like erysipelas. Tumefied. *Small papules on a raised base.* Skin symptoms accompanied by febrile symptoms.

**Relationship:** Compare: *Rhus-t., Fago.* (antidotal). *Humea elegans,* similar skin symptoms.

---

## PRIMULA VERIS

(Cowship) **Prim-v.**

Cerebral congestion with neuralgia; migraine; rheumatic and gouty pain.

**Head:** Sensation of a band around the head; cannot keep a hat on (*Carb-ac.*). Skin of forehead tense. Fear of falling when standing, violent vertigo, as if everything turned around.

**Ears:** Bugging; better, in open air.

**Urinary:** Urine smells strongly of violets (*Ter.*).

**Respiratory:** Cough with burning and pricking in respiratory tract. Weak voice.

**Extremities:** Right axillary muscles painful. Weight and lassitude in limbs, especially shoulders. Burning in hallow of right hand. Drawing pain in thumb and big toe (gout).

**Relationship:** Compare: *Cycl., Ran-b., Oenothera biennis*— Evening primrose (exhausting, watery diarrhea; cholera infantum; hydrocephalus); *Primula farinosa*—Wild primrose (dermatitis, especially on index finger and thumb).

**Dose:** Third potency.

---

## PROPYLAMINUM—TRIMETHYLAMINUM

(Distilled Herring Brine) **Prop.**

In acute rheumatism, dissipates fever and pain in a day or two. Rheumatic prosopalgia and rheumatic metastasis, especially heart lesions.

**Extremities:** *Pain in wrists and ankles;* worse, slightest motion (*Bry.*). Great restlessness and thirst. Rheumatism, needle held in fingers gets too heavy. *Tingling and numbness of fingers.* Pain in wrist and ankle, unable to stand.

**Relationship:** *Chenopodium vulvaria,* the plant has an odor of decaying fish and contains a large amount of propylamine. Weakness in the lumbar and lower dorsal region.

**Dose:** Ten to fifteen drops, in about six ounces of water; teaspoonful doses every two hours.

---

## PRUNUS SPINOSA

(Black-thorn) **Prun.**

Special action on the urinary organs and head. Very valuable in certain neuralgias, anasarca, especially edema pedum. Ankle and foot feel sprained. *Ciliary neuralgia* (*Spig.*).

**Head:** Pressing asunder pain beneath the skull. *Shooting pain from the right frontal bone through the brain to the occiput* (migraine).

**Eyes:** *Ciliary neuralgia.* Bursting pain in the right eyeball. Shooting pains like lightening through the brain extending to the occiput. *Sudden pain in the right eye, as if it would burst,* better by lachrymation. Irido-choroiditis. Opacity in the vitreous humor. Eyes feel as if they would burst (glaucoma).

**Mouth:** Piercing toothache, as if teeth were pulled out; worse, taking anything warm.

**Abdomen:** Ascites. Cramp-like pain in the bladder region; worse, walking.

**Rectum:** Hard, nodular stool with rectal pain, as if an angular body was pressed inward. Burning in the anus after slimy diarrhea.

**Urinary:** Tenesmus of the bladder. Ineffectual effort to micturate. *Must hurry, impelled to micturate; the urine seems to pass as far as the glans and then returns causing pain in the urethra.* Neuralgic dysuria. *Must press for a long time before urine appears.*

**Chest:** Wheezing when walking. Oppression of the chest; anxious, short respiration. Angina pectoris. Furious beating of heart; worse, slightest motion.

**Skin:** Herpes zoster. *Dropsy.* Itching of finger tips, as if frozen.

**Relationship:** Compare: *Laur., Prunus padus*—Birdcherry (sore throat, pressure behind sternum and sticking pain in the rectum); *Prunus virginiana*—Wild cherry (*heart tonic;* relieves the flagging and distended ventricle; irritable heart; dilatation of the right heart; *cough, worse at night on lying down;* weak digestion, especially in elderly people; chronic bronchitis; increases muscular tone); *Pyrus americana*—Mountain ash (irritation of eyes; constriction around the waist; spasmodic pains in uterus, bladder, heart, sensation of cold water in stomach, coldness extends up the esophagus; neuralgic and gouty pains).

**Dose:** Third to sixth potency.

---

## PSORINUM

(Scabies Vesicle) **Psor.**

The therapeutic field of this remedy is found in the so called psoric manifestations. *Psorinum* is a cold medicine; wants the head kept warm, *wants warm clothing* even in summers. *Extreme sensitiveness to cold. Debility,* independent of any organic disease, especially in weakness after an acute disease. *Lack of reaction,* i.e., phagocytes defective; when well chosen remedies fail to act. Scrofulous patients. Secretions *have a filthy smell.* Profuse sweating. Cardiac weakness. Skin symptoms very prominent. Often gives immunity from catching cold. Easy perspiration when walking. Syphilis, inherited and tertiary. *Offensive discharges.*

**Mind:** Hopeless; despairs of recovery. *Melancholy,* deep and persistent; religious. Suicidal tendency.

**Head:** Wakes up at night with pain, as if from a blow on the head. Chronic headaches; hungry during attacks; with vertigo. Hammering pain; brain feels too large; worse, change of weather. Dull, pressure, pain in the occiput. Humid eruptions on the scalp (crusta lactea); hair matted (plica plonica). Hair dry.

**Eyes:** Agglutinated. Blepharitis. *Chronic ophthalmia, that constantly recurs.* Edges of lids red. Secretion acrid.

**Ears:** Raw, red, *oozing scabs around the ears.* Sore pain behind the ears. Herpes extends from the temples over the ears to the cheeks. *Offensive discharge from eczema around the ears. Intolerable itching.* Chronic otorrhea. *Very fetid pus from ears,* brownish, offensive.

**Nose:** Dry, coryza, with stoppage of nose. Chronic catarrh; dropping from posterior nares. Acne rosacea.

**Face:** Swelling of the upper lip. Pale, delicate. *Humid eruptions on the face.* Sickly.

**Mouth:** Obstinate rhagades at corners. Tongue, gums ulcerated; tough mucus of a foul taste adheres to the soft palate.

**Throat:** Tonsils greatly swollen (tonsillitis); dysphagia, with pain in ears. Profuse, offensive saliva; tough mucus in the throat. Recurring quinsy. *Eradicates tendency to quinsy.* Hawking up of cheesy, pea- like balls with a disgusting smell and taste (*Agar.*).

**Stomach**: Eructations like bad eggs. *Very hungry all the time; must have something to eat in the middle of the night.* Nausea; vomiting of pregnancy. Pain in abdomen after eating.

**Stool:** Mucoid, *bloody, excessively fetid, dark fluid.* Hard, difficult stool, with blood from the rectum and burning piles. *Constipation in infants,* in pale, sickly scrofulous children.

**Female:** *Leucorrhea* fetid, lumpy with severe backache and *debility.* Mammae swollen and painful (mastitis). Pimples oozing an acrid fluid that burns and excoriates the glands.

**Respiratory:** Asthma with dyspnea; worse, sitting up; better, lying down and keeping arms spread wide apart. Dry, hard cough, with great weakness of chest. *Sensation of ulceration under sternum.* Pain in the chest; better, lying down. Cough returns every winter, from suppressed eruption. *Hay fever* returning irregularly every year.

**Extremities:** Weakness of joints, as if they would not hold together. *Eruptions around finger nails.* Fetid foot sweats.

**Sleep:** Sleepless from intolerable itching. Easily startled.

**Fever:** Profuse, offensive perspiration; night sweats.

**Skin:** Dirty, dingy look. Dry, lustreless, rough hair. *Intolerable itching.* Herpetic eruptions, especially on the scalp and in the bends of joints with itching; worse, from warmth of bed. Enlarged glands. Sebaceous glands secrete excessively; oily skin. Indolent ulcers, slow to heal. Eczema behind the ears. Crusty eruptions all over. Urticaria after every exertion. Pustules near finger nails.

**Modalities:** *Worse,* coffee; *Psorinum* patient does not improve while using coffee. *Worse,* changes of weather, in hot sunshine, from cold. *Dread of the least cold air or draft. Better,* heat, warm clothing, even in summer.

**Relationship:** Complementary: *Sulph.*

Compare: *Pediculus capitis*—Head louse (psoric manifestations in children. Eruptions on the dorsum of hand, feet, neck. Prurigo; pellagra. Unusual aptitude for study and work. *Pediculus* transmits typhus and trench fever-Cooties). In lack of reaction compare *Calc.* and *Nat-ars. Bacillus Gaertner* (pessimistic, lack of confidence, subjective, troublesome eye symptoms, fear of heights. Urticaria. Use 30th and 200th-Wheeler).

**Dose:** Two hundredth and higher potencies. Should not be repeated too often. *Psorinum* requires something like 9 days before it manifests its action and even a single dose may elicit other symptoms lasting for weeks (Aegedi).

---

## PTELEA TRIFOLIATA

(Wafer-ash) **Ptel.**

Is a remarkable remedy in stomach and liver affections. The aching and heaviness in the region of the liver is *greatly aggravated by lying* on the left side. *Atonic states of stomach.* Asthma.

**Head:** Feels dull and stupid. *Pain from the forehead to the root of the nose; pain pressing outwards. Frontal headache;* worse, noise, motion, night, rubbing eyes, with acidity. Temples as if pressed together.

**Mouth:** *Excess of saliva* with a dry *bitter taste.* Tongue coated white or yellow; feels rough, swollen (glossitis). Papillae *red, prominent* (*Arg-n.*). Coating may be brownish-yellow.

**Stomach:** Weight and fullness. Griping in the epigastric region with dryness of the mouth. Eructations, nausea, vomiting. Constant sensation of corrosion, heat and burning in the stomach (dyspepsia). Stomach feels empty after eating. *Stomach and liver symptoms associated with pain in the limbs.*

**Abdomen:** Weight and pain on the right side; heavy, aching feeling, relieved by lying on the right side. Liver sore, swollen, sensitive to pressure (hepatomegaly; jaundice). Retraction of the abdomen.

**Respiratory:** Sensation of pressure on the lungs and of suffocation, when lying on the back. *Asthma;* dyspnea; Cramp-like pains in the cardiac region.

**Sleep:** Restless, with frightful dreams; nightmares, wakes up languid and unrefreshed.

**Modalities:** *Worse,* lying on the left side; early morning. *Better,* eating sour things.

**Relationship:** Compare: *Merc., Mag-m., Nux-v., Chel.*

**Dose:** First to thirtieth potency.

---

## PULEX IRRITANS

(Common Flea) **Pul.**

Marked urinary and female symptoms.

**Head:** Very impatient, cross and irritable. Frontal headache with *sensation as if the eyes were enlarged. Face wrinkled and old looking.*

**Mouth:** Metallic taste. Sensation of a thread in the throat. Thirsty, especially during headache.

**Stomach:** Foul breath and taste. Intense nausea with vomiting, purging and faintness.

**Abdomen:** Abdomen bloated. Stool very offensive.

**Urinary:** Scanty with frequent urging, pressure on the bladder and burning in the urethra (urethritis). Flow stops suddenly followed by pain. Urine foul. Cannot retain urine; must attend to the call without delay (cystitis). Irritable bladder before menses.

**Female:** Menses delayed. Increased flow of saliva during menses. Intense burning in the vagina. Leucorrhea, profuse, foul, greenish yellow in color; stains of menses and leucorrhea very hard to wash out. Backache (*Ox-ac.*).

**Back:** Aches, weak; drawing of muscles below the scapulae.

**Fever:** Sensation of a glow all over the body, like being over steam; *chilly,* while sitting besides the fire.

**Skin:** Prickly itching. Sore spots all over. Skin emits a foul odor.

**Modalities:** *Better,* sitting or lying down. *Worse,* left side; moving about.

**Dose:** The higher potencies.

---

## PULSATILLA PRATENSIS

(Wind Flower) **Puls.**

The weather cock among remedies.

The disposition and mental state are the chief guiding symptoms to the selection of *Puls.* It is pre-eminently a female remedy, especially for a mild, gentle, yielding disposition. Sad, cries readily; weeps when talking; *changeable,* contradictory. *The patient seeks open air; always feels better there,* even though she is chilly. All mucous membranes are affected. *Discharges are thick, bland and yellowish-green.* Often indicated after abuse of iron tonics and after a case of badly managed measles. *Symptoms always changing. Thirstless, peevish and chilly.* When the first serious impairment of health is referred to the age of puberty. Great sensitiveness. Wants to hold the head high. Feels uncomfortable with only one pillow. Lies with hands above the head.

**Mind:** Weeps easily. Timid, irresolute. Fears in the evening of being alone, ghosts. Likes sympathy. Children like fuss and caresses. Easily discouraged. Morbid dread of the opposite sex. Religious melancholy. Given to extremes of pleasure and pain. Highly emotional. Mentally, like an April day.

**Head:** Wandering stitches around the head; pain extends to the face and teeth; vertigo; better in open air. Frontal and supra-orbital pain. Neuralgic pain, commencing in the *right temporal* region (migraine), *with scalding lachrymation from the affected side. Headache from overwork.* Pressure on the vertex.

**Eyes:** *Thick, profuse, yellow, bland discharges.* Itching and burning in eyes. Profuse lachrymation and secretion of mucus. *Lids inflamed, agglutinated* (blepharitis). *Styes.* Veins of fundus oculi greatly enlarged. Ophthalmia neonatorum. Subacute conjunctivitis, with dyspepsia; worse, in a warm room.

**Ears:** Sensation as if something was being forced outward. Hearing difficult, as if the ear were stuffed. Otorrhea. Thick, bland discharge; offensive odor. External ear swollen and red. Catarrhal otitis. Otalgia, worse at night. Diminished acuteness of hearing.

**Nose:** Coryza; stoppage of the right nostril, pressing pain at the root of nose. Anosmia. Large green fetid scales in the nose. Stoppage in the evening. Yellow mucus; abundant in the morning. Bad smells, as of old catarrh. Nasal bones sore.

**Face:** Right sided neuralgia with profuse lachrymation. Swelling of the lower lip, which is cracked in the middle. Prosopalgia towards evening till midnight; chilly, with pain.

**Mouth:** Greasy taste. *Dry mouth, without thirst;* wants it washed frequently. Frequently licks the lips dry. *Crack in the middle of the lower lip. Yellow or white coated tongue, covered with tenacious mucus.* Toothache; relieved by holding cold water in the mouth (*Coff.*). Halitosis (*Merc., Aur.*). Food, especially bread, tastes bitter. Profuse, *sweet* saliva. *Alterations in taste,* bitter, bilious, greasy, salty, *foul.* Loss of taste. Desire for tonics.

**Stomach:** *Aversion to fatty food, warm food and drink.* Eructations; *taste of food remains a long time;* after ices, fruits, pastry. *Bitter taste,* diminished taste of all food. Pain as if from subcutaneous ulceration. *Flatulence.* Dislikes butter (*Sang.*). Heartburn. Dyspepsia with great tightness after a meal; must loosen clothing. *Thirstlessness* with nearly all complaints. Vomiting of food eaten long before. Pain in the stomach an hour after eating (*Nux-v.*). Weight as if from a stone, especially in the morning on waking up. Gnawing, hungry feeling (*Abies-c.*). Perceptible pulsations in the pit of the stomach (*Asaf.*). All gone sensation, especially in tea drinkers. Waterbrash, with a foul taste in the morning.

**Abdomen:** Painful, distended; loud rumbling. Pressure, as if from a stone. Colic, with chilliness in the evening.

**Rectum:** Rumbling, watery; worse, night. *No two stools alike.* After fruit (*Ars., Chin.*). Blind hemorrhoids with itching and sticking pains. Dysentery; mucus and blood, with chilliness (*Merc., Rheum*). *Two or three normal stools daily.*

**Urinary:** Increased desire; *worse when lying down.* Burning in the urethral orifice, during and after micturition. Involuntary micturition at night, while coughing or passing flatus. After micturating, spasmodic pain in the bladder.

**Male:** Orchitis; pain from the abdomen to the testicles. Thick, yellow discharge from the urethra; late stage of gonorrhea. Stricture; urine is passed only in drops, stream is interrupted (*Clem.*). *Acute prostatitis.* Pain and tenesmus during micturition, *worse lying on the back.*

**Female:** Amenorrhea (*Cimic., Senec., Polyg.*). Suppressed menses from wet feet, nervous debility, or chlorosis. Tardy menses. Too late, scanty, thick, dark, *clotted, changeable, intermittent.* Chilliness, nausea with a downward pressure and pain. Flow intermits. Leucorrhea acrid, burning, creamy. Pain in the back; tired feeling. Diarrhea during or after menses.

**Respiratory:** Capricious hoarseness; comes and goes. *Dry cough in the evening and at night; must sit up in bed to get relief; loose cough in the morning,* with copious mucoid expectoration. *Pressure on the chest with soreness.* Great soreness in the epigastrium. Urine emitted with cough (*Caust.*). Pain as if from an ulcer in the middle of the chest. Expectoration bland, thick, bitter, greenish. Short breath, anxiety and palpitations when lying on the left side (*Phos.*). Smothering sensation on lying down (asthma).

**Back:** Shooting pain in the nape and back, between the shoulders; in the sacrum after sitting.

**Extremities:** Drawing, tensive pain in thighs and legs, with restlessness, sleeplessness and *chilliness. Pain in limbs, shifting rapidly;* tensive pain, *letting up with a snap.* Numbness around the elbow. Hip joint painful. Knees swollen, with tearing, drawing pains (osteoarthritis). Boring pain in the heels towards the evening; *suffering worse from letting the affected limb hang down* (*Vip.*). Veins of forearms and hands swollen. Feet red, inflamed, swollen (varices). Legs feel heavy and weary.

**Sleep**: *Wide awake in the evening;* first sleep restless. Wakes up languid, unrefreshed. Irresistible sleepiness in afternoon. Sleeps with hands over the head.

**Fever:** *Chilliness,* even in a warm room, *without thirst.* Chilly with pain, in spots, worse evening. Chills around 4 p.m. Intolerable burning heat at night, with distended veins; heat in parts of the body, coldness in other parts. One sided sweat; pain during sweat. *External heat is intolerable, veins are distended* (varices). During apyrexia, headache, diarrhea, loss of appetite, nausea.

**Skin:** Urticaria, after rich food, with diarrhea, from delayed menses, worse undressing. *Measles.* Acne at puberty. Varicose veins.

**Modalities:** *Worse,* from heat, rich fatty food, after eating, towards the evening, in a warm room, lying on the left or on the painless side, when allowing feet to hang down. *Better,* open air, motion, cold applications, cold food and drinks, though not thirsty.

**Relationship:** *Pent.* often indicated after *Puls.* in later colds. *Janosia asoca—Saraca indica (amenorrhea,* menorrhagia, acts powerfully on the female organs. Abdominal pain). *Atriplex hortensis* (uterine symptoms, amenorrhea; hysteria, coldness between shoulders, dislike for warm food, craves strange foods, palpitations, sleeplessness). *Pulsatilla nuttaliana,* identical effects.

Compare: *Cycl., Kali-bi., Kali-s., Sulph. Pimenta officinalis*—Allspice (one sided neuralgias, parts of body hot and cold).

*Anagyris foetida* (headache, amenorrhea).

Antidotes: *Coff., Cham., Nux-v.*

**Dose:** Third to thirtieth attenuation.

---

# PYROGENIUM

(Artificial Sepsin) **Pyrog.**

This remedy was introduced by English homeopaths, prepared from decomposed lean beef allowed to stand in the sun for two weeks and then potentized. The provings and most of the clinical experience has been obtained from this preparation. But subsequently, Dr. Swan potentized some septic pus, which has also been proved and clinically applied. There does not seem to be any marked difference in their effects.

*Pyrog.* is a great remedy for *septic states,* with intense restlessness. "In septic fevers, especially puerperal, *Pyrogenium* has demonstrated its great value as a homeopathic dynamic antiseptic" (H. C. Allen). Hectic, typhoid, typhus, ptomaine poisoning, diphtheria, dissecting wounds, sewer gas poisoning, chronic malaria, after effects of miscarriage, all these conditions, at times may present symptoms calling for this unique medicine. *All discharges are horribly offensive—menstrual,* lochial, diarrhea, vomit, sweat, breath, etc. Great pain and violent burning in abscesses. Chronic complaints that date back to septic conditions. Threatening heart failure in zymotic and septic fevers. Influenza, typhoid symptoms.

**Mind:** Full of anxiety and insane notions. Loquacious. Thinks he is very wealthy. *Restless.* Feels as if crowded with arms and legs. Cannot tell whether dreaming while awake or asleep.

**Head:** Painless throbbing. Fan-like motion of alae nasi (*Lyc., Phos.*). Bursting headache with restlessness.

**Mouth:** Tongue red and *dry,* clean, cracked, smooth, as though varnished (glossitis). Throat dry, articulation difficult. Nausea and vomiting. Taste terribly fetid. Breath horrible.

**Stomach:** Coffee grounds vomiting (hematemesis). Vomits water, when it becomes warm in stomach.

**Abdomen:** Intolerable tenesmus of both bladder and rectum. Bloated, sore, cutting pain (peritonitis).

**Stool:** Diarrhea; horribly offensive, brown-black, painless, involuntary. Constipation with complete inertia (*Op.*); obstinate from of impaction. Stools large, black, carrion-like, or small black balls.

**Female:** Puerperal peritonitis, with extreme fetor. Septicemia following abortion. Menses horribly offensive. Uterine hemorrhages. Fever at each menstrual period, consequent upon latent pelvic inflammation. *Septic puerperal infection.* Pelvic inflammatory disease. Inflammatory exudate. Post-operative cases, with overwhelming sepsis.

**Heart:** Tired feeling around the heart. *Palpitations.* Sensation as if the heart was too full. Can always hear her heart beat. Pulse abnormally rapid, *out of proportion to the temperature.* Pain in the region of left nipple. Conscious of the heart.

**Extremities:** Throbbing in the vessels of the neck. Numbness of hands, arms, feet. Aching in all limbs and bones. *Bed feels too hard* (*Arn.*). Great debility in the morning. Soreness; better by motion (*Rhus-t.*). Rapid decubitus of a septic origin.

**Sleep:** Seems to be in semi-sleep. Dreams all night.

**Fever:** Coldness and chilliness. *Septic fevers.* Latent pyogenic condition. Chills begin in the back. Temperature rises rapidly. Great heat with profuse, hot sweat, but *sweating does not cause a fall in temperature.*

**Skin:** A small cut or injury becomes very swollen and inflamed, discolored. Dry.

**Modalities**: Relief from motion.

**Relationship:** Compare: *Streptococcinum* (anti-febrile action; septic symptoms in infectious diseases. Rapid in its action, especially in its effect on temperature); *Staphylococcinum* in diseases where staphylococcus is the chief bacterial factor, as acne, abscess, furuncle; empyema, endocarditis, etc.); *Sepsinum* a toxin of Proteus vulgaris, prepared by Dr. Shedd, same symptoms as *Pyrog.* of which it is the main constituent; *Echi., Carb-v., Ars., Lach., Rhus-t., Bapt.*

Complementary: *Bry.*

**Dose:** Sixth to thirtieth and higher potencies. Should not be repeated too frequently.

## QUASSIA AMARA—PICRAENA EXCELSA

(Quassia Wood) **Quas.**

Acts on the gastric organs as a tonic (*Gent-l., Hydr.*). Seems to possess a marked action on the eyes, producing amblyopia and cataract. Pain in the right intercostal muscles above the liver. Pressure and stitches in the liver, vagina and sympathetically in the splenic region.

**Stomach:** Atonic dyspepsia, with gas and acidity. Heartburn and gastralgia. Regurgitation of food. Abdomen feels empty and retracted. Dyspepsia after infectious diseases; especially influenza, dysentery. Tongue dry or with a brown sticky coating. Cirrhosis of the liver with ascites.

**Urinary:** Excessive desire, impossible to retain urine; copious micturition day and night. As soon as the child wakes up the bed is drenched.

**Extremities:** Inclination to yawn and stretch (*Rhus-t.*). Sensation of coldness over the back. Prostration, with hunger. Cold extremities, with sensation of internal coldness (*Helo.*).

**Dose:** First to third potency, or spoonful doses of Aqua Quassiae.

---

## QUERCUS GLANDIUM SPIRITUS

(Spirit Distilled from Tincture of Acorn Kernels) **Querc.**

First used by Rademacher for chronic spleen affections; *splenic dropsy.* Antidotes effects of alcohol. Vertigo; deafness, with noises in the head. *Takes away the craving for alcohol;* give dose as low, for several months. Dropsy and liver affections. Useful in gout, old malarial cases with flatulence.

**Relationship:** Compare: *Angelica atropurpurea* (in tincture, five drops, three times daily, produces disgust for liquor; also for atony of different organs, dyspepsia, nervous headache, etc., chronic bronchitis to increase expectoration). *Cean., Lach., Nat-m., Helianthus annuus* (spleen enlarged and painful).

**Dose:** Ten drops to a teaspoonful of the distilled spirit, three to four times a day. A passing diarrhea often appears for a time when using it. Curative effect. *Querc.* acts well in trituration of the acorn 3x in splenic cases, flatulence, old malaria and alcoholic history (Clarke).

---

## QUILLAYA SAPONARIA

(Chile Soap Bark) **Quill.**

Produces and cures symptoms of acute catarrh, sneezing and sore throat. *Most effective in the beginning of coryza,* frequently checking its further development. Colds with a sore throat; heat and dryness of the throat. Cough with difficult expectoration. Squamous skin.

**Relationship:** Compare: *Kali-i., Gels., All-c., Squil. Saponaria officinalis* (sore throat, involuntary micturition). *Seneg.*

**Dose:** Tincture and first potency.

## RADIUM BROMATUM

(Radium Bromide) **Rad-br.**

An important addition to the materia medica, especially since the provings by Diffenbach have precisionized its use. *Rad-br.* of 1,800,000 radioactivity was employed. It is found effective in the treatment of rheumatism and gout, in skin affections generally, acne rosacea, nevi, moles, ulcers and cancers. Lowered blood pressure. *Severe aching pains all over,* with restlessness, better moving about. Chronic rheumatic arthritis. Delay in the appearance of symptoms. Ulcers due to Radium burns, take a long time to heal. Marked increase in the polymorphonuclear neutrophils. Great weakness.

**Mind:** Apprehensive, depressed; fear of being alone in the dark; great desire to be with people. Tired and irritable.

**Head:** Vertigo, with pain in the back of the head, left sided pain when in bed. Pain in occiput and vertex, accompanying severe lumbar ache. Severe pain over the right eye, spreading backwards to the occiput and vertex, better in open air. Head feels heavy. Frontal headache. Both eyes ache. Itching and dryness in the nasal cavities, better in the open air. Aching pain in the angle of right lower jaw. Violent trigeminal neuralgia.

**Mouth:** Dryness of the mouth. Metallic taste. Prickling sensation on the tip of the tongue.

**Stomach:** Empty feeling in the stomach. Warm sensation in the stomach. Aversion to sweets, ice-cream. Nausea and sinking sensation, belching of gas.

**Abdomen:** Pain, violent cramps, rumbling, full of gas; pain over McBurney's point (appendicitis) and at the location of sigmoid flexure. Marked flatulence. Alternating constipation and diarrhea. Pruritus ani and piles.

**Urinary:** Increased elimination of solids, particularly of chlorides. Renal irritation, albuminuria, granular and hyaline casts. Nephritis with rheumatic symptoms. Enuresis.

**Female:** Pruritus vulvae. Delayed and irregular menstruation and backache. Aching pains in the abdomen, over pubes when flow comes on (dysmenorrhea). Right breast sore, relieved by hard rubbing.

**Respiratory:** Persistent cough with tickling in the suprasternal fossa (bronchitis). Dry, spasmodic cough. Throat dry, sore, chest constricted.

**Back:** Aching in the back of neck. Pain and lameness of the cervical vertebrae, worse dropping head forward, better standing, or sitting erect (cervical spondylosis). *Lumbar and sacral* backache, pain appears to be in the *bone,* continuous motion relieves. Backache between shoulders and lumbosacral region, better after walking.

**Extremities:** Severe pain in all the limbs, *joints,* especially in the knee and ankle joints, sharp pain in the shoulders, arms, hands and fingers. Legs, arms and neck feel hard and brittle, as though they would break on moving. Arms feel heavy. Cracking in shoulder. *Pain in toes,* calves, hip joint, popliteal spaces. Muscles of legs and hips sore. *Arthritis,* aching pains, *worse* at night. Dermatitis of the fingers. Trophic changes in the finger nails.

**Sleep:** Restless. Sleepiness with lethargy. Dreams vivid, busy. Dreams of fire.

**Fever:** Cold sensation internally, with chattering of teeth until noon. Internal chilliness followed by heat of the skin, associated with bowel movements and flatulence.

**Skin:** Small pimples. Erythema and dermatitis, with itching, burning, swelling and redness. Necrosis and ulceration. *Itching all over the body,* burning of skin, as on fire. Epithelioma.

**Modalities:** *Better,* open air, continuous motion, hot bath, lying down, pressure. *Worse,* getting up.

**Relationship:** Compare: *Anac.* (the ulceration produced by it is like *Rad-br.* It may appear elsewhere other than on the place of contact; appears late).

Compare: *X-Ray; Rhus-t., Sep., Uran-n., Ars., Puls., Caust.*

Antidotes: *Rhus-v., Tell.*

**Dose:** Thirtieth and twelfth trituration.

---

# RANUNCULUS BULBOSUS

(Buttercup) **Ran-b.**

Acts especially upon the muscular tissue and skin. Its most characteristic effects are upon the chest walls, like pleurodynia. *Bad effects of alcohol; delirium tremens.* Spasmodic hiccough. Hydrothorax. Shocks throughout the body. Sensitive to air and touch. Chronic sciatica.

**Head:** Irritable, pain in the forehead and eye balls. Creeping sensation in the scalp. Pressing pain in the forehead from within outward.

**Eyes:** Day blindness (hemeralopia); mist before the eyes; pressure (glaucoma) and smarting in eyes, as if from smoke. Pain over the right eye; better, standing and walking. Herpes on the cornea. Vesicles on the cornea with intense pain, photophobia and lachrymation.

**Chest:** Various kinds of pains and *soreness, as if the sternum,* ribs, intercostal spaces and both the hypochondria *are bruised. Intercostal rheumatism. Chilliness in the chest when walking in open air.* Stitches in the chest, between shoulder blades; worse, inspiring, moving (pleuritic adhisions). Rheumatic pain in the chest, as if from subcutaneous ulceration. *Tenderness of the abdomen on pressure. Muscular pain along the lower margin of shoulder blade;* burning in small spots from sedentary employment.

**Skin:** *Burning and intense itching* (chilblains)*; worse, contact.* Hard excrescences. *Herpetic eruptions,* with great itching. *Shingles; bluish vesicles.* Itching in palms. Blister-like eruptions on the palms. Corns, sensitive. Horny skin. Finger tips and palms chapped. Vesicular and pustular eruptions.

**Modalities:** *Worse,* open air, motion, contact, atmospheric changes, wet, stormy weather, evening. Cold air brings on all sorts of ailments.

**Relationship:** Incompatible: *Sulph., Staph.*

Compare: *Ranunculus acris* (pain in the lumbar muscles and joints on bending and turning the body); *Ranunculus glacialis*—Reindeer flower Carlina (pulmonary affections; broncho-pneumonical influenza, enormous weight on the head with vertigo and sensation of impending apoplexy; night sweats, more on thighs); *Ranunculus repens* (crawling sensation in the forehead and scalp, in the evening in bed); *Ranunculus flammula* (ulceration; gangrene of arm). Compare, also: *Bry., Crot-t., Mez., Euph.*

Antidotes: *Bry., Camph., Rhus-t.*

**Dose:** Mother tincture, in ten to thirty drop doses in delirium tremens; third to thirtieth potency generally. Chronic sciatica, apply tincture to the heel of the affected leg (M. Jousset).

---

## RANUNCULUS SCELERATUS

(Marsh Buttercup) **Ran-s.**

Is more irritating than others of this botanical family, as seen in the skin symptoms. *Boring, gnawing pain* very marked. *Pemphigus.* Periodical complaints. Fainting with pain in the stomach.

**Head:** Gnawing in one spot, left of the vertex. Frightful dreams about corpses, serpents, battles, etc.

**Nose:** Fluent coryza, with sneezing and burning micturition.

**Mouth:** Teeth and gums sensitive. *Tongue mapped.* Denuded patches. Mouth sore and raw (stomatitis). *Burning and rawness of tongue* (glossitis).

**Abdomen:** Sensation of a plug behind the umbilicus. *Pain over the region of liver, with sensation as if diarrhea would set in.* Pressure as if a plug behind the right false ribs; worse, deep inspiration.

**Chest:** Integument sensitive. Bruised pain and weakness in the chest every evening. *Sore burning behind the xiphoid cartilage.*

**Extremities:** *Boring pain.* Sudden burning, sticking pain *in the right toe.* Corns, with burning and soreness, especially when feet hang down. Gout in fingers and toes.

**Skin:** *Vesicular eruption, with a tendency to form large blisters. Acrid exudation, which makes the surrounding parts sore.*

**Dose:** First to third potency.

---

## RAPHANUS SATIVUS

(Black Garden Radish) **Raph.**

Produces pain and stitches in the liver and spleen. Increases bile and salivary secretions. Symptoms will not appear if salt is used with the radish. Great accumulation and incarceration of flatulence. "Globus" symptoms. Seborrhea, with a greasy skin. Pemphigus. Hysteria; chilliness in the back and arms. Sexual insomnia (*Kali-br.*). Nymphomania. *Post-operative gas pains.*

**Head:** Sadness, aversion to children, especially girls. Headache, brain feels tender and sore.

**Eyes:** Edema of lower eyelids.

**Nose:** Mucus in posterior nares.

**Throat:** Sensation as if a hot ball (globus) rising from the uterus to the throat and the stopping there. Heat and burning in the throat.

**Stomach:** Putrid eructations. Burning in the epigastrium, followed by hot eructation.

**Abdomen:** Retching and vomiting, loss of appetite. Distended, *tympanitic, hard. No flatus emitted upward or downwards.* Griping around the navel. Stool liquidy, frothy, profuse, brown, with colic, and a pad-like swelling of intestines. Vomiting of fecal matter.

**Urinary:** Turbid with yeast-like sediment. Urine more copious, thick like milk.

**Female:** Nervous irritation of genitals. Menses very profuse and long lasting (menorrhagia). *Nymphomania,* with an aversion to her own sex and to children; sexual insomnia.

**Chest:** Pain in the chest extends to the back and throat. Sensation of a heavy lump and coldness in the center of the chest.

**Relationship:** Compare: *Momordica balsamina* (worse, near splenic flexure); *Carb-v., Anac., Arg-n., Brassica napus oleifera.*

**Dose:** Third to thirtieth potency.

---

## RATANHIA PERUVIANA

(Krameria, Mapato) **Rat.**

The rectal symptoms are most important, and have received much clinical confirmation. It has cured pterygium. *Violent hiccough.* Cracked nipples (*Graph., Eup-a.*). *Pin worms.*

**Head:** Bursting in the head after stool, and when sitting with head bent forward. Sensation as if the scalp from the nose to vertex was stretched.

**Stomach:** Pain like knives cutting the stomach.

**Rectum**: Aches, as if full of broken glass. Anus aches and burns for hours after stool. Feels constricted. Dry heat in the anus with sudden knife like stitches. Stools must be forced with a great effort; protrusion of hemorrhoids. *Fissures of the anus, with great constriction, burning like fire,* like hemorrhoids, temporarily relieved by cold water. Fetid, thin diarrhea; stools burn; burning pains before and after stools. Oozing from the anus. *Pin worms* (*Santin., Teucr., Spig.*). Itching in the anus.

**Relationship:** Compare; *Paeon., Crot-t.* (rectal neuralgia); *Sang-n.* (diseases of rectum); *Mucuna pruriens—Dolichos pruriens* (*piles, with* burning; hemorrhoidal diathesis); *Silico-sulphocalcite of Alumina; Slag*—blast iron furnace cindre (anal itching, piles, and constipation; housemaid's knee; abdominal flatulent distention and lumbago). Analogue to *Lyc.*

**Dose:** Third to sixth potency. Locally, the cerate has proved invaluable in many rectal complaints.

---

## RHAMNUS CALIFORNICA

(California Coffee Tree) **Rham-cal.**

One of the most positive remedies for rheumatism and *muscular pains.* Pleurodynia, lumbago, gastralgia. Cystitis; *dysmenorrhea* of myalgic origin; pain in the head, neck and face. *Inflammatory rheumatism,* joints swollen, painful; tendency to metastasis; profuse sweat. Rheumatic heart (Webster).

Provings of students. 2x potency.

**Mind:** Nervous, restless, irritable. Lassitude; mentally dull and dazed; unable to concentrate on studies.

**Head:** *Dizzy* full feeling. Heavy bruised sensation; better, from pressure. *Bursting* sensation with every step. Soreness, especially in the occiput and vertex, worse, bending over. Dull pain in the left temple. Dull aching in the frontal region (left), extending backwards and over the forehead. Deep, right sided frontal headache. Twitching eyelids.

**Ears:** *Dullness of hearing.* Soreness, deep, under the right tragus on swallowing.

**Face:** Flushed, hot and glowing. Outward pressure from malar processes.

**Mouth:** Canker sore between gums and lips. Tongue coated, with a clean, pink central patch.

**Throat:** Dry, rough. Soreness on the right side and tonsil.

**Rectum:** *Constipation* with flatus. Tenesmus and dry stool. Flatulent diarrhea.

**Urinary:** Increased micturition. Tickling in the anterior part of urethra, small morning drop (no previous gonorrhea). Sexual desire increased.

**Respiratory:** Substernal oppression. Tenderness on pressure over the right intercostal muscles.

**Heart:** Variation of pulse. Slow pulse.

**Extremities:** Unable to control the muscular action. Legs sore. Walks like a drunken man.

**Modalities:** Symptoms worse in the evening.

**Relationship:** *Rhamnus cathartica* or *Rhamnus frangula*—European buckthorn, a rheumatic remedy (abdominal symptoms, colic, diarrhea; hemorrhoids, especially chronic). *Rhamnus purshiana—Cascara sagrada* (palliative in constipation, as an intestinal tonic, and dyspepsia dependent thereon. 10-15 drops of tincture).

**Dose:** Tincture in 15 drop doses every four hours.

---

## RHEUM PALMATUM

(Rhubarb) **Rheum**

Of frequent use in children with sour diarrhea; difficult dentition. *The child smells sour.*

**Mind:** Impatient and vehement; desires many things and cries (*Cina*).

**Head:** Sweat on the hairy scalp; constant and profuse. *Cool sweat on the face, especially around the mouth and nose.*

**Mouth:** Profuse saliva. Sensation of coolness in the teeth. Difficult dentition; restless and irritable. Breath smells sour (*Cham.*).

**Stomach:** Desire for various kinds of food, but soon gets tired of all. Throbbing in the pit. Feels full.

**Abdomen:** Colicky pain around the navel. Colic when uncovering. Wind seems to rise up to the chest.

**Rectum:** Before stool, unsuccessful urging to micturate. *Stools smell sour,* pasty, with shivering, tenesmus, and burning in the anus. Sour diarrhea during dentition. Colicky, even ineffectual urging to evacuate altered fecal stools.

**Modalities:** *Worse,* uncovering, after eating, moving about.

**Relationship:** Compare: *Mag-p., Hep., Podo., Cham., Ip.*

Antidotes: *Camph., Cham.*

Complementary: *Mag-c.*

**Dose**: Third to sixth potency.

---

## RHODIUM METALLICUM

(Metal, Chemical, Element) **Rhodi.**

(Proved by MacFarlan in the 200th potency.)

Nervous and tearful. Frontal headache; shocks through the head. Fleeting neuralgic pains in the head, over the eyes, in the ear, on both sides of the nose, teeth. Loose cold in the head. Lips dry. Nausea especially from sweets. Dull headache. Stiff neck and rheumatic pains down the left shoulder and arm. Itching in arms, palms and face. Loose stools with griping pain in the abdomen. Hyperactive peristalsis, tenesmus after stool. Profuse micturition. Cough scratchy, wheezy. Thick, yellow mucus from the chest. Feels week, dizzy with a tired feeling.

---

## RHODODENDRON CHRYSANTHUM

(Snow-rose) **Rhod.**

Rheumatic and gouty symptoms well marked. Rheumatism in the hot season. The modality, worse before a storm is a true guiding symptom.

**Mind:** Dread of a storm; particularly afraid of thunder. Forgetful.

**Head:** Aching in temples. Tearing pain in bones. Headache; worse, wine, wind, cold and wet weather.

**Eyes:** Pain in eyes before a storm. *Ciliary neuralgia,* involving the eyeball, orbit, and head. Sensation of heat in eyes when using them. Muscular asthenopia; darting pains through the eyes from the head, worse before a storm.

**Ears:** Difficulty in hearing, with whizzing and ringing in ears (tinnitus). Hearing better in the morning; noises come on after the patient has been up for a few hours.

**Face:** Prosopalgia; violent jerking pains involving the dental nerves, from the temple to the lower jaw and chin; *better, warmth and eating.* Toothache in damp weather and before a storm. Swollen gums. Stumps of teeth are loosened.

**Male:** Testicles, worse left, swollen, painful, drawn up. Orchitis; glands feel crushed. Induration and swelling of testes after gonorrhea. *Hydrocele* (*Sil.*).

**Chest:** Violent pleuritic pains running downward in the left anterior chest. Breathless and speechless from violent pleuritic pains. Stitches in the spleen from walking fast. Crampy pain under the short ribs.

**Extremities:** Joints swollen. Gouty inflammation of the great toe joint. *Rheumatic tearing in all limbs,* especially right side; worse, at rest and in stormy weather. Stiffness in the neck. Pain in the shoulders, arms, wrists; worse when at rest. Pains in the bones in spots, reappears with change of weather. *Cannot sleep unless legs are crossed.*

**Modalities:** *Worse,* before a storm. *All symptoms reappear in rough weather,* at night, towards the morning. *Better,* after the storm breaks, warmth, and eating.

**Relationship:** Compare: *Ampelopsis* (hydrocele and renal dropsy); *Dulc., Rhus-t., Nat-s.*

**Dose:** First to sixth potency.

---

## RHUS AROMATICA

(Fragrant Sumach) **Rhus-a.**

Renal and urinary affections, especially *diabetes.* Enuresis due to vesical atony; senile incontinence. Hematuria and cystitis come within the range of this remedy.

**Urinary:** *Pale,* albuminous. *Incontinence. Severe pain at the beginning or before micturition,* causing great agony in children. Constant dribbling. *Diabetes,* large quantities of urine with low specific gravity (*Ph-ac., Acet-ac.*).

**Dose:** Tincture, in rather material doses.

---

## RHUS GLABRA

(Smooth Sumach) **Rhus-g.**

Epistaxis and *occipital headache. Fetid flatus.* Ulceration of the mouth. *Dreams of flying through the air* (*Stict.*). *Profuse perspiration arising from debility* (*Chin.*). It is claimed that this remedy will so disinfect the bowels that the flatus and stools will be free from odor. It acts well in putrescent conditions with a tendency to ulceration.

**Mouth:** Scurvy; nursing sore mouth (*Vero-o.*). Aphthous stomatitis.

**Relationship:** Said to be antidotal to the action of mercury and has been employed in the treatment of secondary syphilis after mercurialization.

**Dose:** Tincture. Usually locally to soft, spongy gums, aphthae, pharyngitis, etc. Internally, first potency.

---

# RHUS TOXICODENDRON

(Poison Ivy) **Rhus-t.**

The effects on the skin, mucous membranes, typhoid type of fever and in rheumatic pains make this remedy frequently indicated. *Rhus-t.* affects the fibrous tissue markedly joints, tendons, sheaths, aponeurosis, etc., producing pain and stiffness. Post-operative complications. *Pains tearing asunder.* Motion always "limbers up" the *Rhus-t.* patient, and hence he feels better for a time from a change of position. Ailments from strains, overlifting, getting wet while perspiring. Septic conditions. Cellulitis and infections, carbuncles in the early stages (*Echi.*). Rheumatism in the cold season. *Septicemia.*

**Mind:** Listless, sad. Thoughts of suicide. *Extreme restlessness, with continuous change of position.* Delirium with fear of being poisoned (*Hyos.*). *Sensorium becomes cloudy. Great apprehension at night, cannot remain in bed.*

**Head:** Feels as if a board was strapped on the forehead. Vertigo on rising. *Heavy* head. Brain feels loose, as if struck against the skull when walking or rising. Scalp sensitive; worse on side lain on. Headache in the occiput (*Rhus-r.*); painful to touch. Pain in the forehead, proceeds backwards. Humid eruptions on the scalp; severe itching (crusta lactea).

**Eyes:** Swollen, red, edematous; *orbital cellulitis. Pustular inflammations.* Photophobia; profuse flow of yellow pus. Edema of lids, suppurative iritis. Lids inflamed, agglutinated, swollen. Old injuries of the eyes. Circumscribed corneal injection. Intensive ulceration of the cornea. Iritis, after exposure to cold and dampness, of rheumatic origin. Eye painful on turning or on pressing, can hardly move it, as in acute retro-bulbar neuritis. Profuse gush of hot, scalding tears on opening the lids.

**Ears:** Pain in the ears (otalgia), with sensation as if something was in them. Lobules swollen. Discharge of bloody pus (otorrhea).

**Nose:** *Sneezing*; coryza from getting wet. Tip of nose red, sore, ulcerated. Swelling of the nose. Epistaxis on stooping.

**Face:** *Jaws crack when chewing.* Easy dislocation of the jaw (*Ign., Petr.*). *Swollen face,* erysipelas. Cheek bones sensitive to touch. Parotitis. Facial neuralgia, with chilliness; worse, evening. *Crusta lactea (Calc., Viol-t.).*

**Mouth**: Teeth feel loose and long; gums sore. Tongue red and cracked; *coated, except for a red triangular space at the tip;* dry and red at edges (glossitis). Corners of mouth ulcerated; fever blisters around the mouth and chin (*Nat-m.*). *Pain in the maxillary joint.*

**Throat**: Sore, with *swollen glands.* Sticking pain on swallowing. Parotitis, left side.

**Stomach**: Want of appetite for any kind of food, with an unquenchable thirst. *Bitter taste* (*Cupr.*). Nausea, vertigo and bloated abdomen after eating. *Desire for milk.* Marked thirst, with a dry mouth and throat. Pressure as if from a stone (*Bry., Ars.*). *Drowsy after eating.*

**Abdomen**: Violent pains, relieved by lying on the abdomen. Swelling of the inguinal glands. Pain in the region of ascending colon. Colic, must walk bent forward. Excessive distention after eating. Rumbling of flatus on first rising, but disappears with continuous motion.

**Rectum**: Diarrhea of blood, slime, and reddish mucus. Dysentery, with tearing pains down the thighs. Stools with a cadaverous odor. Frothy, painless stools. Will often abort the beginning of a suppurative process near the rectum.

**Urinary**: Dark, turbid, high colored, *scanty* urine, with a white sediment. Dysuria, with loss of blood (hematuria).

**Male**: Swelling of glands and prepuce (balanitis), dark red erysipelatous; scrotum thick, swollen, *edematous* (hydrocele). *Itching intense.*

**Female**: Swelling, with intense itching of vulva (pruritus vulva). Pelvic articulations stiff when beginning to move. Menses early, profuse, and prolonged, acrid (menorrhagia, metrorrhagia). *Lochia thin, protracted, offensive, diminished* (*Puls., Sec.*), *with shooting pains, extending upwards in the vagina* (*Sep.*).

**Respiratory:** Tickling behind upper sternum. *Dry, teasing cough* from midnight till morning, *during a chill, or when putting hands out of bed. Hemoptysis* from overexertion; blood bright red. Influenza, with aching in all the bones (*Eup-per.*). Hoarseness from overstraining the voice (*Arn.*). Oppression of the chest, cannot get breath with sticking pains (pleurisy). Bronchial cough in old people, worse on waking up with expectoration of small plugs of mucus.

**Heart:** Hypertrophy from overexertion. Pulse quick, weak, irregular, intermittent, with numbness of the left arm. *Trembling and palpitations when sitting still.*

**Back**: Pain between the shoulders on swallowing. *Pain and stiffness in the lumbosacral region; better, motion, or lying on something hard;* worse, while sitting. Stiffness in the nape of neck.

**Extremities:** Hot, painful swelling of joints (osteoarthritis). *Pain tearing in tendons, ligaments and fasciae.* Rheumatic pains spread over a large surface at the nape of neck, loins, and extremities; better motion (*Agar.*). Soreness of the condyles in bones. *Limbs stiff, paralyzed. The cold fresh air is not tolerated; it makes the skin painful.* Pain along the ulnar nerve. Tearing down the thighs. *Sciatica;* worse, cold, damp weather, at night. Numbness and formication, after overwork and exposure. Paralysis; trembling after exertion. Tenderness around knee joint. Loss of power in forearm and fingers; crawling sensation in the tips of fingers. Tingling in feet.

**Sleep:** *Dreams of great exertion.* Heavy sleep, as from stupor. Sleepless before midnight.

**Fever:** Adynamic; restless, trembling. Typhoid; tongue dry and brown; sordes; bowels loose; great restlessness. Intermittent; chills, with a dry cough and restlessness. During heat, urticaria. Hydroa. Chilly, as if cold water was poured over him followed by heat and an inclination to stretch the limbs.

**Skin:** Red, swollen; *itching intense.* Vesicles, herpes; *urticaria;* pemphigus; erysipelas; vesicular suppurative forms. Glands swollen. *Cellulitis.* Burning eczematous eruptions with tendency to scale formation

**Modalities:** *Worse,* during sleep, cold, wet rainy weather and after rain; at night, *during rest,* drenching, when lying on the back or in the right side. *Better,* warmth, dry weather, motion; walking, change of position, rubbing, warm applications, from stretching out limbs.

**Relationship:** Complementary: *Bry., Calc-f., Phyt.* (rheumatism).In urticaria follow with *Bov.*

Inimical: *Apis.*

Antidotes: Bathing with milk and Grindelia lotion very effective. *Ampelopsis trifoliata*—Three-leaf woodbine (toxic dermatitis due to vegetable poisons, 30 and 200. Very similar to Rhus poisoning. Desensitizing against Ivy poisoning by using the ascending doses of the tincture by mouth or by hypodermic injections is recommended by the old school authorities, but is not as effective as the homeopathic remedies especially *Rhus-t.* 30 and 200 and *Anac.,* etc.). *Anac., Crot-t., Grin., Mez., Cypr., Plumbg.* (eczema of vulva); *Graph.*

Compare: *Rhus radicans* (almost identical action; characteristics are, burning in the tongue, tip feels sore, pains are often semilateral and in various parts, often remote and successive. Many symptoms are better after a storm has thoroughly set in, especially after an electric storm. Has pronounced *yearly* aggravation (*Lach.*). *Rhus radicans* has *occipital headache,* and pain in the nape of neck, pains draw the head *forward*). *Rhus diversiloba*—California Poison oak (antidote to *Rhus-t.*, violent skin symptoms, with intense itching; marked swelling of the face, hands and genitals; skin very sensitive; eczema and erysipelas, great nervous weakness, tired from the least effort; goes to sleep from sheer exhaustion); *Xero.* (dysmenorrhea and skin symptoms).

Compare, also: *Arn., Bapt., Lach., Ars., Hyos., Op.* (stupefaction more profound). *Mimosa humilis*—Sensitive plant (rheumatism, knee stiff, lancinating pains in back and limbs. Swelling of ankles. Legs tremble).

**Dose:** Sixth to thirtieth potency. The 200th and higher are antidotal to poisoning with the plant and tincture.

---

## RHUS VENENATA

(Poison Elder) **Rhus-v.**

The skin symptoms of this species of Rhus are very severe.

**Mind:** Great melancholy; no desire to live, gloomy.

**Head:** Heavy, frontal headache; worse, walking or stooping.

**Eyes:** Eyes almost closed with marked swelling of lids.

**Ears:** Inflammation (otitis).

**Nose:** Nose red and shiny. Face swollen.

**Face:** Swollen especially under the right eye.

**Mouth:** Tongue red at the tip. Fissured in the middle. Vesicles on the under surface.

**Abdomen:** Profuse, watery, white stools in the morning, 4 a. m., with colicky pains; expelled with force. Pain in the hypogastrium before every stool.

**Extremities:** Paralytic drawing in the right arm, especially wrist, extending to the fingers. paraplegia.

**Skin:** Itching; relieved by hot water (chilblains). *Vesicles* (herpes). *Erysipelas; skin dark red.* Erythema nodosum, with nocturnal itching and pains in the long bones.

**Relationship:** Antidote: *Clem.* The California Poison oak (*Rhus diversiloba*) is identical to it. It antidotes *Rad-br.* and follows it well.

Compare: *Anac.*

**Dose:** Sixth to thirtieth potency.

---

## RICINUS COMMUNIS—BOFAREIRA

(Castor Oil) **Ric.**

Has a marked action on the gastro-intestinal tract. *Increases the quantity of milk* in nursing women. Vomiting and purging. Languor and weakness.

**Head:** Vertigo, occipital pain, congestive symptoms, buzzing in the ears. Face pale, twitching of mouth.

**Stomach:** Anorexia with great thirst, burning in the stomach, pyrosis, nausea, *profuse vomiting,* pit of stomach sensitive. Mouth dry.

**Abdomen:** Rumbling with contraction of recti muscles, colic, incessant diarrhea with purging (gastroenteritis). Rice water stools with cramps and chilliness (cholera).

**Stool:** Loose, incessant, painless, with painful cramps in muscles of extremities. Anus inflamed. Stools green, slimy, and bloody (dysentery). Fever, emaciation, somnolence.

**Relationship:** Compare: *Resorcinum* (summer complaint with vomiting); destroys organic germs of putrifaction; *Cholas terrapina* (cramps of muscles). *Ars., Verat-a.*

**Dose:** Third potency. Five drops every four hours for increasing the flow of milk; also locally a poultice of the leaves.

---

## ROBINIA PSEUDACACIA

(Yellow Locust) **Rob.**

A remedy for hyperchlorhydria. In cases where albuminoid digestion is too rapid and starch digestion is perverted. Gastric symptoms with the most *pronounced acidity* are well authenticated, and are the guiding symptoms. The acidity of *Rob.* is accompanied by frontal headache. *Intensely acrid eructations.* Acrid and greenish vomiting, colic and flatulence, nocturnal burning pains in stomach and constipation with an urgent desire. *Acidity in children.* Stools and perspiration sour. Incarcerated flatus.

**Head:** Dull, throbbing, frontal pain; worse, motion and reading. Gastric headache with acid vomiting.

**Stomach:** Dull, heavy aching. Nausea; *sour* eructations; profuse vomiting of an *intensely sour* fluid (*Sul-ac.*). Great distension of the stomach and bowels. Flatulent colic (*Cham., Dios.*). Sour stools; child smells sour.

**Female:** Nymphomania. Acrid, fetid leucorrhea. Discharge of blood between menstrual periods (metrorrhagia). Herpes on vagina and vulva.

**Relationship:** *Mag-p., Arg-n., Orexine tannate* (hyperchlorhydria; deficient acid and slow digestion; 14 hourly doses).

**Dose:** Third potency. Must be continued for a long time.

---

# ROSA DAMASCENA

(Damask Rose) **Ros-d.**

Useful in the beginning of hay fever, with involvement of the eustachian tube.

**Ears:** Hardness of hearing; tinnitus, *Eustachian catarrh* (*Hydr., Merc-d.*).

**Relationship:** Compare: in hay fever: *Phleum pratense*—Timothy grass (hay fever with asthma; watery coryza, itching in the nose and eyes; frequent sneezing, dyspnea. Use 6-30 potency—Rabe). *Succ-ac., Sabad., Euph., Psor., Kali-i., Naphtin.*

**Dose:** Lower potencies.

---

# RUMEX CRISPUS

(Yellow Dock) **Rumx.**

Is characterized by pains, numerous and varied, neither fixed nor constant anywhere. Cough caused by an incessant tickling in the throat pit, tickling extends down to the bifurcation of the bronchial tubes. Touching the throat pit brings on cough. Worse from the least cold air; cough ceases by covering the entire body and head with bed clothes. *Rumx.* diminishes the secretions of mucous membranes, and at the same time exalts sensitivity of the mucous membranes in the larynx and trachea. Its action on the skin is marked, producing an intense itching. *Lymphatics enlarged* (adenitis) and secretions perverted.

**Stomach:** Tongue sore at edges; coated; sensation of a hard substance in the pit of the stomach; hiccough, pyrosis, nausea; *cannot eat meat; it causes eructations, pruritus.* Jaundice after excessive use of alcohol. Chronic gastritis; aching pain in pit of stomach with shooting pain in the chest; extends towards the throat pit, worse motion or talking. Pain in the left breast after meals; *flatulence.*

**Rectum:** Brown, watery, diarrhea *early in the morning,* with cough, driving him out of bed. Valuable in advanced phthisis (*Seneg., Puls., Lyc., Ars.*). Itching in the anus, with sensation of a stick in the rectum. Piles.

**Respiratory:** Nose dry. *Tickling in the throat pit causes cough. Copious mucus discharge* from nose and trachea. *Dry, teasing cough* (bronchitis), *preventing sleep. Aggravated by pressure, talking and especially by inspiring cool air and at night.* Thin, watery, frothy expectoration by the mouthful; later, stringy and tough. Rawness of larynx and trachea. Soreness behind the sternum, especially in the left side and in the area around the left shoulder. *Raw pain under the clavicle.* Lump in throat.

**Skin:** Intense itching of skin, especially of *lower extremities; worse, exposure to cold air when undressing.* Urticaria; contagious prurigo.

**Modalities:** Worse, in the evening, from inhaling cold air; left chest; uncovering.

**Relationship:** Compare: *Caust., Sulph., Bell., Rumx.* contains chrysophanic acid to which the skin symptoms correspond. *Rumex acetosa*—Sheep sorrel (gathered in June and dried, used locally for epithelioma of the face (Cowperthwaite). Dry, unremitting short cough, and violent pain in the bowels; uvula elongated; inflammation of the esophagus; also cancer); *Rumex obtusifolius—Lapathum*—Broad leaf dock (epistaxis and headache following; pain in kidneys; leucorrhea).

**Dose:** Third to sixth potency.

---

## RUTA GRAVEOLENS

(Rue Bitterwort) **Ruta**

Acts on the periosteum and cartilages, eyes and uterus. Complaints from straining, *especially the flexor tendons*. Tendency to the formation of deposits on the periosteum, tendons and around the joints, especially in the wrist. Overstraining of ocular muscles. All parts of the body are painful, *as if bruised.* Sprains (after *Arn.*). Lameness after sprains. Jaundice. *Feeling of intense lassitude, weakness and despair.* Injured "bruised" bones.

**Head:** Pain, as if from a nail; after an excess of intoxicating drinks. Periosteum sore. Epistaxis.

**Eyes:** *Eye strain followed by headache. Eyes red, hot, and painful from sewing or reading fine print* (hypermetropic) (*Nat-m., Arg-n.*). *Disturbances of accommodation.* Weary pain while reading. Pressure deep in the orbits (glaucoma). Tarsal cartilage feels bruised. Pressure over the eyebrow. Asthenopia.

**Stomach:** Gastralgia of a aching, gnawing character.

**Rectum:** *Difficult feces,* evacuated only after straining. Constipation, alternating with mucoid, frothy stools; discharge of blood with stool. When sitting, tearing stitches in the rectum. *Carcinoma affecting the lower bowel. Prolapsus ani* every time the bowels move, after confinement. Frequent, unsuccessful urging to stool. Protrusion of rectum when stooping.

**Urinary:** Pressure in the neck of bladder after micturating; painful closure (*Apis*). Constant urging to micturate, feels as if bladder is full.

**Respiratory:** Cough with copious, thick, yellow expectoration; chest feels weak. Painful spot on the sternum; short breath with tightness of chest (asthma).

**Back:** Pain in the nape, back and loins. Backache better pressure and lying on back. Lumbago worse morning before rising.

**Extremities:** Spine and limbs feel bruised. Lumbosacral region and loins painful. Legs give out on rising from a chair, hips and thighs, weak (*Phos., Con.*). Contraction of fingers. Pain and stiffness in wrists and hands. Ganglion (*Benz-ac.*). Sciatica; worse, lying down at night; pain from the back extending down to hips and thighs. Hamstrings feel shortened (*Graph.*). *Tendons sore.* Aching pain in tendo-Achilles. *Thighs pain on stretching the limbs.* Pain in bones of feet and ankles (periostitis, perichondritis). Great restlessness.

**Modalities:** *Worse,* lying down, from cold, wet weather.

**Relationship:** Compare: *Rat., Card-m.* (rectal irritation); *Jab., Phyt., Rhus-t., Sil., Arn.*

Antidote: *Camph.*

Complementary: *Calc-p.*

**Dose:** First to sixth potency. Locally, the tincture for ganglia and as a lotion for the eyes.

---

## SABADILLA

(Cevadilla Seed, Asagraea Officialis) **Sabad.**

Action on mucous membrane of the nose and the lachrymal glands, producing coryza and symptoms like *hay fever,* which have been utilized homeopathically. *Chilliness;* sensitive to cold. Ascarides, with reflex symptoms (nymphomania; convulsive symptoms). Children's diarrhea with constant cutting pains.

**Mind:** Nervous, timid, easily startled. Has erroneous notions about himself. Imagines that he is very sick; that parts are shrunken; that she is pregnant; that she has cancer; delirium during intermittent fever.

**Head:** Vertigo with sensation as though all things were turning around each other, accompanied by blackness before eyes and sensation of fainting. Dullness and oppression. Oversensitiveness to odors. *Thinking* produces headache and sleeplessness.

**Eyes:** *Eyelids red, burning* (blepharitis). *Lachrymation.*

**Ears:** Difficult hearing.

**Nose:** *Spasmodic sneezing, with a running nose. Coryza,* with severe frontal pains and redness of eyes and lachrymation. Copious, watery, nasal discharge.

**Throat:** Sore; *begins on left side* (*Lach.*). Much tough phlegm. Sensation of skin hanging loosely; must swallow it. *Warm food and drink relieve.* Empty swallowing very painful. Dry fauces and throat. Sensation of a lump in the throat with *a constant* necessity to swallow. Chronic sore throat; worse, from cold air. Tongue as if burnt.

**Stomach:** Spasmodic pain in the stomach with dry cough and difficult breathing. *No thirst.* Loathing for strong food. Canine appetite for sweets and farinaceous food. Pyrosis; copious salivation. Cold, empty feeling in the stomach. *Desire for hot things. Sweetish* taste.

**Female:** Menses too late; comes by fits and starts. *Intermits* (*Kreos., Puls.*) (due to transient and localized congestion of womb alternating with chronic anemic state).

**Extremities:** Cracking of skin under and beneath the toes; inflammation under the toe nails (paronychia).

**Fever:** *Chill predominates;* from below upwards. Heat in the head and face; hands and feet icy cold, with chill. Lachrymation during paroxysm. Thirstless.

**Skin:** Dry, like parchment. Horny, deformed, *thickened nails.* Hot, burning, creeping, crawling sensation. Itching in the anus.

**Modalities:** *Worse,* cold and cold drinks, full moon. *Better,* warm food and drink, wrapped up.

**Relationship:** Complementary: *Sep.*

Compare: *Veratrinum* (is an alkaloid of *Sabadilla,* not of *Verat.*, locally in neuralgias, and for removal of dropsy. Five grains to two drams lanolin, rubbed on the inside of thighs, causes diuresis). *Colch., Nux-v., Arund.* and *Pollatinum. Phleum pratense*—Timothy (hay fever. Potentized l2, specific to many cases and evidently acts in a desensitizing manner. Rabe); *Cumarinum* (hay fever).

Antidotes: *Puls., Lyc., Con., Lach.*

**Dose:** Third to thirtieth potency.

---

# SABAL SERRULATA

(Saw Palmetto) **Sabal**

*Sabal* is homeopathic to irritability of the genito-urinary organs. General and sexual debility. Promotes nutrition and tissue building. Head, stomach and ovarian symptoms marked. Of unquestioned value in prostatic enlargement, *epididymitis* and difficulties in passing urine. Acts on the membrano-prostatic portion of urethra. Iritis, with prostatic problems. *Valuable for undeveloped mammary glands. Fear of going to sleep.* Languor, apathy and indifference.

**Head:** Confused, full; dislikes sympathy; makes her angry. Vertigo, with headache. Neuralgia in feeble patients. Pain runs up from the nose and centers in the forehead.

**Stomach:** Belching and acidity. Desire for milk (*Rhus-t., Apis*).

**Urinary:** Constant desire to pass water at night. *Enuresis;* paresis of sphincter vesicae. Chronic gonorrhea. Difficulty in passing urine (dysuria). Cystitis with prostatic hypertrophy.

**Male:** *Prostatic problems;* enlargement; discharge of prostatic fluid. Wasting of testes (atrophy) and *loss of sexual power.* Coitus painful at the time of emission. *Sexual neurotics.* Organs feel cold (impotence).

**Female:** Ovaries tender and enlarged (ovaritis); *breasts shrivel* (atrophy) (*Iod., Kali-i.*). Young female neurotics; suppressed or perverted sexual inclination.

**Respiratory:** Copious expectoration, with catarrh of nose. Chronic bronchitis (*Stann., Hep.*).

**Relationship:** Compare: *Ph-ac., Stigmata maydis; Santal., Apis.* In prostatic symptoms: *Ferr-pic., Thuj., Pic-ac.* (more sexual erethism). *Populus tremuloides* (prostatic enlargement with cystitis).

**Dose:** Mother tincture, ten to thirty drops. Third potency often better. The tincture must be prepared from the *fresh berries* to be effective.

---

## SABINA

(Savine) **Sabin.**

Has a special action on the uterus; also upon serous and fibrous membranes; hence its use in gout. *Pain from sacrum to the pubis. Hemorrhages, where blood is fluid and clots together.* Tendency to miscarriage, especially at third month. *Violent pulsations;* wants windows open.

**Mind:** *Music is intolerable,* produces nervousness.

**Head:** Vertigo with suppressed menses. Bursting headache, suddenly coming and going slowly. Rush of blood to head and face. Drawing pain in the masseter muscles. Toothache when chewing.

**Stomach:** Heartburn. Desire for lemonade. Bitter taste (*Rhus-t.*). Lancinating pain from the pit of stomach to the back.

**Abdomen:** Bearing down, constrictive pain. Colic, mostly in the hypogastric region. Tympanitic distention.

**Rectum:** Sense of fullness. Constipation. *Pain from back to pubis.* Hemorrhoids, with bright red blood; bleeds copiously.

**Urinary:** Burning and throbbing in the region of kidneys. Hematuria; much urging. Bladder inflamed (cystitis). with throbbing all over. Inflammation of urethra (uretritis).

**Male:** Inflammatory gonorrhea, with pus-like discharge. Sycotic excrescences. Burning, sore pain in glans. Prepuce painful with difficulty in retracting it (phimosis). Increased desire.

**Female:** *Menses profuse, bright.* Uterine pains extend to the thighs. Threatened miscarriage. Sexual desire increased (nymphomania). Leucorrhea after menses, corrosive, offensive. Discharge of blood between periods (metrorrhagia), with sexual excitement (*Ambr.*). Retained placenta; intense after-pains. Menorrhagia in women who abort readily. Inflammation of ovaries and uterus after abortion. Promotes expulsion of moles from the uterus (*Canth.*). *Pain from sacrum to pubis, and from below upwards, shooting up the vagina.* Hemorrhage; partly clotted; worse from *least motion.* Atony of uterus.

**Back:** *Pain between sacrum and pubis from one bone to another.* Paralytic pain in small of back.

**Extremities:** Bruised pains in the anterior portion of the thighs. Shooting in heels and metatarsal bones. *Arthritic pain in joints.* Gout; worse, in a heated room. Red, shining swelling. Gouty nodosities (*Am-p.*).

**Skin:** Fig warts with intolerable itching and burning. Exuberant granulations (*Thuj., Nit-ac.*). *Warts.* Black pores in skin (comedones).

**Modalities:** *Worse,* from least motion, heat, warm air. *Better,* in cool fresh air.

**Relationship:** Complementary: *Thuj.*

Compare: *Sanguisorba officinalis* (venous congestion and passive hemorrhages; varices of lower extremities; dysentery. *Long lasting, profuse menses* with congestion to head and limbs in sensitive, irritable patients. *Climacteric* hemorrhages. Use 2x attenuation). *Sanguisuga officinalis*—Leech (hemorrhages, especially bleeding from anus. Use 6x). *Rosmarinus officinalis* (menses too early; violent pains followed by uterine hemorrhage. Head heavy, *drowsy.* Chilly with icy coldness of lower extremities without thirst, followed by heat. Memory deficient). *Croc., Calc., Tril-p., Ip., Mill., Erig.*

Antidote: *Puls.*

**Dose:** Locally, for warts, tincture. Internally, third to thirtieth potency.

---

## SACCHARUM OFFICINALE—SUCROSE

(Cane-sugar) **Sacch.**

According to the great Dr. Hering, a large proportion of chronic diseases of women and children are developed by using too much sugar.

Sugar is an antiseptic. Combats infection and putrefaction; has a solvent action on fibrin and stimulates secretion by the intense osmotic changes induced, thus rinsing out the wound with serum from within outward, favoring healing. Leg ulcers.

Sugar must be considered as a sustainer and developer of the musculature of the heart and is hence useful in failure of compensation and a variety of cardio-vascular problems. Acts as a nutrient and tonic, in wasting disorders, anemia, neurasthenia, etc., increasing weight and power.

Corneal opacity. Dim sight (cataract): *Acidity and anal itching.* Cold expectoration. Myocardial degeneration.

Fat, bloated, large limbed children, who are *cross, peevish,* whining; capricious; want dainty things, tidbits, and refuse substantial food. Edema of feet. Headache every seven days.

**Relationship:** Compare: *Saccharum lactis*—Sugar of milk-lactose (diuresis; amblyopia; *cold pains,* as if produced by fine, icy cold needles with tingling, as if frost bitten; great physical exhaustion. *Sugar of milk* in large doses to develop the Bacillus acidophilus to correct putrefactive intestinal conditions and also constipation).

Compare: *Saccharinum* (hinders both the salivary and peptic fermenting actions with consequent dyspepsia. Prof. Lewin believes its action to be on the secretory cells themselves and it causes pain (right hypogastrium), loss of appetite, diarrhea and wasting).

**Dose:** Thirtieth potency and higher. Locally in gangrene. One ounce of sugar lump, morning and evening is a valuable adjunct in the treatment of obstinate cases of heart failure due to deficient heart muscle without a valvular lesion. Epilepsy; blood with reduced sugar content irritates the nervous system, tending to convulsions.

*Sugar* as an oxytocic has its most suitable application towards the end of labor when there is no mechanical obstruction and delay is due to uterine inertia. 25 grammes dissolved in water, several times, every half hour.

---

# SALICYLICUM ACIDUM

(Salicylic Acid) **Sal-ac.**

The symptoms point to its use in rheumatism, dyspepsia and *Meniere's disease.* Prostration after influenza; also tinnitus aurium and deafness. Hematuria.

**Head:** Vertigo; tendency to fall on the left side. Headache; confusion in the head on rising suddenly. Incipient coryza. Piercing pain in temples.

**Eyes:** Retinal hemorrhage. Retinitis after influenza, also albuminuric.

**Ears:** *Roaring and ringing in ears.* Deafness with vertigo.

**Throat:** Sore, red and swollen. Pharyngitis; dysphagia.

**Stomach:** *Canker sores,* with burning soreness and halitosis. *Flatulence; hot, sour belching.* Putrid fermentation. *Fermentative dyspepsia.* Tongue purplish, leaden colored.

**Rectum:** Putrid diarrhea; gastro-intestinal derangements, especially in children; stools like green frog's spawn (*Mag-c.*). Pruritus ani.

**Extremities:** Knees swollen and painful. Acute articular rheumatism; worse, touch and motion, profuse sweat. Pain shifts. Sciatica, burning pain; worse at night. Copious footsweat and its ill effects when suppressed.

**Skin:** Itching vesicles and pustules; better by scratching. Sweat without sleep. Urticaria. Hot and burning skin. Purpura. Herpes zoster. Necrosis and softening of bones.

**Relationship:** Compare: *Salolum* (rheumatic pain in joints, with soreness and stiffness, headache over the eyes; urine violet smelling); *Colch., Chin., Lac-ac. Spirae.* and *Gaul.* contain Salicylic acid.

**Dose:** Third decimal trituration. In acute articular rheumatism, 5 grains every 3 hours (old school dose).

---

# SALIX NIGRA

(Black-willow) **Sal-n.**

Has a positive action on the generative organs of both sexes. Hysteria and nervousness. Libidinous thoughts and lascivious dreams. Controls genital irritability. Moderates sexual passion. Satyriasis and erotomania. In acute gonorrhea, with marked erotic trouble; chordee. After masturbation; spermatorrhea.

**Face:** Red, swollen, especially the tip of nose, eyes bloodshot and sore to touch and on motion. Roots of hair hurt. Epistaxis.

**Male:** Painful movement of the testicles (orchitis).

**Female:** Before and during menses, marked nervous disturbance, pain in ovaries; difficult menstruation. Ovarian congestion and neuralgia. Menorrhagia. Bleeding with uterine fibroid. Nymphomania.

**Back:** Pain across the sacral and lumbar region. Unable to step quickly.

**Relationship**: Compare: *Yohim., Canth.*

**Dose:** Material doses of the tincture, thirty drops.

---

# SALVIA OFFICINALIS

(Sage) **Salv.**

Controls excessive sweating when circulation is enfeebled; of less use in phthisis *with night sweats* and suffocating, tickling cough. Galactorrhea. Exerts a tonic influence on the skin.

**Respiratory:** Tickling cough, especially in consumption.

**Skin:** Soft, relaxed, with enfeebled circulation and cold extremities. *Colliquative perspiration.*

**Relationship:** Compare *Chrysanthemum leucanthemum*—Ox-eye daisy (has a specific action on sudoriparous glands. Quietens the nervous system like *Cypripedium pubessens.* Right sided tearing pain in bones of the jaw and temple. Pain in teeth and gums, worse touch, better warmth. Irritable and tearful. Here use 12x. *Insomnia and night sweats.* For colliquative sweating and hyperesthesia of nervous system. Material doses of tincture). *Phel., Tub., Salvia sclerea* (tonic influence on the nervous system; dose, teaspoonful to one pint on hot water, as inhalent for sponging). *Rubia tinctorum*—Madder: A remedy for the spleen (*Cean.*). Chlorosis and amenorrhea; tuberculosis. Anemia; undernourished conditions; splenic anemia. Dose, 10 drops of tincture).

**Dose:** Tincture, in twenty drop doses, in a little water. The effects manifest themselves quickly, two hours after taking a dose, and they persist for from two to six days.

---

# SAMBUCUS NIGRA

(Elder) **Samb.**

Acts especially on the respiratory organs. Dry coryza of infants, snuffles, edematous swellings. *Profuse sweat* accompanies many affections.

**Mind:** Sees images on shutting the eyes. *Constant fretfulness.* Very easily frightened. Fright followed by suffocative attacks.

**Face:** Turns blue with cough. Red, burning spots on cheeks. Heat and perspiration on face.

**Abdomen:** Colic with nausea and flatulence; frequent watery, slimy stools.

**Urinary:** Profuse urine with dry heat of the skin. Frequent micturition with scanty urine. Acute nephritis; dropsical symptoms with vomiting.

**Respiratory:** Chest oppressed with pressure in the stomach, and nausea. Hoarseness with tenacious mucus in the larynx (laryngitis). Paroxysmal, *suffocative cough* (bronchitis), *coming on around midnight,* with crying and dyspnea. Spasmodic croup (whooping cough). Dry coryza. *Snuffles in infants;* nose dry and obstructed. Loose choking cough. When nursing, child must let go of nipple, nose blocked, cannot breathe. *Child wakes up suddenly, nearly suffocated, sits up, turns blue* (cyanosed). *Cannot expire* (*Meph.*). Millar's asthma.

**Extremities:** Hands turn blue. Edematous swelling in legs, insteps, and feet. Feet icy cold. Debilitating night sweats (*Salvia, Acet-ac.*).

**Fever:** Dry heat while sleeping. *Dreads uncovering. Profuse sweat over the entire body during waking hours.* Dry, deep cough precedes the fever paroxysm.

**Skin:** Dry heat of skin during sleep. Bloated and swollen; general dropsy; *profuse sweat on waking.*

**Modalities:** *Worse,* sleep, during rest, after eating fruit. *Better,* sitting up in bed, motion.

**Relationship:** Compare: *Ip., Meph., Op., Samb-c.* (of great value in dropsies; large doses required—fluid extract, 1/4 to 1 teaspoonful three times daily).

Antidotes: *Ars., Camph.*

**Dose**: Tincture to sixth potency.

---

## SANGUINARIA CANADENSIS

(Blood Root) **Sang.**

Is a right sided remedy pre-eminently, and chiefly affects the mucous membranes, especially that of the respiratory tract. It has marked vasomotor disturbances, as seen in the circumscribed redness of the cheeks; flashes of heat, rush of blood to head and chest, distention of temporal veins, burning in palms and soles, and has been found very applicable to climacteric disorders. *Burning* sensations, as if from hot water. Influenzal coughs. Phthisis. *Sudden stopping of catarrh from the respiratory tract followed by diarrhea. Burning* in various parts is characteristic.

**Head:** Worse *right* side, sun headache. Periodical sick headache; pain begins in the occiput, spreads upwards, and *settles over the eyes, especially right* (migraine). *Veins is the temples are distended.* Pain better lying down and sleep. Headaches return at climacteric; every seventh day (*Sulph., Sabad.*). Pain in a small spot over the upper left parietal bone. Burning in eyes. Pain in the back of head "like a flash of lightening."

**Ears:** Burning in ears. Otalgia with headache. Humming and roaring (tinnitus). Aural polypus.

**Nose:** Hay fever. Ozena with profuse, offensive yellowish discharges. *Nasal polypi.* Coryza, followed by diarrhea. Chronic rhinitis; membrane *dry* and congested.

**Face:** Flushed. Neuralgia; pain extends in all directions from the upper jaw. *Redness and burning of cheeks. Hectic flush.* Fullness and tenderness behind the angle of jaws.

**Throat:** Swollen; worse, right side. Dry and constricted. Ulceration of mouth and fauces, with a dry, burning sensation. Tongue white; feels scalded. Tonsillitis (quinsy).

**Stomach:** Aversion to butter. Craving for piquant things. Unquenchable thirst. Burning, vomiting. Nausea, with salivation. Sinking, faint, all gone feeling (*Phos., Sep.*). Spitting up of bile; gastro-duodenal catarrh.

**Abdomen:** Diarrhea as coryza improves. Pain over the liver region. Diarrhea; bilious, liquid, gushing stool (*Nat-s., Lyc.*). Cancer of rectum.

**Female:** Leucorrhea fetid, corrosive. Menses offensive, profuse. Soreness of breasts. Uterine polypi. Before menses, itching in axillae. Climacteric disorders.

**Respiratory:** Edema of the larynx. Trachea sore. Heat and tension behind the sternum. Aphonia. *Cough of gastric origin;* relieved by eructation. Cough, with burning pains in the chest; worse, right side. Sputum tough, *rust colored,* offensive, almost impossible to raise. Spasmodic cough after influenza and *after whooping cough.* Cough returns with every fresh cold. Tickling behind the sternum, produces a constant hacking cough; worse at night on lying down. Must sit up in bed. Burning soreness on the right side of the chest, extends to the right shoulder. Severe soreness under the right nipple. Hemoptysis from suppressed menses. *Severe dyspnea* and constriction of chest. Offensive breath and purulent expectoration. Burning in chest as if from hot steam going from the chest to the abdomen. Fibrous stage of phthisis. Pneumonia; better, lying on the back. Asthma with stomach disorders (*Nux-v.*). Valvular disease with lung disease, hydrothorax, phosphates in urine and loss of flesh. Sudden stoppage of catarrh in air passages brings on diarrhea.

**Extremities:** Rheumatism of the right shoulder, left hip joint and nape of neck. *Burning in soles and palms.* Rheumatic pain in places least covered by flesh; not in joints. Toes and soles of feet burn. Right sided neuritis; better touching the part.

**Skin:** Antidotes *Rhus poisoning.* Red, blotchy eruptions; worse in spring. Burning and itching; worse by heat. Acne with scanty menses. Circumscribed red spots over malar bones.

**Modalities:** *Worse,* sweets, right side, motion, touch. *Better,* acids, sleep, darkness.

**Relationship:** Complementary: *Ant-t.*

Compare: *Justicia adhatoda* (bronchial catarrh, coryza, hoarseness; oversensitive). *Dig.* (migraine). *Bell., Iris, Meli., Lach., Ferr., Op.*

**Dose:** Tincture in headaches; sixth potency in rheumatism.

---

# SANGUINARINUM NITRICUM

(Nitrate of Sanguinarine) **Sangin-n.**

Is of use in polypus of the nose. Acute and chronic catarrh. Acute pharyngitis (*Wye.*). Smarting and burning in throat and chest especially under the sternum. *Influenza.* Lachrymation, pains in eyes and head, sore scalp; *sense of obstruction.* Chronic follicular pharyngitis (quinsy).

**Nose:** *Feels obstructed. Profuse, watery mucus with burning pain.* Enlarged turbinates (adenoids) at the beginning of the hypertrophic process. Secretion scant, tendency to dryness. Small crusts which bleed when removed. Post-nasal secretions adherent to the nasopharynx, dislodged with difficulty. Dry and burning nostrils; watery mucus, with pressure over the root of nose. Nostrils plugged with thick, yellow, bloody mucus. *Sneezing.* Rawness and soreness in posterior nares.

**Mouth:** Ulceration on the *side* of the tongue.

**Throat:** Rough, dry, *constricted, burning.* Right tonsil sore, dysphagia.

**Respiratory**: Short, hacking cough, with expectoration of thick, yellow, sweetish mucus. *Pressure behind the center of sternum.* Dryness and burning in the throat and bronchi. *Tickling cough.* Chronic nasal, laryngeal and bronchial catarrh. Voice altered, deep, hoarse.

**Relationship:** Compare: *Sanguinarinum tartaricum* (exopthalmos; *mydriasis,* dim vision); *Arum-t., Psor., Kali-bi.*

**Dose:** Third trituration.

---

# SANICULA AQUA

(The Water of Sanicula Springs, Ottawa, Ill) **Sanic.**

Has been found to be a useful remedy in enuresis, seasickness, constipation, etc. Rickets.

**Head:** Dread of downward motion (*Borx.*). *Profuse sweat on occiput* and in the nape of neck, during sleep (*Calc., Sil.*). Profuse, scaly dandruff. Soreness behind the ears.

**Eyes:** Photophobia. Lachrymation in cold air or from cold application.

**Mouth:** Tongue large, flabby, burning; must protrude it to keep it cool. Ringworm on the tongue.

**Throat:** Thick, ropy, tenacious mucus.

**Stomach:** Nausea and vomiting from car riding. Thirst; drinks little and often (*Ars., Chin.*). Is vomited as soon as it reaches the stomach.

**Rectum:** Stools large, heavy and painful. *Pain in the whole perineum.* No desire till there is a large accumulation. After great straining only partially expelled; recedes, crumbles at the verge of anus (*Mag-m.*). Very offensive odor. Excoriation of skin around the anus, perineum and genitals. Diarrhea; changeable in character and color; after eating.

**Female:** Bearing down, as if the contents of pelvis would escape (prolapse); better, rest. Desire to support parts. Soreness of the uterus. Leucorrhea with *odor of fish brine or old cheese* (*Hep.*). Vagina feels large.

**Back:** Sensation as if sacrum dislocated better lying on right side.

**Extremities:** Burning of soles of feet (*Sulph., Lach.*). *Offensive foot sweat* (*Sil., Psor.*). Cold, clammy sweat on extremities.

**Skin:** Dirty, greasy, brownish, wrinkled. Eczema, fissured hands and fingers (*Petr., Graph.*).

**Modalities:** *Worse, moving arms backward.*

**Relationship**: Compare: *Abrot., Alum., Calc., Sil., Sulph., Sanicula aqua* must not be confounded with the Sanicle (poolroot or wood marsh), also called *Sanic.* This is used in various nervous affections, resembling *Valer*. It is used as a resolvent for sanguineous extravasations, and as an astringent. Has not been proved.

**Dose:** Thirtieth potency.

---

# SANTONINUM

(Santonin) **Santin.**

Is the active principle of Santonica, the unexpanded flower heads of *Artemisia maritima—Cina.*

The eye stymptoms and those of the urinary tract are most prominent. It is of unquestioned value in the treatment of worm diseases, gastro-intestinal irritation, *itching in the nose,* restless sleep, twitching of muscles. Ascaris lumbricoides and thread worms, but not tapeworms. *Nocturnal cough* in children. *Chronic cystitis.* Laryngeal crisis and lightening pains of tabes.

**Head:** Occipital headache, with *chromatic hallucinations.*

**Eyes:** Sudden dimness of sight (amblyopia, cataract). *Color blindness;* Xanthopsia. Strabismus due to worms. Dark rings around the eyes.

**Nose:** *Itching on the nose.* Bores into the nostrils.

**Mouth:** Halitosis depraved appetite; thirsty. Tongue deep red. *Grinding of teeth.* Nausea; better after eating. Choking sensation.

**Urinary:** Urine greenish if acidic and reddish purple if alkaline. *Incontinence and dysuria. Enuresis.* Sensation of fullness in the bladder. Nephritis.

**Relationship:** Compare: *Cina; Teucr., Naphtin., Nat-p., Spig.*

**Dose:** Second to third trituration. Lower preparations are often toxic. Do not give to a child with fever or constipation.

---

## SAPONARIA OFFICINALIS

(Soap Root) **Sapo.**

Of great use in the treatment of acute colds, coryza, sore throat, etc. Will often "break up" a cold.

**Mind:** Utter indifference to pain or possible death. Apathetic, *depressed with sleepiness.*

**Head:** Stitching pain, *supraorbital;* worse, left side, evening, motion (migraine). Throbbing over orbits. Congestions of head; tired feeling in the nape. *Coryza.* Sensation of drunkeness with a constant endeavor to go towards the left. Left sided trigeminal neuralgia, especially supraorbital. Stopped up feeling in the nose, also itching and sneezing.

**Eyes:** Violent pain in the eye. Hot stitches deep in the eyeball. Ciliary neuralgia; worse, left side. Photophobia. Exophthalmos, worse reading and writing. Increased intraocular pressure, glaucoma.

**Stomach:** Dysphagia. Nausea, heartburn; full feeling not relieved by eructation.

**Heart:** Impulse weak; pulse less frequent. Palpitations, with anxiety.

**Modalities:** *Worse,* at night, mental exertion, left side.

**Relationship**: Compare: *Saponinum*—a glucosidal principle found in *Quill., Yuc., Seneg., Dios.* and other plants (tired, indifferent. *Pain in the left temple, eye,* photophobia, hot stitches deep in the eye. Facial nerve affections. Migraine. Severe pain *before* menstrual flow; severe sore throat, worse right side; tonsils swollen, worse in a warm room. Sharp burning taste and violent sneezing).

Compare, also: *Verb., Cocc.* (both containing Saponin). *Quill., (Anag., Agro., Helon., Sars., Par., Cycl.* and others contain Saponin).

# SARCOLACTICUM ACIDUM

**Sarcol-ac.**

Is apparently formed in muscle tissue during the stage of muscle exhaustion. Differs from ordinary lactic acid in its relation to polarized light.

It represents a much broader and more profoundly acting drug and its pathogenesis is quite dissimilar from the normal acid. Proved by Wm. B. Griggs, M.D., who found it of great value in the most violent form of *epidemic influenza, especially with violent retching and great prostration,* when *Ars.* fails. Spinal neurasthenia, muscular weakness, dyspnea with myocardial weakness.

Tired feeling with *muscular prostration,* worse after any exertion. Sore feeling all over, worse in the afternoon. Restless at night. Difficulty in getting sleep. Tired feeling in the morning on getting up.

**Throat:** Constriction in the pharynx. Sore throat with tightness in the naso-pharynx. Tickling in throat.

**Stomach:** Nausea. Uncontrollable vomiting, even of water followed by extreme weakness.

**Back and Extremities:** Tired feeling in the back, neck and shoulders. Paralytic weakness. Wrist tires easily from writing. Extreme weakness from climbing stairs. Stiffness of thigh and calves. Arms feel as if there is no strength in them. Cramps in the calves.

**Dose:** Sixth to 30th potency. The 15x has the most marked action (Griggs).

# SARRACENIA PURPUREA

(Pitcher Plant)

**Sarr.**

A remedy for variola. Visual disorders. Congestion of head with irregular heart action. Chlorosis. Contains a very active proteolytic enzyme. Sick headache; throbbing in various parts, especially in neck, shoulders and head, which feels full, as if bursting.

**Eyes:** Photophobia. Eyes feel swollen and sore. Pain in the orbits. Black objects move with the eye.

**Stomach:** Hungry all the time, even after a meal. Sleepy during meals. Copious, painful vomiting.

**Back:** Pains shooting in a *zig-zag* manner from the lumbar region to middle of the scapula.

**Extremities:** Limbs weak; bruised pain in knees and hip joints. Bones of arm, pain. *Weak between shoulders.*

**Skin:** Variola, aborts the disease, arrests pustulation.

**Relationship**: Compare: *Ant-t., Variol., Maland.*

**Dose**: Third to sixth potency.

---

# SARSAPARILLA OFFICINALIS

(Smilax) **Sars.**

Renal colic; marasmus and periosteal pains due to venereal disease. Eruptions following hot weather and vaccinations; boils and eczema. Urinary symptoms well marked.

**Mind:** Despondent, sensitive, easily offended, ill humored and taciturn.

**Head:** *Pain causes depression.* Shooting pain from above the right temporal region. Pain *from occiput to eyes.* Words reverberate in the ear to the root of nose. Periosteal pain due to venereal disease. Influenza. Scalp sensitive. *Eruptions on the face and upper lip.* Moist eruptions on the scalp (plica plonica). Crusta lactea beginning on the face.

**Mouth:** Tongue white; *aphthae; salivation;* metallic taste; no thirst. Fetid breath (halitosis).

**Abdomen:** Rumbling and fermentation. *Colic and backache at the same time.* Much flatus; cholera infantum.

**Urinary:** Urine scanty, slimy, flaky, sandy, *bloody* (hematuria, Bright's disease). Gravel. Renal colic (calculi). *Severe pain at the conclusion of micturition. Urine dribbles while sitting.* Bladder distended and tender (cystitis). *Child screams before and while passing urine.* Sand on diaper. Renal colic and dysuria in infants. *Pain from the right kidney extends downward.* Tenesmus of bladder; urine passes in a thin, feeble stream. Pain at meatus.

**Male:** Bloody, seminal emissions. Intolerable stench on genitals. Herpetic eruptions on genitals. Itching of scrotum and perineum. Syphilis; squamous eruption and bone pains.

**Female:** Nipples small, withered, *retracted. Before menstruation, itching and humid eruptions of the forehead.* Menses late and scanty. Moist eruptions in the right groin before menses.

**Extremities:** Paralytic, tearing pains. Trembling of hands and feet. Burning on sides of fingers and toes. Onychia, ulceration around finger tips, cutting sensation under the nails. Rheumatism, bone pains; worse at night. Deep rhagades on fingers and toes; burning under the nails. Tetter on hands; ulceration around finger tips (*Psor.*). Cutting sensation under nails (*Petr.*). Rheumatic pains after gonorrhea.

**Skin:** *Emaciated, shrivelled, lies in folds* (*Abrot., Sanic.*), dry, flabby.

Herpetic eruptions; ulcers. Rash from exposure to open air; dry, itching; *comes on in spring;* becomes crusty. Rhagades; skin cracked on hands and feet. Skin hard, indurated. Summer cutaneous affections.

**Modalities:** *Worse,* dampness, at night, after micturating, when yawning, in spring, before menses.

**Relationship:** Complementary: *Merc., Sep.*

Compare: *Berb., Lyc., Nat-m., Petr., Sassafras officinalis, Saururus cernuus*—Lizard's tail (irritation of kidneys, bladder, prostate and urinary passages. Painful and difficult micturition; cystitis with strangury). *Cucurbita citrullus*—Watermelon (infusion of the seed acts promptly in dysuria with constriction and backache, relieves pain and stimulates flow).

Antidote: *Bell.*

**Dose:** First to sixth potency.

---

## SCROPHULARIA NODOSA

(Knotted Figwort) **Scroph-n.**

A powerful medicine whenever *enlarged glands* are present. Hodgkin's disease.

A valuable skin remedy. Has a specific affinity for the breast; very useful in the dissipation of breast tumors. *Eczema of the ear.* Pruritus vaginae. Lupoid ulceration. *Scrofulous swellings* (*Cist.*). *Painful hemorrhoids.* Tubercular testis. Ephithelioma. Nodosities in the breasts (*Scir.*). Pain in all flexor muscles.

**Head:** Vertigo felt in the vertex, greater when standing; drowsiness; pain from the forehead to the back of head. Eczema behind the ear. Crusta lactea.

**Eyes:** Distressing photophobia (*Con.*). Spots before eyes. Stitches in eyebrows. Sore eyeballs.

**Ears:** Inflammation around the auricle. Deep ulcerated auricle. Eczema around the ear.

**Abdomen:** *Pain in the liver* on pressure. Colic below the navel. Pain in the sigmoid flexure and *rectum. Painful,* bleeding, protruding *piles.*

**Respiratory:** Violent dyspnea, oppression of chest with trembling. Pain in the area above the bifurcation of trachea. Asthma in scrofulous patients.

**Sleep:** *Great drowsiness;* in the morning and before and after meals with weariness.

**Skin:** Prickling, itching, worse at the back of the hand.

**Modalities:** *Worse* lying on right side.

Compare: *Lobelia erinus, Ruta, Carc., Con., Aster.*

**Dose:** Tincture and first potency. Apply locally on cancerous glands also *Semp-v.*

# SCUTELLARIA LATERIFOLIA

(Skullcap) **Scut.**

This is a nervous sedative, where *nervous fear* predominates. *Cardiac irritability. Chorea.* Nervous irritation and spasms of children, during dentition. *Twitching of muscles.* Nervous weakness after influenza.

**Mind:** *Fear of some calamity.* Inability to fix attention (*Aeth.*). Confusion.

**Head:** *Dull, frontal headache.* Eyes feel pressed outwards. Flushed face. Restless sleep and frightful dreams. *Must move around* . Night terrors. Migraine; worse, over the right eye; *aching in eyeballs.* Explosive headaches of school teachers with frequent micturition; headaches in front and at the base of brain. Nervous sick headaches, worse noise, odor, light, better night; rest, 5 drops of tincture.

**Stomach:** Nausea; sour eructations; hiccough; pain and distress.

**Abdomen:** Gas, fullness and distention, colicky pain and uneasiness. Light colored diarrhea.

**Male:** Seminal emissions and impotency, with fear of never getting better.

**Extremities:** Twitchings of muscles; must be moving. Chorea. Tremors. Sharp stinging pains in upper extremities. Nocturnal restlessness. Weakness and aching.

**Sleep:** Night terrors; sleeplessness; sudden wakefulness; frightful dreams.

**Relationship:** Compare: *Cypr., Lycps-v.*

**Dose:** Tincture and lower potencies.

---

# SECALE CORNUTUM—CLAVICEPS PURPUREA

(Ergot) **Sec.**

Produces contraction of the unstriped muscular fibres; hence a constringent feeling throughout the body. This produces an anemic condition, coldness, numbness, petechiae, mortification, gangrene. A useful remedy for old people with shrivelled skin, thin, scrawny old women. All the *Sec.* conditions are *better from cold;* the whole body is prevaded by a sense of great heat. Hemorrhages; continuous oozing; *thin,* fetid, watery black blood. *Debility, anxiety, emaciation, though appetite and thirst may be excessive.* Facial and abdominal muscles twitch. *Sec.* decreases the flow of pancreatic juice by raising the blood pressure (Hinsdale).

**Head:** Passive, congestive pain (rises from back of head), with a pale face. Head drawn back (epilepsy). Falling of hair; dry and gray. *Epistaxis,* dark, oozing.

**Eyes:** Pupils dilated. Incipient cataract, senile especially in women. *Eyes sunken and surrounded by a blue margin.*

**Face:** *Pale, pinched, sunken.* Cramps commence in the face and spread all over the body. Livid spots on the face. *Spasmodic distortion.*

**Mouth:** Tongue dry, *cracked; blood-like ink exudes,* coated thick; viscid, yellowish, cold, livid. *Tingling at the tip of the tongue, which is stiff.* Tongue swollen, paralyzed.

**Stomach:** *Unnatural ravenous appetite; craves* acids. *Thirst* unquenchable. Singultus, nausea; vomiting of blood and coffee ground fluid (hematemesis). Burning in the stomach and abdomen; tympanites. Eructations of bad odor.

**Stool:** Cholera-like stools, with coldness and cramps. *Olive green, thin, putrid, bloody, with icy coldness and an intolerance to being covered, with great exhaustion. Involuntary stools;* no sensation of passing feces, anus wide open.

**Urinary:** Paralysis of the bladder. Retention, with unsuccessful urging. Discharge of black blood from the bladder (hematuria). Enuresis in old people.

**Female:** Menstrual colic, with coldness and intolerance to heat. Passive hemorrhages in feeble, cachectic women. Burning pains in the uterus. *Brownish, offensive leucorrhea.* Menses irregular, copious, dark; *continuous oozing of watery blood* till the next period. Threatened abortion around the *third* month (*Sabin.*). During labor no expulsive action, as though everything is relaxed. After-pains. Suppression of milk; breasts do not fill properly. Dark, offensive lochia. Puerperal fever, putrid discharges, tympanites, coldness, suppressed urine.

**Chest:** Angina pectoris. Dyspnea and oppression, with cramps in the diaphragm. Boring pain in chest. Precordial tenderness. Palpitations, with contracted and intermittent pulse.

**Back:** Spinal irritation, tingling in lower extremities; can only bear the slightest covering. *Locomotor ataxia.* Formication and numbness. Myelitis.

**Extremities:** Cold, dry hands and feet in excessive smokers with sensation of fuzziness in the fingers. Trembling, staggering gait. Formication, pain and spasmodic movements. Numbness. Fingers and feet bluish (cyanosis) shrivelled, *spread apart or bent backwards,* numb. *Violent, cramps. Icy coldness of extremities.* Violent pain in finger tips, tingling in toes.

**Sleep:** Profound and long. Insomnia with restlessness, fever, anxious dreams. *Insomnia in drug and liquor habitues.*

**Fever:** *Coldness;* cold, dry skin; cold, clammy sweat; excessive thirst. Sense of internal heat.

**Skin:** Shrivelled, numb; mottled dusky-blue tinge. Sclerema and edema neonatorum. Raynaud's disease. Blue color (cyanosis). *Dry gangrene,* developing slowly. *Varicose ulcers. Burning sensation;* better by cold; *wants parts uncovered,* though cold to touch. Formication; petechiae. Small wounds continue to bleed. Livid spots. Boils, small, painful, with green contents; mature slowly. *Skin feels cold to touch,* yet covering is not tolerated. *Great aversion to heat. Formication under the skin.*

**Modalities:** *Worse,* heat, *warm covering. Better,* cold, *uncovering,* rubbing, stretching out of limbs.

**Relationship:** Compare: *Ergotinum* (beginning arteriosclerosis progressing rather rapidly. Increased blood pressure: 2x trituration. Edema, gangrene and purpura hemorrhagia; when *Sec.,* though indicated, fails); *Pedicularis canadensis* (symptoms of locomotor ataxia; spinal irritation); *Brassica napus oleifera*—Rape seed (dropsical swellings, scorbutic mouth, voracious appetite, tympanites, dropping of nails, gangrene); *Cinnm., Colch., Ars., Aur-m. 2x* (locomotor ataxia); *Agrostema glithago*—Corn cockle—active constituent is *Saponinum,* which causes violent sneezing and sharp burning taste; burning in the stomach, extends to the esophagus, neck and breast; (vertigo, headache, difficult locomotion, burning sensation); *Ustilago, Carb-v., Pituitrinum* (dilated os, little pain, no progress. Dose, ½ c.c., repeat in half hour, if necessary. Hypodermically contraindicated in first stage of labor, valvular lesions or deformed pelvis).

Antidotes: *Camph., Op.*

**Non-homeopathic Uses:** In hemorrhages of puerperium, after the uterus is entirely emptied, when it fails to contract satisfactorily and in secondary puerperal hemorrhage the result of incomplete involution of the uterus, give one-half to one dram of the fluid extract. Remember Pagot's law. "As long as the uterus contains anything, be it child, placenta, membranes, clots, never administer ergot."

**Dose:** First to thirtieth potency.

---

# SEDUM ACRE

(Small Houseleek) **Sed-ac.**

Hemorrhoidal pains, like those of anal fissures; constricting pains, worse for hours after stool. *Fissures.*

**Relationship:** Compare: *Mucuna urens* (hemorrhoidal diathesis and diseases depending thereon); *Sedum telephium* (uterine hemorrhages, also of bowels and rectum; *menorrhagia, especially at climacteric); Sedum repens—Sedum alpestre* (*cancer;* specific action on abdominal organs; pain, loss of strength).

**Dose:** Tincture to sixth potency.

# SELENIUM METALLICUM

(The Element Selenium) **Sel.**

*Sel.* is a constant constituent of bones and teeth.

Marked effects on the genito-urinary organs, and is often indicated in elderly men, especially for prostatitis and sexual atony. *Great debility;* worse, heat. Easy exhaustion, mental and physical, in old age. Debility after exhausting diseases.

**Mind:** Lascivious thoughts, with impotency. Mental labor fatigues. *Extreme sadness.* Abject despair, uncompromising melancholy.

**Head:** Hair falls out. *Pain over the left eye; worse, walking in sun, strong odors and tea.* Scalp feels tense. Headache from tea drinking.

**Throat:** Incipient tubercular laryngitis. Hawking and raising transparent lumps of mucus every morning. *Hoarseness.* Cough in the morning, with expectoration of bloody mucus (hemoptysis). Hoarseness of singers. Very clear, starchy mucus (*Stann.*).

**Stomach:** Desire for brandy and other strong drinks. Sweetish taste. Hiccough and eructations after smoking. After eating, pulsations all over, especially in the abdomen.

**Abdomen:** Chronic liver affections; liver painful, *enlarged with a fine rash over the liver region.* Stool constipated, hard and accumulated in the rectum.

**Urinary:** Sensation at the tip of urethra as if a biting drop was forcing its way out. Involuntary dribbling.

**Male:** Dribbling of semen during sleep (spermatorrhea). Dribbling of prostatic fluid (prostatorrhea). Irritability after coitus. *Loss of sexual power,* with lascivious fancies. *Increased desire, decreased ability.* Semen thin, odorless. Sexual neurasthenia. On attempting coition, penis relaxes (impotence). *Hydrocele.*

**Extremities:** Paralytic pains in the lumbosacral region, in the morning. Tearing pain in hands, at night.

**Sleep:** *Sleep prevented by pulsations in all vessels,* worse abdomen. Sleepless till midnight, wakes up early and always at the same hour.

**Skin:** Dry, scaly eruptions on palms, with itching (psoriasis palmaris). *Itching around the ankles* and folds of skin, between fingers. Hair falls out from brows, beard, and genitals. Itching around finger joints and between fingers; in palms (scabies). Vesicular eruptions between fingers (*Rhus-t., Anac.*). Seborrhea oleosa; comedones *with an oily surface of the skin;* alopecia. *Acne.*

**Modalities:** *Worse,* after sleep, in hot weather, from Cinchona, draught of air, coition.

**Relationship:** Incompatible: *Chin., Wine.*

Compare: *Agn., Calad., Sulph., Tell., Ph-ac.*

Antidotes: *Ign., Puls.*

**Dose:** Sixth to thirtieth potency. Colloidal *Sel.* injection for inoperable cancer. Pain, sleeplessness, ulceration and discharge are markedly diminished.

---

## SEMPERVIVUM TECTORUM

(Houseleek) **Semp.**

Is recommended for herpes zoster and *cancerous tumors.* Scirrhous induration of tongue. Mammary carcinoma. Ringworm. Hemorrhoids.

**Mouth:** Malignant ulcers of the mouth. Cancer of tongue (*Gali.*). Tongue has ulcers; *bleed easily,* especially at night; marked soreness of the tongue with *stabbing* pains. The whole mouth is very tender (stomatitis).

**Skin:** Erysipelatous affections. *Warts* and corns. Aphthae. Flushed surface and stinging pain.

**Relationship:** Compare: *Sedum acre*—Small house leek (scorbutic conditions; ulcers, intermittent fever) (*Gali., Kali-cy.*); *Oxalis acetosella*—Wood sorrel (the inspissated juice is used as cautery to remove cancerous growths of the lips); *Cotyledon umbilicus; Ficus carica* (Fig): The milky juice of the freshly broken stalk applied to warts; causes their disappearance.

**Dose:** Tincture and 2 decimal, also fresh juice of plant. Locally for bites of insects, stings of bees and poisoned wounds, *warts.*

---

## SENECIO AUREUS

(Golden Ragwort) **Senec.**

Its action on the female organism has been clinically verified. Urinary organs also affected in a marked degree. Backaches with congested kidneys. Early cirrhosis of liver.

**Mind:** Inability to fix mind on one subject. Despondent. Nervous and irritable.

**Head:** Dull, stupefying headache. *Wave like dizziness* from occiput to sinciput. *Sharp pain over the left eye, and through the left temple.* Fullness of nasal passages; burning; *sneezing;* profuse flow.

**Face:** Teeth very sensitive. *Sharp, cutting pain* on the left side. *Dryness* of fauces, throat and mouth.

**Throat:** Dry mouth, throat, and fauces. Burning in the pharynx, raw feeling in the naso-pharynx, must swallow, though painful.

**Stomach:** Sour eructations; nausea.

**Abdomen:** Pain around the umbilicus; spreads all over the abdomen; better, stool. Thin, watery stool, intermingled with hard lumps of feces (*Ant-c.*). *Straining at stool; thin, dark, bloody with tenesmus.*

**Urinary:** Scanty, high colored, *bloody* with profuse mucus and *tenesmus. Great heat and constant urging.* Nephritis. Irritable bladder of children with headache. Renal colic (*Pareir., Ocim., Berb.*).

**Male:** Lascivious dreams with involuntary emissions. *Prostate enlarged.* Dull, heavy pain in the spermatic cord, extending to testicles.

**Female:** *Menses retarded,* suppressed. *Functional amenorrhea in young girls* with backache. Before menses, inflammatory conditions of throat, chest and bladder. After menstruation commences, these improve. Anemic dysmenorrhea with urinary disturbances. Premature and very profuse menses (*Calc., Erig.*).

**Respiratory:** Acute inflammatory conditions of the upper respiratory tract. Hoarseness. *Cough loose,* with labored inspiration. Chest sore and raw. Dyspnea on ascending (*Calc.*). Dry teasing cough, stitching chest pains.

**Sleep:** Great drowsiness, with unpleasant dreams. Nervousness and sleeplessness.

**Relationship:** Compare: *Senecio jacobaea* (cerebro-spinal irritation, rigid muscles, chiefly of neck and shoulders; also, in cancer); *Alet., Caul., Sep.*

**Dose:** Tincture to third potency. *Senecin,* first trituration.

---

# SENEGA

(Snakewort) **Seneg.**

Catarrhal symptoms, especially of the respiratory tract, and distinct eye symptoms of a paralytic type, are most characteristic. Circumscribed spots in the chest left after inflammations.

**Mind:** Suddenly remembers unimportant regions which he saw long ago. Inclined to quarrel.

**Head:** Dullness, with pressure and weakness of eyes. Pain in temples. *Bursting* pain in forehead.

**Eyes:** Hyperphoria, better by bending head backwards. Acts on the rectus superior. Blepharitis; lids dry and crusty (*Graph.*). Dryness, with sensation as *if too large for the orbits.* Staring. Lachrymation. Flickering; must wipe eyes frequently. Objects look shaded (amblyopia). Muscular asthenopia (*Caust.*). Diplopia; better only by bending head backward. Opacities in vitreous humor. Promotes absorption of lens fragments after operation.

**Nose:** Dry. Coryza; profuse watery mucus and sneezing. Nostrils feel peppery.

**Face:** Paralysis of the left side of face. Heat in face. Burning vesicles at the corners of mouth and lips.

**Throat:** Catarrhal inflammation of the throat and fauces, with scraping hoarseness. Burning and rawness. Sensation as if the membrane had been abraded.

**Urinary:** Greatly diminished; loaded with shreds and mucus; scalding before and after micturition. *Back,* bursting distending pain in kidney region (nephritis).

**Respiratory:** Hoarseness. Hurts to talk. Bursting pain in the back on coughing. Catarrh of larynx (laryngitis). Aphonia. Hacking cough (whooping cough). Thorax feels too narrow. *Cough often ends in a sneeze. Rattling in chest* (*Ant-t.*). Chest oppressed on ascending. Bronchial catarrh, *with sore chest walls;* profuse mucus; sensation of oppression and weight on chest (pneumonia). *Difficulty in raising tough, profuse mucus,* in the aged. Asthenic bronchitis in old people with chronic interstitial nephritis or chronic emphysema. Old asthmatics with congestive attacks. *Exudations in pleura* (pleurisy). Hydrothorax (*Merc-sul.*). Pressure on the chest as though the lungs were forced back to the spine. Voice unsteady, vocal cords partially paralyzed.

**Modalities:** *Worse,* walking in open air, during rest. *Better,* from sweat; *bending head backwards.*

**Relationship:** Compare: *Caust., Phos., Saponin., Ammc., Calc., Nepeta cataria*—Catnip (to break up a cold; infantile colic; hysteria).

**Dose:** Tincture to thirtieth potency.

---

# SENNA

(Cassia Acutifolia) **Senn.**

Is of a lot of use in infantile colics, when the child seems to be *full of wind.* Oxaluria, with excess of urea; increased specific gravity. Where the system is broken down, bowels constipated, muscular weakness and waste of nitrogenous materials, *Senna* will act as a tonic. Ebullitions of blood at night. *Acetonemia,* prostration, fainting, constipation with colic and flatulence. Liver enlarged and tender.

**Rectum:** Fluid yellowish, with pinching pains before. Greenish mucus; never-get-done sensation (*Merc.*). Burning in the rectum, with strangury of bladder. *Constipation,* with colic and flatulence. Liver enlarged and tender, stools hard and dark, with loss of appetite, coated tongue, bad taste and *weakness* (jaundice).

**Urinary:** Specific gravity and density increased; hyperazoturia, oxaluria, phosphaturia and acetonuria.

**Relationship:** Compare: *Kali-c., Jal.*

Antidotes: *Nux-v., Cham.*

**Dose:** Third to sixth potency.

---

## SEPIA OFFICINALIS

(Inky Juice of Cuttlefish) **Sep.**

Acts specially on the portal system, with venous congestion. Stasis and thereby ptosis of viscera, weariness and misery. Weakness, yellow complexion, bearing down sensation, especially in women, upon whose organism it has the most pronounced effect. Pains extend down to the back, chills easily. Tendency to abortion. Hot flushes at menopause with weakness and perspiration. Symptoms travel upwards. Easy fainting. Ball-like sensation in inner parts. *Sep.* acts best on brunettes. All pains are from below up. One of the most important uterine remedies. Tubercular patients with chronic hepatic problems and uterine reflexes. *Feels cold* even in a warm room. Pulsating headache in the cerebellum.

**Mind:** *Indifferent* to those loved best. Averse to occupation, *to family.* Irritable; easily offended. Dreads to be alone. *Very sad.* Weeps when telling symptoms. Miserly. Anxious towards evening; indolent.

**Head:** Vertigo, with sensation of something rolling around in the head. Prodromal symptoms of apoplexy. Stinging pain from within outward and upwards mostly on the left side, or in the forehead, with nausea, vomiting (migraine); worse indoors and when lying on the painful side. Jerking of head backwards and forwards. Coldness of the vertex. Headache in *terrible shocks* at menstrual nisus, with scanty flow. Hair falls out (dandruff). Open fontanelles. Roots of hair sensitive. Pimples on forehead near the hair margine.

**Eyes:** Muscular asthenopia; black spots in the field of vision; asthenic inflammations, in connection with uterine problems. Aggravation of eye problems in the morning and evening. Tarsal tumors (styes). Ptosis, ciliary irritation. Venous congestion of the fundus.

**Ears:** *Herpes behind ears on the nape of neck.* Pain as if from sub cutaneous ulceration. Swelling and eruptions on the external ear.

**Nose:** *Thick, greenish discharge* (ozena); thick plugs and crusts. *Yellowish saddle across the nose.* Atrophic catarrh with greenish crusts from anterior nose and pain at the root of nose. Chronic nasal catarrh, especially post-nasal dropping of heavy, lumpy discharges; must be hawked through the mouth.

**Face:** Yellow blotches (chloasma); pale or sallow; yellow around the mouth. Rosacea; saddle-like brownish distribution on nose and cheeks.

**Mouth:** Tongue white. Taste salty, putrid. Tongue foul, but clears during menses. Swelling and cracking of lower lip. Pain in teeth from 6 p.m. till midnight; worse on lying.

**Stomach:** *Feeling of goneness; not relieved by eating* (*Carb-an.*). Nausea at smell or sight of food. Nausea worse lying on side. *Tobacco dyspepsia.* Everything tastes too salty (*Carb-v., Chin.*). Band of pain around four inches wide encircling the hypochondria. *Nausea in the morning before eating.* Disposition to vomit after eating. Burning in the pit of the stomach. Longing for *vinegar,* acids and pickles. Worse, after milk, especially when boiled. Acid dyspepsia with a bloated abdomen, sour eructations. Loathes fat.

**Abdomen:** *Flatulent,* with headache. *Liver sore and painful* (jaundice); *relieved by lying on right side.* Many brown spots on the abdomen (liver spots). Sensation of relaxation and bearing down in the abdomen.

**Rectum:** Bleeding with stools and fullness of the rectum. Constipation; large, hard stools; *sensation of a ball in rectum;* cannot strain; great tenesmus and pains shooting *upwards.* Dark brown, round balls glued together with mucus. Soft stool, difficult. Prolapsus ani (*Podo.*). *Almost constant oozing from anus.* Infantile diarrhea, *worse from boiled milk* and rapid exhaustion. *Pains shoot up* in rectum and vagina.

**Urinary:** Red, *adhesive,* sand in urine (hematuria). Enuresis, *during first sleep.* Chronic cystitis, slow micturition with bearing down sensation above the pubis.

**Male:** Organs cold. Offensive perspiration. Gleet; discharge from urethra only at night; no pain. Condylomata surrounds head of penis (gonorrhea). Complaints from coition.

**Female:** Pelvic organs relaxed. *Bearing down sensation as if everything would escape through the vulva* (*Bell., Kreos., Lac-c., Lit-t., Nat-c., Podo.*); must cross limbs to prevent protrusion, or press against vulva. Leucorrhea yellow, greenish; with much itching. Menses *too late and scanty,* irregular; *early and profuse;* sharp clutching pains. Violent stitches upward in the vagina, from the uterus to the umbilicus. *Prolapse* of uterus and vagina. Morning sickness. Vagina painful, especially during coition (dysparunia).

**Respiratory:** Dry, fatiguing cough, apparently coming from the stomach. Taste of rotten eggs with coughing. Oppression of chest, morning and evening. Dyspnea; worse, after sleep; better, rapid motion. Cough in the morning, with profuse expectoration, tasting salty (*Phos., Ambr.*). Hypostatic pleuritis. Whooping cough that drags on. Cough excited by tickling in the larynx or chest.

**Heart:** Violent, intermittent palpitations. Pulsations in all arteries. Tremulous sensations with flushes.

**Back:** *Weakness in the lumbosacral region. Pains extend to the back.* Coldness between shoulders.

**Extremities:** Lower extremities lame and stiff, tension as if too short. Heaviness and bruised feeling. *Restlessness in all limbs,* twitching and jerkings night and day (chorea). Pain in heel. Coldness of legs and feet.

**Fever:** Frequent flushes of heat; sweat from least motion. General lack of warmth in the body. Feet cold and wet. Shivering, with thirst; worse, towards evening.

**Skin:** Herpes circinatus in isolated spots. Itching; not relieved by scratching; worse in bends of elbows and knees. Chloasma; herpetic eruptions on lips, around the mouth and nose. Ringworm like eruption every spring. Urticaria on going in open air; better in a warm room. Hyperidrosis and bromidrosis. Foots sweat, worse on toes; intolerable odor. Lentigo in young women. Ichthyosis with offensive odor of skin.

**Modalities:** *Worse,* forenoons and evenings; washing, laundry work, dampness, left side, after sweat; cold air, before a thunderstorm. *Better,* by *exercise,* pressure, warmth of bed, hot applications, drawing limbs up, cold bathing, after sleep.

**Relationship:** Complementary: *Nat-m., Phos. Nux-v.* intensifies action. *Guaj.* often beneficial after *Sep.*

Inimical: *Lach., Puls.*

Compare: *Lil-t., Murx., Sil., Sulph., Asperula odorata*—Nacent oxygen—Distilled water charged with the gas (leucorrhea in young girls and uterine catarrh); *Ozone (sacral* pain; tired feeling through the pelvic viscera and perineum); *Dictamnus albus*—Burning bush (soothes labor pains; metrorrhagia, leucorrhea and constipation; also somnambulism). *Lapathum acutum* (leucorrhea with constriction and expulsive effort through the womb and pain in kidneys).

**Dose:** Twelfth, 30th and 200th potency. Should not be used too low or be repeated too frequently. On the other hand Dr. Jousset's unique experience is that it should be continued for some time in strong doses. 1x twice a day.

---

## SERUM ANGUILLAE

(Eel Serum) **Ser-ang.**

The *Serum of Eel* has a toxic action on the blood, rapidly destroying its globules. The presence of albumin and renal elements in urine, hemoglobinuria, prolonged anuria (24 and 26 hours), together with the results of autopsy, plainly demonstrate its elective action on the kidneys. Secondarily, the liver and the heart are affected, and the alterations observed are those usually present in infectious diseases.

From all these facts it is easy to infer, *a priori,* the therapeutical indications of *Eel serum.* Whenever the kidney becomes acutely affected, either from cold, infection or intoxication, and the attack is characterized by *oliguria, anuria* and *albuminuria,* we will find *Eel's serum* eminently efficacious to re-establish diuresis, and it rapidly arrests albuminuria. When, in a *heart disease* with cardiac irregularities and a marked state of asystole the kidney becomes affected and its function is inhibited, we may expect good results from this serum. But to determine the choice of remedy is not an easy matter. While *Dig.* is indicated, in the well known symptomatic trilogy: *Arterial hypertension, oliguria and edema; Serum of the Eel* seems better adapted to cases of *hypertension and oliguria, without edema.* We should bear in mind that the elective action of the *Eel's serum* is on the kidney, and I believe we can well assert that if *Dig.* is a cardiac remedy, the *Eel's serum* is a renal remedy. So far, at least, the clinical observations published seem to confirm this distinction. The *Serum of Eel* has given very small results in attacks of asystolia; but it has been very efficacious in *cardiac uremia.* There, where *Dig.* is powerless, *Serum of Eel* has put an end to the renal obstruction and produced an abundant diuresis. But its really specific indication seems to be for *acute nephritis a frigori* (Jousset).

Subacute nephritis. Heart diseases, *in* cases of failure of compensation and impending asytole. The experiments of Dr. Jousset have amply demonstrated the rapid hematuria, albuminuria and oliguria caused by it. In the presence of acute nephritis with threatening uremia, we should always think of this serum. Very efficacious in functional heart diseases. Mitral insufficiency, asystolia with or without edema, dyspnea and difficult urinary secretion.

**Relationship:** Great analogy exists between *Eel serum* and the venom of *Vipera.*

Compare, also: *Pelias berus; Lach.*

**Dose:** Attenuations are made with glycerine or distilled water, the lower 1x to 3 in heart disease, the higher in sudden renal attacks.

---

# SILICEA TERRA

(Silica, Pure Flint) **Sil.**

Imperfect assimilation and consequent defective nutrition. It goes further and produces neurasthenic states in consequence, with an increased susceptibility to nervous stimuli and exaggerated reflexes. Diseases of bones, caries and necrosis. *Sil.* can stimulate the organism to re-absorb fibrotic conditions and scar tissue. In phthisis, it must be used with care, for here it may cause the absorption of scar tissue, liberate the disease, walled in, to new activities (J. Weir). Organic changes; it is deep and slow in action. Periodical states; abscesses, quinsy, headaches, spasms, epilepsy, sensation of coldness before an attack. Keloid growth. Scrofulous, rachitic children, with a large head, open fontanelles and sutures, distended abdomen, slow in walking. *Ill effects of vaccination. Suppurative processes.* It is related to all fistulous burrowings. Ripens abscesses since it promotes suppuration. *Sil.* patient is cold, chilly, hugs the fire, wants plenty of warm clothing, hates drafts, hands and feet cold, worse in winter. Lack of vital heat. Prostration of mind and body. Great sensitiveness to taking cold. *Intolerance to alcoholic stimulants.* Ailments attended with *pus formation.* Epilepsy. *Want of grit,* moral or physical.

**Mind:** Yielding, *faint-hearted, anxious.* Nervous and excitable. *Sensitive* to all impressions. Brain fag. Obstinate, headstrong children. Abstracted. Fixed ideas; thinks only of *pins,* fears them, searches and counts them.

**Head:** Aches from fasting. Vertigo from looking up; *better, wrapping up warmly; when lying on the left side* (*Mag-m., Stront-c.*). *Profuse sweat on head,* offensive, and extends to the neck. Pain begins in the occiput, and spreads all over the head and settles over the eyes. Swelling in the glabella.

**Eyes:** Angles of eyes affected. *Swelling of lachrymal duct.* Aversion to light, especially daylight; it produces dazzling, sharp pain through eyes (photophobia); eyes tender to touch; worse when closed. Vision confused; letters run together on reading. *Styes.* Iritis and irido-choroiditis, with pus in the anterior chamber. *Perforating* or sloughing corneal ulcer. Abscess in the cornea after a traumatic injury. Cataract in office workers. After effects of keratitis and leucoma, clearing the opacity (cataract). Use 30th potency for months.

**Ears:** Fetid discharge (otorrhea). Caries in the mastoid. Loud pistol-like retort. Sensitive to noise. *Roaring in ears* (tinnitus).

**Nose:** Itching on the tip of nose. Dry, hard crusts form, *bleeding when loosened.* Nasal bones sensitive. Sneezing in the morning. Obstructed and anosmia. Perforation of septum.

**Face:** Skin cracked on margin of lips. Eruptions on chin. Facial neuralgia, throbbing, tearing; face red; worse, cold damp.

**Mouth:** *Sensation of a hair on the tongue.* Gums sensitive to cold air. Boils on gums. Abscess at the root of teeth (caries). Pyorrhea (*Merc-c.*). Sensitive to cold water.

**Throat:** Periodical quinsy. *Pricking as of a pin in tonsil.* Colds settle in throat. *Parotid glands swollen* (*Bell., Rhus-t., Calc.*). Stinging pain on swallowing (mumps, parotiditis). Hard, cold swelling of cervical glands (cervical adenitis).

**Stomach:** Disgust for meat and *warm food.* On swallowing food, it easily gets into posterior nares. Want of appetite; thirst excessive. Sour eructations after eating (*Sep., Calc.*). Pit of stomach painful to pressure. Vomiting after drinking (*Ars., Verat.*).

**Abdomen:** Pain or a painful cold feeling in the abdomen, better external heat. Hard, bloated. Colic; cutting pain with constipation; yellow hands (jaundice) and blue nails. Much rumbling in bowels. Inguinal glands swollen and painful. Hepatic abscess.

**Rectum:** Feels paralyzed. *Fistula in ano* (*Berb., Lach.*). Fissures and hemorrhoids, *painful, with spasm of sphincter. Stool comes down with difficulty; when partly expelled, recedes again.* Great straining; rectum stings; closes on stool. Feces remain for a long time in the rectum. *Constipation always before and during menses;* with an irritable sphincter ani. Diarrhea with a cadaverous odor.

**Urinary:** Hematuria, enuresis with red or yellow sediment. Prostatic fluid discharged when straining at stool. Nocturnal enuresis in children with worms.

**Male:** Burning and soreness of genitals, with eruptions on the inner surface of thighs. Chronic gonorrhea, with thick, fetid discharge. Elephantiasis of scrotum. Sexual erethism; nocturnal emissions. Hydrocele.

**Female:** A milky (*Calc., Puls., Sep.*), acrid leucorrhea, during micturition. Itching of vulva and vagina; very sensitive. Discharge of blood between menstrual periods (metrorrhagia). Profuse menses, with paroxysms of *icy coldness over the entire body.* Nipples very sore; ulcerate easily; drawn in. Fistulous ulcers of breast (*Phos.*). Abscess of labia. Discharge of blood from the vagina, every time the child is nursed. Vaginal cysts (*Lyc., Puls., Rhod.*). Hard lumps in breast (carcinoma) (*Con.*).

**Respiratory:** Colds fail to yield; sputum persistently mucopurulent and profuse. Slow recovery after pneumonia. Cough and sore throat, with expectoration of little granules like shot, which, when broken, smell very offensive. Cough with expectoration during the day, bloody (hemoptysis) or purulent. Stitches in the chest extending to back. *Violent cough as lying down, with thick, yellow lumpy expectoration;* suppurative stage of expectoration (*Bals-p.*).

**Back:** Weak spine; very susceptible to draughts on back. Pain in coccyx. Spinal irritation after injuries to spine; diseases of vertebrae. Potts' disease.

**Extremities:** Sciatica, pain through hips, legs and feet. Cramps in calves and soles. Loss of power in legs. Hand tremulous when using them. Paralytic weakness of forearm. *Affections of finger nails,* especially if white spots are present on the nails. Ingrowing toe nails. *Icy cold and sweaty feet. The parts lain on go to sleep. Offensive sweat on feet,* hands and axillae. Suppurating sensation in finger tips. Panaritium. Pain in knee, as if tightly bound. Calves tense and contracted. Pain beneath the toes. Soles sore (bunion) (*Ruta*). *Soreness in feet from instep, through out to the sole. Suppuration.*

**Sleep:** *Night walking;* gets up while asleep (somnambulism). Sleeplessness, with great orgasm of blood and heat in head. Frequent starts in sleep. Anxious dreams. Excessive gaping.

**Fever:** Chilliness; very sensitive to cold air. Creeping, shivering over the whole body. Cold extremities, even in a warm room. Sweat at night; worse towards the morning. *Suffering parts feel cold.*

**Skin:** *Felons, abscesses, boils, old fistulous ulcers.* Delicate, pale, waxy. Cracks on finger tips. Painless swelling of glands. Rose colored blotches. Scars (cicatrix) suddenly become painful. Pus offensive. *Promotes expulsion of foreign bodies from tissues.* Every littlc injury suppurates. Long lasting suppuration and fistulous tracts. Dry finger tips. Eruptions itch only during daytime and in the evening. *Crippled nails.* Indurated tumors. Abscesses of joints. After impure vaccination. Bursa. Lepra, nodes and coppery spots. *Keloid growths.*

**Modalities:** *Worse,* new moon, in the morning, from washing, during menses, uncovering, lying down, damp, lying on left side, cold. *Better,* warmth, wrapping up the head, summer; in wet or humid weather.

**Relationship:** Complementary: *Thuj., Sanic., Puls., Fl-ac. Merc.* and *Sil.* do not follow each other well.

Compare: Black Gunpowder 3x (abscesses, boils, carbuncles, limb purple. Wounds that refuse to heal; accident from bad food or water: Clarke). *Hep., Kali-p., Pic-ac., Calc., Phos., Tabasheer; Nat-sil.* (tumors, hemophilia, arthritis; dose, three drops three times daily, in milk); *Ferr-cy.* (epilepsy; neuroses, with irritable weakness and hypersensitiveness, especially of a periodical character). *Silica marina*—Sea sand (*Sil.* and *Nat-m.* symptoms. *Inflamed glands* and commencing of suppuration. Constipation. Use for sometime 3x trituration). *Vitrum*—Crown glass (Potts' disease, after *Sil.*, necrosis, discharge thin, watery, fetid. Severe pain, fine *grinding* and *grating* like grit). *Arund-d.* (acts on excretory and generative organs; suppuration, especially chronic, and where the ulceration is fistulous, especially in long bones. Itching eruption on chest, upper extremities and behind the ear).

**Dose:** Sixth to thirtieth potency. The 200th and higher of unquestioned activity. In malignant affections, the lowest potencies are needed at times.

---

## SILPHIUM LANCINATUM

(Rosin-weed) **Silphu.**

Is used in various forms of asthma and chronic bronchitis. Catarrh of the bladder. Catarrhal influenza. Dysentery; attack preceded by constipated stools covered with white mucus.

**Respiratory:** Cough with expectoration, *profuse,* stringy, forthy, light colored. Excited by the sense of mucus rattling in the chest and worse by drafts of air. Constriction of lungs. Catarrh, with copious, stringy, mucus discharges. Desire to hawk and scrape the throat. Irritation of posterior nares, involving the mucous membranes of nasal passages with constriction of supra-orbital region.

**Relationship:** Compare: *Aral., Cop., Ter., Cub., Samb., Silphion cyrenaicum* (phthisis pulmonum with incessant cough, profuse night sweats, emaciation, etc.); *Polygonum aviculare* (has been found useful in phthisis, when given in material doses of the mother tincture); *Salv.* (tickling cough). *Arum-d.* (loose cough at night on lying down). *Just.* (bronchial catarrh, hoarseness, oversensitive).

**Dose:** Third potency. Lower triturations preferred by some.

---

## SINAPIS NIGRA—BRASSICA NIGRA

(Black Mustard) **Sin-n.**

Is of use in hay fever, coryza, and pharyngitis. Dry nares and pharynx, with thick, lumpy secretion. Small pox.

**Head:** Scalp hot and itchy. *Sweat on the upper lip and forehead.* Tongue feels blistered.

**Nose:** Mucus from posterior nares feels *cold.* Scanty, *acrid* discharge. *Stoppage of left nostril all day,* or in the afternoon and evening. Dry, hot, with lachrymation, sneezing; hacking cough; better lying down. *Nostrils alternately stopped.* Dryness of anterior nares.

**Throat:** Feels scalded, hot, inflamed. Asthmatic breathing. Loud coughing spells with barking expiration.

**Stomach:** *Offensive breath,* smelling like onions (*Asaf., Coch.*). Burning in the stomach, extending up to the esophagus, throat, and mouth, which is full of canker sores. Hot sour eructations. *Colic; pains come on when bent forward; better, sitting up straight.* Sweat better when nausea comes on.

**Urinary:** Pain in the bladder, frequent *copious* flow, day and night.

**Respiratory:** Cough is relieved by lying down.

**Back:** Rheumatic pain in the intercostal and lumbar muscles; sleeplessness from pain in the back and hips.

**Relationship:** Compare: *Sulph., Caps., Coloc., Sinapis alba*—White mustard (throat symptoms marked, especially *pressure and burning, with obstruction in the esophagus;* sensation of a lump in the esophagus behind the manubrium sterni with several eructations; similar symptoms of the rectum).

*Mustard oil* by inhalation (acts on the sensory nerve endings of the trigeminal. Relieves pain in middle ear disease and in painful conditions of the nose, nasal cavities, and tonsils).

**Dose:** Third potency.

---

## SKATOLUM

**Skat.**

Represents the ultimate end of proteid decomposition and is a constituent of human feces.

Acne with auto-intoxication dependent upon intestinal decomposition. Stomach and abdominal symptoms; frontal headache.

**Mind:** Lack of concentration; impossible to study; *despondent;* desire to be with people. Sluggishness with no ambition. Irritable. Feels mean towards everyone. Desire to curse and swear.

**Head:** Frontal headache, worse over the left eye, in the evening, *better by a short sleep.*

**Mouth:** Tongue coated, *foul taste.* Salty taste of all cereals. *Belching.* Appetite increased.

**Rectum:** Light yellow, *very offensive* stool. Intestinal dyspepsia.

**Urinary:** Frequent, scanty, burning, difficult.

**Sleep:** Increased desire to sleep; wakes up unrefreshed, half doped feeling.

**Relationship:** Compare: *Indol., Bapt., Sulph.*

**Dose:** Sixth potency.

---

## SKOOKUM-CHUCK

(Strong Medicinal Water. Salts From Water of Medicinal Lake near Spokane, Wash.) **Skook.**

Has a strong affinity for skin and mucous membranes. An anti-psoric medicine.

Otitis media. Profuse, ichorous, cadaverously smelling discharge. Lithemia. *Catarrh.* Urticaria. *Skin affections. Eczema. Dry skin. Hay fever.* Profuse coryza and constant sneezing.

**Relationship:** *Saxonitum* (appears to have remarkable cleansing, deodorizing and soothing properties for the skin—Cowperthwaite. Eczema, scalds, burns, sores and hemorrhoids).

**Dose:** Third trituration.

# SOLANUM NIGRUM

(Black Nightshade) **Sol-n.**

Used with success in ergotism, with tetanic spasms and stiffness of the whole body, mania. Marked action on the head and eyes. *Meningitis.* Chronic intestinal toxemia. Brain irritation during dentition. Restlessness of a violent and convulsive nature. Formication with contraction of extremities.

**Head:** Furious delirium. Vertigo; terrible headache and complete cessation of the mental faculties. Hydrocephalus. Night terrors. *Congestive* headache.

**Eyes:** Pain over both the eyes. Alternate dilatation and contraction of pupils; weak sight (amaurosis); floating spots.

**Nose:** Acute coryza; *profuse, watery discharge from the right nostril;* left stopped up, with chilly sensation, alternating with heat.

**Respiratory:** Constrictive feeling in the chest, with difficult breathing; cough with tickling in the throat. Expectoration *thick, yellow.* Pain in the *left* chest, sore to touch.

**Fever:** Alternation of coldness and heat. Scarlet fever; eruptions in spots, large and vivid.

**Relationship:** Compare: *Bell., Solanum carolinense*—Horse nettle (convulsions and epilepsy, twenty to forty drop dose; is of great value in grand mal of the idiopathic type, where the disease has begun beyond age of childhood; hystero-epilepsy, also in whooping cough); *Solanum mammosum*—Apple of Sodom (pain in the left hip joint); *Solanum oleraceum* (swelling of the mammary gland with profuse secretion of milk); *Solanum tuberosum*—Potato berries (cramps in calves and contraction of fingers; spitting through closed teeth); *Solanum vesicarium* (recommended in facial paralysis); *Solaninum aceticum* (threatening paralysis of the lungs in the course of bronchitis in the aged and children must cough a long time before able to raise expectoration); *Solanum pseudocapsicum* (acute pain, in lower abdomen); *Solanum tuberosum aegrotans*—Diseased potato (prolapse of the rectum, patulous anus; offensive breath and odor of body; tumors of rectum look like decayed potato; dreams of pools of blood).

**Dose:** Second to thirtieth potency.

---

# SOLIDAGO VIRGAUREA

(Golden-rod) **Solid.**

Inhalation of the pollen has caused hemorrhage from the lungs in phthisis. *Repeated colds of tuberculosis* (2x). *Sensation of weakness,* chills alternating with heat; naso-pharyngeal catarrh, burning in the throat, pain in limbs and thoracic oppression. Pain in the region of kidneys with dysuria. *Kidneys sensitive to pressure.* Bright's disease. Hay fever when Solidago is the exciting cause. Here give 30th potency or higher.

**Eyes:** Injected, watery, burning, stinging (ophthalmia).

**Nose:** Nares irritated with abundant mucus secretion; paroxysms of sneezing.

**Stomach:** Bitter taste, especially at night; coated tongue with very scanty brown and sour urine.

**Urinary:** Scanty, reddish-brown, thick sediment, dysuria, gravel. *Difficult and scanty.* Albumen, blood and slime in urine (albuminuria, hematuria). Pain in kidneys extends forward to the abdomen and bladder (calculus) (*Berb.*). *Clear and offensive urine.* Sometimes makes the use of the catheter unnecessary.

**Female:** Uterine enlargement, organ pressed down upon the bladder. *Fibroid tumors.*

**Respiratory:** Bronchitis, cough with profuse purulent expectoration, blood streaked; oppressed breathing. Continuous dyspnea. Asthma, with nocturnal dysuria.

**Back:** Backache, due to renal congestion (*Senec.*).

**Skin:** Blotches, especially on the lower extremities; *itch.* Exanthema of lower extremities, with urinary disturbances, dropsy and threatened gangrene.

**Relationship:** *Iodoformium* 2x antidotes poison of Golden-rod. *Ars., Agrimonia eupatoria* (pain in region of kidneys).

**Dose:** Tincture to third potency. Oil of Solidago, 1 oz. to 8 oz. Alcohol. 15 drops doses to promote expectoration in bronchitis and bronchial asthma in old people (Eli G. Jones).

---

# SPARTIUM SCOPARIUM—CYSTISUS SCOPARIUS

(Broom) **Saroth.**

Spartein sulphate increases the strength of the heart, slows it and reduces the blood pressure. It continues the good effects of *Verat.* and *Dig.* without any of the undesirable effects of either (Hindale).

Spartein sulphate (the alkaloid of Broom) lowered the systolic and diastolic pressures in the provers. Sphygmograms also show a condition of lowered blood pressure. It depresses the heart by it's poisonous action on the myocardium and by its stimulating action on the vagus. This accounts for the lowered blood pressure and reduced pulse rate. It weakens the cardiac contraction. The total amount of urine is increased. The drug has, therefore, diuretic properties and is useful in dropsy.

Albuminuria. Cheyne-Stokes respiration. Irregular heart following influenza and various infections. Hypotension. Used palliatively in physiological dosage to combat arterial hypertention, arteriosclerosis. Very useful hypodermically 1/10 to 1/4 grain in sustaining the heart after stopping habit of Morphia. *Saroth.* is indicated when primarily the muscles of the heart and especially the nervous apparatus is affected. Acts rapidly and its action lasts for three to four days. Does not disturb digestion. Nephritis.

**Stomach:** Great accumulation of gas in the gastro-intestinal canal, with mental depression.

**Urinary:** Burning along the urinary tract or in pudendum. *Profuse flow of urine.*

**Heart:** Tobacco heart. Angina pectoris. Irregular action, disturbed rhythm due to gas, etc., feeble in nervous hysterical patients. Myocardial degeneration, failing compensation. Hypotension. *Saroth.* in 2 gr. doses for water logged cases, cannot lie down. Here it produces much comfort. Has a specific action on the kidneys, enabling them to eliminate and relieve the cardiac distress.

**Dose:** Homeopathically, first to third trituration.

**Non-homeopathic Uses:** (Palliative as above), one to two grains t.i.d. by mouth, exerts a definite action upon the kidneys that will enable them to relieve the distress of the heart. It is a safe drug and prompt in its action. Hypodermically, not less than ¼ of a grain. Doses as high as 2 grains by mouth, three times a day is safe (Hinsdale).

---

## SPIGELIA ANTHELMIA

(Pinkroot) **Spig.**

*Spig.* is an important remedy in pericarditis and other diseases of the heart, because the provings were conducted with the greatest regard for objective symptoms and the subjective symptoms have by innumerable confirmations, proved to be correct (C. Hering).

Has a marked elective affinity for the eye, heart and nervous system. Neuralgia of the fifth facial nerve is very prominent in its effects. Is especially adapted to anemic, debilitated, rheumatic and scrofulous subjects. Stabbing pains. Heart affections and neuralgia. *Very sensitive to touch. Parts feel chilly; send a shudder through the frame.* A remedy for symptoms due to the presence of worms. *Child refers to the navel as the most painful part* (*Gran., Nux-m.*).

**Mind:** Afraid of sharp, pointed things, pins, needles, etc.

**Head:** *Pain beneath the frontal eminence and temples, extending to the eyes* (*Onos.*). Semi-lateral, involving the left eye (migraine); pain violent, throbbing; worse, making a false step. Pain as if a band around the head (*Carb-ac., Cact., Gels.*). Vertigo, hearing exalted.

**Eyes:** Feel too large; *pressive pain on turning them* (glaucoma). Pupils dilated; photophobia; rheumatic ophthalmia. *Severe pain in and around the eyes, extending deep into the socket.* Ciliary neuralgia, a true neuritis.

**Nose:** Forepart of the nose is always dry; *discharge through the posterior nares. Chronic catarrh* with post-nasal dropping of bland mucus.

**Face:** *Prosopalgia, involving the eye, zygoma, cheek, teeth, temple,* worse, stooping, touch, from morning till sunset.

**Mouth:** Tongue fissured, painful. Tearing toothache; worse, after eating and cold. *Foul odor from the mouth* (halitosis). Offensive taste.

**Rectum:** Itching and crawling. Frequent ineffectual urging to stool. Ascarides.

**Heart:** Violent palpitations. Precordial pain and great aggravation from movement. Frequent attacks of palpitations, especially with halitosis. Pulse weak and irregular. Pericarditis with sticking pains, palpitations, dyspnea. Neuralgia extending to one arm or both arms. Angina pectoris. Craving for hot water which relieves. Rheumatic carditis, trembling pulse; entire left side sore. *Dyspnea; must lie on the right side with head high.*

**Fever:** Chilliness on the slightest motion.

**Modalities:** *Worse,* from touch, motion, noise, turning, washing, concussion. *Better,* lying on the right side with head high; inspiring.

**Relationship:** Compare: *Spigelia marylandica* (maniacal excitement, paroxysmal laughing and crying, loud, disconnected talking, vertigo, dilated pupils, congestions); *Acon., Cact., Cimic., Arn.* (*Spig.* is the chronic of *Arn.*); *Cinnb.* (supra-orbital pain); *Naja, Spong.* (heart); *Sabad., Teucr., Cina* (worm symptoms).

Antidote: *Puls.*

**Dose:** Sixth to thirtieth potency for neuralgic symptoms; second to third potency for inflammatory symptoms.

---

## SPIRAEA ULMARIA

(Hardhack) **Spirae.**

Burning and pressure in esophagus, feels contracted, but not made worse by swallowing. *Morbidly conscientious.* Relieves irritation of the urinary passages; influences the prostate gland; checks gleet and prostatorrhea; has been used for eclampsia, epilepsy and hydrophobia. Bites of mad animals. Heat in various parts. (Salicylic acid is found in *Spirae.*)

# SPIRANTHES AUTUMNALIS

(Lady's Tresses) **Spira.**

Has been used for milk flow in nursing women, lumbago and rheumatism, colic, with drowsiness and spasmodic yawning. Is an anti-phlogistic (anti-inflammatory) remedy akin to *Acon.* its symptoms show congestion and inflammation. Acidity and burning in the esophagus with eructation.

**Female:** Pruritus; vulva red; dryness and burning in the vagina. Burning pain in vagina during coition (dysparunia). Leucorrhea, bloody.

**Extremities:** Sciatic pain, especially on the right side. Pain in the shoulders. Swelling of veins of hands. Pain in all articulations of hands (rheumatism). Coldness of feet and toes.

**Fever:** Flushes of heat. Sweat on palms. Hands alternately hot and cold.

**Dose:** Third potency.

---

# SPONGIA TOSTA

(Roasted Sponge) **Spong.**

A remedy especially marked in the symptoms of the respiratory organs, cough, croup, etc. Heart affections and is often indicated for the tubercular diathesis, Children with fair complexion, lax fibre; swollen glands (adenitis). *Exhaustion and heaviness of the body after slight exertion, with orgasm of blood to chest, face. Anxiety and difficult breathing.*

**Mind:** Anxiety and fear. Every excitement increases the cough.

**Head:** Rush of blood; bursting headache; worse, forehead.

**Eyes:** Watering; gummy or mucoid discharge.

**Nose:** Fluent coryza, alternating with stoppage. Dryness; chronic, dry, nasal catarrh.

**Mouth:** Tongue dry and brown; full of vesicles.

**Throat:** Thyroid gland swollen (exopthalmic goitre). Stitches and dryness. Burning and stinging. Sore throat; worse after eating sweet things. Tickling causes cough. Clears throat constantly.

**Stomach:** Excessive thirst, *great hunger.* Cannot bear tight clothing around the trunk. Hiccough.

**Male:** *Swelling of spermatic cord and testicles, with pain and tenderness. Orchitis.* Epididymitis. Heat in parts.

**Female:** Before menses, pain in the sacrum, hunger, *palpitations. During menses,* wakes up with suffocative spells (*Cupr., Iod., Lach.*). Amenorrhea, with asthma (*Puls.*).

**Respiratory:** Great dryness of all air passages. *Hoarseness; larynx dry, burns, constricted* (laryngismus, laryngitis). Cough, *dry, barking, croupy;* larynx sensitive to touch. *Croup* (whooping cough); *worse, during inspiration and before midnight.* Respiration short, panting, *difficult; sensation of a plug in the larynx. Cough abates after eating or drinking,* especially warm drinks. The dry, chronic sympathetic cough or organic heart disease is relieved by *Spong.* (*Naja*). Irrepressible cough from a spot, deep in the chest, as if raw and sore. Chest weak; can scarcely talk. Laryngeal phthisis. Goitre with suffocative spells. Bronchial catarrh with wheezing, asthmatic cough, worse cold air, with profuse expectoration and suffocation (asthma); worse, lying with head low and in a hot room. Oppression and heat of chest, with sudden weakness.

**Heart:** Rapid and violent palpitations, with dyspnea; cannot lie down; also feels best resting in a horizontal position. *Awakened suddenly after midnight with pain and suffocation;* is flushed, hot and frightened to death (*Acon.*). Valvular insufficiency. Angina pectoris; faintness, and anxious sweat. Ebullition of blood, veins distended. *Surging of blood into the chest, as if it would force out upward.* Hypertrophy of the heart, especially right, with asthmatic symptoms.

**Sleep:** *Wakes up in a fright and feels suffocated.* Generally worse after sleep, or sleeps into an aggravation (*Lach.*).

**Fever:** *Attacks of heat with anxiety;* heat and redness of face and perspiration.

**Skin:** *Swelling and induration of glands;* also exophthalmic; cervical glands swollen with tensive pain on turning the head, painful on pressure; goitre. Itching; measles.

**Modalities:** *Worse,* ascending, wind, before midnight. *Better,* descending, lying with head low.

**Relationship:** Compare: *Acon., Hep., Brom., Lach., Merc-i-f.* (goitre).

**Dose:** Second trituration or tincture to third potency.

---

# SQUILLA MARITIMA

(Sea Onion) **Squil.**

A slow acting remedy. Corresponds to ailments requiring several days to reach their maximum. Persistent, dull, rheumatic pains permeate the body. A splenic remedy; stitches under the left free ribs. Important heart and kidney medicine. *Broncho-pneumonia.*

Acts especially on the mucous membranes of the respiratory and digestive tracts, and also upon the kidneys. Valuable in chronic bronchitis of old people with mucus rales, dyspnea and scanty urine.

**Eyes:** Feels irritable; child bores into them with fists. Sensation as if swimming in cold water.

**Stomach:** Pressure-like a stone.

**Urinary:** Great urging; *profuse watery urine. Involuntary* spurting of urine when coughing (*Caust., Puls.*).

**Respiratory:** Fluent coryza; margins of nostrils feel sore. Sneezing; throat irritated; short, dry cough; must take a deep breath. *Dyspnea, stitches in the chest* and painful contraction of abdominal muscles. *Violent,* furious, exhausting cough, with profuse mucus; salty, slimy expectoration, and with *involuntary spurting of urine and sneezing. Child rubs face with fist during cough* (*Caust., Puls.*). Cough provoked by taking a deep breath or cold drinks, from exertion, change from warm to cold air. Cough of measles. Frequent calls to micturate at night, passing large quantities (*Ph-ac.*). *Sneezing with coughing.*

**Heart:** A cardiac stimulant affecting the peripheral vessels and coronary arteries.

**Extremities:** Icy cold hands and feet, with warmth of the rest of the body (*Meny.*). Feet get sore from standing. Tender feet in shop girls.

**Skin:** Small, red spots all over the body, with a prickling pain.

**Modalities:** *Better,* rest; *worse,* motion.

**Relationship:** Compare: *Dig., Stroph-h., Apoc-h., Bry., Kali-c., Squil.* follows *Dig.,* if it fails to relieve water logged cases.

**Dose:** First to third potency.

---

# STANNUM METALLICUM

(Tin) **Stann.**

Chief action is centered upon the nervous system and respiratory organs. Debility is very marked when *Stann.* is the remedy, especially the debility of chronic bronchial and pulmonary conditions, characterized by profuse muco-purulent discharges on a tubercular base. *Talking causes a very weak feeling in the throat and chest. Pains that come and go gradually,* call unmistakably for *Stann.* Paralytic weakness; spasms; paralysis.

**Mind:** Sad, anxious. *Discouraged.* Dread of seeing people.

**Head:** Aching in temples and forehead. Obstinate acute coryza and influenza with cough. Pain worse motion; *gradually increasing and decreasing* as if constricted by a band; forehead feels as if pressed inwards. Jarring of walking resounds painfully in the head. Drawing pains in the malar bones and orbits. Ulceration of the ring hole in the lobe of ear.

**Throat:** Much adhesive mucus, difficult to detach; efforts to detach causes nausea. Throat dry and stings.

**Stomach:** Hunger. *Smell of cooking causes vomiting.* Bitter taste. Pain better pressure, but sore to touch. Sensation of *emptiness in the stomach.*

**Abdomen:** Cramp-like colic around the navel with a feeling of emptiness (worms). *Colic relieved by hard pressure.*

**Female:** *Bearing down sensation.* Prolapsus, with *a weak, sinking feeling in the stomach* (*Sep.*). *Menses early and profuse.* Pain in vagina, upward and back to the spine. Leucorrhea, with great debility.

**Respiratory:** Hoarse; mucus expelled by a forcible cough. Violent, dry cough in the evening lasting till midnight (bronchitis). Cough excited by *laughing,* singing, talking; worse lying on right side. During the day, with *copious green, sweetish,* expectoration. Chest feels sore. *Chest feels weak;* can hardly talk. Influenzal cough from noon to midnight with scanty expectoration. Respiration short, oppressive (asthma); stitches on the left side when breathing and lying on the same side. *Phthisis mucosa. Hectic fever.*

**Extremities:** Paralytic weakness; drops things. Ankles swollen. Limbs suddenly *give out when attempting to sit down.* Dizziness and weakness *when descending.* Spasmodic twitching in muscles of forearm and hand. Fingers jerk when holding a pen. Neuritis. Typewriter's paralysis.

**Sleep:** Sleeps with one leg drawn up and the other stretched out.

**Fever:** Heat in the evening; *exhausting night sweats,* especially towards morning. Hectic. Perspiration, principally on the forehead and nape of neck; debilitating; musty smelling or offensive.

**Modalities:** *Worse,* using voice (i.e., laughing, talking, singing), lying on right side, warm drinks. *Better,* coughing or expectorating, hard pressure.

**Relationship:** Complementary: *Puls.*

Compare: *Stann-i.* 3x. (valuable in chronic chest diseases characterized by plastic tissue changes. Persistent inclination to cough, excited by a tickling dry spot in the throat, apparently at the root of the tongue. Dryness of throat. Trachial and bronchial irritation of smokers. Pulmonary symptoms; cough, loud, hollow, ending with expectoration (*Phel.*). State of purulent infiltration. *Advanced* phthisis, sometimes when *Stann-i.* has not taken effect, an additional dose of *Iod.* in milk caused the drug to have its usual beneficial effect—Stonham).

Compare: *Caust., Calc., Sil., Tub., Bac., Helon. Myrtus chekan* (chronic bronchitis, cough of phthisis, emphysema, with gastric catarrhal complications and thick, yellow difficult sputum. Old people with weakened power of expectoration).

**Dose:** Third to thirtieth potency.

# STAPHYSAGRIA

(Stavesacre) **Staph.**

Nervous affections with marked irritability, diseases of the genito-urinary tract and skin, most frequently give symptoms calling for this drug. Acts on teeth and alveolar periosteum. Ill effects of anger and insults. *Sexual sins and excesses. Very sensitive.* Lacerated tissues. Pain and nervousness after extraction of teeth. Sphincters lacerated or stretched.

**Mind:** Impetuous, *violent outbursts of passion,* hypochondriacal, sad. *Very sensitive* as to what others say about her. Dwells on sexual matters; prefers solitude. Peevish. Child cries for many things, and refuses them when offered.

**Head:** Stupefying headache; passes off with yawning. Brain feels squeezed. Sensation of a ball of lead in the forehead. Itching eruption above and behind the ears (*Olnd.*).

**Eyes:** Heat in eyeballs, dims spectacles. *Recurrent styes. Chalazion* (*Platan.*). Eyes sunken, with blue rings. Margin of lids itch (blepharitis). Affections of canthi, particularly the inner. Lacerated or incised wounds of cornea. Bursting pain in eyeballs of syphilitic iritis.

**Mouth:** Toothache during menses. *Teeth black and crumbling* (caries). Salivation, spongy gums, bleed easily (scurvy) (*Merc., Kreos.*). Submaxillary glands swollen. After eating feels sleepy. Pyorrhea (*Plan.*).

**Throat:** *Stitches flying to the ear on swallowing, especially left.*

**Stomach:** Flabby and weak. Desire for stimulants. Stomach feels relaxed. *Craving for tobacco.* Canine hunger, even when stomach is full. Nausea after abdominal surgery.

**Abdomen:** Colic after anger. Hot flatus. Swollen abdomen in children with much flatus. Colic with pelvic tenesmus. *Severe pain following an abdominal surgery.* Incarcerated flatus. Diarrhea after drinking cold water, with tenesmus. *Constipation* (2 drops of tincture at night and in the morning), hemorrhoids with an enlarged prostate.

**Urinary:** *Cystocele* (locally and internally). Cystitis in lying-in patients. Ineffectual urging to micturate in *newly married* women. Pressure upon the bladder; feels as if it did not empty. *Sensation as if a drop of urine was continuously rolling along the channel.* Burning in urethra during micturition. Prostatic problems; frequent micturition, burning in the urethra *when not micturating* (urethritis) (*Thuj., Sabal, Ferr-pic.*). Urging and pain *after* micturating. Pain after lithotomy.

**Male:** Especially after self abuse; persistent dwelling on sexual subjects. Spermatorrhea, with sunken features; guilty look; emissions, with backache, weakness and sexual neurasthenia. Dyspnea after coition.

**Female:** *Parts very sensitive* (nymphomania), worse sitting down (*Berb., Kreos.*). *Irritable bladder in young married women.* Leucorrhea. Prolapsus, with sinking in the abdomen; aching around the hips.

**Extremities:** Muscles, especially of calves, feel bruised. *Backache; worse in morning before rising.* Extremities feel beaten and painful. Joints stiff. *Crural neuralgia.* Dull aching of nates extending to the hip joint and lumbosacral region.

**Skin:** Eczema of head, ears, face and body; thick scabs, dry and itch violently; *scratching changes location of itching.* Fig warts pedunculated (*Thuj.*). Arthritic nodes. Inflammation of phalanges (rheumatism). Night sweats.

**Modalities:** Worse, anger, indignation, grief, mortification, loss of fluids, onanism, sexual excesses, tobacco: least touch on affected parts. *Better,* after breakfast, warmth, rest at night.

**Relationship:** Inimical: *Ran-b.*

Complementary: *Caust., Coloc.*

Compare: *Ferrum pyrophosphoricum* (tarsal cysts); *Coloc., Caust., Ign., Ph-ac., Calad.*

Antidote: *Camph.*

**Dose:** Third to thirtieth potency.

---

# STELLARIA MEDIA

(Chickweed) **Stell.**

Induces a condition of stasis, congestion and sluggishness of all functions. Morning aggravation.

Sharp, *shifting,* rheumatic pain in all parts very pronounced. *Rheumatism;* darting pain in almost every part; stiffness of joints; parts sore to touch; worse, motion. *Chronic rheumatism. Shifting pains* (*Puls., Kali-s.*). Psoriasis. Enlarged and inflamed gouty finger joints.

**Head:** General irritability. Lassitude, indisposition to work. Dull, frontal headache; worse in the morning and on the left side with sleepiness. Neck muscles stiff and sore.

**Eyes:** Smarting and burning in eyes, feel protruded.

**Abdomen:** *Liver engorged, swollen, with stitching pain and sensitive to pressure.* Clay colored stools (jaundice). Hepatic torpor. Constipation or alternating constipation and diarrhea.

**Extremities:** Rheumatoid pains in different parts of the body. Sharp pain in the small of back, over the kidneys, in the gluteal region, extending down the thigh. Pain in shoulders and arms. *Synovitis.* Bruised feeling. Rheumatic pain in calves of legs.

**Modalities:** *Worse,* mornings, warmth, tobacco. *Better,* evenings, cold air, motion.

**Relationship:** Compare: *Puls.* (similar in rheumatism, pains shifting, worse rest, warmth; better cold air).

**Dose:** Tincture, externally. Internally, 2x potency.

---

# STICTA PULMONARIA

(Lungwort) **Stict.**

Offers a set of symptoms like coryza, bronchial catarrh and influenza, together with nervous and *rheumatic* disturbances. There is a general feeling of dullness and malaise, as when a cold is coming on; dull, heavy pressure in the forehead, catarrhal conjunctivitis, etc. *Rheumatic stiffness of the neck* (cervical spondylosis).

**Mind:** *Feels as if floating in air* (*Dat-a., Lac-c.*). Confusion of ideas; *patient must talk.*

**Head:** Dull headache, with a dull heavy pressure in the forehead and *root of nose. Catarrhal headache before discharge appears.* Burning in eyes and soreness of balls. Sensation as if the scalp was too small. Burning in the eyelids.

**Nose:** *Sensation of fullness at the root of the nose* (*Nux-v.*). Atrophic rhinitis (*Calc-f.*). *Dryness of nasal membrane. Constant need to blow the nose, but no discharge.* Dry scabs, especially in the evening and at night. *Hay fever;* incessant sneezing (*Sabad.*).

**Abdomen:** Diarrhea; stools profuse, frothy; worse, morning.

**Urinary:** Urine increased, with soreness and aching in bladder.

**Female:** Scanty flow of milk (agalactia).

**Respiratory:** Throat raw; dropping of mucus posteriorly. *Dry, hacking cough at night; worse, inspiration* (bronchitis). Tracheitis, facilitates expectoration. Loose cough in the morning. Pain through the chest from the sternum to the spinal column (angina pectoris). Cough after measles (*Sang.*); *worse towards evening and when tired. Pulsations from the right side of sternum, down to the abdomen.*

**Extremities:** Rheumatic pain in the right shoulder joint, deltoid and biceps. Swelling, heat, redness of joints. *Spot of inflammation and redness over affected joint.* Pain severe and drawing. Chorea-like spasms; legs feel as if floating in air. *Housemaid's knee* (*Rhus-t., Kali-i., Slag*). Shooting pain in knees. Joints and neighboring muscles red, swollen, painful. Rheumatic pains precede catarrhal symptoms.

**Modalities:** *Worse,* sudden changes in temperature.

**Relationship:** Compare: *Dat-a., Bougmanica* (cannot concentrate on thoughts; brain floats in thousands of problems and grand ideas. Floating sensation, as if ideas were floating outside of brain. Headache, heartburn. Burning sensation around the cardiac end of stomach, extending to the esophagus with a sense of constriction. Heat and fullness over the liver region). *Cetraria*—Iceland moss (chronic diarrhea, phthisis, hemoptysis. Is used as a decoction and boiled with milk as an expectorant and nutrient in bronchorrhea, catarrh, etc.). Also compare: *Eryngium, Dros., Still., Rumx., Samb.*

**Dose:** Tincture to sixth potency.

---

## STIGMATA MAYDIS—ZEA MAYDIS

(Corn-silk) **Stigm.**

Has marked urinary symptoms, and has been used with success in organic heart disease, with marked edema of the lower extremities and scanty micturition. Enlarged prostate and retention of urine. Uric and phosphatic diathesis. Gonorrhea. Cystitis.

**Urinary:** Suppression and *retention.* Dysuria. Renal lithiasis; nephritic colic; blood and red sand in urine (hematuria). Tenesmus after micturating. Vesical catarrh. Gonorrhea. Cystitis.

**Relationship:** Compare: *Shucks* (as a decoction used for chronic malaria, teaspoonful doses freely. Dr. E.C. Lowe, England).

**Dose:** Tincture in ten to fifty drop doses.

---

## STILLINGIA SILVATICA

(Queen's Root) **Still.**

Chronic periosteal rheumatism, syphilitic and scrofulous affections. Respiratory symptoms well marked. Torpor of lymphatics; torpid liver with jaundice and constipation.

**Mind:** *Gloomy forebodings;* depressed.

**Urinary:** Urine colorless. *Deposits white sediment;* urine milky and thick.

**Respiratory:** Dry, spasmodic cough. Larynx constricted with stinging in the fauces. Trachea feels sore when pressed. *Hoarseness* and chronic laryngeal affections in public speakers.

**Extremities:** Aching pains in *bones* of extremities and back.

**Skin:** Ulcers; chronic eruptions on hands and fingers. *Enlarged cervical glands.* Burning, itching of legs; worse, exposure to air. Exostosis.

Scrofuloderma; syphilis, secondary eruption and later symptoms. Valuable for intercurrent use.

**Modalities:** *Worse,* in the afternoon, damp air, motion. *Better,* in the morning, dry air.

**Relationship:** Compare: *Staph., Merc., Syph., Aur., Cory.* (syphilitic nodes).

**Dose:** Tincture and first potency.

---

## STRAMONIUM

(Thorn-apple) **Stram.**

The entire force of this drug seems to be expended on the brain, though the skin and throat show some disturbance. Suppressed secretions and excretions. Sensation as if limbs were separated from the body. Delirium tremens. Absence of pain and muscular mobility especially in muscles of expression and of locomotion. Gyratory and graceful motions. Parkinsonism.

**Mind:** *Devout, earnest, beseeching and ceaseless talking.* Loquacious, garrulous, laughing, singing, swearing, praying, rhyming. Sees ghosts, hears voices, talks with spirits. Rapid changes from joy to sadness. Violent and lewd. Delusions about his identity; thinks himself to be tall, double, as if a part is missing. Religious mania. Cannot bear solitude or darkness; *must have light and company.* Sight of water or anything glittering brings on spasms (hydrophobia). Delirium, with a desire to escape (*Bell., Bry., Rhus-t.*).

**Head:** *Raises head frequently from the pillow.* Pain in the forehead and over the eyebrows, beginning at 9 a.m., worse until noon. Boring pain, preceded by obscure vision. Rush of blood to head; staggers, with a tendency to fall forward and to the left. Auditory hallucinations.

**Eyes:** Seem prominent, *staring wide open;* pupils dilated (meningitis). Loss of vision; complains that it is dark, *and calls for light. Small objects look large.* Parts of the body seem enormously swollen. Strabismus. All objects look black.

**Face:** Hot, red; circumscribed redness of cheeks. Blood rushes to the face; distorted (epilepsy). *Expression of terror.* Pale face.

**Mouth:** Dry; dribbling of viscid saliva. Aversion to water. *Stammering.* Risus sardonicus. Cannot swallow on account of spasm. Chewing motion.

**Stomach:** Food tastes like straw. Violent thirst. Vomiting of mucus and *green* bile.

**Urinary:** *Suppression,* bladder empty.

**Male:** *Sexual erethism,* with indecent speech and action. Hands constantly on the genitals.

**Female:** *Metrorrhagia,* with *loquacity, singing,* praying. Puerperal mania, with characteristic mental symptoms and profuse sweatings. Convulsions after labor.

**Extremities:** *Graceful, rhythmic motions.* Convulsions of upper extremities and of isolated groups of muscles. *Chorea;* spasms partial, constantly changing (tetanus, trismus). *Violent pain in left hip.* Trembling, twitching of tendons, staggering gait (locomotor ataxia).

**Sleep:** Awakens terrified; screams with fright. Deep snoring sleep. Sleepy but cannot sleep (*Bell.*).

**Fever:** Profuse sweat, which does not relieve. Violent fever.

**Skin:** Shining red flash. *Effects of suppressed eruptions in scarlatina* with delirium, etc.

**Modalities:** *Worse,* in dark room, when alone, looking at bright or shining objects, after sleep, on swallowing. *Better,* from bright light, company, warmth.

**Relationship:** Compare especially: *Hyos.* and *Bell.* It has less fever than *Bell.*, but more than *Hyos.* It causes more functional excitement of the brain, but never approaches the true inflammatory condition of *Bell.*

Antidotes: *Bell., Tab., Nux-v.*

**Dose:** Thirtieth potency and lower.

---

# STRONTIUM CARBONICUM

(Carbonate of Strontia) **Stront-c.**

Rheumatic pains, chronic sprains, stenosis of esophagus. Pains make patient faint or sick all over. Chronic *sequelae of hemorrhages,* after surgery with much oozing of blood, coldness and prostration. Arteriosclerosis. High blood pressure with a flushed face, pulsating arteries and threatened apoplexy. Violent involuntary starts. Affections of bones, especially femur. Restlessness at night, smothering feeling. *For shock after surgery. Neuritis,* great sensitiveness to cold.

**Head:** *Vertigo with headache and nausea.* Distensive pressure. Aches from nape of neck, spreading upwards; better wrapping the head up warmly (*Sil.*). Flushes in the face; violent pulsating pain. Supraorbital neuralgia; pain increases and decreases slowly (*Stann.*). Face red; burns, itches.

**Eyes:** Burning and hyperemia of eyes. Pain and lachrymation on using eyes (asthenopia), with dancing and chromatic alterations of objects looked at.

**Nose:** Bloody crusts in nose. Itching, redness and burning of nose.

**Stomach:** Loss of appetite, aversion to meat, craves bread and beer. Food tasteless. Eructations after eating. Hiccough causes chest pains; cardialgia.

**Abdomen:** Sticking pain in the abdominal ring. Uncomfortable fullness and swelling of abdomen (flatulence).

**Rectum:** Diarrhea; *worse at night; continuous urging;* better towards morning. Burning in the anus lasts a long time after stool (*Rat.*).

**Extremities:** Sciatica with edema of the ankle. Rheumatic pain in the right shoulder. Rheumatism with diarrhea. Gnawing as if in the marrow of bones. Cramps in calves and soles. *Chronic* spasms, particularly of the ankle joint. Edematous swelling. Icy cold feet. Rheumatic pains, especially in joints. Veins of hands engorged (varicose veins).

**Fever:** Heat, with an aversion to uncover or undress.

**Skin:** Moist, itching, burning eruption; better in open air, especially warm sunshine. *Sprains of ankle joint, with edema.* Violent perspiration at night.

**Modalities:** *Better* immersing in *hot water; worse,* change of weather; from being quiet; when beginning to move; great sensitiveness to cold.

**Relationship:** Compare: *Arn., Ruta, Sil., Bar-c., Carb-v., Stront-i.* (arteriosclerosis). *Stront-br.* (often gives excellent results where a bromide is indicated. Vomiting of pregnancy. Nervous dyspepsia. It is anti-fermentative and neutralizes excessive acidity). *Stront-n.* (morbid cravings; headache and eczema behind ears).

**Dose:** Sixth trituration and thirtieth potency.

---

# STROPHANTHUS HISPIDUS

(Kombe Seed) **Stroph-h.**

*Stroph-h.* is a muscle poison; it increases the contractile power of all striped muscles. Acts on the heart, *increasing the systole and diminishes the rapidity.* Maybe used with advantage to tone the heart, and run off dropsical accumulations. In small doses for a weak heart; it feels enlarged. In mitral regurgitation, where edema and dropsy have supervened (*Dig.*). *Stroph-h.* occasions no gastric distress, has no cumulative effects, is a greater diuretic and is safer for the aged, as it does not affect the vasomotors. In pneumonia and in severe prostration from hemorrhage after surgery and acute diseases. After a long use of stimulants; *irritable heart* of tobacco smokers. Arteriosclerosis; rigid arteries of aged. Restores tone to *brittle* tissues, especially of the heart muscle and valves. Especially useful in failing compensation dependent upon a fatty heart. *Hives.* Anemia with palpitations and breathlessness. Exophthalmic goitre. Corpulent people.

**Head:** Temporal pain with diplopia, impaired vision; brilliant eyes and a flushed face. Senile vertigo.

**Stomach:** Nausea with a special disgust for alcohol and thus aids in the treatment of dipsomania. Seven drops of tincture.

**Urinary:** Increased secretion; scanty and albuminous.

**Female:** Menorrhagia; uterine hemorrhage; uterus heavily congested. Aching pain through hips and thighs during climacteric.

**Respiratory:** *Dyspnea,* especially on ascending. Lungs congested. Edema of lungs. Bronchial and cardiac asthma.

**Heart:** Pulse quickened. Heart's action is weak, rapid, irregular, due to muscular *debility;* and *insufficiency.* Cardiac pain (angina pectoris).

**Extremities:** Swollen, dropsical. Anasarca.

**Skin:** Urticaria, especially the more chronic forms.

**Relationship:** Compare: *Dig.* (but is slower than *Stroph-h.* in its action); *Ph-ac.* (weak heart, irregular pulse, fluttering sensation in the cardiac region, palpitations during sleep, fainting).

**Dose:** Tincture and 6x potency. In more acute cases, five to ten drops of the tincture, three times a day.

---

## STRYCHNINUM PURUM

(Alkaloid of Nux Vomica) **Stry.**

Its primary function is to stimulate the motor centers and the reflex action of the spinal cord. Homeopathic to spasms of muscles, cramps from an undue reflex excitability of the cord, spasms of the bladder, etc. *Stry.* stimulates the central nervous system, mental activities and the special senses are rendered more acute. Respiration increased. All reflexes are made more active. Stiffness in muscles, face and neck. Opisthotonos. Tetanic convulsions with opisthotonos. The muscles relax between paroxysms; worse slightest touch, sound, odor. Influences the spinal cord more directly and is less appropriate in visceral derangements than *Nux-v. Tetanus.* Explosive nervousness. Pain and sensations come *suddenly* and return at *intervals.*

**Head:** Restless. *Over irritability.* Full and bursting headache, with heat in eyes. Vertigo, with roaring in ears. Jerking of head forward. Scalp sore. Itching of scalp and nape.

**Eyes:** Hot, painful, protruding (expohthalmos), staring. Pupils dilated. Sparks before eyes. Spasmodic contraction of ocular muscles; trembling of lids (chorea).

**Ears:** Hearing very acute; burning, itching and roaring

**Face:** Pale, anxious, livid. Jaws stiffened; lower jaw spasmodically closed (tetnus).

**Throat:** Dry, contracted; sensation of a lump. Deglutition impossible. Burning along the oesophgus with spasms of the esophagus. Violent itching in the roof of mouth.

**Stomach:** Constant retching. Violent vomiting. Nausea of pregnancy.

**Abdomen:** Sharp pain in abdominal muscles, gripping pain in bowels.

**Rectum:** Feces discharged involuntarily during spasms. Very obstinate constipation.

**Female:** Desire for coitus (*Canth., Camph., Fl-ac., Lach., Phos., Plat.*). Any touch on the body excites a voluptuous sensation (nymphomania).

**Respiratory:** *Spasm of muscles* around the larynx. Excessive dyspnea. Sharp, contractive pains in muscles of chest. Persistent cough, recurring after influenza.

**Back:** *Rigidity of cervical muscles.* Sharp pains in the nape and down the spine. *Back stiff;* violent jerks in the spinal column. *Icy sensation down the spine.*

**Extremities:** Limbs stiff. Rheumatism with stiff joints. *Violent jerking* (athetosis), *twitching, and trembling* (chorea). Tetanic convulsions and opisthotonos; spasms provoked by the slightest touch and by any attempt to move. Shocks in the muscles. *Cramp-like pains.*

**Fever:** Cold chills flowing down the spine. Perspiration in a stream down head and chest. Lower extremities cold.

**Skin:** Itching in the whole body, especially nose. Icy sensation down the spine.

**Modalities:** *Worse,* morning; touch; noise; motion: after meals. *Better,* lying on the back.

**Relationship:** Compare: *Eucalyptus globulus* (neutralizes ill effects *of Stry*). *Strychninum arsenicosum* (paresis in the aged, relaxed musculature. Prostration. Psoriasis; chronic diarrhea with paralytic symptoms; compensatory hypertrophy of heart with beginning of fatty degeneration; marked dyspnea on lying down; edema of lower extremities, urine scanty, high specific gravity, heavily loaded with glucose. Diabetes. 6x trituraton). *Strychnini et ferri citras* (chlorotic and paralytic conditions; dyspepsia with vomiting of ingesta; 2x and 3x trituration); *Strychninum nitricum* (2x and 3x. Said to remove craving for alcohol. Use for weeks); *Strychninum sulphuricum* (gastric atony); *Strychninum valerianicum* (exhaustion of brain power: women of high nervous erethism).

**Non-homeopathic Uses:** To produce its direct physiological effects in paralysis, the dose will range from one-fiftieth to one-twentieth of a grain, repeated three times a day. Under twelve years of age, fiftieth to one two-hundredth of a grain. *Stry.*, hypodermically, is capable of arresting progressive muscular atrophy, is a stimulant to the respiratory centers and is useful in embarrassed breathing, in the course of pneumonia especially. Is an antidote to *Chlol.*, used in asphyxia from gas and chloroform and early stages of opium poisoning. Dose one one-hundredth to one-sixtieth grain every three hours.

**Dose:** Third to thirtieth potency.

---

## STRYCHNINUM PHOSPHORICUM

(Phosphate of Strychnin) **Stry-p.**

This drug acts through the cerebro-spinal system upon muscles, causing twitching, stiffness, weakness and loss of power; upon circulation, producing irregularity of pulse, and upon the mind, producing lack of control, *an uncontrollable desire to laugh* and disinclination to use the brain. Very irregular pulse. Tachycardia. Rapid and weak pulse. Useful in chorea, hysteria, acute asthenia after acute fevers. Symptoms *worse* motion, *better* rest and in open air. An excellent remedy in anemia of spinal cord; paralysis (paraplegia, hemiplegia); burning, aching, and weakness of spine (locomotor ataxia); pain extends to the front of chest; tenderness on pressure in the mid-dorsal region; cold, clammy feet; hands and *axillae covered with clammy perspiration.* Atelectasis and break in the compensation of a hypertrophied heart; beginning of fatty degeneration of the heart muscle (Royal).

**Dose:** Third trituration.

---

## SUCCINUM

(Electron, Amber—A Fossil Resin) **Succ.**

Nervous and hysterical symptoms. Asthma. Affections of spleen.

**Head:** Fear of trains and closed places. Headache, lachrymation, sneezing.

**Respiratory:** Asthma, incipient phthisis, chronic bronchitis, pains in chest. Whooping cough.

**Relationship:** Compare: Do not confound with *Ambr. Succinicum acidum* (hay fever. Paroxysmal sneezing, dropping of watery mucus from nostrils; asthma. Inflammation through respiratory tract; causing asthma, chest pains, etc., itching of eyelids, canthi and nose worse drafts. Use 6 to 30th potency).

Compare: *Arund., Wye., Sabad., Sin-n.*

**Dose:** Third trituration. Five drop doses of the oil.

---

# SULFONALUM

(A Coal Tar Product) **Sulfon.**

Vertigo of cerebral origin, cerebellar disease, ataxic symptoms and chorea, present a field for the homeopathic employment of this drug. *Profound weakness,* all gone, faint feeling and despondency. Loss of control of sphincters. Muscular inco-ordination.

**Mind:** Mental confusion, incoherency, illusions; apathetic. *Alternation of happy, hopeful states with depression and weakness.* Extreme irritability.

**Head:** Dropsy, stupid; pain on attempting to raise head. Vertigo, unable to rise.

**Eyes:** Diplopia. *Eyes bloodshot and restless. Ptosis.*

**Ears:** Tinnitus.

**Mouth:** Aphasia; *tongue as if paralysed.* Dysphagia.

**Urinary:** Albuminuria with casts. Scanty. Pink color. Constant desire to micturate; scanty, brownish-red. Hematoporphyrinuria.

**Respiratory:** Congestion of lungs; stertorous breathing. Sighing dyspnea.

**Extremities:** Ataxic movements, *staggering gait* (locomotor ataxia); cold, weak, trembling; legs seem too heavy. Extreme restlessness; muscular twitchings (chorea). Knee jerks disappear. Stiffness and paralysis of both legs (paraplegia). Anesthesia of legs.

**Sleep:** Fidgety, wakeful, drowsy. Insomnia.

**Skin:** Itching, bluish purpura. Erythema.

**Relationship:** *Trional* (insomnia associated with physical excitement; vertigo, loss of equilibrium, ataxia, nausea, vomiting, diarrhea, stertorous breathing, cyanosis, tinnitus, hallucinations).

**Non-homeopathic Uses:** As a hypnotic. Dose, ten to thirty grains in hot water. Takes about two hours to act.

**Dose:** Third trituration.

---

# SULPHUR

(Sublimated Sulphur) **Sulph.**

This is the great Hahnemannian anti-psoric. Its action is centrifugal, from within outward having an elective affinity for the skin, where it produces heat and *burning* with itching; worse by heat of bed. Inertia and relaxation of fibre; hence feebleness of tone characterizes its symptoms. *Ebullitions of heat, dislike for water, dry and hard hair and skin, red orifices, sinking feeling in the stomach around* 11 a.m., *and cat-nap sleep;* always indicate *Sulphur* homeopathically.

*Standing* is the worst position for *Sulphur* patients, it is always uncomfortable. Dirty, filthy people, prone to skin affections. Aversion to being washed. *When carefully selected remedies fail to act, especially in acute diseases,* it frequently arouses the reacting powers of the organism. *Complaints that relapse. General offensive character of discharges and exhalations.* Extremely red lips and face, flushing easily. Often of great use in beginning the treatment of chronic cases and in finishing acute ones.

**Mind:** Very forgetful. Difficulty, in thinking. Delusions; thinks rags are beautiful things; that he is immensely wealthy. Busy all the time. Childish peevishness in grown people. Irritable. Affections vitiated; *very selfish,* no regard for others. Religious melancholy. Averse to business; loafs; too lazy to arouse himself. Imagines giving wrong things to people, causing their death. *Sulphur* subjects are nearly always irritable, depressed, thin and weak, even with a good appetite.

**Head:** Constant *heat on top of the head* (*Cupr-s., Graph.*). Heaviness and fullness, pressure in the temples. Throbbing headache (meningitis); worse, stooping, with vertigo. Sick headache, recurring periodically. Tinea capitis, dry form. *Scalp dry,* falling of hair; worse, washing. *Itching; scratching causes burning.*

**Eyes:** *Burning* ulceration on the margin of lids (ulcerative blepharitis). Halo around lamp light. Heat and *burning in eyes* (*Ars., Bell.*). Black motes before eyes. First stage of corneal ulceration. Chronic ophthalmia with severe burning and itching. Parenchymatous keratitis. Cornea like ground glass.

**Ears:** Whizzing in ears (tinnitus). Bad effects from the suppression of otorrhea. Oversensitive to odors. Deafness, preceded by exceedingly sensitive hearing; catarrhal deafness.

**Nose:** Herpes across the nose. Nose stuffed indoors. Imaginary foul smells. *Alae red and scabby. Chronic dry catarrh; dry scabs and readily bleeding.* Polypus and adenoids.

**Mouth:** Lips dry, *bright red,* burning. *Bitter taste* in the morning. Jerks through teeth. Swelling of gums; throbbing pain. Tongue white, with a red tip and borders (stomatitis).

**Throat:** Pressure, as if from a lump, from a splinter, or of a hair. Burning, redness and dryness. A ball seems to rise and close the pharynx (globus hystericus).

**Stomach:** Complete loss of, or excessive appetite. Putrid eructation. Food tastes too salty. Drinks a lot, eats little. *Milk disagrees.* Great desire for sweets (*Arg-n.*). *Great acidity,* sour eructation. Burning, painful, weight-like pressure. *Very weak and faint around* 11 a.m., must have something to eat. Nausea during gestation. Water fills the patient up.

**Abdomen:** Very sensitive to pressure; sensation of rawness and soreness internally. Movements as if something alive in the abdomen (*Croc., Thuj.*). Pain and soreness over the liver region (jaundice). Colic after drinking.

**Rectum:** Itching and burning in the anus; piles dependent on abdominal plethora. Frequent, unsuccessful desire; hard, knotty, insufficient. Child afraid, on account of pain. *Redness around the anus* with itching. *Morning diarrhea, painless, drives him out of bed* with prolapsus recti. Hemorrhoids, oozing and belching

**Urinary:** Frequent micturition, especially at night. *Enuresis,* especially in scrofulous, untidy children. Burning in urethra during micturition, lasts long after (urethritis). Mucus and pus in urine; *parts sore over which it passes* (Bright's disease). *Must hurry,* sudden call to micturate. *Great quantities of colorless urine.*

**Male:** Stitches in the penis. Involuntary emissions. Itching in genitals when going to bed. Organs cold, relaxed and powerless (impotence).

**Female:** Pudenda *itches. Vagina burns.* Profuse offensive perspiration. Menses too late, short, scanty and difficult; thick, black, *acrid, making parts sore.* Menses preceded by headache. Leucorrhea, burning, excoriating. Nipples cracked; smart and burn.

**Respiratory:** Oppression and burning sensation in chest. *Difficult respiration; wants windows open.* Aphonia. Sensation of heat throughout the chest. Red, brown spots all over the chest. Loose cough (bronchitis); worse talking, morning, greenish, purulent, sweetish expectoration. *Much rattling of mucus* (pneumonia). Chest feels heavy; stitches, heart feels too large and palpitating. *Pleuritic exudations.* Use *Tinctura Sulphuris.* Stitching pains extending to the back, worse lying on back or breathing deeply (pleurisy). Flushes of heat in the chest, rising to the head. *Oppression, as if a load was put on the chest. Dyspnea* in the middle of the night, relieved by sitting up (asthma, hydrothorax). *Pulse more rapid in the morning* than in the evening.

**Back:** Drawing pain between shoulders. Stiffness of nape. Sensation as if vertebrae glided over each other

**Extremities:** Trembling of hands. *Hot, sweaty hands.* Rheumatic pain in left shoulder. Heaviness; paretic feeling. Rheumatic gout, with itching. *Burning in soles and hands at night.* Sweat in armpits, smelling like garlic. Drawing and tearing in arms and hands. Stiffness of knees and ankles. Cannot walk erect; *stoop shouldered.* Ganglion.

**Sleep:** Talks, jerks and twitches during sleep. Vivid dreams. Wakes up singing. Wakes up frequently and becomes wide awake suddenly. *Catnaps;* slightest noise awakens. Cannot sleep between 2 and 5 a.m.

**Fever:** *Frequent flashes of heat. Violent ebullitions of heat throughout the entire body.* Dry skin and great thirst. Night sweat on the nape and occiput. Perspiration of single parts. Disgusting sweats. Remittent type.

**Skin:** *Dry, scaly, unhealthy; every little injury suppurates.* Freckles. *Itching, burning; worse scratching and washing.* Pimply eruption, pustules, rhagades, hang-nails. Excoriation, especially in folds (*Lyc.*). Sensation of a band around the bones. Skin affections after local medication. *Pruritus,* especially from warmth, in the evening, often recurs in springtime, in damp weather.

**Modalities:** *Worse,* at rest, when standing, *warmth of bed,* washing, bathing in the morning, 11 a.m., night, from alcoholic stimulants, periodically. *Better, dry, warm weather,* lying on the right side, from drawing up the affected limbs.

**Relationship:** Complementary: *Aloe; Psor., Acon., Pyrarara* (a fish caught in the Amazon, clinically used for various skin affections). Lepra, tuberculides, syphilides, varicosities, etc.

Compare: *Acon.* (*Sulph.* often follows in acute diseases); *Merc.* and *Calc.* are frequently useful *after Sulphur,* not before. *Lyc., Sep., Sars., Puls., Sulphur hydrogenisatum* (delirium, mania, asphyxia); *Sulphur terebinthinatum* (chronic rheumatic arthritis; chorea); *Tannicum acidum* (nasal hemorrhage; elongated uvula; gargle; constipation). *Magnes artificialis* (great hunger in the evening, profuse sweat on face, bruised pain in joints, rectal constriction after stool).

*Magnetis polus articus* (anxious, *coldness of eyes as if a piece ice lay in the orbit,* increased flow of saliva, constipation, sopor, trembling, abdominal flatulence).

*Magnetis polus australis* (dryness of lids, easy dislocation of ankle, *ingrowing toe nails,* aching in patella, shooting in soles).

Compare in adenoids: *Agraphis nutans.*

**Dose:** Acts in all potencies from the lowest to the highest. Some of the best results are obtained from the higher and not too frequent doses. The twelfth potency is a good one to begin treatment with, going higher or lower according to the susceptibility of the patient. In chronic diseases, 200th and upward. In *torpid* eruptions the *lowest* potencies.

---

## SULPHUR IODATUM

(Iodide of Sulphur) **Sul-i.**

Obstinate skin affections, notably in *barber's itch* and *hyperemia.* Weeping eczema.

**Throat:** Uvula and tonsils enlarged and reddened. Swollen. Tongue thick. Parotid hypertropied (parotiditis).

**Skin:** Itching on ears, nose, and in the urethra. Papular eruption on the face. Cold sores on lips. Boils on the neck. Barber's itch. *Acne.* Lichen planus. Arms covered with an itching rash. Hair feels as if erect.

**Dose:** Third trituration.

# SULPHURICUM ACIDUM

(Sulphuric Acid) **Sul-ac.**

The "debility" common to acids shows itself here, especially in the digestive tract, giving a very relaxed feeling in the stomach with a craving for stimulants. *Tremor and weakness;* everything must be done in a hurry. *Hot flushes,* followed by perspiration with trembling. Tendency to gangrene following mechanical injuries. Writer's cramp. Lead poisoning. Gastralgia and hypochlorhydria. Purpura hemorrhagica.

**Mind:** Fretful, impatient. Unwilling to answer questions; hurried.

**Head:** Right sided neuralgia (migraine); painful shocks; skin feels pinched. Sensation as if the brain was loose in the forehead and falling from side to side (*Bell., Rhus-t.*). Concussion of brain where skin is cold, body bathed in cold sweat. Compressive pain in the side of occiput; *relieved by holding the hands near the head.* Pain of outer parts, as if there were subcutaneous ulcers; painful to touch. *Thrust in right temple as if a plug was pressed in.*

**Eyes:** Intra-ocular hemorrhage following traumatism. Great chemosis with aching and sharp pain.

**Mouth:** Aphthae; gums bleed readily (scorbutic). Halitosis. Pyorrhea.

**Stomach:** Heartburn; *sour eructations; sets teeth on edge* (*Rob.*). *Craving for alcohol. Water causes coldness of the stomach;* must be mixed with liquors. *Relaxed feeling in the stomach.* Averse to the smell of coffee. Sour vomiting. Desire for fresh food. *Hiccough.* Coldness in the stomach relieved by applied heat. Nausea with chilliness.

**Abdomen:** Weak feeling, with a dragging sensation in the hips and lumboscral region. *Sensation as if the hernia would protrude,* especially left side.

**Rectum:** Piles; oozing dampness. Rectum feels as if it had a big ball. Diarrhea, fetid, black, with sour odor of the body and an empty faint feeling in the abdomen.

**Female:** Menstruation early and profuse. Erosion of the cervix in the aged; easily bleeding. Acrid, burning leucorrhea, often with bloody mucus.

**Respiratory:** Respiration rapid with shooting in the cervical muscles and movement of alae nasi; *larynx moves up and down violently.* Bronchitis in children with a short, teasing cough.

**Extremities:** Cramp-like paralytic contraction in arms, hands; jerking of fingers while writing.

**Skin:** Bad effects from mechanical injuries with bruises and livid skin. Ecchymosis. Petechiae, *Purpura hemorrhagica.* Livid, red, itchy blotches. Hemorrhage of black blood from all outlets. Cicatrices turn red and blue and become painful. Chilblains with a gangrenous tendency. Carbuncles, boils and other staphylococcal and streptococcal infections.

**Modalities:** *Worse,* from excess of heat or cold, in the forenoon and evening. *Better,* from warmth, and lying on the affected side.

**Relationship:** Complementary: *Puls.*

Compare: *Arn., Calen., Led., Sep., Calc.*

**Dose:** *Sul-ac.* mixed with three parts of alcohol, ten to fifteen drops three times daily for several weeks, has been successfully used to subdue the craving for liquor. For homeopathic purposes, second to thirtieth potency.

---

## SULPHUROSUM ACIDUM

(Sulphurous Acid, $H_2SO_3$) **Sulo-ac.**

*Sulphurous acid,* tonsillitis (as a spray), acne rosacea, *ulcerative stomatitis,* pityriasis versicolor.

**Head:** Anxious, furious, disposed to fight. Headache better by vomiting. Ringing in ears.

**Mouth:** Ulcerative inflammation of mouth. Tongue red or bluish-red. Coated.

**Stomach:** Loss of appetite. Obstinate constipation.

**Female:** Fluor albus (leucorrhea). Debility.

**Respiratory:** Persistent choking cough with copious expectoration. Hoarseness, constriction of chest. Difficult breathing.

**Dose:** As a spray in tonsillitis. According to Ringer, ten to fifteen minims taken ten minutes before each meal will remedy pyrosis and prevent fermentation and flatulence. It also removes thrush. Homeopathically, third attenuation.

---

## SUMBULUS MOSCHATUS— FERULA SUMBUL

(Musk-root) **Sumb.**

Has many hysterical and nervous symptoms and is of use in neuralgic affections and anomalous, functional, cardiac disorders. *Numbness on becoming cold.* Numbness of the left side. *Insomnia* of delirium tremens (fifteen drops of tincture). Sensation as if water was dropping down the spine. Asthma. A tissue remedy for sclerosed arteries.

**Head:** Emotional and fidgety. Dull in the morning, clear in the evening. Mistakes in writing and adding. Comedones.

**Nose:** Tenacious, yellow mucus in the nose.

**Throat:** Choking constriction; constant swallowing. Belching of gas from the stomach. Spasm of pharyngeal muscles. Tenacious mucus in the throat.

**Urinary:** *Oily pellicle on the surface of urine.*

**Female:** Ovarian neuralgia. *Abdomen full, distended and painful.* Climacteric flushes.

**Heart:** *Nervous palpitations.* Neuralgia around the left breast and left hypochondrial region (angina pectoris). *Cardiac asthma.* Aching in the left arm, heavy, numb and weary. Loses breath on slightest exertion. Pulse irregular.

**Modalities:** *Worse,* active exercise; left side.

**Relationship:** Compare: *Asaf., Mosch.*

**Dose:** Tincture to third potency. Dr. W. McGeorge advises 2x every 3 hours for arteriosclerosis.

---

# SYMPHORICARPUS RACEMOSA

(Snowberry) **Sym-r.**

This drug is highly recommended for the persistent *vomiting of pregnancy.* Gastric disturbances, fickle appetite, nausea, waterbrash, bitter taste. *Constipation.* Nausea during menstruation. Nausea, *worse any motion. Averse to all food. Better,* lying on back.

**Dose:** Second and third potency. 200th has proved curative.

---

# SYMPHYTUM OFFICINALE

(Comfrey, Knitbone) **Symph.**

The root contains a crystalline solid, that stimulates the growth of epithelium on ulcerated surfaces. It may be administered internally in the treatment of gastric and duodenal ulcers. Also in gastralgia and externally in pruritus ani. Injuries to sinews, tendons and periosteum. Acts on joints generally. Neuralgia of knee.

Of great use in wounds penetrating the perineum and bones, *and in non-union of fractures;* irritable stump after amputation, irritable bone at point of fracture. Psoas abscess. *Pricking pain* and soreness in periosteum.

**Head:** Pain in the occiput, top and forehead; changing places. Pain comes down to the nasal bone. Inflammation of inferior maxillary bone, hard, red, swelling.

**Eyes:** *Pain in the eye after a blow from an obtuse object* (black eye). For traumatic injuries of the eyes no remedy equals this.

**Relationship:** Compare: *Arn., Calc-p.*

**Dose:** Tincture. Externally as a dressing for sores, ulcers and pruritus ani.

---

## SYPHILINUM

(The Syphilitic Virus—A Nosode) **Syph.**

Utter prostration and debility in the morning.

Shifting rheumatic pains. Chronic eruptions and rheumatism.

Ichthyosis. Syphilitic affections. Pains from darkness to daylight; decrease and increase gradually. Hereditary tendency to alcoholism. *Ulceration of* mouth, nose, genitals, skin. *Succession of abscesses.*

**Mind:** Loss of memory; remembers everything previous to his illness. Apathetic; *feels as if going insane or being paralyzed. Fears the night* and the suffering from exhaustion on awakening. Hopeless; *despair of recovery.*

**Head:** Linear pains from temple, across, or from eyes, backward; cause sleeplessness and delirium at night. *Falling of hair.* Pain in bones of head. Top of head feels as if coming off. Stupefying cephalgia.

**Eyes:** *Chronic, recurrent, phlyctenular inflammation of cornea;* successive crops of phyctenules and abrasions of epithelial layer of cornea; photophobia intense, lachrymation profuse. Lids swollen; *pain intense at night;* ptosis. Tubercular iritis. Diplopia; one image seen below the other. Sensation of cold air blowing on the eye (*Fl-ac.*).

**Ears:** Caries in ossicles of the ear of a syphilitic origin.

**Nose:** Caries of nasal bones, hard palate and septum, with perforation; ozena.

**Mouth:** Teeth decay at gum; edges serrated, dwarfed. Tongue coated, teeth indented; deep longitudnal cracks. Ulcers smart and burn (stomatitis). *Excessive flow of saliva; it runs out of the mouth when sleeping.*

**Stomach:** *Craves alcohol.*

**Rectum:** Feels tied up with strictures. Enemas very painful. Fissures, prolapse.

**Female:** Ulcers on the labia. Leucorrhea *profuse, thin, watery, acrid,* with sharp, knife-like pain in ovaries.

**Respiratory:** Aphonia; chronic asthma in summer, wheezing and rattling (*Ant-t.*). Cough dry, hard; worse at night; windpipe sensitive to touch (*Lach.*). Lancinating pains from the base of the heart to the apex at night.

**Extremities:** Sciatica; worse at night; better around day break. Rheumatism of shoulder joint, at insertion of deltoid. Runaround[1]. Severe pain in long bones. Redness and rawness between toes (*Sil.*). Rheumatism, muscles are caked in hard knots or lumps. *Always washing the hands.* Indolent ulcers. Muscles contracted in hard knots.

**Skin:** Reddish-brown eruption, with a disagreeable odor. Extreme emaciation.

**Modalities:** *Worse,* at night, sundown to sunrise, seashore, in summer. *Better,* inland and mountains, during day, moving about slowly.

**Relationship:** Compare: *Merc., Kali-i., Nit-ac., Aur., Alum.*

**Dose:** The highest potencies only and in infrequent doses.

---

# SYZYGIUM JAMBOLANUM

(Jambol Seeds—Enlexing, Active Principle) **Syzyg.**

Has an immediate effect of increasing the blood sugar, glycosuria results.

A very useful remedy in diabetes mellitus. *No other remedy causes such a marked degree of diminution and disappearance of sugar in the urine. Prickly heat in the upper part of the body;* small red pimples itch violently. Great thirst, weakness, emaciation. A very large amount of urine with high specific gravity. Old ulcers of skin. Diabetic ulceration. The seeds powdered, ten grains three times a day: also, the tincture.

**Relationship:** Compare: *Insulinum*—An aqueous solution of the active principle from the pancreas which affects sugar metabolism. If administered at suitable intervals in diabetes mellitus, the blood sugar is maintained at a normal level and the urine remains free of sugar. Over dosage is followed by weakness, fatigue, tremulousness and profuse sweating.

**Dose:** Mother tincture, 2x, 3x.

---

# TABACUM

(Tobacco) **Tab.**

The symptomatology of *Tabacum* is exceedingly well marked. The nausea, giddiness, death-like pallor, vomiting, icy coldness and sweat, with the intermittent pulse, are all very characteristic. Has marked antiseptic qualities and is antidotal to cholera germs. Complete prostration of the entire muscular

[1] Fingers and thumbs have run arounds (infantile syphilis) (Clarke — Dictionary of Practical Materia Medica).

system. Collapse. Gastralgia, enteralgia, *seasickness,* cholera infantum; cold, but *wants abdomen uncovered.* Vigorous peristaltic activity. Diarrhea. Produces high tension and arteriosclerosis of the coronary arteries. Should prove the most well indicated homeopathic drug for angina pectoris, with coronaritis and hypertension (Cartier). Constriction of the throat, chest, bladder, rectum. Pallor, breathlessness, hard cord-like pulse.

**Mind:** Sensation of excessive wretchedness. *Very despondent.* Forgetful. Discontented.

**Head:** Vertigo *on opening the eyes;* sick headache with deathly nausea; periodical. Tight feeling, as if from a band. Sudden pain, as if struck by a hammer. Nervous deafness. Secretion from eyes, nose and mouth increased.

**Eyes:** Dim sight; sees as if through a veil; strabismus. *Amaurosis;* muscae volitantes. Central scotoma. Rapid blindness without a lesion, followed by venous hyperemia and atrophy of optic nerve.

**Face:** Pale (anemia), blue, pinched, sunken, collapsed, covered with cold sweat (*Ars., Verat.*). Freckles.

**Throat:** Nasopharyngitis and tracheitis, *hemming,* morning cough, sometimes with vomiting. Hoarseness of public speakers.

**Stomach:** Incessant nausea; worse, smell of tobacco smoke (*Phos.*); vomiting on least motion, sometimes of fecal matter, *during pregnancy with much spitting. Seasickness; feels terribly faint, sinking feeling in the pit of the stomach.* Sense of relaxation in the stomach with nausea (*Ip.*). Gastralgia; pain from the cardiac end extending to the left arm.

**Abdomen:** Cold. *Wants abdomen uncovered.* It lessens the nausea and vomiting. Painful distention. Incarcerated hernia.

**Rectum:** Constipation; rectum paralyzed, prolapsed. Diarrhea, sudden, watery with nausea, vomiting, prostration and cold sweat (cholera); discharges look like sour milk, thick, curdled, watery. Rectal tenesmus.

**Urinary:** Renal colic; violent pain along the ureter, left side.

**Respiratory:** Difficult, violent constriction of chest. Precordial oppression, with palpitations and pain between the shoulders. Cough followed by hiccough. Cough dry, teasing, must take a swallow of cold water (*Caust., Phos.*). Dyspnea with tingling down the left arm when lying on the left side.

**Heart:** Palpitations when lying on the left side. Pulse intermits, feeble, imperceptible. Angina pectoris, pain in the precordial region. Pain radiates from the center of sternum. Tachycardia. Bradycardia. *Acute dilatation* caused by shock or violent physical exertion (Royal).

**Extremities:** Legs and hands icy cold; limbs tremble. Paralysis following apoplexy (*Plb.*). Gait shuffling, unsteady. Feebleness of arms.

**Sleep:** Insomnia with a dilated heart, cold, clammy skin and anxiety.

**Fever:** Chills with *cold sweat.*

**Modalities:** *Worse,* opening eyes; evening; extremes of heat and cold. *Better,* uncovering, open fresh air.

**Relationship:** Compare: *Hydrobromicum acidum, Camph., Verat., Ars.* Compare: *Nicotinum* (alternate tonic and clonic spasms, followed by general relaxation and trembling; nausea, cold sweat and speedy collapse; head drawn back, contraction of eyelids and masseter muscles; muscles of neck and back rigid (tetnus); hissing respiration from spasm of laryngeal and bronchial muscles).

Antidote: Vinegar; sour apples. *Camph.* is the physiological antagonist. *Ars.* (chewing tobacco); *Ign.* (smoking); *Sep.* (neuralgia and dyspepsia); *Lyc.* (impotency); *Nux-v.* (bad taste due to tobacco); *Calad.* and *Plan.* (causes aversion to tobacco); *Phos.* (tobacco heart, sexual weakness).

**Dose:** Third to thirtieth and higher potencies.

---

# TANACETUM VULGARE

(Tansy) **Tanac.**

Abnormal lassitude. Nervous and tired feeling. "Half dead, half alive feeling" all over. Of use in chorea and reflex spasms (worms). Said to be a specific against effects of poison ivy.

**Mind:** Irritable, sensitive to noise. Mental fatigue, nausea and vertigo, worse in a closed room.

**Head:** Heavy, dull, confused. Headache on least exertion.

**Ears:** Roaring and ringing (tinnitus); voice sounds strange; *ears seem to close up suddenly.*

**Abdomen:** Pain in bowels; relieved by stool. Desire for stool immediately after eating. *Dysentery.*

**Female:** Dysmenorrhea, with bearing down pains, tenderness, drawing in groins. Menses suppressed; later, profuse.

**Respiratory:** Hurried, labored, stertorous respiration. Frothy mucus obstructs the air passages.

**Relationship:** Compare: *Cimic., Cina, Absin., Nux-v.* follows well.

**Dose:** Tincture to third potency.

---

# TANNICUM ACIDUM

(Tannin, Digallic Acid) **Tann-ac.**

Mostly used locally against excessive secretion of mucous membranes, to contract tissues and check hemorrhages. In osmidrosis (bromhidrosis), corrects fetor of perspiration. Obstinate nervous coughs. Hematuria. Obstinate constipation. Pain in abdomen, sensitive to pressure. Intestines can be felt like cylindrical enlargements. One-half percent solution.

**Relationship:** *Gallicum acidum q.v.*

---

## TARAXACUM OFFICINALE

(Dandelion) **Tarax.**

For gastric headaches, bilious attacks with characteristically mapped tongue and jaundiced skin. Cancer of the bladder. Flatulence. *Hysterical tympanites.*

**Head:** Sensation of great heat on top of the head. *Sternomastoid* muscle is very painful to touch.

**Mouth:** Mapped tongue. Tongue covered with a white film (typhoid fever); feels raw; comes off in patches, leaving *red, sensitive spots.* Loss of appetite. Bitter taste and eructations. Salivation.

**Abdomen:** Liver enlarged and indurated (jaundice). Sharp stitches in the left side (cholelithiasis). Sensation of bubbles bursting in bowels. Tympanites. Evacuation difficult.

**Extremities:** Very restless limbs. *Neuralgia of the knee; better, pressure.* Limbs painful to touch.

**Fever:** Chilliness after eating, worse drinking; *finger tips cold. Bitter taste.* Heat without thirst, in the face, *toes.* Sweat on falling asleep.

**Skin:** *Profuse night sweats.*

**Modalities:** *Worse,* resting, lying down, sitting. *Better,* touch.

**Relationship:** Compare: *Cholinum,* a constituent of Taraxacum root, has given encouraging results in the treatment of cancer. *Cholinum* is closely related to *Neurinum,* it is the "Cancronie" of Prof. Adamkiewicz (E. Schlegel), *Bry., Hydr., Nux-v. Tela araneae* (nervous asthma and sleeplessness).

**Dose:** Tincture to third potency. In cancer 1-2 drams fluid extract.

---

## TARENTULA CUBENSIS

(Cuban Spider) **Tarent-c.**

A toxemic medicine, septic conditions. *Diphtheria.* Adapted to the most severe types of inflammation and pain, early and persistent prostration. Various forms of malignant suppuration. Purplish hue and burning, stinging pains. Bubo. It is the remedy for *pain of death; soothes the last struggles. Pruritus, especially around the genitals.* Restless feet. Intermittent septic chills. Bubonic plague. As a curative and preventive remedy especially during the period of invasion.

**Head:** Dizziness after heat and hot perspiration. Dull ache on top of the head. Shooting pains through the left eye, across the frontal region.

**Stomach:** Stomach feels hard, sore. Loss of appetite, except for breakfast.

**Urinary:** Retention. Cannot hold urine on coughing.

**Back:** Itching across the kidney region.

**Extremities:** Hands tremble (chorea), turgid with blood.

**Sleep:** Drowsiness. Sleep restless. Sleep prevented by harsh cough.

**Skin:** Red spots and pimples. Feels puffed all over. *Carbuncles,* burning, stinging pains. Purplish hue. Gangrene. Abscesses, where pain and inflammation predominate. Scirrhus of breasts. "Senile" ulcers.

**Modalities:** *Better,* smoking. *Worse,* night.

**Relationship:** Compare: *Ars., Pyrog., Crot-h., Echi., Anthraci., Bell., Apis.*

**Dose:** Sixth to thirtieth potency.

---

# TARENTULA HISPANICA

(Spanish Spider) **Tarent.**

Remarkable nervous phenomena; hysteria with chlorosis; *chorea,* dysmenorrhea, spinal irritability. Bladder tenesmus (cystitis). *Constrictive* sensations. Formication. *Extreme restlessness;* must keep in constant motion even though walking aggravates. Hysterical epilepsy. Intense sexual excitement.

**Mind:** Sudden alteration of mood. Foxy. Destructive impulses; *moral relaxation.* Must constantly busy herself or walk. *Sensitive to music.* Averse to company, but wants someone present. Ungrateful, discontented. Guided by whims.

**Head:** Intense pain, as if thousands of needles were pricking the brain. *Vertigo.* Wants hair brushed or head rubbed.

**Male:** Sexual excitement; lasciviousness reaching almost to insanity; seminal emissions.

**Female:** Vulva dry and hot with severe itching. Profuse menstruation, with frequent erotic spasms. *Pruritus vulvae, nymphomania.* Dysmenorrhea with very sensitive ovaries.

**Heart:** Palpitations; precordial anguish, sensation as if the heart was twisted and turned around.

**Extremities:** Weakness of legs; choreic movements. Numbness of legs. Multiple sclerosis with trembling. *Twitching and jerking.* Yawning with uneasiness in the legs, must move them constantly. Extraordinary contractions and movements (locomotor ataxia).

**Modalities:** *Worse,* motion, contact, noise. *Better,* in open air, *music,* bright colors, rubbing affected parts. *Worse,* seeing others in trouble.

**Relationship:** Compare: *Agar., Ars., Cupr., Mag-p.*
Antidotes: *Lach.*
**Dose:** Sixth to thirtieth potency.

---

## TARTARICUM ACIDUM

(Tartaric Acid) **Tart-ac.**

Found in grapes, pineapple, sorrel and other fruits. It is an antiscorbutic antiseptic, stimulating the mucous and salivary secretions.

Dullness and lassitude. Great weakness with diarrhea, and a dry and brown tongue. Pain in heels (*Phyt.*).

**Stomach:** Excessive thirst, continuous vomiting causes burning in the throat and stomach. Dyspepsia with copious secretion of mucus.

**Abdomen:** Pain around the umbilicus and in the region of loins. Stool coffee ground in color (worse at night), with a brown and dry tongue and dark green (bilious) vomiting.

**Dose:** Third trituration. The pure acid, 10-30 grains dissolved in water.

---

## TAXUS BACCATA

(Yew) **Tax.**

In pustular diseases of skin and night sweats. Also in gout and chronic rheumatism.

**Head:** Supra-orbital and temporal pain on the right side, with lachrymation. Pupils dilated. Face puffy and pale.

**Stomach:** *Saliva hot,* acrid. Nausea. Pain in the pit of the stomach and region of navel. After eating, cough. Sensation of pins and needles in the pit of the stomach; of *emptiness,* must eat frequently (compare the coniferae).

**Skin:** Large, flat, itchy pustules. Offensive smelling night sweats. Podagra. Erysipelas.

**Dose:** Tincture to third potency.

---

## TELLURIUM METALLICUM

(The Metal Tellurium) **Tell.**

Marked skin (herpes circinatus), spinal, eye and ear symptoms. A very *sensitive back.* Pains all over the body. Offensive discharges. Slow development of symptoms (*Rad-br.*). Sacral and sciatic pains.

**Head:** Neglectful and forgetful. Pain on the left side of head and forehead above the left eye. Distortion and twitching of left facial muscles; when speaking, left angle of mouth drawn upwards and to the left (facial palsy). Fear of being touched in sensitive places. Congestion to head and nape of neck, followed by weakness and faintness in the stomach. Itching of scalp; red spots.

**Eyes:** Lids *thickened, inflamed,* itching (blepharitis). Pterygium; pustular conjunctivitis. Cataract, following ocular lesions; aids the absorption of infiltrations in the iris and choroid.

**Ears:** *Eczema behind the ear. Catarrh of the middle ear* (otitis media), *discharge acrid, smells like fish pickle* (otorrhea). *Itching, swelling, throbbing in the meatus.* Deafness.

**Nose:** Coryza, lachrymation and hoarseness; better in open air (*All-c.*). Obstructed; hawks salty phlegm from posterior nares.

**Stomach:** Craving for apples. Empty and weak feeling. Heartburn.

**Rectum:** Pruritus ani et perinei after every stool.

**Back:** Pain in the sacrum. *Pain from the last cervical to fifth dorsal vertebra,* very sensitive; worse touch (*Chinin-s., Phos.*). *Sciatica;* worse right side, *coughing, straining* and at night, with a sensitive vertebral column. *Contraction of tendons in bends of knees.*

**Skin:** Itching of hands and feet. Herpetic spots; *ringworm* (*Tub.*). *Ring-shape lesions,* offensive odors from affected parts. Barber's itch. Stinging in the skin. *Fetid exhalations* (*Sulph.*). Offensive foot sweat. Eczema, behind the ears and occiput. Circular patches of eczema (eczema circinata).

**Modalities:** *Worse,* while at rest at night, cold weather, from friction, coughing, laughing, lying on painful side, touch.

**Relationship:** Compare: *Rad-br., Sel., Tetradymitum*—crystals from Georgia and North Carolina containing *Bismuth, Tellurium* and *Sulphur* (coccygodynia, ulceration of nails; pains in hands, in small spots, ankles, heels, and tendo-Achilles); *Sep., Ars., Rhus-t.*

**Dose:** Sixth potency and higher. Takes a long time to develop its action, which is very prolonged.

---

## TEREBINTHINIAE OLEUM

(Turpentine) **Ter.**

Has a selective affinity for *bleeding mucous membranes.* Tympanites and urinary symptoms are very marked. Inflammation of the kidneys with hemorrhages—dark, passive, fetid. Bright's disease preceded by dropsy (Goullon). Drowsiness and strangury. Coma. *Unbroken chilblains.*

**Head:** Dull pain as from a band around the head (*Carb-ac.*). Vertigo with vanishing of vision. Disturbed sense of equilibrium. Tired and difficult concentration of thoughts. Cold in the head with sore nostrils and disposition to epistaxis.

**Eyes:** Ciliary neuralgia over right eye. Intense pain in the eye and side of head. Amblyopia from alcohol.

**Ears:** Own voice sounds unnatural; humming as in a seashell, talking loudly is painful. Otalgia.

**Mouth:** Tongue *dry, red, sore, shining;* burning in the tip, with prominent papillae (glossitis) (*Arg-n., Bell., Kali-bi., Nux-m.*). Breath cold, foul. Choking sensation in the throat. Stomatitis. Dentition.

**Stomach:** Nausea and vomiting; heat in the epigastric region.

**Abdomen:** *Enormous distention.* Diarrhea; stools watery, greenish, fetid, bloody. Pain before flatus with relief after stools. Hemorrhage from bowels. Worms; lumbricoides. Abdominal dropsy; pelvic peritonitis. Fainting after every stool. Enterocolitis, with hemorrhage and ulceration of the bowels.

**Urinary:** *Strangury with hematuria.* Scanty, suppressed, *odor of violets.* Urethritis with painful erections (*Canth.*). Nephritis following any acute disease. Constant tenesmus.

**Female:** Intense *burning in the uterine region.* Metritis; puerperal peritonitis. Metrorrhagia with burning in the uterus.

**Respiratory:** Difficult breathing; lungs feel distended; hemoptysis.

**Heart:** Pulse rapid, small, thready, intermittent.

**Back:** *Burning pain in the region of kidneys.* Drawing pain in the right kidney extending to the hip.

**Fever:** Heat, with violent thirst, dry tongue, profuse cold, clammy sweat. Typhoid with tympanites, hemorrhages, stupor, delirium. Prostration.

**Skin:** Acne. Erythema; itching pustular, vesicular eruption; urticaria. Purpura, ecchymosis, dropsies. Scarlatina. Chilblains; with excessive itching and pulsative pains. Aching soreness of the muscles.

**Relationship:** Compare: *Alumn., Sec., Canth., Nit-ac., Terebenum* 1x; (chronic bronchitis and winter coughs; subacute stages of inflammation of the respiratory tract. Loosens secretion, relieves the tightened feeling, makes expectoration easy. *Neurotic coughs.* Huskiness in public speakers, and singers. Cystitis when urine is alkaline and offensive).

*Ononis spinosa*—Rest harrow (diuretic, lithotriptic. Chronic nephritis; diuretic effects like *Juniper;* calculus, epistaxis, worse washing face).

Antidote: *Phos.*

**Dose:** First to sixth potency.

---

# TEUCRIUM MARUM VERUM

(Cat-thyme) **Teucr.**

Nasal and rectal symptoms marked. *Polypi.* Affections of children. Suitable after too much medicine has been taken. Oversensitiveness. *Desire to stretch.* A remedy of first importance in chronic nasal catarrh with atrophy; large, offensive crusts and clinkers. *Ozena. Loss of sense of smell* (anosmia).

**Head:** Excited, tremulous feeling. Frontal pain; worse, stooping. Strengthens the brain after delirium tremens.

**Eyes:** Smarting in the canthi; lids red and puffy; tarsal tumor. (*Staph.*).

**Ears:** Hissing and ringing otalgia.

**Nose:** Catarrhal condition of both anterior and posterior nostrils. *Mucus polypus.* Chronic catarrh; *discharge of large, irregular clinkers.* Halitosis. *Crawling in the nostrils,* with lachrymation and sneezing. Coryza, with stoppage of nostrils.

**Stomach:** Vomiting of large quantities of dark green masses. Constant hiccough, attended with pain in the back. Unnatural appetite. Hiccough on eating, after nursing.

**Rectum:** *Itching in the anus and constant irritation in the evening in bed. Ascarides with nocturnal restlessness.* Crawling sensation in the rectum after stool.

**Respiratory:** Dry cough, tickling in the trachea; *mouldy taste in the throat* when hawking up mucus, expectoration profuse.

**Extremities:** Affection of finger tips and joints of toes. Tearing pain in arms and legs. *Pain in toe nails,* as if they had grown into the flesh (ingrown toe nails).

**Sleep:** Restless, with twitching, choking, and starting up frightened.

**Skin:** Itching causes tossing about all night. Very dry skin. Suppurating grooves in the nails.

**Relationship:** Compare: *Teucrium scorodonia:* Woodsage (in tuberculosis with muco-purulent expectoration; dropsy; orchitis and *tuberculous epidymitis; especially* in young, thin individuals with tuberculosis of the lungs, glands; bones and urogenitals, 3x). *Cina, Ign., Sang., Sil.*

**Dose:** First to sixth potency. Locally for polypi, dry powder.

---

# THALLIUM METALLICUM

(The Metal Thallium) **Thal.**

*Thal.* seems to influence the endocrines, especially the thyroid and adrenalin. Most horrible neuralgic, spasmodic, shooting pains. Muscular atrophy. Tremors. Relieves the violent pains in locomotor ataxia. *Paralysis of lower limbs.* Pain in stomach and bowels, like electric shocks. Paraplegia. *Alopecia* following acute, exhausting diseases. Night sweats. Polyneuritis. Dermal trophic lesions.

**Extremities:** *Trembling. Paralytic feeling.* Lancinating pains, like electric shocks. Very tired. Chronic myelitis. Numbness in fingers and toes, which extension upto the lower limbs, involving the lower abdomen and perineum. *Paralysis of the lower limbs.* Cyanosis of extremities. Formication, beginning in fingers and extending through the pelvis, perineum and inner thighs to the feet.

**Relationship:** Compare: *Lath., Caust., Arg-n., Plb.*

**Dose:** Lower trituration to thirtieth potency.

---

## THEA CHINENSIS

(Tea) **Thea**

Nervous sleeplessness, heart problems, palpitations, and dyspepsia of old tea drinkers. Produces most of the sick headaches. *Tabacum* antidotal (Allen).

**Head:** Temporary mental exaltation. Ill humored. Sick headache radiating from one point. Sleepless and restless. Hallucinations of hearing. Cold damp feeling at the back of head.

**Stomach:** Sinking sensation in the epigastrium. *Faint, all gone feeling* (*Sep., Hydr., Olnd.*). Craves acids. Sudden production of wind in large quantities.

**Abdomen:** Borborygmi. Liability to hernia.

**Female:** Soreness and tenderness in the ovaries.

**Heart:** Anxious oppression. Precordial distress. Palpitations; unable to lie on the left side. Fluttering. Pulse rapid, irregular, intermittent.

**Sleep:** Sleepy during daytime; sleepiness at night, with vascular excitement and restlessness, dry skin. Horrible dreams cause no horror.

**Modalities:** *Worse,* night, on walking in open air, after meals. *Better* warmth; warm bath.

**Relationship:** Antidote: *Kali-hp., Thuj., Ferr., Kali-i.* (material doses for tea taster's cough.)

**Dose:** Third to thirtieth potency.

Theine ¼ - ½ grain hypodermically for sciatica and supraorbital neuralgia.

---

# THERIDION CURASSAVICUM

(Orange Spider) **Ther.**

Nervous hyperesthesia. Has an affinity for the tubercular diathesis. Vertigo, sick headache, peculiar pain around the heart region, phthisis florida, scrofula have all been treated successfully with this remedy. *Sensitive to noise; it penetrates the body, especially teeth.* Noises seem to strike on painful spots over the body. Rachitis, caries, necrosis. Phthisis, stitch high up in the left apex (*Anthraci.*). Where the indicated remedy does not hold long.

**Mind:** Restless; finds pleasure in nothing. Time passes too quickly.

**Head:** Pain worse anyone walking over the floor. *Vertigo, with nausea and vomiting on least motion,* particularly on closing eyes.

**Eyes:** Luminous vibrations before the eyes; sensitive to light. Pressure behind the eyeballs. Throbbing over the left eye.

**Nose:** Discharge yellowish, thick, offensive; ozena (*Puls., Thuj.*).

**Stomach:** Seasickness. Nausea and vomiting on closing eyes and on motion (*Tab.*). Stinging pain on left side over the anterior aspect of spleen. Burning in the liver region.

**Respiratory:** Pain in the upper left chest (*Myrt-c., Pix, Anis.*). *Pain in the left floating ribs. Cardiac anxiety with pain* (angina pectoris). Pinching in left pectoral muscle.

**Back:** Sensitiveness between the vertebrae; avoids pressure on the spine. Stinging pains.

**Skin:** *Stinging thrusts everywhere.* Sensitive skin of thighs. *Itching sensations.*

**Modalities:** *Worse,* touch; pressure; on shipboard; riding in a carriage; closing the eyes; jar; noise. coitus; left side.

**Dose:** Thirtieth potency.

---

# THIOSINAMINUM—RHODALLINUM

(A Chemical Derived from Oil of Mustard Seed) **Thiosin.**

A resolvent, externally and internally, for *dissolving scar tissue,* tumors, enlarged glands; lupus, strictures, adhesions. Ectropion, opacities of the cornea, cataract, ankylosis, fibroids, scleroderma. Noises in ear. Suggested by Dr. A.S. Hard for retarding old age. A remedy for tabes dorsalis, improving the lightening pains. Gastric, vesicle and rectal crises. Stricture in the rectum, 2 grains twice daily.

**Ears:** Arteriosclerotic *vertigo; tinnitus.* Catarrhal deafness with cicatricial thickening. Subacute suppurative otitis media, formation of fibrous bands impeding free movement of the ossicles. Thickened drum. Deafness due to some fibrous change in the nerve.

**Dose:** Inject, a 10 percent solution in glycerine and water, 15-30 drops twice a week under the skin or into the lesion. Internally in capsules of ½ grain daily. In obstinate cases of arteriosclerosis doses of ½ grain, never more, 3 times a day. Vertigo and arthritis (Bartlett). 2x attenuation.

---

## THLASPI BURSA PASTORIS—CAPSELLA

(Shepherd's Purse) **Thlas.**

Is an anti-hemorrhagic and anti-uric acid remedy. Albuminuria during gestation. Chronic neuralgia. Renal (nephritis) and vesical irritation. Hemorrhage from uterine fibroid, with aching in the back or a general bruised soreness. Aching between the scapulae. Uterine hemorrhage, with cramps and expulsion of clots. Craves buttermilk. Effects of suppressed uterine diseases (Burnett).

**Head:** Eyes and face puffy. Vertigo; worse, rising. Frontal pain; worse towards the evening. Scaly eruptions behind the ears. Tongue coated, white. Sharp pain over the right eye drawing the eye upwards.

**Nose:** Bleeding in nasal surgeries. Especially passive hemorrhage. Frequent epistaxis.

**Mouth:** Mouth and lips cracked.

**Urinary:** Frequent desire; *urine heavy,* phosphatic. Chronic cystitis. Dysuria and spasmodic retention. Hematuria. Accumulation of gravel. Renal colic (calculi). *Brick dust sediment.* Urethritis; urine runs away in little jets. Often replaces the use of the catheter.

**Male:** Spermatic cord sensitive to concussion of walking or riding.

**Female:** Metrorrhagia; too frequent and copious menses. Hemorrhage with violent uterine colic (fibroid miscarriage). Every alternate period is very profuse. Leucorrhea before and after menses; bloody, dark, offensive; *stains indelibly. Sore pain in the womb on rising.* Scarcely recovers from one period before another begins.

**Relationship:** Compare: *Urt-u., Croc., Tril-p., Mill.*

**Dose:** Tincture to sixth potency.

---

# THUJA OCCIDENTALIS

(Arbor Vitae) **Thuj.**

Acts on the skin, blood, gastro-intestinal tract, kidneys and brain. Its relation to the production of pathological vegetations, condylomata, warty excrescences, spongy tumors is very important. Moist mucus tubercles. Bleeding fungus growths. Nevus. Excess of venosity.

The main action of *Thuj.* is on the skin and genito-urinary organs, producing conditions that correspond with Hahnemann's sycotic dyscrasia, whose chief manifestation is the formation of wart-like excrescences upon mucous and cutaneous surfaces, fig warts and condylomata. Has a specific antibacterial action, as in gonorrhea and vaccination. Suppressed gonorrhea, salpingitis. *Ill effects of vaccination.* Sycotic pains, i.e., tearing in muscles and joints, worse at rest, better in dry weather, worse damp humid atmosphere; lameness. *Hydrogenoid constitutions,* whose blood is morbidly hydroscopic, so that damp air and water are inimical. Complaints from moonlight. *Rapid exhaustion and emaciation.* Left sided and a chilly medicine. Variola, aborts the pustule and prevents the suppurating fever. *Vaccinosis,* viz., inveterable skin problems, neuralgia, etc.

**Mind:** *Fixed ideas,* as if a strange person was at his side; as if soul and body were separated; as if something was alive in the abdomen (*Croc.*). Emotional sensitiveness; music causes weeping and trembling.

**Head:** Pain as if pierced by a nail (*Coff., Ign.*). Neuralgia from tea (*Sel.*). Left sided headache (migraine). White, scaly dandruff; hair dry and falling out. Greasy skin of face.

**Eyes:** Ciliary neuralgia; iritis. Eyelids agglutinated at night; dry, scaly. Styes and tarsal tumors (*Staph.*). Acute and subacute inflammation of the sclera. Sclera raised in patches and looks bluish-red. Large, flat phlyctenules; *indolent.* Recurring episcleritis. Chronic scleritis.

**Ears:** Chronic otitis; discharge purulent (otorrhea). Creaking when swallowing. Polypi.

**Nose:** Chronic catarrh; thick, green mucus; blood and pus (ozena). On blowing the nose, pain in teeth. Ulcerations within the nostrils. Dryness of nasal cavities. Painful pressure at the root.

**Mouth:** Tip of tongue very painful. *White blisters on the side close to the root, painfully sore.* Teeth decay next to gums; very sensitive; gums retract (scorbutic). Drinks fall audibly into the stomach. Ranula; varicose veins on the tongue and the mouth. Pyorrhea alveolaris.

**Stomach:** Complete loss of appetite. Dislike for fresh meat and potatoes. Rancid eructations after fatty food. Cutting pain in the epigastrium. Cannot eat onions. Flatulence; pain after food; sinking sensation in the epigastrium before food; thirst. Tea drinker's dyspepsia.

**Abdomen:** Distended; indurations in the abdomen (cancer). Chronic diarrhea, worse after breakfast. Discharges forcibly expelled; gurgling sound. Brown spots. *Flatulence and distention; protruding here and there* (hernia). Rumbling and colic. Constipation with violent rectal pain, causing the stool to recede (*Sil., Sanic.*). Piles swollen; pain worse sitting with stitching, burning pains in the anus. Anus fissured; painful to touch with warts. *Movements as if something living* (*Croc.*), without pain.

**Urinary:** Urethra swollen, inflamed (urethritis). Urinary stream splits and small. Sensation of trickling after micturition. Severe cutting *pains after* (*Sars.*). Frequent micturition accompanying pains. Desire sudden and urgent, but cannot be controlled. Paralysis of sphincter vesicae.

**Male:** Inflammation of the prepuce and glans; pain in the penis. Balanitis. *Gonorrheal rheumatism. Gonorrhea.* Chronic induration of testicles. Pain and burning felt near the neck of the bladder; with a frequent and urgent desire to micturate. Prostatic enlargement (*Ferr-pic., Thiosin., Iod., Sabal*).

**Female:** Vagina *very sensitive* (vaginitis) (*Berb., Kreos., Lyss.*). Warty excrescences on the vulva and perineum. Profuse leucorrhea; thick, greenish. Severe pain in the left ovary and left inguinal region. Menses scanty, retarded. *Polypi; fleshy* excrescences. Ovaritis; worse left side, at every menstrual period (*Lach.*). Profuse perspiration before menses.

**Respiratory:** Dry, hacking cough in the afternoon, with pain in the pit of the stomach. Stitches in the chest; worse, cold drinks. *Asthma in children* (*Nat-s.*). Papilloma of the larynx. Chronic laryngitis.

**Extremities:** When walking, limbs feel as if made of wood or glass, and would break easily. Tips of fingers swollen, red, feel dead. Muscular twitchings, weakness and trembling (chorea). Cracking in joints. Pain in heels and tendo-Achilles. Nails brittle. Ingrowing toe nail.

**Sleep:** Persistent insomnia.

**Fever:** Chill beginning in thighs. Sweat *only on uncovered parts,* or all over except head when sleeping; profuse, sour smelling like honey. Orgasms of blood in the evening, with throbbing in the blood vessels.

**Skin:** Polypi, tubercles, *warts,* epithelioma, naevi, carbuncles, ulcers, especially in the ano-genital region. Freckles and blotches. Perspiration sweetish and strong. Dry skin with brown spots. Zona; herpetic eruptions. Tearing pain in glands. Glandular enlargement. Nails crippled; brittle and soft. *Eruptions only on covered parts;* worse after scratching. Very sensitive to touch. Coldness of one side. Sarcoma; polypi. *Brown spots on hands and arms.*

**Modalities:** *Worse,* at night, from heat of bed; at 3 a.m. and 3 p. m., from cold, damp air; after breakfast; fat, coffee; vaccination. *Better,* left side; while drawing up a limb.

**Relationship:** Compare: (Hydrogenoid constitution: *Calc., Sil., Nat-s.,*

*Aran., Apis, Puls.). Cupressus australis* (sharp, prickling pain; general feeling of warmth; rheumatism and gonorrhea). *Cupressus lawsoniana* (acts like *Thuj., terrible pains in the stomach). Sphingurus martini* (falling out of hair from beard; pain in the jaw joint and zygoma); *Sil., Maland.* (vaccination); *Med.* (suppressed gonorrhea); *Merc., Cinnab., Ter., Juniperus, Sabin., Sil., Canth., Cann-s., Nit-ac., Puls., Ant-t., Arborin* is a non-alcoholic preparation of *Thuj.*

Antidotes: *Merc., Camph., Sabin.* (warts).

Complementary: *Sabin., Ars., Nat-s., Sil.*

**Dose:** Locally, for warts and excrescences, tincture or cerate. Internally, tincture to thirtieth potency.

---

# THYMOLUM

(Thyme Camphor) **Thymol.**

A remedy having a wide field in genito-urinary diseases. It is indicated in pathological emissions, priapism and prostatorrhea. The provings show an action limited to the sexual organs, producing a typical sexual neurasthenia. Specific for hookworm disease (*Chen-a.*).

**Mind:** Irritable, arbitrary, must have his own way. Craves company. Energy gone.

**Male:** Profuse, nocturnal, seminal emissions with lascivious dreams of a perverted character. Priapism. Urine burning with subsequent dribbling of urine. Polyuria. Urates increased. Phosphates decreased.

**Back:** Tired, aching feeling throughout the lumbar region. *Worse,* mental and physical labor.

**Sleep:** Wakes up tired and unrefreshed. Lascivious and fantastic dreams.

**Modalities:** *Worse,* mental and physical labor.

**Relationship:** Compare: *Carbn-tm.* as a remedy for hookworms, according to Dr. Lambert, Suva, Fiji who employed it in 50,000 cases.

"1. *Carbn-tm.* is a vermifuge and vermicide of great potency, and has shown itself to be the best vermifuge in the treatment of hookworms in a country where the disease predominates.

"2. It gives little discomfort to the patient, is palatable, requires no preparation of the patient, and even when in the pure form is apparently not toxic, all of these features are of an advantage in a popular campaign.

"W. G. Smillie, and S.B. Pessoa, of Sao Paulo, Brazil, also found *Carbn-tm.* to be extremely efficient in removing hookworms. A single dose of 3 c.c., given to adults has removed 95 percent of all the hookworms harbored."

**Dose:** Sixth attenuation.

# THYMUS SERPYLLUM

(Wild Thyme) **Thymu.**

Respiratory infections in children; dry nervous asthma, whooping cough, severe spasms but little sputum.

Ringing in the ears (tinnitus) with sensation of pressure in the head. Burning in the pharynx, sore throat worse, empty swallowing; blood vessels distended, dark.

**Dose:** Tincture.

---

# THYREOIDINUM

(Dried Thyroid Gland of the Sheep) **Thyr.**

*Thyr.* produces anemia, emaciation, muscular weakness, sweating, headache, nervous tremor of face and limbs, tingling sensations and paralysis. Heart rate increased, exophthalmus and dilatation of pupils. *In myxedema and cretinism* its effects are striking. Rheumatoid arthritis. Infantile wasting. Rickets. Delayed union of fractures. In half grain doses, twice a day over a considerable period is said to be *effective in undescended testicles* in boys. Thyroid exercises a general regulating influence over the mechanism of the organs of nutrition, growth and development. Thyroid weakness causes a decided craving for a large amount of sweets.

Of use in psoriasis; and *tachycardia.* Arrested development in children. Improves the memory. *Goitre.* Excessive obesity. Acts better with pale patients, rather than those of high color. Amblyopia. *Mammary tumors. Uterine fibroid.* Great weakness and hunger, yet loses flesh. *Nocturnal enuresis. Agalactea.* Begin treatment, early in pregnancy. Dose 1 1/2 gr. 2 to 3 times daily. *Vomiting of pregnancy* (give early in the morning before patient gets up). *Fibroid tumors of the breast,* 2x trituration. Dilates arterioles (*Adrenalinum* contracts them). Sensation of faintness and nausea. Marked sensitiveness to cold. Hypothyroidism after acute diseases, i.e., weakness. Easy fatigue, weak pulse, tendency to fainting, palpitations, cold hands and feet, low blood pressure, chilliness and sensitive to cold (*Thyr.* 1x, 3 times daily). Has a powerful diuretic action in myxedema and various types of edemas.

**Mind:** Stupor, alternating with restless melancholy. Irritable, worse least opposition; goes into a rage over trifles.

**Head:** Brain feels light. *Persistent frontal* headache.

**Eyes:** Progressive diminution of sight (amblyopia) with central scotoma (*Carbn-s.*). Eyeballs prominent (exopthalmic goitre).

**Mouth:** Lips burn. Tongue thickly coated. Bad taste in the mouth.

**Throat:** Dry, congested, raw, burning; worse, left side.

**Stomach:** Desire for sweets and thirst for cold water. Nausea worse riding in a car. Flatulence, marked flatus in abdomen.

**Urinary:** Increased flow; polyuria; with albumen and sugar. *Enuresis* in weak children who are nervous and irritable (1/2 gr. night and morning). Urine smells of violets, burning along the urethra, increase of uric acid in urine.

**Respiratory:** Dry, painful cough with scanty, difficult expectoration and burning in the pharynx.

**Heart:** Weak, frequent pulse, with an inability to lie down. *Tachycardia* (*Naja*). Anxiety around the chest, *as if constricted. Palpitations from least exertion.* Severe heart pain. Ready excitability of heart. Heart's action weak, with numbness of fingers (angina pectoris).

**Extremities:** Rheumatic arthritis with a tendency to obesity, coldness and cramps in the extremities. Peeling of skin in lower limbs. Cold extremities. Aching pains. Edema of legs. Trembling of limbs and the entire body.

**Skin:** *Psoriasis* associated with adiposity (*not* in developing stage). Skin *dry,* impoverished. Cold hands and feet. *Eczema.* Uterine fibroids. *Browny swelling.* Swelling of glands with stony hardness (adenitis). Sluggish cases. Jaundice with pruritus. Ichthyosis, lupus. Itching without eruption, worse night.

**Relationship:** Compare: *Spong., Calc., Fuc., Lycps-v., Iodothyrinum* (the active principle isolated from the thyroid gland, a substance rich in iodine and nitrogen, affects metabolism, reducing weight, may produce glycosuria. Use cautiously in obesity, for a fatty heart may not be able to maintain the accelerated rhythm. Milk contains the internal secretion of the thyroid). *Thymus gland extract* (arthritis deformans; metabolic osteoarthritis, 5 grain tablets, 3 times daily). High potencies very efficient in exophthalmic goitre.

**Dose:** Crude *Thyr.* at times; better sixth to thirtieth potency. If the crude *Thyr.* is taken (two to three grains or more daily); the pulse should be watched. Must not be given in physiological doses where with feeble heart with high blood pressure and is contraindicated in tubercular patients.

---

## TILIA EUROPAEA

(Linden) **Til.**

Of value in muscular weakness of the eye; hemorrhage of thin, pale blood (anemia). Puerperal metritis. Diseases of the antrum (*Kali-i., Chel.*).

**Head:** *Neuralgia* (first right, then left side), *with a veil before the eyes.* Confusion, with dimness of vision.

**Eyes:** Sensation of a gauze before the eyes (*Calc., Caust., Nat-m.*). Binocular vision imperfect.

**Nose:** Much sneezing, with fluent coryza. Epistaxis.

**Female:** *Intense, sore feeling around the uterus;* bearing down pain with hot sweat, but without relief. Profuse slimy leucorrhea when walking (*Bov., Carb-an., Graph.*). Soreness and hyperemia of the external genitals (*Thuj., Sulph.*). Pelvic inflammation, tympanites, abdominal tenderness and hot sweat which does not relieve.

**Skin:** Urticaria. Violent itching, and burning like fire after scratching. Eruptions of small, red itchy pimples. *Sweat warm and profuse* soon after falling asleep. Sweat increases as rheumatic pains increase.

**Modalities:** *Worse,* in the afternoon and evening; in a warm room, heat of bed. *Better,* cool room, motion.

**Relationship:** Compare: *Lil-t., Bell.*

**Dose:** Tincture to sixth potency.

---

## TITANIUM METALLICUM

(The Metal) **Titan.**

Is found in the bones and muscles. Has been used in lupus and tuberculous processes externally, also in skin disease, nasal catarrh, etc. Apples contain 0.11 percent of *Titan.* Imperfect vision, the peculiarity being that only *half an object* can be seen at one time . Giddiness with *vertical hemiopia.* Also sexual weakness with *very early ejaculation* of semen during coitus. Bright's disease. Eczema, lupus, rhinitis.

**Dose:** Lower and middle potencies.

---

## TONGO ODORATA—DIPTRIX ODORATA

(Seeds of Coumarouna—A Tree in Guiana) **Tong.**

Useful in neuralgia; pertussis.

**Head:** Tearing pains in the supra-orbital nerve, with heat and throbbing pain in the head and epiphora (migraine). Confused, especially in the occiput, with somnolence and a sort of intoxication.

**Eyes:** Trembling in right upper lid.

**Nose:** Coryza; nose stopped, must breathe through the mouth.

**Extremities:** Tearing pains in hip joints, femur and knees, especially on the left side.

**Relationship:** *Meli., Antho., Asper.* and *Tong.*, contains Coumarin, the active principle. Compare them in hay fever; also, *Trif-p., Naphtin., Sabad.*

**Dose:** Tincture and lower potencies.

---

# TORULA CEREVISIAE

(Saccharomyces, Yeast Plant) **Tor.**

Introduced by Drs. Lehman and Yingling. Not proved, hence clinical symptoms only, but many have been verified. Sycotic remedy. Anaphylactic states produced by proteins and enzymes (Yingling).

**Head:** Aching in the back of the head and neck. Headache, sharp pains all over. Worse from constipation. Irritable and nervous.

**Nose:** Sneezing and wheezing. Catarrhal discharge from posterior nares.

**Abdomen:** Bad taste. Nausea. Poor digestion. Belching of gas in the stomach and abdomen. Soreness all over the abdomen. Sense of fullness. Rumbling, pains shift, flatulence. *Constipation.* Sour, yeasty, mouldy odor from discharges.

**Extremities:** Backache, tired and weak from elbows and knees down. Hands cold like ice and go to sleep easily.

**Sleep:** Disturbed with much restlessness.

**Skin:** Boils, recurrent. Itching eczema around the ankles. Tinea versicolor.

**Dose:** Pure yeast cake or potencies from 3rd to higher ones. Yeast poultices are used in skin diseases, boils and swellings.

---

# TRIBULUS TERRESTRIS

(Ikshugandha) **Trib.**

An East Indian drug useful in urinary affections, especially dysuria, and in debilitated states of the sexual organs, as expressed in seminal weakness, ready emissions and impoverished semen. Prostatitis, calculus affections and sexual neurasthenia. It meets the auto-traumatism of masturbation, correcting the emissions and spermatorrhea. Partial impotence caused by over indulgence of advancing age, or when accompanied by urinary symptoms, incontinence, painful micturition, etc.

**Dose:** Ten to twenty drops of the tincture, three times daily.

---

# TRIFOLIUM PRATENSE

(Red Clover) **Trif-p.**

*Produces the most marked ptyalism.* Feeling of fullness with congestion of the salivary glands, followed by an increased, copious flow of saliva. Sensation as if mumps was coming on. *Crusta lactea;* dry, scaly crusts. Stiff neck. *Cancerous diathesis.*

**Head:** Confusion and headache on awaking. Dullness in the anterior brain. Mental failure, loss of memory.

**Mouth:** *Increased flow of saliva* (*Merc., Syph.*). Sore throat with hoarseness.

**Respiratory:** Coryza like the one which precedes hay fever; thin mucus, with marked irritation. *Hoarseness and choking; chills with cough at night.* Cough on exposure to open air. Hay fever. Spasmodic cough; *whooping cough,* paroxysms; worse at night.

**Back:** Neck stiff; cramps in the sternocleido muscles; relieved by heat and rubbing.

**Extremities:** Tingling in palms. Hands and feet cold. Tibial ulcers.

**Relationship:** Compare: *Trifolium repens*—White clover (prophylactic against mumps, sensation of congestion in the salivary glands, pain and hardening, especially submaxillary; worse, lying down. Mouth filled with watery saliva, *worse lying down.* Taste of blood in the mouth and throat. Sensation as if the heart would stop, with great fear, better sitting up or moving about; worse, when alone, with cold sweat on the face).

**Dose:** Tincture.

---

# TRILLIUM PENDULUM

(White Beth-root) **Tril-p.**

A general hemorrhagic medicine, *with great faintness* and *dizziness.* Chronic diarrhea of bloody mucus. Uterine hemorrhage. Threatened abortion. *Relaxation of the pelvic region.* Cramp-like pains. Phthisis with purulent and copious expectoration and spitting of blood.

**Head:** Pain in the forehead; worse, noise. Confused.

**Eyes:** Eyeballs feel too large. Vision blurred (amaurosis); everything looks bluish.

**Nose:** *Epistaxis* (*Mill., Meli.*).

**Mouth:** Hemorrhage from the gums (scurvy). *Bleeding after tooth extraction.*

**Stomach:** Heat and burning in the stomach, rising up in the esophagus (hyperchlorhydria). Hematemesis.

**Stool:** Chronic diarrhea; discharge bloody. Dysentery; passes almost pure blood.

**Female:** Uterine hemorrhages *with sensation as though the hips and back were falling to pieces; better tight bandages.* Gushing of bright red blood on least movement. Hemorrhage from fibroids (*Calc., Nit-ac., Phos., Sul-ac.*). Prolapse, with great bearing down sensation. Leucorrhea copious, yellow, stringy (*Hydr., Kali-bi., Sabin.*). Metrorrhagia at climacteric. *Lochia suddenly becomes sanguinous.* Dribbling of urine after labor.

**Respiratory:** Cough, with hemoptysis (phthisis). Copious, purulent expectoration. Aching at the end of the sternum. Suffocative attacks of irregular breathing with sneezing. Shooting pains through the chest.

**Relationship:** Compare: *Trillium cernuum* (eye symptoms, everything looks bluish; greasy feeling in the mouth); *Fic-r.* (hemorrhages; menorrhagia, hematuria, epistaxis, hematemesis, bleeding piles); *Sanguisuga officinalis*—Leech (hemorrhages; bleeding from the anus). *Ip., Sabin., Lach., Ham.*

**Dose:** Tincture and lower potencies.

---

# TRINITROTOLUENUM

(T.N.T.) **Trinit.**

Symptoms found in immunition workers handling T.N.T. who inhale, ingest and also absorb some through the skin. They were compiled by Dr. Conrad Wesselhoeft and published in December, 1926, Journal of the American Institute of Homeopathy.

The destructive action of T.N.T. on the red blood corpuscles is responsible for anemia and jaundice with their secondary symptoms. The hemoglobin is changed so it cannot act satisfactorily as an oxygen carrier and as a result we have breathlessness, dizziness, headache, faintness, palpitation, undue fatigue, muscle cramps and cyanosis; also drowsiness, depression and insomnia. Later stages of poisoning produce toxic jaundice and aplastic anemia. Jaundice is the result of cellular destruction in contrast to obstructive jaundice.

**Head:** Depression and headache (frontal). Aversion to company, apathetic and weeps easily. Faintness, dizziness, mental sluggishness; delirium, convulsions, coma. Face very dark.

**Mouth:** Bitter taste, marked thirst, sour regurgitation; dull burning behind ensiform; nausea, vomiting.

**Stool:** Constipation followed by diarrhea and cramps.

**Urinary:** Highly colored urine, burning micturition, sudden desire, incontinence and retention.

**Respiratory:** Nose dry with a stuffed sensation. Sneezing, coryza, burning in the trachea, choking, weight on chest; dry, convulsive cough, raises mucus plugs.

**Heart:** Palpitations, tachycardia, bradycardia, intermittent pulse.

**Skin:** Hands stained yellow (jaundice). Dermatitis, nodular erythema, vesicles, itching and burning; puffiness. *Tendency to hemorrhage* under the skin (purpura), and from the nose (epistaxis). *Tired pain in the poplitial fossa.*

**Modalities:** *Worse,* alcohol (falls after one or two drinks of whisky), *tea* (marked aversion).

**Relationship:** Compare: *Zinc., Phos., Cina, Ars., Plb.*

**Dose:** Thirtieth potency has been used with success.

---

## TRIOSTEUM PERFOLIATUM

(Fever Foot) **Trios.**

*Trios.* is a very valuable remedy in diarrhea attended with colicky pain and nausea, *numbness of lower limbs after stool* and increased flow of urine; also in influenza. Quietens nervous symptoms (*Coff., Hyos.*). Biliousness. Bilious colic.

**Head:** Occipital pain with nausea on rising, followed by vomiting. Influenza, with aching pains all over, and heat in the limbs. *Ozena;* frontal pain.

**Stomach:** Loathing of food; nausea on rising, followed by vomiting and cramps. Stools watery, frothy (gastroenteritis).

**Extremities:** Stiffness of all joints; calves numb; aching in bones. Rheumatic pain in the back. Pain in limbs.

**Skin:** Itching welts (eruptions). *Urticaria* from gastric derangement.

**Dose:** Sixth potency.

---

## TRITICUM REPENS—AGROPYRUM REPENS

(Couch Grass) **Tritic.**

An excellent remedy for excessive irritability of the bladder, dysuria, cystitis, gonorrhea.

**Nose:** Always blowing the nose.

**Urinary:** Frequent, *difficult* and painful micturition (*Pop.*). Gravelly deposits. Catarrhal and purulent discharges (*Pareir.*). Strangury, pyelitis; enlarged prostate. Chronic cystic irritability. Incontinence; constant desire. Urine is dense and causes irritation of the mucous surfaces.

**Relationship:** Compare: *Tradescantia diuretica* (hemorrhage from ear and upper air passages; dysuria, urethral discharge; scrotum inflamed). *Chim., Senec., Pop., Baros., Uva.*

*Polytrichum juniperinum*—Ground moss (dysuria in old people; dropsy, urinary obstruction and suppression).

**Dose:** Tincture or infusion by boiling two ounces in a quart of water until it is reduced to a pint. To be taken as four doses in 24 hours.

---

# TROMBIDIUM MUSCAE DOMESTICAE

(Red Acarus of the Fly) **Trom.**

Has a specific place in the treatment of dysentery. Symptoms *are worse by food and drink.*

**Abdomen:** Severe pain before and after stool; stool only after eating. Gripping in the hypochondrium, in the morning. Congestion of the liver, with urgent, loose, stools on rising. Brown, thin, bloody stools with tenesmus (dysentery). During stool, sharp pain on the left side, shooting downward. Burning in the anus.

**Dose:** Sixth to thirtieth potency.

---

# TUBERCULINUM BOVINUM KENT

(A Nucleo-protein, a Nosode from Tubercular Abscess) **Tub.**

*Tub.* is indicated in renal affections, but caution is necessary, for where skin and intestines do not perform normally even high potencies are dangerous. In chronic cystitis, brilliant and permanent results are obtained (Dr. Nebel Montreux).

Of undoubted value in the treatment of *incipient tuberculosis.* Especially adapted to the light complexioned, narrow chested subjects. Lax fibre, low recuperative powers and very susceptible to changes in weather. Patient is always tired; motion causes intense fatigue; aversion to work; wants constant changes. When *symptoms are constantly changing and well selected remedies fail to improve; also the patient takes cold from the slightest exposure.* Rapid emaciation. Of great value in epilepsy, neurasthenia and in nervous children. Diarrhea in children lasting for weeks, extreme wasting, bluish pallor, exhaustion. Mentally deficient children. Enlarged tonsils. Skin affections, *acute articular rheumatism.* Very sensitive, mentally and physically. General exhaustion. Nervous weakness. Trembling. Epilepsy. Arthritis.

**Mind:** Contradictory characteristics of *Tub.* are mania and melancholia; insomnia and sopor. Irritable, especially on waking up. *Depressed,* melancholic. *Fear of dogs, animals especially.* Desire to use foul language, curse and swear.

**Head:** Subject to deep brain headaches and intense neuralgias. Everything seems strange. Intense pain, as if an iron band was around the head. Meningitis. When critical discharges appear, sweat, polyuria, diarrhea, exanthema, repeat the dose only when crisis comes on. Nocturnal hallucinations, wakes up frightened. Plica polonica (*Vinc.*).

**Ears:** Persistent, offensive otorrhea. *Perforation in membrana tympani, with ragged edges.*

**Nose:** Crops of small boils, intensely painful, successively appear in the nose; *green, fetid pus* (ozena).

**Stomach:** Averse to meat. All gone, hungry sensation (*Sulph.*). Desire for cold milk.

**Abdomen:** Early morning, sudden diarrhea (*Sulph.*). Stools dark brown, offensive, discharged with much force. Tabes mesenterica.

**Female:** *Benign mammary tumors.* Menses too early, too profuse, long lasting (menorrhagia). *Dysmenorrhea. Pain increases with the establishment of the flow.*

**Respiratory:** *Enlarged tonsils.* Hard, dry cough during sleep. Expectoration thick, easy; profuse bronchorrhea. Shortness of breath. Sensation of suffocation, even with plenty of fresh air. Longs for cold air. Broncho-pneumonia in children. Hard, hacking cough, profuse sweating and loss of weight, rales all over the chest. Deposits begin in the apex of the lung (repeated doses).

**Back:** Tension in the nape of the neck and down the spine. Chilliness between shoulders or up the back.

**Sleep:** Poor; wakes early. Overpowering sleepiness in daytime. Dreams vivid and distressing.

**Fever:** Post-critical temperature of a remittent type. Here repeat dose every two hours (MacFarlan). Profuse sweat. General chilliness.

**Skin:** Chronic eczema; itching intense; worse at night. *Acne* in tuberculous children. Measles; psoriasis (*Thyr.*).

**Modalities:** *Worse,* motion, music; before a storm; standing; dampness; from draught; early morning, and after sleep. *Better,* open air.

**Relationship:** Compare: *Koch's lymph (acute and chronic* *parenchymatous nephritis;* produces pneumonia, broncho-pneumonia and congestion of the lungs in tuberculous patients, is a remarkably efficacious remedy in lobular pneumonia, *broncho-pneumonia); Aviare*—Tuberculin from birds (acts on the apices of the lungs; has proved to be an excellent remedy in influenzal bronchitis; symptoms similar to tuberculosis; relieves the debility, diminishes the cough, improves the appetite and braces up the whole organism; acute broncho-pulmonary diseases in children; itching of palms and ears; *cough,* acute, inflammatory, irritating, incessant, and tickling; loss of strength and appetite); *Hydr.* (to fatten patients after Tub.); *Form-ac.* (tuberculosis, chronic nephritis, malignant tumors; pulmonary tuberculosis, not in the third stage, however; lupus; carcinoma of the breast and stomach; Dr. Krull uses injections of solutions corresponding to the third centesimal potency; these must not be repeated before six months).

Compare: *Bac., Psor., Lach. Kalagua* (tuberculosis; garlicky odor of all secretions and breath). *Teucrium scorodonia.* Compare: *Thuj.* (vaccinosis may block the way of action of *Tub.* until *Thuj.* has been given and then acts brilliantly-Burnett).

Complementary: *Calc., Chin., Bry.*

**Dose:** *Tub.* needs more frequent repetition in children's complaints than nearly every other chronic remedy (H. Fergie Woods). Thirtieth and much higher, in infrequent doses. When *Tub.* fails *Syphilinum* often follows advantageously, producing a reaction

"The use of *Tub.* in phthisis pulmonalis demands attention on the following points: In apyretics, purely tubercular phthisis results are marked, provided the eliminative organs are in a good order but nothing below the 1000th should be used unless absolutely necessary. In patients with strepto-staphylo-pneumococci in the bronchi; where, also after washing the sputum, a pure "T.B" bacilli mass remains, the same treatment is indicated. In mixed infection, found in a majority of cases where the sputum swarms with virulent micro-organisms in addition to the "T.B", other procedures are necessary. If the heart is in a good shape, a single dose of *Tub.* 1000-2000 is given, provided there are no marked indications for other remedies. With due attention to temperature and possible excretions, the dose is allowed to work until effects are no longer observed, eight days to eight weeks. Usually a syndrome then presents, permitting the accurate choice of an antipsoric *Sil., Lyc., Phos.*, etc. After a while the picture again darkens and a high potency of the isopathic remedy corresponding to the most virulent and prominent micro-organism found in the sputum is now given: *Staphylo-, Strepto-,* or *Pneumococcinum.* The accurate bacteriological analysis of the sputum is absolutely essential; the choice of the ison again clears the picture, and thus we proceed on one side, etiologically (where these isopathica have not yet been proved); and on the other side symptomatically with antipsoric remedies, and the disease is dominated.

My own experience warns, against the use of *Strepto-*, *Staphylo-* or *Pneumococcinum* below the 500th in cases of mixed infection. I use them only from 1000 to 2000, having seen terrible aggravations from the 30, 100, 200, with a lowering of temperature from 104 to 96. Hence the admonition, which need not concern scoffers, but for those who wish to avail themselves of a potent weapon. The toxins used as remedies are, like *Tub.*, prepared from pure and virulent cultures.

And cases, seemingly condemned to speedy death, are brought a year or two back with normal temperature after of course, sacrificing a large portion of the lung tissue. This result is sure when the patient can and will take care of himself, where the heart has withstood the toxin and the stomach and liver are in good function. Further, climatic variations must be avoided. With the great mineral metabolism of the phthisic, diet regulation is imperative and should predominently consist of vegetables, with the addition of psysiological salts in low potency, *Calc.*, 3x, 5x, *Calc-p.*, 2x, 6x, and intercurrently according to indications, organ remedies like *Cact. Tr.* 30, *Chel.* Tr. 30, *Tarax.* Tr., *Nast.* Tr., *Urt-u.* Tr., *Tuss-far.* Tr., *Lysimachia numularia* Tr., for short periods.

The first dose of *Tub.* in any difficult case is, however, the most weighty prescription. The remedy should not be given without a very careful cardiac examination. As the surgeon before the anesthetic, so must the physician know the heart before administering this drug, especially to children, and seniles—and to young seniles. He who observes this rule will have fewer clinical reproaches on his conscience. When *Tub.* is contraindicated, recourse must be had to the nearest antipsoric.

The above caution applies also in asthma, pleuritis, peritonitis in scrofulous (tuberculous) subjects" (Dr. Nebel Montreux).

---

# TUSSILAGO PETASITES

(Butter-burr) **Tus-p.**

Has some action on the urinary organs and is found useful in gonorrhea. Affections of the pylorus.

**Urinary:** Crawling sensation in the urethra.

**Male:** Gonorrhea; yellowish, thick discharge. Erections with urethral crawling. Pain in the spermatic cord.

**Relationship:** Compare: *Tussilago fragrans* (pylorus pain, plethora and corpulency); *Tussilago farfara* (coughs; as an intercurrent medicine in phthisis pulmonalis. See *Tuberculinum*).

**Dose:** Tincture.

# UPAS TIEUT

(Upas Tree, Strychnos Tiente) **Upa.**

Produces *tonic spasms, tetanus and asphyxia.*

**Head:** Disinclined for mental work. Irritable. Dull headache deep in the brain.

**Eyes:** *Pain in the eyes and orbits with conjunctivitis.* Dull sunken eyes. Styes.

**Mouth:** Herpes labialis. Burning of the tongue. Pain in the mouth, as if from a splinter (*Nit-ac.*).

**Male:** Desire increased, with loss of power (impotence). *Dull backache,* as after excessive coitus.

**Chest:** Lancinating pain throughout the right lung, towards the liver, stopping breathing. Violent palpitations; sensation of heaviness in the stomach.

**Skin:** Numb hands and feet. Hangnails inflamed; itching and redness of roots of nails (paronychia).

**Relationship:** Compare: *Upas antiaris*—resinous exudation of *Antiarus toxicaria* (a deadly poison for the muscular system. It suspends both voluntary muscular action and that of the heart without causing convulsions. Used in Java as an arrow poison (Merrell). Differs in producing *clonic spasms,* violent vomiting, diarrhea, great prostration). *Ox-ac. Upa.* when *Bry.* fails (typhoid).

Antidote: *Cur.*

**Dose:** Third to sixth potency.

---

# URANIUM NITRICUM

(Nitrate of Uranium) **Uran-n.**

Causes glycosuria and polyuria. Is known to produce nephritis, diabetes, degeneration of the liver, hypertension and dropsy. Its therapeutic keynotes are *great emaciation, debility and a tendency to ascites with general dropsy.* Backache and delayed menses. Dry mucous membranes and skin.

**Head:** Ill tempered; dull, heavy pain. Mental depression.

**Eyes:** Lids inflamed (blepharitis) and agglutinated; *styes.*

**Nose:** Nostrils sore with purulent, acrid discharge (ozena).

**Stomach:** Excessive thirst; nausea; *vomiting. Ravenous appetite;* eating followed by flatulence. *Boring pain in pyloric region. Gastric and duodenal ulcers.* Burning pain. *Abdomen bloated.* Flatulence, second only to *Lyc.*

**Urinary:** Copious micturition. *Diuresis.* Incontinence of urine. *Diabetes* (mellitus and insipidus). Emaciation and tympanites. *Burning in urethra* with very acrid urine. *Unable to* retain urine without pain. *Enuresis* (*Mullein oil*).

**Male:** Complete impotency with nocturnal emissions. Organs cold, relaxed, sweaty.

**Relationship:** Compare: *Syzyg., Ph-ac., Lac-ac., Arg-n., Kali-bi., Ars., Phlorizinum* (a glucosidal principle obtained from the bark of the root of the apple and other fruit trees. Produces diabetes and fatty degeneraion of the liver; intermittent fever. Daily doses, 15 grains. Phlorizin causes glycosuria. No hyperglycemia results. It compels the secretory epithelium of the kidney to break down serum albumin into sugar. There is no increase in blood sugar).

**Dose:** Second trituration.

---

## UREA PURA

(Carbamide) **Urea**

Tuberculosis. Lumps. Enlarged glands. Renal dropsy with symptoms of general intoxication. Gouty eczema. Albuminuria, diabetes; uremia. Urine thin and of low specific gravity. A hydrogogue diuretic in the treatment of dropsies. 10 grains every 6 hours.

**Relationship:** Compare: *Uricum acidum* (gout, gouty eczema, rheumatism, lipoma); *Urinum* (acne, boils, scurvy, dropsy); *Urt-u., Tub., Thyr.*

---

## URTICA URENS

(Stinging Nettle) **Urt-u.**

A remedy for agalactia and *lithiasis.* Profuse discharge from mucous membranes. Enuresis and urticaria. Splenic affections. *Antidotes ill effects of eating shellfish.* Symptoms return at the same time every year. Gout and uric acid diathesis. Favors elimination.

*Rheumatism associated with urticaria like eruptions. Neuritis.*

**Head:** Vertigo, headache with splenic pains (anemia).

**Abdomen:** Diarrhea, chronic diseases of the large intestine characterized by profuse secretion of mucus.

**Male:** Itching in the scrotum, keeps him awake; scrotum swollen.

**Female:** *Diminished secretion of milk* (agalactia). Uterine hemorrhage. Acrid and excoriating leucorrhea. *Pruritus vulvae with stinging, itching* and edema. Arrests flow of milk after weaning. Excessive swelling of breasts.

**Extremities:** Pain of acute gout; deltoid; pain in ankles, wrists.

**Fever:** General heat in bed with soreness over the abdomen. Fever of gout. Tropical fever.

**Skin:** *Itching blotches. Urticaria,* burning heat with formication; violent itching. Consequences of suppressed nettle rash. Rheumatism alternates with nettle rash. Burns confined to the skin. Urticaria nodosa (*Bov.*). Erythema, with burning and stinging. *Burns and scalds. Chicken-pox* (*Dulc.*). Angioneurotic edema. Herpes labialis with sensation of heat and itching. Itching and stinging in the scrotum.

**Modalities:** *Worse,* from snow-air; water, cool moist air, touch.

**Relationship:** Compare: *Medus., Nat-m., Lac-c., Ric.* (diminished mammary secretion); *Bomb-pr., Rhus-t., Apis; Chlol., Astac., Puls.* (urticaria); *Boletus luridus* and *Anac.* (urticaria tuberosa); *Lyc.* and *Hedeo.* (uric acid conditions); *Form.*

**Dose:** Tincture and lower potencies.

---

# USNEA BARBATA

(Tree Moss) **Usn.**

Is a remedy in some forms of congestive headache; sunstroke.

**Head:** Bursting feeling, *as if the temples would burst, or the eyes would burst out of the sockets.* Throbbing carotids.

**Relationship:** Compare: *Glon., Bell.*

**Dose:** Tincture, drop doses.

---

# USTILAGO MAYDIS

(Corn-smut) **Ust.**

Flabby condition of the uterus. Hemorrhage. Congestion of various parts, especially at climacteric. Crusta lactea (*Viol-t.*).

**Head:** Very depressed. Feels full. Nervous headache from menstrual irregularities.

**Eyes:** Aching in eyeballs with marked lachrymation.

**Male:** Uncontrollable masturbation. Spermatorrhea with erotic fancies and amorous dreams. Emissions with irresistible tendency to masturbation. Dull pain in lumbar region, with great despondency and mental irritability.

**Female:** Vicarious menstruation. Ovaries burn, painful and swollen (ovaritis). Profuse menses after miscarriage; discharge of blood from the slightest provocation; bright red; partly clotted. Menorrhagia at climaxis (*Calc., Lach.*). Oozing of dark blood, clotted, forming long black strings. Uterus hypertrophied (fibroids). *Cervix bleeds easily.* Postpartum hemorrhage. Profuse lochia.

**Extremities:** Muscular debility, *sensation as if boiling water is running along the back.* Clonic and tetanic movements. Muscular contractions, especially of lower limbs.

**Fever:** Abundant sweat. Pulse at first accelerated then enfeebled. Palpitations.

**Skin:** Alopecia. Tendency to small boils. Skin dry; eczema; copper colored spots. Pruritus; sunburn. Psoriasis (internally and externally).

**Relationship:** Compare: *Sec., Sabin., Zea italica* (possess curative properties in skin diseases, particularly in psoriasis and eczema rubrum. Mania for bathing. Impulse for suicide, particularly by drowning. Easily angered. Appetite increased, voracious, alternating with disgust for food. Pyrosis, nausea, vomiting, better drinking wine).

**Dose:** Tincture to third potency.

---

## UVA URSI

(Bearberry) **Uva**

Urinary symptoms are most important. Cystitis with hematuria. Uterine hemorrhage. Chronic cystitis with pain, tenesmus and catarrhal discharges. *Burning after discharge of slimy urine. Pyelitis.* Calculus inflammation. Dyspnea, nausea, vomiting; pulse small and irregular. Cyanosis. Urticaria without itching.

**Urinary:** Frequent urging with severe spasms of the bladder; burning and tearing pain. Urine contains blood (hematuria), pus (pyuria), and a lot of tenacious mucus, with clots in large masses. Involuntary; green urine. Painful dysuria.

**Relationship:** Compare: *Arbutinum* (a crystallized glucoside of *Uva;* found also in *Kalm., Gaul.* and other genera of the family of *Eriaceae;* given in doses of 3 to 8 grains with sugar three times a day. Used as an urinary antiseptic and diuretic). *Arctosphylos manzanita* (acts on renal and reproductive organs. Gonorrhea, cystitis, diabetes, menorrhagia. Tincture of leaves). *Vaccinum myrtillus*—Huckleberries (dysentery; typhoid, keeps intestines aseptic and prevents absorption and reinfection).

**Dose:** Tincture, five to thirty drops. In pyelitis a trituration of the leaves.

---

## VACCININUM

(Nosode From Vaccine Matter) **Vac.**

Vaccine poison is capable of setting up a morbid state of extreme chronicity, named after Burnett Vaccinosis, symptoms are like those of Hahnemann's sycosis. Neuralgias, inveterate skin eruptions, chilliness, indigestion with great flatulent distention (Clarke). Whooping cough.

**Mind:** Irritable, impatient, ill humored, nervous.

**Head:** Frontal headache. Forehead and eyes feel as if split.

**Eyes:** Inflamed and red lids (blepharitis).

**Skin:** Hot and dry. Pimples and blotches. Eruptions like variola.

**Relationship:** Compare: anti-vaccinal remedies; *Vario.*, *Maland.*, *Thuj.*, powerful adjuvants in treatment of malignant disease.

**Dose:** Sixth to 200th potency.

---

# VALERIANA OFFICINALIS

(Valerian) **Valer.**

Hysteria, over sensitiveness, nervous affections, when apparently well chosen remedies fail. Hysterical spasms and affections generally. *Hysterical flatulence* (flatulence in hysterical people).

**Mind:** Changeable disposition. Feels light, as if floating in air. Over sensitiveness (*Staph.*). Hallucinations at night. *Irritable.* Tremulous.

**Head:** Sensation of great coldness. Pressure in the forehead. Feeling of intoxication.

**Ears:** *Otalgia from exposure to draughts and cold.* Nervous noises. Hyperesthesia.

**Throat:** *Sensation as if a thread was hanging down the throat.* Nausea felt in the throat. Pharynx feels constricted.

**Stomach:** Hunger with nausea. Erucatations foul. Heartburn with gulping of rancid fluid.[1] Nausea with faintness. *Child vomits curdled milk in large lumps after nursing.*

**Abdomen:** Bloated. Hysterical cramps[2]. Thin, watery diarrhea, *with lumps of coagulated milk and violent screaming in children.* Greenish, papescent, bloody stool. Spasms in bowels after food and at night, in bed.

**Female:** Menses late and scanty (*Puls.*).

**Respiratory:** Choking on falling asleep. Spasmodic asthma; convulsive movements of the diaphragm.

**Extremities:** Rheumatic pain in limbs. *Constant jerking.* Heaviness. Sciatica; *pain worse standing and resting on the floor* (*Bell.*); better walking. Pain in the heels *when sitting.*

---

1 Frequent, empty or rancid and burning rising (Clarke — Dictionary of Practical Materia Medica).

2 Spasms of stomach and abdomen in incurable cases of hysteria and hypochondriasis (Clarke — Dictionary of Practical Materia Medica).

**Sleep:** Sleepless, with nocturnal itching and muscular spasms. Worse on waking up.

**Fever:** Long lasting heat, often with sweat on the face. *Heat predominates.* Sensation of icy coldness (*Helo., Camph., Abies-c.*).

**Relationship:** Compare: *Asaf., Ign., Croc., Castm., Am-val.* (in neuralgia, gastric disturbance and great nervous agitation. Insomnia especially during pregnancy and menopause. Feeble, hysterical nervous patients).

**Dose:** Tincture.

---

## VANADIUM METALLICUM

(The Metal) **Vanad.**

Its action is that of an oxygen carrier and a catalyzer, hence its use in wasting diseases. Increases amount of hemoglobin, also combines its oxygen with toxins and destroys their virulence. Also increases and stimulates phagocytes.

A remedy in degenerative conditions of the liver and arteries. Anorexia and symptoms of gastrointestinal irritation; albumen, casts and blood in urine. Tremors; vertigo; hysteria and melancholia; neuro-retinitis and blindness. Anemia, emaciation. Cough dry, irritating and paroxysmal, sometimes with hemorrhages. Irritation of nose, eyes and throat. Tuberculosis, chronic rheumatism, diabetes. *Acts as a tonic for digestive function* and in early tuberculosis. Arteriosclerosis, sensation as if the heart was compressed, as if blood had no room in the aorta. Anxious pressure on the whole chest. Fatty heart. Generative states, has brain softening. Atheroma in arteries of brain and liver. Compare: *Ars., Phos. Am-van.* (fatty degeneration of liver).

**Dose:** 6-12 potency. The best form is *Natrium vanadicum* 2 mg. daily, by mouth.

---

## VANILLA PLANIFOLIA

(Vanilla) **Vanil.**

Marked skin irritation resembling Poison oak; is sometimes produced by handling the beans, also by local use of vanilla essence in a hair wash. Vanilla is supposed to stimulate the brain and sexual propensities. Do not use the synthetic vanilla extract. Various disorders of the nervous system and circulation are produced in workers with vanilla. Is an emmanagogue and aphrodisiac. Menses prolonged.

**Dose:** *Vanil.* 6th to 30th, has been found effective in curing the skin affection.

## VARIOLINUM

(Lymph From Small Pox Pustule) **Vario.**

Used for "internal vaccination." Seems to be efficacious in protecting against, modifying and aiding in the cure of small pox.

**Head:** Morbid fear of small pox. Pain in the occiput.

**Eyes:** Inflamed eyelids (blepharitis).

**Ears:** Deafness.

**Respiratory:** Oppressed breathing. Throat feels closed. Cough with thick viscid, bloody mucus (hemoptysis). Sensation of a lump in the right side of throat.

**Back:** *Excruciating backache.* Pain shifts from the back to the abdomen.

**Extremities:** *Aching in legs.* Tired all over with restlessness. Wrists painful.

**Fever:** Hot fever, with intense radiating heat. Profuse, bad smelling sweat.

**Skin:** Hot, dry. Eruption of pustules. *Shingles* (herpes zoster).

**Relationship:** Compare: *Vac.* (same action); *Maland.:* The morbid product of the grease of the horse (a prophylactic of small pox and a remedy for the ill effects of vaccination; chronic eczema following vaccination).

**Dose:** Sixth to thirtieth potency.

---

## VERATRUM ALBUM

(White Hellebore) **Verat.**

A perfect picture of *collapse* with *extreme coldness, blueness, and weakness,* is offered by this drug. Post-operative shock with cold sweat on the forehead a pale face and rapid, feeble pulse. *Cold perspiration on the forehead,* with nearly all complaints. *Vomiting, purging, and cramps in extremities. Profuse,* violent retching and vomiting is most characteristic. Surgical shock. Excessive dryness of all mucous membranes. *"Coprophagia"* violent mania alternates with silence and a refusal to talk.

**Mind:** Melancholy, with stupor and mania. Sits in a stupid manner; notices nothing; *Sullen indifference.* Frenzy of excitement; shrieks, curses. Puerperal mania. Aimless wandering from home. *Delusions of impending misfortunes.* Mania, with a desire to cut and tear things (*Tarent.*). Attacks of pain, with delirium driving *the patient to* madness. Cursing, howling all night.

**Head:** Contracted features. *Cold sweat on the forhead. Sensation of a lump of ice on the vertex* (apoplexy). Headache with nausea, vomiting, diarrhea and a pale face. Neck too weak to hold head up.

**Eyes:** Surrounded by dark rings. Staring; turned upwards (epilepsy, meningitis). Without lustre. Lachrymation with hyperemia. Lids, dry heavy.

**Face:** Features sunken. *Icy coldness of the tip of the nose and face.* Nose grows more pointed. Tearing in cheeks, temples and eyes. *Face very pale, blue, collapsed, cold.*

**Mouth:** Tongue pale, cold; cool sensation, as from peppermint. Dry in the center, not relieved by water. Salty saliva. Toothache, teeth feel heavy, as if filled with lead.

**Stomach:** *Voracious* appetite. *Thirst for cold water, but is vomited as soon as it is swallowed.* Averse to warm food. Hiccough. *Copious vomiting and nausea; aggravated by drinking and least motion.* Craves fruits, juicy and cold things, ice, salt. Anguish in the pit of the stomach. Great weakness after vomiting. Gastric irritability with *chronic* vomiting of food.

**Abdomen:** Sinking and empty feeling. *Cold feeling* in the stomach and abdomen. Pain in the abdomen preceding stool. Cramps, knotting abdomen and legs. Sensation as if hernia would protrude (*Nux-v.*). Abdomen sensitive to pressure, swollen with terrible colic.

**Stool:** Constipation from inactivity of the rectum, with heat and headache. Constipation in babies due to very cold weather. *Stools large, with much straining till exhausted, with cold sweat.* Diarrhea, very painful, watery, *copious and forcibly evacuated,* followed by great prostration. Evacuations of cholera morbus and true cholera when vomiting accompanies the purging.

**Female:** Menses too early; profuse and exhausting. *Dysmenorrhea with coldness,* purging, *cold sweat. Faints from least exertion.* Sexual mania precedes menses.

**Respiratory:** Hoarse, weak voice. Rattling in the chest. Abundant mucus in the bronchial tubes, that cannot be coughed up. Coarse rales. Chronic bronchitis in the aged (*Hippoz.*). Loud, barking, stomach cough, followed by eructation of gas; worse in a warm room. Hollow cough, tickling low down, with a blue face (cyanosed). Cough comes on from drinking, especially cold water; urine escapes when coughing. Cough on entering a warm room from cold air (*Bry.*).

**Heart:** Palpitations with anxiety (angina pectoris), and rapid audible respiration. Pulse irregular, feeble. Tobacco heart from chewing tobacco. Intermittent action of heart in feeble people with some hepatic obstruction. One of the best heart stimulants in homeopathic doses (J. S. Mitchell).

**Extremities:** Soreness and tenderness of joints. Sciatica; pains like electric flashes. *Cramps in calves.* Neuralgia in the brachial plexus; arms feel swollen, cold, paralytic.

**Fever:** Chill *with extreme coldness* and thirst.

**Skin:** Blue, cold, clammy, inelastic; *cold as death.* Cold sweat. Wrinkling of skin of hands and feet.

**Modalities:** *Worse,* at night; wet, cold weather. *Better,* walking and warmth.

**Relationship:** Compare: *Veratrinum*—alkaloid from the seeds of Sabadilla (electric pains, electric shocks in muscles, fibrillary twitchings); *Cholas terrepina* (cramps in calves); *Camph., Cupr., Ars., Cupr-ar.* (*intermittent, cold, clammy sweat*); *Narcissus poeticus* (gastroenteritis with severe griping and cutting pain in bowels. Fainting, trembling, cold limbs, small and irregular pulse); *Trychosanthes dioica* (diarrhea, pain in liver, dizziness after every stool); *Agaricus emeticus* (vertigo; longing for ice cold water; burning pain in stomach); *Agaricus phalloides* (cholera, cramps in stomach, cold extremities, urine suppressed). *Veratrinum* (increased vascular tension. It relaxes it and stimulates the elimination of toxins by skin, kidneys, and liver).

**Dose:** First to thirtieth potency. In diarrhea, not below the sixth.

---

## VERATRUM VIRIDE

(White American Hellebore) **Verat-v.**

Paroxysms of auricular fibrillation. Induces fall of both systolic and diastolic blood pressure. Congestions, especially lungs and base of the brain, with nausea and vomiting. Twitchings and convulsions. Especially adapted to full blooded, plethoric people. Great prostration. Rheumatism of the heart. *Bloated, livid face.* Furious delirium. Effects of sunstroke. *Esophagitis* (Farrington). *Verat-v.* will raise the opsonic index against the *diploccus pneumonia,* 70 to 109 percent. Congestive stage and early manifestations of hepatization in pneumonia. Zigzag temperature. Clinically, it is known that diseases such as Tiegel's contracture, Thompson's disease, athetosis and pseudo-hypertrophic muscular paralysis present a symptomatology quite similar to that produced by *Verat-v.* on muscular tissue (A. E. Hinsdale, M.D.).

**Mind:** Quarrelsome and delirious.

**Head:** Congestion intense, almost apoplectic. Hot head, bloodshot eyes. Bloated, livid face. Hippocratic face. Head retracted, *pupils dilated,* diplopia. Meningitis. *Pain from the nape of neck;* cannot hold head up. Sunstroke; head feels full, throbbing arteries (*Bell., Glon., Usn.*). *Face flushed.* Convulsive twitching of facial muscles (*Agar.*). Vertigo with nausea.

**Mouth:** Tongue white or yellow, *with a red streak down the middle.* Feels scalded. Increased saliva.

**Stomach:** Thirsty. Nausea and vomiting. Smallest quantity of food or drink is immediately rejected. Constrictive pain; increased by warm drinks. *Hiccough;* excessive and painful, *with spasms of esophagus.* Burning in the stomach and esophagus.

**Abdomen:** Pain above the pelvis with soreness.

**Urinary:** Scanty with cloudy sediment.

**Female:** Rigid os (*Bell., Gels.*). Puerperal fever. Suppressed menstruation, with congestion of the head (*Bell.*). Menstrual colic before the appearance of discharge with strangury

**Respiratory:** Congestion of lungs. Difficulty in breathing. Sensation of a heavy load on the chest. Pneumonia with a faint feeling in the stomach and violent congestion. *Croup.*

**Heart:** Pulse *slow, soft, weak,* irregular, intermittent. Rapid pulse, low tension (*Tab., Dig.*). Constant, dull, burning pain in the region of heart Valvular diseases. *Beating of pulses throughout the body,* especially in the right thigh.

**Extremities:** Aching pains in the back of the neck and shoulders. Severe pain in joints and muscles. Violent electric shock-like pain in limbs. Convulsive twitchings (chorea). *Acute rheumatism. Fever.*

**Fever:** Hyperthermy in the evening and hypothermy in the morning. Suppurative fevers with great variation of temperature.

**Skin:** Erysipelas with cerebral symptoms. Erythema. Itching in various parts. *Hot sweat.*

**Relationship:** Compare: *Gels., Bapt., Bell., Acon., Ferr-p.*

Antidotes: *Strychninum*: fluid extract, 20-40 drops.

**Dose:** First to sixth potency.

---

# VERBASCUM THAPSUS

(Mullein) **Verb.**

Has a pronounced action on the inferior maxillary branch of the fifth pair of cranial nerves; on the ear; respiratory tract and bladder. *Catarrhs* and colds, *with periodical prosopalgia.* Quietens nervous, bronchial and urinary irritation and cough.

**Ears:** Otalgia with a sense of obstruction. Deafness. Dry, scaly condition of the meatus (use locally).

**Face:** Neuralgia affecting the zygoma, temporo-maxillary joint and ear (*Meny.*), particularly of the left side, with lachrymation, coryza and sensation *as if the parts were crushed with tongs.* Talking, sneezing and change of temperature aggravate the pain; also, pressing teeth together. Pain seems to come in flashes, excited by least movement, occurring periodically at the same hour in the morning and afternoon everyday.

**Abdomen:** Pain extends deep down, causing contraction of the sphincter ani.

**Rectum:** Many movements a day, with twisting pains around the navel. Hemorrhoids with obstructed, hard stool. Inflamed and painful piles.

**Urinary:** Constant dribbling. *Enuresis.* Burning micturition. Increases with pressure in bladder.

**Respiratory:** *Hoarse;* voice deep, harsh; sounds like a trumpet; "basso profundo." Cough; worse at night. Asthma. Soreness in pharynx, cough during sleep.

**Extremities:** Cramp-like pain in soles, right foot and knee. Lower extremities feel heavy. Thumb feels numb. Neuralgic pain in the left ankle. Stiffness *and soreness of joints of the lower extremities.*

**Modalities:** *Worse,* change of temperature, talking, sneezing, biting hard (inferior dental nerve); from 9 a.m. to 4 p.m.

**Relationship:** Compare: *Rhus-a., Caust., Plat., Sphingurus maritini* (pain in zygoma).

**Dose:** *Mullein oil* (locally for otalgia and dry, scaly conditions of the meatus. Also for teasing cough at night on lying down. Internally, tincture and lower potencies. *Enuresis,* five drop doses at night and in the morning).

---

## VERBENA HASTATA

(Blue Vervain) **Verbe-h.**

Affects the skin and *nervous system.* Nervous depression, weakness, irritation and spasms. Promotes the absorption of blood and allays pain in bruises. Vesicular erysipelas. Passive congestion and intermittent fever. One of the remedies for Poison oak. *Epilepsy,* insomnia, mental exhaustion. In epilepsy, it *brightens up the patient's mental powers* and helps the constipation.

**Dose:** Single dose of the tincture. In epilepsy must be continued for a long time. *Verbe-h.* in the form of a tea as a diuretic drink is used by Vannier (Paris) to aid elimination in tubercular therapy.

---

## VESPA CRABRO

(Live Wasp) **Vesp.**

Skin and female symptoms marked. Indurated feeling. Vasomotor symptoms of skin and mucous membranes.

Dizzy, better lying on back. Fainting. Numbness and blindness. Nausea and vomiting, followed by creeping chills from feet upward. Cramping pain in bowels. Axillary glands swollen with soreness of upper arms. Perspiration on parts laid on with itching.

**Eyes:** Erysipelatous inflammation of lids. *Chemosis.*

**Face:** Painful and swollen (cellutitis). Swelling of mouth and throat, with violent burning pain.

**Urinary:** *Burning* with micturition; also itching.

**Female:** Menstruation, preceded by depression, pain, pressure, and constipation. *Left ovary markedly affected,* with *frequent burning, micturition;* sacral pains extending up the back. *Erosions around the external os.*

**Skin:** Erythema; *intense itching;* burning. *Boils;* stinging and soreness, relieved by bathing with vinegar. Wheals, macules and swellings with burning, stinging and soreness. Erythema multiforme, *relieved* by bathing with vinegar.

**Relationship:** Compare: *Scorpio europaeus* (salivation; strabismus; tetanus); *Apis.*

Antidote; *Semp.,* locally.

**Dose:** Third to thirtieth potency.

# VIBURNUM OPULUS

(High Cranberry) **Vib.**

A general remedy for cramps. Colicky pains in pelvic organs. Superconscious of the internal sexual organs. Female symptoms most important. *Often prevents miscarriage.* False labor pains. Spasmodic and congestive affections of ovarian or uterine origin.

**Head:** Irritable. Vertigo; sensation as if falling forward. Severe pain in the temporal region. Sore feeling in the eyeballs.

**Stomach:** Constant nausea; relieved by eating. No appetite.

**Abdomen:** *Sudden cramps and colicy pain.* Tender to pressure around the umbilicus.

**Rectum:** Stools large and hard with cutting pain in the rectum and soreness of the anus.

**Urinary:** Frequent urging. Copious, pale, light colored urine. Cannot hold water on coughing or walking.

**Female:** Menses *too late, scanty, lasting for a few hours,* offensive in odor, with crampy pains, cramps extend down the thighs (*Bell.*). Bearing down pains before menses. Ovarian region feels heavy and congested (ovaritis). Aching in sacrum and pubes, with pain in anterior muscles of thighs (*Xan.*); *spasmodic and membranous dysmenorrhea* (*Borx.*). Leucorrhea, excoriating. Smarting and itching of genitals. Faints on attempting to sit up. *Frequent and very early miscarriage,* seeming like sterility. Pain from the back to the loins and womb, worse early morning.

**Extremities:** Stiff, sore feeling in the nape of neck. Feels as if the back would break. Sacral backache. Lower extremities weak and heavy.

**Modalities:** *Worse,* lying on the affected side, in a warm room, evening and night. *Better,* in open air and resting.

**Relationship:** Compare: *Viburnum prunifolium*—Black haw (habitual miscarriage; *after-pains;* cancer of the tongue; obstinate hiccough; supposed to be a uterine tonic. Morning sickness; menstrual irregularities in sterile females with uterine displacements). *Cimic., Caul., Sep., Xan.*

**Dose:** Tincture and lower potencies.

## VINCA MINOR

(Lesser Periwinkle) **Vinc.**

A remedy for skin affections, eczema and especially plica polonica; also for hemorrhages and diphtheria.

**Head:** Tearing pain in the vertex, ringing and whistling in ears. Whirling vertigo, with flickering before eyes. *Spots on scalp, oozing moisture, matting hair together. Corrosive itching of scalp.* Bald spots (alopecia). *Plica polonica.* Irresistible desire to scratch.

**Nose:** Tip gets red easily. Moist eruptions on the septum. Stoppage of one nostril. *Sores in the nose.* Seborrhea of upper lip and base of nose.

**Throat:** Dysphagia. Ulcers. Frequent hawking. *Diphtheria.*

**Female:** Excessive menstruation with great weakness. *Passive uterine hemorrhages* (*Ust., Tril-p., Sec.*). Menorrhagia; continuous flow, particulary at climacteric (*Lach.*). Hemorrhages from fibroids.

**Skin:** Corrosive itching. *Great sensitiveness of the skin, with redness and soreness* from slight rubbing. Eczema of head (crusta lactea) and face; pustules, itching, burning and offensive odor. Hair matted together.

**Relationship:** Compare: *Olnd., Staph.*

**Dose:** First to third potency.

## VIOLA ODORATA

(Violet) **Viol-o.**

Has a specific action on the ear. Especially affects dark haired patients; supra-orbital and orbital regions. Rheumatism in the upper parts of the body especially when on the *right* side. *Worm affections* in children (*Teucr.*). Locally, for pain due to uterine fibroids. Also against snake bites, bee stings. *Tension* extends to upper half of face and ears[1].

**Head:** *Burning in the forehead.* Vertigo; everything in the head seems to whirl around. Heaviness of head, with sensation of weakness in the muscles of the nape of neck. *Scalp tense; must knit the brows. Tendency to pain immediately above the eyebrows.* Throbbing under the eye and temple. *Headache across the forehead.* Acts upon frontal sinuses. Hysterical attacks in tuberculous patients.

**Eyes:** Heaviness of lids. Eyeball feels compressed. Flames before the eyes. Myopia. Choroiditis. Illusions of vision; fiery, serpentine circles.

**Ears:** Shooting in ears. Aversion to music. Roaring and tickling. Deep stitches beneath the ears. Deafness; *otorrhea.* Ear affections with pain in eyeballs.

**Urinary:** *Milky urine;* smells strong. Enuresis in nervous children.

**Respiratory:** Torpor at the end of nose, as if from a blow. Dry, short, spasmodic cough and dyspnea; worse at daytime. Oppression of chest. Pertussis with hoarseness. *Dyspnea during pregnancy.* Difficulty in breathing, anxiety and palpitations, with hysteria.

**Extremities:** Rheumatism of the deltoid muscle. Trembling of limbs. *Pressing pain in right carpal and metacarpal joints* (rheumatism) (Ulm.).

**Modalities:** *Worse,* cool air.

**Relationship:** Compare: *Ulmus* (formication in feet, numb, creeping pain in legs and feet; rheumatic pains above wrists; numbness, tingling and full soreness where gastrocnemius gives off its tendon); *Chen-a.* (*ears; serous or bloody effusion in the labyrinth;* chronic otitis media; progressive *deafness to the voice, but sensitive to sounds* of passing vehicles and other noises; buzzing; absent or deficient bone conduction; consciousness of the ear; hearing better for shrill, high pitched sounds than for low ones); *Aur., Puls., Sep., Ign., Cina; Caul.* (in rheumatism of small joints).

**Dose:** First to sixth potency.

---

## VIOLA TRICOLOR

(Pansy) **Viol-t.**

The principal use of this remedy is for eczema in childhood and nocturnal emissions accompanied by very vivid dreams.

---

[1] A keynote symptoms of *Viol-o.* is *tension.* Tension which at times extends to the upper half of face especially the nose thence to forehead and temples, as far as the ears, alternating with a similar sensation in the occiput and cervical muscles. Tension in the integuments of face (Clarke — Dictionary of Practical Materia Medica).

**Head:** Heavy pain, pressing outward. Eczema of the scalp (plica plonica, crusta lactea), with swollen glands. Face hot and sweaty after eating.

**Throat:** Increased phlegm, causes hawking; worse in open air. Dysphagia.

**Urinary:** Copious; disagreeable, cat like odor.

**Male:** Swelling of prepuce, burning in glans (balanitis). Itching. Involuntary, seminal emissions at stool.

**Skin:** *Impetigo.* Intolerable itching. Eruptions, particularly over the face and head with burning, itching; worse at night. Thick scabs, which cracks, exude a tenacious yellow pus. Eczema impetigonoides of the face. Sycosis.

**Modalities:** *Worse,* winter; 11 a.m.

**Relationship:** Compare: *Rhus-t., Calc., Sep.*

**Dose:** Lower potencies.

---

# VIPERA BERUS

(The German Viper) **Vip.**

Viper poisoning causes a temporary increase in reflexes, paresis supervenes with paraplegia of the lower extremities extending upwards. Resembles acute ascending paralysis of Landry (Wells). Has a special action on kidneys and induces hematuria. Cardiac dropsy.

Indicated in inflammation of veins with great swelling; *bursting sensation. Hepatomegaly.* Ailments of menopause. Edema of glottis. Polyneuritis, poliomyelitis.

**Face:** Excessively swollen. Lips and tongue swollen, livid, protruding. Tongue dry, brown, black. Speech difficult.

**Abdomen:** Violent pain in enlarged liver, with jaundice and fever; extends to the shoulder and hip.

**Extremities:** Patient is obliged to keep the extremities elevated, but if *allowed to hang down, it seems as if they would burst and the pain is unbearable* (phlegmasia alba dolens) (*Aran.*). *Varicose veins* and acute phlebitis. Veins swollen, sensitive; bursting pain. Severe cramps in lower extremities.

**Skin:** Livid. Skin peels in large plates. Lymphangioma, boils, carbuncles, with *a bursting* sensation, relieved by elevating parts.

**Relationship:** *Pelius berus*—Adder (prostration and fainting, faltering pulse, skin yellow, *pain around the navel.* Swelling of arm, tongue, right eye; giddiness, nervousness, faintness, sickness, compression of chest, can not breathe properly or take a deep breath; aching and stiffness of limbs, joints stiff, collapsed feeling, great thirst); *Ser-ang.* (heart and kidney diseases. Failure of compensation and impending asystole).

**Dose:** Twelfth potency.

# VISCUM ALBUM

(Mistletoe) **Visc.**

Low blood pressure. Dilated blood vessels but does not act on the centers in the medulla. Pulse is slow due to central irritation of the vagus.

The symptoms point especially to rheumatic and gouty complaints; neuralgia, especially sciatica. Epilepsy, *chorea* and metrorrhagia. *Rheumatic deafness. Asthma.* Spinal pain, due to uterine disease. Rheumatism with *tearing pain.* Hypertensive albuminuria. Valvular disease with disturbances in the sexual sphere. Symptoms of epileptic aura and petit mal.

**Head:** Sensation as if the whole vault of skull was lifted up. Persistent vertigo.

**Eyes:** Blue rings around the eyes. Diplopia. Buzzing and stopped up feeling in ear. Deafness from cold. Facial muscles in constant agitation.

**Ears:** Buzzing (tinnitus) and stopped up sensation. Deafness from exposure to cold.

**Face:** Facial muscles in consistant agitation.

**Female:** Hemorrhage with pain (dysmenorrhea, menorrhagia); blood partly clotted and partly bright red. Climacteric complaints (*Lach., Sulph.*). Pain from sacrum to pelvis, with tearing, shooting pains from above downwards. Retained placenta (*Sec.*). Chronic endometritis. Metrorrhagia. Ovaralgia, especially on left side.

**Respiratory:** Dyspnea; *feeling of suffocation when lying on the left side.* Spasmodic cough. *Asthma,* if connected with gout or rheumatism. Stertorous breathing.

**Heart:** Hypertrophy with valvular insufficiency; pulse small and weak; unable to rest in a reclining position. Palpitations during coitus. Low tension. Failing compensation, dyspnea worse lying on left side. Weight and oppression of the heart; as if a hand was squeezing it; tickling sensation around the heart.

**Extremities:** Pain alternates in the knee and ankle with shoulder and elbow. *Sciatica. Tearing,* shooting pain in both thighs and upper extremities. A *glow* rises from the feet to the head; seems to be on fire. Periodic pain from sacrum to pelvis, *worse in bed,* with pain in thighs and upper extremities. General tremor, as if all muscles were in a state of fibrillary contraction (chorea). Dropsy of extremities. Sensation of a spider crawling over the back of hand and foot. Itching all over. Compressing pain in feet.

**Modalities:** *Worse,* winter, cold, stormy weather; in bed. Movement; lying on left side.

**Relationship:** Compare: *Sec., Conv., Bry., Puls., Rhod. Guipsine*—active principle (exalts the hypotensive properties of *Visc.*). *Hedera helix*—Common Ivy (intracranial pressure).

**Dose:** Tincture and lower potencies.

## WYETHIA HELENOIDES

(Poison Weed) **Wye.**

Has marked effects on the throat and has proven to be an excellent remedy in *pharyngitis,* especially of the follicular form. Irritable throat of singers and public speakers. Useful also in hemorrhoids. Symptoms of hay fever; *itching in posterior nares.*

**Head:** Nervous, uneasy, depressed. Dizzy. Rush of blood to the head. Sharp pain in forehead.

**Mouth:** Feels as if scalded; sensation of heat down the esophagus. Itching in the palate.

**Throat:** Constant clearing and hemming. *Dry,* posterior nares; no relief from clearing. *Throat feels swollen;* epiglottis dry and burning. Dysphagia. Constant desire to swallow saliva. Uvula feels elongated.

**Stomach:** Sense of weight. Belching of wind alternating with hiccough. Nausea and vomiting.

**Abdomen:** Pain below the ribs of right side (pain in the liver region).

**Rectum:** Loose, dark stools at night. Itching in the anus. Constipation, *with hemorrhoids;* not bleeding.

**Female:** Pain in the left ovary, shooting down to the knee. Pain in the uterus; can outline its contour.

**Respiratory:** *Dry, hacking cough,* caused by tickling of the epiglottis. Burning sensation in the bronchial tubes. Tendency to get hoarse on talking or singing; throat hot, dry. Dry asthma.

**Extremities:** Pain in the back; extends to the tip of spine. Pain, right arm, stiffness of wrist and hand. Aching pains all over.

**Fever:** Chill at 11 a.m. Thirst for ice water during chill. No thirst with heat. Profuse sweat all night. Terrific headache during sweat.

**Relationship:** Compare: *Arum-d., Sang., Lach.*

**Dose:** First to sixth potency.

---

## XANTOXYLUM FRAXINEUM

(Prickly Ash) **Xan.**

Its specific action is on the nervous system and mucous membranes. Paralysis, especially *hemiplegia.* Painful hemorrhages, after-pains, *neuralgic dysmenorrhea* and rheumatic affections, offer a therapeutic field for this remedy, especially in patients of spare habit and nervous, delicate organization. Indigestion from over eating or from too much fluid. Sluggish capillary circulation. Neurasthenia, poor assimilation, insomnia, occipital headache. Increases mucus secretion of the mouth and stimulates the secretion from all the glands with ducts opening in the mouth.

**Mind:** Nervous, frightened. Mental depression.

**Head:** Feels full. Weight and pain on the vertex. Pain over eyes, throbbing pressure over nose, pressure in the forehead; head seems divided; ringing in the ears. Occipital headache. Sick headache with dizziness and flatulence.

**Mouth:** Dryness of the mouth and fauces, pharyngitis (*Wye.*).

**Face:** Neuralgia of the lower jaw.

**Rectum:** Griping with diarrhea. Dysentery with *tympanites,* tenesmus; inodorous discharges.

**Female:** Menses too early and painful. Ovarian neuralgia with pain in the loins and lower abdomen; worse, *left side,* extending down the thigh, along the genito-crural nerves. *Neuralgic dysmenorrhea* with neuralgic headaches; pain in the *back and down the legs.* Menses thick, almost black. *After-pains* (*Arn., Cupr., Cham.*). Leucorrhea at time of menses. Neurasthenic patients who are thin, emaciated; poor assimilation with insomnia and occipital headache.

**Respiratory:** Aphonia. Constant desire to take a long breath (asthma); oppression of chest. Dry cough, day and night.

**Extremities:** Paralysis of the left side following spinal disorders (multiple sclerosis). Numbness of the left side; impairment of nerves of motion (motor nerves). Hemiplegia. Pain in nape, extending down the back (coccygodynia). Sciatica; worse, hot weather. Anterior, crural neuralgia (*Staph.*). Left arm numb. Neuralgic shooting pain, as if from electricity, all over the limbs.

**Sleep:** Hard and unrefreshing; dreams of flying. Sleepleesness in neurasthenics.

**Relationship:** Compare: *Gnaph., Cimic., Staph., Mez., Piscidia erythmia*—White dogwood (a nerve sedative. *Insomnia due* to worry, nervous excitement, spasmodic cough; pain of irregular menstruation; regulates the flow. Neuralgic and spasmodic affections. Use tincture in rather material doses).

**Dose:** First to sixth potency.

---

## XEROPHYLLUM

(Tamalpais Lily, Basket Grass Flower) **Xero.**

Should prove curative in eczematous conditions, Poison oak, early typhoid states, etc.

**Mind:** Dull, cannot concentrate on studies; forgets names; *writes last letters of words first;* misspells common words.

**Head:** Feels full, stuffed up, pain across the forehead and above the eyes. Great pressure at the root of the nose. Bewildered. Loss of consciousness. Pulsating headache.

**Eyes:** Painful, sensation of sand in the eyes, smarting; difficult to focus on close work (hypermetropia). Eyes feel sore, burn.

**Nose:** Stuffed; tightness at the bridge of nose; acute nasal catarrh.

**Face:** Bloated in the morning. Puffy under the eyes.

**Throat:** Stitching pain upon swallowing.

**Stomach:** Feels full and heavy. Eructations sour; offensive, an hour after luncheon and dinner. Vomiting at 2 p.m.

**Abdomen:** Intestinal flatulence. In the morning, rumbling in bowels, with desire for stool.

**Rectum:** Constipation, stools hard, like small lumps. Difficult, soft stools, with much straining. Much flatus. Bearing down pain in the rectum.

**Urinary:** Difficulty of retaining; dribbling when walking. Frequent micturition at night.

**Female:** Bearing down sensation. Vulva inflamed (vulvitis), with furious itching. Increased sexual desire (nymphomania), with ovarian and uterine pains, and leucorrhea.

**Respiratory:** Posterior nares raw; discharge thick, yellow mucus. Sneezing. Trachea sore; lungs feel constricted.

**Back:** Sensation of heat from the sacrum to the scapulae. Backache, extending down the legs. Pain over the kidney region. Sensation of heat deep in the spine.

**Extremities:** Muscular lameness, trembling. Pain in the knees. Limbs feel stiff (*Rhus-t.*).

**Skin:** Erythema with vesication and intense itching, stinging and burning. Blisters like little lumps. Skin rough and cracked; feels like leather. Dermatitis, especially around the knees. Inflammation resembling Poison oak. Inguinal glands and popliteal fossa swollen.

**Modalities:** *Worse,* application of cold water, in the afternoon and evening. *Better,* application of hot water, in the morning, moving affected parts.

**Relationship:** Compare: *Rhus-t., Anac., Grin.*

**Dose:** Sixth potency or higher.

---

# X-RAY

(Vial Containing Alcohol Exposed to X-Ray) **X-ray**

Repeated exposure to Roentgen (*X-ray*) has produced skin lesions often followed by cancer. Distressing pain. Sexual glands are particularly affected. Atrophy of ovaries and testicles. Sterility. Changes take place in the blood lymphatics and bone marrow. Anemia and leukemia. Corresponds to stubbornness as in burns, they refuse to heal. Psoriasis.

Has the property of stimulating cellular metabolism. Arouses the reactive vitality, mentally and physically. Brings to surface, suppressed symptoms, especially sycotic and those due to mixed infections. Its homeopathic action is thus centrifugal, towards the periphery.

**Head:** Sticking pains in different parts of the head and face. Dull pain in right upper jaw. Stiff neck. Sudden cricks in the neck, pains more severe behind the ears. Pain in the muscles of neck when lifting the head from the pillow.

**Ears:** Sensation of fullness in ears, ringing (tinnitus).

**Mouth:** Tongue dry, rough, sore. Nausea. Dysphagia.

**Male:** Lewd dreams. Sexual desire lost. Re-establishes suppressed gonorrhea.

**Extremities:** Rheumatic pains. General tired and sick feeling.

**Skin:** Dry, itching eczema. Erythema around roots of nails. Skin dry, wrinkled. Painful cracks. Warty growths. Nails thicken. Psoriasis. Palms rough and scaly.

**Modalities:** *Worse,* in bed, afternoon, evening and night; open air.

**Relantionship:** Compare: *Electricitas*: Sugar of milk saturated with the current (anxiety, nervous tremors, restlessness, palpitations, headache. Dreads approach of thunderstorms; heaviness of limbs).

*Magnetis poli ambo*—Magnet: Sugar of milk or distilled water exposed to the influence of entire mass (burning lancinations throughout the body; pains as in broken joints, when cartilages of two bones touch; shooting and jerkings; headache as if a nail was driven in; tendency of old wounds to bleed afresh).

*Magnetis polus arcticus*—North pole of the magnet: Disturbed sleep, somnambulism, cracking in cervical vertebrae, sensation of coldness; toothache.

*Magnetis polus australis*—South pole of the magnet: Severe pain in the inner side of nail of the big toe, *ingrowing toe;* easy dislocation of foot joints; feet are painful on hanging down.

**Dose:** Twelfth potency and higher.

---

# YOHIMBINUM

(Corynanthe Yohimbe) **Yohim.**

Excites sexual organs and acts on the central nervous system and respiratory centre. An aphrodisiac, used in physiological doses, but contraindicated in all acute and chronic inflammations of abdominal organs. Homeopathically, should be of service in congestive conditions of the sexual organs. Causes hyperemia of the milk glands and stimulates the function of lactation. Menorrhagia.

**Head:** Agitation, with flying sensations of heat in face.

**Mouth:** Disagreeable, metallic taste. Copious salivation. Nausea and eructation.

**Rectum:** Bleeding piles. Intestinal hemorrhage.

**Male:** *Strong and lasting erections.* Neurasthenic impotence. Urethritis.

**Sleep:** *Sleepless.* Thoughts of events from the entire past life keep him awake.

**Fever:** Rigor; intense heat, waves of heat and chilliness. tendency to sweat.

**Dose:** As a sexual stimulant, ten drops of a one percent solution, or hypodermic tablets of 0.005 gm. Homeopathic dose, third potency.

---

# YUCCA FILAMENTOSA

(Bear Grass) **Yuc.**

So called bilious symptoms with headache. Despondent and irritable.

**Head:** Aches, as if the top of head would fly off. Arteries of the forehead throb. Nose red.

**Mouth:** Yellow; tongue yellow, coated with imprint of teeth (*Merc., Podo., Rhus-t.*). Taste as of rotten eggs (*Arn.*).

**Throat:** Sensation as if something was hanging down from the posterior nares; cannot get it up or down.

**Abdomen:** Deep pain on the right side, over the liver, extending to the back. Stool yellowish brown, with bile (jaundice).

**Male:** Burning and swelling of the prepuce, with redness of meatus. Gonorrhea (*Cann-s., Tus-p.*).

**Skin:** Erythematous redness.

**Dose:** Tincture to third potency.

---

# ZINCUM METALLICUM

(Zinc) **Zinc.**

The provings picture cerebral depression. The word "fag" covers a large part of the action of *Zinc.* Tissues are worn out faster than they are repaired. Poisoning from suppressed eruptions or discharges. The nervous symptoms are of most importance. Defective vitality. Impending brain paralysis. *Period of depression in disease.* Spinal affections. Twitchings. Pain, as if between skin and flesh. Great relief from discharges. Chorea from fright or suppressed eruptions. *Convulsions, with a pale face and no heat.* Marked anemia with profound prostration. It causes destruction and a decrease in the number of red blood corpuscles. Repercussed eruptive diseases. In chronic diseases with brain and spinal symptoms, trembling, convulsive twitching and fidgety feet are guiding symptoms.

**Mind:** Weak memory. *Very sensitive to noise.* Aversion to work, talking. *Child repeats everything that is said to it.* Fears arrest on account of a supposed crime. Melancholia. *Lethargic, stupid.* Paresis.

**Head:** Feels as if he would fall to the left side. Headache from the smallest quantity of wine. Hydrocephalus. Rolls head from side to side. Bores head into the pillow (meningitis). *Occipital* pain, with weight on the vertex. Automatic motion of head and hands. Brainfag; headaches in overtaxed school children. *Forehead cool; base of brain hot.* Roaring in the head. Starting from fright.

**Eyes:** Pterygium; smarting, lachrymation, itching. Pressure as if pressed into the head. Itching and soreness of lids and *inner angles* (blepharitis). Ptosis. *Rolling of eyes* (strabismus). Blurring of one-half of vision (hemiopia); worse, stimulants. *Squinting.* Amaurosis with severe headache. Red and inflamed conjunctiva; *worse, inner canthus* (conjunctivitis).

**Ears:** Tearing and stitching pain (otalgia), with external swelling. Discharge of fetid pus (otorrhea).

**Nose:** Sore feeling high up; pressure on the root.

**Face:** *Pale* lips and corners of mouth cracked. Redness and itching eruptions on the chin. Tearing in facial bones.

**Mouth:** Teeth loose. Gums bleed (scorbutic). Gnashing of teeth. Bloody taste. Blisters on the tongue (aphthae). Difficult dentition in weak children with cold and restless feet.

**Throat:** Dry; constant inclination to hawk up tenacious mucus. Rawness and dryness in the throat and larynx. Pain in the muscles of throat when swallowing.

**Stomach:** Hiccough, nausea, vomiting of bitter mucus. Burning in stomach, heartburn from sweet things. *Cannot stand the smallest quantity of wine. Ravenous hunger* around 11 a.m (*Sulph.*). Great greediness when eating; cannot eat fast enough. Atonic dyspepsia, sensation as if the stomach had collapsed.

**Abdomen:** Pain after a light meal with tympanites. Pain in a spot beneath the navel. Gurgling and griping; distended. Faltulent colic with retraction of abdomen (*Plb.*). Enlarged, indurated sore liver. Reflex symptoms from a floating kidney. *Griping after eating.*

**Rectum:** Hard, small, constipated stool. *Cholera infantum* with tenesmus; green mucoid discharges. Sudden cessation of diarrhea, followed by cerebral symptoms.

**Urinary:** Can only void urine when sitting bent backwards. Hysterical retention. Involuntary micturition when walking, coughing or sneezing.

**Male:** Testicles swollen (orchitis), drawn up. Erections violent. Emissions with hypochondriasis. Falling off of hair (pubic). Drawing in of testicles, up to the spermatic cord.

**Female:** Ovarian pain, *especially on the left side; can't keep still* (*Vib.*). Nymphomania of lying-in women. Menses too late, suppressed; lochia suppressed (*Puls.*). Breasts painful. Nipples sore. Menses flow more at night (*Bov.*). All complaints *better during menstrual flow* (*Eupi., Lach.*). *All the female symptoms are associated with restlessness, depression, coldness, spinal tenderness and restless feet.* Dry cough before and during menses.

**Respiratory:** Burning pressure beneath the sternum. Constriction and cutting in the chest. Hoarseness. Debilitating, spasmodic cough; worse, eating sweet things. Child grasps genitals during cough. Asthmatic bronchitis with constriction of the chest. *Dyspnea better as soon as expectoration appears.*

**Back:** Pain in the lumbosacral region. Cannot bear to be *touched on the back* (*Sulph., Ther., Chin.*). Tension and stinging between shoulders. Spinal irritation (myelitis). *Dull aching around the last dorsal or first lumbar vertebrae; worse sitting. Burning along the spine. Nape of neck weary from writing or any exertion.* Tearing in the shoulder blades.

**Extremities:** Lameness, *weakness, trembling and twitching* of various muscles (chorea). Chilblains (*Agar.*). *Feet in continuous motion; cannot keep still. Large varicose veins on the legs.* Sweaty. Convulsions, *with a pale face. Transverse pains,* especially in the upper extremity. *Soles of feet sensitive.* Steps with the entire sole on the floor.

**Sleep:** Cries out during sleep; body jerks; wakes up frightened, startled. Nervous motion of feet when asleep. Screams out loudly at night in sleep without being aware of it. Somnambulism (*Kali-p.*).

**Fever:** Frequent, febrile shiverings down the back. Cold extremities. Night sweat. Profuse foot sweat.

**Skin:** *Varicose veins,* especially of lower extremities (*Puls.*). Formication in feet and legs, as if bugs crawling all over the skin, preventing sleep. Eczema, especially in the anaemic and neurotic. Itching of thighs and *in hollow of knees. Retrocession of eruptions.*

**Modalities:** *Worse,* at menstrual period, from touch, between 5 to 7 p.m., after dinner, from wine. *Better,* while eating, discharges and appearance of eruptions.

**Relationship:** Compare: *Agar., Ign., Plb., Arg-met., Puls., Hell., Tub.*

Inimical: *Nux-v., Cham.* Compare in amelioration by secretions: *Lach., Stann., Mosch.*

Compare: *Zincum aceticum* (effects of night watching and erysipelas; brain feels sore; *Rademacher's solution,* five drop doses, three times a day in water, *for those who are compelled to work, on an insufficient amount of sleep); Zincum bromatum* (dentition, chorea, hydrocephalus); *Zincum oxydatum* (nausea and sour taste. Sudden vomiting in children. Vomiting of bile and diarrhea. Flatulent abdomen. Watery stools with tenesmus. Debility after influenza. Fiery red face, *great drowsiness* with a dream-like, unrefreshing sleep. Effects similar to effects of night watching. Mental and physical exertion-Rademacher); *Zincum sulphuricum* (not repeated frequently (high potency) will clear up opacities of the cornea—McFarland. Corneitis; granular lids; tongue paralyzed; cramps in arms and legs; trembling and convulsions. Hypochrondriasis due to masturbation; nervous headaches); *Zincum cyanatum* (as a remedy for meningitis and cerebro-spinal meningitis, paralysis agitans, chorea and hysteria, it has received some attention); *Zincum arsenicosum* (chorea, anemia, *profound exhaustion* on slight exertion. Depression and marked involvement of lower extremities); *Zincum carbonicum* (post-gonorrheal throat affections, tonsils swollen, bluish superficial spots); *Zincum phosphoricum* (herpes zoster 1x); *Zincum muriaticum* (disposition to pick the bed clothes; sense of smell and taste perverted; bluish-green tint of skin; cold and sweaty); *Zincum phosphoricum* (neuralgia of head and face; lightening like pains in locomotor ataxia, brainfag, nervousness and vertigo; sexual excitement and sleeplessness); *Ammonium valerianicum* (violent neuralgia with great nervous agitation); *Zincum picricum* (facial paralysis; brain fag, headache in Bright's disease; seminal emissions; loss of memory and energy). *Zincum oxydatum* is used locally as an astringent and stimulant, for application to unhealthy ulcers, fissures, intertrigo, burns, etc.

**Dose:** Second to sixth potency.

# ZINCUM VALERIANICUM

(Valerinate of Zinc) **Zinc-val.**

A remedy for *neuralgia,* hysteria, angina pectoris and other *painful* affections, especially the *ovarian affections.* Epilepsy without an aura. Hysterical angina pectoris[1]. *Facial* neuralgia, violent in the left temple and inferior maxillary. Sleeplessness in children. Obstinate *hiccough.*

**Head:** Violent, neuralgic, *intermittent headaches.* Becomes almost insane with pain, which is piercing and stabbing. Uncontrollable sleeplessness from pain in the head with melancholy.

**Female:** *Ovaralgia; pain shoots down the limbs,* even to the foot.

**Extremities:** Severe pain in the neck and spine. Cannot sit still; legs in constant motion. Sciatica.

**Dose:** First and second trituration. Must be continued for some time in treatment of neuralgia.

---

# ZINGIBER OFFICINALE

(Ginger) **Zing.**

Debilitated state of the digestive tract, sexual system and respiratory diseases, call for this remedy. Complete cessation of renal function.

**Head:** Hemicrania (migraine); sudden glimmering before the eyes; feels confused and empty. Pain over the eyebrows.

**Nose:** Feels obstructed and dry. Intolerable itching; red pimples.

**Stomach:** Taste of food remains long, especially of bread and toast. Feels heavy, as if from a stone. *Complaints from eating melons and drinking impure water. Acidity* (*Calc., Rob.*). Heaviness in the stomach on wakening up with wind and rumbling, great thirst and emptiness. Pain from the pit to under the sternum, worse eating.

**Abdomen:** Colic, diarrhea, extremely loose bowels. Diarrhea from drinking contaminated water, with much flatulence, cutting pain and relaxation of the sphincter. Chronic intestinal catarrh.

**Rectum:** Anus, hot, sore and painful during pregnancy. Hemorrhoids hot, sore and painful (*Aloe*). Anus hyperemic and inflamed.

**Urinary:** Frequent desire to micturate. Stinging and burning in the orifice. Yellow discharge from urethra. Urine thick, turbid, with a strong odor,

---

[1] A favourite anti-hysterical medicine (Clarke — Dictionary of Practical Materia Medica).

suppressed (albuminuria). Complete suppression after typhoid. After micturating, continues to ooze in drops.

**Male:** Itching of prepuce. Sexual desire excited; painful erections. Emissions.

**Respiratory:** Hoarseness. *Smarting below the larynx;* breathing difficult. *Asthma,* without anxiety, *worse* towards the morning. Scratching sensation in the throat; stitches in the chest. Cough dry, hacking; copious morning sputa.

**Extremities:** All the joints are very weak. Back lame. Cramps in soles and palms.

**Relationship:** Compare: *Calad.*

Antidote: *Nux-v.*

**Dose:** First to sixth potency.

---

# ZIZIA AUREA

(Thaspium Aureum, Medow Parsnip) **Ziz.**

Hysteria, epilepsy, chorea, hypochondriasis, come within the sphere of this remedy.

**Mind:** Suicidal; depressed; laughing and lachrymose moods alternate.

**Head:** Pressure on top, in the right temple, associated with backache.

**Male:** Great lassitude following coitus. Sexual power increased.

**Female:** Intermittent neuralgia of the left ovary. Acrid, profuse leucorrhea, with retarded menses.

**Respiratory:** Dry cough, with stitches in the chest (pleurisy) Dyspnea.

**Extremities:** Unusual tired feeling. *Chorea, especially during sleep. Fidgety legs* (epilepsy, convulsions) (*Tarent-c.*). Lameness in arms and spasmodic twitching.

**Modalities:** Worse, *during sleep.*

**Relationship:** Compare: *Agar., Stram., Tarent-c., Cic., Aeth.*

**Dose:** Tincture to third potency.

# REPERTORY

# MIND

**AWKWARD, Lets things fall from hand:** Aeth., *Apis, Bov.,* Hell., Ign., Lach., *Nat-m.,* Nux-v., Tarent.

**BRAIN FAG:** *Aeth.,* Ail., Alf., *Anac.,* Anh., *Arg-n.,* Aven., Bapt., *Calc., Calc-p.,* Coca, *Cocc.,* Cupr., *Gels.,* Kali-br., *Kali-p.,* Lec., Nat-m., Nux-v., *Ph-ac., Phos., Pic-ac.;* Sil., *Stry-p.,* Zinc., *Zinc-p., Zinc-pic.* (See **Neurasthenia, NERVOUS SYSTEM.**)

**CATALEPSY, Trance:** *Acon.,* Art-v., Camph-mbr., *Cann-i.,* Cham., Cic., *Crot-c.,* Cur., Gels., Graph., Hydr-ac., Hyos., Lach., Merc., *Morph., Mosch.,* Nux-m., *Op.,* Sabad., Stram.

**CLAIRVOYANCE:** *Acon., Anac.,* Anh., Cann-i., Nabal., Nux-m., *Phos.* (See **Hallucinations.**)

**COMPREHENSION, Difficult:** Agn., *Ail., Anac., Bapt.,* Cocc., *Gels., Hell.,* Lyc., Nat-c., *Nux-m.,* Olnd., *Op., Ph-ac.,* Phos., Plb., Xero., *Zinc.* (See **Memory.**)

**COMPREHENSION, Easy:** Bell., *Coff.,* Lach.

**CONSCIOUSNESS, Loss of:** Absin., *Ail.,* Arn., Atro., *Bell., Cann-i.,* Carb-ac., *Cic.,* Cupr-act., Gels., Glon., *Hell., Hydr-ac., Hyos.,* Mur-ac., Nux-m., Oena., *Op.,* Stram., Xero., *Zinc.*

**CRETINISM, Imbecility, idiocy:** Absin., *Aeth., Anac.,* Arn., Bac., *Bar-c.,* Bar-m., *Bufo,* Calc-p., Hell., Ign., Iod., Lol., Nat-c., Oxyt., Ph-ac., Plb., Sulph., *Thyr.*

**DELIRIUM, Alcoholic (delirium tremens):** Acon., *Agar.,* Ant-t., *Atro., Bell., Cann-i., Caps.,* Chinin-s., Cimic., Dig., Hyos., *Hyosin-hbr., Kali-br.,* Kali-p., Lach., Lup., *Nux-v.,* Op., Passi., Past., *Ran-b., Stram.,* Stry-n., Sumb., Teucr.

**Carphologia (picking at bed clothes, flocks):** Agar., Atro., *Bell.,* Hell., *Hyos.,* Mur-ac., Op., *Stram.,* Zinc-m.

**Coma vigil:** Cur., *Hyos.,* Mur-ac., Op., Phos.

**Destructive (desire to bark, bite, strike, tear things):** *Bell., Canth.,* Cupr., Hyos., Sec., *Stram., Verat.,* Verat-v.

**Effort to escape from bed, or hide:** Acon., *Agar., Bell., Bry.,* Cupr., Hell., *Hyos.,* Oper., Op., Rhus-t., *Stram., Verat.*

**Furor, frenzy, ravings:** Acon., Agar., *Bell., Canth.,* Cic., Cupr., *Hyos.,* Merc-cy., Oena., Sol-n., *Stram., Verat.*

**Lascivious furor:** *Canth., Hyos.,* Phos., Stram., Verat.

**Loquacity, talks incessantly:** *Agar., Bell.*, Cann-i., *Cimic., Hyos., Lach.*, Merc-cy., Op., Oper., *Stram.,* Verat.

**Merry, dancing, singing:** Agar., *Bell., Hyos.,* Stram., Verat.

**Muttering, low, incoherently:** Agar., *Ail.,* Apis, Arn., Bapt., Bell., Crot-h., Hell., *Hyos.,* Lach., *Mur-ac., Ph-ac.,* Phos., *Rhus-t.,* Stram., Verat.

**Rapid answering:** Cimic., *Lach.,* Stram., Verat.

**Slow answering, relapses:** Arn., Bapt., Diph., *Hell.,* Hyos., *Ph-ac.,* Phos., Sulph.

**Sopor, stupor, coma:** Aeth., Agar., *Ail.,* Am-c., *Ant-t., Apis,* Arn., *Bapt.,* Bell., Ben-n., *Camph., Carb-ac.,* Diph., Gels., *Hell., Hyos.,* Lach., Laur., Lob-p., Mur-ac., Nit-s-d., Nux-m., *Op., Ph-ac.,* Phos., Pilo., *Rhus-t.,* Stram., Ter., Thyr., Verat., *Zinc.*

**DEMENTIA:** *Agar., Anac.,* Apisin., *Bell.,* Calc., Calc-p., Cann-i., Con., Hell., *Hyos.,* Ign., *Lil-t.,* Merc., *Nat-sal.,* Op., *Ph-ac., Phos., Pic-ac.,* Sulph., *Verat.*

**Epileptic:** Acon., *Bell.,* Cimic., Cupr., *Cupr-act.*, Laur., *Oena., Sil.,* Sol-c., Stram., Verat-v.

**Masturbatic:** *Agn.,* Calc-p., Canth., Caust., Dam., Nux-v., Op., *Ph-ac.,* Phos., Pic-ac., *Staph.*

**Paretic:** *Acon., Aesc-g.,* Agar., Ars., *Bad.,* Bell., Cann-i., Cimic., Cupr., Hyos., Ign., Iodof., Merc., *Phos., Plb.,* Stram., Verat-v., Zinc.

**Senile:** Anac., *Aur-i.,* Bar-act., *Bar-c.,* Calc-p., Con., Nat-i., *Phos.,* Sec.

**Syphilitic:** Aur-i., *Kali-i.,* Mercuries, Nit-ac., Sulph.

**EMOTIONS, Effects, Anger, bad news, disappointment, vexation:** Acon., Apis, Ars., Aur., *Bry.,* Caust., *Cham.,* Cocc., Colch., *Coloc., Gels.,* Grat., Hyos., Ign., Lach., Nat-m., *Nux-v.,* Ph-ac., Puls., Sep., *Staph.*

**Fright, fear:** *Acon.,* Apis, Aur., Bell., *Gels.,* Hyos., Hyper., Ign., Nat-m., Morph., *Op.,* Puls., Samb., Verat.

**Grief, sorrow:** Am-m., Ant-c., Apis, Aur., Calc-p., Caust., *Cocc.,* Cycl., Hyos., *Ign.,* Lach., Nat-m., *Ph-ac.,* Plat., Samb.

**Jealousy:** Apis, Hyos., *Lach.,* Staph.

**Joy, excessive:** Caust., *Coff.,* Croc.

**Nostalgia (homesickness):** *Caps.,* Eup-pur., Hell., *Ign.,* Mag-m., *Ph-ac.,* Senec.

**Shame, mortification, reserved displeasure:** Aur., Ign., Nat-m., *Staph.*

**FEARS, Dread, Being carried or raised:** *Borx.,* Bry., Sanic.

**Crossing streets, crowds, excitement:** *Acon.,* Hydr-ac., Plat.

**Dark, ghosts:** *Acon., Ars.,* Bell., Carb-v., Caust., Hyos., Lyc., Med., Op., *Phos., Puls.,* Rad-br., Rhus-t., *Stram.*

**Death, fatal diseases, impending evil:** *Acon; Agn.,* Anac., *Apis,* Arg-n.,

*Ars., Aur., Cact.,* Calc., Cann-i., *Cimic., Dig.,* Gels., Graph., Hydr., Ign., Kali-c., Lac-c., *Lil-t.,* Med., Naja, Nat-m., *Nit-ac., Nux-v.,* Phase., *Phos., Plat.,* Podo., *Psor.,* Puls., Rhus-t., Sabad., *Sec.,* Sep., Stann., Staph., Still., Syph., Verat.

**Downward motion, falling:** *Borx.,* Gels., Hyper., *Sanic.*

**Heart ceases beating, must move:** Gels. (reverse Dig.).

**Lectophobia:** Cann-s.

**Loss of reason:** *Acon.,* Alum., *Arg-n., Calc.,* Cann-i., Chlor., *Cimic.,* Iod., Kali-br., Lac-c., *Lil-t.,* Lyss., *Manc.,* Med., Plat., Sep., Syph., Verat.

**Motion:** *Bry.,* Calad., Gels., Mag-p.

**Music:** *Acon., Ambr.,* Bufo, *Nat-c.,* Nux-v., *Sabin.,* Tarent., Thuj.

**Noises:** Acon., *Asar., Bell., Borx.,* Calad., *Cham.,* Cocc., Ferr., Ign., Kali-c., Mag-m., Med., Nat-c., Nit-ac., *Nux-v., Phos.,* Sil., Tanac., Tarent., *Ther.,* Zinc.

**People (anthropophobia):** *Acon.,* Ambr., Anac., *Aur., Bar-c.,* Con., Gels., Ign., Iod., Kali-p., Lyc., Meli., Nat-c., Nat-m., *Sep.,* Stann., *Staph.*

**Places, closed:** Succ.

**Pointed objects:** Sil., Spig

**Poison:** *Hyos.,* Kali-br., Lach., Rhus-t., Verat-v.

**Rain:** Naja.

**Solitude, aversion to:** Ant-t., Ars., *Bism.,* Con., *Hyos., Kali-c.,* Lac-c., Lil-t., *Lyc.,* Naja, *Phos.,* Puls., Rad-br., Sep., *Stram.,* Thymol., Verat.

**Solitude, desire for:** Ambr., Arag., *Ars-met.,* Aur., *Bar-c.,* Bry., *Bufo,* Cact., Caps., *Carb-an.,* Cimic., *Coca,* Cycl., *Gels., Ign.,* Iod., Nat-c., Nat-m., *Nux-v.,* Oxyt., Ph-ac., *Staph.,* Thuj.

**Space (agoraphobia):** *Acon.,* Arg-n., Arn., *Calc.,* Hydr-ac., Nux-v.

**Stage fright:** Anac., Arg-n., *Gels.*

**Syphilis:** Hyos.

**Thunderstorms:** Borx., Elec., *Nat-c., Phos.,* Psor., Rhod., Sil.

**Touch, contact:** *Acon., Ant-c.,* Ant-t., Apis, *Arn., Bell.,* Bruc., *Cham., Chin.,* Cina, *Colch., Hep.,* Iod., *Kali-c., Lach.,* Mag-p., Nit-ac., Nux-m., *Nux-v.,* Phos., *Plb.,* Sanic., Sep., *Spig.,* Stram., Sulph., *Tarent.,* Thuj.

**Water (hydrophobia):** Agav-a., Anag., Ant-c., *Bell., Canth.,* Cocc-s., Fagu., *Hyos., Lach.,* Laur., *Lyss.,* Spirae., *Stram.,* Sulph., Tanac., Verat., Xanth.

**HYPOCHONDRIASIS:** Alf., Aloe, Alum., *Anac., Arg-n., Ars., Aur.,* Aur-m., Aven., Cact., *Calc., Cimic., Con.,* Ferr., Helon., Hydr-ac., Hyos., *Ign.,* Kali-br., *Kali-p., Lyc.,* Merc., Nat-c., *Nat-m., Nux-v., Ph-ac.,* Plb., Podo., Puls., Stann., *Staph., Sulph.,* Sumb., Tarent., Thuj., Valer., *Verat.,* Zinc., Zinc-o., Ziz.

**HYSTERIA:** Acon., Agn., *Ambr.,* Am-val., Apis, Aqui., *Asaf.,* Aster., Bell.,

Cact., Caj., Camph-mbr., Cann-i., Castm., Caul., Cham., *Cimic., Cocc.,* Con., *Croc., Eup-a., Gels.,* Hyos., Ictod., *Ign., Kali-p.,* Lil-t., Mag-m., *Mosch.,* Mygal., *Nux-m.,* Orig., Ph-ac., *Phos., Plat., Puls.,* Scut., Senec., *Sep.,* Stram., Stry-p., *Sumb., Tarent.,* Ther., *Valer., Zinc-val.*

**IMAGINATION: Fancies, hallucinations, illusions: Acute vivid:** *Absin.,* Acon., Agar., Ambr., *Bell., Cann-i.,* Dub., *Hyos.,* Kali-c., *Lach., Op.,* Rhus-t., Scop., *Stram.,* Sulph., *Verat.* (See **Hallucinations.**)

**Away from home, must get there:** *Bry.,* Calc-p., Cimic., Hyos., *Op.*

**Bed occupied by another person:** Petr.

**Bed sinking:** Bapt., Bell., *Benz.,* Kali-c.

**Bed too hard:** *Arn., Bapt.,* Bry., *Morph., Pyrog.,* Ruta.

**Being abused or criticized:** *Bar-c.,* Cocain., Hyos., Ign., Pall., Staph.

**Being assassinated:** Absin., Kali-br., Plb.

**Being broken in fragments, scattered about:** *Bapt.,* Daph., *Petr.,* Phos., Stram.

**Being crushed by houses:** Arg-n.

**Being dead:** Apis, *Lach.,* Mosch., *Op.*

**Being demon, curses, swears:** Anac.

**Being doomed, lost to salvation:** Acon., Ars., Aur., Cycl., Lach., *Lil-t.,* Lyc., Meli., Op., *Plat.,* Psor., Puls., Stram., Sulph., *Verat.*

**Being double (dual personality):** *Anac; Bapt., Cann-i.,* Petr., *Stram.,* Thuj., Valer.

**Being enveloped in dark cloud, world black and sinister:** Arg-n., *Cimic., Lac-c.,* Puls.

**Being frightened by a mouse running from under a chair:** *Aeth., Cimic.,* Lac-c.

**Being guilty of some committed crime:** Ars., Cina, *Cycl., Ign.,* Nux-v., Ruta, Staph., *Verat.,* Zinc.

**Being hollow in organs:** *Cocc.,* Oxyt.

**Being in strange surroundings:** *Cic.,* Hyos., Plat., Tub.

**Being light, spirit-like, hovering in the air:** *Asar., Dat-a.,* Hyper., *Lac-c.,* Lat-h., Nat-ar., Op.; Rhus-g., *Stict., Valer.*

**Being made of glass, wood, etc.:** Eupi., Rhus-t., *Thuj.*

**Being occupied about business:** *Bry.,* Op.

**Being persecuted by his enemies:** *Anac.,* Chin., *Cocain., Hyos.,* Kali-br., *Lach.,* Nux-v., Plb., Rhus-t., Stram.

**Being poisoned:** *Hyos.,* Lach., Rhus-t., Verat-v.

**Being possessed of two wills:** *Anac.,* Lach.

**Being possessed of brain in stomach:** Acon.

**Being possessed of two noses:** Merl.

**Being pregnant, or something alive in the abdomen:** *Croc.*, Cycl., *Op.*, Sabad., Sulph., *Thuj.*, Verat.

**Being pursued:** *Anac.*, Hyos., Stram.

**Being separated body and soul:** *Anac.*, Nit-ac., Thuj.

**Being swollen:** Acon., *Aran.*, *Arg-n.*, Asaf., Bapt., *Bov.*, *Cann-i.*, Glon., Op., Plat.

**Being under superhuman control:** *Anac.*, *Lach.*, Op., Plat., Thuj.

**Being very sick:** Ars., Podo., Sabad.

**Being very wealthy:** Phos., *Plat.*, Pyrog., *Sulph.*, Verat.

**Dimensions of things larger:** Acon., Agar., *Arg-n.*, Atro., Bov., *Cann-i.*, *Gels.*, Glon., *Hyos.*, Op., Par.

**Dimensions of things reversed:** Camph-mbr.

**Dimensions of things smaller:** Plat.

**Duration of time and space lost or confused:** Anh., *Cann-i.*, Cic., *Glon.*, Lach.

**Duration of time changed, it passes too rapidly:** *Cocc.*, Ther.

**Duration of time changed, it passes too slowly:** *Alum.*, Ambr., Anh., *Arg-n.*, *Cann-i.*, Med., Nux m., Nux-v.

**Hallucinations: Remedies in general:** *Absin.*, *Agar.*, Ambr., *Anac.*, Anh., *Antip.*, Ars., Atro., *Bell.*, *Cann-i.*, Canth., Cham., Chlol., Cimic., Cocain., *Crot-c.*, *Hyos.*, Kali-br., Lach., Nat-sal., Nux-v., *Op.*, Phos., *Stram.*, Sulph., Thea, Trion., Zinc-m.

**Hallucinations, auditory (bells, music, voices):** Agar., *Anac.*, *Antip.*, Ars., Bell., *Cann-i.*, Carbn-s., *Cham.*, Cocain, Elaps, Merc., Naja, Nat-p., Puls., *Stram.*, Thea.

**Hallucinations, olfactory:** *Agn.*, *Anac.*, Ars., Euph-a., *Op.*, Par., Puls., Zinc-m.

**Hallucinations, tactile:** *Anac.*, Canth., *Op.*, Stram.

**Hallucinations, visual (animals, bugs, faces):** *Absin.*, Agar., Ambr., Anh., *Antip.*, Ars., *Atro.*, *Bell.*, Calc., *Cann-i.*, Cimic., Cocain., *Hyos.*, Kali-br., Lach., *Morph.*, Nat-sal., *Op.*, Past., Phos., Plat., Puls., Sant., *Stram.*, Sulph., Valer., Verat.

**INSANITY,** (See **Mania, Melancholia, Dementia.**)

**LOQUACITY:** *Agar.*, Ambr., Bell., Cann-i., *Cimic.*, Cocain., Eug., *Hyos.*, *Lach.*, Op., Past., Physal., *Stram.*, Tarent., Valer., Verat.

**MANIA, Remedies in general:** Absin., *Acon.*, Agar., *Anac.*, Arn., Ars., Atro., Bapt., *Bell.*, Bry., *Cann-i.*, *Canth.*, Chin., Chlol., *Cimic.*, Croc., *Crot-c.*, Cupr., Cupr-act., Glon., *Hyos.*, Kali-br., *Lach.*, Laur., Lil-t., Lyc., Merc., Nat-m., Nux-v., *Op.*, Orig., Passi., Phos., Pic-ac., Pisc., *Plat.*, Puls., Rhus-t., Sec., *Sol-n.*, Spig-m., Spong., Sul-h., Sulph., *Stram.*, Tarent., Ust., *Verat.*, Verat-v.

**Erotomania (nymphomania, satyriasis):** Ambr., Apis, Bar-m., Calc-p., *Cann-i., Canth.,* Ferul., Gins., Grat., *Hyos.,* Lil-t., Manc., *Murx.,* Orig., *Phos.,* Pic-ac., Plat., Rob., Sal-n., *Stram., Tarent.,* Verat.

**Lypemania:** Ars., *Aur.,* Caust., Cic., *Ign.,* Nux-v., *Puls.*

**Monomania (kleptomania, etc.):** *Absin.,* Cic., Hyos., Oxyt., Plat., Tarent.

**Puerperal:** Agn., Bell., *Cimic.,* Hyos., Plat., Sec., Senec., *Stram., Verat., Verat-v.*

**MELANCHOLIA, Remedies in general:** Acon., *Agn.,* Alum., *Anac.,* Arg-n., *Ars., Aur.,* Bapt., Bell., Cact., Calc., Camph., Caust., Chin., *Cimic.,* Coca, Coff., *Con., Cycl.,* Dig., Ferr., Gels., Hell., *Helon., Ign.,* Iod., Kali-br., Lac-c., Lach., *Lil-t.,* Lyc., Merc., *Nat-m.,* Nux-m., *Nux-v.,* Op., *Ph-ac.,* Phos., Pic-ac., *Plat.,* Plb., Plb-act., Podo., *Puls.,* Sep., Sil., Sol-c., Stram., Sulph., Tarent., Thuj., *Verat.,* Verat-v., Zinc.

**Pubertal:** Ant-c., *Hell.,* Manc., Nat-m.

**Puerperal:** Agn., Bell., *Cimic.,* Nat-m., Plat., *Verat-v.*

**Religious:** Ars., *Aur., Aur-m.,* Kali-br., Lil-t., Meli., Plb., Psor., Puls., *Stram., Sulph., Verat.*

**Sexual:** Agn., Aur., *Cimic.,* Con., *Lil-t.,* Nux-v., Pic-ac., Plat., Sep.

**MEMORY, Forgetful, weak or lost:** Absin., Acon., *Aeth., Agn., Alum.,* Ambr., *Anac.,* Anh., *Arg-n.,* Arn., *Aur.,* Aza., *Bar-c.,* Calad., *Calc.,* Calc-p., Camph., *Cann-i.,* Carb-v., Cocc., *Con.,* Glyc., Ichth., *Kali-br.,* Kali-c., *Kali-p., Lac-c.,* Lach., Lec., *Lyc.,* Med., Merc., *Nat-c., Nat-m.,* Nit-ac., *Nux-m., Nux-v.,* Olnd., Op., *Ph-ac., Phos., Pic-ac.,* Plb., Rhod., Rhus-t., *Sel.,* Sep., Sil., *Sulph.,* Syph., Tell., Thyr., *Zinc., Zinc-p.,* Zinc-pic.

**Cannot remember familiar streets:** Cann-i., *Glon.,* Lach., Nux m.

**Cannot remember names:** *Anac.,* Bar-act., *Chlor., Euon.,* Guaj., Hep., Lyc., Med., *Sulph.,* Syph., Xero.

**Cannot remember right words (amnesic aphasia, paraphasia):** Agar., Alum., *Anac.,* Arag., Arg-*n.,* Arn., Calc., Calc-p., Cann-i., Cham., Chin., Dios., Dulc., *Kali-br.,* Lac-c., Lil-t., *Lyc., Nux- m.,* Ph-ac., *Plb.,* Sumb., Xero.

**Difficulty or inability of fixing attention:** *Aeth.,* Agar., *Agn.,* Aloe, Alum., *Anac.,* Apis, Arag., Arg-n., Bapt., Bar-c., Cann-i., Caust., *Con.,* Fago., *Gels.,* Glon., Glyc., Hell., Ichth., Indol., Irid-met., Lac-c., Lyc., Op., Nat-c., *Nux-m., Nux*-v., *Ph-ac., Phos., Pic-ac.,* Pitu., Sep., Sil., Staph., Sulph., Syph., Xero., *Zinc.*

**Omits letters, words:** Benz-ac., Cere-s., Cham., *Kali-br.,* Lac-c., Lach., *Lyc.,* Meli., *Nux-m.,* Nux-v.

**Thoughts, rapid:** Anac., Bell., *Cann-i.,* Chin., Cimic., *Coff., Ign.,* Lac-c., Lach., *Phys.*

**Thoughts, slow:** Agn., Caps., *Carb-v.,* Lyc., Med., *Nux-m.,* Op., *Ph-ac., Phos.,* Plb., Sec., Thuj.

**Thoughts vanish while reading, talking, writing:** *Anac.,* Asar., Camph., *Cann-i.,* Lach., Lyc., *Nux-m.,* Pic-ac., Staph.

**Unable to think:** Abies-n., *Aeth.,* Alum., *Anac.,* Arg-*n.,* Aur., Bapt., Calc., Cann-i., Caps., *Con.,* Dig., *Gels.,* Glyc., *Kali-p.,* Lyc., *Nat-c.,* Nat-m., *Nux-m., Nux-v.,* Olnd., Petr., *Ph-ac., Phos., Pic-ac.,* Rhus-t., Sep., Sil., Zinc.

**Weak from sexual abuse:** *Agn., Anac.,* Arg-n., Aur., Chin., Nat-m., Nux-v., *Ph-ac., Staph.*

**MIND, Absence:** *Acon., Agn., Anac.,* Apis, Arag., Arn., Bar-c., *Cann-i.,* Ictod., *Kali-br.,* Kreos., *Lac-c.,* Lach., Merc., Nat-m., *Nux- m.,* Ph-ac., Rhus-t., Tell., Zinc.

**Absence of moral and will power:** Abrot., Acetan., *Anac.,* Cere- s., *Coca, Cocain.,* Kali-br., *Morph.,* Op., Pic-ac., Stry-p., *Tarent.*

**Cloudiness, confusion, depression, dullness:** *Abies n.,* Acon., Aesc., Agar., *Ail.,* Alf., Alum., *Anac., Apis,* Arag., Arg-n., Arn., *Bapt.,* Bar-c., Bell., Calc., Cann-i., Cann-s., Carbn-s., Cic., Cocc., Colch., Euon., Ferr., *Gels., Glon.,* Glyc., *Hell.,* Hyos., Hyper., Indol., Irid-met., Kali-br., Kali-p., Lac-c., Lec., Lyc., Manc., Nat-c., *Nux-m., Nux-v., Op., Ph-ac.,* Phos., Pic-ac., Pisc., *Rhus-t., Sel.,* Staph., Stram., Sulfon., Xero., *Zinc.,* Zinc-val.

**Excitement, exhilaration:** Acon., Agar., *Bell., Cann-i., Canth.,* Coca, Cocain., *Coff.,* Croc., Eucal., *Hyos., Lach.,* Merc-cy., Nux-v., Op., Paul., Phys., Pisc., *Stram.,* Thea, *Verat.*

**MOOD, DISPOSITION, Anxiety felt during thunderstorm:** Nat-c., *Phos.*

**Anxiety felt in stomach:** *Ars., Dig.,* Ip., Kali-c., *Puls.,* Verat.

**Anxious:** *Acon.,* Aeth., *Agn.,* Aml-ns., Anac., Ant-c., Arg-n., *Ars.,* Asaf., *Aur.,* Bell., *Bism.,* Borx., Cact., *Calc.,* Camph., Cann-i., Cham., Chin., Cimic., Coff., Con., Cupr., *Dig.,* Hep., *Ign., Kali-c., Lach., Lil-t.,* Med., Nat-c., Nat-m., Nit-ac., *Nux-v.,* Op., *Phos., Plat.,* Psor., *Puls.,* Rhus-t., Sec., *Sep.,* Sil., Staph., Stram., Sulph., Tab., *Verat.*

**Apathetic, indifferent to everything:** Agar., Agn., *Apis,* Arg-n., Arn., Ars., *Bapt.,* Bry., *Chin., Cimic.,* Con., Cyt-l., Fl-ac., *Gels.,* Glyc., *Hell.,* Hydr-ac., *Ign.,* Indol; Lach., Lil-t., Merc., Nat-m., Nux-m., Nux-v., *Op., Ph-ac.,* Phos., Phyt., *Pic-ac.,* Plat., Puls., Sec., *Sep., Staph.,* Thuj., Verat.

**Aversion to mental and physical work:** Agar., Alf., *Aloe, Anac.,* Arag., Aur-m., Bapt., *Bar-c., Calc., Caps., Carb-ac.,* Caust., *Chin.,* Coca, Con., Cycl., *Gels.,* Glon., Hell., Indol., *Kali-p.,* Lec., Mag-p., Nat-c., Nicc-s., Nit-ac., *Nux-v.,* Oxyt., *Ph-ac.,* Phos., *Pic-ac.,* Puls., Rham-cal., Sel., Sep., Sil., Stry-p., Tanac., Thymol., *Zinc.*

**Bashful, timid:** *Ambr.,* Aur., *Bar-c.,* Calc., Calc-sil., Caust., Coca, Con., Graph., *Ign.,* Kali-p., Lil-t., Manc., Meli., Phos., *Puls.,* Sil., *Staph.*

**Complaining, discontented, dissatisfied:** Aloe, *Ant-c.,* Ars., Bism., Borx., Bry., Caps., *Cham., Cina,* Colch., Indol., Kali-c., Mag-p., Nit-ac., *Nux-v.,* Plat., Psor., *Puls.,* Staph., Sulph., Tab.

**Despairing, hopeless, discouraged easily, lack of confidence:** *Acon., Agn.,* Alum., *Anac.,* Ant-c., Arg-n., Arn., *Ars., Aur.,* Bar-c., Calc., Calc-sil., Caust., Con., Gels., Hell., *Ign.,* Iod., Lil-t., Nat-m., Nit-ac., Nux-v., Op., *Ph-ac.,* Phos., Pic-ac., Psor., *Puls.,* Ruta, Sel., *Sep.,* Sil., Staph., Syph., Thymol., Verat.

**Fault finding, finicky, cautious:** Apis, *Ars., Cham.,* Graph., Helon., Morph., *Nux-v., Plat.,* Sep., Staph., Sulph., Tarent., Verat.

**Fearlessness, daring:** *Agar.,* Bell., Cocain., *Op.,* Sil.

**Fretful, cross, irritable, peevish, quarrelsome, whining:** Abrot., *Acon., Aesc.,* Aeth., Agar., Alf., Anac., *Ant-c., Ant-t.,* Apis, Ars., Aur., *Bry.,* Bufo, Calc., Calc-br., *Caps.,* Caust., *Cham.,* Chin., *Cina, Colch., Coloc.,* Con., Croc., Ferr., Helon., Hep., Iber., *Ign.,* Indol., Ip., Kali-c., *Kali-p., Kreos.,* Lac-c., Lil-t., Lyc., *Nat-m., Nit-ac., Nux-v.,* Plat., Puls., Rad-br., Rheum, Sars., *Sep.,* Sil., *Staph.,* Sulfon., Sulph., Syph., Thuj., Thymol., Tub., *Valer.,* Verat., Verat-v., Zinc.

**Fretful day and night:** *Cham.,* Ign., Ip., Lac-c., *Psor., Stram.*

**Fretful day only:** Lyc.

**Fretful night only:** Ant-t., *Jal.,* Nux-v., Rheum.

**Fretful so that child cannot bear to be touched, looked at, or spoken to:** *Ant-c.,* Ant-t., *Cham., Cina,* Gels., *Nux-v.,* Sanic., *Sil.,* Thuj.

**Fretful so that child wants different things, but petulantly rejects them:** Ant-t., Bry., *Cham., Cina,* Ip., Kreos., Rheum, *Staph.*

**Gay, frolicsome, hilarious:** Anag., Bell., *Cann-i., Coff., Croc.,* Cypr., Eucal., *Form., Hyos.,* Lach., Nux-m., Plat., Spong., Stram., Thea, Valer.

**Grieving, introspective, sighing:** Ail., Calc-p., *Cimic.,* Dig., *Iber., Ign., Lyc., Mur-ac.,* Nat-m., *Ph-ac., Puls.*

**Haughty, arrogant, proud:** Bell., Con., Cupr., Lach., Lyc., *Pall.,* Phos., *Plat.,* Staph., *Stram.,* Verat.

**Haughty, contempt of others:** Ip., *Plat.*

**Haughty, contempt of self:** *Agn., Aur.,* Lac-c., Thuj.

**Hypersensitive, cannot bear contradiction, vexed at trifles:** Acon., *Anac., Ant-c.,* Arn., Ars., Asaf., Asar., Aster., *Aur.,* Bell., *Bry.,* Canth., *Caps., Cham.,* Chin., *Cina,* Cocc., *Colch.,* Coloc., Con., Ferr., Glon., Hell., Helon., Hep., *Ign.,* Lach., Lyc., Mez., Morph., Mur-ac., *Nat-m.,* Nit-ac., *Nux-v.,* Pall., Petr., Phos., *Plat.,* Puls., Sars., *Sep.,* Sil., *Staph.,* Thuj., Thyr.

**Hysterical (changeable, vacillatory):** *Acon., Alum., Ambr., Asaf.,* Camph-mbr., Cast., Caust., *Cimic.,* Cob., Cocc., Coff., *Croc.,* Gels., *Ign.,* Kali-p., Lil-t., Mang-act., *Mosch.,* Nat-m., *Nux-m.,* Phos., *Plat.,* Puls., Sep., *Sumb.,* Tarent., *Valer., Zinc-val.,* Ziz.

**Impatient, impulsive:** Acon., *Anac.,* Ant-c., Arg-n., *Cham., Coloc.,* Hep., Ign., Ip., Med., *Nat-m., Nux-v.,* Puls., Rheum, Sep., *Staph.,* Sulph.

**Impudent, insulting, malicious, revengeful, spiteful:** *Anac.,* Ars., Bufo, *Cham.,* Chin., Cupr., Lac-c., Lyc., *Nit-ac., Nux-v., Staph.,* Tarent.

**Impudent, teasing, laugh at reproof:** Graph.

**Inclined to quarrel:** Seneg.

**Indecisive, irresolute:** Arg-n., Aur., *Bar-c., Calc-sil.,* Caust., *Graph., Ign.,* Nux-m., Nux-v., *Puls.*

**Indolent, listless, lethargic, ambitionless:** Alet., Aloe, Anac., *Apis,* Aur., *Bapt.,* Bar-c., Berb-a., *Bry.,* Calc., *Caps.,* Carb-ac., Carb-v., Con., Cycl., Dig., Euphr., Ferr., *Gels.,* Glon., Helon., Indol., Kali-p., Lec., Lil-t., Merc., Nat-m., Nux-v., *Ph-ac.,* Phos., *Pic-ac.,* Puls., Ruta, Sarcol-ac., *Sep.,* Stann., Sulph., Thymol., Zinc.

**Jealous:** *Apis,* Hyos., Ign., *Lach.,* Nux-v.

**Melancholic, despondent, depressed, low spirited, gloomy, apprehensive, "blues":** Abies-n., *Acon., Aesc., Agn.,* Alf., *Alum.,* Am-c., Am-m., *Anac.,* Ant-c., Apis, Arg-met., Arg-n., *Ars.,* Ars-met., *Aur.,* Bry., But-ac., Cact., Calc., Calc-ar., Caust., *Chin., Cimic.,* Cocc., *Con.,* Cupr., *Cycl.,* Dig., Euon., Euphr., *Graph.,* Hell., *Helon.,* Hep., *Hydr.,* Iber., *Ign., Indg.,* Indol., Iod., Kali-br., Kali-p., Lac-c., Lach., *Lil-t., Lyc.,* Med., Merc., Mygal., Myric., Naja, Nat-c., *Nat-m.,* Nat-s., Nit-ac., Nux-m., *Nux-v., Ph-ac., Phos., Plat., Plb.,* Podo., *Psor., Puls.,* Rad-br., Rhus-t., Sarcol-ac., Sars., Senec., *Sep.,* Sil., Spig., *Stann., Staph.,* Still., Sulph., Tab., Thuj., *Tub.,* Verat., Zinc., Zinc-p.

**Mild, gentle, yielding:** Alum., *Ign.,* Murx., Ph-ac., *Puls.,* Sep., Sil.

**Misanthropic, miserly, selfish:** Ars., *Lyc.,* Pall., Plat., Sep., *Sulph.*

**Nervous, excited, fidgety, worried:** Absin., *Acon., Ambr., Anac.,* Ap-g., Apis, *Arg-n., Ars.,* Asaf., *Asar.,* Aur., *Bell., Borx.,* Bov., But-ac., Calc-br., *Camph-mbr.,* Caust., Cedr., *Cham., Cimic.,* Cina, *Coff.,* Con., Ferr., *Gels.,* Helon., Hyos., *Hyos-hbr.,* Iber., *Ign.,* Kali-br., Kali-p., Lac-c., Lach., Lil-t., Mag-c., Med., Morph., Nat-c., Nux-m., *Nux-v., Phos.,* Psor., Puls., Sec., *Sep., Sil.,* Staph., *Stram., Sumb.,* Tarent., Thea, *Valer.,* Zinc., Zinc-p., Zinc-val.

**Obscene, amative:** *Canth.,* Hyos., Lil-t., Murx., *Phos.,* Puls., Staph., Stram., *Verat.*

**Restless (mentally and physically):** Absin., *Acon.,* Agar., Ambr., Arag., *Ars.,* Aur., Bell., *Bism.,* Camph., Cann-i., Canth., Caust., Cench., *Cham.,*

*Cimic.*, *Coff.*, *Hyos.*, *Ign.*, Iod., *Kali-br.*, Lac-c., Lach., Laur., Lil-t., Med., *Morph.*, Mur-ac., Mygal., Nat-c., Nat-m., Nux-v., Op., *Phos.*, Phyt., Plat., Psor., *Pyrog.*, Rad-br., *Rhus-t.*, Ruta, Sil., *Stram.*, *Tarent.*, Urt-u., Valer., Verat., Verat-v., Zinc., Zinc-val.

**Sad, sentimental, sighing:** *Agn.*, Am-c., Am-m., *Ant-c.*, *Aur.*, Cact., Calc-p., Carb-an., Cimic., Cocc., Con., *Cycl.*, Dig., *Graph.*, Iber., *Ign.*, *Indg.*, Kali-p., Lach., Lil-t., Mur-ac., Naja, Nat-c., *Nat-m.*, Nat-s., Nit-ac., Nux-v., Ph-ac., Phos., Plat., Psor., *Puls.*, Rhus-t., Sec., *Sel.*, *Sep.*, *Stann.*, Staph., Sulph., Thuj., Zinc.

**Sad, weeping from music:** Acon., *Ambr.*, *Graph.*, *Nat-c.*, Nat-s., *Sabin.*, Tarent., *Thuj.*

**Slovenly, filthy:** Am-c., *Caps.*, Merc., *Psor.*, *Sulph.*, Verat.

**Stubborn, obstinate, self willed:** Agar., Ant-c., *Bry.*, Caps., *Cham.*, Chin., Kali-c., *Nit-ac.*, *Nux-v.*, Sanic., Sil., *Staph.*

**Stupid:** Aesc-g., *Anac.*, *Apis*, Arn., *Bapt.*, Bell., Bry., Cocc., *Gels.*, *Hell.*, Hyos., Indol., Lach., *Nux-m.*, *Op.*, *Ph-ac.*, Phos., Rhus-t., Sec., Stram., Verat.

**Suicidal:** Alum., Anac., *Ant-c.*, *Ars.*, *Aur.*, Chin., Fuli., Ign., Iod., Kali-br., *Naja*, Nat-s., Nit-ac., *Nux-v.*, Psor., Puls., Rhus-t., Sec., Sep., Sil., Ust., Verat.

**Suspicious, mistrustful:** *Anac.*, Anh., Caust., *Cimic.*, *Hyos.*, Lach., Merc., *Nux-v.*, Puls., *Staph.*, Verat., Verat-v.

**Sympathetic:** *Caust.*, Cocc., Puls.

**Taciturn, disinclined to be disturbed, or answer questions:** Agar., *Ant-c.*, Ant-t., Arn., Bell., *Bry.*, Cact., Carb-an., *Cham.*, *Coloc.*, *Gels.*, Hell., Ign., Iod., Mur-ac., Naja, *Nat-m.*, Nat-s., *Nux-v.*, Oxyt., *Ph-ac.*, Phos., Sars., Sil., Sulph.

**Taciturn, morose, sulky, sullen, unsociable:** *Ant-c.*, Ant-t., Arn., Aur., *Bry.*, *Cham.*, *Chin.*, Cimic., Coloc., Con., Cupr., Ign., Lyc., Nat-m., *Nux-v.*, *Plat.*, Puls., Sanic., Sil., Sulph., Tub., *Verat.*, Verat-v.

**Tearful, weeping:** *Am-m.*, Ant-c., *Apis*, Ars., Aur., Cact., Calc., Caust., *Cimic.*, Cocc., Croc., *Cycl.*, Dig., *Graph.*, *Ign.*, Lac-c., Lach., Lil-t., Lyc., Mag-m., *Nat-m.*, Nit-ac., Nux m., Ph-ac., Plat., *Puls.*, Rhus-t., *Sep.*, Sil., *Stann.*, Sulph.

**NIGHT TERRORS:** Acon., *Aur-br.*, Calc., Cham., Cic., *Cina*, Chlol., Cypr., *Kali-br.*, Kali-p., Scut., Sol-n., *Stram.*, Tub., Zinc.

**PROPENSITY, To be abusive, curse, swear:** *Anac.*, Bell., Canth., Cere-s., *Lac-c.*, Lil-t., *Nit-ac.*, Pall., *Stram.*, *Tub.*, Verat.

**To be aimlessly busy:** Absin., *Arg-n.*, Ars., Canth., *Lil-t.*, Sulph., Tarent.

**To be carried:** Ant-t., Ars., Benz-ac., *Cham.*, Cina, Ip.

**To be cruel, violent, inhuman:** Abrot., *Absin., Anac.,* Bell., Bry., Canth., Croc., *Nit-ac., Nux-v.,* Plat., Staph., *Stram.,* Tarent., Verat.

**To be destructive, bite, strike, tear clothes:** *Bell.,* Bufo, *Canth.,* Cupr., *Hyos.,* Lil-t., Sec., *Stram.,* Tarent., *Verat.*

**To be dirty, untidy, filthy:** Caps., *Psor.,* Sil.

**To be magnetized:** Calc., *Phos.,* Sil.

**To be obscene:** Anac., *Canth., Hyos.,* Lach., Lil-t., *Phos.,* Plat., Stram., Verat.

**To commit suicide:** Alum., *Ant-c., Ars., Aur.,* Caps., Cimic., *Ign.,* Kali-br., Merc., *Naja,* Nat-s., *Nux-v.,* Psor., Puls., Rhus-t., Ust., Verat., Ziz.

**To dance:** *Agar.,* Bell., Cic., *Croc.,* Hyos., Stict., Stram., *Tarent.*

**To do absurd things:** Bell., Cann-i., Cic., *Hyos.,* Lach., Stram., Tarent.

**To eat greedily:** Lyc., Zinc.

**To handle organs:** Bufo, Canth., Hyos., Ust., Zinc.

**To hurry:** Acon., Alum., Apis, *Arg-n., Aur.,* Bell., Coff., Ign., *Lil-t.,* Med., Nat-m., *Sul-ac.,* Thuj., Zinc-val.

**To hurry others:** Arg-n., Cann-i., *Nux-m.*

**To kill beloved ones:** Ars., Chin., Merc., *Nux-v., Plat.*

**To laugh immoderately at trifles:** Anac., *Cann-i., Croc., Hyos.,* Ign., *Mosch.,* Nux-m., *Plat., Stram., Stry-p.,* Tarent., Zinc-o.

**To lie:** *Morph.,* Op., Verat.

**To mutilate body:** Agar., *Ars.,* Bell., Hyos., Stram.

**To perform great things:** Cocain.

**To pray, beseech, entreat:** Aur., Puls., *Stram.,* Verat.

**To repeat everything:** Zinc.

**To scold:** *Con.,* Dulc., Lyc., *Mosch., Nux-v.,* Pall., *Petr.,* Verat.

**To sing:** *Agar.,* Bell., Cann-i., Cic., *Croc., Hyos.,* Spong., *Stram.,* Tarent., Verat.

**To slide down in bed:** Mur-ac.

**To stretch and yawn incessantly:** Aml-ns., Plb.

**To talk in rhymes, repeat verses, prophecy:** Agar., Ant-c., Lach., Stram.

**To tear things:** Agar., *Bell., Cimx.,* Cupr., *Stram.,* Tarent., *Verat.*

**To tease, laugh at reproofs:** Graph.

**To theorize or meditate:** *Cann-i.,* Cocc., Coff., *Sulph.*

**To touch different things:** Bell., Sulph., *Thuj.*

**To wander from home:** Arag., *Bry.,* Elat., Lach., Verat.

**To work:** Aeth., Aur., Cere-b., *Cocain.,* Coff., *Eucal.,* Fl-ac., *Helon., Lacer.,* Ped., Pisc.

**SCREAMS, Shrill, sudden, piercing:** *Apis, Bell.,* Borx., Bry., Calc., Cham., *Chin., Cic., Cina,* Cypr., Gels., *Hell.,* Iodof., Kali-br., *Stram.,* Tub., Verat., *Zinc.*

**SENSES, Dulled:** Ail., *Anac., Bapt.,* Caps., Dig., *Gels., Hell.,* Ph-ac., Rhus-t.

**Hyperacute:** *Acon.,* Asaf., *Asar.,* Atro., Aur., *Bell.,* Borx., *Cham.,* Chin., *Coff., Colch.,* Ferr., *Ign.,* Lyss., Morph., *Nux-v., Op., Phos.,* Sil., *Stry.,* Sulph., Tarent., Valer., Zinc.

**SPEECH, Hurried:** Anac., Aur., *Bell., Bry.,* Cocc., *Hep., Hyos.,* Lil-t., Merc., *Verat.*

**Lost or paralysis (aphasia):** Bar-act., *Bar-c., Both., Caust.,* Cham., Chen-a., *Colch.,* Con., Glon., *Kali-br.,* Kali-cy., Lach., *Lyc.,* Mez., Phos., Plb., *Stram.,* Sulfon. (See **NERVOUS SYSTEM.**)

**Nasal:** Bar-m., Bell., Lach., Ph-ac.

**Slow, difficult enunciation, inarticulate, stammering:** *Aesc-g.,* Agar., Anac., Anh., Atro., Bar-c., Bell., *Both., Bov.,* Bufo, Cann-i., *Cann-s., Caust.,* Cere-s., Cic., *Cupr.,* Gels., Hyos., *Ign.,* Kali-br., Kali-cy., Lach., Laur., Merc., Mygal., Naja, Nat-m., Nux-m., Olnd., *Op., Phos., Stram.,* Sulfon., Thuj, Vip.

**Slow, monotonous, economical:** Mang-act., Mang-o.

**SOMNAMBULISM:** Acon., *Art-v., Cann-i.,* Cur., Ign., *Kali-br.,* Kali-p., Phos., *Sil., Zinc.*

**STARTLES, easily frightened:** *Acon.,* Agar., Apis, *Asar., Bell., Borx.,* Calad., Calc., Carb-v., *Cham.,* Cimic., Cypr., *Ign., Kali-br.,* Kali-c., Kali-p., Nat-c., *Nux-v.,* Op., *Phos.,* Psor., Samb., *Scut.,* Sep., *Sil., Stram.,* Sulph., *Tarent.,* Ther., Tub., Zinc.

**TAEDIUM VITAE (disgust of life):** *Ant-c.,* Ars., *Aur., Chin.,* Hydr., Lac-c., Lac-d., Kali-br., Naja, Nat-s., Nit-ac., *Phos.,* Plat., Podo., Rhus-t., Sulph., Tab., *Thuj.,* Verat.

■

# HEAD

**BRAIN, Abscess:** Arn., Bell., Crot-h., Iod., Lach., Op., Vip.

**Anemia:** Alum., *Ars., Calc-p.,* Camph., *Chin., Ferr.,* Ferr-p., Kali- c., *Kali-p., Nux-v., Phos.,* Sec., Tab., Verat., *Zinc.*

**Atrophy:** *Aur., Bar-c.,* Fl-ac., Iod., *Phos., Plb.,* Zinc.

**Concussion:** *Acon., Arn., Bell.,* Cic., Ham., *Hyper.,* Kali-i., *Nat-s., Op.,* Sul-ac.

**Congestion, (rush of blood to head):** Absin., *Acon.,* Act-sp., Agar., Ambr., *Aml-ns.,* Arn., Aster., Aur., *Bell., Bry.,* Cact., Calc-ar., Carb-v., Cham., *Chin., Chinin-s.,* Cinnb., Coff., Croc., Cupr., Cupr-act., Ferr-p., *Ferr-py.,* Gels., *Glon.,* Hyos., Ign., Iod., Lach., Lyc., Lycpr., *Meli.,* Nat-s., *Nux-v., Op.,* Sang., Sep., Sil., Stram., *Sulph., Verat-v.*

**Congestion, passive:** Aesc., Chlol., *Chin.,* Dig., *Ferr-py., Gels.,* Hell., *Op.,* Phos.

**Inflammation (meningitis), Cerebral (acute and chronic):** Acon., Aeth., *Apis,* Apoc., Arn., Ars., Bapt., *Bell., Bry.,* Calc., Calc-br., Calc-p., Camph., Carb-ac., Chin., Chinin-s., Chr-o., *Cic.,* Cimic., Crot-h., *Cupr., Cupr-act.,* Dig., Gels., Glon., *Hell.,* Hydr-ac., Hyper., Iod., Iodof., Kali-i., Kreos., Lach., Merc-c., Merc-d., Mosch., *Op.,* Ox-ac., Phys., Plb., Phos., Rhus-t., *Sil.,* Sol-n., *Sulph., Stram., Tub.,* Verat-v., Vip., *Zinc.* (See **Hydrocephalus.**)

**Inflammation, basilar:** *Cupr-cy.,* Dig., Hell., Iod., Sec., Tub., *Verat-v.*

**Inflammation, cerebro-spinal:** *Agar.,* Ail., *Apis,* Arg-n., Atro., *Bell.,* Bry., *Cic., Cimic.,* Cocc., *Crot-h., Cupr-act.,* Cyt-l., Echi., *Gels.,* Glon., *Hell.,* Hyos., Ip., Kali-i., Nat-s., Op., Oreo., Phys., Sil., Stram., Sulph., Verat-v., Zinc., *Zinc-cy.*

**Inflammation, traumatic:** Acon., *Arn.,* Bell., *Hyper.,* Nat-s., Sil.

**Inflammation, tubercular:** *Apis, Bac.,* Bell., Bry., Calc., *Calc-p.,* Cocc., *Cupr-cy.,* Dig., Glon., *Hell.,* Hyos., Iod., *Iodof.,* Kali-i., Op., Stram., *Sulph.,* Tub., *Verat-v.,* Zinc., Zinc-o.

**Paralysis:** Alumn., Con., Cupr., Gels., Hell., Lyc., Op., *Plb., Sec., Zinc.* (See **Apoplexy, CIRCULATORY SYSTEM.**)

**Sclerosis (softening, degeneration):** Agar., Arg-n., *Aur., Bar-c.,* Cann-i., Con., Kali-br., Kali-i., Kali-p., Lach., Lyc., Nux-m., Nux-v., *Phos.,* Pic-ac., *Plb.,* Salam., Vanad., *Zinc.* (See **Arteriosclerosis, CIRCULATORY SYSTEM.**)

**Tumors:** Apom., Arn., *Bar-c.,* Bell., Calc., *Con.,* Glon., Graph., Hydr., *Kali-i., Plb.,* Sep.

**CEREBELLAR DISEASE:** Helo., Sulfon.

**FONTANELLES, Tardy closure:** Apis, Apoc., *Calc., Calc-p.,* Merc., Sep., *Sil., Sulph.,* Zinc.

**HEADACHE (cephalagia), CAUSE, Altitude high:** Coca.

**Bathing:** Ant-c.

**Beer:** Rhus-t.

**Bright's disease:** Am-val., Zinc-pic.

**Candy, sweets:** Ant-c.

**Catarrh:** *All-c.,* Hydr., Merc., Puls., *Stict.*

**Catarrh suppressed:** Bell., *Kali-bi.,* Lach.

**Coffee:** Arum-t., Ign., *Nux-v.,* Paull.

**Constipation:** *Aloe,* Alum., *Bry.,* Coll., Hydr., Nit-ac., *Nux*-v., Op., Rat.

**Dancing:** Arg-n.

**Diarrhea alternating:** *Aloe,* Podo.

**Effete matter in system:** Asc-c.

**Emotional disturbances:** Acetan., Arg-n., Cham., Cimic., Coff., *Epiph., Gels., Ign.,* Mez., Ph-ac., *Pic-ac.,* Plat., Rhus-t., Sil.

**Eruptions suppressed:** Ant-c., Psor., Sulph.

**Eye strain:** Acetan., *Cimic., Epiph., Gels., Nat-m., Onos.,* Ph-ac., *Ruta,* Tub.

**Fasting:** Ars., Cact., Lach., *Lyc.,* Sil.

**Gastralgia alternating or attending:** Bism.

**Gastro-intestinal derangements:** *Ant-c.,* Bry., Carb-v., *Chin.,* Ip., *Iris,* Nux-m., *Nux-v., Puls.,* Rham-cal., Rob.

**Hair cut:** Bell., Bry.

**Hat, pressure:** Calc-p., Carb-v., *Hep.,* Nat-m., Nit-ac.

**Hemorrhage, excesses or vital losses:** Carb-v., *Chin.,* Ferr., Ferr-py., Ph-ac., Sil.

**Hemorrhoids:** Coll., Nux-v.

**Ice water:** Dig.

**Influenza:** Camph., Lob-p.

**Ironing:** *Bry.,* Sep.

**Lemonade, tea, wine:** Sel.

**Liver derangements:** Lept., Nux-v., Ptel.

**Lumbago, alternating with it:** Aloe.

**Malaria:** *Ars.,* Caps., Cedr., Chin., *Chinin-s.,* Cupr-act., *Eup-per.,* Gels., *Nat-m.*

**Mental exertion or nervous exhaustion:** Acetan., Agar., *Anac., Arg-n.,* Aur-br., Chion., Cimic., Coff., *Epiph., Gels.,* Ign., *Kali-p.,* Mag-p., *Nat-c.,* Nicc., *Nux-v.,* Phase., Ph-ac., *Pic-ac.,* Sabad., Scut., Sil., Zinc.

**Mercury:** Still.
**Narcotics, abuse:** Acet-ac.
**Over-lifting:** Calc.
**Perspiration, suppressed:** Asc-c., Bry.
**Riding against wind:** Calc-i., *Kali-c.*
**Riding in cars:** *Cocc.,* Graph., Med., *Nit-ac.*
**Sexual excitement, weakness:** Chin., Nux-v., Onos., *Ph-ac., Sil.*
**Sleep, damp room:** Bry.
**Sleep, loss:** Cimic., Cocc., *Nux-v.*
**Spinal disease, chorea:** Agar.
**Spirituous liquors:** Agar., *Ant-c.,* Lob., *Nux-v.,* Paull., Rhod., Ruta, *Zinc.*
**Sunlight or heat:** *Bell.,* Cact., Ferr-p., *Gels., Glon.,* Kalm., Lach., *Nat-c.,* Nux-v., Sang., Stram.
**Syphilis:** Ars., *Aur.,* Aur-ar., Sars., Still., Syph.
**Tea:** Nux-v., Paull., *Sel.,* Thuj.
**Tobacco:** Ant-c., Calad., Carb-ac., *Gels., Ign.,* Lob., Nux-v.
**Traumatism:** *Arn.,* Hyper., Nat-s.
**Uremia:** Arn., Bapt., Cann-i., *Glon.,* Hyper., *Sang.*
**Uterine disease, reflex:** Aloe, Bell., *Cimic.,* Gels., Ign., Puls., *Sep.,* Zinc-p.
**Vaccination:** Thuj.
**Weather changes:** *Calc-p.,* Phyt.

**TYPE: Anemic:** Ars., Calc-p., *Chin.,* Cycl., Ferr., *Ferr-p., Ferr-r.,* Kalm., Nat-m., *Ph-ac.,* Zinc.
**Catarrhal:** *All-c.,* Ars., *Bell.,* Bry., Camph., Eup-per., Euphr., *Gels., Kali-bi.,* Lyc., Menth., *Merc.,* Nux-v., *Puls.,* Sabad., Sang., *Stict.,* Sulph.
**Chronic:** *Arg-n.,* Chinin-s., Cocc., Lach., *Nat-m.,* Phos., Plb., *Psor.,* Sep., *Sil.,* Thuj., Tub., *Zinc.*
**Chronic, old people:** Bar-c., Calc-p., Iod., Phos.
**Chronic, school girls:** *Calc-p.,* Kali-p., *Nat-m., Ph-ac., Pic-ac.,* Psor., Tub., Zinc.
**Chronic, sedentary persons:** Anac., *Arg-n.,* Bry., *Nux-v.*
**Climacteric:** Aml-ns., Cact., *Cimic.,* Croc., *Cycl., Glon.,* Lach., *Sang.,* Sulph.
**Congestive:** *Acon.,* Aml-ns., Arg-n., *Bell., Bry., Cact.,* Chinin-s., *Ferr-p., Gels., Glon.,* Glyc., Joan., Lach., *Meli.,* Nat-m., Nux-v., Op., Phase., *Sang.,* Sil., Sol-n., Sulph., Usn., *Verat-v.*
**Congestive, passive:** *Chinin-s.,* Ferr-p., *Ferr-py.,* Gels., Op., Sil.

**Gastric, bilious:** Am-pic., Anac., *Arg-n.,* Bapt., *Bry.,* Cham., Chel., *Chion.,* Cycl., Eup-per., *Ip., Iris,* Lob., Merc., *Nux-v.,* Podo., *Puls.,* Rob., *Sang.,* Strych., Tarax.

**Hysterical (clavus):** Agar., Aqui., *Coff.,* Euon., Hep., *Ign.,* Kali- c., Mag-m., Nat-m., Nux-*v., Plat.,* Puls., Thuj.

**Menstrual:** Aeth., Aven., Bell., Cact., Cann-i., Cann-s., Chin., Chion., *Cimic.,* Cocc., *Croc., Cycl.,* Ferr., *Glon.,* Glyc., Kali-p., Lac-d., Lach., Lil-t., *Nat-m., Plat-m., Puls., Sang., Sep.,* Ust., Vib., Xan.

**Migraine, megrim, nervous:** Am-c., Am-val., *Anac.,* Anh., *Arg-n.,* Aspar., Aven., *Bell.,* Bry., Calc., *Calc-act., Cann-i.,* Carb-ac., Cedr., Chion., *Cimic.,* Cit-v., *Cocc., Coff.,* Crot-c., *Cycl., Epiph., Gels., Guar., Ign.,* Indg., *Iris,* Kali-bi., *Kali-c., Lac-d., Lach., Meli., Menis.,* Nat-m., Nicc., *Nux-v., Onos.,* Paul., Plat-m., *Puls., Sang.,* Sapin., *Scut., Sep.,* Sil., Spig., Stann., Sulph., Tab., Thea, Ther., Verb., Xan., *Zinc-s., Zinc-val.,* Ziz.

**Neuralgic:** *Aconin.,* Aesc., All-c., Arg-n., *Ars., Bell.,* Bism., *Cedr.,* Chel., *Chinin-s.,* Cimic., Coloc., Der., *Gels., Mag-p.,* Meli., Mentho., Oreo., Pall., Phos., *Spig.,* Tarent., Zinc-val.

**Rheumatic, gouty:** Act-sp., Bell., Bry., Calc., Colch., Coloc., Der., *Guaj.,* Hep., Ip., Kali-s., Kalm., Lyc., Nux-v., *Phyt., Rhus-t.,* Sep., Sil., Sulph.

**Uremic:** Arn., *Glon.,* Hyper., Sang.

**Utero-ovarian:** Bell., *Cimic., Gels.,* Helon., Ign., Joan., Lil-t., Plat., *Puls., Sep.,* Zinc.

**LOCATION: Frontal:** *Acon.,* Aesc., Alf., Agar., Ail., *All-c., Aloe,* Am-c., *Anac.,* Antip., Arg-n., Ars., Aur., *Bell., Bry.,* Calc., Carb-ac., Cedr., *Chinin-s.,* Chion., Eup-per., Euphr., Gels., *Glon., Hydr.,* Ign., Indol., Iris, *Kali-bi., Lept.,* Meli., Menis., Nat-m., *Nux-v.,* Phos., Pic-ac., Prun., *Ptel.,* Puls., Rob., Rhus-t., *Scut.,* Sil., Stell., Stict., *Viol-o.*

**Frontal, extending to eyes, root of nose, face, etc.:** Acon., *Agar.,* All-c., *Aloe,* Ars-met., Bad., *Bry.,* Caps., Cedr., Cere-b., *Cimic.,* Hep., Ign., Kali-i., *Lach.,* Mag-m., Mentho., Onos., *Plat.,* Prun., *Ptel., Spig., Stict.*

**Frontal, extending to occiput, nape of neck and spine:** *Bry.,* Euon., Gels., Lac-d., Menis., Nux-v., *Oreo.,* Prun., Sep., Tub.

**Occipital:** Aeth., Alf., Anac., Aven., *Bry.,* Camph., Cann-i., Carb-v., *Cimic., Cocc.,* Euon., Eup-per., Ferr., *Gels.,* Gins., Jug-c., Lac-c., Lach., Lec., Nicc-s., *Nux-v.,* Onos., Oreo., *Petr.,* Ph-ac., *Pic-ac.,* Plat-m., Rad-br., *Rhus g., Sang.,* Sep., *Sil.,* Sulph., Xan., Zinc.

**Occipital, extending to eyes and forehead:** Arund., Bell., Carb-v., Chin., Cimic., *Gels.,* Glyc., Indol., Lac-c., Mag-m., Onos., Ph-ac., Pic-ac., *Rhus-r., Sang., Sars., Sil.,* Spig.

**Semilateral (hemicrania):** Arg-n., *Ars., Bell., Bry.,* Cedr., Cham., *Coff.,* Coloc., *Cycl.,* Gins., Glon., *Ign.,* Joan., Kali-bi., Lach., Nat-m., Ol-an., *Onos.,* Phos., Prun., *Puls., Sang.,* Sep., *Sil., Spig., Stann.,* Thuj.

**Semilateral, left side:** Nat-m., Nux-v., *Onos.*, Sapin., *Spig.*

**Semilateral, right side:** *Cedr.*, Chel., Iris, Kali-bi., Rad-br., *Sang.*, Sil., Tab.

**Spinal and cervical:** Bell., *Cimic., Cocc.*, Dulc., *Gels., Goss., Hell.*, Nat-m., Nat-s., Nicc-s., *Oreo., Ph-ac., Pic-ac.*, Scut., *Sil.*, Verat-v.

**Supraorbital:** Acon., Aconin., Aloe, *Ars.*, Carb-ac., *Cedr.*, Cere-b., *Chinin-s.*, Cimic., Cinnb., Coloc., Glon., Ign., Indol., Iris, *Kali-bi.*, Lyc., Meli., Mentho., *Nux-v.*, Phel., Puls., Viol-o.

**Supraorbital, left:** Act-sp., Arg-n., Bry., Carb-v., *Cedr.*, Cocc., Euon., Mentho., Nux-v., Oreo., Oxyt., Sapo., Sel., Senec., *Spig.*, Tell., Xan.

**Supraorbital, right:** Arund., *Bell., Bism., Chel., Iris,* Kali-bi., Meli., Plat., Sang., Sil.

**Sutures, along:** Calc-p.

**Temples:** *Acon., Anac.*, Arn., *Bell., Bry.*, Caps., Cedr., *Carb-ac., Chin.*, Chinin-s., Epiph., Gels., *Glon.*, Ign., Lach., Naja, *Onos.*, Oreo., *Phel.*, Ph-ac., Plat., Rhus-t., *Sang., Senec.*, Sep., Spig., *Stann.*, Sul-ac., Usn.

**Temples, ear to ear:** Antip., Calc-ar., Mentho., Pall., Syph.

**Vertex (crown of head):** Alumn., Anac., Act-sp., Ars., *Cact.*, Calc-p., Chin., *Cimic.*, Gels., Glon., Hyper., *Lach., Meny.*, Naja, Nux-v., Pall., *Phel., Ph-ac.*, Plat., Puls., Rad-met., Sep., *Sulph.*, Verat.

**CHARACTER OF PAIN: Aching, dull:** Acon., *Aesc.*, Alf., All-c., *Aloe,* Ant-c., *Arg-n.*, Ars., Aza., Bapt., Bell., But-ac., Caps., Carb-ac., Carb-v., Card-m., *Chin., Cimic.*, Cocc., Euon., *Gels., Hell., Hydr.*, Ichth., *Ign.*, Indol., Iris, Kali-bi., *Lept.*, Lil-t., Mentho., Myrt., Naja, Nat-ar., *Nux-v., Nyct.*, Onos., Oreo., *Phel.*, Pic-ac., *Plb.*, Scut., *Sil., Stann., Stel.*

**Boring, digging:** *Arg-n., Asaf.*, Aur., Bell., *Clem., Coloc., Hep.*, Nat-s., Sep., Stram.

**Bruised, battered, sore:** Arn., *Bapt.*, Bell-p., *Chin.*, Coff., Euon., *Eup-per., Gels.*, Guar., *Ign.*, Ip., Lyc., Mentho., *Nux-v.*, Phel., Ph-ac., *Rhus-t.*, Sil., Tab.

**Burning, heat:** *Acon.*, Alumn., *Apis,* Arn., *Ars.*, Aster., Bell., Calc-p., *Glon.*, Helon., *Lach.*, Lil-t., Merc., Ox-ac., Phel., *Phos.*, Sil., Tong., Verat-v., Viol-o.

**Bursting, splitting:** *Acon.*, Bell., *Bry.*, Cact., *Caps., Chin.*, Daph., Gels., *Glon.*, Lycpr., Mag-m., Meli., *Nat-m.*, Nux-m., Nux-v., Olnd., Puls., Sang., Sep., Stry., *Usn.*, Verat.

**Constrictive, band-like, squeezing:** Acon., *Anac., Ant-t.*, Antip., *Cact., Carb-ac.*, Carb-v., Card-m., Coca, Cocc., Eup-per., *Gels.*, Glon., Guan., Iod., Lept., *Merc.*, Merl., *Nit-ac.*, Osm., *Plat.*, Spig., *Stann., Sulph.*, Tarent., Tub.

**Distensive, full:** *Acon.*, Aml-ns., Arg-n., Bapt., *Bell.*, Bov., *Bry.*, Cact., *Caps.*, Chin., Chinin-ar., Cimic., *Gels.*, *Glon.*, Glyc., Kali-bi., Mentho., Nux-v., Stry., *Sulph.*, Verat-v.

**Drawing:** Bism., *Bry.*, *Caps.*, Carb-v., Caul., *Caust.*, *Cham.*, Kali-c., Nux-v.

**Excruciating, violent:** Agar., Aml-ns., *Anac.*, Arg-n., Aur., *Bell.*, Bry., *Chin.*, *Cimic.*, *Glon.*, Kali-i., Meli., Oreo., Plat-m., *Sang.*, Scut., Sil., *Spig.*, Stry., Zinc-val.

**Heaviness:** *Acon.*, *Aloe*, Arg-n., *Bapt.*, Bar-m., Bell., *Bry.*, Cact., Calc., Carb-v., *Cocc.*, *Gels.*, *Glon.*, Glyc., Hydr., Hyper., *Ign.*, Iris, *Lach.*, Lil-t., Meli., *Meny.*, Merc., *Nux-v.*, Onos., *Op.*, Oreo., Petr., *Phel.*, *Ph-ac.*, Phos., Pic-ac., Plat., Puls., Rhus-t., *Sep.*, *Sulph.*, Ther.

**Periodical, intermittent:** Acon., Am-pic., Arg-n., *Ars.*, *Bell.*, Cact., *Cedr.*, Chel., *Chin.*, Eup-per., Gels., Ign., Kali-cy., Mag-m., Nicc., Nicc-s., *Sang.*, Sep., *Spig.*, Tab., Tela, Zinc-val.

**Periodical, intermittent, alternate days:** *Anh.*, *Chin.*

**Periodical, intermittent, every third day: seventh day:** Eup-per.

**Periodical, intermittent, every seventh day:** Calc-ar., Sabad., *Sang.*, Sil., Sulph.

**Periodical, intermittent, every eighth day:** Iris.

**Periodical, intermittent, every week or two:** Sulph.

**Periodical, intermittent, every two-three weeks:** Ferr.

**Periodical, intermittent, every six weeks:** Mag-m.

**Periodical, intermittent, lasting several days:** Tab.

**Periodical, with increase and decrease of sun:** Glon., Kalm., Nat-c., *Nat-m.*, *Sang.*, *Spig.*, Tab.

**Piercing, as from nail:** *Agar.*, Anan., Aqui., *Coff.*, *Hep.*, *Ign.*, M-ambo., *Nux-v.*, Paraf., Ruta, Sil., *Thuj*, Zinc-val.

**Pressing:** *Acon.*, *Aloe*, *Anac.*, *Bell.*, *Bry.*, Cact., *Caps.*, *Carb-ac.*, *Cham.*, *Chel.*, Chion., Cimic., Epiph., *Eup-per.*, Ferr., *Glon.*, Hydr-ac., *Ign.*, Kali-c., Lach., Meli., *Meny.*, *Nux-v.*, Onos., Op., Oreo., Petr., *Ph-ac.*, *Plat.*, Podo., Puls., Rhus-t., Sang., Sep., Stann., Stict., Sul-ac., *Sulph.*, Verat., *Zinc.*

**Pressing, as from pincers, or vise:** Act-sp., Bism., *Cact.*, Cham., Lyc., Menis., *Meny.*, Ph-ac., *Plat.*, Puls., *Verb.*, Viol-t.

**Pressing asunder:** Arg-n., *Asaf.*, Aur., *Bry.*, Carb-an., Chin., *Cimic.*, Cor-r., Erio., *Fago.*, *Menis.*, Prun., *Ptel.*, Stront-c.

**Pressing, dull as from weight:** Aloe, Alumn., *Anac.*, *Cact.*, Carb-v., *Cimic.*, Eup-per., Hyper., *Lach.*, Meny., *Naja*, *Nux-v.*, Op., Petr., *Phel.*, *Ph-ac.*, Puls., *Sep.*, *Sulph.*, Ther.

**Pressing, in small spots:** Arg-n., Ictod., *Ign., Kali-bi.,* Plat., Thuj.

**Shifting, shooting, stinging, tearing:** Acon., Aesc., Apis, Arn., Ars., *Bell., Caps., Cedr., Chin.,* Cimic., Coloc., Ign., *Iris,* Kali-bi., Kali-c., Lac-c., *Prun.,* Puls., Sang., Sil., Spig., Vinc.

**Shock (electric)-like stabbing:** Apis, *Aster., Bell.,* Cann-i., Cic., Cocc., *Glon.,* Rhod., *Sang., Sep.,* Tab., Zinc-val.

**Stitching, sticking:** Acon., Aesc., Arn., Ars., Bell., *Bry.,* Cann-i., *Caps.,* Cycl., *Kali-c.,* Nicc., Puls., Tarent.

**Stupefying:** Arg-n., *Bell.,* Bry., Gels., *Glon.,* Senec., Staph., Syph.

**Throbbing, beating, hammering, pulsating:** *Acon.,* Act-sp., Aml-ns., Arg-n., Ars., *Bell.,* Bry., Cact., Cann-i., *Caps., Chin.,* Chinin-ar., Chinin-s., Cimic., Croc., Eup-per., *Ferr.,* Ferr-p., Gels., *Glon.,* Glyc., Hyper., *Iris, Lac-d.,* Lach., Lyc., *Meli., Nat-m.,* Nux-v., Paull., Psor., Puls., Sang., Sep., Sil., *Spig., Sulph.,* Tong., Verat-v.

**CONCOMITANTS: Anguish, anxiety:** Acon., Ars., Plat.

**Arterial excitement, tension:** Acon., *Bell., Glon.,* Glyc., Ictod., Meli., Usn., *Verat-v.*

**Burning along spine:** Pic-ac.

**Chilliness:** *Arg-n.,* Camph., Lact-v., Mang-m., *Puls., Sang.,* Sil.

**Coldness in back and occiput:** Berb.

**Coldness in head:** Calc., Calc-act., Sep., Verat.

**Coldness of hands and feet:** Bell., *Calc.,* Ferr., Lach., Meli., *Meny.,* Naja, Sep., Sulph., Verat.

**Colic:** Aloe, Cocc.

**Constipation:** Aloe, Alum., *Bry.,* Euon., *Hydr.,* Lac d., Nicc., *Nux.v.,* Op., Plb.

**Coryza:** Agar., All-c., Camph.

**Cough:** Arn., Caps., Lyc.

**Delirium:** Agar., Bell., Syph., Verat.

**Diarrhea:** Aloe, Cham., Podo., Verat.

**Drowsiness:** *Ail.,* Ant-t., Bran., Chel., Dub., *Gels., Ind.,* Lept., Myric., Stel.

**Ears, burning:** Rhus-t.

**Ears, deafness:** Chinin-s., Verb.

**Ears, roaring:** Aur., *Chin., Chinin-s.,* Ferr., Sang., Sulfon.

**Ears, stitching:** Caps.

**Empty feeling in stomach:** *Ign.,* Kali-p., *Sep.*

**Excitement, emotional:** Cann-i., Pall.

**Excitement, sexual:** Apis, Plat-m.

**Exhaustion, asthenia:** *Ars.,* Aur-br., *Chin., Gels.,* Ign., Ind., Lac d., Lob., *Pic-ac.,* Sang., Sulph.

**Eyes, blindness, or visual disturbances, precede or attend:** Anh., Bell., *Cycl.,* Epiph., *Gels.,* Ign., *Iris, Kali-bi.,* Kali-c., Lac-c., *Lac-d., Nat-m.,* Nicc., Nux-v., Pic-ac., Podo., Psor., *Sang.,* Sil., Spig., *Ther., Zinc-s.*

**Eyes, enlarged feeling:** Arg-n.

**Eyes, heaviness:** Aloe.

**Eyes, heaviness of, and lids:** Bell., Gels.

**Eyes, injection:** *Bell.,* Meli., Nux-v.

**Eyes, lachrymation:** Chel., Phel., Rhus-t., Spig., Tax.

**Eyes, soreness, pain:** Aloe, Cedr., *Cimic., Eup-per., Gels.,* Hom., Mentho., Myrt-c., Nat-m., Phel., *Scut.,* Sil., *Spig.*

**Eyes, vision returns as headache comes on:** *Iris,* Lac-d., Nat-m.

**Face, flushed, hot:** *Acon.,* Aml-ns., *Bell.,* Cham., Ferr-p., Gels., *Glon.,* Mag-p., *Meli.,* Naja, Nat-m., Nux-v., Podo., *Sang.,* Sep.

**Face, pale:** Acon., *Calc.,* Chin., Ign., *Lach.,* Lob., Meli., Nat-m., Sil., Spig., Tab., *Verat.*

**Faintness:** Nux-v., Verat.

**Fever:** Acon., Ars., *Bell.,* Ferr-p.

**Flatulence:** Asc-t., Calc-act., Calc-p., Cann-i., *Carb-v.,* Xan.

**Gastralgia, attending or following:** Bism.

**Gastro-intestinal derangements:** Agar., Aloe, Arg-n., Ars., *Bry.,* Cann-i., *Carb-v., Chin.,* Iris, *Nux-v.,* Podo., *Puls.*

**Hair, falling out:** Ant-c., Nit-ac., Sil.

**Head, nodding:** Lam., Sep.

**Head, retracted:** Bell., Cocc., *Goss.*

**Heart's action labored:** Lycps-v.

**Hemorrhoids:** Nux-v.

**Hunger:** Anac., Cact., *Epiph.,* Ign., *Lyc., Psor.*

**Hypochondrium, right, stitches:** Aesc.

**Irritability:** Anac., *Bry., Cham.,* Ign., *Nux-v.*

**Liver disturbance:** Chel., Jug-c., *Lept.,* Nux-v.

**Loquacity:** Cann-i.

**Lumbago, alternating:** Aloe.

**Mental depression, despondency:** Aloe, *Arg-n.,* Aur., *Ign.,* Indol., Iris, Lac d., Naja, Pic-ac., Plb., *Puls., Sars.,* Sep., Zinc.

**Mental weakness:** Arg-n., Nux-v., Sil.

**Muscular soreness:** Gels., Rhus-t.

**Nausea:** Aloe, *Ant-c.,* Ars., *Bry., Cocc.,* Ferr., Gels., Indol., *Ip., Iris,* Lac-c., Lac d., Lob., Lob-p., Naja, Nat-m., *Nux-v.,* Paull., Petr., *Puls., Sang., Sep.,* Sil., *Tab.*

**Nodules, gouty of scalp:** Sil.

**Nosebleed:** Agar., Aml-ns., Ant-c., Ham., *Meli.*
**Nose, dry, neuralgia:** Dulc.
**Numbness, tingling, of lips, tongue, nose:** Nat-m.
**Numbness:** Chel., Indol., Plat.
**Occipital soreness:** Cimic., Sil.
**Oversensitiveness:** Ars., *Bell., Cham.,* Chin., Coff., *Ign., Nux-v., Sil.,* Spig., Tela.
**Pains in abdomen:** Cina, Coloc., Verat.
**Pains in limbs:** Sang.
**Pains in lumbar region:** Rad-br.
**Palpitation:** Cact., Spig.
**Polyuria:** Asc-c., *Gels., Ign.,* Lac-d., *Sang.,* Scut., Sil.
**Ptyalism:** Fagu., Iris.
**Respiratory affections:** Lact-v.
**Restlessness:** *Ars.,* Hell., Ign., Pyrog., Spig.
**Scalp, bruised feeling:** Aesc., *Chin.,* Coloc., Sil.
**Scotoma:** Aspar.
**Sleeplessness:** *Coff.,* Ind., Syph., Zinc-val.
**Spasmodic symptoms:** Ign.
**Sweat profuse:** Lob., Tab.
**Temporal veins engorged:** Carl., Gels.
**Thirst:** Pulx.
**Tongue coated, fetor oris, etc:** Calc-act., Card-m., Euon., Gymno., *Puls.*
**Toothache:** Sang.
**Trembling all over:** *Arg-n.,* Borx., *Gels.*
**Vertigo:** Acon., Agro., Bry., *Chin.,* Chinin-s., *Cocc., Eup-pur., Gels.,* Glon., Ign., Lept., Lob-p., *Nux-v.,* Podo., Sep., Xan.
**Vomiting:** Arg-n., *Ars., Bry.,* Calc-act., Cham., Chin., Cocc., Glon., *Ip., Iris,* Lac-c., *Lac-d.,* Lob., Meli., Nat-m., *Nux-v.,* Puls., Rob., *Sang.,* Sep., Sil., Tab., Verat., Zinc-s.
**Yawning:** Kali-c., Staph.

**MODALITIES: Aggravation; After drugging:** Nux-v.
**After midnight:** Ferr.
**Afternoon:** Anan., Bad., *Bell.,* Cycl., Eup-pur., Indol., Lob., Meli., Sel.
**Air, open:** *Ars.,* Bov., Bran., *Chin.,* Cocc., Coff., Mag-m., *Nux-v.,* Sep.
**Anger:** Nux-v.
**Ascending:** Ant-c., Bell., But-ac., *Calc.,* Conv., *Meny.*
**Attention, close:** Ign.
**Awaking from sleep:** Lach.

**Beating time:** Anh.
**Bending head backward:** Glon.
**Bending head forward:** Bell., Cob.
**Closing teeth:** Am-c.
**Cold, draft of air:** *Ars.,* Bell., *Chin.,* Eup-pur., Ferr-p., Ichth., Ign., Iris, Nux-v., Rhod., Rhus-t., Sil.
**Contact, touch:** *Bell., Chin.,* Ferr-p., Rhus-t., *Tarent.*
**Coughing:** Acon., Arn., *Bell., Bry., Caps.,* Carb-v., Iris, Kali-c., *Nat-m., Nux-v.,* Petr., Phos., Sep., Sulph.
**Drinking coffee:** Act-sp., Ign., Nux-v.
**Drinking milk:** Brom.
**Eating:** Am-c., Arn., *Ars.,* Atro., *Bry.,* Cact., Cocc., Coff., Gels., Ign., Lach., *Lyc., Nux-v.*
**Evening:** *All-c.,* Aur., Caust., Cycl., Eup-pur., Indol., Kali-s., *Puls.,* Thlas.
**Exertion, mental or physical:** Aloe, *Anac., Arg-n.,* Cocc., *Epiph.,* Gels., Nat-c., *Nux-v.,* Ph-ac., Phos., *Pic-ac.,* Sep., Sil., Tub.
**Gradually, crescendo, decrescendo:** Plat., Stann.
**Hawking:** Conv.
**Jar, misstep, etc.:** Aloe, *Bell.,* Bry., Chin., Crot-h., Ferr-p., *Glon.,* Lach., Lyc., Meny., Rhus-t., Sil., *Spig., Ther.*
**Left side:** Anac., Ars-met., *Brom.,* Chinin-s., *Cycl.,* Epiph., Eup-pur., *Lach.,* Nicc., Oreo., Paraf., Sapo., *Senec.,* Sep., *Spig.,* Thuj.
**Light:** *Bell.,* Ferr., *Ign.,* Kali-bi., Kali-c., Lac-d., Lyss., *Nux-v.,* Oreo., Phel., Sang., Scut., Sil., Tarent.
**Lying down:** Ars-met., *Bell.,* Bov., Chin., Coloc., Eup-per., Gels., *Glon.,* Lach., Lyc., Rhus-t., Sang., Ther.
**Lying on back of head:** Cocc., Coloc.
**Lying on painful side:** Sep.
**Menses:** Croc., Lac d., *Nat-m.,* Sep.
**Morning:** Aesc., Alum., *Am-m.,* Aspar., Cycl., Hep., *Lac-d.,* Myric., *Nat-m.,* Nicc., *Nux-v.,* Ph-ac., Podo., Sang., Spig., Stel., Sulph.
**Morning, on awaking, opening eyes:** Bov., *Bry.,* Graph., *Nat-m., Nux-v.,* Onos., Stry., Tab.
**Motion:** Acon., Anac., *Apis, Bell., Bry.,* But-ac., Chin., Cocc., *Gels., Glon.,* Glyc., Ign., Iris, Lach., Mag-m., Mentho., Nat-m., *Nux-v., Ph-ac.,* Ptel., Rhus-t., Sep., *Sil., Spig.,* Stann., Ther.
**Motion of eyes:** Bell., *Bry.,* Cimic., Coloc., Cupr., Gels., Ichth., Ign., *Nux-v., Phys.,* Puls., Rhus-t., Spig.
**Muscular strain:** Calc.
**Narcotics:** Coff.

**Night:** Ars., *Aur.,* Bov., Merc-d., Ptel., *Puls.,* Stry., Sulph., Syph., Tarent.

**Noises:** Acon., Ars., *Bell.,* Coff., Ferr-p., *Ign.,* Lac-d., Lachn., Nit-ac., *Nux-v.,* Phel., *Ph-ac.,* Ptel., Sang., Scut., *Sil.,* Spig., Tab., Tarent.

**Noon:** Chinin-s., Sang., Tab.

**Nosebleed:** Aml-ns., Ant-c.

**Objects, bright:** *Bell.,* Oreo., Ph-ac., *Sil.,* Spig.

**Odors:** Coff., Ign., Scut., *Sel.*

**Overheating:** Carb-v., Sil., Thuj.

**Pressure:** Dios., Hep., Lach., Nat-ar., Ptel., Sil.

**Riding in cars:** Cocc., Kali-c., Petr.

**Right side:** *Bell.,* Bry., *Cact.,* Carb-ac., *Chel.,* Crot-h., Hep., Iris, *Lyc.,* Mez., *Sang.,* Tax.

**Rising in bed:** *Bry.,* Cocc.

**Sitting:** Chin., Rhus-t.

**Sleep after:** Crot-c., Ign., *Lach.*

**Stimulants, abuse:** Ign., *Nux-v.*

**Stool:** Aloe, Ign., Ox-ac.

**Stooping:** Acon., Ars-met., *Bell., Bry.,* Glon., *Ign.,* Lach., *Nux-v.,* Puls., Rhus-v., Sep., Sil., *Spig.,* Sulph.

**Sun:** *Bell.,* Gels., *Glon.,* Kali-bi., Lach., *Nat-c.,* Nux-v., *Sang., Sel.,* Spig.

**Talking:** Cact., Coff., Ign., Mez.

**Tobacco:** Carb-ac., Gels., Hep., *Ign.,* Lob., Nat-ar.

**Warmth in general:** *All-c.,* Aloe, Bry., Euphr., *Glon.,* Hyper., *Led.,* Nicc., Phos., *Puls.,* Sep.

**Water, sight of:** Lyss.

**Weather changes:** *Calc-p.,* Dulc., Guaj., *Phyt.,* Psor., Rhod., Spig.

**Wine:** Nux-v., Rhod., Zinc.

**Winter:** Aloe, Bism., Carb-v., Nux-v., Sabad., Sulph.

**Working in black:** Cedr.

**MODALITIES: Ameloration; After rising:** Kali-p.

**Bending head backward:** *Bell.,* Murx.

**Bending head forward:** Cimic., Hyos., Ign.

**Closing eyes:** Ant-t., Bell.

**Cold in general:** *All-c.,* Aloe, Alumn., Ars., Bism., Cycl., Ferr-p., Ictod., Lyc., Phos., *Puls.,* Spig., *Tab.*

**Conversation:** Dulc.

**Dark room:** Sang., Sil.

**Eating:** Alum., *Anac.,* Ap-g., Carl., *Chel.,* Coca, Kali-p., *Lith-c., Psor.*

**Holding hands near head:** Carb-an., Glon., Petr., Sul-ac.

**Lying:** Anac., *Bry., Chin.,* Ferr., Gels., Ign., Lach., Mag-m., Nux-v., Ph-ac., *Sang., Sil.,* Ther.

**Lying on painful side:** Calc-ar., Ign.

**Lying on painful side with head high:** *Bell.,* Gels.

**Lying on painful side with head low:** Absin., Aeth.

**Menses, during:** All-c., Bell., Glyc., Joan., Lach., *Meli.,* Zinc.

**Mental exertion:** *Helon.,* Pic-ac.

**Motion, gentle:** Chin., Glon., Helon., Iris, Kali p., *Puls.*

**Motion, hard, continued:** Indg., Rhus-t., Sep.

**Nosebleed:** Bry., Bufo, Ferr-p., Mag-s., *Meli.,* Psor., Rhus-t.

**Open air:** Acon., Act-sp., *All-c., Coca,* Indol., Joan., *Puls.,* Rad-met., Sep., Thuj.

**Partially closing eyes:** *Aloe,* Cocc-s., Oreo.

**Polyuria:** Acon., *Gels., Ign., Ph-ac.,* Sang., Sil., Verat.

**Pressure:** *Apis, Arg-n., Bell.,* Bry., Carb-an., *Chin.,* Coloc., Gels., *Glon., Ign.,* Indg., Lac-c., Lac-d., *Mag-m.,* Mag-p., *Meny.,* Nux-m., Nux-v., Par., *Puls.,* Sang., Sep., Sil., Spig., Thuj., *Verat.*

**Raising head:** Sulfon.

**Rest, quiet:** Bell., *Bry.,* Cocc., *Gels.,* Lith-c., Meny., Nux-v., Oreo., Puls., *Sang., Sil.,* Spig.

**Rubbing:** Indg., Tarent.

**Semierect posture:** Bell.

**Sleep:** Cocc-s., Gels., Nat-m., *Sang.,* Scut., Sil.

**Smoking:** Aran.

**Stimulants:** Gels.

**Stool and expelling flatus:** Aeth., Sang.

**Stooping:** Cina, Ign., Meny.

**Sweating:** Nat-m.

**Tea:** Carb-ac.

**Thinking of pain:** Camph., Helon., *Ox-ac.*

**Turning head forward:** Ign.

**Uncovering head:** Glon., Lyc.

**Warmth in general:** Am-c., Chin., Coloc., Ichth., *Mag-p.,* Nux-v., *Phos.,* Rhus-t., *Sil.*

**Wrapping or bandaging tightly:** Agar., *Apis, Arg-n.,* Bell., Glon., Ign., Lac-d., Mag-m., *Pic-ac.,* Puls., *Sil.,* Stront-c.

**HYDROCEPHALUS (acute and chronic); hydrocephaloid:** Acon., *Apis, Apoc., Arg-n.,* Arn., Ars., *Bac.,* Bar-c., *Bell., Bry., Calc., Calc-p.,* Canth., Carb-ac., *Chin.,* Chinin-s., *Cupr-act.,* Cypr., Cyt-l., Dig., Gels., *Hell., Iod., Iodof.,* Ip., Kali-br., Kali-i., Merc., Oeno., Op., Phos., Podo., *Sil.,* Sol-n., *Sulph.,* Tub., Verat., *Zinc.,* Zinc-br., Zinc-m.

**MOTION: POSITION OF HEAD: Boring back into pillow or rolling sideways:** *Apis,* Arum-t., *Bell., Hell., Podo.,* Zinc.

**Cannot hold head up, neck so weak:** Abrot., *Aeth.,* Cocc., Nat-m., Verat.

**Drawn back, retracted:** *Agar.,* Art-v., *Bell.,* Camph-mbr., *Cic.,* Cur., Hydr-ac., Iodof., Morph., Nat-s., Sec., Stram., Sulph., *Verat-v.*

**Motion constant, jerking trembling:** *Agar.,* Ant-t., Ars., *Bell.,* Cann-i., Cham., *Hyos.,* Lam., Mygal., Nux-m., Op., *Stram.,* Stry., Verat-v., Zinc.

**SCALP, Dandruff (seborrhea):** Am-m., *Ars., Bar-c.,* Bran., Bry., Fl-ac., *Graph.,* Hep., Hera., Iod., *Kali-s.,* Lyc., Nat-m., Phos., Sanic., *Sep.,* Sil., Sul-i., Sulph., Thuj.

**ERUPTIONS: Boils:** Anac., *Ant-t.,* Aur., *Calc-m.,* Calc-s., Dulc., *Hep.,* Jug-r., Scroph-n., *Sil.*

**Crusta lactea:** Astac., Bar-c., *Calc.,* Calc-i., Calc-s., Cic., Clem., *Dulc.,* Graph., *Hep.,* Kali-m., Lappa, *Lyc.,* Merc., *Mez.,* Olnd., Petr., Psor., Rhus-t., Sars., Scroph-n., *Sep.,* Sil., Sulph., *Trif-p., Vinc., Viol-t.*

**Eczema:** Astac., *Calc.,* Clem., *Graph., Lappa,* Hydr., Lyc., Mez., *Olnd., Petr.,* Psor., Sel., Sulph., Tell., Viol-o.

**Erysipelas:** Bell., Euph., Rhus-t.

**Favus (prurigo, scald head):** Aethi-m., Ars., Ars-i., Calc., Calc-i., *Calc-m.,* Calc-s., *Dulc.,* Ferr-i., Graph., *Hep.,* Jug-r., Kali s., Nit-ac., Sep., *Sil.,* Sulph., Viol-t.

**Growths, tumors, exostoses:** Anan., Aur-m., *Calc-f.,* Cupr., Fl-ac., *Hecla, Kali-i.,* Merc., Merc-p., Sil., Still.

**Herpes:** Anan., Chrysar., Nat-m., Olnd., *Rhus-t.*

**Itching eruptions:** Clem., *Olnd.,* Sil., Staph., *Sulph.*

**Moist, humid eruptions:** *Calc-s., Clem., Graph., Hep.,* Lyc., Merc., *Mez., Olnd., Petr.,* Psor., *Rhus-t., Sep.,* Sil., Staph., *Vinc.*

**Moist, humid eruptions, behind ears:** *Graph.,* Lyc., *Olnd., Petr.,* Staph., Thlas., Tub.

**Moist, humid eruptions, on margin of hair, nape of neck:** *Clem.,* Hydr., Nat-m., *Olnd.,* Sulph.

**Plica polonica:** Ant-t., Bar-c., Borx., Graph., *Lyc.,* Nat-m., Psor., Sars., Tub., *Vinc.,* Viol-t.

**Pustules:** Arund., Cic., *Clem.,* Graph., Iris, Jug-c., Mez.

**Ringworm (tinea capitis):** Ars., *Bac.,* Bar-m., Calc., Chrysar., Dulc., *Graph.,* Kali s., *Mez.,* Petr., *Psor., Sep.,* Sil., Sulph., *Tell.,* Tub., Viol-t. (See **SKIN.**)

**Scabs, crusts:** Ant-c., Ars., Calc-s., Cic., *Dulc., Graph.,* Hep., Lyc., *Mez.,* Sulph., Trif-p.

**Scales, dry:** *Ars.,* Kali-s., Mez., *Nat-m.,* Phos., Phyt., Psor., Sanic., Thlas.

**Spots, red:** Tell.

**Wens:** *Bar-c., Benz-ac.,* Graph., Hep., *Kali-i.,* Nit-ac., Phyt.

**HAIR: Brittle, harsh, dry:** Bad., Bell., Borx., Graph., *Kali-c.,* Plb., *Psor.,* Sec., Staph., Thuj.

**Falling out (alopecia):** *Alum.,* Ant-c., *Ars.,* Arund., Aur., Bac., Bar-c., Calc., Calc-i., Carb-v., Chrysar., *Fl-ac., Graph.,* Hyper., Kali-c., Lyc., Manc., Mez., *Nat-m., Nit-ac.,* Petr., *Ph-ac., Phos.,* Pix., *Sel., Sep.,* Sil., Stry-ar., *Syph., Thal.,* Thuj., Thyr., Sphing., *Vinc.,* Zinc.

**Greasy:** Ben-n., Bry., Merc.

**Gray, premature:** Lyc., *Ph-ac.,* Sec., Sul-ac.

**Tangled, in bunches:** *Borx.,* Fl-ac., Lyc., *Psor.,* Tub., Vinc.

**SCALP, itching:** Alum., Ant-c., *Ars.,* Arund., *Bov., Calc.,* Carb-v., Clem., Graph., Hera., Iod., Jug-r., Mag-*c.,* Manc., Menis., Nit-ac., *Olnd.,* Phos., Sep., Sil., Stry., *Sulph.,* Tell., *Vinc.*

**Neuralgia:** *Acon., Cimic.,* Hydr., Phyt.

**Numbness:** *Acon.,* Alum., Ferr-br., *Graph., Petr.*

**Sensitive to touch, combing:** *Acon.,* Apis, Arn., Ars., Azar., *Bell.,* Bov., *Bry.,* Carb-v., Caust., *Chin.,* Euon., *Eup-per., Gels., Hep.,* Kali-bi., Lachn., Meli., Merc., Nat-m., Nit-ac., Nux-m., *Nux-v.,* Olnd., *Par.,* Rhus-t., Sep., *Sil.,* Stry., Sulph.

**Sweat:** *Calc.,* Calc-p., *Cham.,* Graph., Hell., Hep., Hera., Hyper., Mag-m., Merc., Podo., *Rheum,* Sanic., *Sil.*

**Tension:** *Acon.,* Arn., Asar., *Bapt.,* Canch., Caust., Iris, *Merc., Par.,* Rat., Sel., Stict., *Viol-o.*

**SENSATIONS: As if a ball, firmly lodged in forehead:** Staph.

**As if brain were frozen:** Indg.

**As if brain were loose, in forehead, falling laterally:** Bell., Bry., Rhus-t., Sul-ac.

**As if hair were pulled, on vertex:** *Acon., Arg-n.,* Kali-n., Lachn., Mag-c., *Phos.*

**As if top would fly off:** Acon., *Cann-i., Cimic.,* Passi., Syph., Visc., Yuc.

**Bewildered, confused, stupid, intoxicated feeling:** *Absin.,* Acon., *Ail.,* Aloe, Anac., *Apis,* Aran., Arn., *Bapt.,* Bell., *Bry.,* Cann-i., Carb-v., Chin., *Cocc., Gels., Glon., Hell.,* Mentho., Nat-c., Nux- m., *Nux-v., Op., Ph-ac., Phos., Querc.,* Rhus-t., Sep., *Sulph.,* Tanac., Xero., Zinc.

**Bruised, sore feeling, of brain:** Arg-met., *Arn., Bapt.,* Bell., *Bell-p.,* Bov., *Chin.,* Eupi., Led., *Nux-v.,* Petr., Rhus-t., Verat. (See **Headache.**)

**Burning, head:** *Acon.,* Alumn., Apis, Arn., *Ars., Aster.,* Bell., Canth., Nux-v., *Phos.,* Zinc.

**Burning on vertex:** Aven., Cupr-s., Daph., *Frax., Graph.,* Helon., *Lach.,* Rhus-t., *Sulph.,* Tarax.

**Bursting:** *Acon.,* Arg-n., *Bell., Bry.,* Caps., Chin., Cocain., Form., *Gels., Glon.,* Nat-c., Nat-m., Nux m.

**Coldness:** Agar., Ars., Bar-c., *Calc.,* Calc-p., Calc-sil., Carb-v., Con., Helo., Laur., Nat-m., *Sep.,* Sil., Valer., *Verat.*

**Coldness in occiput:** Berb., Calc-p., Dulc., Ferul., *Helo., Phos.*

**Compressed in vise:** *Anac.,* Antip., Arg-n., *Berb., Cact.,* Cann-i., *Carb-ac.,* Cimic., Coca, *Eup-per.,* Franc., Gels., Hyper., Mag-p., Nit-ac., *Plat.,* Stann., Sulph., Tub. (See **Headache.**)

**Crawling, formication:** *Acon.,* Calc., Petr., Ran-b., Ran-r., Sulph.

**Emptiness, hollowness:** *Arg-met.,* Caust., *Cocc.,* Cupr., Cupr-act., Gran., *Ign.,* Manc., *Phos.,* Puls., Zinc.

**Enlarged, full, expanded feeling:** Acetan., *Acon., Arg-n.,* Ars-met., *Bapt., Bell.,* Bov., Bry., Cimic., Cocc., *Gels., Glon.,* Jug-c., Just., Lachn., *Meli.,* Mentho., Nat-c., *Nux-v.,* Oxyt., Par., Rhus-t., Usn., *Verat-v.*

**Gnawing in spot:** Nat-s., Ran-s.

**Heaviness:** *Acon.,* Agar., *Aloe,* Arn., Apis, *Bapt.,* Calc., Chel., Chin., Cimic., *Gels.,* Mur-ac., Op., Oreo., *Petr.,* Ph-ac., Plat., Rhus-t., Sep. (See **Headache.**)

**Lightness:** Abies-c., Hyos., *Jug-c.,* Manc., Nat-ar., Nat-hchls.

**Looseness of brain:** *Am-c.,* Ars., Bell., Bry., Chin., Hyos., Kali-c., *Rhus-t.,* Spig., Sul-ac., Sulph.

**Numbness:** Alum., *Bapt.,* Bufo, Calc-ar., Cocc., Con., Graph., *Kali-br.,* Olnd., Par., Petr., *Plat.*

**Opening and shutting:** *Cann-i., Cimic.,* Cocc., Lac-c.

**Tired feeling:** *Apis,* Arn., Chinin-ar., Con., Ferr-p., *Phos.,* Zinc-val.

**Undulating, surging, wave-like:** *Acon.,* Aur., *Bell.,* Canth., *Chin.,* Chinin-s., Cimic., *Glon.,* Hep., Hyos., Ind., Lach., Mag-p., *Meli.,* Nux-v., Pall., Rhus-t., Senec., Sulph.

**Wild, crazy feeling on vertex:** Lil-t.

**VERTIGO, Dizziness, Remedies in general:** *Absin., Acon.,* Adren., Aesc-g., Aeth., *Agar., Alum.,* Ambr., Ant-c., *Apis,* Apom., *Arg-n.,* Arn., Ars-i., Aur-m., Bapt., *Bell.,* Bism., Borx., *Bry., Calc.,* Cann-i., *Carb-ac., Carb-v.,* Chen-a., *Chin., Chinin-s.,* Cimic., *Coca, Cocc., Con.,* Cycl., Cyt-l., Dig., Eup-per., Ferr., Formal., *Gels.,* Gins., *Glon., Gran., Hydr-ac.,* Iod., Kali-c., Lach., *Lith m.,* Lol., Lup., Merc., *Morph.,* Mosch., Nat-sal., Nicot., *Nux-v., Op.,* Ox-ac., Petr., *Phos., Pic-ac.,* Podo., *Puls.,* Querc., Rad-br., Sal-ac., Senec., Sep., *Sil.,* Spig., Stront-c., Stry., Sulph., *Tab.,* Tarent., *Ther.,* Wye.

**CAUSE AND TYPE, Anemia of brain:** Arn., Bar-m., Calc., *Chin.,* Chinin-s., Con., Dig., *Ferr.,* Ferr-c., Hydr-ac., Nat-m., Sil.

**Cerebral origin:** Bell., *Cocc.,* Gels., Sulfon., Tab.

**Congestion of brain:** *Acon.,* Arn., *Bell.,* Chin., *Cupr., Glon.,* Hydr-ac., *Iod., Nux-v.,* Op., Stram., *Sulph.*

**Epileptic:** Arg-n., Calc., *Cupr.,* Kalm., Nux-v., *Sil.*

**Gastro-enteric derangement:** Aloe, *Bry.,* Chin., *Cocc.,* Ip., Kali-c., *Nux-v., Puls.,* Rham-cal., *Tab.*

**Hysterical:** *Asaf., Ign.,* Valer.

**Labyrinthic origin (Meniere's disease):** Arn., Bar-m., Bry., Carbn-s., Caust., *Chen-a.,* Chin., *Chinin-s., Chinin-scl.,* Con., Ferr-p., Gels., Hydrobr-ac., Kali-i., *Nat-sal.,* Onos., Petr., Pilo., Pyrus, *Sal-ac.,* Sil., Tab., *Ther.*

**Mal-de-mer:** Apom., *Cocc.,* Petr., Staph., Tab.

**Mental exertion:** *Arg-n.,* Nat-c., *Nux-v.*

**Nervous origin:** Ambr., Arg-n., Cocc., Nux-v., *Phos.,* Rhus-t., Ther.

**Noises:** Nux-v., *Ther.*

**Odor of flowers:** Nux-v., Phos.

**Old age (senile changes):** *Ambr., Ars-i.,* Bar-m., Bell-p., *Con.,* Dig., *Iod.,* Op., *Phos.,* Rhus-t., Sulph.

**Open air:** Arn., Calc-act., Canth., Cycl., *Nux-v.*

**Optical disturbances:** Con., *Gels.,* Pilo.

**Pelvic troubles:** Aloe, Con.

**Sunlight:** Agar., Nat-c.

**Worms:** Cina, Spig.

**OCCURRENCE, Alternates with colic:** Coloc., Mag-c., Spig.

**Beginning in nape of neck, or occiput:** *Gels.,* Iber., Petr., *Sil.*

**When ascending stairs:** Ars-h., *Calc.*

**When closing eyes:** Apis, Arn., *Lach.,* Mag-p., *Ther.,* Thuj.

**When coughing:** Ant-t.

**When descending stairs:** *Borx.,* Con., Ferr., Meph., *Sanic.*

**When eating:** Am-c., Cocc., Mag-m., *Nux-v.,* Puls.

**When entering warm room:** Ars., *Iod.,* Plat., Tab.

**When frightened:** Op.

**When in high ceilinged room:** Cupr-act.

**When looking at colored light:** Art-v.

**When looking at running water:** Arg-met., Brom., *Ferr., Verat.*

**When looking down:** *Borx.,* Olnd., Kalm., *Spig.*

**When looking fixedly:** Caust., Con., Lach., Olnd.

**When looking up:** Calc., Chinin-ar., *Gran.,* Kali-p., Petr., *Puls., Sil.,* Tab.

**When lying down:** Adon., Apis, Calad., *Con.,* Lach., Nat-m., Nux-v., Rhod., Rhus-t., Sil., Staph., *Ther.,* Thuj.

**When opening eyes:** Lach., *Tab.*

**When reading:** Am-c., Arn., Cupr., Nat-m.

**When riding in carriage:** *Cocc.,* Hep., Lac-d., Petr.

**When rising from bed or chair:** *Acon.,* Adon., Bell., *Bry.,* Cann-i., *Cocc.,* Con., Ferr., *Nat-sal., Nux-v.,* Olnd., Op., Petr., Phos., Rhus-t., Sulph.

**When rising in morning:** *Alum., Bry.,* Jac-c., *Lach.,* Lyc., *Nux-v.,* Op., Phos., Podo., Puls.

**When shaking, or turning head:** *Acon.,* Calc., *Con.,* Hep., Kali-c., *Morph.,* Nat-ar.

**When standing with eyes closed:** Arg-n., Lath.

**When stooping:** *Acon.,* Bar-c., Bell., Bry., Glon., Iod., *Kalm.,* Nux-v., Oreo., *Puls., Sulph.,* Ther.

**When turning eyes:** Con.

**When turning head:** Bry., Calc., Coloc., *Con.,* Kali-c., Mentho., *Morph.,* Nat-ar.

**When turning head to left:** *Coloc.,* Con.

**When turning in bed:** Bell., *Con.*

**When walking:** Acon., Agar., *Bell., Caust.,* Chin., Dig., *Gels.,* Kali-c., Lach., Mag-p., Nit-ac., Nux-m., *Oreo.,* Petr., *Ph-ac.,* Rhus-t., *Ther.*

**When walking in dark:** Stram.

**When walking in open air:** Agar., Arn., *Cycl.,* Dros., *Nux-v.,* Sep., *Sulph.*

**When walking over bridge or water:** Ferr., Lyss.

**CONCOMITANTS: Buzzing, tinnitus:** Arg-n., Bell., Carb-v., Chen-a., *Chinin-s., Gels.,* Pic-ac., *Stry.,* Valer.

**Deathly pallor:** *Dub.,* Puls., *Tab.*

**Debility, prostration:** Ambr., *Arg-n.,* Bapt., Chin., Con., Echi., Gels., *Tab.,* Verat.

**Dim vision, diplopia, etc.:** Arg-n., Bell., *Gels.,* Glon., Nux-v., Valer., Vinc.

**Drowsiness, hot head:** Aeth.

**Fainting, unconscious:** Acon., Alet., Berb., *Bry.,* Camph., *Carb- v.,* Glon., *Nux-v.,* Phos., Sabad., Tab.

**Gastralgia, spasms:** Cic.

**Head feels elongated, urging to urinate:** Hyper.

**Headache:** Acon., Agro., Apis, Cocc., *Nux-v.*

**Intoxicated feeling:** Abies-c., Arg-met., Bell., Chin., *Cocc.,* Con., *Gels., Nux-v.,* Op., Oxyt., Petr.

**Liver disturbances:** Bry., Card-m., Chel.

**Nausea, vomiting:** Acon., *Bry., Cocc.,* Euon., *Kali-bi., Nux-v., Petr.,* Pilo., *Podo.,* Puls., Stront-c., *Tab.,* Ther.

**Nervous phenomena:** Ambr., Cocc., *Gels., Ign.,* Phos.

**Nosebleed:** Bell., Bry., Carb-an.

**Opisthotonos:** Cic.

**Palpitation, heart symptoms:** Aeth., Bell., *Cact.,* Dig., Spig.

**Pressure at root of nose:** Bapt.

**Relief from closing eyes:** Aloe, Lol.

**Relief from food:** Alum.

**Relief from holding head perfectly still:** Con.

**Relief from lying down:** Apis, Atha., Aur., Bry., Chin., *Cocc.,* Nit-ac., Puls.

**Relief from nosebleed:** Brom.

**Relief from rest:** Arn., Colch., Cycl., Spig.

**Relief from vomiting:** Tab.

**Relief from walking in open air:** Am-m., Kali-c., Mag-p., *Puls., Rhus-t.,* Tab.

**Relief from warmth:** Mang-m., Sil., Stront-c.

**With balancing sensation:** Ferr.

**With staggering, trembling, weakness:** *Arg-n.,* Crot-h., *Gels.,* Nux-v., Ph-ac., Phos., Stram.

**With tendancy to fall backward:** *Absin.,* Bell., Bry., Kali-n., Nux-v.

**With tendancy to fall forward:** Alum., *Bry.,* Card-m., Caust., Chel., Elaps., Guar., Mag-p., Petr., *Podo.,* Spig., Stram., Urt-u., Vib.

**With tendancy to fall to left:** Aur., Bell., *Con., Dros.,* Eup-per., Iod., Sal-ac., Sil., Stram., Zinc.

**With tendancy to fall to right:** Helo., Kali-n.

■

# EYES

**BROWS, Hair falls out:** *Alum.,* Borx., Merc., *Nit-ac.,* Plb-act., Sanic., *Sel.,* Sil.

**Pimples on:** Fl-ac., Sil., Thuj.

**Warty growths on:** Anan.

**CANTHI (angles), Itching, smarting:** Alum., Ap-g., Ars., Carb-v., Fl-ac., *Gamb., Hep.,* Lyc., Nat-m., Nux-v., Phos., Succ-ac., Sulph., *Zinc.*

**Sore, raw, fissured:** *Ant-c.,* Borx., *Graph.,* Petr., *Sil.,* Staph., Zinc.

**Swollen, red:** Agar., *Arg-n.,* Cinnb., Graph., Zinc.

**CATARACT:** Am-c., Arg-i., Calc., *Calc-f.,* Cann-s., *Caust.,* Chim., *Cine.,* Coch., Colch., *Con., Euphr.,* Iod., Kali-m., Led., Mag-c., *Naphtin.,* Nat-m., *Phos.,* Platan-oc., Puls., Quas., Santin., Sec., Seneg., Sep., *Sil., Sulph.,* Tell., *Thiosin.,* Zinc.

**CHAMBER, anterior, pus in:** Hep., Sil.

**Chamber, hemorrhage after iridectomy:** Led.

**CHOROID: Congestion:** Agar., Phos., Rhod., Ruta, *Santin.*

**Choroid, detachment:** Acon., Arn., Nux-v.

**Choroid, extravasation:** Ham.

**Choroid, inflammation (choroiditis), atrophic:** Nux-v., Phos., *Pilo.*

**Choroiditis, disseminated and simple:** Ars., *Bell.,* Bry., Cedr., Gels., Ip., *Kali-i., Merc.,* Merc-i-r., Naphtin., Phos., *Prun.,* Santin., Tab., Tell., Thuj.

**Choroiditis, suppurative:** Hep., Rhus-t.

**Choroiditis, suppurative, with iris involvement:** Kali-i., *Prun.,* Sil.

**Choroiditis, suppurative, with retinal involvement (syphilitic):** Aur., *Kali-i.,* Kali-m., Merc-c., *Merc-i-r.*

**CILIARY MUSCLE: Accommodation disturbed:** Ip., Ruta.

**Ciliary muscle, paretic condition:** *Arg-n.,* Atro., Caust., Dub., *Gels.,* Par., Phys.

**Ciliary muscle, spasm:** *Agar.,* Esin., Ip., Jab., Lil-t., *Phys.,* Pilo.

**CILIARY NEURALGIA:** Ars., *Cedr.,* Chel., Chen-a., Chin., *Cimic., Cinnb.,* Coloc., Com., Croc., Crot-t., *Gels.,* Lach., Mez., Nat-m., Par., Phos., Plan., *Prun., Rhod.,* Sapo., Spig. (See **Pain.**)

**CONJUNCTIVA: Chemosis:** *Apis,* Guare., Hep., *Kali-i.,* Rhus-t., Sul-ac., *Vesp.*

**Discharge, acrid:** Ars., Arum-t., *Euphr., Merc.,* Merc-c., Psor., Rhus-t.

**Discharge, clear mucus:** Ip., Kali-m.

**Discharge, creamy, profuse:** *Arg-n., Calc-s.,* Dulc., Hep., *Nat-p.,* Nat-s., Pic-ac., *Puls.,* Rhus-t., Syph.

**Discharge, ropy:** Kali-bi.

**Ecchymoses and injuries:** Acon., *Arn., Ham.,* Lach., Led., Nux-v.

**Foreign bodies, irritation:** *Acon.,* Sulph.

**Granulations, blisters or wart-like:** Thuj.

**Hyperemia:** *Acon.,* All-c., Ars., *Bell.,* Ip., *Nux-v.,* Rhus-t., Sulph., *Thuj.*

**Inflammation (conjunctivitis): Acute and sub-acute catarrhal:** *Acon., Apis, Arg-n., Ars., Bell., Canth., Chlol.,* Dub., Dulc., *Euphr., Ferr-p.,* Guare., *Hep.,* Kali-m., *Merc.,* Merc-c., Merl., Nat-ar., Op., Pic-ac., *Puls.,* Rhus-t., Sep., Stict., Sulph., Upa.

**Inflammation, chronic:** *Alum., Ant-c.,* Arg-n., *Ars., Aur-m.,* Bell., Euphr., *Kali-bi.,* Merc., Pic-ac., Psor., *Puls., Sulph.,* Thuj., Zinc.

**Inflammation, croupous, diphtheritic:** Acet-ac., Apis, Guare., Iod., *Kali-bi., Merc-cy.*

**Inflammation, follicular (granular):** Abr., Apis, Arg-n., *Ars.,* Aur., *Aur-m.,* Calc-i., Crot-t., *Kali-bi.,* Nat-m., Phyt., Puls., *Thuj.,* Zinc-s.

**Inflammation, gonorrheal:** *Acon.,* Ant-t., Apis, *Arg-n.,* Calc-hp., *Hep.,* Kali-bi., *Merc.,* Merc-c., *Puls.,* Rhus-t., Verat-v.

**Inflammation, gonorrheal, sympathetic form:** *Arg-n.,* Euphr., Merc., Puls. (See **Purulent**.)

**Inflammation, phlyctenular:** Ant-t., *Calc., Calc-pic.,* Con., Euphr., Graph., Ign., Merc-c., Puls., *Rhus-t.,* Sil., Sulph.

**Inflammation, purulent:** *Arg-n.,* Calc-hp., Hep., Merc., *Merc-c .,* Puls., *Rhus-t.,* Sil.

**Inflammation, pustular:** Abr., *Ant-t.,* Arg-n., Ars., Calc., Graph., *Hep.,* Kali-bi., *Merc-c.,* Merc-n., Puls., Rhus-t.

**Inflammation, traumatic:** *Acon., Arn.,* Bell., *Calen.,* Canth., Euphr., *Ham.,* Led., Symph.

**CORNEA: Abscess of:** Calc-s., *Hep.,* Kali-s., Merc-c., Sil., Sulph.

**Ectasia:** Calc-p.

**Exudation, serous:** Apis.

**Foreign bodies:** *Acon.,* Calc-hp., Hep., Rhus-t., Sulph.

**Inflammation (keratitis):** Acon., Apis, Ars., Ars-i., *Aur-m.,* Bell., Cann-s., Con., Euphr., Hep., Ilx-a., *Kali-bi.,* Kali-m., *Merc-c.,* Nux-v., Phos., Sang., Sulph., Thuj.

**Inflammation, arthritic:** Clem., Colch., Coloc.

**Inflammation, herpetic, vesicular:** *Apis, Ars.,* Calc-p., Euphr., Ran-b., Tell.

**Inflammation, interstitial, in persons of hereditary syphilis:** Aur., *Aur-m.,* Cann-s., Merc-c., Merc-cy.

**Inflammation, parenchymatous, syphilitic origin:** *Aur-m.*, Calc-hp., *Kali-i.*, Kali-m., Merc., Sulph.

**Inflammation, phlyctenular:** *Apis,* Bell., Calc., *Calc-f.,* Calc-p., Con., *Graph.,* Hep., Ip., *Merc-c.,* Puls., Rhus-t., Syph., Thuj.

**Onyx:** Hep.

**Opacities:** Arg-n., Aur., Aur-m., Bar-c., Cadm-s., Calc., *Calc-f.,* Calc-hp., Calc-i., *Caust., Cann-s., Cine.,* Con., *Euphr.,* Hep., Kali-bi., Kali-m., Merc., Merc-c., *Naphtin.,* Nit-ac., Phos., Puls., Sacch., Seneg., *Sil.,* Sulph., Thiosin., Zinc., Zinc-s.

**Pustules:** *Ant-c.,* Calc., Con., Crot-t., Euphr., *Hep.,* Kali-bi., Kali- i., Merc-n., Nit-ac.

**Staphyloma, after suppurative inflammation:** *Apis,* Euphr., Ilx-a., Phys.

**Ulcers:** Aethi-a., Apis, *Arg-n.,* Ars., Aur-m., *Calc.,* Calc-hp., Calc-i., Calc-sil., *Euphr.,* Graph., *Hep., Kali-bi.,* Kali-m., *Merc-c.,* Merc-i-f., Nat-m., Nit-ac., Rhus-t., *Sil.,* Sulph., Thuj., Zinc.

**Ulcers, deep:** Ars., Euphr., *Kali-bi., Merc-c.,* Merc-i-f., Merc-i-r., Sil.

**Ulcers, indolent:** Calc., *Kali-bi., Sil.,* Sulph.

**Ulcers, superficial, flat:** Ars., Asaf., Euphr., Kali-m., Merc., Nit-ac.

**Ulcers, vascular:** Aur.

**Wounds, incised, lacerated:** Staph.

**EYEBALLS: Bad effects from exposure to snow:** Acon., Cic.

**Bad effects from electric or artificial light:** Glon., Jab.

**Bad effects from glare of fire:** Acon., Canth., Glon., Merc.

**Bad effects from operations:** *Acon.,* Arn., Asar., Bry., Croc., Ign., *Led.,* Rhus-t., Seneg., Stront-c., Thuj.

**Bad effects from sight seeing, moving pictures:** Arn.

**Burning, smarting:** *Acon., All-c., Ars.,* Aur-m., Ars-met., *Bell.,* Calc., Canth., Croc., *Euphr.,* Fago., Ferr-p., Lept., Lyc., Mag-p., *Merc-c., Nat-ar., Nat-m.,* Op., Phyt., Pilo., Puls., Ran-b., Sang., *Sulph., Thuj., Zinc.*

**Coldness:** Alum., Asar., Con., Mez., Nat-m., Plat.

**Coldness, as if wind blowing under lids:** *Croc.,* Fl-ac., Syph., Thuj.

**Dryness, heat:** *Acon.,* Alum., Ars., *Bell.,* Berb., Clem., Croc., Grat., *Lyc., Merc-c.,* Nat-ar., Nat-c., Nat-m., Nat-s., Nux-m., Op., Seneg., Sep., Stict., *Sulph.,* Zinc.

**Edema of ocular conjunctiva, translucent:** Apis.

**Enlarged, swollen feeling:** Acon., *Bell.,* Ox-ac., Par., Ph-ac., *Rhus-t.,* Sarr., *Seneg., Spig.,* Tril-p.

**Eruptions about:** Ant-t., Crot-t., Guaj.

**Heat:** Aesc., Carb-v., Indol., Lil-t., Meph., Op., Phos., *Ruta,* Sapo., Stry., *Sulph.*

**Heat, and flickering, worse in damp weather:** Aran.

**Heat, and sensitive to air:** Clem., Cor-r.

**Heaviness:** Bapt., *Gels.,* Lycpr., Meli., *Onos.,* Op., Par., Parth., Sep., Sulfon.

**Hemorrhage (intra-ocular):** Arn., *Ham.,* Lach., Led., *Sul-ac.,* Suprar.

**Injuries:** Acon., *Arn.,* Calen., Canth., Coch., *Ham.,* Led., Phys., *Rhus-t.,* Sul-ac., *Symph.*

**Itching:** Agar., *Agn.,* All-c., Ant-c., Ars-met., *Aur-m.,* Calc., Caust., Croc., *Fago.,* Gamb., *Merc.,* Nux-v., Puls., *Rhus-t.,* Squil., *Sulph.,* Zinc.

**LOOK: CONDITION: Dull:** Ant-c., *Ant-t.,* Bapt., Diph., Merc., Lycpr., Onos.

**Fixed, staring, distorted:** *Bell.,* Cann-i., *Cic.,* Cupr., Glon., *Hell.,* Hyos., *Morph.,* Oena., Op., Ph-ac., Pisc., *Stram.,* Stry.

**Glazed, death-like:** *Op.,* Ph-ac., Zinc. (See **FACE**.)

**Glistening, dazzling, brilliant:** *Bell.,* Bry., *Canth.,* Cupr., Hyos., Merc-*c.,* *Stram.,* Verat-v.

**Looking downwards:** *Aeth., Hyos.*

**Protruding, bulging (exophthalmos):** Aml-ns., *Bell.,* Clem., Com., Ferr-p., Glon., Helo., *Lycps-v.,* Par., Sangin-t., Sapo., Spong., Stel., *Stram.,* Stry., *Thyr.*

**Red, blood-shot, suffused:** *Acon.,* Aesc., Ail., *All-c., Bell.,* Cinnb., Dulc., *Gels.,* Ham., Hyos., *Merc-c.,* Morph., Op., Ruta, Sil., Sulfon., Sulph., *Thuj,* Verat-v.

**Red, inflamed:** *Acon.,* Ant-c., Arg-n., Ars., Aur-m., *Bell.,* Caust., Clem., *Euphr.,* Ferr-p., Hep., Indol., Ip., Jac-c., Lyc., Merc., Nat-m., Rhus-t., Sangin-n.

**Red, raw:** Arg-n., Crot-t.

**Red, with yellow vision:** Aloe.

**Rolling downwards:** *Aeth.,* Hyos.

**Rolling in vertical axis:** *Ben-n.,* Zinc.

**Rolling on falling asleep:** Aeth.

**Rolling quickly with closed eyes:** Cupr.

**Rolling upwards:** Bell., *Cic.,* Hell., Mur-ac., Oena.

**Sensation as if fat on eyes:** Paraf.

**Sensation as if sand or sticks in:** *Acon.,* Alum., Ars., *Caust.,* Coc-c., Euphr., Ferr-p., Graph., *Nat-m.,* Phos., Phyt., *Sulph.,* Xero.

**Sensation as if wind blowing in eyes:** Fl-ac.

**Squinting to relieve pain in forehead:** Aloe.

**Stiffness:** Asar., Aur., *Kalm.,* Med., Nat-ar., Rhus-t.

**Sunken, surrounded by blue rings:** Acet-ac., Ant-c., Ap-g., *Ars., Camph., Chin.,* Cupr., Gran., Hell., Ip., Nat-c., *Ph*-ac., Phos., Sec., *Staph.,* Upa, *Verat.,* Visc. (See **FACE**.)

**Syphilitic diseases:** Jac-g., Kali-i., Merc-i-f., Nit-ac., Thuj.

**Trembling (nystagmus):** *Agar.,* Ben-n., Carbn-h., *Cic., Gels.,* Iod., Kali-i., Mag-p., Phys.

**Unable to keep eyes fixed steadily:** Arg-n., Par.

**Whites of, yellow:** Brass., Cham., *Chel., Chin.,* Crot-h., Dig., Euon-a., Iod., Lach., Merc., Myrt-s., Nat-p., Nat-s., *Podo.,* Plb., Sep. (See **FACE.**)

**EYELIDS AND MARGINS: Agglutination:** Agar., Alum., *Ant-c.,* Apis, Arg-n., Borx., Calc., Caust., Dig., *Euphr., Graph.,* Kali- bi., Kali-c., Lyc., *Merc.,* Nat-ar., Nat-m., Psor., *Puls.,* Rhus-t., Sep., *Sulph.,* Thuj., Uran-n., Zinc.

**Blueness:** Dig., Morph.

**Drooping (ptosis):** Alum., Caul., *Caust., Con.,* Dulc., *Gels.,* Graph., Haem., Helo., Kalm., *Morph.,* Naja, Nat-ar., Nit-ac., Nux-m., Nux-v., Op., Phos., Plb., Rhus-t., *Sep.,* Spig., Stram., Sulfon., Syph., Upa, Verat., *Zinc.*

**Dryness:** *Acon.,* Alum., Ars., *Bell., Graph.,* Lith-c., Nux-v., Puls., Seneg., Sep., Sulph., Zinc.

**Dryness, scaliness:** *Ars.,* Borx., Sep., Tell., Thuj.

**Ectropion:** Apis, Graph., Thiosin.

**Entropion:** *Borx.,* Graph., Nat-m., Tell.

**ERUPTIONS, growths, blisters, vesicles:** Canth., *Nat-s.,* Pall., *Rhus-t.,* Sep., *Thuj.*

**Chalazae, tarsal tumors:** Ant-t., Calc., Caust., *Con.,* Ferr-py., *Kali- i.,* Platan-oc., Sil., *Staph., Thuj.,* Zinc.

**Cysts, sebaceous:** *Benz-ac.,* Calc., *Calc-f.,* Iod., *Kali-i.,* Merc., Platan-oc., *Staph.*

**Eczema, fissures:** Bac., Chrysar., *Graph., Petr.,* Staph., Sulph., Tell.

**Granular lids (trachoma):** Abr., *Alum.,* Ars., Aur-m., *Calc.,* Cinnb., Dulc., *Euphr.,* Graph., Hep., *Kali-bi.,* Kali-m., Merl., Nat-ar., Nat-s., Puls., Sep., Sulph., *Thuj,* Zinc-s.

**Pustules:** Ant-c., Hep.

**Scabs, crusts, scurfs:** Arg-n., *Ars.,* Borx., Calc., *Graph.,* Kali-m., Lyc., Seneg., *Sep.*

**Styes (hordeolum):** Agar., Apis, Aur-m-n., *Calc-pic.,* Con., *Graph., Hep.,* Lyc., Merc., *Puls., Sep., Sil., Staph., Sulph.,* Thuj., Uran-n.

**Styes followed by hard nodosities:** Con., Staph., Thuj.

**Ulcers:** Arg-n., *Ars., Caust.,* Euphr., *Graph.,* Hep., Lappa, Lyc., *Sulph., Tell.* (See **Tissues, GENERALITIES.**)

**Inflammation (blepharitis): Acute:** *Acon.,* Apis, Arg-n., *Ars.,* Cham., Dig., Dulc., *Euphr.,* Hep., Kreos., *Merc.,* Merc-i-f., *Merc-pr-r.,* Nat-ar., Petr., *Puls.,* Rhus-t., Sulph., Upa, Uran-n.

**Inflammation, chronic:** *Alum.*, Ant-c., *Arg-n.*, Aur., Bar-c., *Borx.*, Calc., Clem., Euphr., *Graph.*, Hep., Jug-c., Merc-c., Merc-pr-r., Petr., Psor., Sep., *Sil.*, *Staph.*, *Sulph.*, *Tell.*

**Inflammation, erysipelatous:** *Apis*, Bell., *Rhus-t.*, Vesp.

**Redness:** Agar., Am-br., *Ant-c.*, Apis, Arg-n., Ars., *Bell.*, Cinnb., Clem., Dig., Euphr., Graph., Hep., Lyc., Merc., *Merc-c.*, Rhus-t., Sabad., *Sulph-* (See **Inflammation.**)

**SENSATIONS: Burning and smarting:** Agar., All-c., Alum., Apis, *Ars.*, Arund., Bell., Calc., Cham., Croc., *Euphr.*, Graph., Kali- bi., Kali-i., Lyc., Merc., Mez., Nat-m., Puls., Sabad., *Sulph.*

**Coldness:** Croc., Ph-ac.

**Heaviness:** Caul., *Gels.*, Haem., Helo., Nat-m., *Sep.* (See **Drooping**.)

**Itching:** Agar., Alum., *Ambro.*, Calc., *Gamb.*, Graph., Lyc., Mez., *Morph.*, *Puls.*, Rhus-t., Staph., Succ-ac., *Sulph.*, Tell., Zinc.

**Pulsation of superciliary muscle:** Cina.

**Rawness and soreness:** *Ant-c.*, Arg-n., Ars., Borx., Euphr., *Graph.*, Hep., Merc-c., Petr., Sulph., Zinc. (See **Blepharitis.**)

**Spasms of eyelids, twitching (blepharospasm, nictitation):** *Agar.*, Ars., Atro., *Bell.*, Calc., Cham., Cic., *Cod.*, Croc., Esin., Gels., Guaj., *Hyos.*, Ign., Lob-p., Mag-p., Nat-m., Nicot., *Nux-v.*, Phys., *Puls.*, Ruta, Stry., Sul-ac.

**Stiffness:** Caust., Gels., Kalm., Rhus-t.

**Swelling (edema):** Am-br., *Apis*, Arg-n., *Ars.*, Ars-met., Aur-m., Bell., Calc., Dig., Euph-l., *Euphr.*, Graph., Hep., *Kali-c.*, Kali-i., Merc-c., Nat-ar., Nat-c., Phos., Puls., *Rhus-t.*, Rhus-v., Sabad., Sep.

**Thickening:** *Alum.*, Arg-n., Calc., *Graph.*, Hep., Merc., *Tell.*

**GLAUCOMA:** *Acon.*, Atro., Aur., *Bell.*, Bry., Caust., Cedr., Cocain., Coloc., Com., Croc., Esin., *Gels.*, Mag-c., Nux-v., Op., *Osm.*, *Phos.*, *Phys.*, Prun., Rhus-t., *Spig.*, Suprar.

**HYPOPION:** Crot-t., *Hep.*, Merc., Merc-c., Plb., *Sil.*

**IRIDO-CHOROIDITIS:** Kali-i., Prun., *Sil.*

**Irido-cyclitis, traumatic, with infection and sequelae:** Nat-sal.

**IRIS: Prolapse:** Ant-s-aur., Phys.

**IRITIS: Remedies in general:** *Acon.*, Ars., Bell., Cedr., *Cinnb.*, *Clem.*, Dub., *Euphr.*, Ferr-p., Gels., Grin., Hep., Iod., Kali-bi., Kali-i., Merc., *Merc-c.*, Puls., *Rhus-t.*, Spig., Sulph., Syph., Tell., Ter., Thuj.

**Plastic:** *Acon.*, Bry., Cinnb., Hep., *Merc-c.*, Rhus-t., Thuj.

**Rheumatic:** Arn., *Bry.*, Clem., Colch., *Euphr.*, Form., Kali-bi., Kalm., Led., Merc-c., *Rhus-t.*, Spig., Ter., *Thuj.*

**Serous:** Apis, *Ars.*, Bry., Cedr., *Gels.*, Merc., Merc-c., Spig.

**Syphilitic:** Asaf., *Aur., Cinnb.,* Clem., Iod., Kali-bi., *Kali-i., Merc-c.,* Merc-cy., Merc-i-f., *Nit-ac.,* Sulph., Thuj.

**Traumatic:** Acon., *Arn.,* Bell., *Ham.,* Led., Rhus-t.

**Tuberculous:** *Ars.,* Kali-bi., Sulph., Syph., Tub.

**LACHRYMAL SAC: Blenorrhea:** Ant-t., Calc., Calen., *Hep., Merc-d.,* Nat-m., Petr., *Puls.,* Sil., Stann.

**Dacryocystitis:** Apis, Fl-ac., *Hep., Iod.,* Merc., Petr., *Puls., Sil., Stann.*

**Duct closed, from cold, exposure:** Calc.

**Duct, stricture:** Nat-m.

**Duct, swollen:** Graph., Sil.

**Epiphora:** Calc., Graph., Hep., Merc., *Merl., Nat-m.,* Squil., Sil., Tang. (See **Lachrymation.**)

**Fistula lachrymalis:** *Calc.,* Caust., *Fl-ac.,* Lach., Merc-c., Nat-m., Nit-ac., Petr., Phos., Phyt., *Sil.,* Stann., Sulph.

**LACHRYMATION:** Acon., *All-c., Ambro.,* Antip., Apis, *Ars.,* Ars-met., Aur., Calc., Caust., Con., Eug., *Euphr.,* Guare., Ip., *Kali- i.,* Lyc., Merc., *Merc-c.,* Merl., Nat-ar., *Nat-m.,* Phos., Phyt., *Puls.,* Rhus-t., *Sabad.,* Sangin-n., Sil., Squil., Stict., Succ., Sulph., Tax.

**Acrid, burning, hot:** Apis, *Ars.,* Cedr., Eug., *Euphr.,* Graph., *Kali-i.,* Kreos., *Merc-c.,* Naphtin., *Nat-m., Rhus-t.,* Sulph.

**Bland:** All-c., *Puls.*

**MODALITIES: Relief in open air:** All-c.

**Worse at night:** Apis.

**Worse from cold application:** Sanic.

**Worse from coughing:** Euphr., *Nat-m.*

**Worse from eating:** Ol-an.

**Worse from foreign bodies in eyes, cold wind, reflection from snow:** Acon.

**Worse in morning, early:** Calc.

**Worse in open air:** Calc., Colch., Lyc., Phos., Sanic., Sil.

**LAGOPHTHALMOS:** Phys.

**MEIBOMIAN GLANDS: Swollen:** *Aeth.,* Bad., Clem., Dig., Graph., Hep., Puls., Rhus-t. (See **Blepharitis.**)

**OCULAR MUSCLES: Contracted spasmodically:** *Agar.,* Cic., Phys., Stry.

**Ocular muscles, pain:** Carb-v., Cimic., *Onos.* (See **Pain.**)

**Ocular muscles, paralysis:** Arg-n., Bell., *Caust., Con.,* Euphr., *Gels.,* Hyos., Lach., Oxyt., Phos., Phys., *Rhus-t., Ruta,* Santin., Seneg., Syph.

**Ocular muscles, paralysis, extrinsic:** Gels., Phos.

**Ocular muscles, paralysis, intrinsic:** Alum., Con., Lach., Nat-m., Onos., Ruta.

**Ocular muscles, paralysis superior rectus:** Seneg.

**Ocular muscles, paralysis, weak:** *Gels.,* Lach., Nat-m., Phys., *Ruta,* Til.

**OCULAR TENSION: Decreased:** Apisin., Cedr., Esin., Nat-m., Osm., Prun., Ran-b., Rhod.

**Increased:** (See **Glaucoma**.)

**OPHTHALMIA: Catarrhal:** *Acon.,* Am-m., Apis, Ars., Bell., Cham., Dulc., *Euphr.,* Gels., *Kali-bi.,* Merc., Merc-c., Nux-v., *Puls.,* Sulph.

**Chronic:** *Alum.,* Arg-n., Ars., Con., Euphr., *Graph.,* Kali-bi., Lyc., *Psor.,* Sep., *Sulph.,* Zinc.

**Follicular, granular:** Abr., Aur-m., Euphr., *Puls.*

**Gonorrheal (neonatorum):** Acon., *Arg-n.,* Bell., Calc-s., Cann-s., *Hep.,* Kali-s., *Merc., Merc-c., Merc-pr-r.,* Nit-ac., *Puls.,* Rhus-t., Syph., Thuj.

**Gonorrheal, constitutional:** Acon., *Clem.,* Nit-ac., Puls.

**Purulent:** Apis, *Arg-n.,* Calen., Grin., *Hep.,* Merc-c., Merc-pr-r., Nat-s., Plb., Puls., *Rhus-t.*

**Rheumatic:** Acon., Bell., *Bry.,* Calc., Caust., Clem., Colch., Euphr., Ilx-a., *Kali-bi.,* Led., Lith-c., Lyc., Merc., Merc-c., Nux-v., Phyt., *Rhus-t.,* Sil., Spig., Sulph.

**Scrofulous:** Aeth., *Aethi-a., Aethi-m.,* Apis, Arg-n., Ars., Ars-i., Aur., Aur-m., Bar-c., Bar-i., Bell., *Calc., Calc-i.,* Cann-s., Cist., Clem., *Coch.,* Colch., Con., *Euphr., Graph., Hep.,* Iod., *Kali-bi., Merc-c.,* Merc-d., Merc-n., Merc-pr-r., Nat-m., *Nit-ac.,* Psor., Puls., Rhus-t., Scroph-n., Sil., *Sulph.,* Thuj., Viol-t., Zinc-s.

**Senile:** Alum.

**Sympathetic:** *Bell.,* Bry., Calen., Merc., *Rhus-t., Sil.* (See **Conjunctivitis**.)

**Syphilitic:** Apis, Asaf., Gels., Kali-i., Merc-c., Nit-ac.

**OPTICAL: Hyperesthesia:** Chrysar.

**OPTIC DISCS: Hyperemic, retinal vessels enlarged:** Bell., Onos.

**Optic discs, pallor, visual field contracted, retinal vessels shrunken:** Acetan.

**OPTIC NERVE: Atrophy:** Agar., Arg-n., Atoxyl, Carbn-s., Iodof., Nux-v., *Phos.,* Santin., *Stry-n.,* Tab.

**Inflammation (neuritis):** *Apis,* Ars., Bell., Carbn-s., Kali-i., *Merc-c.,* Nux-v., Pic-ac., Plb., Puls., Rhus-t., Santin., Tab., Thyr.

**Neuritis, choked:** Bell., Bry., Dub., Gels., Hell., Nux-v., Puls., Verat-v.

**Neuritis, descending:** Ars., Cupr., Merc-c.

**Paralysis:** Nux-v., Oxyt., Ph-ac.

**ORBITS: Bony tumors:** Kali-i.

**Cellulitis:** *Apis,* Hep., Kali-i., Phyt., *Rhus-t.,* Sil.

**Injuries:** Acon., *Arn.,* Ham., Symph.

**Pain around:** Apis, *Asaf.,* Aur., Bell., *Cinnb.,* Hep., Hydrc., Ilx-a., Plat., Plb., Spig.

**Pain, deep in:** *Aloe,* Gels., Merc-c., Phos., Phyt., Plat., Ruta, Sarr., *Spig.,* Stann., Upa (See **Pain.**)

**Periostitis:** Asaf., *Aur., Kali-i.,* Merc., Sil.

**PAIN: LOCATION: Ciliary body:** Ars., *Cedr.,* Chen-a., Chr-o., *Cimic., Cinnb., Com.,* Crot-t., *Gels.,* Par., Phos., Plan., *Prun.,* Rhod., *Spig.,* Thuj.

**Eyeballs:** *Acon.,* Alf., Am-br., Asaf., Aur., Aza., Bapt., *Bell., Bry., Cedr.,* Chel., Chim., Chin., *Cimic., Clem.,* Cocc., Coloc., *Com.,* Con., Crot-t., Esin., *Eup-per., Euphr., Gels.,* Grin., Guare., Hep., Indol., Jab., Kali-i., Kalm., *Lycps-v.,* Mentho., *Merc-c.,* Nat-m., Nicc-s., Nit-ac., Olnd., Onos., Osm., Par., Passi., Ph-ac., Phos., Phys., Plat., *Prun., Puls.,* Rhod., Rhus-t., *Ruta,* Sang., *Spig.,* Staph., Symph., Syph., Ter., Ther., Thuj., Upa, Viol-o.

**Orbits:** Aloe, Am-pic., *Asaf.,* Aur., Chel., Cimic., Cinnb., Crot-t., Gels., Ilx-a., *Kali-i.,* Mentho., *Phos.,* Ruta, *Spig.,* Ther., *Upa.*

**Supra-orbital:** Asaf., *Bry.,* Carb-ac., *Cedr., Chinin-s.,* Dub., *Gels., Kali-bi.,* Mag-p., Meli., Mentho., Merc-c., Plat., Ruta, *Spig.,* Thuj.

**TYPE: Aching, sore:** Aesc., Alf., Aloe, Arn., Arg-n., Bapt., *Bry.,* Cimic., *Eup-per.,* Euphr., Esin., Gels., *Ham.,* Led., Lept., Mentho., *Nat-m.,* Nicc-s., Nit-ac., Onos., Rad-met., Rhus-t., *Ruta,* Sep., *Spig.*

**Boring:** Asaf., *Aur., Coloc., Crot-t.,* Hep., Merc-c.

**Bruised:** *Arn.,* Aur-m., Cimic., Cupr., *Gels.,* Hep., Nat-m.

**Burning, smarting:** *Acon.,* All-c., Ammc., *Ars.,* Asaf., Carb-v., Clem., Euphr., Ilx-a., Indol., Iod., Jab., Lyc., Merc-c., *Nat-m., Phos.,* Ran-b., *Ruta,* Sil.

**Enlarged feeling, bursting:** Am-br., Bry., *Cimic., Com.,* Par., *Prun., Spig.*

**Neuralgic:** *Ars.,* Asaf., Bell., *Cedr.,* Chin., Chinin-s., *Cimic., Cinnb.,* Coloc., Com., Crot-t., *Gels.,* Kali-i., Kalm., Mag-p., Meli., Mez., Osm., Phos., Phys., *Prun.,* Rhod., *Spig.*

**Periodically, intermittent:** Ars., Asaf., *Cedr.,* Chin., Chinin-s., *Spig.*

**Piercing, penetrating:** Apis, Aur., Mill., Rhus-t.

**Pressing inwards, as if retracted:** Aur-m., *Crot-t.,* Hep., Olnd., *Par., Ph-ac.*

**Pressing outwards:** Asar., *Bry.,* Cimic., *Cocc.,* Coloc., Com., Guare., *Lycps-v.,* Merc-c., Passi., *Spig.,* Ther.

**Pressive, crushing:** Acon., Asaf., Aur-m., Chin., Clem., Crot-t., Cupr., Euphr., Hep., Mentho., Nit-ac., Olnd., *Par., Ph-ac.,* Phos., *Prun.,* Ran-b., Rhus-t., *Ruta,* Sang., Sep., *Spig.*

**Sensitive to touch:** *Acon.,* Arn., Ars., Aur., *Bell., Bry.,* Cimic., Clem., Eup-per., *Ham., Hep.,* Lept., Rhus-t., Sil., *Spig.,* Thuj. (See **Aching.**)

**Shooting, stitching, darting, cutting:** Acon., Asaf., *Bry.,* Calc., Chim., *Cimic., Cinnb.,* Clem., *Coloc.,* Euphr., Graph., Hell., Hep., *Kali-c.,* Kalm., Mag-p., Merc-c., *Nit-ac.,* Phys., Prun., Rhod., Rhus-t., Sil., *Spig.*

**Splinter-like:** Apis, Aur., *Hep.,* Med., Merc., *Nit-ac.,* Sulph., Thuj.

**Stinging:** *Apis,* Euphr., Hep., Kali-c., Puls., Thuj.

**Strained, stiff feeling:** *Guaj.,* Jab., *Kalm.,* Med., *Nat-m.,* Onos., Rhus-t., *Ruta.*

**Tearing:** Ars., Asaf., *Aur-m.,* Bell., Chel., Colch., Crot-t., Guare., Merc-c., *Puls.,* Sil.

**Throbbing:** Asaf., *Bell.,* Bry., Cimic., *Hep.,* Merc., Ther.

**MODALITIES: Aggravation: At night:** *Ars.,* Asaf., Cinnb., Con., Euphr., Hep., *Kali-i.,* Lyc., *Merc.,* Merc-c., Puls., Rhus-t., Sep., Spig., *Syph.,* Thuj.

**Before a storm:** Rhod.

**From closing eyes:** Sil.

**From cold air:** *Asar., Clem.,* Hep., Mag-p.

**From damp, cold, rainy weather:** Merc-c., *Rhus-t., Spig.*

**From glare of light:** Asar., Con., Merc.

**From looking down:** Nat-m.

**From looking up:** Chel.

**From lying down:** Bell.

**From motion:** Ars., *Bry.,* Cimic., Crot-t., Grin., Indol., Kalm., Rhus-t., *Spig.*

**From motion, or use of eyes:** *Arg-n.,* Arn., *Bry.,* Cimic., Euphr., Kalm., *Nat-m.,* Onos., Phys., Rhus-t., *Ruta, Spig.*

**From sunlight:** Asar., Merc.

**From sunrise to sunset:** Kalm., Nat-m.

**From touch:** *Bry., Hep.,* Phos.: Plan.

**From warmth:** Arg-n., *Com.,* Puls., Sulph., Thuj.

**Worse on left side:** Mentho., Onos., *Spig.,* Ther.

**Worse on right side:** *Bell.,* Cedr., *Chel.,* Com., Kalm., *Mag-p.,* Prun., Ran-b., Ruta.

**MODALITIES: Amelioration: Cold air, applications:** Arg-n., *Asar.,* Puls.

**Darkness:** Con., Lil-t.

**Lying down on back:** Puls.

**Motion:** Kali-i.

**Pressure:** Arg-n., Asaf., Chel., *Chinin-s., Coloc.,* Con., Lil-t.

**Rest:** Asaf., Bry., Cimic.

**Touch, pressure:** Asaf., Chel.

**Warmth:** Ars., *Hep.,* Mag-p., *Thuj.*

**PANNUS:** Apis, *Aur-m.,* Chinin-m., *Hep.,* Kali-bi., Merc-i-r., Nit-ac. (See Cornea.)

**PAN-OPHTHALMITIS:** Hep., Rhus-t.

**PERCEPTIVE POWER, lost:** Kali p.

**PHOTOPHOBIA:** *Acon.,* Agn., Ail., All-c., Ant-t., Apis, *Arg-n., Ars.,* Ars-met., Asar., Aur-m., *Bell., Benzol.,* Calc., Calc-p., Cimic., Clem., *Con.,* Croc., Elaps, *Euphr., Graph.,* Hep., *Ign.,* Kali-c., Lil-t., Lyc., *Merc., Merc*-c., Nat-s., Nux-m., *Nux-v.,* Op., Ph-ac., Phos., Psor., *Puls., Rhus-t.,* Scroph-n., Sil., Spig., *Sulph.,* Ther., Zinc.

**PTERYGIUM:** Am-br., Apis, Calc., *Cann-s.,* Guare., Lach., *Rat.,* Spig., *Sulph.,* Tell., *Zinc.*

**PUPILS: Contracted (myosis):** Acon., Cina, *Esin.,* Gels., Hell., Ign., Iodof., Lon-x., Merc-c., *Morph., Op.,* Oxyt., Phos., *Phys.,* Pilo., Sol-n.

**Dilated (mydriasis):** Acetan., Agar., *Agn., Ail., Atro., Bell.,* Calc., Camph., *Cic., Cocain.,* Dig., *Dub.,* Gels., Glon., Hell., *Hyos., Iodof.,* Nit-ac., *Nux m.,* Oena., Sec., *Stram.,* Verat-v., Zinc.

**Insensible, poor reaction:** Bell., Benzol., Camph., *Cic., Gels.,* Hell., Hydr-ac., Hyos., Laur., Nit-ac., Op., Phos., Pilo., Stram., *Zinc.*

**RETINA: Anemia:** Lith-c.

**Apoplexy (hemorrhage from, traumatism, cough, etc.):** Acon., *Arn.,* Bell., Both., Croc., *Crot-h., Ham.,* Lach., *Led.,* Nat-sal., Phos., Symph.

**Artery, spasm:** Nux-v.

**Congestion:** Acon., *Aur., Bell.,* Carbn-s., *Dub.,* Ferr-p., Gels., Phos., Puls., *Santin.*

**Congestion from cardiac disease:** Cact.

**Congestion from light, artificial, brilliant:** Glon.

**Congestion from menstrual suppression:** Bell., Puls.

**Congestion from overuse of eyes:** *Ruta,* Santin.

**Detachment:** *Aur-m.,* Dig., *Gels.,* Naphtin., Pilo.

**Edema:** *Apis,* Bell., Canth., *Kali-i.,* Phos.

**Hyperesthesia (optical):** *Bell.,* Cimic., Con., Lil-t., Macro., *Nux-v., Ox-ac.,* Phos., Stry.

**Inflammation (retinitis), albuminuric and chronic:** Crot-h., Gels., Kalm., *Merc-c.,* Nat-sal., Phos., *Plb.,* Sal-ac.

**Inflammation, apoplectic:** Glon., Lach.

**Inflammation, leukemic:** Nat-s., Thuj.

**Inflammation, pigmentary:** Nux-v., Phos.

**Inflammation, proliferating:** Kali-i., Thuj.

**Inflammation punctata albescens:** Bell., Kali-i., Merc-c., Merc-i-r., Naphtin., Sulph.

**Inflammation, simple and serous:** *Aur.,* Bell., *Ben-d.,* Bry., *Dub.,* Gels., *Merc.,* Pic-ac., Puls., Santin.

**Inflammation, syphilitic:** Iod., *Kali-i.*

**Injuries:** Acon., *Arn.,* Bell., *Ham.,* Lach., Led., Phos.

**Thrombosis and degeneration:** Ham., Phos.

**SCLEROTICA: Degeneration:** Aur., Bar-m., Plb.

**Ecchymosis:** *Arn.,* Bell., Cham., Ham., Lach., *Led.,* Nux-v., Seneg.

**Inflammation, deep (scleritis):** *Acon., Ars.,* Aur-m., Ery-a., Hep., Kalm., *Merc-c.,* Sep., *Spig.,* Thuj.

**Inflammation, superficial (episcleritis):** *Acon.,* Bell., Bry., Kali-i., Merc-c., Rhus-t., Ter., *Thuj.*

**STRABISMUS (squinting):** Alum., Alumn., Apis, Apoc., *Bell.,* Ben-d., Calc p., *Cic.,* Cina, Cupr-act., Cycl., *Gels., Hyos.,* Nux-v., *Santin.,* Sec., Spig., *Stram.,* Tab., *Zinc.*

**Convergent:** Cycl., Jab.

**Dependent on convulsions:** Bell., *Cic.,* Hyos.

**Dependent on injuries:** Cic.

**Dependent on worms:** Bell., *Cina,* Cycl., Hyos., Merc., *Santin.,* Spig.

**Divergent:** Morph., Nat-sal.

**VISION: AMAUROSIS (blindness):** Acon., Apis, *Aur.,* Bell., Calc., Caust., Chin., Chinin-s., *Con.,* Cycl., Dulc., *Gels.,* Hep., Hyos., Manc., *Merc.,* Mom-b., Naphtin., Nat-m., Nux m., Nux-v., *Phos.,* Plb., *Plb-act.,* Santin., Sep., Sil., Stram., Stry., Tab., Vanad., Zinc.

**Colors:** *Ben-d.,* Carbn-s., Phys., *Santin.*

**Day:** Acon., *Both.,* Castm., Lyc., Phos., Ran-b., Sil.

**Hysterical:** Phos., Plat., Sep.

**Night:** *Bell.,* Cadm-s., Chin., Hell., Hep., Hyos., Lyc., *Nux-v.,* Phys., Puls., Stry.

**Retro-bulbar neuritis:** Iodof.

**Tobacco:** *Nux-v.,* Phos., Pilo., Plb-act.

**AMBLYOPIA (blurred, weak vision):** Acon., *Agar., Anac.,* Arn., *Aur.,* Bapt., *Ben-d., Caust.,* Chin., Colch., *Con., Cycl.,* Dig., Elaps, Esin., Euphr., *Gels.,* Hep., *Jab., Kali-c.,* Kali-p., Lil-t., *Lith-m.,* Lyc., Mag-p., Naphtin., *Nat-m.,* Nux-m., Nux-v., *Onos.,* Ox-ac., Osm., Ph-ac., *Phos.,* Phys., Pilo., *Puls.,* Ran-b., Rhus-t., *Ruta, Santin.,* Seneg., Sep., Sil., Stront-c., *Tab.,* Thuj., Titan., Zinc.

**Objects appear as looking through mist or veil:** Agar., Calc., *Caust.,* Cina, *Croc., Cycl., Gels.,* Kali-c., Lil-t., *Mom-b., Nat-m., Phos.,* Phys., Plb., *Puls., Ruta, Sep., Tab.*

**Objects appear elongated:** Bell.

**Objects appear inverted:** Bell., Guare.

**Objects appear too large:** Bov., Hep., *Hyos.,* Nicc., Nux-m., *Ox-ac.*

**Objects appear too small:** Ben-d., Glon., Nicot., *Plat.,* Stram.

**Retinal images persist:** Jab.

**When reading, eyes easily fatigued:** Ammc., Calc., Cina, *Jab.,* Nat-ar., Nat-m., Phos., *Ruta,* Sep., Sulph.

**When reading, eyes feel pressed asunder or outward, relieved by cold bathing:** Asar.

**When reading, letters appear red:** Phos.

**When reading, letters disappear:** Cic., Cocc.

**When reading, letters run together:** *Agar.,* Bell., *Calc.,* Cann-i., Chin., Cina, Con., Elaps, Ferr., Hyos., Lyc., *Nat-m.,* Sil.

**ASTHENOPIA (eye strain, with spasm of accommodation):** *Agar.,* Alum., Am-c., Ammc., Apis, Arg-n., Arn., Art-v., Bell., Carbn-s., *Caust., Cimic.,* Cina, Croc., *Gels.,* Ign., *Jab.,* Kali-c., Kalm., *Lac-f., Macro., Nat-m.,* Nicc-s., Nicot., Nux-v., Onos., Par., *Phos., Phys.,* Rhod., *Ruta,* Santin., Seneg., Sep., Stront-c.

**External recti:** Cupr-act., Gels.

**Internal recti:** Jab., Muscin., Nat-m., Phys., Pilo.

**Myopic:** Esin., Lil-t.

**ASTIGMATISM:** Gels., *Lil-t.,* Phys.

**DIPLOPIA (double vision):** Agar., Aur., *Bell.,* Cic., Con., *Cycl.,* Dig., *Gels.,* Gins., *Hyos.,* Nat-m., *Nit-ac.,* Olnd., Onos., Phos., Phys., Plb., Sec., Stram., Sulfon., Sulph., Syph., Verat-v.

**HEMIOPIA:** Calc-s., Glon., Hep., *Lith c.,* Lyc., Mur-ac., Nat-m., *Titan.,* Verat-v.

**Left half:** Calc., Lith-c., Lyc.

**Lower half:** Aur., Dig.

**Vertical:** Ferr-p., *Lith-c.,* Morph., Mur-ac., *Titan.*

**HYPERMETROPIA:** Calc., Con., *Jab.,* Nat-m., Petr., Ruta, Sep., Sil.

**MYOPIA:** Acon., *Agar.,* Aur-m., Bell., Carbn-s., Euphr., Gels., Lil-t., Nit-ac., Phos., *Phys., Pilo.,* Ruta, Viol-o.

**OPTICAL ILLUSIONS (chromopsia, photopsia): Black before eyes:** Agar., *Atro.,* Bell., *Carb-v., Carbn-s.,* Chin., Cycl., Dig., Lach., Lyc., Mag-c., Mag-p., Merc., Nat-m., Phos., Phys., Sep., Stront-c., *Tab.,* Zinc.

**Blue before eyes:** Crot-h., Tril-c., Tril-p.

**Confusion of colors:** *Bell.,* Calc., Croc., Merc., *Puls.,* Ruta, Staph., Stram.

**Flashes, flames, flickering:** Agar., Aloe, *Bell.,* Calc-f., Caust., Clem., *Cycl.,* Glon., Hep., Ign., *Iris,* Lyc., Phos., Phys., *Puls.,* Seneg., Viol-o.

**Gray:** Arg-n., Conv., Guare.

**Green:** Dig., *Osm., Phos.*

**Halo around light:** Bell., Chlol., Hyos., Sulph.

**Objects appear white:** Chlol.

**Object, brilliant, fantastic, colored, fiery:** *Anh., Aur., Bell.,* Chin., *Cycl.,* Nat-m., Sep.

**Red before eyes:** Antip., Apis, *Bell., Dub.,* Elaps, Hep., *Phos.,* Stront-c.

**Sparks, stars:** Aur., *Bell.,* Calc-f., Caust., Croc., *Cycl.,* Glon., Lyc., Naphtin., Sil., Stry.

**Spots (muscae volitantes):** *Agar.,* Anac., *Atro.,* Aur., Carb-v., Caust., *Chin.,* Colch., Con., *Cycl.,* Cypr., Kali-c., Meli., *Merc., Nit-ac., Nux-v., Phos.,* Phys., Sep., Sil., Sulph., Tab.

**Yellow before eyes:** *Aloe,* Canth., Cina, Digox., *Santin.*

**VITREOUS OPACITIES: Diffused:** Ham., Hep., Kali-i., Merc-c., Merc-i-r., Thuj.

**Turbid:** Chol., *Kali-i.,* Phos., Prun., *Seneg.,* Sol-n., Sulph.

■

# EARS

**AUDITORY NERVE, Torpor:** *Chen-a.*

**AURICLE (external ear), Burning, as if frost bitten:** Agar., Caust., Sang.

**ERUPTIONS, Remedies in general:** *Ant-c.,* Bar-c., *Calc.,* Calc-s., *Graph.,* Lyc., *Mez.,* Petr., Rhus-t., Tell.

**Acne:** Calc-s.

**Eczema around:** *Ars.,* Arund., Bov., Chrysar., *Clem.,* Crot-t., *Graph.,* Hep., Kali-m., *Mez.,* Olnd., Petr., Psor., *Rhus-t.,* Sanic., Scroph-n., Tell.

**Erysipelas:** *Apis,* Bell., Rhus-t., Rhus-v.

**Fissures:** Calc., Graph.

**Frost bites:** Agar., *Apis,* Bell., Rhus-t.

**Intertrigo:** Petr.

**Herpes:** Cist., Graph., Psor., Rhus-t., *Sep.,* Tell.

**Moist, oozing:** Ant-c., Calc., *Graph.,* Hep., *Mez.,* Petr., *Psor.,* Sanic.

**Pustules:** Ars., *Hep.,* Psor.

**Scabs, scurfs:** Chrysar., Hep., *Psor.*

**Glands, swollen, painful, around:** *Bar-c.,* Bell., *Calc.,* Caps., Graph., Iod., *Merc.*

**Itching:** *Agar.,* Ars., Hep., Nat-p., *Sul-i.,* Tub.

**Lobe, eruption on:** Bar-c.

**Lobe, ulceration of ring hole:** Stann.

**Numbness:** Mag-c., Plat., Verb.

**Pain, tearing, with tophi:** Berb.

**Red, raw, sore:** Graph., Petr., Sulph.

**Red, swollen:** *Acon., Agar.,* Anac., Apis, *Bell.,* Chin., Graph., Hep., Kali-bi., Medus., Merc., Puls., *Rhus-t.,* Scroph-n., Sulph.

**Sensitive to touch:** Arn., *Bell.,* Bry., *Caps., Chin.,* Ferr-p., *Hep.,* Psor., Sanic., Sep.

**CERUMEN:** Carb-v., Caust., *Con.,* Elaps, Graph., Lach., Puls., Sep., Spong.

**DEAFNESS, HARDNESS OF HEARING, Remedies in general:** Agar., *Agra.,* Am-c., *Ambr.,* Arn., Ars-i., *Bar-c., Bar-m.,* Bell., Calc., Calc-f., Calen., Carb-an., Carbn-s., *Caust.,* Cheir., *Chen-a., Chin., Chinin-s.,* Con., Dig., Dulc., Elaps, Ferr-p., Ferr-pic., *Graph.,* Hep., Hydr., Hydrobr-ac., Iod., Kali-ar., Kali-c., *Kali-m.,* Lob., *Lyc.,* Mang-act., Merc., *Merc-d.,* Mez., Nat-c., *Nat-sal., Nit-ac., Petr.,* Ph-ac., *Phos.,* Psor., Puls., Rham-cal., Sal-ac., Sangin-n., Sep., *Sil.,* Tell., *Thiosin., Verb.,* Viol-o.

**CAUSE: Abuse of mercury:** Hep., Nit-ac.

**Adenoids and hypertrophied tonsils:** *Agra.,* Aur., Bar-c., Calc-p., Merc., Nit ac., Staph.

**Alternate with sensibility of ear:** Sil.

**Apoplexy:** Arn., Bell., Caust., Hyos., Rhus-t.

**Bone conduction, deficient, or absent:** Chen-a.

**Catarrh (eustachian, middle ear):** Ars-i., Asar., *Calcareas,* Caust., Gels., Graph., *Hep.,* Hydr., *Iod.,* Kali-bi., *Kali-m.,* Kali- s., Mang-act., Mentho., Merc., *Merc-d.,* Petr., *Puls,* Ros-d., Sang., Sep., Sil., Thiosin.

**Cerebral:** Chen-a., Mur-ac.

**Cold exposure:** Acon., Kali-m., Visc.

**Concussion:** Arn., Chinin-s.

**Damp weather:** Mang-act.

**Discharge suppressed or eczema:** Lob.

**Eruption of scalp, suppressed:** Mez.

**Human voice, difficult to hear:** Calc., *Chen-a.,* Ign., Phos., Sil., Sulph.

**Infectious diseases:** Arn., *Bapt., Gels.,* Hep., Lyc., Petr., Phos., Puls.

**Nervous exhaustion, and nervous origin:** *Ambr.,* Anac., Aur., *Bell.,* Caust., Chin., Chinin-s., *Gels., Ign., Lach.,* Ph-ac., Phos., Plat., Tab., *Valer.*

**Nutritional disturbance, in growing children:** Calc., Merc-i-r.

**Old age:** Kali-m., Merc-d., Phos.

**Rheumatico-gouty diathesis:** *Ferr-pic.,* Ham., Kali-i., Led., Sil., Sulph., Visc.

**Sclerotic condition of conducting media:** Ferr-pic., Thiosin.

**Scrofulous diathesis:** *Aethi-m.,* Calc., Merc., Mez., Sil., *Sulph.*

**Sounds, low toned:** Chen-a.

**Syphilis:** Kreos.

**Working in water:** Calc.

**MODALITIES: Aggravated before menses:** Ferr-pic., Kreos.

**Ameliorated from noise, riding in cars:** Calen., *Graph.,* Nit-ac.

**EUSTACHIAN TUBES (catarrh or closure):** Alf., Alum., Bar-m., *Calcareas,* Caps., *Caust.,* Ferr-i., Ferr-p., Gels., *Graph.,* Hep., Hydr., *Iod.,* Kali-bi., Kali-chl., *Kali-m.,* Lach., Lob-c., Mentho., Merc., *Merc-d.,* Nit-ac., Pen., Petr., Phyt., *Puls.,* Ros-d., Sangin-n., *Sil.,* Visc.

**Eustachian tube inflamed, sub-acute, great pain:** Bell., Caps.

**Eustachian tube, tickling inducing swallowing, cough:** Gels., Nux-v., Sil.

**EXTERNAL AUDITORY CANAL; Boils, pimples:** Bell., *Calc-pic.,* Hep., *Merc., Pic-ac., Sil.,* Sulph.

**Burning:** Ars., Arund., *Caps.,* Sang., Stry.

**Digging and scratching into:** Cina, Psor.

**Dryness:** Calc-pic., Carb-v., Ferr-pic., *Graph.,* Nux-v., Petr., Verb.

**Exostoses:** Calc-f., *Hecla,* Kali-i.

**Feels, as if distended by air:** Mez., Puls.

**Fissures:** *Graph.,* Petr.

**Inflammation and pain:** *Acon.,* Apis, Ars-i., *Bell.,* Borx., Brach., *Calc-pic., Cham., Ferr-p.,* Hep., Kali-bi., *Kali-m., Merc.,* Nit-ac., Psor., *Puls.,* Rhus-t., *Tell.*

**Itching:** *Alum.,* Anac., Calc., Caust., Elaps, Hep., Kali-bi., Kali-c., Psor., *Puls.,* Sabad., *Sep.,* Sil., *Sulph., Tell.,* Viol-o.

**Polypoid excrescenses, granulations:** Alum., Calc., *Calc-i.,* Calc-p., Form., Kali-bi., Kali-i., *Kali-m.,* Merc., *Nit-ac.,* Phos., *Sang.,* Sil., Staph., Teucr., *Thuj.*

**Scales, epithelial, exfoliated, with scurfy accumulation:** Calc-pic.

**Sensation, as if drop of water in left ear:** Acon.

**Sensation, as if heat emanated from:** *Aeth.,* Caust.

**Sensation, as if obstructed:** Aeth., *Anac.,* Asar., Carbn-s., *Cham.,* Crot-h., Glon., Merc., Nit-ac., *Puls., Verb.*

**Sensation, as if open too much:** Mez.

**Sensitive to air, touch:** Ars., Bell., *Borx.,* Caps., *Cham.,* Ferr-p., *Hep.,* Merc., Mez., Nux-v., Petr., Tell.

**HYPERSENSITIVE; to noises, sounds, voices:** Acon., Anh., *Asar.,* Aur., *Bell., Borx.,* Chen-a., *Chin.,* Cimic., *Coff.,* Ferr-p., Ign., Iod., Lach., Mag-m., *Nat-c.,* Nit-ac., Nux m., *Nux-v.,* Op., Petr., Ph-ac., Phos., Plan., Puls., Sang., Sep., *Sil.,* Spig., Ter., *Ther.*

**LABYRINTH; Bloody, serous effusion, in:** Chen-a.

**Inflamed (otitis interna):** Aur., Kali-i., Merc-i-r.

**MASTOID PROCESS, Caries:** *Aur.,* Caps., Fl-ac., *Nit-ac.,* Sil.

**Inflammation (mastoiditis):** *Am pic.,* Asaf., *Aur., Bell.,* Benz-ac., Canth., *Caps.,* Hep., Kali-m., Mag-p., Mentho., *Onos.,* Onis., Tell.

**MEMBRANA TYMPANI: Calcareous deposits:** Calc-f.

**Inflammation (myringitis):** *Acon.,* Atro., Bell., Bry., Chin., *Hep.* (See **Otitis.**)

**Perforated:** Aur., Calc., Caps., Kali-bi., Merc., *Sil.,* Tell., *Tub.*

**Thickened:** Ars-i., Merc-d., Thiosin.

**Thin, white, scaly deposit:** Graph.

**Ulceration:** Kali-bi.

**OSSICLES; Caries:** Asaf., *Aur.,* Calc., Caps., Fl-ac., Hep., Iod., *Sil.,* Syph.

**Petrous bone, tender to touch:** Caps., Onos.

**Sclerosis, also petrous portion of temporal bone:** Calc-f.

**TYMPANUM (middle ear): Inflammation (otitis):**

**Catarrhal, acute:** *Acon., Bell.,* Cham., *Ferr-p.,* Gels., Hep., *Kali-m., Merc., Puls.,* Rhus-t., Sil.

**Catarrhal, chronic:** Agar., Ars., *Bar-m., Calc., Caust.,* Chin., Graph., *Hydr., Iod.,* Jab., Kali-bi., Kali-i., *Kali-m., Merc-d.,* Nit-ac., Phos., Sang., Teucr. (See **Eustachian tubes**.)

**Suppurative, acute (otitis media suppurative, acute):** *Acon.,* Ars., Ars-i., *Bell.,* Borx., Bov., Calc-s., *Caps., Cham., Ferr-p.,* Gels., Guaj., *Hep.,* Kali-bi., Kali-m., *Merc.,* Myris., *Plan., Puls.,* Sil., Thiosin.

**Suppurative, chronic:** *Aethi-m.,* Alum., *Ars-i.,* Aur., Bar-m., *Calc.,* Calc-f., *Calc-i.,* Caps., *Caust.,* Chen-a., Elaps, *Hep.,* Hydr., Iod., *Kali-bi.,* Kali-i., Kali-m., Kali-p., *Kali-s.,* Kino, Lap-a., Lyc., *Merc.,* Naja, Nit-ac., *Psor., Puls., Sil., Sulph.,* Tell., *Thuj.,* Viol-o.

**TYPE OF DISCHARGE (otorrhea), Bloody:** Ars., Ferr-p., Hep., Kali-i., *Merc.,* Psor., Rhus-t., Skook.

**Excoriating, thin:** *Alum.,* Ars., Ars-i., Calc-i., Calc-p., Cist., *Iod.,* Merc., Syph., *Tell.*

**Muco-purulent, fetid, acrid or bland:** Aethi-a., Ars-i., Asaf., Aur., Borx., *Calc., Calc-s.,* Caps., *Carb-v.,* Elaps, Ferr-p., Graph., *Hep.,* Hydr., Kali-bi., *Kali-s.,* Kino, Lyc., *Merc.,* Merc-pr-r., Nat-m., Psor., *Puls., Sil.,* Sulph., *Tell.,* Thuj., Tub.

**PAIN (otalgia):** *Acon.,* Antip., Apis, *Bell.,* Borx., *Caps., Cham.,* Chinin-s., Coff., Dulc., *Ferr-p.,* Gels., *Hep.,* Iod., Kali-bi., Kali-i., Mag-p., Mentho., *Merc.,* Naja, *Plan., Puls.,* Sang., Ter., Valer., Viol-o., Visc., *Verb.*

**TYPE; Aching, constant:** Caps., Guaj., Merc.

**Boring:** Am-pic., *Asaf.,* Aur., Bell., *Caps.,* Kali-i., Sil., Spig.

**Burning:** *Ars.,* Caps., Kreos., Sang., Sulph.

**Cramp-like, pressing, piercing:** *Anac.,* Calc., *Cham.,* Kali-bi., Merc., *Puls.*

**Neuralgic, lancinating, shifting, shooting, paroxysmal:** Acon., All-c., *Bell.,* Caps., *Cham.,* Chin., Ferr-p., Kali-c., *Mag-p.,* Nit-ac., *Puls.,* Sil., *Spig.,* Viol-o.

**Pulsating, throbbing:** Acon., *Bell.,* Cact., Calc., *Ferr-p., Glon.,* Merc., Merc-c., Puls., Rhus-t., Tell.

**Stinging:** Acon., Apis, Caps.

**Stitching:** Borx., *Cham.,* Ferr-p., Hep., Kali-bi., *Kali-c.,* Merc., Nit-ac., *Plan.,* Puls., Viol-o.

**Tearing:** *Bell.,* Caps., *Cham.,* Kali-bi., Kali-i., Merc., Plan., *Puls.*

**MODALITIES; Aggravation, At night:** *Acon.,* Ars., Bell., Calc-p., *Cham.,* Dulc., Ferr-p., Hep., Kali-i., *Merc., Puls.,* Rhus-t.

**From cold air:** Calc-p., Caps., *Cham., Hep.,* Kali-m., Mag-p., Sang.

**Noise:** Bell., Cham.

**Pressure, motion:** Mentho.

**Warmth:** Acon., Borx., Calc-p., *Cham.,* Dulc., *Merc.,* Nux-v., *Puls.*

**Washing face and neck with cold water:** Mag-p.

**AMELIORATION: During day:** Acon.

**From being carried, motion:** Cham.

**From cold applications:** Puls.

**From motion, covering:** Aur.

**From sipping cold water:** Bar-m

**From warmth:** *Bell.,* Caps., Cham., Dulc., Hep., *Mag-p.*

**In open air:** Acon., Aur., Ferr-p., *Puls.*

**TINNITUS AURIUM (noises in ears), Remedies in general:** Adren., Am-c., Antip., Aphis, Ars., *Bar-c., Bar-m.,* Bell., Canch., Carbn-s., *Caust., Chen-a., Chin., Chinin-s., Chinin-sal.,* Cimic., Cit-d., Con., Dig., Ferr-p., Ferr-pic., *Graph.,* Hep., Hydr., Jab., Kali-c., Kali-i., *Kali-m.,* Kali-p., Lach., Lec., Lith-m., Merc., Merc-d., Nat-m., *Nat-sal.,* Parth., Petr., Phos., Pilo., Plat., Plb., *Puls., Sal-ac.,* Sang., *Sangin-n.,* Sil., Sulfon., Sulph., *Viol-o.*

**Buzzing:** Am.c., Anac., Antip., *Bar-m.,* Calc., Canch., Caust., *Chen-a.,* Chin., *Chinin-s.,* Dig., Dios., Ferr-p., Form., Graph., Iod., Iris, Kali-p., Kreos., Lach.

**Cracking, snapping, when blowing nose, chewing, swallowing, sneezing:** Ambr., Aphis, *Bar-c., Bar-m.,* Calc., Form., Gels., *Graph.,* Kali-c., *Kali-m.,* Lach., *Nit-ac.,* Petr., Puls., Sil., Thuj.

**Hissing:** Cann-i., *Chinin-s.,* Dig., *Graph.,* Teucr.

**Humming:** Alum., Anac., Calc., *Caust.,* Chin., Ferr-p., *Kali-p.,* Kreos., *Lyc.,* Petr., Puls., Sang., Sep., Ter.

**Intolerance of music:** *Acon.,* Ambr., Bufo, Viol-o.

**Pulsating, throbbing:** Calc., Caust., *Ferr-p., Glon.,* Hep., Hydrobr-ac., Lach., Merc., *Morph.,* Nit-ac., *Puls.*

**Re-echoing of voice, sounds:** Bar-c., *Bar-m.,* Bell., *Caust.,* Coloc., Lyc., Phos., Ter.

**Ringing, as of bells:** *Bell.,* Calc-f., Carbn-s., Caust., Cham., *Chin., Chinin-s.,* Form., *Graph.,* Iris, Lach., Mez., *Nat-sal.,* Petr.

**Roaring:** Aur., Calc., Caust., Chin., *Chinin-s.,* Elaps, Ferr-p., *Graph.,* Kreos., *Lyc.,* Merc., Merc-d., Nat-m., Nat-sal., Nit-ac., Petr., Ph-ac., *Puls., Sal-ac.,* Sang., *Sil.,* Stry., Viol-o.

**Roaring, relieved by music:** Ign.

**Rushing:** Ferr-p., Gels., Puls.

**Singing:** *Chinin-s.,* Dig., Graph., Lach., Puls.

**Whizzing:** Bar-m., Bell., *Hep.,* Rhod., Sulph.

■

# NOSE

**AFFECTIONS, Syphilitic:** Asaf., *Aur.,* Aur-m., *Cinnb.,* Fl-ac., *Kali-bi., Kali-i.,* Merc-c., Sil.

**BONES, Caries:** Asaf., *Aur.,* Aur-m., Cadm-s., Kali-bi., Merc., Merc-i-r., Phos. (See **Tissues, GENERALITIES.**)

**Pain:** *Asaf., Aur.,* Cinnb., *Hep.,* Kali-i., Lach., *Merc.,* Puls., *Sil.*

**Periostitis:** Asaf., *Aur.,* Merc., *Phos.* (See **Tissues.**)

**Ulceration:** Asaf., *Hecla,* Hep., Kali-bi. (See **Tissues.**)

**EXTERNAL NOSE; ERUPTIONS, growths: Acne:** Ars., *Ars-br.,* Aster., Borx., *Caust.,* Clem., Elaps, Kali-br., Nat-c., Sil., Zing.

**Eczema:** Bals-p., Iris, Sars.

**Erysipelas:** Bell., Canth., Rhus-t.

**Freckles:** Phos., Sulph.

**Furuncles:** Cadm-s., Cur., *Hep.,* Sil.

**Herpes:** Acon-l., Alum., Bell., Mur-ac., Nat-m., *Sep.,* Sulph.

**Lupus:** Ars., Aur-m., Kali-bi., Kreos., Thuj., X-ray.

**Pustules:** *Hep.,* Petr., Psor., Sil.

**Scales:** *Caust.*

**Warts:** Caust., Thuj. (See **SKIN.**)

**Inflammation:** Acon., Agar., *Apis, Aur.,* Aur-m., *Bell.,* Borx., Carb-an., Ferr-i., *Ferr-pic.,* Fl-ac., Graph., *Hep.,* Hippoz., *Kali-i.,* Medus., Merc-c., Naphtin., Nat-c., *Nit-ac.,* Sil., Sulph.

**Itching:** *Agar., Cina,* Fil., *Ign.,* Iod., Ph-ac., Pin-s., Teucr., Zing.

**Numbness:** Nat-m.

**Redness:** Agar., Alum., *Apis,* Ars., Bell., *Borx.,* Iod., *Kali-i.,* Nat-c., Psor., Rhus-t., Rhus-v., Yuc., Zinc.

**Soreness to touch:** Alum., Aur., Bry., Calc., *Cinnb.,* Con., Graph., *Hep.,* Kali-bi., Lachn., Lith-m., *Merc., Nit-ac.,* Rhus-t., Sil.

**Varicose veins:** Carb-v.

**Yellow saddle:** Sep.

**ALAE (wings), Burning, hot, biting:** Aphis, Ars., *Sangin-n.,* Seneg., Sin-n., Sulph.

**Dryness:** Chlor., Hell., *Sangin-n.*

**Eczema:** *Ant-c.,* Bals-p., Bar-c., *Graph., Petr.*

**Eruptions, growths, cracks, crusts, ulcerations:** Alum., *Ant-c., Arum-t.,* Aur., Aur-m-n., Bov., *Calc.,* Caust., Cor-r., Cund., *Graph.,* Ign., *Kali-bi.,* Kali-c., Lyc., Merc., *Nit-ac., Petr.,* Sulph., Ter., *Thuj.*

**Fanning:** Ant-*t.,* Brom., *Chel.,* Gad., Kali-br., *Lyc., Phos.,* Pyrog., Sul-ac.

**Herpes:** Dulc., Nat-m., Phys., Sil.

**Itching:** Carb-v., *Cina,* Nat-p., *Santin.,* Sil., Sulph.

**Red, inner angles:** Agar., Merc., Plb-act., Sulph.

**Soreness to touch:** *Alum., Ant-c.,* Ars., *Arum-t.,* Aur-m., Calc., Cop., Cor-r., Fago., *Graph., Hep., Kali-bi.,* Merc., Merc-c., *Nit-ac.,* Petr., Squil., Uran-n.

**Sooty, dirty nostrils:** Hell.

**Throbbing:** Acon., Brom.

**TIP, Blueness:** Carb-an., *Dig.*

**Burning:** Bell., Borx., Ox-ac., Rhus-t.

**Cold, pale, pointed:** Apis, *Ars.,* Calc-p., *Camph.,* Carb-v., *Chin.,* Hell., *Tab., Verat.* (See **FACE.**)

**Congestion:** Am-c.

**ERUPTIONS, growths, Acne:** Am-c., Caust., Sep.

**Cracks:** Alum., *Graph.,* Petr.

**Furuncles:** Anan., Borx.

**Herpes:** Aeth., Clem., Conv., Dulc., Nat-m.

**Knobby:** Aur.

**Pustules:** Kali-br.

**Scales:** Caust., Nat-c.

**Ulcers:** Borx., Rhus-t.

**Tumors:** Anan., Carb-an.

**Warts:** Caust.

**Inflammation:** Bell., Borx., Cist., Euph., Nicc., Nit-ac., Rhus-t., Sep.

**Itching:** Carb-an., Caust., *Cina, Morph.,* Petr., *Santin.,* Sil.

**Redness:** Bell., *Borx.,* Calc., *Caps.,* Kali-i., Kali-n., Nicc., Nit-ac., *Rhus-t.,* Sal-n., *Sil.,* Sulph., Vinc.

**Soreness to touch:** Borx., *Hep., Menth.,* Rhus-t.

**Tingling:** Bell., *Morph.*

**Torpor, as from blow:** Viol-o.

**INTERNAL NOSE: Abscess of septum:** Acon., *Bell.,* Calc., *Hep.,* Sil.

**Bleeding (epistaxis), Remedies in general:** Abrot., *Acon.,* Agar., Am-c., Ambro., *Arn.,* Ars., *Bell., Bry.,* Cact., Calc., Carb-v., *Chin.,* Croc., Crot-c., Elaps, Ferr-act., *Ferr-p., Ferr-pic.,* Fic-r., *Ham., Ip.,* Kali-c., Kali-chl., Lach., *Meli.,* Merc., *Mill.,* Mur-ac., Nat-n., Nat-sal., *Nit-ac.,* Nux-v., Onis., Osm., *Phos.,* Puls., Sec., Sep., Sulph., *Thlas.,* Til., *Tril-p.,* Vip.

**CAUSE, Blowing nose:** Agar., Aur., Bov., *Carb-v.,* Caust., Graph., *Phos., Sec.,* Sep., Sulph.

**Cough:** Arn.

**Eating:** Am-c.

**Hemophilia:** Ars., Crot-h., Ham., Ip., *Lach., Phos.*

**Hemorrhoids, suppressed:** Nux-v.

**Menses, absent (vicarious):** *Bry., Ham.,* Lach., Nat-s., *Phos., Puls.,* Sep.

**Motion, noise, light:** Bell.

**Operations:** Thlas.

**Recurrent cases:** Ars., Ferr-p., Mill., Phos.

**Stooping:** Rhus-t.

**Straining:** Carb-v.

**Symptomatic (fevers, purpura):** Arn., Ham., Ip., Lach., Phos., Rhus-t.

**Traumatism:** Acet-ac., *Arn.,* Ham., Mill.

**Washing:** *Am-c., Ant-s-aur.,* Arn., Kali-c., Mag-c.

**OCCURRENCE AND CONCOMITANTS: At night during sleep:** *Merc.,* Nux-v.

**In children growing rapidly:** Abrot., Arn., *Calc.,* Croc., Phos.

**In daily attacks:** Carb-v.

**In morning from washing face:** Am-c., Arn., *Kali-c.,* Onis.

**In morning on awaking, arising, etc.:** Aloe, Ambr., Bov., *Bry.,* Chin., Lach., *Nux-v.*

**In old people:** Agar., *Carb-v.*

**Persistent, with goose flesh:** Camph.

**Preceded by heat and pain in head:** Nux-v.

**With biliousness:** Chel.

**With chest affections:** Ham., Nit-ac.

**With chronic vertigo:** Sulph.

**With face congested, red:** Bell., *Meli.,* Nux-v.

**With face pale:** Carb-v., Ip.

**With prostration:** Carb-v., Chin., Diph.

**With relief of chest symptoms:** Bov.

**With relief of headache:** Ham., *Meli.*

**WIth tightness, pressure at root of nose:** Ham.

**TYPE OF BLOOD: Black, stringy:** *Croc.,* Crot-h., Merc.

**Bright red:** *Acon.,* Bell., Bry., Carb-v., Erech., *Ferr-p.,* Ip., *Mill., Tril-p.*

**Coagulated:** Chin., Nat-chlor., Nux-v.

**Dark, fluid:** Arn., *Ham.,* Lach., Mur-ac., *Sec.*

**Non-coagulable, passive, profuse:** Bry., Carb-v., Crot-h., Thlas., Tril-p.

**BLOWS NOSE continually:** Am-c., Borx., Hydr., Lac-c., Mag-m., *Stict.*, Tritic.

**Boring, digging into:** *Arum-t., Cina,* Hell., Ph-ac., *Santin.,* Teucr., Zinc.

**Burning, smarting:** Acon., Aesc., All-c., Alum-sil., Am-m., *Ars., Ars-i.,* Arum-t., Bar-c., Brom., Caps., Cop., Hep., *Hydr., Merc.,* Merc-c., Penth., Sabad., *Sang.,* Sangin-n., Sin-n.

**Coldness:** *Aesc., Camph., Cist.,* Cor-r., Hydr., Lith-c., Verat.

**Congestion, violent:** Bell., Cupr., *Meli.*

**Dryness:** *Acon.,* Aesc., *Am-c.,* Bell., Calc., *Camph.,* Con., Cop., Glyc., *Graph.,* Kali-bi., Kali-c., Kali-i., Lem-m., *Lyc.,* Nat-m., Nit-ac., Nux-m., *Nux-v.,* Onos., Petr., *Phos.,* Rumx., *Samb., Sang.,* Sangin-n., Senec., Sep., Sil., Sin-n., *Stict.,* Sulph. (See **Stoppage.**)

**ERUPTIONS, growths: Furuncle, pimples:** Sil., Tub., Vinc.

**Lupus:** *Ars.,* Calc., Cic., Hydr., *Hydrc.,* Merc., Rhus-t., Sulph., Tub.

**Nodular swelling:** Ars.

**Papilloma:** Caust., Nit.ac., *Thuj.*

**Polypi:** *All-c.,* Cadm-s., *Calc.,* Calc-i., Calc-p., Caust., Con., Form., Kali-bi., Kali-n., Lem-m., Merc-i-r., Nit-ac., *Phos.,* Psor., *Sang., Sangin-n.,* Staph., *Teucr., Thuj.,* Wye.

**Scabs, crusts, plugs, clinkers:** *Alum.,* Ant-c., *Arum-t.,* Aur., Borx., Cadm-s., Calc-f., Cop., Dulc., Elaps, *Graph.,* Hep., *Hydr., Kali-bi.,* Lem-m., *Lyc.,* Nat-ar., Nat-m., Nit-ac., *Puls.,* Sangin-n., *Sep.,* Sil., Stict., Sulph., *Teucr.,* Thuj.

**Ulcerations, excoriations:** All-c., Alum., Ars., Ars-i., Arum-t., Aur., Borx., *Graph., Hep., Hydr., Kali-bi.,* Kali-c., Kreos., Merc., Merc-c., *Nit-ac.,* Ran-s., *Sil.,* Thuj., *Vinc.*

**HARDNESS (rhino-scleroma):** Aur-m-n., Calc-f., Con.

**INFLAMMATION (rhinitis); Acute, catarrhal from pollen irritation, HAY FEVER, rose cold, summer catarrh:** All-c., *Ambro., Aral., Ars., Ars-i.,* Arum-t., Arund., Benz-ac., Chinin-ar., Cocain., Cupr-act., Dulc., Euph-pi., *Euphr.,* Gels., Hep., Ip., Kali-i., Kali s-chr., *Lach.,* Linu-u., Merc-i-f., *Naphtin.,* Nat-i., Nat-m., Nux-v., Poll., *Psor., Ran-b.,* Ros-d., *Sabad.,* Sang., *Sangin-n.,* Sil., *Sin-n.,* Skook., Solid., *Stict.,* Suprar., Trif-p., Tub.

**Inflammation, acute, catarrhal, ordinary cold in head:** *All-c., Acon.,* Aesc., Am-c., Am-m., *Ars., Ars-i., Arum-t.,* Aven., Bell., Brom., *Bry., Camph.,* Cham., *Dulc.,* Eup-per., *Euphr.,* Ferr-p., *Gels.,* Glyc., Hep., *Hydr.,* Hydrc-ac., *Iod., Just., Kali-bi., Kali-i.,* Lach., Mentho., *Merc., Nat-ar., Nat-m., Nux-v.,* Phos., Puls., *Quill.,* Sabad., Samb., Sang., *Sangin-n.,* Solid., *Stict.,* Ter., Ther., Trom.

**CONCOMITANTS, Aching in limbs:** Acon., Bry., *Eup-per., Gels.*

**Chilliness (initial stage):** *Acon.*, Bapt., *Camph.*, Caps., Ferr-p., *Gels.*, Merc-i-r., *Nat-m.*, Nux-v., Phyt., *Quill.*, Sapo.

**Predisposition to colds:** Agra., Alum., Ars., Bac., Bar-c., *Calc.*, Calc-i., Calc-p., Calen., Dulc., Ferr-p., Gels., *Hep.*, Hydr., Kali-c., Merc., *Nat-m.*, Nux-v., Phos., *Psor.*, Sep., Solid., *Sulph.*, *Tub.*

**CORYZA; Dry (stuffy colds, snuffles):** Acon., Ambro., *Am-c.*, Am-m., Arum-t., *Calc.*, Camph., Caust., *Cham.*, Cist., Con., Dulc., Elaps, Glyc., Graph., *Hep.*, Iod., *Kali-bi.*, *Kali-c.*, Lach., *Lyc.*, Mentho., *Nat-m.*, Nit-ac., *Nux-v.*, Osm., Puls., *Samb.*, Sep., Sil., Sin-n., *Stict.*, Teucr. (See **Stoppage**.)

**Alternately dry and fluent:** Am-c., *Ars.*, *Lac-c.*, Lach., Mag-m., *Nat-ar.*, *Nux-v.*, Puls., Quill., *Sin-n.*, Sol-n., Spong.

**Coryza, fluent, watery (running cold):** Aesc., Agra., *Ail.*, *All-c.*, Am-m., Am-p., *Ambro.*, *Aral.*, *Ars.*, *Ars-i.*, *Arum-t.*, *Brom.*, Cycl., Eucal., Eup-per., *Euphr.*, *Gels.*, Hydr., Iod., Ip., *Just.*, Kali-chl., *Kali-i.*, *Merc.*, Merc-c., Narc-po., *Nat-ar.*, *Nat-m.*, *Quill.*, *Sabad.*, *Sangin-n.*, Sil., Sol-n., Squil., Trif-p.

**Coryza, periodic:** Ars., Chin., Nat-m., Sang.

**Coryza, with chronic tendency:** Am-c., Calc., Calc-i., *Con.*, Graph., Hep., *Kali-bi.*, Kali-i., *Puls.*, *Sars.*, *Sil.*, Sulph.

**Coryza, with palpitation, especially in aged:** Anac.

**Coryza with thick mucus:** *Aur.*, Ferr-i., *Hep.*, *Kali-bi.*, Kali-s., *Merc.*, Penth., *Puls.*, Sangin-n., Sep., *Stict.*

**Coryza, worse in evening:** All-c., Glyc., Puls.

**Coryza, worse in newborn:** Dulc.

**Coryza, worse in warm room, better in open air:** All-c., Ars., Nux-v.

**Cough:** *All-c.*, Alum., *Bell.*, Bry., Dros., Euphr., *Just.*, Lyc., Nux-v., Sang., Sin-n., *Stict.*

**Fever, low type, in old people:** Bapt.

**Headache:** Acon., All-c., Ars., Bell., *Bry.*, Camph., Chin., Eup-per., *Gels.*, Kali-bi., *Kali-i.*, Nat-ar., *Nux-v.*, Sabad., Sang.

**Hoarseness, aphonia:** All-c., Ars., *Caust.*, *Hep.*, Osm., Phos., Pop-c., Tell., Verb.

**Infants, with snuffles:** Acon., *Am-c.*, Bell., *Cham.*, Dulc., Elaps, *Hep.*, Merc-i-f., *Nux-v.*, *Samb.*, Stict., Sulph.

**Insomnia:** Ars., Cham.

**Lachrymation, sneezing:** Acon., *All-c.*, Am-p., Ambro., Aral., *Ars.*, Ars-i., Camph., Cham., *Cycl.*, Eup-per., *Euphr.*, *Gels.*, Ip., *Just.*, Kali-chlr., *Kali-i.*, Mentho., Merc., Naphtin., *Nat-m.*, *Nux-v.*, Quill., *Sabad.*, Sin-n., Solid., Squil., Stict. (See **Lachrymation**.)

**Photophobia:** All-c., Ars., Bell., *Euphr.*

**Prostration, lassitude:** Ars., Ars-i., Bapt., Gels., Quill.

**Respiration, asthmatic:** Ant-t., *Aral., Ars-i.,* Bad., *Ip.,* Naphtin.

**Inflammation, acute, croupous, fibrinous:** *Am-caust.,* Apis, Ars., Echi., Hep., *Kali-bi.,* Lach., Merc., Nit-ac.

**Inflammation, chronic atrophic (sicca):** *Alum.,* Am-c., Aur., *Calc-f.,* Cinnb., Elaps, Fl-ac., Graph., *Hep., Kali-bi.,* Kali-i., Kali-s-chr., *Lem-m., Lyc.,* Merc., Sabal, *Sep., Stict., Sulph.,* Teucr., Wye.

**Inflammation, chronic catarrhal:** *Alum.,* Am-br., *Am-m.,* Ars-i., Aur-m., Bals-p., Brom., *Calc.,* Calc-p., Cub., Elaps, *Eucal., Hep., Hippoz., Hydr., Kali-bi.,* Kali-c., Kali-i., Kreos., Lem-m., Med., *Merc.,* Merc-i-r., *Nat-c.,* Nat-m., Nat-s., Nit-ac., Phos., Psor., *Puls.,* Sabad., Sang., Sangin-n., *Sep.,* Sil., Spig., Stict., Teucr., Ther., Thuj.

**Inflammation, purulent in children:** Alum., Arg-n., *Calc.,* Cycl., Hep., Iod., *Kali-bi., Lyc.,* Nat-c., Nit-ac.

**TYPE OF DISCHARGE IN RHINITIS; Acrid, watery, fluent, hot, or thin mucus:** *All-c.,* Am-caust., *Am-m., Ambro., Aral., Ars., Ars-i.,* Arum-t., Bell., Carb-v., Cham., Eucal., *Gels.,* Glyc., *Iod., Kali-i.,* Kreos., Lach., Merc., *Merc-c.,* Mur-ac., Naphtin., *Nat-ar., Nat-m.,* Nit-ac., *Sabad.,* Sang., *Sangin-n.,* Squil., Sulph., Trif-p.

**Albuminous, clear mucus:** Aesc., Calc., Camph., Graph., Hydr., Kali-bi., Kali-i., *Kali-m.,* Lac-c., Mentho., *Nat-m.,* Phos.

**Bland mucus:** *Euphr.,* Jug-c., Kali-i., *Puls.,* Sep.

**Bloody mucus:** Ail., Arg-n., Ars., *Arum-t.,* Aur., Echi., *Hep.,* Hydr., Kali-bi., Merc-c., *Merc-i-r.,* Penth., *Phos.,* Sangin-n., Sil., Thuj.

**Green, yellow, fetid (purulent or muco-purulent):** Alum., Ars., Ars-i., Arum-t., Aur., *Bals-p., Calc.,* Calc-i., Calc-s., *Dulc.,* Eucal., *Hep., Hydr., Kali-bi.,* Kali-i., *Kali-s., Lyc.,* Med., *Merc.,* Nat-c., *Nat-s.,* Nit-ac., Pen., Phos., *Puls.,* Sangin-n., Sep., Sil., Ther., Thuj., Tub.

**Membranous formation:** *Am-caust.,* Echi., Hep., *Kali-bi.* (See **Croupous Rhinitis.**)

**Offensive, fetid:** Ars-i., Asaf., *Aur.,* Bals-p., *Calc.,* Echi., Elaps, Eucal., Graph., *Hep., Hydr., Kali-bi.,* Kali-i., Merc., Nat-c., Nit-ac., Psor., *Puls.,* Sang., Sep., *Sil., Sulph.,* Ther., Tub.

**Profuse:** Ail., *All-c.,* Am-m., Aral., *Ars., Ars-i.,* Arum-t., Bals-p., Calc-i., *Euphr., Hep., Hydr., Kali-bi., Kali-i., Merc.,* Nux-v., *Puls.,* Sang., Sangin-n., Sep., Thuj.

**Salty tasting:** Aral., Tell.

**Scabs, crusts, plugs:** *Alum.,* Alum-sil., Ant-c., Aur., Aur-m., Borx., Calc-f., Calc-sil., Caust., Elaps, Fago., *Graph.,* Hep., *Hydr., Kali-bi.,* Lem-m., *Lyc.,* Merc-i-f., Nat-ar., Nit-ac., Petr., Psor., *Puls., Sep.,* Sil., Stict., *Sulph., Teucr.,* Ther., Thuj.

**Thick:** Alum., Am-br., *Calc.,* Hep., Hydr., *Kali-bi., Merc., Merc-c.,* Nat-c., Pen., *Puls.,* Sep., Ther., Thuj.

**Unilateral:** Calc-s., Calen., Phyt.

**Viscid, ropy, stringy:** *Bov.,* Gal-ac., *Hydr., Kali-bi.,* Myrt-c., Stict., Sumb.

**ITCHING in nose:** *Agn.,* All-c., Am-c., Ars-i., *Arund.,* Aur., Brom., *Cina,* Fago., Glyc., *Hydr.,* Nat-m., Ran-b., Ros-d., Sabad., Sang., *Santin.,* Sep., Sil., *Teucr., Wye.*

**Nervous disturbance:** Agar.

**Numbness, tingling:** Acon., Jug-c., *Nat-m.,* Plat., Ran-b., Sabad., Sang., Sil., *Stict.*

**OZENA, Odor:** Alum., Ars-i., *Asaf.,* Aur., *Aur-m., Cadm-s.,* Calc., Calc-f., Carb-ac., Diph., Elaps, Ferr-i., Graph., *Hep.,* Hippoz., *Hydr.,* Hydrin-m., *Iod., Kali-bi.,* Kali-c., Kali-chr., Kali-i., Kali-p., Kreos., Lach., Lem-m., *Merc.,* Merc-i-f., Merc-pr-r., *Nit-ac.,* Ph-ac., Phos., *Psor., Puls., Sep.,* Sil., Teucr., Ther., Thuj, *Trios.*

**Syphilitic:** Asaf., *Aur.,* Aur-m., Crot-h., *Fl-ac.,* Kali-bi., Kali-i., *Nit-ac.,* Syph.

**PAIN in: Aching in dorsum, better from pressure:** Agn.

**Boring, gnawing:** Asaf., *Aur.,* Brom., Kali-i., Merc-i-r.

**Burning:** Aesc., *Ars., Ars-i.,* Arum-t., Chr-ac., *Kali-i.,* Lach., Merc-c., *Sang.* (See **Burning.**)

**Cramp-like:** Plat., Sabad.

**Pressing at root of nose:** *Acon., All-c.,* Alum., Arum-t., Caps., Cinnb., Gels., Hep., Iod., *Kali-bi.,* Kali-i., Meny., Nat-ar., *Nux-v.,* Onis., *Par.,* Plat., Puls., Ran-b., Ruta, *Sangin-n., Sep., Stict.,* Ther.

**Pressing in frontal sinuses:** Gels., Ign., Iod., Kali-bi., *Kali-i.,* Merc., Nux-v., Sang., *Stict.*

**Sharp to ears:** Merc-c.

**Splinter-like, sticking:** *Aur., Hep.,* Kali-bi., *Nit-ac.*

**String like to ear:** Lem-m.

**Throbbing:** Bell., *Hep.,* Kali-i.

**Violent shooting, from occiput to root of nose, from suppressed discharge:** Kali-bi.

**POSTERIOR NARES (naso-pharynx), Inflammation of, Acute:** *Acon.,* Camph., Cist., Gels., Kali-bi., Mentho., *Merc-c.,* Nat-ar., Wye. (See **Rhinitis, Pharyngitis.**)

**Chronic:** Aur., Calc-f., Elaps, Fago., *Hydr., Kali-bi., Kali-*c., Merc-c., Pen., Sep., *Spig., Stict.,* Sulph., Thuj.

**Chronic with dropping of mucus, Remedies in general:** *Alum.,* Am-br., Ant-c., Ars-i., Aur., Calc-sil., *Cor-r.,* Echi., Glyc., *Hydr.,* Irid., *Kali-bi.,*

Kali-m., *Lem-m.,* Merc-i-r., Nat-c., *Pen., Phyt., Sangin-n.,* Sin-n., Spig., Stict., Teucr., Ther., Wye.

**Clear, acrid, thin mucus:** Ars-i.

**Clear mucus:** All-c., *Kali-m.,* Nat-m., Lycpr.

**Lumpy:** Osm., Teucr.

**Thick, tenacious, yellow, or white mucus:** Alum., Am-br., Ant-c., Calc-sil., Cor-r., *Hydr., Kali-bi.,* Lem-m., Mentho., Merc-i-f., Nat-c., Sangin-n., Sep., Spig.

**Tumors:** Chr-ac., Osm.

**Wet, raw feellng:** Pen.

**SENSE OF SMELL, Diminished:** *Alum., Cycl.,* Hell., *Hep., Kali*-c., Mentho., Mez., Rhod., Sil., Tab.

**Hypersensitive:** *Acon.,* Agar., Aur., *Bell., Carb-ac.,* Carb-v., *Cham.,* Chin., Coff., *Colch.,* Graph., Ign., Lyc., Mag-m., *Nux-v., Phos.,* Sang., Sabad., *Sep.,* Sulph.

**Hypersensitive to flowers:** Graph.

**Hypersensitive to food:** Ars., Colch., Sep.

**Hypersensitive to tobacco:** Bell.

**Lost (anosmia) or perverted:** *Alum.,* Am-m., Amgd-p., *Anac.,* Apoc-a., Aur., Bell., Calc., *Hep.,* Ign., Iod., Just., *Kali-bi.,* Lem-m., *Mag-m., Nat-m.,* Nit-ac., *Puls.,* Sang., Sep., Sil., Sulph., Teucr., Zinc-m.

**Parosmia (illusions):** Agn., *Anac.,* Apoc-a., Ars., Aur., *Bell.,* Calc., Cor-r., Dios., Graph., Ign., *Kali-bi.,* Mag-m., *Merc.,* Nit-ac., Nux-v., *Phos., Puls.,* Sang., Sulph.

**SENSITIVENESS of nose to air, touch:** *Aesc.,* Alum., Alum-sil., *Ant-c.,* Aral., Ars., *Arum-t.,* Aur., Aur-m., Bell., Calc., Camph., *Hep.,* Kali-bi., *Merc.,* Nat-m., Osm., Sil.

**SINUSES, (antrum, frontal, sphenoidal), Affections in general:** Ars., *Asaf.,* Aur., Bell., Calc., Camph., Eucal., *Hep., Iod.,* Kali-bi., *Kali-i.,* Kali-m., Lyc., Merc., *Merc-i-f.,* Mez., Ph-ac., *Phos., Sil.,* Spig., *Stict.,* Teucr.

**Catarrh of frontal sinuses:** Ammc., Ign., Iod., *Kali-bi., Kali-i.,* Lyc., Mentho., Merc-i-f., Nat-m., Nux-v., Sabad., Stict., Thuj.

**Pain and swelling of antrum:** Phos., Spig.

**Syphilitic affections:** Aur., *Kali-i.,* Nit-ac.

**SNEEZING (sternutation):** Acon., *All-c.,* Am-m., Ambro., *Aral., Ars., Ars-i.,* Arum-t., Arund., Calc., Camph., *Cycl.,* Eup-per., Euph., *Euphr., Gels.,* Ichth., Iod., *Ip.,* Kali-bi., *Kali-i.,* Lob-c., Mentho., Merc., Napht., Nat-m., Nit-ac., Nux-v., Ros-d., Rhus-t., *Sabad.,* Sang., *Sangin-n.,* Sapo., Senec., Seneg., Sin-n., Squil., *Stict.,* Succ-ac.

**Sneezing, chronic tendency:** Sil.

**Sneezing, ineffectual:** *Ars.,* Carb-v., Sil.

**Sneezing, worse coming into warm room; rising from bed; handling peaches:** All-c.

**Sneezing, worse in cool air:** Ars., Hep., Sabad.

**Sneezing, worse in evening:** Glyc.

**Sneezing, worse in morning:** Camph., Caust., *Nux-v.,* Sil.

**Sneezing, worse immersing hands in water:** Lac-d., Phos.

**STOPPAGE, Stuffiness:** *Acon., Am-c.,* Am-m., Ambro., Anac., Apoc., Ars., Ars-i., *Arum-t., Aur.,* Aur-m-n., *Calc.,* Campn., Caust., *Cham.,* Con., Cop., Elaps, Eucal., Fl-ac., *Form.,* Glyc., Graph., Helia., *Hep., Kali-bi.,* Kali-c., Kali-i., Lem-m., *Lyc.,* Mentho., Nat-ar., Nat-c., Nat-m., Nit-ac., *Nux-v.,* Par., Pen., Petr., *Puls.,* Rad-br., Sabad., *Samb., Sangin-n.,* Sapo., Sep., Sil., *Sin-n.,* Spong., *Stict.*

**Stoppage, alternating nostrils:** Acon., Am-c., Borx., *Lac-c.,* Mag-m., *Nux-v.*

**Swelling:** Antip., Ars., *Ars-i., Aur.,* Aur-s-a., Bar-c., Bell., Calc., Hep., *Kali-bi., Lem-m., Merc-c.,* Merc-i-r., *Nit.ac.,* Sabad., Sang., Sep. (See **Inflammation.**)

**ULCERATION OF SEPTUM:** Alum., Aur., Brom., Calc., Carb-ac., Fl-ac., Hippoz., *Hydr., Kali-bi.,* Kali-i., Merc-c., Nit-ac., Sil., Vinc.

**Ulceration, syphilitic:** *Aur.,* Aur-m., Cor-r., Kali-bi., *Kali-i.,* Lach., Merc-aur., *Nit-ac.*

**Wet feeling not relieved by blowing:** Pen.

■

# FACE

**APPEARANCE; CONDITION, Anemic, alabaster-like, waxen:** *Acet-ac., Apis, Ars.,* Calc-p., Ferr., Lach., Merc-c., Nat-c., Sep., Sil.

**Bloated, puffy:** Aeth., *Am-be., Apis, Ars.,* Bor-ac., Both., Calc., Ferr., *Kali-c.,* Hell., Hyos., Lach., Medus., *Merc-c., Op.,* Tax., Xero.

**Bloated about eyes:** *Am-be.,* Ars., Bor-ac., Elaps, *Merc-c.,* Nat-c., *Phos.,* Rhus-t., Thlas., Xero.

**Bloated about lower eyelids:** *Apis,* Xero.

**Bloated about upper eyelids:** Kali-c.

**Blue, livid (cyanosis):** Absin., Am-c., *Ant-t.,* Arg-n., *Ars.,* Aur., *Camph.,* Carb-an., *Carb-v.,* Chlor., *Cic.,* Cina, Cinnb., Crot-h., Cupr., *Cupr-act., Dig.,* Ferr., *Hydr-ac., Ip.,* Lach., *Laur., Morph.,* Oena., Op., Phenac., Rhus-t., *Samb.,* Sec., Stry., *Tab., Verat.* (See **CIRCULATORY SYSTEM.**)

**Blue rings around, dull looking eyes:** *Abrot.,* Acet-ac., *Ars.,* Berb., Bism., Calc., *Camph., Chin., Cina,* Cycl., Ip., Nat-c., *Oena., Ph-ac., Phos., Santin.,* Sec., Sep., Spig., Stann., *Staph.,* Tab., *Verat.,* Zinc.

**Blushing:** Ambr., *Aml-ns.,* Carb-an., Carl., *Coca,* Ferr., Stram., Sulph.

**Bronzed:** Ant-c., Nit-ac., Sec., Spig.

**Brown spots on:** Caul., Sep.

**Coppery look:** Alum., Nit-ac.

**Distorted:** Absin., Art-v., Bell., Camph., *Cic., Cupr.,* Cupr-act., Crot-h., Hell., Hyos., Nux-v., *Op.,* Sec., *Stram.*

**Earthy, dirty, sallow, cachectic:** *Acet-ac., Ars.,* Berb., Calc-p., Camph., *Carb-v., Caust.,* Chel., *Chin.,* Ferr., Glyc., Hydr., Iod., *Lyc.,* Merc., Merc-c., *Nat-m.,* Nux-v., Ph-ac., Phos., Pic-ac., *Plb.,* Psor., *Sanic., Sec., Sep.,* Spig., *Staph.,* Sulph.

**Expression, anxious, suffering:** *Acon., Aeth., Ars.,* Borx., *Camph.,* Canth., Chin., Cina, Iod., Kreos., Merc-c., Plb., *Stram.,* Stry., *Tab., Verat.*

**Expression, drowsy, stupid:** Ail., Apis, *Bapt.,* Cann-i., *Gels.,* Hell., *Op.,* Rhus-t.

**Expression, stolid, mask-like:** Mang-act.

**Greasy, shiny, oily:** *Nat-m., Plb.,* Psor., Sanic., Sel., Thuj.

**Hippocratic (sickly, sunken, deathly cold):** Acon., Aeth., *Ant-t.,* Arn., *Ars.,* Berb., *Camph., Carb-v.,* Chin., Cypr., Hell., Lach., Merc-cy., Plb., Pyrog., *Sec., Tab., Verat.,* Zinc.

**Jaundiced, yellow:** *Ars.,* Berb., Blatta-a., Bry., Calc., Carb-v., *Chel., Chin., Chion.,* Crot-h., *Dig.,* Hep., Hydr., Iod., Kali-c., Lach., Lyc., Merc., *Merc-d.,* Myric., Nat-m., Nat-p., Nat-s., *Nux-v.,* Ol-j., Petr., Pic-ac., *Plb.,* Podo., *Sep., Tarax.,* Yuc. (See **Jaundice**.)

**Pale:** Abrot., *Acet-ac., Ant-t.,* Apis, Arg-n., *Ars.,* Bell., Berb., Borx., Calc., Calc-p., *Camph., Carb-v.,* Chin., *Cina,* Cupr., *Cycl.,* Dig., *Ferr., Ferr-act., Ferr-m.,* Ferr-r., Glon., Hell., *Ip.,* Kali-c., Lach., Lec., Med., *Merc-c.,* Merc-d., *Morph.,* Nat-c., Nat-m., Nit-ac., Ph-ac., Phos., *Plb., Puls.,* Pyrog., *Santin., Sec.,* Sep., Sil., Spig., Stann., Staph., *Tab., Verat.,* Zinc.

**Parchment-like:** Ars.

**Red, becomes deathly pale on rising:** *Acon.,* Verat.

**Red, dark, dusky besotted, bloated:** *Ail.,* Apis, Ars-met., *Bapt.,* Both., Bry., Carb-ac., Diph., *Gels.,* Hyos., Lach., *Morph.,* Nux-v., *Op.,* Rhus-t., Stram.

**Red, distorted:** Bell., *Cic., Cupr.,* Cupr-act., Crot-h., Hyos., Op., *Stram.*

**Red, flushed after eating:** Alum., Carb-an., Carl., Cor-r., Stront-c.

**Red, flushed, from emotion, pain, exertion:** Acon., *Ferr.,* Ign., Meli.

**Red, flushed, hot, florid:** Acet-ac., *Acon.,* Agar., *Aml-ns., Aster.,* Bapt., *Bell.,* Canth., Caps., *Ferr-p.,* Gels., *Glon.,* Glyc., Kreos., *Meli.,* Mygal., Op., Querc., Rham-cal., *Sang., Stram.,* Sulph., *Verat-v.*

**Red, semi-lateral:** Acon., *Cham., Cina,* Dros., Ip., *Nux-v.*

**Red, though cold:** Asaf., Caps.

**Sensitive, after neuralgia:** Cod.

**Sweating:** *Acet-ac.,* Aml-ns., *Ant-t.,* Ars., *Cham.,* Glon., Samb., Sil., *Tab., Verat.,* Viol-t.

**Sweating, cold:** *Ant-t., Ars.,* Camph., *Carb-v.,* Cina, Euph., *Lob., Tab., Verat.,* Zinc-m.

**Sweating in small spots, while eating:** Ign.

**Sweating on forehead:** Cham., Euph., Op., *Verat.*

**Swelling:** *Acon.,* All-c., Ant-ar., Antip., *Apis,* Ars., Ars-met., *Bell.,* Colch., *Hell.,* Lach., *Merc-c.,* Oena., Op., Phos., *Rhus-t.,* Rhus- v., Verat., Vesp., Vip.

**Swelling, from toothache:** *Bell.,* Cham., Coff., Mag-c., *Merc.*

**Wrinkled, shrivelled, old looking:** Abrot., *Arg-n., Bar-c.,* Borx., Calc-p., Con., *Fl-ac.,* Iod., Kreos., Lyc., *Nat-m.,* Op., *Psor., Pulx., Sanic.,* Sars., Sec., Sil., Sulph.

**BONES (facial), Caries:** Aur., Cist., Fl-ac., Hecla.

**Exostoses:** Fl-ac., Hecla.

**Inflammation:** Aur.

**Pains:** Alum., Arg-n., Astra-m., *Aur.,* Carb-an., Caust., Dulc., *Hep., Merc.,* Nit-s-d., *Phos., Sil.,* Zinc.

**Sensitive:** Aur., *Hep.,* Kali-bi., Mez. (See **Jaws.**)

**CHEEKS; Bites when chewing, talking:** Caust., *Ign.,* Ol-an.

**Burning:** Agar., Euph., Ferr-p., Nit-s-d., Ph-ac., Phos., Sulph. (See **Sensation.**)

**Eruptions:** *Ant-c.,* Dulc., Graph., *Led., Mez.* (See **Eruptions on Face.**)

**Lumpy:** Antip.

**Pains:** Agar., Ang., Verat. (See **Prosopalgia.**)

**Redness:** Brom., *Caps.,* Cic., Coff., Colch., Euph., Euphr., *Meli.* (See **Red Face.**)

**Redness, unilateral:** *Acon., Cham.,* Cina, Dros., Ip., *Nux-v.*

**Spots, circumscribed, red, burning:** Benz-ac., Bry., *Cina,* Ferr-m., Lachn., *Phos.,* Samb., *Sang.,* Stram., Sulph.

**Swelling:** *Acon.,* Bell., Bov., *Calc-f.,* Euph., Kali-m., *Plan.,* Plat. (See **Swelling of Face.**)

**Tingling, numbness**: *Acon.,* Plat.

**Ulcers, wart-like:** Ars.

**Yellow saddle in uterine disease:** Sep.

**CHIN, Eruptions:** *Ant-c.,* Aster., *Cic.,* Dulc., *Graph., Hep.,* Nat-m., Ph-ac., Rhus-t., Sep., Sil., *Sul-i.,* Zinc.

**ERUPTIONS ON FACE, Acne rosacea:** *Ars-br.,* Carb-an., Chrysar., *Eug., Kreos.,* Ov., Psor., Sul-ac., Sulph.

**Acne simplex:** Ambr., *Ant-c., Bell., Berb-a.,* Calc-p., Calc-s., Carb-v., Cimic., Clem., Con., Crot-t., *Eug.,* Graph., Ind., *Jug-r.,* Kali-ar., Kali-br., Kali-c., *Led.,* Med., Nat-m., *Nux-v.,* Ph-ac., *Sulph.,* Thuj.

**Angioma:** Abrot.

**Blotches:** *Berb-a.,* Kali-c., Nux-v.

**Cancer, open, bleeding:** Cist.

**Chilblains:** Agar.

**Comedones:** *Abrot.,* Eug., Jug-r., Nit-ac., *Sulph.*

**Crusta lactea:** Calc., Hep., Merc-pr-r., *Rhus-t.,* Sil., Viol-t. (See **Scalp.**)

**Eczema:** Anac., *Ant-c., Ars.,* Calc., Carb-ac., *Crot-t.,* Dulc., *Graph.,* Hep., Led., Merc-pr-r., *Mez.,* Nat-m., Sep., Sil., Sul-i., Sulph., *Vinc.,* Viol-t.

**Epithelioma:** Ars., Kali-s., Lob-e.

**Erysipelas:** Anac-oc., Anan., *Apis, Bell.,* Borx., *Canth.,* Carb-an., *Euph.,* Ferr-m., *Graph.,* Gymno., Hep., *Rhus-t.,* Sep., Sol-crl., Verat-v.

**Erythema:** Ars-i., *Bell.,* Cund., Echi., Euph., *Graph.,* Nux-v.

**Furuncles:** Alum., *Ant-c.,* Calc-p., *Hep., Led.,* Med.

**Herpes (tetter):** Anac-oc., Canth., Clem., *Dulc.,* Euph., Lim., Lyc., *Nat-m., Rhus-t.,* Sep.

**Humid, moist:** Ant-c., Cic., Dulc., *Graph.,* Hep., Mez., Psor., Rhus-t., Viol-t.

**Itching eruption on forehead during menses:** Eug., Psor., Sang., Sars.

**Lentigo (freckles):** Am-c., Iris-g., Graph., Lyc., *Mur-ac.,* Nat-c., *Nit-ac.,* Phos., Sep., *Sulph.,* Tab., Thuj.

**Lupus:** Cist.

**Pustules:** *Ant-c.,* Bell., Calc., *Calc-s., Cic.,* Graph., *Hep.,* Ind., Merc., Psor.

**Rough, harsh:** *Berb-a.,* Kali-c., *Petr.,* Sulph.

**Scabs, crusts, scurfs:** Ars., Cic., Cist., Dulc., Graph., Hep., Mez., Rhus-t.

**Scales:** Ars., Euph.

**Spots, copper colored:** Benz-ac., *Carb-an.,* Lyc., Nit-ac.

**Spots, red:** *Berb-a.,* Euph., Kali-bi., *Kali-c.,* Oena., Petr.

**Spots, yellow:** Nat-c., *Sep.*

**SYPHILIDAE; Areolae, papules:** Kali-i.

**Copper spots:** Carb-an., Lyc., *Nit-ac.*

**Crusts, areolae:** Nit-ac.

**Pustules:** Kali-i., Nit-ac.

**Tubercles:** Alum., Carb-an., Fl-ac.

**Ulcer, eroding:** Con.

**Warts:** Calc-s., Castm., *Caust.,* Kali-c.

**Whiskers, eruptions:** Hep.

**Whiskers, falling out:** Graph., Sel. (See **Scalp.**)

**Whiskers, itching:** Calc. (See **SKIN.**)

**FOREHEAD feels contracted, wrinkled:** Bapt., Bell-p., Grat., *Hell.,* Lyc., Phos., Prim-v.

**Glabella, swelling:** Sil.

**JAWS, Cracking when chewing:** Am-c., Gran., Lac-c., *Nit-ac., Rhus-t.*

**Dislocated easy:** Ign., *Petr., Rhus-t.,* Staph.

**Growths, swelling:** Amph., *Calc-f.,* Hecla, Plb., Thuj.

**Pain:** Acon., Agar., Alum., Am-m., Am-pic., *Amph.,* Ang., Arum-t., Astr., Aur., Bapt-c., Calc-caust., Carb-an., *Caust.,* Merc., Phos., Rhus-t., Sang., *Sphing.,* Spig., Xan.

**Stiffness (trismus, lockjaw):** Absin., *Acon.,* Arn., Bell., Carbn-o., Caust., Cham., *Cic., Cupr., Cupr-act.,* Cur., Dulc., Hydr-ac., *Hyper., Ign.,* Merc-c., *Morph.,* Nicot., *Nux-v.,* Oena., Olnd., Phys., Sol-n., Stram., *Stry.,* Verat.

**Trembling:** Alum., *Ant-t.,* Cadm-s., *Gels.*

**LOWER JAW, Caries, necrosis:** Amph., Ang., *Phos.,* Sil.

**Chewing motion:** Acon., Bell., *Bry., Hell.,* Stram.

**Epulis:** Plb-act., Thuj.

**Hanging down, relaxed:** Arn., Ars., Gels., *Hell.,* Hyos., Lach., Lyc., *Mur-ac., Op.*

**Nodes, painful:** Graph.

**Pain:** Caust., Chin., Chinin-s., Sil., Spig., Xan. (See **Jaws.**)

**Swelling:** Amph., Aur-m-n., Merc., *Phos.,* Sil., Symph.

**UPPER JAW, Affections of Antrum of Highmore:** Arn., Bell., Chel., Com., Euph-a., Hep., *Kali-i.,* Kali-s., Mag-c., Merc-c., Par., *Phos.,* Sil., Til.

**Pain:** Astra-m., Calc-p., Euph., *Fl-ac.,* Merc-i-r., *Phos.,* Polyg-h., *Spig.*

**Tumor:** Hecla.

**MUSCLES (facial) Distortion (risus sardonicus):** *Cic.,* Cupr-act., Hydr-ac., Op., *Sec.,* Stram., Stry., Tell.

**Pain:** Anac., Ang., Cocc., Colch., Oxyt., Sabin. (See **Prosopalgia.**)

**Paralysis: Bell's palsy:** *Acon.,* Aethi-m., Alum., *Am-p.,* Bell., Cadm-s., *Caust.,* Cocc., Cur., *Dulc.,* Form., *Gels., Graph.,* Hyper., *Kali chl., Kali-i.,* Physal-al., *Rhus-t.,* Ruta, *Seneg.,* Zinc-pic.

**Left side:** Cadm-s., Seneg.

**Right side:** Bell., Caust.

**Stiffness:** Absin., Acon., *Agar.,* Bapt., *Caust.,* Gels., Helo., Nux-v., Rhus-t. (See **Trismus.**)

**Twitching, spasmodic:** Agar., Arg-n., *Bell.,* Caust., Cham., *Cic., Cina,* Cyt-l., *Gels., Hyos., Ign.,* Laur., Meny., *Mygal.,* Nux-v., *Oean.,* Op., Sec., Stram., Tell., Visc.

**PROSOPALGIA, Pain (face-ache):**

**TYPE: Congestive, inflammatory, neuralgic:** *Acon., Agar.,* All-c., Aran., Arg-n., *Ars., Bell.,* Cact., *Caps.,* Caust., *Cedr., Cham., Chin.,* Chinin-ar., *Chinin-s.,* Cimic., Coff., *Coloc.,* Ferr., *Gels.,* Hecla, *Kali-i.,* Kali-p., Kalm., *Mag-p.,* Mentho., Merc., Merc-c., *Mez.,* Nit-s-d., Phos., *Plan., Plat.,* Puls., Rad-br., Rhod., *Rhus-t.,* Sang., Sil., *Spig.,* Stann., Sulph., Thuj., Til., *Verb.,* Zinc-p., *Zinc-val.*

**Reflex, from decayed teeth:** Coff-t., Hecla, Merc., *Mez.,* Staph.

**Rheumatic**: *Acon.,* Act-sp., *Caust.,* Cham., Colch., Coloc., *Dulc.,* Puls., *Rhod., Rhus-t.,* Spig.

**Syphilitic (mercurial):** *Kali-i.,* Mez., Nit-ac.

**Toxic (malarial, quinine):** Ars., Chin., Ip., Nat-m.

**LOCATION, Eyes:** Ars., *Cimic.,* Clem., Nux-v., Par., *Spig.,* Thuj. (See **EYES.**)

**Jaw, lower**: *Amph.,* Calc., Lach., Nit-s-d., Plat., Rad-br., *Rhod.,* Xan., Zinc-val.

**Jaw, upper**: *Amph.,* Bism., *Calc-caust., Cham.,* Coloc., Dulc., *Euph-a.,* Graph., Iris, *Kali-cy., Kali-i.,* Kalm., *Kreos.,* Mez., Par., Sang., Thuj., *Verb.*

**Jaw, upper, (infra-orbital):** Colch., Iris, Mag-p., *Mez.,* Nux-v., *Phos.,* Verb.

**Jaw, upper, to teeth, temples, ears, eyes, malar bones:** *Act-sp.,* Arg-n., Ars., Bell., Bism., *Cham.,* Clem., *Coff., Coloc.,* Dulc., *Kali-cy., Mez.,* Phos., Plan., Rhod., Sang., *Spig.,* Thuj., *Verb.*

**Malar bones (zygoma):** Ang., Arg-met., Aur., *Calc-caust.,* Caps., *Cimic.,* Coloc., Hydrc., Lec., Mentho., Ol-an., Mag-c., Mez., Par., *Plat.,* Rhus-t., *Sphing., Spig.,* Stry., Thuj., *Verb.,* Zinc.

**Unilateral, left**: *Acon.,* Arg-n., *Coloc.,* Cor-r., Hydrc., *Lach.,* Par., Plat., Sapo., Senec., *Spig., Verb.,* Zinc-val.

**Unilateral, right:** Aran., *Cact.,* Caps., Cedr., Clem., Coff., Colch., Hyper., *Kalm., Mag-p., Mez., Puls.*

**TYPE OF PAIN; Cramp-like drawing, pressing:** Ang., Bism., Bry., *Cact.,* Cocc., Coloc., *Mez., Plat.,* Thuj., Verat., *Verb.*

**Cutting, tearing, jerking, stitching, rending:** Acon., Amph., *Ars.,* Aur., Caust., *Cham.,* Chin., *Coloc.,* Dulc., Hyper., Mag-p., Merc., Mez., Nux-v., Phos., *Puls.,* Rhod., Rhodi., Senec., Sil., *Spig.*

**Fine line of pain coursing along the nerve:** All-c., Caps.

**Gradual onset and cessation:** Plat., *Stann.*

**Gradual onset and sudden cessation:** Arg-met., *Bell.,* Puls.

**Hot needles, penetrating:** Ars.

**Icy needles, penetrating:** Agar.

**Lancinating, paroxysmal, lightening-like, radiating:** Arg-n., Ars., *Bell.,* Cocc., *Coloc.,* Gels., Graph., Hep., *Kali-i.,* Kreos., Mag-p., *Nux-v.,* Phos., Plan., *Rhodi.,* Sang., *Spig., Stry.,* Zinc.

**Periodical, intermittent:** Cact., Cedr., *Chin.,* Chinin-s., *Coloc.,* Graph., Mag-p., Plan., *Spig.,* Verat., Verb.

**CONCOMITANTS; Acid, sour eructations:** Arg-n., Nux-v., Verb.

**Canine hunger, preceded by coldness:** Dulc.

**Catarrh (coryza, lachrymation):** Verb.

**Cheek, dark red:** Spig.

**Chilliness:** Coloc., Dulc., *Mez., Puls.,* Rhus-t.

**Gastralgia, alternating:** Bism.

**Lachrymation:** Bell., Ip., Nux-v., Plan., *Puls.,* Verb.

**Mental irritability:** Cham., Coff., Kreos., Nux-v.

**Numbness**: *Acon.,* Mentho., Mez., Plat., Rhus-t.

**Photophobia:** Nit-s-d., Plan.
**Ptosis:** Gels.
**Restlessness, palpitation:** Spig.
**Salivation, stiff neck:** Mez.
**Tenderness to touch:** Acon., *Bell., Chin.,* Coloc., *Hep.,* Mez., Par., Spig., Verb.
**Twitching about face:** Agar., Bell., *Colch.,* Kali-c., Nux-v., Thuj., *Zinc.*
**Vision veiled:** Til.

**MODALITIES; Aggravation, From acids, motion, emotion:** Kali-c.
**From chewing, opening mouth:** Ang., Cocc., Hell., Hep., Mez.
**From cold, dry exposure:** *Acon.,* Coff., Kalm., Mag-c., Mag-p., Nit-s-d.
**From cold, wet exposure:** Coloc., *Dulc.,* Mag-m., Rhus-t., *Sil., Spig.,* Thuj.
**From contact, touch:** *Bell.,* Caps., *Chin.,* Coloc., *Cupr., Hep.,* Mag-p., *Mez.,* Par., *Spig.,* Verb.
**From eating, drinking:** Bism., Iris, *Mez.*
**From eating, motion:** Coloc., Phos., Verb.
**From eating, motion, stooping, jar, etc.:** *Bell.,* Ferr-p., *Spig.*
**From morning until sunset:** Spig.
**From motion, noise:** Ars., Chin., Chinin-s., *Spig.*
**From pressure:** Caps.
**From rest:** Mag-c., Plat., Rhus-t.
**From talking, motion, sitting or lying on unaffected side:** Kreos.
**From talking, sneezing, change of temperature, pressure of teeth:** Verb.
**From tea:** Sel., Spig., Thuj.
**From thinking of pain:** Aur.
**From tobacco:** Sep.
**From warmth:** Cham., Glon., Kali-s., Merc., Mez., *Puls.*
**In afternoon:** Cocc.
**In daytime:** Cedr., Plan., Spig.
**In evening, night:** *Ars.,* Caps., Mag-c., Merc., Mez., *Puls.,* Rhus-t.

**AMELIORATION: From chewing:** Cupr-act.
**From cold applications, cold:** Bism., *Clem.,* Kali-p., Phos., *Puls.*
**From eating:** Rhod.
**From kneeling, and pressing head firmly against floor:** Sang.
**From motion, open air:** Thuj.
**From pressure:** Chin., Coloc., Mag-m., *Rhod.*
**From rest:** Coloc., Nux-v.
**From rubbing:** Acon., *Plat.*

**From warmth:** Ars., Calc., *Coloc.*, Cupr-act., Mag-m., *Mag-p.*, Mez., Thuj. (See **MODALITIES.**)

**SENSATIONS: Burning heat:** *Agar.*, Agro., Ant-c., *Ars.*, Arum-t., *Canth.*, *Caps.*, *Cham.*, *Euph.*, Kali-c., Nat-c., Sang., Seneg., Sil., Stront-c., *Sulph.*, Viol-t.

**Cobwebs dried on, as if:** Alum., *Bar-c.*, *Borx.*, Brom., Euph., *Graph.*, Ph-ac., *Ran-s.*

**Coldness:** Abrot., *Agar.*, *Ant-t.*, *Camph.*, Carb-v., Dros., *Helo.*, Ph-ac., *Plat.*, *Verat.* (See **Hippocratic Face.**)

**Contracted, wrinkled feeling, in forehead:** *Bapt.*, *Bell-p.*, Grat., *Hell.*, Phos., Prim-v.

**Formication (numbness, tingling, crawling):** *Acon.*, Agar., Colch., Gymno., Helo., Myric., Nux-v., *Plat.*

**Itching**: *Agar.*, Ant-c., *Mez.*, Myric., Nat-m., Rhus-t., Sep., Stront-c.

**TIC-DOULOUREUX:** *Acon.*, *Aconin.*, Anan., Arg-n., *Ars.*, *Bell.*, Caps., Cimic., *Cocc-s.*, *Colch.*, Cupr., *Gels.*, Glon., Graph., Kali-c., Kali-chl., *Kali-i.*, *Mag-p.*, *Mez.*, Nat-s., Nux-v., *Phos.*, Rhus-t., Sep., Stann., Staph., Sulph., *Stry.*, *Thuj*, *Verb.*, *Zinc.* (See **Prosopalgia, Trifacial Neuralgia.**)

■

# MOUTH

**BREATH, cold:** Ant-t., Ars., *Camph., Carb-v.,* Cist., Cupr., Euph-l., *Helo.,* Jatr., *Tab.,* Ter., *Verat.*

**Breath offensive (fetor oris):** Abies-n., Alum., Ambr., Anac., *Ant-c., Arn., Ars., Aur., Bapt.,* Borx., Bry., Calag., Calc., Caps., *Carb-ac.,* Carb-v., Chel., Chin., Cist., Daph., *Diph.,* Graph., Hell., *Hep.,* Indol., *Iod.,* Kali-chl., Kali-p., Kali-perm., *Kali-tel.,* Kreos., Lach., *Merc.,* Merc-c., Merc-cy., *Merc-d.,* Mur-ac., *Nat-tel., Nit-ac., Nux-v., Petr.,* Phyt., Psor., *Puls., Querc.,* Rheum, *Sep.,* Sin-n., Spig., Stann., Sul-ac., Ter.

**Breath offensive, after meals only:** Cham., *Nux-v.,* Sulph.

**Breath offensive, in evening or night:** Puls., Sulph.

**Breath offensive, in girls at puberty:** Aur.

**Breath offensive, in morning only:** *Arn.,* Bell., *Nux-v.,* Sil., Sulph.

**EXTERNAL MOUTH; Commissures (corners), Color, pearly white about:** Aeth., *Cina,* Santin.

**Color, yellow about:** Sep.

**Cracks, ulcerations:** Am-m., *Ant-c.,* Ars., *Arum-t.,* Arund., Bov., Cund., Echi., Eup-per., *Graph.,* Hell., *Hep.,* Nat-m., *Nit-ac.,* Petr., Rhus-t., Sec.

**Eruptions around:** Ant-c., *Ars.,* Aster., Echi., *Graph., Hep.,* Naphtin., Mez., Mur-ac., *Nat-m.,* Petr., Seneg.

**LIPS, Black:** *Ars.,* Bry., *Merc-c.,* Vip.

**Blue, cyanosed:** Ars., *Camph.,* Carb-an., Carb-v., *Cupr.,* Cupr-s., *Dig.,* Hydr-ac., Sec., *Verat., Zinc.* (See **FACE.**)

**Burning, hot, parched:** Acon., Anis., Arn., *Ars.,* Arum-t., *Bry.,* Caps., Nat-m., Phos., Rhus-t., *Sulph.,* Thyr.

**Cancer:** Acet-ac., *Ars.,* Ars-i., Clem., Com., Con., Cund., *Hydr.,* Kreos., Lyc., *Sep.,* Tab., Thuj.

**Chewing motion:** Acon., *Bell., Bry.,* Hell., Stram.

**Cold sores, herpes, hydroa:** Agar., Ars., Calc-f., *Caps.,* Dulc., Frax., Hep., Med., *Nat-m., Rhus-t.,* Rhus-v., *Sep.,* Sul-i., Upa.

**Cracks, ulcerations:** Ant-c., *Ars., Arum-t.,* Bry., Carb-v., Carbn-s., *Clem., Cund.,* Echi., Glyc., *Graph.,* Kali-bi., Merc-pr-r., Mur-ac., Nat-m., *Nit-ac.,* Phos., *Rhus-t.,* Sil.

**Cracks, ulcerations in middle of lower lip:** Am-c., Graph., *Hep., Nat-m.,* Puls., Sep.

**Distortion:** *Art-v.,* Cadm-s., *Cic., Cupr-act.,* Cur., Stram.

**Dryness:** Acon., Ant-c., *Bry.,* Chion., Chin., Euon., Glyc., Hell., Helon., Mur-ac., *Nat-m., Nux-m.,* Ph-ac., Puls., Rhus-t., Senec., Sep., *Sulph., Zinc.* (See **Burning.**)

**Eczema:** *Ant-c.,* Aur-m., Bov., Calc., Graph., Lyc., *Mez., Rhus-v.*

**Eruptions; Acne:** Borx., Psor., Sars., *Sul-i.*

**Exfoliation:** Con., Sep.

**Foam at the mouth:** Absin., Cic., *Cupr.,* Cupr-act., *Hydr-ac.,* Hyos., Lyss., *Oean.,* Op. (See **Convulsions, NERVOUS SYSTEM.**)

**Glued together:** Cann-i., *Helon.*

**Licks them frequently:** Puls.

**Numbness, tingling**: *Acon.,* Crot-h., Echi., *Nat-m.*

**Pain, soreness**: Anis., *Arum-t.,* Borx., Calc., Nat-m., *Rhus-t., Rhus-* v., Sep.

**Picks them until they bleed:** *Arum-t.,* Hell., Zinc.

**Red, bleeding**: *Arum-t.,* Kreos.

**Red, crimson:** Aloe, *Sulph.,* Tub.

**Swelling:** Antip., *Apis,* Bov., Bry., Caps., Medus., Merc-c., *Rhus- v., Vip.*

**Swelling of lower:** Puls., Sep.

**Swelling of upper:** Apis, *Bell.,* Calc., *Hep.,* Nat-c., *Nat-m.,* Psor., *Rhus-t.*

**Twitching, spasmodic**: *Agar., Art-*v., Cimic., *Gels., Ign.,* Mygal., Nicc., Op., Stry.

**Ulcer, cancerous:** Ars.

**INNER MOUTH (buccal cavity), Bleeding, after tooth extraction:** Arn., Bov., Chin., *Ham.*

**Burning, smarting:** Acon., Aesc., Apis, *Ars., Arum-t.,* Bell., Borx., Bry., Caps., *Canth.,* Carb-ac., Carb-v., Colch., Ferr-p., *Iris,* Merc-c., Sang., Sulph., *Tarax.,* Vesp.

**Canker-sores:** Agav-a., *Ant-c., Arg-n.,* Ars., *Borx.,* Caps., Carb-v., Echi., Hydr., Kali-bi., *Kali-chl.,* Lach., Lyc., Merc., *Merc-c.,* Mur-ac., Nat-hchls., *Nat-m., Nit-ac.,* Phyt., Sal-ac., *Sul-ac.,* Sulph. (See **Aphthous Stomatitis.**)

**Coldness:** Camph., *Cist.,* Cocc-s., Sin-n., Verat.

**Dryness**: *Acon.,* Aesc., Alum., *Apis, Ars., Bell.,* Borx., *Bry.,* Cupr., Dub., Hyos., Iris-t., Kali-bi., Kali-p., Lach., *Lyc.,* Merc-c., Merl., *Morph.,* Mur-ac., Nat-m., Nat-s., *Nux-m.,* Op., Phos., *Puls., Rad-br.,* Rhus-t., Sang., Senec., Sep., Ter.

**Dryness with great thirst:** Acon., *Ars., Bry.,* Rhus-t., Sulph., Verat.

**Dryness, yet no thirst**: *Apis,* Lach., *Lyc., Nux-m.,* Par., *Puls.,* Sabad.

**Glands, salivary cellular tissue inflamed:** Anthraci., Bry., *Hep., Merc.,* Mur-ac.

**Inflammation (stomatitis), In general:** Acon., Alum., Arg-n., Arum-t., *Bapt.*, Bell., *Borx.*, Caps., Corn., *Hydr.*, *Kali-chl.*, Kali-m., *Merc.*, *Merc-c.*, Nat-m., *Nit-ac.*, Nux-v., Ran-s., Sep., Sin-n., *Sul-ac.*, Sulph., Vesp.

**Inflammation, aphthous (thrush):** Aeth., Ant-t., Ars., Bapt., *Borx.*, Bry., Carb-v., Eup-a., Hydr., *Hydrin-m.*, *Kali-chl.*, Kali-m., *Merc.*, *Merc-c.*, *Mur-ac.*, Nat-m., Nit-ac., Rhus-g., Sars., *Semp.*, *Sul-ac.*, *Sulph.*

**Inflammation, follicular, vesicular:** Anac., Anan., Canth., *Caps.*, Kali-chl., *Hydrin-m.*, Mag-c., Nat-m., *Mur-ac.*, *Rhus-t.*, Sulph.

**Inflammation, gangrenous (noma, cancrum oris):** *Ars.*, Bapt., Hydr., *Kali-chl.*, Kali-p., *Kreos.*, *Lach.*, Merc., *Merc-c.*, *Mur-ac.*, Sec., Sul ac.

**Inflammation, mercurial:** Bapt., Carb-v., Hep., Hydr., Mur-ac., *Nit-ac.*

**Inflammation, ulcerative:** Agav-a., Aln., *Arg-n.*, *Ars.*, Arum-t., Bapt., Borx., Chlor., *Cinnb.*, Cory., *Hep.*, *Hydrin-m.*, Kali-bi., *Kali-chl.*, Kali-cy., Mag-c., Mentho., *Merc.*, *Merc-c.*, *Mur-ac.*, *Nit-ac.*, Nit-m-ac., Phos., *Rhus-g.*, Sul-ac., Sulo-ac., Tarax.

**Itching:** Arund., Borx., Kali-bi.

**Mucous membrane glossy, as if varnished:** Apis, Nit-ac., Ter.

**Mucous membrane inflamed from burns:** Apis, Canth.

**Mucous membrane pallid:** Ferr., Morph.

**Mucous membrane red, dusky**: *Bapt.*, Lach., Morph., *Phyt.*

**Mucous membrane red, tumid, with gray based ulcers:** Kali- chl. (See **Stomatitis.**)

**Pain:** Apis, *Arum-t.*, Bell., Borx., Hep., *Merc.*, *Nit-ac.*, Upa (See **Stomatitis.**)

**Pain from plate of teeth, worse on touch, eating:** Alumn., Borx.

**PALATE: Aphthae:** Agav-a.

**Blisters:** Nat-s.

**Coating, creamy:** Nat-p.

**Constriction, scratching:** Acon.

**Dryness:** Carb-an.

**Edema:** Apis.

**Elongated:** Stry. (See **Uvula.**)

**Itching, tickling**: *Arund.*, Gels., Wye.

**Necrosis, caries**: *Aur.*, Merc-cy.

**Red, swollen:** Acon., *Apis*, Aur., Bell., Fl-ac., *Kali-i.*, Merc-c.

**Ulceration, rawness:** Ant-c., *Arum-t.*, *Cinnb.*, Hep., Merc-c., Merl., *Nit-ac.*, Sul-ac., Tarax. (See **THROAT**.)

**Wrinkled, pain on chewing, nursing:** Borx.

**PTYALISM; Saliva, increased:** *Acet-ac.*, All-s., Anac., Ant-c., *Arum-t.*, Bapt., Bism., Bry., Cham., Chin., Chion., Colch., Cupr., Daph., Dig., Dulc.,

*Epiph., Euph.,* Gran., Hep., *Iod., Ip., Iris, Jab.,* Kali-chl., *Kali-i.,* Kali-perm., Lac-c., Lac-ac., *Lob., Merc., Merc-c.,* Merc-cy., Merc-d., Merc-i-r., Mez., Muscin., Nat-m., *Nit-ac., Nit-m-ac.,* Phos., *Pilo.,* Podo., Ptel., *Puls.,* Rhus-t., Sang., Sars., Sep., Sulph., *Syph.,* Tab., Trif-p.

**After eating:** All-s.

**During pregnancy:** Acet-ac., *Gran., Iod., Jab.,* Lac-ac., *Merc.,* Muscin., Nit-ac., Pilo., Sep. (See **Pregnancy, FEMALE SEXUAL SYSTEM**.)

**During sleep:** *Cham.,* Cocc-s., Lac-ac., *Merc.,* Rheum, *Syph.*

**From mercurialization:** *Hep.,* Iod., *Iris,* Kali-chl., Nit-ac.

**Saliva acrid, hot:** Ars., *Arum-t.,* Borx., Daph., *Kali-chl.,* Kreos., Merc., *Nit-ac.,* Tax.

**Bitter:** *Ars.,* Atha., Bry., Kali-s., *Puls.,* Sulph.

**Bloody:** Antip., *Ars.,* Mag-c., *Merc., Nit-ac.,* Nux-v.

**Fetid, offensive:** Ars., *Iod.,* Kreos., Manc., *Merc.,* Merc-d., Nit.ac., Psor., Rheum.

**Frothy, cotton-like:** Alet., Aq-mar., *Berb.,* Bry., Canth., Lyss., *Nux-m., Nux-v.,* Ph-ac., Sulph.

**Metallic:** Bism., Cham., Cocc., *Cupr., Merc., Nit-ac.,* Zinc.

**Milky:** Plb-o.

**Mucus:** Bell., Colch., *Dulc., Nit-ac.,* Ph-ac., *Phos.,* Puls.

**Ropy, tenacious, slimy, soapy:** Am-m., Ant-c., Arg-n., Dulc., *Epiph.,* Hydr., *Hydrin-m.,* Iod., Iris, *Kali-bi.,* Kali-chl., Lyss., *Merc.,* Myric., Nat-m., Pilo., *Puls.,* Tarax.

**Salty:** Ant-c., *Euph.,* Lac-ac., *Merc-c., Nat-m.,* Phos., Sep., Verat.

**Sour:** Iris, *Nit-ac.,* Nux-v., Par., Podo.

**Sweetish:** Cupr., Merc., Plb-act., *Puls.,* Stann.

**Watery:** Asar., Bism., Iod., Jab., Lob., *Nat-m.,* Phos., Trif-r.

**ULCERATIONS, Soreness of mouth:** Alum., *Arg-n., Ars., Arum-t., Borx.,* Caps., *Hep.,* Hydr., *Hydrin-m.,* Kali-chl., *Merc., Merc-c., Mur-ac., Nit-ac.,* Nux-m., Phyt., *Ran-s., Rhus-g.,* Semp., Sin-n., Sul-ac., Tarax. (See **Stomatitis, Ulcerative**.)

**Ulcerations, syphilitic mucus patches:** *Cinnb.,* Kali-bi., Merc., *Merc-c.,* Merc-n., Merc-pr-r., *Nit-ac.,* Still., *Thuj.* (See **MALE SEXUAL SYSTEM**.)

**Varicose veins:** Ambr., Thuj.

■

# TONGUE

**COATING; COLOR, Blackish:** *Ars.,* Bapt., Camph., Lach., Lyc., Merc., Merc-c., *Merc-cy.,* Merc-d., *Op.,* Phos., Rhus-t., Vip.

**Bluish, livid, pale:** Ars., Cupr-s., *Dig., Gymno.,* Merc-cy., *Morph.,* Op., Mur-ac., *Sec., Verat.,* Vip.

**Brownish:** Am-c., Ant-t., *Ars.,* Bapt., *Bry.,* Cupr-ar., Echi., Hyos., Med., *Merc-cy.,* Morph., Mur-ac., Nat-s., Phos., Sec., Vip.

**Brown center:** *Bapt.,* Phos., Plb.

**Brownish, dry:** *Ail.,* Ant-t., *Ars., Bapt., Bry.,* Kali-p., *Lach., Rhus-t.,* Spong., Tart-ac., Vip.

**Clean:** *Ars., Asar.,* Chin., *Cina,* Cory., Dig., *Ip.,* Mag-p., Nit-ac., *Pyrog., Rhus-t.,* Sep.

**Clean anteriorly, coated posteriorly:** Nux-v.

**Clean at menstrual nisus, foul after flow ceases:** Sep.

**Dark streak in center, typhoid tongue:** Arn., Bapt., Mur-ac.

**Flabby, moist, with imprints of teeth:** Ars., Chel., *Hydr.,* Kali-bi., *Merc.,* Merc-c., *Merc-d.,* Nat-p., *Podo.,* Pyrog., *Rhus-t.,* Sanic., Stram., Yuc.

**Frothy, with bubbles on side:** Nat-m.

**Furred:** Ant-t., Ars., *Bapt.,* Canth., *Card-m.,* Chinin-ar., Coca, Ferr-pic., Gels., Guaj., Lyc., Myric., *Nux-v.,* Puls., Rumx. (See **White.**)

**Grayish-white base:** Kali-m.

**Greenish:** Nat-s., Plb-act.

**Mapped:** Ant-c., *Ars., Kali-bi.,* Lach., Merc., *Nat-m.,* Nit-ac., Ox-ac., Phyt., Ran-s., Rhus-t., *Tarax.,* Ter.

**Mapped, with red, insular patches:** Nat-m.

**Red:** *Acon., Apis, Ars., Bell., Bor-ac., Canth.,* Crot-h., Diph., Gels., Hyos., *Kali-bi.,* Lach., Merc-c., Mez., Nux-v., *Pyrog., Rhus-t.,* Ter.

**Red, dry, especially center:** Ant-t., Rhus-t.

**Red edges:** Amgd-p., Ant-t., Ars., Bapt., *Bell.,* Canth., Card-m., *Chel.,* Echi., Kali-bi., Lac-c., Lach., *Merc.,* Merc-c., Merc-i-f., Nit-ac., Podo., *Rhus-t.,* Rhus-v., Sulph., Tarax.

**Red edges, white center:** Bell., Rhus-t.

**Red in center, or streaks:** Ant-t., *Ars.,* Caust., Crot-h., *Verat-v.*

**Red, papillae pale, effaced:** All-s.

**Red, papillae prominent:** Ant-t., *Arg-n.,* Ars., *Bell.,* Kali-bi., Lyc., Mez., Nux-m., *Ptel., Ter.*

**Red, raw:** Ars., *Arum-t.,* Canth., Tarax.

**Red, shining, glossy, as if varnished:** Apis, *Canth.,* Crot-h., Jal., *Kali-bi.,* Lach., *Nit-ac.,* Phos., *Pyrog.,* Rhus-t., *Ter.*

**Red spots, sensitive:** Ran-s., *Tarax.,* Ter.

**Red tip:** Amygd-p., *Arg-n., Ars.,* Cycl., Merc-i-f., Phyt., *Rhus-t.,* Rhus-v., Sulph.

**Red, wet, central furrow:** Nit-ac.

**Strawberry**: *Bell.,* Frag., Sapo.

**Unilateral**: *Daph.,* Lob., Rhus-t.

**White-furred, slimy, pasty:** Acon., Aesc., *Ant-c., Ant-t.,* Arg-n., Arn., *Bapt.,* Bell., *Bism., Bry.,* Calc., Carb-v., Card-m., *Chel.,* Chin., *Cycl.,* Ferr., Glon., Hedeo., *Hydr.,* Ip., Kali-c., Kali-chl., Kali-m., Lac-c., Lob., Lyc., *Merc.,* Merc-c., Mez., Nat-m., Nux-v., Ox-ac., Par., Petr., Phos., *Puls., Sep.,* Sulph., Tarax., Verat-v.

**Yellow, dirty, thick coating:** *Aesc., Bapt.,* Bry., Carb-v., Cham., *Chel., Chin.,* Chion., Ferr., *Hydr.,* Indol., *Kali-bi.,* Kali-s., Lept., Lyc., *Merc., Merc-d., Merc-i-f.,* Myric., Nat-p., *Nat-s.,* Nux-v., *Ost.,* Podo., *Puls.,* Sang., Sulph., *Yuc.*

**Yellow patch in center:** *Bapt.,* Phyt.

**CONDITIONS, Anesthesia:** Carbn-s.

**Atrophy:** Mur-ac.

**Biting:** Absin., Anis., Hydr., Hyos., *Ign.,* Ph-ac., Sec.

**Burning, smarting scalded feeling:** *Acon.,* Apis, *Ars.,* Arum-t., Bapt., Bell., Berb., Canth., Caps., Carb-an., Caust., Coloc., *Iris,* Lyc., Merc-c., Mez., *Mur-ac.,* Nat-m., Ph-ac., Podo., *Ran-s., Sang.,* Sanic., Sin-n., Sulph.

**Burning tip:** *Ars.,* Bar-c., Calc., Caps., *Iris,* Lath., Phys., *Sang.,* Ter.

**Coldness:** Acet-ac., *Camph.,* Carb-v., *Cist., Helo.,* Hydr-ac., Sec., *Verat.*

**Dryness:** *Acon.,* Ail., Ant-t., Apis, *Ars.,* Bapt., *Bell., Bry.,* Calc., Colch., Hyos., Kali-bi., Kali-c., Lach., Leon., Merc., Merc-c., *Morph., Mur-ac.,* Nat-m., *Nux-m., Par.,* Ph-ac., Phos., Puls., Pyrog., *Rhus-t., Sulph., Ter., Verat-v.,* Vip.

**ERUPTIONS, growths, Cancer:** Alumn., Apis, *Ars., Aur.,* Aur-m-n., Crot-h., Gali., Kali-chl., *Kali-cy., Mur-ac.,* Semp., *Strych-g., Thuj.,* Vib-p.

**Cracks, excoriations:** Anan., *Ars., Arum-t.,* Arund., Bapt., Bell., Bor-ac., Borx., Bry., Cham., *Kali-bi.,* Lach., Leon., Nat-m., *Nit-ac.,* Phyt., Plb-act., Pyrog., Ran-s., *Rhus-t.,* Rhus-v., Semp. (See **Ulcerations**.)

**Epithelioma:** Ars., Carb-ac., Chr-ac., *Hydr., Kali-cy.,* Mur-ac., *Thuj.*

**Furrows lengthwise, in upper part:** Merc.

**Growths, nodules:** Ars-h., *Aur.,* Aur-m-n., Castm., *Gali.,* Mur-ac., Nit-ac., *Thuj.*

**Psoriasis**: *Castor-eq.,* Kali-bi., *Mur-ac.*

**Ranula:** Ambr., *Calc.,* Ferr-p., Fl-ac., Merc., Nit-ac., *Thuj.*

**Ringworm:** Nat-m., Sanic. (See **Red edges**.)

**Ulcerations:** Apis, *Arg-n.,* Ars., Ars-h., Bapt., Fl-ac., Kali-bi., Lyc., *Merc.,* Mur-ac., *Nit-ac., Nit-m-ac.,* Sangin-n., Semp., Syph., Thuj.

**Ulcerations, syphilitic:** Aur., *Cinnb.,* Fl-ac., *Kali-bi.,* Lach., Merc., Mez., *Nit-ac.*

**Veins, varicose:** Ambr., *Ham.,* Thuj.

**Vesicles, blisters:** Am-c., Apis, Berb., Borx., *Canth.,* Carb-an., Lacer., *Lyc.,* Merl., Mur-ac., *Nat-p., Nat-m.,* Nit-ac., Phyt., Rhus-t., Sul-ac., *Sulph.,* Thuj.

**Warts:** Aur-m., Mang-act.

**HARD, induration of:** Alumn., Aur., *Calc-f.,* Mur-ac., Semp., *Sil.*

**HEAVINESS:** Caust., Colch., Gels., Gua., Merl., Mur-ac., Nux-v.

**INFLAMMATION (glossitis):** *Acon., Apis,* Ars., Bell., Canth., Crot-h., *Lach.,* Merc., *Merc-c., Mur-ac., Ox-ac.,* Phyt., Ran-s., *Sul-ac., Vip.* (See **Swelling.**)

**NUMBNESS, tingling:** *Acon.,* Con., Echi., *Gels.,* Ign., Lath., Merl., *Nat-m.,* Nux m., Nux-v., Plat., Rad-br., Rheum, Sec.

**PAIN:** Acon., *Ars.,* Arum-t., Bell., Kali-ar., Kali-i., Merc., *Nit-ac., Phyt.,* Ruta, Semp., *Thuj.* (See **Soreness.**)

**PARALYSIS:** Acon., Acon-c., Anac., Arn., Ars., Bar-c., *Bell., Both.,* Cann-i., *Caust.,* Cocc., *Con.,* Cupr., *Cur., Dulc., Gels.,* Gua., Hyos., Lach., Lob-p., *Mur-ac.,* Nux-m., Olnd., Op., *Plb.,* Sec., Stram., Zinc-s. (See **NERVOUS SYSTEM.**)

**PROTRUSION, difficult:** Anac., *Apis,* Ars., Calc., *Caust.,* Crot-h., Dulc., *Gua., Gels., Hyos., Lach.,* Merc., Mur-ac., *Mygal.,* Nat-m., Pyrog., Plb., Stram., Sulfon., Ter.

**Snake, like:** Absin., Crot-h., *Cupr., Lach.,* Lyc., *Merc.,* Sanic., *Vip.*

**RAWNESS, roughness:** Apis, *Ars., Arum-t., Canth.,* Dulc., *Nit-ac.,* Phyt., *Ran-s.,* Tarax.

**SENSATION, as if hair on tongue:** All-s., Kali-bi., Nat-m., *Sil.*

**as if swollen, enlarged:** Absin., Aeth., *Anac.,* Crot-h., Nux-v., Ptel., Puls.

**SORENESS:** *Apis, Arum-t.,* Cist., Kali-c., Merc-c., Mur-ac., *Nit-ac.,* Ox-ac., Phel., Phys., *Ran-s., Rhus-t.,* Semp., Sep., Sil., *Ter.,* Thuj.

**SPASM:** Acon., Bell., Ruta, Sec. (See **Trembling.**)

**STIFFNESS:** Con., *Dulc.,* Hyos., Lac-c., Merc-i-r., Nicc., Sec., Stram.

**SWELLING:** *Acon., Apis,* Ars., Arum-t., Aster., Bapt., *Bell.,* Bism., Caj., *Canth., Crot-h.,* Diph., Frag., Kali-tel., Lach., Mag-p., *Merc-c., Mez., Mur-ac.,* Oena., Ox-ac., Ruta, Thuj., *Vesp., Vip.,* Vip-t.

**TREMBLING:** *Absin., Agar., Agri.,* Apis, Ars., Bell., Camph., Caust., Cham., *Gels., Lach., Merc.,* Plb., Stram.

■

# TASTE

**LOST**: *Amgd-p., Ant-c.,* Bry., Cycl., Form., Gymne., Just., Lyc., Mag-c., *Mag-m., Nat-m.,* Podo., *Puls.,* Sang., Sil., Sulph.

**PERVERTED; ALTERED, In general:** Aesc., *Alum.,* Ant-t., *Arg-n.,* Arn., Ars., Calc., Camph., Carb-v., Chel., *Chin.,* Cycl., Fago., *Gymne., Hydr.,* Kali-c., Lyc., Mag-c., Mag-m., *Merc.,* Merc-c., *Nat-m.,* Nit-ac., *Nux-v.,* Par., Podo., *Puls.,* Rheum, *Sep., Sulph.,* Zinc-m.

**After eating:** Ars., Carb-v., *Nat-m.,* Nit, ac., Zinc.

**After sleep:** Rheum.

**Acid, astringent, sour:** Aloe, Am-c., *Calc.,* Carb-v., Cham., Chin., Euph., Hep., *Hydr.,* Ign., Iris, Kali-c., Lob., *Lyc., Mag-c.,* Nat-p., Nit-ac., *Nux-v.,* Ph-ac., Phos., *Puls.,* Sep., *Sulph.*

**Bitter, bilious:** *Acon.,* Aloe, Ars., *Atha.,* Bapt., *Bry.,* Camph., *Card-m., Cham., Chel., Chin., Coloc.,* Cupr., Dig., *Hydr.,* Ip., Kali-c., *Lyc.,* Merc-c., *Myric.,* Nat-m., Nat-s., *Nux-v.,* Par., *Podo.,* Ptel., *Puls.,* Rhus-t., Sabad., *Sep.,* Stann., *Sulph., Tarax.*

**Bitter from tobacco:** *Asar.,* Euphr., Puls.

**Bloody-like:** *Alum.,* Chel., Kali-c., Manc., *Nit-ac.,* Sil., Sulph., Trif-p., Zinc.

**Coppery, metallic:** Aesc., Arg-n., Ars., Bism., Cocc., *Cupr., Cupr-ar.,* Lac-ac., *Lob., Merc-c.,* Nit-m-ac., Nux-v., *Rhus-t.,* Sulph.

**Delicate, changeable:** Coff., *Puls.*

**Disgusting, putrid, foul, slimy:** *Arn.,* Aur-m., Borx., Calc., *Carb-v.,* Chel., Ferr., Graph., Hep., Indol, Led., Lem-m., Lyc., *Merc.,* Merc-c., Nat-m., Nat-s., Nux-v., Petr., Phos., Podo., *Puls., Pyrog.,* Sep., Yuc.

**Flat, insipid, straw-like, pappy:** *Ant-c.,* Ant-t., *Ars.,* Bapt., Borx., *Chin., Cycl.,* Euph-a., *Ferr.,* Glyc., Ign., Kali-s., Nux-m., *Puls.*

**Greasy, fatty, pasty:** Arn., Carb-v., Caust., Euon., Ol-an., Phos., *Puls.,* Tril-c.

**Peppery:** Hydr.

**Perverted in morning:** Fago., Graph., Hydr., *Nux-v.,* Puls.

**Salty:** Ant-c., Ars., *Bell.,* Cadm-s., *Carb-v.,* Chin., *Cycl., Merc.,* Merc-c., *Puls., Sep.,* Sulph., Zinc.

**Sweet:** Agar., *Apoc-a.,* Bism., Chel., Cupr., Dig., Glyc., *Merc., Nit-ac.,* Phel., *Plb.,* Puls., *Pyrog., Sabad.,* Sel., Stann.

■

# GUMS

**BLEEDING easily:** *Agav-a., Alum.,* Ambr., Ant-c., *Arg-n., Arn., Ars.,* Bapt., Benz-ac., Borx., Calc., *Carb-v.,* Cist., Crot-h., Echi., Hep., *Iod., Kreos.,* Lach., *Merc.,* Merc-c., *Nit-ac., Phos.,* Plan., Sep., Sil., Staph., Sul-ac., Sulph., Zinc.

**Bleeding protractedly, after tooth extraction:** Ars., Bov., *Ham., Kreos.,* Phos., Tril-p.

**BLUE line along margin:** Plb.

**BURNING:** Antip. (See **Pain.**)

**COLD feeling:** Cocc-s.

**DESIRE to press teeth together:** Phyt., Podo.

**EPULIS:** Calc., Plb., *Thuj.*

**INFLAMMATION (gumboil):** *Acon., Bell.,* Borx., *Calc-f.,* Calc-s., Cham., *Hecla,* Hep., Kreos., *Merc.,* Merc-c., Phos., Rhus-t., *Sil.* (See **Pain, Swelling.**)

**PAINFUL after tooth extraction:** Arn., Sep.

**Sore, sensitive:** Alum., Am-c., Arg-n., *Bapt.,* Bell., Borx., Calc., *Carb-v.,* Caust., *Cham.,* Dol., *Hep., Kreos., Merc., Nit-ac.,* Plan., Rhus-t., *Sil.,* Sulph., Thuj.

**RED seam (strophulus):** *Ant-c.,* Apis, *Cham.,* Kali-p., *Puls.,* Rhus-t.

**SCORBUTIC (soft, spongy, receding):** *Agav-a.,* Alum., Ant-c., Arn., *Ars.,* Bapt., *Carb-v.,* Cist., Echi., Hep., *Iod.,* Kali-c., Kali-chl., Kali-p., *Kreos., Merc., Mur-ac.,* Nat-m., *Nit-ac., Phos., Staph.,* Sulph., Thuj.

**SWELLING**: *Apis,* Bell., Bism., Calc., Caust., *Cham.,* Cist., Graph., Kreos., Lach., Mag-m., *Merc.,* Merc-c., Merc-d., *Merc-i-r.,* Mur-ac., Nit-ac., *Phos.,* Plb., Rhod., Sep., Sil., Staph., Sulph., Ter.

**ULCERATION (pyorrhea alveolaris):** Aur., *Bapt.,* Carb-v., *Caust., Cist.,* Emetin., Kali-c., Kreos., *Merc., Merc-c., Nit-ac.,* Phos., *Plan., Sep., Sil., Staph.,* Sul-ac., Thuj.

■

# TEETH

**ALVEOLAR abscess:** Hep., Merc., Sil.

**BLACK, dark, crumbling:** Ant-c., *Kreos.,* Merc., Phos-h., *Staph.,* Syph., Thuj.

**CARIES, decay, premature:** Calc., Calc-f., *Calc-p.,* Cocc., Fl-ac., Hecla, *Kreos.,* Merc., *Mez.,* Phos., *Plan.,* Sil., *Staph.,* Tub.

**Caries, at crown:** Merc., *Staph.*

**Caries, at root:** *Merc.,* Mez., Sil., Syph., *Thuj.*

**CUPPED, dwarfed, serrated:** Staph., *Syph.*

**DENTITION (teething difficult, delayed):** *Acon., Bell., Borx., Calc., Calc-p.,* Caust., *Cham.,* Cheir., *Coff., Cupr.,* Gels., *Hecla, Kali- br., Kreos.,* Mag-p., Merc., Nux-v., Passi., Phyt., *Podo.,* Puls., *Sil.,* Sol-n., Staph., Sulph., *Ter.,* Zinc., Zinc-br.

**With cerebral, nervous symptoms:** Acon., Agar., *Bell., Cham.,* Cimic., Cypr., Dol., *Hell.,* Kali-br., *Podo.,* Sol-n., Ter., *Zinc.*

**With compression of gums:** Cic., Phyt., Podo.

**With constipation, general irritation, cachexia:** *Kreos.,* Nux-v., Op.

**With convulsions**: *Bell.,* Calc., *Cham., Cic.,* Cupr., Glon., Kali- br., *Mag-p.,* Sol-n., Stann., *Zinc-br.*

**With cough:** Acon., Bell., Ferr-p., Kreos.

**With deafness, otorrhea, stuffiness of nose:** Cheir.

**With diarrhea:** Aeth., *Calc., Calc-p., Cham.,* Ferr-p., Ip., Kreos., Mag-c., Merc., Olnd., Phos., *Podo.,* Puls., Rheum, *Sil.*

**With effusion threatened, in brain:** *Apis,* Hell., Tub., *Zinc.*

**With eye symptoms:** Bell., Calc., Puls.

**With insomnia:** Bell., Cham., *Coff., Cypr.,* Kreos., Passi., Scut., Ter.

**With intertrigo:** Caust., Lyc.

**With milk indigestion:** Aeth., Calc., *Mag-m.*

**With salivation:** Borx.

**With sour smell of body, pale face, irritability:** Kreos.

**With weakness, pallor, fretfulness, must be carried rapidly:** Ars.

**With worms:** *Cina,* Merc., Stann.

**FEEL cold:** *Cocc-s.,* Gamb., Ph-ac., Rheum.

**Feel loose:** Alum., Am-c., Arn., Bism., Calc-f., Carb-v., Hyos., Lyc., *Merc., Merc-c., Nit-ac., Plan.,* Rhus-t., Sil., *Zinc.*

**Feel numb:** Plat.

**Feel sensitive to cold, chewing, touch:** *Acon.,* Ars., Bell., Carb-v., Cham., *Coff., Fl-ac.,* Gymno., Merc., Parth., Plan., *Staph.* (See **Pain**.)

**Feel too long:** Bry., Carb-v., Caust., *Cham.,* Clem., Lyc., Mag-c., *Merc., Mez.,* Parth., Plan., Rat., Rhus-t.

**Feel warm:** Fl-ac.

**FISTULA DENTALIS:** Calc-f., Caust., *Fl-ac.,* Nat-m., *Sil.,* Staph., Sulph.

**GRINDING:** Apis, *Bell.,* Cann-i., *Cic.,* Cina, Hell., Mygal., *Phys.,* Plan., *Podo., Santin.,* Spig., Zinc.

**ODONTALGIA: Toothache: Remedies in general:** *Acon.,* Agar., Ant-c., Antip., Apis, *Ars.,* Atro., *Bell., Bry.,* Calc., Carb-ac., Carb-v., *Cham., Clem.,* Cocc-s., *Coff.,* Coloc., Ferr., Gels., Glon., Hecla, Ign., Kali-c., *Kreos.,* Lach., *Mag-c., Mag-p., Merc., Nux*-v., Ox-ac., Phos., Phyt., *Plan., Puls.,* Sep., Spig., *Staph.,* Tab., Ther., Thuj.

**CAUSE: Coffee:** Cham., Ign.

**Cold bathing:** Ant-c.

**Decayed teeth:** Cham., *Kreos., Merc.,* Mez., Staph.

**Dental pulp, inflamed:** Bell.

**Drafts, or cold exposure:** *Acon.,* Bell., Bry., *Calc.,* Cham., Merc., *Puls., Rhod.,* Sil.

**Extraction of teeth:** Arn., Staph.

**Menses, during:** Bar-c., Cham., Sep., *Staph.*

**Nursing baby:** Chin.

**Pregnancy:** Alum., *Calc.,* Cham., *Mag-c.,* Nux m., Puls., Rat., Tab. (See **FEMALE SEXUAL SYSTEM.**)

**Tea:** Thuj.

**Tobacco smoking:** *Clem.,* Ign., Plan., *Spig.*

**Washing clothes:** Phos.

**LOCATION: Decayed teeth:** *Ant-c., Cham., Kreos.,* Mag-c., *Merc., Mez.,* Nux-v., Staph., Thuj.

**Eye-teeth:** Ther.

**Lower:** Antip., Caust., Merc., Staph., Verb.

**Molars:** Antip., Bry., Caust.

**Roots of teeth:** Meph., *Merc.,* Staph.

**Sound teeth:** Arg-n., Caust., Cham., Plan., Spig., Staph.

**Upper teeth:** Bell., Fl-ac

**TYPE: Neuralgic, congestive:** *Acon.,* Aran., Ars., *Bell.,* Cedr., *Cham., Coff.,* Dol., Ferr-pic., *Ign.,* Mag-c., Mag-p., Merc., Plan., *Spig.* (See **Odontalgia.**)

**Rheumatic:** Acon., *Bry.,* Cham., Chinin-s., Colch., Guaj., Merc., *Puls., Rhod.*

**TYPE OF PAIN: Aching:** Cham., Kreos., Merc., Mez., Staph.

**Burning:** *Ars.,* Bell., Sil.

**Drawing, jerking, tearing:** *Bell., Cham.,* Chim., Coff., Cycl., Kreos., Meph., *Merc., Nux-v., Prun., Puls.,* Rhod., Sep., Sil., *Spig.,* Sulph.

**Gnawing, boring:** Calc., Carb-v., Mez., Nux-v., Plan., Puls., Sil., Staph.

**Periodical:** Ars., Chinin-s., Coff.

**Shock like:** Am-c., Aran., Nux-v.

**Shooting:** Calc., *Cham.,* Kali-c., Mag-*c., Nux-v.,* Phos., Sep., Sil.

**Stitching:** *Bry.,* Cham., Nit-ac., Puls.

**Throbbing:** Acon., *Bell.,* Cocc-s., Glon., Kali-c., Mag-c., Merc., *Sil.* (See **Odontalgia.**)

**CONCOMITANTS: Distraction of the mind:** Acon., Cham.

**Heat, thirst, fainting:** Cham.

**Neuralgia of lids, reflex:** Plan.

**Rush of blood to head, loose feeling of teeth:** Hyos.

**Soreness of teeth:** Bell., Merc., Plan., Zinc.

**Swelling about jaws, cheeks:** Bell., Borx., Cham., *Hecla,* Hep., Lyc., *Merc., Sil.* (See **Gumboil.**)

**MODALITIES: AGGRAVATION: After midnight:** Ars.

**At night:** Ant-c., Aran., *Bell.,* Caust., *Cham., Clem., Mag-c.,* Mag-p., *Merc.,* Mez., *Puls.,* Sep., Sil., Sulph.

**From blowing nose:** Culx., Thuj.

**From change of weather:** Aran., Merc., *Rhod.*

**From cold foods, drinks:** *Calc.,* Lach., Mag-p., *Merc., Nux-v.,* Staph., Sulph.

**From cold in general:** *Ant-c., Calc.,* Hyos., Lyc., Mag-c., Merc., *Nux-v.,* Plan., *Sil.,* Spig., Sulph.

**From contact, touch:** Bell., Calc-f., Caust., Chin., Kali-c., Mag-m., Mez., Plan., *Staph.*

**From eating:** Ant-c., Bell., Bry., *Calc.,* Cham., Chim., *Kali-c.,* Mag-p., Mez., Nux-v., *Puls.,* Sil., *Spig.,* Staph., Zinc.

**From exertion of mind or body:** Chim., Nux-v.

**From lying down, rest, quiet:** *Aran.,* Mag-c., Nat-s., *Rat., Sep.*

**From shrill sounds:** Ther.

**From smoking tobacco:** Clem., Ign., *Spig.*

**From warm food:** *Bism.,* Bry., Calc., *Caust., Clem., Coff.,* Merc., *Puls.,* Sil.

**In intervals between meals:** Ign.

**In morning:** Hyos.

**Warmth in general:** *Cham., Merc.,* Prun., *Puls.,* Sep.

**Windy weather, thunderstorms:** Rhod.

**AMELIORATION: Cold air:** Nat-s., Puls.

**Cold drinks:** *Bism., Bry.,* Chim., *Coff.,* Ferr., Ferr-p., Nat-s., *Puls.*

**Eating:** Ign., Plan., *Spig.*

**Hot liquids:** *Mag-p.*

**Lying down:** Spig.

**Mouth open, sucking in air:** Mez.

**Pressure external:** Bry., Chin.

**Pressure of teeth:** Chin., *Ol-an.,* Staph.

**Rubbing cheek:** Merc.

**Sweat in general:** *Aphis,* Cham., *Chen-g.*

**Walking about:** Mag-c., Rat.

**Warmth:** *Ars.,* Chin., Lyc., *Mag-p.,* Merc., Nux-v.

**Wet finger:** Cham.

**RIGG'S DISEASE:** Cal-ren., Merc., Sil-mar.

**SORDES and deposits:** *Ail.,* Alum., Ars., *Bapt., Echi.,* Hyos., Iod., Kali-p., Merc-c., *Mur-ac.,* Ph-ac., Plan., *Rhus-t.*

■

# THROAT

**ADENOID VEGETATIONS:** *Agra.,* Bar-c., Calc., *Calc-f., Calc-i., Calc-p.,* Chr-ac., Iod., Kali-s., Lob-s., Mez., Psor., *Sangin-n.,* Sulph., Thuj.

**DIPHTHERIA; Remedies in general:** Ail., *Apis, Ars.,* Ars-i., Arum-t., *Bapt., Bell., Brom.,* Calc-chl., *Canth.,* Carb-ac., *Crot-h., Diph.,* Echi., Guaj., *Kali-bi.,* Kali-chl., *Kali-m., Kali-perm.,* Lac-c., *Lach.,* Lachn., Led., Lob., *Lyc., Merc-c., Merc-cy.,* Merc-i-f., Merc-i-r., *Mur-ac.,* Naja, *Nit-ac., Phyt.,* Rhus-t., Sang., Sulph., Tarent-c., Vinc., Zinc.

**TYPE, Ataxic:** Ars., Bell., Lach., Mosch., Phos.

**Laryngeal:** Apis, *Brom.,* Canth., Chlor., Diph., *Hep.,* Iod., *Kali-bi.,* Lac-c., *Merc-cy.,* Petr., Phos., Samb., Spong.

**Malignant:** *Ail.,* Apis, Ars., *Carb-ac.,* Chinin-ar., Crot-h., Diph., *Echi.,* Kali-p., Lac-c., *Lach., Merc-cy.,* Mur-ac., Pyrog.

**Nasal:** *Am-c.,* Am-caust., *Kali-bi.,* Lyc., Merc-cy., *Nit-ac.*

**CONDITIONS, Extension downwards:** Iod., *Kali-bi.,* Lac-c., Merc-cy.

**Extension left to right:** Lac-c., *Lach.,* Sabad.

**Extension right to left:** Lyc.

**Extension upward:** Brom.

**With croup:** Acet-ac., *Brom.,* Hep., *Iod., Kali-bi.,* Kali-m., Lach., Merc-cy., Phos., Samb., Spong.

**With drooling:** Lac-c., Merc-cy.

**With objective symptom only; painless type; deficient reaction; sopor, stupor, epistaxis:** Diph.

**With post-diphtheritic paralysis:** *Arg-n., Caust.,* Cocc., Con., Cur., Diph., *Gels.,* Kali-p., Lach., Olnd., *Phos., Plb.,* Rhus-t., Sec.

**With prostration from beginning:** Ail., *Apis, Ars.,* Bapt., Canth., *Carb-ac.,* Crot-h., *Diph.,* Kali-perm., *Lach., Merc-cy.,* Mur-ac., Phyt.

**With spasm of glottis:** Mosch., Samb.

**With urine scanty:** Apis, Ars., Canth., Lac-c., Merc-cy., Naja.

**ESOPHAGUS; Burning, smarting:** Acon., *Am-caust.,* Asaf., Ars., *Canth.,* Caps., Carb-ac., *Crot-t.,* Gels., *Iris, Merc-c.,* Mez., Ox-ac., *Phos.,* Sang., Sin-a., Stry.

**Constriction:** Abies-n., *Alum.,* Am-m., *Asaf., Bapt., Bell.,* Cact., *Caj.,* Caps., *Cic.,* Cund., Gels., Hyos., Ign., *Lyss.,* Merc-c., Naja, *Phos.,* Plat., Plb., Rhus-t., Stram., Verat-v.

**Dryness:** *Acon., Bell.,* Cocc., *Mez., Naja.*

**Inflammation (esophagitis):** Acon., Alum., Ars., *Bell.,* Merc-c., Naja, *Phos.,* Sul-ac., Verat.

**Pain:** *Am-caust.,* Cocc., Gels., *Phos.*

**Spasm (esophagismus):** Aconin., Arg-cy., Asaf., *Bapt.,* Bar-c., *Bell.,* Canth., Cic., Hyos., *Ign.,* Lach., Lyss., Merc-c., *Naja,* Stram., Stry., *Verat-v.* (See **Pharynx.**)

**FAUCES, Anesthesia:** Kali-br.

**Burning heat:** *Acon.,* Aesc., Bell., *Canth., Caps.,* Carb-ac., Gels., *Phos., Phyt.,* Sin-n., Still.

**Dryness:** Acon., *Aesc., Bell.,* Canth., Caps., Gels., Jug-c., *Nux-m., Phos., Phyt., Sabad.,* Senec.

**Inflammation:** Ail., Apis, *Bell.,* Ferr-p., *Kali-bi.,* Mentho., Merc., Merc-i-f.

**Necrosis:** Merc-cy.

**Redness:** *Bell.,* Carb-ac., Ferr-p., Gymno., Mentho., *Merc-cy., Merc-i-r.,* Mez., Naja, Puls.

**Roughness, sensitive:** Aesc., Coc-c., Dros., *Nux-v.,* Phos., *Phyt.*

**Tingling:** *Acon.,* Echi., Phyt.

**Ulceration:** Cory., *Kali-bi.,* Merc-i-r., *Nit-ac.,* Sang. (See **Pharynx.**)

**PHARYNX; Abscess (retro-pharyngeal):** Antip., Bell., Bry., *Hep.,* Lach., *Merc.,* Nit-ac., Phos., *Sil* .

**Abscess, predisposition to:** Calc., *Calc-i.,* Ferr-p., *Kali-i., Sil.*

**Adherent crusts:** Elaps, Kali-bi., Kali-m.

**Anesthesia:** Gels., *Kali-br.*

**Burning, smarting, scalded feeling:** Acon., *Aesc., Am-caust.,* Apis, *Ars.,* Ars-i., *Arum-t., Aur.,* Bar-c., Bell., Camph., *Canth., Caps.,* Carb-ac., *Caust.,* Cocain., Con., Glyc., Guaj., Hydr., *Iris,* Kali-bi., *Kali-perm.,* Kreos., Lyc., Merc., *Merc-c.,* Merc-i-f., *Mez.,* Nat-ar., Nit-ac., *Phos., Phyt.,* Pop-c., Quill., *Sang.,* Sangin-n., Senec., *Sulph.,* Wye.

**Coldness:** Cist.

**Constriction, spasmodic:** *Acon.,* Aesc., Agar., Alum., Apis, *Arg-n.,* Ars., Arum-t., Asaf., *Bapt., Bell.,* Both., Cact., Calc., Caj., *Canth., Caps., Cic.,* Cocain., Cupr., *Hyos., Ign.,* Lach., *Merc-c.,* Mez., Morph., Nux-v., *Phyt.,* Plb., Puls., Rat., Sang., *Sangin-n.,* Sarcol-ac., *Stram., Stry.,* Sumb., Valer.

**DYSPHAGIA; Deglutition painful, difficult, Remedies in general:** *Agar.,* Ail., Alum., Amgd-p., Anac., Apis, Ars., Atro., *Bapt., Bell.,* Both., Bry., *Caj., Canth., Caps.,* Carb-ac., *Cic.,* Cocc., Con., Cocain., Cur., Dub., Fl-ac., Grat., Hep., Hydr-ac., *Hyos., Ign.,* Iod., Kali-bi., Kali-br., Kali-c., Kali-chl., Kali-m., Kali- perm., *Lac-c., Lach.,* Lyc., Lyss., *Merc., Merc-c.,* Merc-cy., Merc-i-f., Merc-i-r., Nat-p., *Nit-ac.,* Phos., *Phyt.,* Pop-c., Psor., Sang., Sangin-n., Senec., *Stram., Stry.*

**Can swallow only liquids:** *Bapt., Bar-c.,* Cham., Nat-m., Plb., *Sil.*

**Can swallow only solids, liquids descend with difficulty:** *Alumn., Bell.,* Both., Bry., Cact., *Canth., Crot-h.,* Gels., *Hyos.,* Ign., Lach., *Lyss., Merc-c.,* Sil.

**Choking when eating, drinking:** Abies-n., *Anac.,* Caj., *Cann-s.,* Glon., *Merc-c.,* Mur-ac., Nicc., Nit-ac., *Phyt., Pip-m.,* Santin., Sumb.

**Food descends "wrong way":** *Anac.,* Cann-s., Kali-c., *Meph.,* Nat-m.

**Food regurgitates, per nasum:** *Bell.,* Diph., Kali-perm., *Lach.,* Lyc., Merc., *Merc-c.*

**Liquids descend with gurgling sound:** Ars., *Cupr-act.,* Hydr-ac., *Laur.,* Thuj.

**Swallows food and drink hastily:** *Anac., Bell.,* Bry., Coff., Hell., *Hep.,* Olnd., Zinc.

**DEPOSITS: Membranous:** *Acet-ac.,* Apis, Brom., Carb-ac., *Kali-bi.,* Kali-m., Kali-perm., Lach., Merc-cy., Mur-ac., *Nit-ac.,* Phyt. (See **Diphtheria**.)

**DRYNESS:** *Acon., Aesc.,* Agar., *Alum., Apis, Ars.,* Asaf., *Atro., Bell., Bry.,* Canth., *Caps.,* Caust., Cist., Cocain., Cocc., Dros., *Dub.,* Ferr-p., *Guaj.,* Hep., Hyos., Just., Kali-bi., Kali-c., Kali-chl., *Lach.,* Lem-m., *Lyc.,* Merc., Merc-c., Merl., Mez., *Morph.,* Nat-m., Nat-s., Nit-ac., *Nux-m.,* Onos., *Phos., Phyt.,* Puls., Quill., Rhus-t., *Sabad., Sang.,* Sangin-n., Sarcol-ac., Sep., *Spong.,* Stry., Sulph., *Wye.*

**EDEMA:** Ail., *Apis,* Ars., Kali-perm., Lach., Mag-p., Mur-ac., *Nat-ar.,* Phos., Phyt., Rhus-t.

**ERYSIPELAS:** *Apis,* Bell., *Canth.,* Euph., Lach., *Rhus-t.*

**GLOBUS HYSTERICUS:** *Ambr., Aqui., Asaf.,* Bell., Gels., Hyos., *Ign.,* Kali-p., Lach., Lob., Mag-m., Manc., *Mosch., Nux-m.,* Plat., Raph., *Valer.* (See **Hysteria**.)

**HAWKING: Hemming (clearing throat):** *Aesc., Alum.,* Am-m., *Arg-met., Arg-n., Arum-t.,* Bry., Calc., Canth., Carb-v., *Caust.,* Cist., *Coc-c.,* Cocc., Con., *Cor-r.,* Eucal., Guaj., Gymno., *Hep.,* Hepat., *Hydr.,* Iber., Just., *Kali-bi.,* Kali-c., *Kali-m.,* Lach., *Lyc.,* Merc-i-f., *Merc-i-r., Nat-c., Nat-m.,* Nit-ac., *Nux-v., Phos., Phyt.,* Psor., *Sel.,* Sep., Silphu., Spong., *Stann., Sulph., Tab.,* Trif-p., Vinc., Viol-t., *Wye.* (See **Chronic Pharyngitis.**)

**Hawking with cheesy, fetid, lumps:** *Agar.,* Kali-bi., Kali-m., Mag-c., Merc-i-r., *Psor.,* Sec., Sil. (See **Follicular Pharyngitis**.)

**Hawking, with fetid pus:** Antip., *Hep.,* Lyc., Sil.

**Hawking, with gelatinous, viscid, gluey mucus; difficult raising:** Aesc., Aloe, *Alum.,* Am-br., Am-m., *Arg-n., Arum-t., Canth.,* Carb-v., *Caust.,* Cist., *Coc-c.,* Coca, Euphr., *Hydr.,* Iber., *Kali-bi.,* Kali-c., Lach., *Merc-*

*i-f., Merc-i-r.,* Myric., Nat-c., Nat-m., Nat-s., Nux-v., Petr., Ph-ac., Phos., *Phyt.,* Psor., *Rumx.,* Sang., *Sel.,* Sep., Silphu., *Stann.*

**HOLLOW feeling, as if pharynx had disappeared:** Lach., Phyt.

**INCLINATION to swallow constantly:** Aesc., Asaf., *Bell.,* Caust., Lac-c., *Lach.,* Lac-ac., Lyss., *Merc., Merc-i-f.,* Myric., Phyt., Sumb., Wye.

**INFLAMMATION (Pharyngitis), Atrophic (sicca):** Aesc., *Alum.,* Dub., Arg-n., Ars-i., Kali-bi., Nux-v., Sabal.

**Inflammation, catarrhal, acute:** *Acon., Aesc.,* Apis, Arg-n., *Bell.,* Bry., Canth., *Caps.,* Caust., Cist., Eucal., Ferr-p., *Gels.,* Glyc., *Guaj.,* Gymno., *Hep.,* Iod., *Just., Kali-bi.,* Kali-c., Kali-m., Lach., Lachn., Led., Mentho., *Merc.,* Merc-c., Merc-i-f., Merc-i-r., Naja, Nat-ar., Nat-i., Nux-v., *Phyt.,* Quill., Sal-ac., *Sang., Sangin-n.,* Squil., *Wye.*

**Inflammation, catarrhal, acute, predisposition to:** Alumn., *Bar-c.,* Graph., Lach., Sulph.

**Inflammation, catarrhal, chronic:** Aesc., *Alum.,* Am-br., *Am-caust.,* Arg-i., *Arg-met., Arg-n.,* Ars., Arum-t., Aur., Bar-c., Brom., Calc-p., Cann-i., Carb-v., Caust., Cinnb., Cist., *Coc-c.,* Cub., Elaps, Ferr-p., Graph., *Hep., Hydr., Iod., Kali-bi.,* Kali-c., Kali-chl., *Lach., Lyc.,* Med., *Merc.,* Merc-c., Merc-i-f., *Nat-c.,* Nat-m., *Nux-v.,* Ox-ac., Pen., Petr., Phos., Puls., *Rumx.,* Sabad., Sabal, *Sang.,* Sec., Seneg., *Sep.,* Stann., Sumb., Tab., *Wye.*

**Inflammation, follicular, acute:** Aesc., Apis, Bell., Caps., *Ferr-p.,* Iod., Kali-bi., *Kali-m.,* Merc., *Phyt.,* Sangin-n., Wye.

**Inflammation, follicular, chronic (Clergymen'a sore throat):** Aesc., *Alum.,* Am-br., *Arg-n.,* Arn., Ars-i., *Arum-t.,* Calc-f., Calc-p., Caps., Caust., Cinnb., Cist., Dros., *Hep., Hydr.,* Ign., *Kali-bi.,* Kali-m., *Lach.,* Merc-cy., *Merc-i-r.,* Nat-m., Nux-v., Phos., *Phyt., Sangin-n.,* Stict., Still., Sulph., *Wye.*

**Inflammation, herpetic:** *Apis,* Ars., Borx., Hydr., Jac-c., *Kali-bi.,* Kali-chl., Lach., Merc-i-f., Nat-s., *Phyt.,* Sal-ac.

**Inflammation, rheumatic:** Acon., Bry., Colch., Guaj., Phyt., Rhus- t.

**Inflammation, septic:** Am-c., *Hep.,* Mur-ac., *Sil.*

**Inflammation, tubercular:** Merc-i-r.

**AGGRAVATIONS: From cold:** *Cist.,* Fl-ac., Hep., *Lyc.*

**From drinks, warm or hot:** *Lach.,* Merc-i-f., Phyt.

**From menses:** Lac-c.

**From pressure:** Lach., Merc-c.

**From sleep:** *Lach.,* Lyc.

**From suppressed foot sweat:** *Bar-c.,* Psor., Sil.

**From swallowing, empty:** Antip., *Bar-c.,* Crot-h., Doli., *Hep., Just.,* Lac-c., *Lach., Merc.,* Merc-i-f., Merc-i-r., Phyt., Sabad.

**From swallowing liquids:** Bell., Bry., Ign., *Lach.*

**From swallowing solids:** Bapt., Merc., Morph. (See **Deglutition**.)

**From swallowing sweet things:** Spong.

**From warmth:** Coc-c., Iod., Lach., *Merc.*

**In afternoon:** Lach.

**In bed:** *Merc.,* Merc-i-f.

**In intervals of swallowing:** Caps., Ign.

**On left side:** *Lach., Merc-i-r.,* Sabad.

**On left to right:** Lac-c., *Lach.,* Sabad.

**On right side:** Bar-c., *Bell.,* Guaj., *Lyc.,* Mag-p., Merc., *Merc-i-f.,* Nicc., Phyt., Podo., *Sang., Sulph.*

**AMELIORATIONS: From inspiring cold air:** Sang.

**From swallowing:** Gels., *Ign.*

**From swallowing liquids:** Cist.

**From swallowing liquids, warm:** *Alum., Ars.,* Calc-f., *Lyc.,* Morph., Sabad.

**From swallowing solids:** *Ign.,* Lach.

**PAPULES:** Hippoz., Iod. (See **Follicular Pharyngitis**.)

**PARALYSIS, neurosis:** *Alum.,* Bar-m., *Bell., Caust.,* Cocc., *Con.,* Cur., Gels., Hep., *Hyos., Ign., Lach.,* Lob., Lyc., Merc., Morph., Nit-ac., *Nux-m.,* Plb., *Pop-c.,* Rhus-t., *Sil.,* Stram., Sulph.

**PERISTALSIS reversed:** Ambr., Asaf.

**PLUG or lump sensation:** Alum., Bar-c., *Bell.,* Carb-v., Graph., *Hep., Ign., Lach.,* Lob., Merc-i-f., Nat-m., *Nux-v.,* Plb-act., Phyt., Puls., Rumx., Sulph., Wye.

**PUSTULES:** Aeth. (See **Ulceration**.)

**RAWNESS, roughness, scraping:** *Acon., Aesc., Alum.,* Am-c., *Am-caust.,* Am-m., *Arg-met., Arg-n., Arum-t.,* Bar-c., Bell., *Bry.,* Brom., *Carb-v., Caust.,* Coc-c., Con., Cub., *Dros.,* Fago., Gels., *Hep., Hepat.,* Hom., Hydr., *Iod., Kali-bi.,* Kali-c., Lac-ac., Merc., Merc-cy., Nit-ac., *Nux-v.,* Onos., Pen., *Phos., Phyt., Pop-c.,* Puls., *Rumx., Sang.,* Sangin-n., *Sep.,* Stict., Sulph.

**REDNESS:** *Acon.,* Aesc., *Bell.,* Ferr-p., Gins., Merc., Merc-i-f., Merc-i-r., Merc-n., Sal-ac., *Sulph.*

**Redness, dark, livid:** *Ail.,* Alum., *Am-c.,* Am-caust., Amgd-p., *Apis,* Arag., *Arg-n.,* Ars., *Bapt.,* Bell., Canth., Caps., Crot-h., Diph., *Gymno., Lach.,* Merc-c., Mur-ac., *Naja,* Nat-ar., Pen., *Phyt.,* Puls., Wye., Zinc-c.

**Redness, glossy, as if varnished:** Alum., *Apis,* Arag., Bell., Cist., Hydr., Kali-bi., *Lac-c.,* Phos.

**RELAXATION:** Aesc., *Alum.,* Alumn., Am-m., Bar-c., *Calc-p.,* Eucal., Pen.

**SENSITIVE, sore, tender:** *Acon., Aesc.,* Ail., *Apis,* Arg-met., *Arg-n.,* Arn., *Arum-t.,* Atro., Bar-c., *Bell.,* Brom., Bry., Calc-p., *Canth., Caps.,* Carb-ac., *Caust.,* Dol., Fago., Ferr-p., Fl-ac., Graph., Gymno., *Hep.,* Hom., Hydr., Ign., *Kali-bi.,* Kali-c., Kali-i., *Kali-perm.,* Lac-c., *Lach.,* Lachn., Led., Lyc., Mentho., *Merc., Merc-c., Merc-cy., Merc-i-f., Merc-i-r.,* Mur-ac., Naja, Nit-ac., *Nux-v.,* Ox-ac., Petr., Phos., *Phyt.,* Pop-c., Quill., Rhus-t., Sabad., *Sang.,* Sangin-n., Spong., Sulph., Trif-p., Verb., Wye.

**SORE, irritable of smokers:** Aesc., Arg-n., Caps., Nat-m., Nux-v.

**SPASM**: *Bell.,* Canth., *Sumb.* (See **Constriction.**)

**STICKING, pricking, splinter-like pains, extending to ears, worse swallowing, yawning, etc.:** Agar., Alum., *Arg-n.,* Dol., Ferr-i., Gels., Guaj., *Hep., Kali-bi., Kali-c.,* Lac-c., *Nit-ac., Phyt.,* Psor., Sil., Staph.

**STIFFNESS:** Aesc., Kali-m., Mag-p., Mez., Nux-m., Phyt., *Rhus-t.* (See **Constriction.**)

**SWELLING:** *Acon.,* Aesc., Ail., *Apis,* Arg-n., Arum-t., Bapt., *Bar-c., Bell.,* Canth., *Caps.,* Crot-h., Gymno., *Hep.,* Kali-bi., *Kali-m., Kali-perm.,* Lac-c., *Lach., Merc.,* Merc-c., *Merc-cy., Merc-i-f., Merc-i-r.,* Naja, Nat-ar., *Phyt.,* Sabad., Sang., Vesp., Wye. (See **Inflammation.**)

**SYPHILIS:** *Aur.,* Bell., Cinnb., Fl-ac., Hydr., *Kali-bi.,* Kali-i., Merc-c., *Merc-i-f., Merc-i-r.,* Merc-n., Mez., *Nit-ac., Phyt.,* Sulph.

**TICKLING, as from hair:** Aesc-g., All-s., Ambr., *Arg-n.,* Caust., Dros., Hepat., *Kali-bi.,* Lach., Nat-m., Nit-ac., Nux-v., Pulx., *Sabad.,* Sang., Sulph., *Valer.,* Yuc.

**ULCERATION:** Ail., Am-c., *Apis,* Aral., Bapt., *Cinnb.,* Hydr., *Hydrin-m., Kali-bi.,* Kali-m., *Lach.,* Merc., *Merc-c.,* Merc-cy., Merc i-f., Merc-i-r., Mur-ac., *Nit-ac., Phyt.,* Sang., Vinc.

**Ulceration, aphthous**: *Canth.,* Eucal., *Hydrin-m.,* Nit-ac.

**Ulceration, gangrenous:** Ail., Am-c., *Ars.,* Bapt., Crot-h., Echi., Kali-chl., Kali-n., Kali-perm., *Lach.,* Merc., *Merc-cy.,* Mur-ac., Sil.

**Ulceration, mercurial:** Hep., Hydr., Lyc., Nit-ac.

**Ulceration, syphilitic:** Aur., Calc-f., *Fl-ac.,* Hippoz., Jac-g., *Kali-bi.,* Kali-i., Lach., Lyc., Merc., *Merc-c.,* Merc-i-f., Merc-i-r., *Nit-ac.,* Phyt., Still.

**VEINS, varicose**: *Aesc.,* Aloe, *Bar-m.,* Ham., Phyt., Puls.

**TONSILS, Abscess (peritonsillar):** Calc-s.

**DEPOSITS ON; Creamy, extends over tonsils, uvula, soft palate:** Nat-p.

**Dark, dry, wrinkled:** Ars.

**Dark, gangrenous:** Bapt.

**Grayish, dirty, like macerated skin, covering tonsils, uvula pharynx:** Phyt.

**Grayish, dirty, thick, with fiery red margins:** Apis.

**Grayish, extends to posterior nares, air passages, later purplish black:** Echi.

**Grayish, patch on tonsils:** Kali-m.

**Grayish, thick; shred like borders, adherent or free:** Merc.

**Grayish-white, in crypts:** Ign.

**Grayish-yellow, slight; easily detached; worse on left:** Merc-i-r.

**Patchy on right tonsil and inflamed fauces, easily detached:** Merc-i-f.

**Plugs of mucus constantly form in crypts:** Calc-f.

**Shining, glazed white or yellow patch:** Lac-c.

**Thick, brownish-yellow like wash leather, or firm, fibrinous, pearly, extends over tonsils, soft palate:** Kali-bi.

**Thick, dark gray, or brownish-black:** Diph.

**Thin, false; on yellowish red tonsils and fauces:** Merc.

**Thin, then dark, gangrenous:** Merc-cy.

**HYPERTROPHY, Induration:** Alumn., Ars-i., Aur., Bac., *Bar-c., Bar-i.,* Bar-m., Brom., Calc., Calc-f., *Calc-i., Calc-p.,* Ferr-p., Hep., *Iod., Kali-bi.,* Kali-m., Merc-i-f., *Merc-i-r.,* Plb-i., Phyt., Sil., Sul-i., Thuj.

**Hypertrophy, with hardness of hearing:** *Bar-c.,* Calc-p., *Hep.,* Lyc., Plb., Psor.

**Inflammation (tonsillitis); Acute Catarrhal and Follicular:** *Acon., Ail.,* Am-m., Amgd-p., *Apis, Bapt.,* Bar-act., *Bar-c.,* Bar-m., *Bell.,* Brom., Caps., Dulc., Eucal., Ferr-p., Gels., Gins., *Guaj., Gymno.,* Hep., *Ign.,* Iod., Kali-bi., *Kali-m.,* Lac-c., *Lach.,* Lyc., *Merc., Merc-i-f., Merc-i-r.,* Naja, Nat-s., *Phyt.,* Rhus-t., Sabad., *Sang., Sil.,* Sulph.

**Inflammation, acute phlegmonous (quinsy):** Acon., Apis, *Bar-c.,* Bar-i., *Bell.,* Caps., Cinnb., Guaj., *Hep.,* Lac-c., Lach., Lyc., *Merc.,* Merc-i-f., Merc-i-r., *Phyt., Psor.,* Sang., Sangin-n., Sil., *Tarent-c.,* Vesp.

**Inflammation, chronic tendency**: *Bar-c.,* Calc-p., Fuc., Hep., Lach., Lyc., Psor., *Sil.*

**Eradicate tendency to quinsy, to**: Psor.

**Redness, dark:** Ail., Amyg., *Bapt.,* Brom., Caps., Diph., Gymno., *Lach.,* Merc., *Phyt.*

**Swelling:** *Acon.,* Am-m., *Apis,* Ars-i., Bar-act., *Bar-c., Bell.,* Brom., Calc., Calc-p., Caps., Cinnb., Cist., Diph., Ferr-p., Gels., Guaj., *Hep.,* Ign., Iod., Kali-bi., Kali-m., *Lach.,* Lyc., *Merc.,* Merc-c., *Merc-i-f., Merc-i-r., Phyt.,* Psor., *Sangin-n.* (See **Tonsillitis.**)

**Ulceration:** *Ars.,* Bar-c., Echi., *Hep.,* Ign., *Kali-bi.,* Lach., Lyc., Merc., Merc-c., Merc-i-f., Merc-i-r., Merl., Nat-s., Nit-ac., Phyt., *Sil.* (See **Follicular Tonsillitis.**)

**Ulceration, gangrenous:** Am-c., Ars., Bapt., Crot-h., *Lach., Merc-cy.,* Mur-ac.

**UVULA: Constricted feeling:** Acon.

**Edematous, sac-like:** *Apis,* Ars., Caps., *Kali-bi., *Mur-ac., *Nat-ar.,* Phos., Phyt., Rhus-t.

**Elongation, relaxation:** Alum., *Alumn.,* Bar-c., Bell., Calc-f., Canth., *Caps., Coc-c.,* Cocc-s., Croc., Fago., Hep., *Hyos., Kali-bi.,* Merc., *Merc-c.,* Nat-m., Nux-v., *Phos., Phyt.,* Rumx-act., Sabad., Wye.

**Inflammation (uvulitis):** *Acon.,* Amgd-p., *Bell.,* Caps., Cist., Iod., *Kali-bi., Kali-perm.,* Merc., *Merc-c.,* Nat-s., Nux-v., Puls., Sul-i.

**Pain:** Trif-p., Tus-p.

**Sore spot behind, better by eating:** Am-m.

**Ulceration:** Ind., *Kali-bi.,* Merc-c.

**Whitened, shrivelled:** Carb-ac.

**White, tenacious, mucus:** Am-caust.

■

# STOMACH

**APPETITE; Defective, lost (anorexia):** *Abies-n.,* Alet., Alf., Am-c., *Ant-c.,* Arn., *Ars., Bapt.,* Bism., But-ac., Calc., Calc-p., Caps., *Carb-ac.,* Carb-v., Card-m., *Chel., Chin., Chinin-ar.,* Chion., Coca, Cocc., Coff., Colch., Cycl., Dig., *Ferr., Gent-l.,* Glyc., Helon., Hydr., *Ign., Ip.,* Iris, Kali-bi., *Lec., Lyc.,* Merc-d., Myric., Nicc., *Nux-v.,* Ph-ac., Phos., Plat., Prun., Prun-v., *Puls.,* Raph., *Rhus-t.,* Sep., Stront-c., Stry-ar., *Stry-p.,* Sulph., Sym-r., Tarax.

**Appetite, increased, ravenous (bulimy):** Abies-c., *Abrot.,* Agar., *Alf.,* All-s., *Anac.,* Ars., Ars-br., Bell., Brass., Bry., Cact., *Calc.,* Calen., Chel., Chin., Cimic., *Cina,* Ferr., Glyc., Gran., Graph., Hep., Ichth., Ign., *Iod.,* Kali-c., Lac-ac., Lap-a., Lob., *Lyc.,* Merc., Nat-c., *Nat-m., Nux-v.,* Olnd., Op., *Petr.,* Petros., *Phos., Psor.,* Rhus-t., Sec., Stann., *Sulph., Thyr., Uran-n., Zinc.*

**Appetite, increased, hungry at night:** Abies-n., Chin., *Cina,* Ign., Lyc., Nat-c., Petr., *Phos., Psor.,* Sel., *Sulph.*

**Appetite, increased, hungry before noon:** Hep., *Sulph.,* Zinc.

**Appetite, increased hungry, even after a meal:** *Alf.,* Calc., Casc., *Cina,* Iod., Indol., Lac-c., *Lyc.,* Med., *Phos.,* Phyt., *Psor.,* Staph., Stront-c., Sulph., Zinc.

**Appetite, inereased, yet loses flesh:** Abrot., Acet-ac., *Iod., Nat-m.,* Sanic., Tub., Uran-n.

**Appetite, increased, yet quickly satiated:** Am-c., Arn., Ars., Bar-c., Carb-v., *Chin., Cycl.,* Ferr., Lith-c., *Lyc.,* Nat-m., Nux-v., Petros., Podo., Prun., *Sep., Sulph.*

**APPETITE PERVERTED; AVERSIONS, Alcoholic beverages:** Ign., Sil.

**Beer:** Asaf., Bell., Chin., Nux-v., Puls.

**Boiled food:** Calc.

**Brandy:** Ign., Lob-e.

**Bread:** Aphis, Cycl., Ign., *Lyc., Nat-m.,* Puls., Sulph.

**Butter:** Cycl., Hep., *Puls.,* Sang.

**Coffee:** *Cham.,* Fl-ac., *Nux-v.,* Sul-ac.

**Drinks in general:** Bell., *Canth.,* Cocc., Ign., Kali-bi., Lyss., Nux-v., Stram. (See **Hydrophobia.**)

**Drinks, warm and hot:** Cham., Kali-s., *Puls.*

**Eggs:** Ferr.

**Fats:** *Calc.,* Carb-an., *Carb-v., Cycl.,* Hep., Nat-m., Petr., *Puls.,* Sep.

**Food cooked:** Graph., Sil.

**Food, in general:** *Ant-c., Ars.,* Canth., *Cocc., Colch.,* Dulc., Erio., Ferr., Ign., *Ip., Kali-bi.,* Kali-c., *Nux-v.,* Podo., Puls., Rheum, Rhus-t., Sabad. (See **Anorexia**.)

**Food, smell, sight of:** Ant-c., *Ars.,* Cocc., *Colch.,* Dig., *Nux-v., Sep.,* Sil., Stann., Sym-r.

**Food warm, hot:** Calc., Ign., Lyc., Petr., *Puls.,* Sil., Verat.

**Meat:** Aloe, *Alum.,* Aphis, *Arn.,* Bell., *Calc., Carb-v.,* Card-m., Chin., Colch., Crot-h., *Cycl.,* Ferr-p., *Graph.,* Lyc., Morph., *Mur-ac., Nit-ac.,* Petr., *Puls., Sep.,* Sil., Stront-c., Sulph., Thuj.

**Milk:** Arn., Bell., *Carb-v.,* Ferr-p., *Guaj.,* Nat-c., Past., Puls., Sep., Sil., *Sulph.*

**Potatoes:** Alum., Thuj.

**Salt food:** Graph., Sel.

**Sour things:** Dros., Ferr., Sulph.

**Sweets:** Bar-c., Caust., *Graph.,* Rad-br., Sulph.

**Tobacco:** Arn., Calc., Canth., Cocc., *Lob.,* Nat-m., *Nux-v.,* Plan.

**Tobacco, odor of:** Casc., *Ign.,* Lob.

**Wine:** Sulph.

**APPETITE PERVERTED; CRAVINGS (pica), Acids, pickles, sour things:** *Abies-c.,* Alum., Am-m., *Ant-c.,* Ant-t., Arn., *Ars.,* Arund., Calc., Carb-an., Chel., *Chin.,* Cod., *Hep.,* Ign., Joan., Kali-bi., Lact., *Mag-c.,* Myric., Nat-m., *Ph-ac., Puls., Sec., Sep.,* Thea, *Verat.*

**Alcoholic beverages:** *Ars., Asar.,* Calc-ar., *Caps., Carb-ac.,* Carb-v., Chin., *Coca,* Cocc., Ferr-p., *Kali-bi.,* Lach., Lec., Med., Mosch., *Nux-v.,* Phos., Psor., Puls., *Sel.,* Staph., Stront-c., *Sul-ac., Sulph., Syph.,* Tub.

**Apples:** Aloe, *Ant-t.,* Guaj., Tell.

**Beer, bitter:** Aloe, Cocc., *Kali-bi.,* Nat-m., Nux-v., Puls.

**Bread:** Ferr., Stront-c.

**Butter:** Ferr.

**Buttermilk:** Elaps.

**Charcoal, coal, chalk, etc.:** *Alum., Calc.,* Cic., Ign., Nit-ac., *Psor.*

**Cheese:** Arg-n., Cist.

**Coffee:** *Ang.,* Ars., Con., Lec., Mosch.

**Drinks, cold:** *Acon., Ant-t.,* Asim., *Ars.,* Bell., *Bry.,* Calc., Cocc., *Cupr.,* Dulc., *Merc.,* Nat-s., Onos., Phos., Rhus-t., *Verat.* (See **Thirst**.)

**Drinks, hot:** Ang., Casc., Castn-v., *Chel., Lyc.,* Med., Sabad., Spig.

**Effervescent beverages:** Colch.

**Eggs:** Calc.

**Farinaceous food:** Calc-p., Sabad.

**Fats:** Mez., Nit-ac., Nux-v., Sulph.

**Food, coarse, raw:** *Abies-c.,* Sil.
**Food, cold:** Bry., *Phos., Puls.,* Sil.
**Food, fish:** Sul-ac.
**Food, warm, hot:** Chel., Cupr., Sabad.
**Fruits, juicy things:** Aloe, *Ant-t.,* Chin., Mag-c., Med., *Ph-ac.,* Phos., Verat.
**Ham rind:** Calc-p.
**Lemonade:** Am-m., Cycl., Puls., Sabin., Sec.
**Meat:** *Abies-c., Calc-p.,* Lil-t., *Mag-c.,* Meny.
**Meat, salt, smoked:** Calc-p.
**Milk:** Apis, Ars., *Ph-ac., Rhus-t.,* Sabal, Sulph.
**Oysters:** Lach.
**Salt:** Calc., Carb-v., *Caust.,* Con., Med., Nat-m., Nit-ac., *Phos.,* Sulph., Verat.
**Spices:** Alum., *Chin.,* Fl-ac., *Hep.,* Nux-m., *Nux-v.,* Phos., Sang., Staph.
**Sweets, candy:** Alf., Am-c., *Arg-n.,* Calc., *Cina,* Coca, *Cocain.,* Crot-h., Joan., *Kali-c., Lyc.,* Mag-m., Med., Sabad., *Sulph.*
**Tea:** Alum., Hep.
**Tobacco:** *Asar., Carb-ac.,* Carb-v., Coca, Daph., *Staph.*
**Tonics:** Puls.
**Various things:** Bry., Cham., *Chin., Cina,* Fl-ac., Rheum, Sang.
**Vegetables:** Abies-c., Mag-c.
**Water, cold:** *Acon.,* Agar-em., *Ant-t.,* Apoc., *Ars.,* Asim., Bell., *Bry., Calc., Eup-per.,* Onos., Op., *Phos., Verat.* (See **Thirst.**)

**APPETITE; THINGS THAT DISAGREE, Beer:** Ferr., *Kali-bi.*
**Bread:** Ant-c., *Hydr.,* Lyc., *Nat-m.,* Nit-ac., Puls.
**Butter:** Carb-an., *Carb-v.,* Nat-m., Puls.
**Cabbage:** *Bry.,* Carb-v., Kali-c., Lyc., Petr.
**Cheese:** Coloc.
**Coffee:** Carb-v., Lyc., *Nux-v.*
**Drinks, cold:** *Ars.,* Calad., Dig., Elaps, Kali-i., *Verat.*
**Drinks, warm, hot:** Bry., Graph., *Phos., Puls.,* Pyrog.
**Eggs:** Colch.
**Fats:** Ant-c., Calc., Carb-v., *Cycl.,* Lyc., *Puls.,* Thuj.
**Fish:** Carb-v.
**Food, cold:** Kali-i.
**Food of any kind:** Alet., Amgd-p., *Carb-v.,* Lach., Mosch., Nat-c.
**Food, warm:** Puls.
**Meat:** Ars., Borx., *Bry.,* Carb-v., *Chin.,* Mag-m., Nat-m., *Puls.,* Sel., Sil., Verat.

**Meat in excess:** All-s.
**Fruits:** *Ars.,* Carb-v., *Caust.,* Ferr., Kali-bi., *Rumx.*
**Melons:** Zing.
**Milk:** *Aeth., Calc., Carb-v.,* Chin., Kali-i., Lact., Mag-c., *Mag-m.,* Nicc., Ol-j., Podo., Rheum, Sep., *Sulph.*
**Mushrooms, poisonous:** Camph.
**Odor of food nauseates:** *Ars.,* Cocc., *Colch.,* Dig., *Sep.*
**Onions:** Brom., Lyc., Thuj.
**Oysters:** Carb-v., Lyc.
**Pastry:** Ant-c., Lyc., *Puls.*
**Pork:** Ant-c., Carb-v., Cycl., *Puls.*
**Potatoes:** *Alum.,* Sep.
**Salt food:** Carb-v.
**Sausage:** Acet-ac., Ars., Puls.
**Soup:** Kali-c.
**Sour foods, drinks:** *Ant-c.,* Carb-v., Dros., Nat-m., Ph-ac.
**Starchy food:** *Carb-v.,* Chin., Lyc., *Nat-c.,* Nat-s., Sulph.
**Strawberries:** Ox-ac.
**Sweets:** *Arg-n.,* Ip., Lyc., Sulph., Zinc.
**Tea:** *Chin.,* Dios., Ferr., Kali-hy., *Sel.,* Thuj.
**Tobacco:** *Ign.,* Kali-bi., Lob., Lyc., Phos., *Sel.,* Tab.
**Vegetables:** Hydr.
**Vinegar:** Ant-c., Carb-v.
**Water:** *Ars.,* Chinin-ar.
**Water, impure:** Zing.
**Wine:** Ant-c., *Zinc.*

**ATONY, (myasthenia):** Bell., Ign., Podoin., *Stry-p.*

**BILIOUSNESS:** Aesc., Aloe, Aq-mar., *Bapt.,* Berb., *Bry.,* Card-m., Cham., *Chel., Chin.,* Chion., Crot-h., Dios., *Euon.,* Eup-per., Ferr., Gent-l., *Hydr., Iris,* Kali-c., *Lept.,* Lyc., Mag-m., *Merc.,* Myric., *Nat-s.,* Nitro-m-ac., *Nux-v., Podo.,* Ptel., *Puls.,* Sep., Sulph., *Tarax., Trios.* (See **Liver.**)

**CANCER:** Acet-ac., Am-m., Arg-n., *Ars.,* Bar-c., *Bell.,* Bism., Cadm-s., Calc-f., Carb-v., Con., *Cund.,* Graph., *Hydr., Kali-bi.,* Kali-c., *Kreos.,* Mag-p., Nux-v., *Orni.,* Phos., Plb., Sec. (See **GENERALITIES.**)

**CARDIAC ORIFICE, Contraction:** Alum., *Bar-m.,* Bry., Dat-a., *Phos.,* Plb.
**Pain (cardialgia):** *Agar., Arg-n.,* Asaf., Bar-c., Bism., Cann-i., *Carb-v.,* Caul., *Cupr., Ferr-cy.,* Ferr-t., Form., Ign., Mag-m., Nat-m., Nit-ac., *Nux-v., Onis.,* Stront-c., Thea. (See **Pain.**)
**Spasmodic contraction, painful, cardio-spasm:** Aeth., *Agar.,* Am-c., *Arg-n.,* Ars., *Bell.,* Calc., Caul., *Con.,* Hyos., *Ign.,* Nat-m., *Nux-v.,* Phos., Puls., Rhus-t., Sep., Sil.

**Dilatation (gastroptosis):** Bism., Graph., *Hydrin-m.,* Kali-bi., *Nux-v.,* Phos., Puls., Xan.

**GASTRALGIA:** (See **Pain.**)

**GASTRIC AFFECTIONS, better in open air:** Adon.

**of cigar makers:** Ign.

**HEMORRHAGE (hematemesis):** Acet-ac., Acon., *Arn., Ars.,* Both., *Cact.,* Canth., Carb-v., *Chin., Cocain,* Crot-h., Cupr., Erig., Ferr-p., Fic-r., *Ger., Ham.,* Hyos., *Ip.,* Kreos., Mangi., *Mill.,* Nit-ac., Nux-v., *Phos., Sec.,* Tril-p., Zinc.

**HICCOUGH (singultus):** Aeth., Agar., Aml-ns., Ars., Bell., *Caj.,* Caps., Carb-an., Carb-v., *Cic.,* Cocain., Cocc., *Cupr., Cycl.,* Dios., Eup-per., *Gins.,* Hep., Hydr-ac., Hyos., *Ign., Kali-br.,* Mag-p., *Morph., Mosch.,* Nat-m., Nicc-met., Nicot., Nux-m., *Nux-v.,* Ol-suc., Ran-b., Stram., *Sul-ac.,* Tab., Verat., Verat-v., Zinc-o., *Zinc-val.*

**Hiccough, after smoking:** Ign., Sel.

**Hiccough, followed by spasm:** Cupr.

**Hiccough, with belching:** Ant-c., *Caj.,* Chin., Cic., *Dios., Nux-v.,* Wye.

**Hiccough, with hysterical, nervous symptoms:** Gels., *Ign., Mosch.,* Nux-m., Zinc-val.

**Hiccough, with pains in back, after eating, nursing:** Teucr.

**Hiccough, with retching, vomiting:** Jatr., Mag-p., Merc., *Nux-v.*

**Hiccough, with spasm of esophagus:** Verat-v.

**Hiccough, with yawning:** Aml-ns., Carls., *Cocc.*

**HYPER-ACIDITY (hyperchlorhydria):** Acet-ac., Anac., Ant-c., *Arg-n., Atro.,* Bism., *Calc.,* Calc-p., *Carb-v.,* Cham., Chin., Chinin-ar., Coffein., Con., Grin., Hydr., Ign., *Iris,* Lob., Lyc., Mag-c., Mur-ac., *Nat-c.,* Nat-p., *Nux-v., Orex-tan.,* Petr., Phos., Prun-v., *Puls., Rob., Sul-ac.,* Sulph.

**HYPERESTHESIA:** *Arg-n.,* Ars., Bism., Chinin-ar.

**HYPERPERISTALSIS:** Ars., Fel., Hyos., *Ign., Phos.*

**INDIGESTION; DYSPEPSIA, Remedies in general:** *Abies c., Abies-n.,* Abrot., Acet-ac., Aesc., Aeth., Agar., Alet., Alf., All-s., Aln., Aloe, Alum., *Anac., Ant-c.,* Ant-t., Apoc., *Arg-n.,* Arist-m., *Arn., Ars.,* Atrop., Bapt., Bar-c., Bell., *Bism.,* Brom., *Bry.,* Calc., Calc-chln., Caps., *Carb-ac., Carb-v., Card-m.,* Cas-s., *Cham., Chel., Chin.,* Cina, *Coca,* Coch., *Colch.,* Coloc., Corn-f., Cupr-act., *Cycl., Dios.,* Fel., Ferr., Gent-l., *Graph.,* Hep., *Hom., Hydr., Ign.,* Iod., *Ip.,* Iris, *Kali-bi., Kali-c.,* Kali-m., *Lach.,* Lept., *Lob., Lyc.,* Merc., *Nat-c.,* Nat-m., Nat-s., Nit-ac., *Nux-m., Nux-v.,* Op., Petr., Ph-ac., *Phos.,* Pic-ac., Podo., Pop., Prun., Prun-v., Ptel., *Puls., Rob.,* Sal-ac., Sang., *Sep.,* Stann., *Stry-af-cit.,* Sul-ac., *Sulph.,* Uran-n., Xero.

**CAUSE, Abuse of drugs:** Nux-v.

**Acids:** *Ant-c.,* Ars., Chin., Nat-m.

**Aged, debilitated:** Abies-n., Ars., Bar-c., *Carb-v.,* Chin., Fl-ac., *Hydr.,* Kali-c.

**Beer:** Ant-t., Bapt., Bry., *Kali-bi.,* Lyc., *Nux-v.*

**Bread:** Ant-c., Bry., Lyc., Nat-m.

**Bright's disease:** Apoc. (See **URINARY SYSTEM.**)

**Buckwheat cakes:** Puls.

**Cheese:** Ars., Carb-v., Coloc., Nux-v.

**Coffee:** Cham., Kali-c., Lyc., *Nux-v.*

**Cold bathing:** Ant-c.

**Debauchery in general:** Ant-t., *Carb-v., Chin.,* Nat-s., *Nux-v.*

**Decayed meat, fish:** Ars., Carb-v.

**Dietetic indiscretions:** All s., *Ant-c., Bry., Carb-v.,* Chin., Coff., *Ip.,* Lyc., Nat-c., *Nux-v., Puls.,* Xan.

**Egg albumen:** Nux-v.

**Excesses:** Carb-v., *Chin.,* Kali-c., *Nux-v.*

**Fat food:** Ant.c., *Calc.,* Carb-v., *Cycl.,* Ip., *Kali-m., Puls.,* Thuj.

**Fatigue, brain fag, in children:** Calc-f.

**Fevers, acute, after:** Chin., Quas.

**Flatulent food:** Chin., Lyc., Puls.

**Fruits:** Ars., *Chin.,* Elaps, *Puls.,* Verat.

**Gastric juice, scanty:** Aln., *Alum.,* Lyc.

**Gout:** Ant-t., Chin., *Colch.,* Nux-m., Thuj.

**Hasty eating, drinking:** Anac., Coff., *Olnd.*

**Hot weather:** Ant-c., *Bry.*

**Ice water, ices:** *Ars.,* Carb-v., Elaps, Ip., Kali-c., Nat-c., *Puls.*

**Lactation:** *Chin.,* Sin-a.

**Meats:** *Caust.,* Ip., Puls., Sil.

**Melons:** Ars., Zing.

**Menstruation:** Arg-n., Cop., Sep. (See **FEMALE SEXUAL SYSTEM.**)

**Milk:** *Aeth.,* Calc., Carb-v., Mag-c., Mag-m., Nit-ac., Sul-ac., Sulph.

**Nervous, from unpleasant emotions:** Cham., Nux-m., Nux-v.

**Night watching:** Nux-v.

**Pastry:** Ant-c., Carb-v., Ip., Kali-m., Lyc., *Puls.*

**Pork sausage:** Chin., Puls.

**Pregnancy:** Sabad., *Sin-a.,* Thea.

**Salt, abuse of:** Phos.

**Sedentary life:** Nux-v.

**Sweets:** Ant-c., *Arg-n.,* Ip., *Lyc.,* Zinc.

**Tea:** Abies-n., *Chin., Dios.,* Puls., Thea, Thuj.

**Tobacco:** Abies-n., *Nux-v.,* Sep.

**Urticaria:** Cop.

**Vegetables, tobacco:** Ars., Asc-t., Nat-c., Nux-v., *Sep.*

**Water:** Ars.

**Wines, liquors**: *Ant-c.,* Caps., Carb-v., Coff., Nat-s., *Nux-v.,* Sul-ac., Sulph., Zinc.

**TYPE; Atonic, nervous, acid:** Alet., *Alf.,* Alst., *Anac.,* Ang., *Arg-n.,* Calc., Caps., Carb-ac., *Carb-v., Chin.,* Ferr., Grin., Hep., *Ign.,* Jug-c., *Kali-p.,* Lob., *Lyc.,* Mag-c., Nat-c., *Nux-v., Phos., Ptel.,* Quas., Rat., Rob., Sul-ac., Sulph., Valer.

**Catarrhal:** Abies-c., Abies-n., Anis., *Ant-c., Arg-n.,* Bals-p., Calc., Carb-ac., Carb-v., Chin., Coll., Cory., Ger., *Hydr.,* Hydr-ac., *Ip., Kali-bi.,* Lyc., Nux-v., Ox-ac., *Puls.,* Sulph. (See **Chronic Catarrhal Gastritis**.)

**Latent or masked:** Cact., Carb-v., Chin., Hydr-ac., *Nat-m., Sep.,* Spig., Tab.

**SYMPTOMS AND CONDITIONS: Acidity:** Arg-n., *Calc.,* Carb-v., Ign., Lob., Lyc., Nat-c., *Nux-v.,* Puls., *Rob.,* Sulph. (See **Hyperchlorhydria**.)

**Cough:** Lob-s., Tax. (See **RESPIRATORY SYSTEM**.)

**Digestion, weak, slow (bradypepsia):** Alst., *Anac., Ant-c., Arg-n.,* Ars., Asaf., Bism., *Bry.,* Caps., *Carb-an., Carb-v., Chin.,* Coch., Coff., Colch., *Cycl., Dios.,* Eucal., Gran., *Graph., Hydr.,* Ip., Kali-bi., *Lyc.,* Merc., *Nat-c.,* Nat-m., *Nux-v.,* Prun-v., *Puls.,* Zing. (See **Indigestion**.)

**Distress from simplest food:** Alet., Amgd-p., *Ant-c.,* Carb-an., Carb-*v.,* *Chin.,* Dig., *Hep., Kali-c., Lach., Nat-c., Nux-v.,* Puls.

**Drowsiness, sleepiness:** Aeth., Ant-c., Bism., *Carb-v., Chin., Epiph., Fel.,* Graph., Grat., Kali-c., *Lyc., Nat-ch., Nat-m., Nux- m.,* Nux-v., Ph-ac., Phos., Sarr., Staph., Sulph.

**Eructations, belching:** *Abies-n.,* Acet-ac., Agar., Alum., *Anac., Ant-c., Arg-n.,* Arn., *Asaf.,* Bism., *Bry., Caj., Calc.,* Calc-p., Caps., Carb-ac., Carb-an., *Carb-v.,* Cham., *Chin., Cycl., Dios.,* Fago., Ferr., Ferr-p., Glyc., *Graph.,* Grat., *Hep.,* Hydr., Ind., *Iod.,* Ip., Jug-c., Kali-bi., *Kali-c.,* Lob., *Lyc.,* Mag-c., *Mosch., Nat-c.,* Nat-p., Nat-m., Nit-ac., *Nux-m., Nux-v.,* Petr., *Phos.,* Podo., *Puls., Rob.,* Rumx., Sal-ac., Sang., *Sep.,* Sil., Sul-ac., *Sulph.,* Uran-n., Valer.

**Eructations, odorless tasteless, empty:** *Agar.,* Aloe, *Ambr.,* Am-m., Anac., Asar., Bism., Calad., Calc-i., Coca, Cocc., Hep., Ign., *Iod., Olnd.,* Plat.

**Eructations, rancid, putrid, foul:** *Arn.,* Asaf., Bism., Calc-i., *Carb-v.,* *Cham.,* Cycl., Dios., *Graph.,* Hydr., *Kali-c.,* Mag-m., *Mag-s.,* Orni., Plb., Psor., *Puls.,* Raph., Sang., *Sep.,* Sulph., Thuj., Valer., Xero.

**Eructations, relieve temporarily:** *Arg-n.,* Asaf., Bar-c., Bry., Calc., *Carb-v.,* Kali-c., Lach., Mosch., *Nux-m.,* Nux-v., Ol-an., Ox-ac., Puls.

**Eructations, sour, burning, acid, bitter:** Acet-ac., Ant-c., Arg-n., Bry., *Calc.,* Calc-i., Calc-p., Carb-ac., Carb-an., *Carb-v.,* Cham., Chin., *Dios.,* Ferr-p., Fl-ac., Graph., Ip., Hep., *Hydr., Kali-c.,* Lac-ac., Lact., *Lyc.,* Mag-c., *Nat-c.,* Nat-m., Nat-n., *Nat-p., Nit-ac.,* Nit-m-ac., *Nux-v.,* Ox-ac., Petr., Ph-ac., *Phos.,* Podo., *Puls.,* Raph., *Rob.,* Sabal, Sal-ac., Senec., *Sep.,* Sil., Sin-n., *Sul-ac., Sulph.,* Xero.

**Eructations, tasting of ingesta:** *Ant-c., Carb-v.,* Chin., Cycl., *Ferr.,* Graph., *Puls., Sep.,* Sil., Sulph.

**Fainting:** Ars., Chin., Mosch., Nux-m., Nux-v., Ph-ac.

**Flatulent distention of stomach, drum-like:** *Abies-c.,* Agar., Ant-c., Apoc., *Arg-n., Asaf.,* Bry., But-ac., *Caj., Calc.,* Calc-f., Caps., Carb-ac., *Carb-v., Chin., Colch.,* Cycl., Dios., Ferr-ma., *Graph.,* Grat., Hydr., *Ign.,* Indol., Iod., Jug-c., Kali-bi., *Kali-c., Lach., Lyc.,* Mosch., *Nux-m., Nux-v.,* Ox-ac., Ph-ac., Phos., Pop-t., *Puls.,* Sil., Sulph., Thuj. (See **Sensation**.)

**Headache:** Arg-n., *Bry.,* Carb-v., Chin., Cycl., Kali-c., Lach., Lept., *Ign.,* Nat-m., Nux-m., *Nux-v.,* Puls., Rob., *Sang.,* Tarax. (See **HEAD**.)

**Heartburn, pyrosis:** Am-c., Ant-c., Apom., *Arg-n.,* Ars., Bism., *Bry.,* Caj., Calc., Calen., Caps., Carb-ac., *Carb-v.,* Chinin-s., Dat-a., *Dios.,* Fago., Gal-ac., Graph., Iod., Kali-c., Lach., Lob., *Lyc.,* Mag-c., Ph-ac., Mag-m., *Nat-m.,* Nit-ac., Nux-m., *Nux-v.,* Ox-ac., *Puls.,* Rob., Sang., Sin-a., Sin-n., *Sul-ac.,* Tab.

**Hiccough:** Bry., Hyos., Ign., *Nux-v.,* Par., Sep.

**Lassitude, weakness:** Act-sp., Ant-t., *Ars.,* Cann-s., Caps., Carb- an., *Carb-v.,* Chin., Graph., Grat., Hydr., *Lyc., Nux-v.,* Phos., Puls., Sep.

**Mental depression, dullness:** Anac., Chin., Cycl., Hydr., Lyc., Nat-c., Nit ac., *Nux-v.,* Puls., Sep., Tab. (See **MIND**.)

**Nausea, vomiting:** Aeth., *Ant-c.,* Ant-t., *Arg-n., Ars.,* Atro., Bism., *Bry., Carb-ac.,* Carb-v., Cham., Cocc., *Ferr.,* Graph., Ign., *Ip., Kali-bi., Kreos.,* Lept., Lob., Lyc., Nat-c., *Nux-v.,* Petr., Phos., *Puls.,* Rhus-t., *Sang.,* Sep., Sil. (See **Vomiting**.)

**Pain:** *Abies-n.,* Aesc., *Arg-n.,* Arn., *Ars., Bry.,* Calc-i., Calc-m., Carb-v., Chin., Coloc., Cupre-l., Dios., Gamb., *Hed.,* Hom., Ip., Kali-m., Nat-m., *Nux-v.,* Paraf., *Phos.,* Puls., Scutel., Sep., *Stann.,* Thuj. (See **Pain**.)

**Pain immediately after eating:** *Abies-n.,* Arn., Ars., Calc., *Carb-v.,* Chin., Cocc., *Kali-bi., Kali-c., Lyc., Nux-m.,* Phys.

**Pain several hours after eating:** Aesc., *Agar.,* Anac., Bry., Calc-hy., Con., *Nux-v.,* Ox-ac., *Puls.*

**Palpitation of the heart:** Abies-c., *Arg-n., Cact., Carb-v.,* Hydr-ac., Lyc.,

*Nat-m., Nux-v., Puls.,* Sep., *Spig.,* Tab. (See **CIRCULATORY SYSTEM**.)

**Pressure as from a stone:** *Abies-n.,* Acon., Aesc., Anac., *Arg-n.,* Arn., *Ars., Bry., Calc.,* Carb-v., Cham., Chin., Dig., Ferr., Graph., Hep., *Kali-bi.,* Lob., *Lyc., Nux-v.,* Ph-ac., *Phos., Puls.,* Rhus-t., Rumx., Sep., Squil., Sulph.

**Pulsation in epigastrium:** *Asaf.,* Eucal., *Hydr.,* Nat-m., *Puls.,* Sel., *Sep.*

**Pulsation in rectum:** Aloe.

**Regurgitation of food:** Aeth., *Alum.,* Am-m., *Ant-c.,* Asaf., *Carb-v.,* Cham., Chin., Ferr., Ferr-i., Graph., Ign., *Ip.,* Merc., Nat-p., *Nux-v., Phos., Puls.,* Quas., *Sulph.*

**Salivation:** Cycl., Lob., *Merc.,* Nat-m., Puls., Sang. (See **MOUTH**.)

**Sweating:** Carb-v., Nat-m., Nit-ac., Sep.

**Toothache:** Cham., Kali-c., Lyc., Nat-c., Nit-ac.

**Vertigo:** Bry., Carb-v., Chin., Cycl., *Grat.,* Ign., *Nux-v.,* Puls., Rhus- t. (See **HEAD**.)

**Waterbrash:** *Abies-n.,* Acet-ac., *Ant-c.,* Ars., Bism., *Bry.,* Calc., *Carb-v.,* Dios., Fag., Graph., Hep., Hydr., Kali-c., Lac-ac., *Lyc.,* Mag-m., Nat-m., Nit-ac., *Nux-v.,* Podo., *Puls.,* Sep., Sulph., Sym-r., Verat.

**INFLAMMATION (gastritis): Acute:** Acon., Agar-em., *Ant-t., Ars., Bell.,* Bism., Bry., Canth., Ferr-p., Hedeo., *Hydr.,* Hyos., *Ip.,* Iris, *Kali-bi.,* Kali-chl., Merc-c., *Nux-v., Ox-ac., Phos.,* Puls., Santin., Sin-a., *Verat.,* Zinc.

**Inflammation, acute, from alcoholic abuse:** Arg-n., *Ars.,* Bism., Crot-h., *Cupr., Gaul.,* Lach., *Nux-v.,* Phos.

**Inflammation, acute, with intestinal involvement (gastroenteritis):** Alumn., *Arg-n., Ars., Bapt.,* Bism., Bry., *Cupr.,* Merc., Merc-c., *Rhus-t.,* Santin., Zinc.

**Inflammation, chronic (catarrh of stomach):** Alum., Anis., *Ant-c., Ant-t., Arg-n.,* Arn., Ars., *Bism.,* Calc., Calc-chln., Caps., Carb-ac., *Carb-v., Chin., Colch.,* Dig., *Graph., Hydr.,* Hydr-ac., Iod., Ip., *Kali-bi.;* Kali-c., Lyc., *Merc-c., Nux-v.,* Op., Ox-ac., *Phos.,* Podo., *Puls.,* Rumx., Sang., Sep., Sil., Sulph., Verat., Zinc.

**NAUSEA (qualmishness):** *Ant-c., Ant-t., Apoc., Apom., Arg-n., Arn.,* Ars., Asar., Bell., Berb., Bism., *Bry., Cadm-s.,* Carb-ac., *Carb-v.,* Card-m., Casc., Cham., Chel., Chion., *Cocc., Colch., Cupr., Cycl.,* Dig., Eug., Fago., *Ferr.,* Glon., Hed., Hyper., Ichth., *Ip., Iris, Kali-bi., Kali-c.,* Kalm., Kreos., Lac-ac., Lach., *Lob.,* Merc., Merc-c., *Morph.,* Nat-c., Nat-m., *Nux-v.,* Ost., *Petr.,* Podo., *Puls.,* Sabad., Sang., Sarcol-ac., *Sep.,* Spig., *Stry., Sym-r., Tab.,* Ther., *Verat.,* Verat-v.

**Nausea after abdominal operations:** Staph.

**Nausea after eating:** Am-c., Asar., Cycl., Graph., Nux-v., Puls., Sil.

**Nausea before breakfast:** Berb., Goss., Nux-v., *Sep.*
**Nausea from beer:** Kali-bi.
**Nausea from closing eyes:** Lach., *Ther.,* Thuj.
**Nausea from coffee:** Cham.
**Nausea from fat:** Nit-ac.
**Nausea from ices, cold:** Ars.
**Nausea from pessaries:** Nux-m.
**Nausea from looking at moving objects:** Asar., Cocc., Ip., Jab.
**Nausea from immersing hands in warm water:** Phos.
**Nausea from nervousness, emotional excitement:** Mentho.
**Nausea from pregnancy:** Cocc., Con., *Lac-ac.,* Lac-v-c., Lob., Mag-c., *Mag-m.,* Ph-ac., Pilo., Sep., *Staph.,* Stry., Sulph. (See **FEMALE SEXUAL SYSTEM.**)
**Nausea from riding in cars, boat:** Arn., *Cocc., Lac-d., Nux-m.,* Nux-v., *Petr.,* Sanic., Ther.
**Nausea from smell or sight of food:** Aeth., *Ars.,* Cocc., *Colch.,* Nux-v., Puls., *Sep.,* Stann., Sym-r.
**Nausea from smoking:** Euphr., Ign., *Ip.,* Nux-v., *Phos.,* Tab.
**Nausea from sweets:** Graph.
**Nausea from water:** Apoc., Ars., Verat.
**Nausea from water, aerated, champagne:** Dig-ox.
**With cramps:** Trios.
**With desire for stool:** Dulc.
**With diarrhea, anxiety:** Ant-t.
**With drowsiness:** Apoc.
**With faintness:** *Bry., Cocc.,* Colch., Hep., Nux-v., Plat., *Puls.,* Tab., Valer.
**With headache:** *Aloe,* Form., Puls.
**With hunger:** *Berb-a.,* Cocc., Ign., Valer.
**With menses:** *Cocc.,* Crot-h., Sym-r.
**With pain, coldness:** Cadm-s., Hep.
**With pale, twitching face, no relief from vomiting:** Ip.
**With pressure downward, in intestines:** Agn.
**With relief from eating:** *Lac-ac.,* Mez., Santin., *Sep.,* Vib.
**With relief from lemonade:** Cycl., Puls.
**With relief from lying down:** Echi., *Kali-c.,* Puls.
**With relief from smoking:** Eug.
**With relief from swallow of cold water:** Cupr.
**With relief from uncovering abdomen; in open air:** Tab.
**With salivation:** *Ip.,* Petr., Sang.

**With vertigo:** *Cocc.,* Hyos., Lach., Puls., Tab., *Ther.*
**With vision dim:** Mygal.
**With weakness, anxiety, recurs periodically:** Ars.
**Worse after eating:** Asar., Berb-a., Dig., *Ip., Nux-v.,* Puls.
**Worse from least sound or noise:** Ther.
**Worse from motion, rising:** Ars., *Bry.,* Cocc., Sym-r., *Tab.,* Trios., *Verat.*
**Worse in morning:** Anac., Calc., Fago., Carb-v., *Graph.,* Lac-ac., Nat-c., *Nux-v.,* Phos., Puls., *Sep.,* Sil., Sulph.

**NERVOUS DISORDERS:** *Agar.,* Bell., Coloc., *Mag-p., Nux*-v., Sang. (See **Pain.**)

**PAIN (gastrodynia), Type, Aching:** Aesc., Anac., *Hydr.,* Ruta.

**Burning, as from ulcer:** *Acet-ac.,* Agar-em., *Arg-n.,* Arn., *Ars.,* Asaf., Bism., Cadm-br., Canth., *Carb-v., Chinin-ar.,* Colch., Con., *Cund.,* Cyt-l., Dat-a., Form., Graph., *Iod.,* Iris, Kali-i., Lac-ac., Lap-a., Manc., Nat-m., *Nux-v., Ox-ac., Phos.,* Rob., Sep., *Sulph.,* Uran-n. (See **Sensations.**)

**Crampy, contractive, colicky, drawing:** *Abies-n.,* Act-sp., *Agar-ph., Arg-n.,* Bapt., *Bell., Bism.,* But-ac., Cact., Calc., Calc-i., *Carb-v., Cham.,* Cocain., *Cocc., Coloc.,* Con., Cupr., Dat-a., Gran., *Graph., Ign.,* Ip., Jatr., Kali-c., Lob., *Mag-p., Nux-v.,* Petr., Phos., Plat., Ptel., Sep., Verat-v. (See **Sensations.**)

**Cutting, lancinating, stitching, spasmodic, paroxysmal, darting, tearing, shooting:** Acon., Act-sp., *Arg-n., Atro., Bell.,* Bism., *Bry.,* Carb-v., Card-m., Caust., *Chinin-ar., Coloc.,* Con., Cupr., *Cupr-act., Cupr-m., Dios.,* Hydr., Ign., Iris, Kali-c., *Mag-p., Nux-v.,* Ox-ac., Rat., Sep., Sulph., Thal.

**Epigastric (pit of stomach):** *Abies-c., Abies-n.,* Act-sp., Aesc., Aloe, Am-m., Anac., *Arg-n.,* Arn., *Ars.,* Bar-m., *Bell.,* Bism., *Bry.,* Calc., Calc-i., Carb-ac., Carb-v., Cina, Coloc., Cupr., *Dios.,* Graph., *Hydr.,* Jatr., Kali-bi., Kali-c., Kalm., Lob., Lyc., Nat-m., *Nux*-v., Ox-ac., Paraf., *Phos., Sep.,* Sang., Verat.

**Gnawing, hungry like:** *Abies-c.,* Abrot., Aesc., *Agar.,* Am-m., *Anac., Arg-n.,* Asar., *Cina,* Ign., *Iod.,* Lach., Phos., *Puls.,* Ruta, Sep., *Uran-n.* (See **Sensations.**)

**Neuralgic (gastralgia):** Abies-n., Acet-ac., Aesc., Alum., Anac, *Arg-n., Ars., Atro., Bell., Bism., Bry., Carb-v., Cham.,* Chel., *Chinin-ar.,* Cina, *Cocc.,* Cod., Colch., *Coloc.,* Cund., *Cupr-ar.,* Dig., *Dios.,* Ferr., Gels., Glon., *Graph., Hydr ac.,* Ign., *Ip.,* Kali-c., Lob., *Mag-p.,* Mentho., Nicc-met., Nux-m., *Nux-v., Ox-ac.,* Petr., *Plb.,* Ptel., Puls., Quas., Rham-cal., Ruta, Spig., Stann., *Stry.,* Sul-ac., Tab., *Verat.,* Zinc.

**CONCOMITANTS to gastralgia, With anemia:** *Ferr.,* Glon., Graph.
**With backache, anxiety, despondency, sallow face:** Nit-ac.

**With chronic gastritis:** Alum., Atro., Bism., Lyc.
**With chronic ulcer:** Arg-n.
**With constipation:** Bry., Graph., Nux-v., Phys., *Plb.*
**With extension to sides, then to back:** Colch.
**With extension to shoulders:** Nicc.
**With gout:** Colch., Urt-u.
**With hysteria:** Asaf., Ign., Plat.
**With lactation:** Carb-v., Chin.
**With menses:** Arg-n., Cocc.
**With nervous depression:** Arg-n., Gaul., *Nux-v.*
**With pain in throat and spine alternately:** Paraf.
**With pregnancy:** Petr.
**With recurrence:** Graph.
**With uterine disorder:** Borx.
**Sickening pain:** Ost.

**MODALITIES TO PAIN; Aggravation, At night:** Anac., Arg-n., Ars., Cham., Cocc., Ign., Kali-bi.
**From beer:** Bapt., *Kali-bi.*
**From bending forward:** Kalm.
**From coffee:** Canth., Cham., Nux-v., Ox-ac.
**From empty stomach:** *Anac.,* Cina, Hydr-ac., *Petr.*
**From food:** *Arg n.,* Bell., *Bry.,* Ign., Kali-bi., *Nux-v.*
**From food, warm:** Bar-c.
**From jar:** Aloe, *Bell.,* Bry.
**From nursing:** Aeth.
**From pressure:** Arg-n., Calc., Coch., Ign.
**From touch:** Bell., Ign., Nux-v., *Ox-ac.*
**From walking, descending stairs:** Bry.
**From water, cold:** Calc.
**From worms:** *Cina,* Gran.

**AMELIORATION: From bending backward, standing erect:** Bell., *Dios.*
**From drinks, cold:** Bism.
**From drinks, warm:** Graph., Verat-v.
**From eating:** *Anac.,* Brom., Calc-p., *Chel.,* Graph., *Hep.,* Hom., Hydr-ac., Ign., *Iod.,* Kreos., Lach., Nat-m., *Petr.,* Puls., Sep.
**From ice cream:** Phos.
**From pressure:** Bry., Fl-ac., *Plb.*
**From sitting erect:** Kalm.
**From vomiting:** Hyos., Plb.

**PYLORUS: Constriction:** Cann-i., *Chin.,* Hep., *Nux-v., Phos.,* Orni., Sil.

**Induration:** Bism., *Cund.,* Graph., *Phos.,* Sep., *Stry-p.*

**Pain:** All-c., Canth., *Hep.,* Lyc., Merc., *Orni.,* Tus-p., *Uran-n.* (See **Constriction.**)

**SENSATION: Anxiety:** Ars., Kali-c., Nit-ac., Phos., Verat.

**As if stomach were full of dry food:** Calad.

**As if stomach were pressed against spine:** Arn.

**As if stomach were swimming in water:** Abrot.

**Burning heat:** Abies-c., Acet-ac., *Acon., Agar.,* Arg-n., *Ars.,* Bism., Calo., *Canth.,* Carb-ac., *Carb-v.,* Caust., Colch., Coloc., Ferr., Glyc., Graph., Hep., *Iris, Lac-ac.,* Merc-c., Nat-m., *Phos.,* Sang., Sep., *Sulph.,* Ter.

**Coldness:** Abrot., Bov., Calc., Calc-sil., *Camph.,* Chin., *Colch.,* Elaps, Hipp., Kali-c., Kreos., *Meny.,* Ol-an., Ox-ac., Pyrus., Sabad., *Sul-ac.,* Tab., *Verat.*

**Distended, drum-like, tightness, clothing intolerable:** *Abies-c.,* Absin., Agar., *Ambr., Anac.,* Ant-c., *Apoc., Arg-n.,* Ars., Asaf., But-ac., *Caj., Calc.,* Calc-f., *Calc-i.,* Calc-p., Caps., *Carb-ac., Carb-v.,* Cham., Chel., *Chin.,* Cocc., *Colch., Dios.,* Euon., Fel., Ferr., *Graph.,* Grat., Ign., *Kali-c., Lach.,* Lec., Lob., *Lyc.,* Merc-c., Mosch., Nat-ch., Nat-m., Nit-ac., *Nux-m., Nux-v.,* Orni., Pop., *Puls.,* Sulph.

**Empty, faint, sinking, "all gone" feeling:** *Abies-c.,* Anac., Apoc., Asaf., Bapt., *Bar-m.,* Caps., Carb-an., *Carb-v., Cimic., Cocc., Dig., Dios.,* Gels., Graph., *Hydr.,* Hydr-ac., *Ign.,* Kali-c., Kali- p., Lac-c., Lat-m., *Lob.,* Lyc., *Merc.,* Morph., *Murx.,* Orni., Petr., *Phos.,* Ptel., *Puls.,* Rad-met., Sang., *Sep.,* Stann., *Sulph., Tab.,* Tell., Thea, Thuj., Tril-p., Vib.

**Empty feeling, aggravated 11 a.m., unable to wait for lunch:** *Sulph.,* Zinc.

**Empty feeling, relieved by eating:** *Anac., Chel.,* Iod., Nat.c., Mur-ac., Phos., *Sep.,* Sulph.

**Empty feeling, relieved by lying down, wine:** Sep.

**Heaviness, pressure, as from stone or lump:** *Abies-n.,* Acon., *Arg-n.,* Arn., *Ars.,* Bism., *Bry., Calc., Carb-v.,* Cham., *Chin.,* Colch., Dig., Ferr., *Graph., Kali-bi.,* Kali-c., Lob., *Lyc., Nux-v.,* Passi., *Phos.,* Pilo., *Puls.,* Rob., Sang., Sep., Spig., *Sulph.,* Xero., Zing.

**Pulsations, throbbing:** *Arg-n.,* Asaf., *Cact.,* Cic., *Crot-h.,* Eucal., *Hydr.,* Iod., *Kali-c.,* Kali-i., Lach., *Nat-m.,* Olnd., *Puls.,* Rheum.

**Relaxed, hanging down feeling:** Agar., *Hydr.,* Ign., *Ip., Staph.,* Sul-ac., *Tab.*

**Tenderness, to contact, pressure, jars:** *Apis, Arg-n.,* Ars., Bell., Bov., *Bry., Calc.,* Calc-i., Canth., Carb-v., Card-m., *Chin.,* Colch., Dig., *Kali-bi.,* Kali-c., *Lach.*, Lec., Lyc., *Merc.*, *Merc-c.*, Nat-c., Nat-m., Nux-m., *Nux-v.*, Phos., Puls., Sang., Sil., Spig., Stann., Sulph.

**Trembling:** Arg-n., Crot-h.

**SOFTENING (gastro-malacia):** Calc., Kreos., Merc-d.

**THIRST:** *Acet-ac.*, *Acon.*, Alf., Ant-c., Ant-t., Apoc., Arn., *Ars.*, Ars-i., Bell., Berb., Bism., *Bry.*, Camph., *Canth.*, *Caps.*, *Cham.*, Chin., Chinin-ar., Cocc., *Colch.*, Crot-h., Cupr-ar., Dulc., *Eup-per.*, Hell., Helon., Ichth., Indol., Iod., Kali-br., Lac-ac., Laur., Lec., Mag-c., Mag-p., Med., *Merc.*, Merc-c., Morph., *Nat-m.*, Nux-v., Op., Petros., Ph-ac., *Phos.*, Podo., Rhus-a., *Rhus-t.*, Sang., Sec., Sep., Squil., Stram., *Sulph.*, Ter., Thuj., Uran-n., *Verat.*, *Verat-v.*

**Constant sipping of cold water:** *Acon.*, Ant-t., *Ars.*, Hyos., Onos., Sanic.

**Drinks seldom, but much:** *Bry.*, Hell., Podo., *Sulph.*, Verat.

**THIRSTLESSNESS:** *Aeth.*, Ant-t., *Apis*, Berb., Chin., Coff., Cycl., *Gels.*, Hell., Meny., Nux-m., *Puls.*, *Sabad.*, *Sars.*

**ULCER OF STOMACH:** *Arg-n.*, *Ars.*, *Atro.*, Bell., Bism., Calc-ar., Crot-h., Cund., Ferr-act., *Ger.*, Graph., Grin., Ham., *Hydr.*, Iod., Ip., *Kali-bi.*, Kali-i., Kreos., Lyc., Merc., *Merc-c.*, Op., *Orni.*, Petr., *Phos.*, Plb-act., Rat., Sin-a., Symph., *Uran-n.*

**VOMITING, retching: Remedies in general:** Abrot., Acon., *Aeth.*, Agar-ph., Alumn., Amgd-p., *Ant-c.*, *Ant-t.*, Apoc., *Apom.*, *Arg-n.*, *Ars.*, Atro., *Bell.*, *Bism.*, Borx., *Bry.*, Cadm-s., Calc., Calc-m., Camph-mbr., Cann-i., Canth., Caps., *Carb-ac.*, Card-m., Casc., *Cer-ox.*, Cham., Chel., Chin., *Cocc.*, *Colch.*, Cupr., *Cupr-act.*, *Cupr-ar.*, Dros., Eup-per., *Ferr.*, Ferr-m., Ferr-p., Gaul., Ger., Gran., Graph., Iod., *Ip.*, *Iris*, Jatr., *Kali-bi.*, Kali-ox., *Kreos.*, Lac-ac., Lach., *Lob.*, *Mag-c.*, Merc-c., *Morph.*, Nat-m., Nat-p., *Nux-v.*, *Op.*, Petr., *Phos.*, Pix., Plb., *Puls.*, Ric., Sang., Sarcol-ac., *Sep.*, Stann., Strych-af-cit., *Sym-r.*, *Tab.*, Uran-n., Valer., *Verat.*, Xero., Zinc.

**CAUSE; Anger in nursing mother, affecting milk:** Valer.

**Anger, with indignation:** Cham., Coloc., Staph.

**Beer:** Cupr., Ip., *Kali-bi.*

**Bowels impacted:** Op., Plb., Pyrog.

**Cancer (hepatic, gastric, uterine):** Carb-ac., Kreos.

**Cerebral:** Apom., Bell., Glon., Plb.

**Clearing throat of mucus in morning:** Bry., Euphr.

**Climacteric:** Aqui.

**Closing eyes:** Ther.

**Cyclic, in infants:** Cupr-ar., Ing., Iris, Kreos., Merc-d.

**Drinks, cold, can only retain hot drinks:** Apoc., *Ars.*, Ars-i., Calad., Casc.,

*Chel.,* Verat.

**Drinks of any kind:** Acon., Apoc., Ant-t., *Ars., Bism., Canth.,* Dulc., *Eup-per.,* Ip., Sanic., Sil., *Verat.*

**Drinks, warm:** *Bry., Phos., Puls.,* Pyrog., Sanic.

**Drunkards in morning:** Ant-t., Ars., Carb-ac., Cupr., *Cupr-ar.,* Ip., Lob., *Nux-v.*

**Eating, drinking:** Acet-ac., *Ant-c.,* Ant-t., *Ars.,* Bism., *Bry.,* Calc-m., Cina, Colch., Crot-h., *Ferr.,* Ferr-p., Hyos., Iod., *Ip.,* Lyc., Nux-v., *Phos., Puls.,* Sil., *Verat.,* Verat-v.

**Eruptions repercussed:** Cupr.

**Gastric irritation:** Ant.c., *Ars.,* Bism., Ferr., Ip., Nux-v., Phos., Puls., Verat.

**Hysterical:** *Aqui.,* Ign., *Kreos.,* Plat., Valer.

**Lying on any side, except right:** Ant-t.

**Lying on right side or back:** Crot-h.

**Menses, after:** Crot-h. (See **FEMALE SEXUAL SYSTEM**.)

**Milk:** *Aeth.,* Ars., Calc., Ferr., Kreos., Mag-c., Mag-m., Merc., Merc-d.

**Motion:** *Bry., Cocc., Colch.,* Dig., Nux-v., *Tab.,* Ther., *Verat.*

**Phthisis:** Kali-br., Kreos.

**Post-operative (laparotomy):** Aeth., *All-c., Bism., Nux-v., Phos.,* Staph., *Stry.*

**Pregnancy:** Acet-ac., Alet., *Amgd-p.,* Ant-t., *Apom.,* Ars., Bism., Carb-ac., *Cer-ox.,* Cocain., *Cocc., Cod.,* Cuc-p., *Cupr-act.,* Ferr., Goss., Graph., Ign., Ing., *Ip.,* Iris, *Kreos., Lac-ac.,* Lac-d., Lob., *Mag-c., Nux-v.,* Petr., Phos., Psor., Puls., *Sep.,* Stront-br., Stry., Sym-r., *Tab.*

**Pressure on spine and cervical region:** Cimic.

**Raising head:** Apom., *Bry.,* Stram.

**Reflex:** Apom., Cer., Cocc., *Ip.,* Kreos., *Valer.*

**Renal origin:** Kreos., Nux-v.

**Riding in cars:** Arn., *Cocc.,* Ip., Kreos., Nux-v., Petr., Sanic., Sil.

**Scarlet fever:** Ail., *Bell.*

**Sea sickness; car sickness:** *Apom.,* Ars., Borx., Carb-ac., Cer., Cocc., Coff., Glon., Ip., *Kreos.,* Nicot., *Nux-v.,* Op., *Petr.,* Sep., *Staph.,* Tab., Ther.

**Water, sight of, must close eyes while bathing:** Lyss., Phos.

**TYPE: Acid, sour:** Ant-c., Ars., Bry., Calad., *Calc.,* Card-m., *Cham., Ferr.,* Ferr-p., Iod., *Iris,* Kali-c., Lac-ac., Lac-d., *Lyc.,* Mag-c., *Nat-p., Nat-s., Nux-v.,* Puls., *Rob.,* Sul-ac., Sulph.

**Bilious (green, yellow):** *Acon.,* Aeth., Ant-c., Ant-t., Ars., Bell., *Bry.,* Carb-ac., *Card-m., Cham., Chel.,* Crot-h., Eup-a., *Eup-per.,* Grat., Ip., *Iris,* Kali-c., Lept., Nux-v., Nyct., Petr., *Podo.,* Puls., Rob., *Sang.,* Sep., Tart-ac.

**Black:** *Ars., Cadm-s., Crot-h.,* Manc., Pix.

**Bloody:** *Acon.,* Arg-n., *Ars.,* Both., Cadm-s., *Canth.,* Crot-h., Ferr., *Ferr-p.,* Fic-r., *Ger., Ham., Ip.,* Iris, Mez., *Phos., Sec.* (See **Hematemesis.**)

**Coffee grounds, like:** *Ars.,* Cadm-s., *Crot-h.,* Lach., *Merc-c.,* Orni., Pyrog., Sec.

**Fecal:** Op., Plb., Pyrog., Raph.

**Food, undigested:** *Ant-c.,* Apoc., Atro., Bals-p., Bism., *Bry.,* Cer., *Chin.,* Colch., Cupr., *Ferr., Ferr-m.,* Ferr-p., Graph., *Ip.,* Iris, Kreos., Lac-c., Nux-v., Petr., Phos., *Puls.,* Sang., Stry-af-cit., Verat.

**Milk, coagula:** *Aeth.,* Ant-c., *Calc.,* Ip., *Mag-c.,* Mag-m., Merc., Merc-d., Podo., Sanic., *Valer.*

**Mucus slimy:** Aeth., Ant-c., *Ant-t., Arg-n.,* Ars., Bals-p., Cadm-s., Carb-v., Colch., *Ip.,* Iris, Jatr., *Kali-bi.,* Kali-m., Kreos., Merc-c., Nux-v., Ox-ac., Petr., *Puls.,* Verat., Zinc.

**Watery:** Abrot., *Ars.,* Bism., Bry., *Euph.,* Euph-c., Iod., Iris, *Kreos.,* Lac-c., *Mag-c.,* Olnd., Verat.

**Yeast, like:** Nat-c., Nat-s.

**CONCOMITANTS: With abdominal rumbling:** Podo.

**With appetite:** Iod., Lob.

**With bowels obstructed, impacted:** Op., Plb., Pyrog.

**With chilliness:** Ars., Dulc., Puls., Tab.

**With cholera:** Ars., Camph. (See **ABDOMEN.**)

**With chronic tendency:** Lob.

**With clavus, fickle appetite, salivation, copious lemon colored urine:** Ign.

**With colic, cramps:** Bism., *Cupr., Cupr-ar.,* Op., Plb., Pix., Sarr., *Verat.* (See **ABDOMEN.**)

**With collapse, weakness:** Aeth., *Ant-t., Ars.,* Cadm-s., Crot-h., Euph-c., *Lob., Tab., Verat.,* Verat-v.

**With constipation:** Nux-v., Op., Plb.

**With depression of spirits:** Nux-v.

**With diarrhea:** Ars., Bism., Calc., Cham., Cupr., *Cupr-ar., Ip.,* Iris, Kreos., Merc-c., Phos., Pulx., Puls., Res., *Verat.* (See **ABDOMEN.**)

**With drowsiness:** *Aeth., Ant-t.,* Ip., Mag-c.

**With fear, heat, thirst, profuse urine and sweat:** Acon.

**With fruitless, anxious retching:** Ars., Bism., Cupr., Podo.

**With headache:** Apom., Iris, Petr. (See **HEAD.**)

**With heart, weak:** Ars., Camph., *Dig.*

**With intervals of days between attacks:** Bism.
**With midnight occurrence; can eat at once after emptying stomach:** Ferr.
**With nausea:** *Aeth.,* Amgd-p., Ant-t., Bry., *Ip.,* Iris, *Lob., Nux-v.,* Petr., *Puls.,* Sang., Sym-r., Verat. (See **Nausea.**)
**With relief of symptoms:** Ant-t., Puls.
**With relief from eating, drinking:** Anac., Tab.
**With relief from cold drinks:** Cupr., *Phos.,* Puls.
**With relief from hot drinks:** Ars., Chel.
**With relief from lying down:** Bry., Colch., Nux-v., Sym-r.
**With relief from lying on right side:** Ant-t.
**With relief from uncovering abdomen; in fresh open air:** Tab.
**With salivation:** Graph., Ign., *Ip.,* Iris, Kreos., Lac-ac., *Lob.,* Puls., Tab.
**With spasms:** *Cupr.,* Hyos., Op.
**With tongue clean:** Cina, Dig., *Ip.*
**With vertigo:** Cocc., Ign., *Nux-v., Tab.*

# ABDOMEN

**APPENDICITIS** (See **Typhilitis.**)

**BURNING heat:** Abies-c., *Acon., Aloe,* Alst., Ant-c., *Apis,* Arg-n., *Ars., Bell.,* Bry., Camph., *Canth.,* Carb-v., Colch., Crot-h., *Iris,* Kali-bi., *Lim.,* Lyc., *Merc-c.,* Nat-s., Nux-v., *Ox-ac.,* Ph-ac., *Phos.,* Podo., Rhus-t., Sang., Sec., Sep., Sulph., Verat.

**CAECUM, affections of:** Ars., *Lach.,* Rhus-v., Verat-v. (See **Appendicitis, Typhilitis.**)

**COLDNESS:** *Aeth.,* Ambr., Aur., Cadm-s., *Calc.,* Camph., Caps., *Chin., Colch.,* Elaps, Grat., *Kali-br., Kali-c.,* Lach., *Meny.,* Phel., Phos., Sec., Sep., *Tab., Verat.*

**COLIC; PAIN, Remedies in general:** *Acon.,* Adren., Aloe, Alum., Anis., *Arg-n.,* Arn., *Ars.,* Bar-c., *Bell., Bry., Caj., Calc-p.,* Carb-ac., Carb-v., *Cham., Chin.,* Chinin-ar., Cic., *Cina, Cocc.,* Coff., Coll., *Colch., Coloc.,* Crot-t., *Cupr., Cupr-act.,* Cycl., Dig., *Dios., Elat.,* Fil., *Gamb.,* Grat., *Ign., Ip.,* Iris, *Iris-t., Jal.,* Lept., *Lim.,* Lyc., *Mag-c., Mag-p.,* Mentho., Merc., *Merc-c., Morph.,* Nat-s., *Nux-v.,* Onis., *Op.,* Ox-ac., Paraf., *Plat., Plb.,* Plb-act., Plb-chr., Podo., Polyg-h., *Puls.,* Raph., *Rheum, Rhus-t.,* Sabin., Samb., Sars., *Senn.,* Sep., *Sil., Sin-n., Stann.,* Staph., Stry., Thuj., *Verat., Vib.,* Zinc.

**CAUSE AND NATURE, Alternates with vertigo:** Coloc., Spig.

**Babies' colic:** Aeth., All-c., *Anis.,* Asaf., Bell., Calc-p., Catar., *Cham., Cina,* Coloc., Jal., Kali-br., Lyc., *Mag-p.,* Menth., Nepet., Rheum, Senn., Staph.

**Biliary, gall stone colic:** Atro., Bell., *Berb.,* Bry., *Calc.,* Card-m., Cham., *Chin.,* Chion., Coloc., Dios., Ip., Iris, Lyc., Menth., Morph-act., Podo., Ric., Ter., Trios. (See **Gall bladder**.)

**Chronic tendency:** Lyc., Staph.

**Flatulent colic:** Absin., Agar., Alf., *Aloe, Anis., Arg-n.,* Asaf., *Bell.,* But-ac., *Caj.,* Calc-p., *Carb-v.,* Carbn-s., *Cham., Chin.,* Cina, *Cocc.,* Coloc., *Dios.,* Hydr-ac., Ip., Iris, *Lyc., Mag-p.,* Mentho., *Nux-v.,* Op., Plb., *Polyg-h.,* Puls., Rad-br., *Raph.,* Rob., Sang., *Senn.,* Zinc.

**From anger:** *Cham.,* Coloc., Staph.

**From carriage riding:** Carb-v., Cocc.

**From cold:** Acon., All-c., Cham., Coloc., Nux-v.

**From eating cheese:** Coloc.

**From eating cucumber salad:** All-c.

**From gastric disorder:** Carb-v., *Chin.,* Coloc., Dios., Ip., Lyc., *Nux-v., Puls.*

**From lithotomy, ovariotomy, attending abdominal section:** Bism., Hep., Nux-v., Raph., *Staph.*

**From uncovering:** Nux-v., Rheum.

**From wet feet:** All-c., Cham., Doli., Dulc.

**From worms:** Art-v., Bism., *Cina,* Fil., Gran., *Indg.,* Merc., Nat-p., Sabad., Spig.

**Hemorrhoidal:** *Aesc.,* All-c., Coloc., *Nux-v.,* Puls., Sulph.

**Hysterical:** Alet., *Asaf.,* Caj., Cocc., *Ign.,* Valer.

**Menstrual:** Bell., Castm., Cham., *Cocc.,* Coloc., Puls. (See **FEMALE SEXUAL ORGANS.**)

**Neuralgic, enteralgic:** Alumn., Ant-t., Ars., *Atro., Bell.,* Cham., *Cocc., Coloc.,* Cupr., Cupr-ar., *Dios.,* Euph., Hydr-ac., Hyos., Kali-c., *Mag-p., Nux-v.,* Op., *Plb.,* Plb-act., Santin., Tab., Verat., Zinc. (See **Type of Pain.**)

**Renal:** *Berb.,* Calc., Dios., Ery-a., *Lyc., Morph-act.,* Oci., Sars., *Tab., Ter.* (See **URINARY SYSTEM.**)

**Rheumatic:** Caust., Coloc., Dios., Phyt., Verat.

**Toxic (lead, copper):** *Alum.,* Alumn., Bell., Ferr., Nat-s., Nux-m., Nux-v., *Op.,* Plat., Sulph., Verat.

**LOCATION: Abdominal muscles:** Acon., *Arn.,* Bell., *Bell-p., Cupr.,* Ham., Mag-m., Nat-n., Plb., *Rhus-t.,* Stry., Sulph.

**Abdominal ring:** Cocc., Graph., Mez., *Nat-m.,* Nux-v., Stront-c.

**Ascending colon:** Rhus-t.

**Groins:** Alum., Am-m., Merc-c., Podo.

**Hypochondria:** Carb-v., *Chin.,* Dios., *Nux-v.,* Pyrus., Sep. (See **Type of Pain.**)

**Hypogastrium:** All-c., *Aloe, Bell.,* Bism., Cocc., *Dios.,* Eucal., Ham., Kali-c., *Lyc.,* Mag c., *Nux-v.,* Pall., Paraf., Plat., *Sabin.,* Sep., Sulph., Trom., Verat-v. (See **SEXUAL SYSTEM.**)

**Ileo-caecal:** Aloe, Bell., Bry., Coff., Ferr-p., *Gamb.,* Iris-t., Kali-m., Lim., Mag-c., *Merc., Merc-c.,* Plb., Rad-met., Rhus-t. (See **Appendicitis.**)

**Inguinal:** Am-m., Ars., Calc., Graph., Sep.

**In small spots:** Bry., Coloc., *Ox-ac.*

**Transverse colon:** *Bell.,* Cham., Colch., Merc-c., Raph.

**Umbilical (about navel):** *Aloe, Benz-ac.,* Berb., *Bov., Bry.,* Calc-p., Carb-v., *Cham.,* Chel., *Cina, Coloc., Dios., Dulc., Gamb., Gran.,* Hyper., Indg., *Ip., Kali-bi.,* Lept., Lyc., *Nux-m.,* Nux-v., Plat., *Plb.,* Puls., Raph., *Rheum,* Senec., *Spig., Stann.,* Sulph., *Verat.,* Verb., Vip.

**TYPE OF PAIN: Bruised:** Aeth., All-s., *Apis,* Apoc., *Arn.,* Ars., *Bell-p.,* Bry.,

Carb-v., Coloc., *Con.,* Eucal., Ferr., *Ham., Merc-c.,* Nat-s., Nit-ac., *Nux-v.,* Phyt., Puls., *Sulph.*

**Colicky, crampy, constricting, cutting, gripping, pinching:** *Acon.,* Aesc., Agar., *Aloe,* Ant-t., Arge., Arg-cy., *Arg-n.,* Arn., Asaf., *Bell.,* Bism., Bry., *Calc-p.,* Catar., *Cham., Chin., Cina, Cocc., Coloc., Colch.,* Con., Crot-t., Cupr., *Cupr-ar., Dios., Dulc., Elat.,* Eup-per., Fil., *Gamb.,* Grat., *Hyper.,* Ign., Iod., *Ip.,* Iris, *Jal., Jatr.,* Kali-bi., Kali-c., Lach., Lept., *Lyc., Mag-c., Mag-p., Merc-c.,* Nat-s., Nicc., Nit-ac., *Nux-v.,* Phos., Phyt., *Plb-act.,* Plb-chr., *Polyg-h.,* Puls., Rad-br., Raph., *Rheum,* Sabin., Sec., *Sep.,* Spig., *Stann.,* Stry., Sulph., Trom., *Verat.,* Vib., Zinc.

**Pressing, plug-like:** *Aloe,* Alum., *Anac., Bell.,* Bry., *Cocc.,* Hyos., Kali-c., Mez., *Nux-v.,* Oena., *Plat.,* Plb., Puls., Ran-s., Sabin., *Sep.*

**Pulsating, bubbling:** Aeth., *Aloe,* Bar-m., *Bell., Berb.,* Calc., Ign., Sang., Sel., Tarax.

**Radiating, shooting, darting, teating, spasmodic:** *Acon.,* Arge., *Bell., Bry.,* Calc., *Cham., Cocc.,* Coch., *Coloc.,* Cupr-act., *Cupr-ar., Dios.,* Graph., Ip., Kali-c., *Lyc., Mag-p.,* Merc., Morph., *Nux-v.,* Ox-ac., Paraf., Plat., *Plb.,* Podo., Puls., Sulph. (See **Enteralgia.**)

**Stitching:** Agar., Apis, Arn., *Bell., Bry.,* Chinin-ar., Hep., *Kali-c.,* Lach., Spig.

**CONCOMITANTS; Abdomen retracted, as if drawn by string:** Chel., *Plb.,* Podo., Tab.

**Abdomen, retracted, tense, scanty urine, desire to stretch:** Plb.

**Abdomen swollen, pad-like:** *Bell.,* Raph.

**Agitation, chill ascending from hypogastrium to cheeks:** Coloc.

**Alternates with coryza:** Calc.

**Alternates with delirium and pain in atrophied limbs:** Plb.

**Alternates with vertigo:** Coloc., Spig.

**Backache:** Cham., *Lyc.,* Morph., Puls., Samb.

**Cheeks red, hot sweat:** Cham.

**Chilliness:** Nux-v., Puls.

**Collapse:** Aeth., Camph., Cupr., *Verat.*

**Constipation:** All-s., *Aloe, Alum.,* Cocc., Coll., Grat., Lyc., *Nux-v.,* Op., *Plb-act.,* Sil.

**Convulsions:** Bell., Cic.

**Cramps in calves:** Coloc., *Cupr-act.,* Plb., Podo.

**Delirium alternating:** Plb.

**Diarrhea:** Ars., Cham., *Coloc.,* Mag-c., Polyg-h., Puls., Samb., Verat.

**Empty feeling, heat, faintness:** *Cocc.,* Hydr.

**Hands yellow, blue nails:** Sil.

**Hiccough, suffocative, in chest and stomach:** Verat.
**Hunger, yet refuses food:** Bar-c.
**Itching of nose, pale, bluish face:** *Cina,* Fil.
**Nausea, frequent, watery, slimy stools:** Cham., Samb.
**Pain and aching in thighs:** Coloc.
**Painful contraction in limbs following:** Abrot.
**Periodical recurrence:** Anis., Aran., *Chin.,* Dios., Kali-br.
**Pulsation in abdominal aorta, epigastric constriction:** Dig.
**Red urine:** Bov., *Lyc.*
**Restlessness, twitching and turning for relief:** Coloc.
**Rumbling of flatus, nausea, liquid feces:** Polyg-h.
**Scanty stools, flatus without relief:** Cina.
**Sour stools:** Rheum.
**Tenesmus (pelvic):** Staph.
**Tossing about, anxiety, no relief from flatus:** *Cham.,* Mag-p.
**Urging to stool:** *Aloe,* Chin., Lept., Nat-s., *Nux-v.,* Op.
**Urine suppressed:** Acon., Plb-act.
**Vomiting:** *Bell.,* Cadm-s., Plb-act.
**Vomiting, hiccough, belching, screaming:** Hyos.
**Yawning, spasmodic, drowsiness:** Spira.

**MODALITIES; Aggravation, about 4 p.m.-5 p.m.:** Coloc., Kali-br., *Lyc.*
**After midnight:** *Ars.,* Cocc.
**At night, after supper:** Grat.
**At night:** Cham., Chin., Cocc., Senn., Sulph.
**From bending, coughing:** Ars., Bell., *Bry.,* Nat-m.
**From bending forward:** Ant-t., *Dios.,* Sin-n.
**From bending forward, lying down, pressure:** Acon., *Dios.*
**From drinking:** Coloc., Sulph.
**From drinking cold water:** Cupr.
**From eating:** Bar-c., *Calc-p.,* Chin., *Coloc.,* Kali-bi., *Nux-v., Psor.,* Zinc.
**From jar, pressure:** Acon., Aloe, *Bell.,* Plb.
**From motion, relief from lying on side:** Bry., Cocc.
**From smoking:** Meny.
**From sweets:** Fil.
**From touch, pressure, motion:** Bry.
**From uncovering arm, leg; standing:** Rheum.
**From warmth, at night:** Cham.

**AMELIORATION: From bending double:** Bov., Chin., *Coloc., Mag-p.,* Podo.,

Sep., *Stann.,* Sulph., Verat.

**From eating:** Bov., Hom.

**From flatus voided per ano:** Aloe, *Carb-v., Chin.,* Cocc., *Coloc.,* Nat-s., Sulph.

**From hot applications or warmth:** Ars., Coloc., *Mag-p.,* Podo., Puls., Sil.

**From lying with knees drawn up:** Lach.

**From pressure:** *Coloc., Mag-p.,* Nit-ac., Plb., Rhus-t., *Stann.*

**From rubbing:** Plb.

**From rubbing, warmth:** Mag-p.

**From sitting erect:** Sin-n.

**From sitting, lying down:** Nux-v.

**From stool:** Aloe, Coloc., Tanac., Verat.

**From straightening body backward or moving about:** Dios.

**From walking about:** All-c., Dios., Mag-p., Puls., *Rhus-t.,* Verat.

**From walking bent over:** Aloe, *Coloc.,* Nux-v., Rhus.t.

**From warm soup:** Acon.

**FLATULENCY; Distention, fullness, heaviness, meteorism, tympanites:** *Abies-n., Abrot.,* Absin., *Acet-ac.,* Acon., Agar., Alf., *Aloe, Anis.,* Ant-c., Apis, *Arg-n.,* Ars., *Asaf.,* Bar-c., *Bell.,* Bov., *Caj., Calc.,* Calc-i., Carb-ac., *Carb-v., Cham.,* Chel., *Chin.,* Cina, *Cocc., Colch.,* Coll., *Coloc.,* Cupr., *Dios.,* Graph., *Ictod.,* Ign., Indol., Iris, *Kali-c., Lach., Lim., Lyc., Mag-c., Mag-p.,* Merc., Merc-c., Mom-b., Mosch., Mur-ac., Napht., Nat-c., Nat-m., *Nat-n., Nat-s., Nux m., Nux-v.,* Onis., *Op., Opun-f., Orni., Ph-ac.,* Podo., *Puls.,* Rad-br., *Raph.,* Rheum, Rhod., *Rhus g.,* Rhus-t., Sars., *Senn., Sep., Sil.,* Stront-c., Sulph., Sumb., *Tarax., Ter.,* Thea, *Thuj.,* Uran-n., Valer., Xan., Zing.

**Flatulence, hysterical:** Alet., *Ambr.,* Arg-n., *Asaf.,* Caj., Cham., Cocc., Ictod., *Ign.,* Kali-p., *Nux m.,* Plat., *Sumb.,* Tarax., Thea, *Valer.*

**Flatulence, incarcerated in flexures:** Am-c., Aur., Bell., Calc., Calc-p., Carb-ac., *Carb-v., Cham., Chin.,* Colch., *Coloc., Graph.,* Hep., Ign., Kali-c., Lim., *Lyc., Mom-b., Nux-v.,* Pall., Phos., Plb., *Puls., Raph.,* Rhus-g., Rob., Staph., Sulph., Thuj.

**Flatulence, offensive, per ano:** *Aloe,* Arn., Bry., *Carb-v.,* Ferr-ma., Graph., Olnd., Sil.

**Flatulence, post operative, no relief from passing it:** Chin.

**Gurgling, rumbling, borborygmus:** *Aloe,* Apoc., Ars., Bapt., Bell., Carb-v., Carbn-s., *Cham.,* Chin., *Cina, Colch.,* Coloc., Conv., Cupr-ar., Crot-t., *Dios., Gamb.,* Glyc., *Graph.,* Grat., Hep., Ip., *Jatr.,* Kali-c., *Lyc.,* Merc., *Nat-s.,* Nux-v., Olnd., *Ph- ac.,* Podo., Puls., Ric., *Rumx.,* Sanic.,

Sep., Sil., Thea, Xero.

**Hardness:** Abrot., Anac., *Bar-c., Calc.,* Carb-v., Chin., *Cina,* Cupr., *Graph., Lyc.,* Nat-c., Nux-v., Op., *Plb-act., Raph., Sil.,* Sulph., Thuj.

**Jumping, as of living thing:** Arund., Brach., Bran., *Croc.,* Cycl., Nux-m., *Op.,* Sabad., Sulph., *Thuj.*

**LARGE, in girls at puberty:** Calc., *Graph.,* Lach., Sulph.

**pendulous in women who have borne many children:** Aur., Aur-m., Bell., Frax., *Helon.,* Phos., *Sep.*

**pot bellied, flabby:** Am-m., *Calc., Calc-p.,* Mez., Podo., Sanic., Sars., *Sep., Sil.,* Sulph., Thuj.

**protrudes here and there:** Croc., Nux-m., Sulph., Thuj.

**RETRACTED, sunken, scow-shaped:** *Calc-p.,* Euph., Iodof., Kali-bi., *Kali-br., Plb., Plb-act.,* Plb-chr., Podo., Ptel., Quas., *Zinc.*

**SENSITIVE, tender to touch, pressure:** Acet-ac., *Acon.,* Aloe, *Apis, Arg-n., Arn.,* Ars., Bapt., *Bell., Bov., Bry.,* Calc., *Carb-v.,* Card-m., Chin., Coff., Coloc., Con., Cupr., Euon., Ferr., Gamb., *Graph., Ham.,* Hed., Hell., Kali-bi., *Lach., Lyc., Merc-c.,* Mur- ac., Nux-v., Podo., *Ran-b.,* Rhus-t., *Sep.,* Sil., *Sumb.,* Sulph., *Ter., Verat.,* Vib.

**SPOTS, brown:** Caul., *Lyc.,* Phos., *Sep.,* Thuj.

**red:** Hyos. (See **SKIN.**)

**TREMBLING in:** Lil-t.

**WEAK, as if diarrhea would ensue:** *Aloe,* Ant-c., Ap-g., Borx., Crot- t., Eucal., Ferr., Form., Nux-v., *Opun.,* Ran-s. (See **Diarrhea**.)

**empty, sinking, relaxed feeling:** Abrot., Acet-ac., *Arn.,* Alst., Ant-c., Cham., *Cocc.,* Euph., Glyc., *Hydr., Ign., Opun.,* Petr., Phys., *Phos.,* Plb-act., *Podo.,* Quas., *Sep., Stann.,* Staph., Sul-ac., Sulfon., *Verat.*

**ANUS; RECTUM, Abscess (peri-rectal):** Calc-s., Rhus-t., Sil.

**Burning, smarting, heat:** Abies-c., *Aesc.,* All-c., *Aloe,* Alum., Alumn., Ambr., Am-m., Ant-c., Aphis, *Ars.,* Bell., Berb., *Canth., Caps., Carb-v., Coll.,* Con., Eucal., Euon., *Gamb.,* Graph., Ham., Hydr., *Iris,* Jug-c., Jug-r., Kali-c., Merc., *Nat-m.,* Nit-ac., *Olnd.,* Paeon., Prun., *Rat.,* Rheum, Sangin-n., Senn., *Sulph.,* Trom.

**Burning before and during stool:** Aloe, Am-m., Ars., Coloc., Con., *Hydr., Iris,* Jug-c., Merc., Ol-an., Rheum.

**Burning after stool:** Aesc., Alumn., Am-m., Aphis., *Ars.,* Aur., Berb., *Canth., Caps., Carb-v., Gamb., Nat-m.,* Nit-ac., Ol-an., *Paeon.,* Prun., *Rat.,* Sil., *Stront-c., Sulph.*

**Congestion:** *Aesc., Aloe,* Alum., *Coll.,* Hyper., Nat-m., Nit-ac., Sabin., *Sep., Sulph.*

**ERUPTIONS, growths; Cancer, scirrhus of, also sigmoid; intolerable pains:**

Alumn., Phyt., Spig.

**Condylomata:** Benz-ac., Kali-br., *Nit-ac., Thuj.*

**Eczema:** Berb., Graph., *Merc-pr-r.* (See **SKIN**.)

**Eminences, studding interior:** Polyg-h.

**Fissures, rhagades, excoriations, ulcerations, soreness, rawness:** *Aesc.*, Agn., *Aloe,* Apis, Arg-n., *Ars., Calc-f., Carb-v.,* Caust., Cimx., *Cund., Graph.,* Ham., *Hydr., Ign.,* Iris, Kali-i., Lach., Led., Merc., *Merc-d.,* Morph., Mur-ac., *Nat-m., Nit-ac.,* Nit-m-ac., *Paeon., Petr.,* Phos., Phyt., Plat., *Plb., Rat.,* Rhus-t., Sangin-n., Sanic., *Sed-ac.,* Sep., *Sil.,* Sulph., Syph., *Thuj.,* Vib.

**Fistula in ano:** Aur-m., Bar-m., *Berb., Calc-p.,* Calc-s., Carb-v., *Caust., Fl-ac.,* Graph., Hydr., Lach., Myris., *Nit-ac.,* Nux-v., *Paeon.,* Phos., Querc., Rat., *Sil.,* Sulph., Thuj.

**Fistula in ano alternates with chest disorders:** Berb., Calc-p., *Sil.*

**Pockets:** Polyg-h.

**Rash, fiery red in babies:** Med.

**Hemorrhage (enterrhagia):** Acal., Acet-ac., *Aesc.,* Aloe, Alum., *Alumn.,* Arn., *Cact., Carb-v.,* Casc., Chin., *Cinnm.,* Cob., Cocain., Crot-h., Erig., *Ham.,* Ign., *Ip.,* Kali-c., *Lach.,* Lycps-v., Mangi., Merc-cy., *Mill., Mur-ac.,* Nat-m., *Nit-ac.,* Ph-ac., *Phos.,* Sed-ac., Sep., Sul-ac., Sulph., *Ter.,* Thuj.

**Hemorrhage during stool:** Alum., *Alumn.,* Carb-v., Ign., Iod., *Ip., Kali-c., Phos.,* Psor., Sep.

**Inflammation (proctitis):** *Aesc., Aloe,* Alum., Ambr., *Ant-c.,* Colch., *Coll., Merc.,* Merc-c., *Nit-ac.,* Paeon., *Phos., Podo.,* Ric., Sabal, Zing.

**Inflammation, syphilitic:** Bell., Merc., *Nit-ac.,* Sulph.

**Itching (pruritus):** Acon., *Aesc.,* Aloe, *Alum., Ambr., Anac., Ant-c., Bar-c.,* Bov., Cadm-i., *Calc.,* Carb-v., Casc., *Caust., Cina, Coll.,* Cop., Ferr., *Ferr-i.,* Gran., Graph., Hom., *Ign., Indg., Lyc., Med., Nit-ac., Paeon.,* Petr., Phos., Pin-s., Plat., Polyg-h., Rad-br., Rat., Rumx., Sabad., *Sacch.,* Sangin-n., Sep., *Spig.,* Staph., *Sulph., Tell.,* Ter., *Teucr.,* Uran-n., Zinc.

**Moisture:** Aloe, Am-m., *Anac., Ant-c.,* Bar-c., *Calc., Carb-v.,* Caust., Graph., *Hep.,* Med., Nit-ac., Nit-m-ac., Paeon., Phos., Rat., *Sep., Sil.,* Sul-ac.

**Operations on, to be given preceding:** Coll.

**PAIN, Aching:** *Aesc.,* Alet., Alumn., Coll., Graph., Lyc., *Rat.*

**Bearing down, pressing:** *Aloe,* Alum., Aphis., Ars., *Cact.,* Cean., Euphr., Hyper., Kali-c., Lach., *Lil-t.,* Med., Op., Prun., *Sep.,* Sul-ac., *Sulph.,* Xero.

**Contraction, spasmodic:** *Aesc.,* Aesc-g., Anac., Arg-n., *Bell.,* Cact., *Caust.,*

Coll., Ferr., Grat., Hydr., *Ign., Lach.,* Lyc., *Med.,* Meli., Merc., Mez., *Nat-m., Nit-ac.,* Nit-m-ac., *Nux-v., Plb-act., Rat.,* Sanic., *Sed-ac.,* Sep., *Syph.,* Tab., Verb.

**Lancinating, even after soft stool:** *Alumn.,* Nat-m., *Nit-ac., Rat.*

**Long lasting, after stool:** *Aesc.,* Aloe, Alumn., Am-m., *Graph., Hydr., Ign.,* Merc-cy., *Mur-ac., Nat-m., Nit-ac.,* Paeon., *Rat., Sed-ac.,* Sep., *Sil.,* Sulph., Thuj., Vib.

**Neuralgic (proctalgia):** *Atro.,* Bar-m., *Bell.,* Colch., *Crot-t.,* Ign., Kali-c., Lach., Lyc., Ox-ac., Phos., Plb., *Stry.,* Tarent.

**Splinter-like, pricking, stinging, stitching, cutting, shooting:** Acon., *Aesc.,* All-c., Alum., Am-m., Bell., Caust., *Coll., Ign., Kali-c., Lach.,* Lyc., Merc., Mez., *Nat-m., Nit-ac.,* Plat., *Rat.,* Ruta, *Sep.,* Sil., *Sulph.,* Thuj.

**Throbbing, pulsating:** Aloe, *Bell.,* Caps., Ham., Lach., *Meli.,* Merc., Nat-m.

**PARETIC, Condition of rectum and sphincters:** *Aloe,* Alum., *Caust., Erig., Gels.,* Graph., Hyos., Mur-ac., Op., Oxyt., Ph-ac., *Phos.,* Plb., Sil., Sulfon., Tab.

**Paretic condition of rectum, feels plugged:** *Aloe, Anac.,* Cann-i., Kali-bi., Med., Plat., Plb., *Sep.,* Sul-ac.

**Paretic condition of rectum, with sense of insecurity of sphincters:** *Aloe,* Alum., Apoc., Erig., Ferr., *Nux-v.,* Sanic., Sec.

**Patulous anus:** *Apis, Phos.,* Sec., Sol-t.

**PROLAPSUS ANI:** *Aesc., Aesc-g., Aloe,* Ant-c., Aral., *Arn., Bell.,* Carb-v., Caust., Colch., *Ferr., Ferr-p.,* Gamb., Ham., Hydr., *Ign.,* Kali-c., Mag-p., *Mur-ac.,* Nux-v., *Phos.,* Plb., *Podo., Polyp-p., Ruta, Sep.,* Sol-t., *Sulph.,* Tab., Trom.

**Prolapsus after confinement, stooping:** Podo., Ruta.

**Prolapsus from debility:** Podo.

**Prolapsus from sneezing:** Podo.

**Prolapsus from straining, overlifting:** Ign., Nit-ac., Podo., Ruta.

**Prolapsus from urinating:** Mur-ac.

**Prolapsus in children:** Bell., Ferr., *Ferr-p.,* Ign., Mur-ac., Nux-v., Podo.

**Prolapsus with diarrhea, stool:** Aesc., *Aloe,* Carb-v., Colch., Crot-t., Fl-ac., *Gamb.,* Ham., *Ign.,* Kali-c., Mur-ac., *Podo.,* Phos., *Ruta, Sulph.*

**Prolapsus with piles, in alcoholics, leading sedentary life:** Aesc-g.

**Prolapsus with stool, rectal spasm:** Ign.

**REDNESS, around:** *Cham.,* Merc-cy., Paeon., *Sulph.,* Zing. (See **Fissures, Proctitis.**)

**Stricture:** *Bell.,* Coff., Hydr., Ign., *Nit-ac.,* Phos., *Sil.,* Tab., Thiosin.(See

**Pain.**)

**Torn, bleeding, after stool:** Lac-d., *Nat-m., Nit-ac.* (See **Fissures.**)

**CATARRH: Gastro-duodenal:** Card-m., *Chin.*, Hydr., Sang. (See **STOMACH.**)

**CHOLERA, ASIATICA:** *Acon.*, Agar-ph., *Ars.*, Bell., Bry., *Camph., Canth., Carb-v.*, Chinin-s., Cic., Colch., *Cupr., Cupr-act., Cupr-ar.*, Dig., Euph-c., Guaj., *Hydr-ac., Ip.*, Jatr., Kali-bi., Lach., Merc-c., Naja, Nux-v., Op., *Ph-ac.*, Phos., Quas., Rhus-t., *Sec.*, Sulph., Tab., Ter., *Verat.*, Zinc.

**CHOLERA INFANTUM, Summer complaint:** *Acon., Aeth.*, Ant-t., *Apis*, Arg-n., *Ars.*, Bell., *Bism.*, Bry., Cadm-s., *Calc.*, Calc-act., *Calc-p.*, Camph., Camph-mbr., Canth., Cham., Chin., Coloc., Crot-t., *Cuph.*, Cupr., Cupr-act., *Cupr-ar.*, Elat., *Euph-c.*, Ferr-p., Graph., Hydr-ac., Indol., *Iodof., Ip.*, Iris, *Kali-br., Kreos., Laur.*, Merc., Nat-m., Ox-ac., Passi., Phos., Phyt., *Podo.*, Psor., Res., Sec., Sep., *Sil.*, Sulph., Tab., *Verat., Zinc.*

**CHOLERA MORBUS:** *Ant-t., Ars.*, Bism., Camph., Chlol., Colch., Coloc., *Crot-t.*, Cupr., *Cupr-ar.*, Elat., Grat., Hydr-ac., *Ip.*, Iris, Op., Oper., *Podo.*, Sec., *Verat.*

**CHOLERINE:** Ant-c., Ars., *Crot-t., Cupr-ar.*, Dios., Elat., Euph-c., *Grat., Ip.*, Iris, *Jatr.*, Nuph., *Ph-ac.*, Sec., *Verat.*

**CONSTIPATION, Remedies in general:** *Abies-n.*, Acon., *Aesc., Aesc-g.*, Agar., Alet., *Aloe, Alum., Alumn.*, Am-c., *Am-m., Anac.*, Apis, *Arn.*, Asar., Berb., *Bry., Calc.*, Calc-f., Carb-ac., *Cas-s., Caust.*, Chel., Chin., Chion., Coca, *Coll., Croc., Dol.*, Eug., Euon., *Euphr.*, Fel., Ferr., Gels., *Glyc., Graph., Grat.*, Guaj., Hep., *Hydr.*, Ign., *Iris, Kali-bi., Kali-c.*, Kali-m., Lac-ac., Lac-d., Lach., *Lyc., Mag-m.*, Mez., Morph., Nabal., *Nat-m., Nit-ac.*, Nit-m-ac., *Nux-v.*, Nyct., *Op., Paraf., Phos.*, Phys., Phyt., *Plat.*, Plb., *Plb-act., Podo., Psor.*, Pyrog., Rat., Rham-cal., Sanic., *Sel.*, Senn., *Sep., Sil.*, Sil-mar., Spig., *Staph.*, Stry., *Sulph., Sym-r., Syph.*, Tab., Tan-ac., Tub., *Verat., Zinc.*, Zinc-m.

**CAUSE AND TYPE, Abuse of enemas:** *Op.*

**After confinement, hepatic and uterine inertia:** Mez.

**Alternating, with diarrhea:** Abrot., Am-m., *Ant-c.*, Bry., Calc-chl., Card-m., Casc., *Chel., Coll.*, Ferr-cy., *Hydr.*, Iod., *Nux-v., Podo.*, Ptel., Rad-br., Ruta, *Sulph.*, Verat.

**From abuse of purgatives:** Aloe, *Hydr., Nux-v.*, Sulph.

**From cheese:** Coloc.

**From gastric derangements:** *Bry.*, Hydr., *Nux-v.*, Puls.

**From going to sea:** Bry., Lyc.

**From gouty acidity:** Grat.

**From hemorrhoids:** *Aesc., Aesc-g.*, Caust., *Coll.*, Hydr., Nat-m., *Nux-v.*,

Podo., *Sulph.* (See **Piles.**)

**From impaction:** Plb., Pyrog., Sel.

**From lead poisoning:** Op., Plat.

**From mechanical injuries:** Arn., Ruta.

**From mental shock, nervous strain:** Mag-c.

**From peristaltic irregularity:** Anac., *Nux-v.*

**From travelling, in emigrants:** Plat.

**From torpor of rectum:** Aloe, *Alum., Anac.,* Caust., Chin., Lach., Lyc., Nat-m., *Op.,* Psor., Sel., *Sep., Sil., Verat.*

**From torpor, inertia, dryness of intestines:** *Aesc.,* Aeth., Alet., *Alum.,* Alumn., *Bry.,* Coffin., *Coll.,* Ferr., Hydr., *Lyc.,* Meli., Mez., *Nat-m.,* Nux-v., *Op.,* Phys., *Plat., Plb act.,* Pyrog., Ruta, Sanic., Sel., *Sulph.,* Verat.

**Infants, bottle fed; artificial food:** Alum., Nux-v., Op.

**Infants, children:** *Aesc., Alum.,* Apis, Bell., *Bry.,* Calc., Caust., *Coll.,* Croc., Hydr., *Lyc., Mag-m., Nux-v.,* Nyct., *Paraf.,* Podo., *Psor.,* Sanic., *Sep., Sil.,* Sulph., *Verat.*

**In old people:** *Alum., Ant-c.,* Hydr., Lyc., *Op.,* Phyt., *Sel., Sulph.*

**In rheumatic subjects, flatulence, indigestion:** Mag-p.

**In women:** *Aesc.,* Alet., *Alum.,* Ambr., Anac., Arn., *Asaf.,* Bry., Calc., *Coll.,* Con., *Graph., Hydr.,* Ign., Lach., Lyc., Mez., *Nat-m.,* Nux-v., Op., *Plat., Plb., Podo.,* Puls., *Sep.,* Sil., Sulph.

**TYPE OF STOOL, Dry, crumbling at verge of anus:** *Am-m., Mag-m., Nat-m.,* Sanic., Zinc.

**Dry, difficult, scanty, knotty, ball or dung like:** Aesc., Aesc-g., *Alum., Alumn.,* Aster., Bar-c., *Card-m.,* Caust., *Chel.,* Coll., Glyc., *Graph.,* Indol., *Lyc., Mag-m.,* Morph., Nit-ac., *Nux-v., Op.,* Petr., *Plat., Plb.,* Pyrog., Sanic., *Sep., Sulph.,* Thuj., Verat., Verb., Xero., Zinc.

**Dry, large, painful:** *Aesc.,* Alet., Aloe, *Alum., Bry.,* Calc., Caust., Glyc., *Graph., Kali-c.,* Lac-d., Meli., Nat-m., Nux-v., *Op.,* Pyrog., Sanic., *Sel.,* Sep., *Sulph., Verat.,* Vib.

**Dry, must be mechanically removed:** Aloe, Alum., Bry., Calc., Indol., *Op., Plb.,* Ruta, Sanic., *Sel.,* Sep., *Sil.,* Verat.

**Dry, with frequent urging:** Alumn., *Anac.,* Aster., Carb-v., *Caust.,* Con., Ferr., Glyc., *Gran., Ign.,* Iod., Lac-d., *Lyc.,* Nit-ac., Nit-m-ac., *Nux-v.,* Paraf., *Plat., Phos.,* Podo., Rob., Ruta, *Sil., Sep.,* Spig., *Sulph.*

**Dry, with partial expulsion and receding:** Op., Sanic., *Sil., Thuj.*

**Frequent, ineffectual urging:** Ambr., Anac., Caust., Ferr., Graph., Lyc., Nat-m., *Nux-v.,* Plat., Sulph.

**Hard:** Aesc., Aloe, *Am-m.,* Ant-c., Bar-c., *Bry.,* Calc., *Chel.,* Con., Glyc., Indol., Iod., Lac-d., *Lyc., Mag-m., Nat-m., Op.,* Phos., *Plb.,* Rat., Sanic.,

Sel., *Sulph.*

**Hard, covered with mucus:** Alum., Am-m., Casc., *Caust., Coll.,* Cop., *Graph., Hydr.,* Nux-v., Sep.

**Hard, then pasty liquid:** Calc., Lyc.

**Large, black, carrion-like:** Pyrog.

**Light colored, grayish, chalky:** Acon., Alumn., *Calc., Chel., Chin.,* Chion., Coll., *Dig.,* Dol., *Hep.,* Hydr., Iber., Indol., Kali-m., *Merc-d., Podo.,* Sanic., Stel.

**No desire or urging:** *Alum., Bry.,* Graph., Hydr., *Op.*

**Pasty, tenacious, adhering to anus:** Alum., Chel., Chion., *Plat.*

**Slender, quill-like:** Arn., *Caust., Phos.,* Staph.

**Soft stool even passed with difficulty:** Agn., Alum., Anac., Chel., Chion., *Plat.,* Rat., Sil.

**CONCOMITANTS: Abdominal weakness, shuddering:** Plat.

**Anus very sore:** Graph., Nat-m., Nit-ac., Sil.

**Backache:** *Aesc.,* Euon., *Ferr.,* Kali-bi., Sulph. (See **Back.**)

**Bleeding:** Alum., Am-m., Anac., Calc-p., *Coll.,* Lac-d., Lam., Morph., Nat-m., *Nit-ac., Nux-v.,* Phos., Psor., Sep., Vib.

**Colic, cramps:** Coll., *Cupr.,* Glon., Op., *Plb-act.*

**Contraction, spasmodic of anus:** Caust., *Lach., Lyc., Nat-m.,* Nit-ac., Plb., Plb-act., Sil. (See **Anus: Rectum.**)

**Enuresis:** Caust.

**Fainting:** Verat.

**Fetor oris:** *Carb-ac.,* Op., Psor.

**Gall stones, jaundice:** Chion. (See **Gall bladder.**)

**Headache:** Bry., Gels., *Hydr.,* Iris, Nux-v., Sep., Verat. (See **HEAD.**)

**Heart weak:** Phyt., Spig.

**Hernia, umbilical:** Cocc., Nux-v.

**Nervous, from presence of others, even nurse:** Ambr.

**Pain, compels child to desist from effort:** Ign., Lyc., *Sulph.,* Thuj.

**Passes better leaning far back:** Med.

**Passes better standing:** Caust.

**Piles:** *Aesc., Aloe,* Alumn., *Calc-f.,* Caust., *Coll.,* Euon., Glon., Graph., Kali-s., Lyc., Nit-ac., *Nux-v.,* Paraf., *Rat.,* Sil., *Sulph.,* Wye. (See **Hemorrhoids.**)

**Prolapsus:** *Aesc.,* Alum., Ferr., *Ign.,* Lyc., Med., *Podo.,* Ruta, Sep., Sulph- (See **Anus: Rectum.**)

**Prolapsus uteri:** Stann.

**Prostate enlarged:** Arn., Sil. (See **MALE SEXUAL SYSTEM.**)

**Prostatic fluid:** Alum., Hep.

**Rectal pain, persistent:** *Aesc.,* Aloe, Alumn., Caust., Hydr., *Ign.,* Lyc., Mur-ac., *Nat-m., Nit-ac.,* Rat., Sep., Sulph., Thuj. (See **Anus, Rectum.**)

**Sensation of light headedness:** Indol.

**Sensation of something remaining behind:** Aloe, Alum., Lyc., Nat-m., *Nux-v.,* Sep., Sil., Sulph.

**Urging absent, no desire:** *Alum., Bry.,* Graph., Hydr., Indol., *Op.,* Sanic., Sulph., Verat.

**Urging felt in lower abdomen:** Aloe. (See **Frequent Urging**.)

**Urging felt in upper abdomen:** Anac., *Ign.,* Verat.

**DIAPHRAGM: Inflammation (diaphragmitis):** Atro., Bell., Bism., *Bry., Cact., Cupr.,* Hep., Hyos., Ign., *Nux-v.,* Ran-b., Stram., Verat-v.

**Pain:** Asaf., Bism., *Bry.,* Cact., *Cimic.,* Nat-m., Nux-v., Sec., Spig., *Stann.,* Stict., *Stry.,* Verat., Zinc-ox.

**Rheumatism:** *Bry.,* Cact., *Cimic.,* Spig., Stict.

**DIARRHEA, Enteritis, Acute:** Acal., Acet-ac., *Acon., Aeth.,* Agar-ph., *Aloe, Alst.,* Andr., *Ant-c.,* Ant-t., *Apis,* Apoc., *Arg-n., Arn., Ars.,* Ars-i., *Asaf., Bapt., Bell.,* Benz-ac., *Bism.,* Bov., *Bry.,* Cadm-s., *Calc.,* Calc-act., *Calc-p., Camph., Canth., Caps., Carb-ac., Carb-v., Cham., Chel., Chin., Chinin-ar.,* Cina, Colch., Coll., *Coloc., Corn., Crot-t.,* Cuph., Cupr-act., Cupr-ar., *Cycl., Dulc.,* Echi., *Elat.,* Epil., *Eucal., Euph.,* Ferr., Ferr-p., Fl-ac., Form., *Gamb., Gels., Grat.,* Hell., Hep., Hyos., Iod., *Ip., Iris,* Jal., *Jatr., Kali-bi.,* Kali-chl., Kali-p., Lept., *Mag-c., Merc., Merc-d.,* Morph., Mur-ac., Nat-m., *Nat-s.,* Nit-ac., *Nuph., Nux-v.,* Olnd., *Op.,* Opun-f., Oreo., Paeon., *Petr., Ph-ac., Phos.,* Phys., *Podo.,* Polyg-h., *Prun.,* Psor., *Puls., Rheum, Rhus-t.,* Rhus-v., Ric., *Rumx.,* Santin., *Sec., Sep., Sil.,* Sul-ac., *Sulph.,* Tab., Ter., *Thuj.,* Valer., *Verat.,* Zinc., Zing.

**Chronic:** Acet-ac., All-s., Aloe, Ang., Ant-c., *Arg-n.,* Arn., *Ars.,* Ars-i., Bapt., *Calc.,* Calc-p., Cetr., *Chap., Chin., Coto.,* Crot-t., *Cupr-ar.,* Elaps, *Ferr.,* Gamb., *Graph.,* Hep., *Iod.,* Iodof., Ip., *Kali-bi.,* Lac-ac., Lach., *Liat.,* Lyc., Mag-m., *Merc.,* Merc-d., Nabal., *Nat-s.,* Nit-ac., Olnd., *Ph-ac., Phos., Podo.,* Psor., Puls., Rhus a., Rhus-t., Rumx., Stry-ar., *Sulph., Thuj.,* Tub., Urt-u.

**CAUSE; OCCURRENCE, Alternates with headache:** Aloe, Podo.

**From acids:** Aloe, *Ant-c.,* Ph-ac., Sulph.

**From acute diseases:** Carb-v., Chin., Psor. (See **Typhoid Fever**.)

**From alcoholic abuse:** Ars., Lach., Nux-v.

**From anger:** *Cham.,* Coloc., Staph.

**From bathing:** *Ant-c.,* Podo.

**From beer, ale:** Aloe, Chin., Ip., *Kali-bi.,* Mur-ac., *Sulph.*

**From cabbage; saurkraut:** Bry., Petr.
**From camping:** *Alst.,* Jug-c., Podo.
**From catarrh, bronchial, suppressed:** Sang.
**From change of weather, draughts:** *Acon., Bry.,* Calc-s., *Caps.,* Colch., *Dulc.,* Ip., *Merc., Nat-s.,* Psor., Rhus-t., Sil.
**From chilling cold drinks, ices:** *Acon.,* Agra., *Ars.,* Bell., *Bry.,* Camph., Carb-v., Caust., Cham., Grat., Nux m., *Puls.,* Staph.
**From coffee:** Cist., *Cycl.,* Ox-ac., Thuj.
**From coryza, ceasing:** Sang.
**From disorganization:** Ars.
**From eggs:** Chinin-ar.
**From emotional excitement, fright:** *Acon., Arg-n., Gels.,* Hyos., *Ign.,* Kali-p., *Op., Ph-ac.,* Puls., Verat., Zinc.
**From eruptions repelled:** Ant-t., Apis, *Bry.,* Dulc., Petr., Psor., *Sulph.*
**From fats:** Cycl., Kali-m., *Puls.,* Thuj.
**From food, crude:** Cham.
**From fruits:** *Ars., Bry.,* Calc-p., *Chin.,* Cist., Coloc., Crot-t., Ip., *Podo., Puls.,* Verat., Zing.
**From gastric derangements:** *Ant-c.,* Bry., Chin., Coloc., Ip., Lyc., *Nux-v., Puls.*
**From high game:** Crot-h., Pyrog.
**From hot weather:** Acon., Aloe, Ambro., *Ant-c.,* Ars., *Bry.,* Camph., Caps., *Cham., Chin.,* Crot-t., *Cuph.,* Ferr-p., Gamb., *Ip.,* Iris, Merc., Nux-m., *Podo.,* Sil., Verat.
**From hydrocephalus, acute:** Hell.
**From hyperacidity:** Cham., Rheum, Rob.
**From intestinal atony, debility:** *Arg-n.,* Caps., *Chin., Ferr.,* Oena., Oreo., *Sec.*
**From jaundice:** *Chion.,* Dig., Nux-v.
**From meat putrescent:** Ars., Crot-h.
**From milk:** *Aeth.,* Calc., Chin., Lyc., *Mag-c., Mag-m.,* Nat-c., Nicc., *Sep.,* Sulph., Valer.
**From milk boiled:** Nux-m.
**From motion:** Apis, *Bry.,* Chin., Colch., Nat-s.
**From motion, downward:** Borx., Cham., Sanic.
**From nephritis:** Ter.
**From noxious effluvia:** Bapt., Carb-ac., *Crot-h.*
**From onions:** Thuj.
**From oysters:** *Brom.,* Lyc., Sul-ac.
**From perspiration checked:** *Acon.,* Cham., Ferr-p.

**From pork:** Acon-l., *Puls.*

**From sweets:** *Arg-n.,* Calc-s., Crot-t., *Gamb.,* Merc.

**From tobacco:** Cham., Tab.

**From tuberculosis:** Acet-ac., Arg-n., *Arn.,* Ars., *Ars-i., Bapt.,* Bism., *Chin.,* Coto., *Cupr-ar.,* Elaps, Ferr., Iod., Iodof., Ph-ac., *Phos.,* Puls., Rumx. (See **Tuberculosis.**)

**From typhoid fever:** *Ars., Bapt.,* Echi., *Epil.,* Eucal., *Hyos.,* Lach., *Mur-ac.,* Nuph., Op., Ph-ac., *Rhus-t.,* Stram. (See **Typhoid Fever.**)

**From ulceration of intestines:** Kali-bi., Merc-c.

**From urination:** Aloe, Alum., Apis.

**From vaccination:** *Sil.,* Thuj.

**From veal:** Kali-n.

**From vegetables, melons:** *Ars., Bry.,* Petr., Zing.

**From water polluted:** *Alst.,* Camph., Zing.

**In infants, children:** *Acon., Aeth.,* Apis, *Arg-n., Ars.,* Arund., Bapt., *Bell.,* Benz-ac., Bism., *Borx., Calc.,* Calc-act., *Calc-p.,* Camph., *Cham.,* Chin., Cina, *Coloc.,* Colos., *Crot-t.,* Dulc., Ferr., Grat., *Hell.,* Hep., *Ip.,* Jal., Kali-br., *Kreos.,* Laur., Lyc., Lyss., *Mag-c.,* Merc., *Merc-c., Merc-d.,* Nit-ac., *Nux-v.,* Paull., *Ph-ac.,* Phos., *Podo., Psor., Rheum,* Sabad., Sep., *Sil., Sulph.,* Valer., *Verat.*

**Infants (dentition):** Acet-ac., *Acon., Aeth.,* Arund., *Bell.,* Benz-ac., Borx., *Calc.,* Calc-act., *Calc p., Cham.,* Ip., Jal., *Kreos., Mag-c.,* Merc., Nux-m., Olnd., Phyt., *Podo.,* Psor., Rheum, *Sil.*

**In old people:** *Ant-c.,* Bov., *Carb-v., Chin.,* Gamb., Op., Phos., *Sulph.*

**In women, before and during menses:** Am-c., *Am-m., Bov.,* Verat. (See **FEMALE SEXUAL SYSTEM.**)

**In women, lying-in period:** *Cham., Hyos.,* Psor., *Sec.,* Stram.

**TYPE OF STOOL: Acrid, excoriating, burning:** *Ars.,* Bry., Carb-v., *Cham.,* Cuph., *Graph.,* Iris, Kreos., Merc., *Merc-c.,* Merc-d., Merc-sul., Podo., *Sulph.,* Ter.

**Bilious:** Ant-t., *Bry.,* Card-m., *Cham.,* Chin., *Corn.,* Crot-t., Fl-ac., Gamb., *Ip., Iris,* Jug-c., *Lept.,* Lyc., Merc., *Merc-d.,* Nat-s., Nyct., *Podo.,* Puls., Sang., Tarax., Yuc.

**Black:** *Ars.,* Brom., Camph., *Caps., Carb-ac.,* Chin., *Crot-h.,* Echi., *Lept.,* Morph., *Op., Psor.,* Pyrog., *Squil.,* Stram., Sul-ac., Verat.

**Blood streaked slime:** Agar., *Aloe,* Arg-n., *Arn.,* Bell., *Canth., Caps.,* Coloc., *Cupr-ar.,* Euph., *Ip.,* Lil-t., Kreos., Mag-c., *Merc., Merc-c.,* Merc-d., *Nux-v.,* Podo., *Psor., Rhus-t., Sulph.,* Tril-p. (See **Dysentery.**)

**Bloody:** Aeth., Ail., Aloe, Am-m., *Arg-n.,* Arn., *Ars., Bapt.,* Both., Cadm-s., *Canth., Caps.,* Carb-ac., *Colch.,* Coloc., Crot-h., Cupr-ar., Dulc., Ferr-p., Ham., *Ip.,* Kali-bi., Kreos., Lach., *Merc., Merc-c., Merc-d., Nux-v., Phos.,* Podo., *Sec., Senec., Sulph., Ter.,* Trom., Valer.

**Brown, dark:** Apis, Arn., *Ars.,* Asaf., *Bapt., Bry.,* Chin., Coloc., Corn., Cupr-act., Cupr-ar., Ferr-m., *Graph.,* Kali-bi., Kreos., *Lept.,* Mur-ac., Nux-v., Podo., *Psor.,* Pyrog., *Raph.,* Rheum, Rumx., *Squil., Sec., Senec.,* Sulph., Tub.

**Changeable:** Am-m., *Cham.,* Euon., Merc., *Podo., Puls.,* Sanic., Sil., *Sulph.*

**Clay colored, chalk-like, light colored:** Aloe, *Bell.,* Benz-ac., Berb., *Calc.,* Chel., *Dig.,* Euph., Gels., *Hep.,* Kali-c., Merc., *Merc-d.,* Myric., *Ph-ac.,* Phos., Podo., Sep.

**Coffee ground-like, mealy:** Crot-h., Dig., *Lach., Podo.,* Tart-ac.

**Colliquative (debilitating):** Acet-ac., Ango., *Ars., Chin., Colch.,* Coto., *Cupr-ar.,* Dios., Elaps, Kali-p., Phell., *Phos., Sec.,* Sep., Serp., *Tab.,* Tart-ac., Upa., *Verat.*

**Fatty, oily:** Caust., *Iod.,* Iris, *Phos.*

**Fermented, flatulent, noisy, spluttering expulsion:** *Acal.,* Agar., Alf., *Aloe,* Apoc., *Arg-n.,* Arn., Benz-ac., Borx., *Calc-p.,* Cham., *Chin.,* Coloc., Corn., *Crot-t., Elat., Gamb.,* Graph., *Grat.,* Iod., *Ip., Jatr.,* Kali-bi., *Mag-c., Nat-s., Nat-sulo.,* Op., *Ph-ac.,* Phos., *Podo.,* Puls., Rheum, Rhus-t., Sanic., Sec., Stict., *Sulph., Thuj.,* Trios., *Verat.,* Yuc.

**Frequent:** Acet-ac., *Acon.,* Aloe, *Ars.,* Calc-act., Caps., *Carb-v., Cham., Chin.,* Crot-t., Cuph., *Cupr-ar.,* Elat., Ip., Mag-c., *Merc., Merc-c.,* Nit-ac., Nux-v., *Ph-ac., Podo.,* Rheum, Rhus-t., Sil., Sulph., Ter., *Verat.*

**Frog spawn or scum-like:** Hell., Mag-c., *Phos.,* Sanic.

**Gelatinous, jelly-like:** *Aloe,* Cadm-s., *Colch., Coloc.,* Euph., *Hell., Kali-bi.,* Oxyt., *Phos.,* Podo., *Rhus-t.*

**Green:** *Acon.,* Aeth., Ant-t., *Apis, Arg-n., Ars., Bell., Borx.,* Bry., Calc., Calc-act., *Calc-p., Cham., Coloc.,* Crot-t., *Dulc., Elat.,* Gamb., *Gels.,* Grat., *Hep.,* Iodof., *Ip.,* Iris, Kreos., Laur., *Mag-c., Merc.,* Merc-c., *Merc-d., Mez., Paull.,* Phos., *Podo., Puls.,* Sal-ac., Sanic., *Sec.,* Sulph., Tab., Valer., Verat.

**Green, turning to blue:** Calc-p., Phos.

**Gurgling, gushing:** Aloe, Apis, *Crot-t., Elat., Gamb.,* Grat., *Jatr.,* Kali-bi., Merc., Nat-s., *Petr., Phos., Podo.,* Sang., Sec., *Thuj.,* Tub., Verat. (See **Fermented.**)

**Hot:** *Calc-p., Cham.,* Dios., Ferr., Merc-c., Merc-sul., Podo., *Sulph.* (See **Acrid.**)

**Involuntary:** *Aloe, Apis,* Apoc., *Arn.,* Ars., *Bapt.,* Camph., Carb-ac., *Carb-v., Gels.,* Hell., *Hyos.,* Op., *Ph ac., Phos.,* Podo., Psor., Pyrog., Rhus-t., *Sec.,* Stry., Sulph., *Verat.,* Zinc.

**Involuntary, as if anus were wide open:** *Apis,* Apoc., *Phos.,* Sec., Trom.

**Involuntary, when passing flatus:** *Aloe,* Calc., Iod., *Mur-ac.,* Nat-m., Nat-s., *Olnd., Ph-ac., Podo.,* Pyrog., Sanic.

**Involuntary, when passing urine:** *Aloe, Alum.,* Apis, Cic., Hyos., *Mur-ac., Squil.,* Sulph., Verat.

**Lumpy, hard:** Aloe, *Ant c.,* Bar-c., Bell., *Bry.,* Cham., Cina, Con., Cub., Glon., *Graph., Mag-c.,* Petr., Phos., *Podo.,* Senec., Trom.

**Mucus, slimy:** *Aloe,* Am-m., *Ant-c.,* Apis, *Arg-n., Arn., Ars., Bell.,* Borx., Calc-act., *Calc-p., Canth., Caps.,* Carb-ac., *Carb-v., Cham.,* Chin., Cina, Cocc., *Colch., Coloc., Cop., Dulc.,* Ferr., Gamb., Graph., Hell., Hep., *Ip.,* Kali-m., Laur., *Mag-c., Merc., Merc-c.,* Merc-d., Nit-ac., *Nux-v.,* Phos., Podo., Prun., *Puls.,* Rheum, Ric., Rhus-t., Ruta, Sep., Spig., *Sulph.,* Tab., Ter., Urt-u. (See **Dysentery**.)

**Non-debilitating:** Calc., Graph., *Ph-ac.,* Puls.

**Offensive, cadaverous:** Ail., Ant-c., Arg-n., *Arn., Ars., Asaf.,* Asc-t., *Bapt., Benz-ac.,* Bism., *Borx., Bry.,* Calc., Calc-p., Carb-ac., *Carb-v., Cham.,* Chin., Coloc., Corn., Crot-h., *Graph., Hep., Kali-p., Kreos.,* Lach., *Lept.,* Merc., *Merc-c., Merc-d.,* Mur-ac., Nit-ac., Nux m., Op., Petr., Ph-ac., *Phos., Podo., Psor.,* Pulx., Pyrog., *Rheum,* Rhus-t., Rumx., Sanic., *Sec.,* Sil., *Squil.,* Stram., Sul-ac., Sulph., *Ter.,* Tub.

**Painless:** Alf., Agar., *Alst., Apis,* Ars., *Bapt.,* Bell-p., Bism., Borx., Chap., *Chin.,* Colch., Crot-t., Dulc., *Ferr., Gels., Graph., Grat.,* Hep., *Hyos.,* Ip., Nit-ac., *Ph-ac., Phos., Podo.,* Psor., *Puls.,* Pyrog., Rhus-t., Ric., Rumx., Sec., Sil., Squil., *Sulph.*

**Papescent:** Aesc., Alf., Aloe, Ars., Bism., *Borx., Bry.,* Chel., *Chin.,* Coloc., *Cycl.,* Gamb., Gels., *Graph., Lept.,* Mag-c., Merc., *Merc-d.,* Nit-ac., Paeon., *Podo.,* Rheum, Sep., Sil., *Sulph.,* Valer., Zinc.

**Profuse:** Acet-ac., Ant-c., *Asaf., Benz-ac.,* Bism., Bry., Calc., Calc-act., Chel., Chin., Coto., *Crot-t., Elat., Euon.,* Euph-c., *Gamb., Jatr.,* Lept., Merc., Nat-n., Oper., Paull., *Phos., Podo.,* Psor., Rhus-t., *Sec.,* Stict., *Ter., Thuj., Verat.*

**Purulent:** Apis, Arn., Calc-s., *Hep., Merc.,* Phos., Sil.

**Rice water:** *Ars.,* Camph., *Jatr.,* Kali-p., Merc., Ric., *Verat.*

**Sago or tallow particles, like:** Phos.

**Scanty:** *Acon., Aloe, Ars., Bell.,* Camph., Canth., Caps., *Colch.,* Coloc., *Merc., Merc-c.,* Merc-d., Nit-ac., *Nux-v.,* Olnd., Sulph. (See **Dysentery**.)

**Shreddy, stringy, membranous, like scrapings of intestines:** Aloe, *Arg-n.,* Ars., Asar., Bol-la., *Canth., Carb-ac., Colch.,* Kali-bi., Kali-n., Merc., *Merc-c.,* Mur-ac., *Nit-ac.,* Podo., Puls., Sul-ac.

**Sour:** *Calc.,* Calc-act., Colch., Coloc., *Colos.,* Graph., *Hep.,* Jal., *Mag-c.,* Merc., Nit-ac., *Podo., Rheum,* Rob., Sulph.

**Spinach chopped, like:** Acon., Arg-n., Cham.
**Sudden, imperative, cannot wait:** *Aloe,* Chin., Cist., *Crot-t., Gamb., Lil-t.,* Nat-c., Paeon., Podo., *Psor., Rumx., Sulph.,* Tab., Trom., Tub., *Verat.*
**Tenacious, glairy:** *Asar., Caps.,* Crot-t., Hell., *Kali-bi.* (See **Mucus.**)
**Undigested, lienteric:** Abrot., Aeth., *Ant-c.,* Arg-n., *Ars., Asar.,* Bry., *Calc., Calc-p.,* Cham., *Chin.,* Crot-t., *Ferr.,* Ferr-act., Ferr-p., *Graph.,* Hep., Iodof., *Mag-c.,* Nit-ac., Nux-m., Nux-v., *Olnd., Ph-ac., Phos., Podo.,* Psor., *Puls.,* Sulph., Valer.
**Watery, like washing of meat:** *Canth.,* Phos., Rhus-t.
**Watery, thin:** Acet-ac., Acon., Aeth., Aloe, *Alst., Ant-c.,* Ant-t., *Apis, Apoc., Ars.,* Asaf., *Bapt., Benz-ac.,* Bism., *Borx., Bry.,* Calc., Calc-act., *Calc-p.,* Carb-v., *Cham.,* Chel., *Chin.,* Colch., *Coloc.,* Crot-h., *Crot-t.,* Cuph., *Cupr-ar.,* Cycl., *Elat.,* Ferr-m., *Gamb.,* Graph., *Grat.,* Hep., Hyos., Iod., Iodof., Ip., *Iris,* Jal., *Jatr.,* Kali-bi., Kali-n., Laur., *Mag-c.,* Mur-ac., Nat-s., Olnd., Oper., Petr., *Ph-ac.,* Phos., *Podo., Psor.,* Puls., *Rheum,* Rhus-t., Rumx., *Sec., Senec., Sulph.,* Tab., Ter., Thuj., Trom., Tub., *Verat.,* Zinc.
**White:** Acon., Ant-c., *Bell., Benz-ac., Calc.,* Caust., Cham., Chel., Cina, Cocc., *Colch.,* Crot-h., Cub., *Dig.,* Dulc., *Hell., Hep.,* Iod., Ip., Kali-m., Mag-c., Merc., *Merc-d.,* Mez., Nux-m., *Ph-ac., Phos., Podo.,* Puls., Trom.
**Yellow:** Aeth., Agar., Alf., Aloe, *Apis, Ars.,* Asar., *Borx., Calc.,* Card-m., Cham., *Chel., Chin.,* Coloc., *Crot-t.,* Cycl., Dulc., *Gamb.,* Gels., Grat., *Hep.,* Hyos., Ip., Merc., *Nat-c.,* Nat-s., *Nuph.,* Nux-m., Petr., Ph-ac., *Podo.,* Puls., Rheum, Rhus-t., Senn., Sep., Sulph., Tab., Thuj.

**CONCOMITANTS, BEFORE STOOL, Chilliness:** Ars., Camph., Elat., *Merc., Phos.,* Verat.
**Colic, cramps:** Aeth., *Aloe,* Alst., *Bell.,* Borx., Casc., *Cham., Chin.,* Cina, *Coloc.,* Crot-t., *Cupr-ar., Dios.,* Dulc., Elat., Gamb., *Ip.,* Iris, Lept., *Mag-c.,* Merc., *Merc-c.,* Merc-d., Nux-v., *Rheum,* Senn., Sulph., Trom., *Verat.* (See **Colic.**)
**Flatulent rumbling:** *Aloe,* Asaf., Carb-v., *Colch.,* Coloc., *Gamb.,* Kali-c., *Nat-s.,* Olnd., *Podo.,* Puls.
**Nausea:** *Bry.,* Chr-ac., *Colch., Ip.,* Merc., Rhus-t., Sep.
**Urging, painful:** *Aloe, Ars., Bell.,* Camph., Cist., *Coloc.,* Con., *Crot-t.,* Form., Gamb., Grat., Hep., *Ign.,* Kali-bi., Lept., Merc., *Merc-c., Merc-d.,* Nat-s., *Nux-v.,* Olnd., Phos., Podo., Rheum, Sil., *Stront-c., Sulph., Verat.*

**DURING STOOL, Backache:** *Aesc.,* Caps., Colch., *Nux-v.,* Puls.
**Burning in anus:** *Aloe,* Aphis, *Ars., Canth.,* Carb-v., Con., *Iris,* Jug-c., *Merc-d., Mur-ac.,* Podo., Prun., *Rat.,* Rheum, Ter., Trom., Verat. (See **Anus.**)

**Chilliness:** Ars., Bell., *Colch.,* Ip., *Jatr., Merc.,* Rheum, Ric., *Sec.,* Trom., *Verat.*

**Colic, cramps:** *Aloe,* Alst., *Ars.,* Bry., Camph., *Canth.,* Caps., Cean., *Cham., Chin., Coloc.,* Crot-t., *Cupr., Cupr-ar.,* Dulc., *Elat.,* Gamb., *Ip.,* Iris, *Jatr.,* Lept., *Merc., Merc-c.,* Merc-d., Podo., Rheum, Ric., Sec., Sil., Sulph., Trios., *Trom., Verat.,* Zing. (See **Colic.**)

**Fainting:** Aloe, *Ars.,* Crot-h., *Merc., Nux-m.,* Sulph.

**Flatus, fetid, expelled:** Agar., *Aloe, Arg-n., Calc-p., Carb-v.,* Chin., Ign., Jatr., *Nat-s.,* Ph-ac., Podo., Thuj.

**Hunger:** Aloe, Ferr., Sec.

**Nausea, vomiting:** Aeth., *Ant-t., Ars., Bism.,* Camph., Carb-ac., Chr-ac., *Colch.,* Crot-t., Cupr., Fil., *Ip., Iris, Jatr.,* Merc., Opun., Phos., *Podo.,* Tab., Trios., *Verat.*

**Pain tearing down posterior limbs:** Rhus-t.

**Stinging pains:** Caps.

**Tenesmus of bladder:** Canth., Lil-t., *Merc-c.*

**Tenesmus, relieved by stool:** Nux-v.

**Tenesmus, urging painful:** *Acon., Aloe,* Ango., Arn., *Ars., Bell.,* Calc., *Canth.,* Caps., Carb-ac., *Colch., Coloc.,* Crot-t., Cuph., Cupr-act., *Cupr-ar.,* Hep., *Ign., Ip., Kali-bi.,* Kali-n., Liat., Mag-c., *Merc., Merc-c.,* Merc-d., Morph., Nat-s., Nit-ac., *Nux-v.,* Op., Phos., Plb-act., *Podo.,* Rheum, Rhus-t., *Senec.,* Sil., *Sulph.,* Tab., Trom., Verat.

**Vomiting, hiccough, suffocative, in stomach and chest:** Verat.

AFTER STOOL: **Anus burning:** Aloe, Apoc., *Ars.,* Bry., *Canth., Caps.,* Carb-v., Coloc., *Gamb.,* Grat., *Iris,* Kali-c., Merc., Merc-c., Nit-ac., Olnd., Prun., *Rat.,* Sulph., Trom., Verat. (See **Anus.**)

**Coldness:** Aloe, *Ars.,* Camph., *Canth.,* Caps., Carb-v., Form., Ip., Merc., *Sec.,* Tab., *Verat.*

**Debility, exhaustion:** Acet-ac., Aeth., Agar., *Ail.,* Aloe, *Arg-n.,* Arn., *Ars.,* Bism., *Camph., Chin., Colch., Con.,* Crot-t., Cupr., Elat., Ferr., Iris, Jatr., *Kali-p.,* Mag-c., Nit-ac., *Phos., Podo., Rhus-t., Sec.,* Sep., Sul-ac., *Tab., Ter.,* Trom., Tub., Upa., *Verat.*

**Fainting:** *Aloe,* Ars., Con., Crot-t., *Merc., Nux-m.,* Paeon., Sars., *Ter.,* Verat.

**Hemorrhoids:** *Aloe,* Ham., Mur-ac., Sulph. (See **Hemorrhoids.**)

**Pains persist in abdomen:** Aloe, *Coloc.,* Crot-t., Dios., *Gamb.,* Grat., Merc., *Merc-c.,* Rheum, Trom., Verat.

**Palpitation, trembling in limbs:** Ars.

**Prolapsus ani:** *Aloe,* Alum., Calc-act., Carb-v., Ham., *Ign.,* Merc., Nit-ac., *Podo.,* Sulph., Trom. (See **Rectum.**)

**Sleep, as soon as tenesmus ceases:** Colch., *Sulph.*

**Stool natural in evening:** Aloe, Podo.

**Sweat:** Acet-ac., Aloe, Ant-t., Ars., Ph-ac., Tab., Tub., *Verat.*

**Tenesmus (never-get-done feeling):** Aeth., Aloe, Ars., *Bell., Canth., Caps.,* Colch., *Gamb.,* Ign., Ip., Kali-bi., Mag-c., *Merc., Merc-c., Merc-d.,* Nit-ac., Nux-v., *Podo.,* Rheum, Senn., Sil., *Sulph.,* Trom.

**Thirst:** Acet-ac., *Caps.,* Dulc.

**Vomiting:** Arg-n., Colch., Cupr., *Ip.,* Iris, *Nux-v.,* Verat.

**Weakness in abdomen and rectum:** Podo.

**MODALITIES, Aggravations, From eating, drinking:** *Aloe, Alst., Apis,* Apoc., *Arg-n., Ars.,* Bry., Canth., *Chin., Coloc., Crot-t., Ferr.,* Kali-p., Lyc., Nux-v., *Phos., Podo.,* Puls., Rheum, Sanic., Sulph., Tanac., Thuj., *Trom., Verat.*

**From motion:** Aloe, Apis, *Bry.,* Chin., *Colch.,* Crot-t., *Nat-s.,* Rheum, Verat.

**From sundown to sunrise:** Colch.

**In afternoon:** Bell., Calc., *Chin.,* Corn., *Lyc.*

**In autumn:** Chin., *Colch., Merc.,* Nux-m., Verat.

**In daytime only:** Hep., *Petr.,* Pilo.

**In evening, night:** *Ars.,* Bell-p., Bov., Calc., Chel., *Chin.,* Dulc., *Ferr.,* Iris, *Merc.,* Nat-n., Nux-m., Podo., *Puls.,* Psor., *Rhus-t., Stront-c.,* Sulph., Wye.

**In morning, early:** Acet-ac., *Aloe,* Ichth., Iris, Lil-t., Med., *Nat-s.,* Nit-ac., *Nuph., Nux-v.,* Petr., Phos., *Podo., Psor.,* Rhus-v., *Rumx.,* Stict., *Sulph.,* Thuj., Trom., Tub.

**In morning:** *Aloe, Apis,* Bov., *Bry.,* Cact., Cist., Crot-t., Ferr., Graph., *Kali-bi.,* Lil-t., Lyc., Nux-v.

**In periodical attacks:** Apis, Ars., *Chin.,* Euph-c., *Kali-bi.,* Iris, Mag-c., Thuj.

**DUODENUM, Catarrhal inflammation (duodenitis):** *Ars.,* Aur., Berb., Cham., Chel., *Chin., Hydr., Kali-bi.,* Lyc., Merc., Merc-d., Nat-s., Nux-v., *Podo.,* Ric., Sang.

**Ulceration:** *Kali-bi.,* Symph., Uran-n.

**DYSENTERY:** *Acon., Aloe,* Alst., Ambro., Ant-t., Apis, *Arg-n., Arn., Ars.,* Asc-t., *Bapt.,* Bell., Calc., *Canth., Caps.,* Carb-ac., Carb-v., Chap., *Chin., Colch.,* Coll., *Coloc.,* Cuph., *Cupr-ar.,* Dulc., Emetin., *Erig., Eucal.,* Ferr-p., Gamb., Ham., Hep., *Ip.,* Iris, *Kali-bi., Kali-chl.,* Kali- m., Kali-p., Lach., Leon., Lept., Lil-t., Lyc., *Mag-c., Merc., Merc-c.,* Merc-d., Nit-ac., *Nux-v., Oper.,* Op., Ph-ac., *Phos.,* Plb-act., *Podo.,* Puls., Rheum, *Rhus-t.,* Sec., *Silphu., Sulph., Tanac.,* Tril-p., *Trom.,* Xan., Vac., Verat., Zinc-s.

**Abuse of local treatment, diphtheritic form:** Nit-ac.

**Chronic, intractable cases:** Aloe, Arg-n., *Ars.,* Chin., Cop., *Dulc.,* Hep., *Merc-c., Nit-ac., Nux-v.,* Ph-ac., Podo., Rhus-a., *Sulph.*

**Hemorrhoidal form:** Aloe, Coll., Ham.

**In old people:** Bapt.

**In plethoric, nervous, climacteric:** Lil-t.

**With nausea from straining pain, little thirst:** Ip.

**With long intervals between:** *Arn.,* Chin.

**With periodical recurrence in spring or early summer:** Kali-bi.

**With rheumatic pains all over:** Asc-t.

**With tearing down thighs:** Rhus-t.

**Worse in autumn:** Acon., *Colch.,* Dulc., *Ip., Merc.,* Merc-c., Sulph. (See **Diarrhea.**)

**ENTERITIS:** (See **Diarrhea.**)

**ENTERO-COLITIS:** (See **Diarrhea.**)

**GALL BLADDER, BILIARY CALCULI (Cholelithiasis):** Aur., Bapt., *Berb.,* Bold., Bry., *Calc., Card-m.,* Chel., *Chin., Chion.,* Chol., *Dios.,* Fab., Fel., Ferr-s., Gels., *Hydr.,* Jug-c., Lach., Lept., Myric., *Nux-v.,* Podo., Ptel., Tarax.

**Biliary colic:** Ars., Atro-s., *Bell., Berb., Calc., Card-m.,* Cham., Chel., *Chin.,* Chion., *Coloc.,* Dig., *Dios.,* Gels., *Hydr.,* Ip., Lyc., Morph-act., *Nux-v.,* Op., Ter.

**HEMORRHOIDS (piles), Remedies in general:** Abrot., *Acon., Aesc., Aesc-g., Aloe, Am-c.,* Am-m., Apis, *Ars.,* Aur., Bar-c., *Bell.,* Brom., *Calc-f., Caps.,* Carb-an., *Carb-v.,* Card-m., Caust., Cham., Chr-ac., *Coll.,* Cop., Dios., Ferr-p., *Fl-ac.,* Grat., *Ham.,* Hep., Hydr., *Hyper.,* Ign., *Kali-m.,* Kali-s., *Lach., Lyc.,* Mag-m., *Mill., Muc-u., Mur-ac.,* Neg., *Nit-ac., Nux-v., Paeon.,* Pin-s., *Podo., Polyg-h.,* Puls., Rad-br., *Rat.,* Sabin., Scroph-n., Sed-ac., Sep., *Semp.,* Sul-ac., *Sulph.,* Thuj., Verb., *Wye.,* Zing.

**Bleeding:** *Acon.,* Aesc., *Aloe, Am-c.,* Bell., Calc-f., *Caps.,* Card-m., Chr-ac., *Coll.,* Erig., Ferr-p., *Fic-r., Ham.,* Hydr., Hyper., Kali-m., Lept., Lycps-v., *Mill.,* Mur-ac., Nit-ac., *Nux-v.,* Oper., *Phos., Sabin.,* Scroph-n., Sep., *Sulph.,* Thlas.

**Bleeding, dark venous blood:** Aloe, *Ham.,* Hydr., Kali-m., *Sulph.*

**Blind:** *Aesc.,* Calc-f., Coll., *Ign.,* Muc-u., *Nux-v.,* Puls., *Sulph.,* Wye.

**Bluish, purplish:** *Aesc., Aesc-g., Aloe,* Ars., Caps., Carb-v., Ham., Lach., Lyc., *Mur-ac.*

**Burning, smarting:** *Aesc.,* Aloe, Am-m., *Ars.,* Calc., *Caps.,* Carb-an., Carb-v., Caust., *Fl-ac.,* Graph., *Ign.,* Mag-m., *Muc-u.,* Neg., *Nux-v.,* Psor., *Rat.,* Sul-ac., *Sulph.*

**Inflamed:** *Acon.,* Aesc., Aloe, Bell., Caust., Cop., Ferr-p., Mur-ac., Verb. (See **Sensitive.**)

**Itching:** *Aesc., Aloe, Caps.,* Carb-v., Caust., Cop., Glon., *Ham.,* Mur-ac., Nit-ac., *Nux-v., Petros.,* Puls., *Sulph.*

**Mucus piles, continually oozing:** *Aloe,* Am-m., *Ant-c.,* Caps., Carb-v., Caust., Puls., Sep., Sul-ac., Sulph.

**Protruding, grape-like, swollen:** Aesc., *Aloe, Am-c.,* Caps., *Carb-v., Caust., Coll., Dios.,* Graph., Ham., Kali-c., Lach., *Mur-ac.,* Nux-m., *Nux-v.,* Rat., Scroph-n., Sep., Sulph., Thuj.

**Protruding when urinating:** Bar-c., *Mur-ac.*

**Sensitive, exquisitely painful:** *Aesc.,* Aesc-g., *Aloe,* Ars., *Bell.,* Cact., *Caps.,* Carb-v., *Caust., Cham., Coll.,* Ferr-p., Graph., *Ham.,* Hyper., Kali-c., *Lach., Lyc.,* Mag-m., *Mur-ac.,* Nat-m., Nit-ac., *Nux-v.,* Plan., Puls., *Rat., Scroph-n., Sed-ac.,* Sep., *Sil.,* Sulph., Thuj., Verb., Zing.

**White piles:** Carb-v.

**CONCOMITANTS: With abdominal plethora:** Aesc., *Aloe,* Coll., Ham., Neg., Nux-v., Sep., *Sulph.*

**With backache:** *Aesc.,* Aesc-g., *Bell.,* Calc-f., Chr-ac., Euon., Ham., Ign., *Nux-v.,* Sulph. (See **Back.**)

**With constipation:** *Aesc.,* Aesc-g., Am-m., Anac., *Coll.,* Euon., Kali-s., *Nux-v.,* Paraf., Sil., *Sulph.,* Verb.

**With debility:** Ars., Chin., Ham., Hydr., Mur-ac.

**With epistaxis:** Carb-v.

**With fissures, soreness of anus:** Caps., Cham., *Nit-ac.,* Rat., *Sed-ac.*

**With heart disease:** Cact., Coll., Dig.

**With hypochondriasis:** Aesc., Grat., *Nux-v.*

**With pelvic congestion:** *Aloe, Coll.,* Ham., Hep., Muc-u., *Podo.,* Nux-v., Sep., *Sulph.*

**With prolapsus ani et uteri:** Podo.

**With spasm of sphincter:** Lach., Sil.

**With stitches in rectum during cough:** Ign., *Kali-c.,* Lach., Nit-ac.

**With sudden development in marastic children:** Mur-ac.

**With tenesmus, anal and visceral, diarrhea:** Caps.

**With tenesmus, constriction, lancinating pains:** Nux-v.

**With tenesmus, dysenteric stools:** Aloe, Sulph.

**With tenesmus, in pregnant females:** Coll.

**With vicarious bleeding:** Ham., Mill.

**AGGRAVATIONS, After confinement,** Aloe, Apis. (See **FEMALE SEXUAL SYSTEM.**)

**After stool for hours:** Aesc., Am-m., Ign., Rat., Sulph.

**As rheumatic symptoms abate:** Abrot.

**During climacteric:** Aesc., Lach. (See **FEMALE SEXUAL SYSTEM.**)

**During menses:** Am-c., Lach.

**During sitting:** Graph., Ign., *Thuj.*

**From alcoholic abuse, in sedentary persons:** Aesc-g., Nux-v.

**From coughing, sneezing:** Caust., *Kali-c.,* Lach.

**From leucorrhea suppressed:** Am-m.

**From talking, thinking of them:** Caust.

**From walking:** Caust., Sep.

**AMELIORATIONS: From cold water:** *Aloe,* Nux-v., Rat.

**From hot water:** *Ars.,* Mur-ac.

**From lying down:** Am-c.

**From walking:** Ign.

**HERNIA:** Aesc., Alum., Am-c., Aur., Calc., Calc-p., *Cocc.,* Cot., Iris-fa., *Lyc.,* Mag-c., *Nux-v.,* Ox-ac., Petr., Phos., Picro., *Sil., Sul-ac.,* Verat., Zinc.

**Incarcerated:** Lob., *Mill.,* Nux-v., *Op.,* Plb.

**In children:** *Calc.,* Lyc., Nit-ac., *Nux-v.,* Sil., Sulph.

**Scrotal, congenital:** Mag-m.

**Strangulated:** Acon., *Bell.,* Lyc., Nux-v., *Op.,* Plb.

**Umbilical:** Calc., Cocc., *Nux-v.,* Plb.

**INTESTINES, Intussusception, obstruction:** Acon., Atro., *Bell.,* Colch., Coloc., *Merc-c., Nux-v., Op., Plb.,* Thuj., Verat.

**Obstruction, post-operative:** Acon., *Arn.,* Bell., Merc-c.

**Paralysis:** Esin-sal., Plb-act.

**Ulceration:** Arg-n., Cupr., *Kali-bi.,* Merc-c., Sul-ac., Sulph., Ter., *Uran-n.*

**JAUNDICE (icterus):** *Acon.,* Aloe, Am-m., Arg-n., Astac., Ars., Aur., *Aur-m-n.,* Barbit., *Berb., Bry., Card-m.,* Cas-s., *Cean., Cham., Chel.,* Chelo., *Chin., Chion.,* Chol., Corn., Crot-h., *Dig.,* Dol., Eup-per., Hep., *Hydr.,* Iod., Jug-c., Kali-bi., Kali-c., Kali-pic., Lach., *Lept., Lyc., Merc.,* Merc-c., *Merc-d., Myric.,* Nat-m., *Nat-p.,* Nat-s., Nit-ac., *Nux-v.,* Ost., *Phos.,* Pic-ac., Plb., *Podo.,* Ptel., Rumx., Ruta, Sep., Still., Sulph., *Tarax., Vip., Yuc.*

**Anaemia, brain disease, pregnancy:** Phos.

**Chronic:** Aur., *Con.,* Iod., *Phos.*

**Extension of catarrhal process:** Am-m., *Chel., Chin.,* Chion., Dig., *Hydr.,* Lob., *Merc.,* Nux-v., Podo.

**From mental emotion:** Bry., *Cham.,* Lach., Nux-v., Vip.

**Infantile:** Cham., *Lup.,* Merc., Merc-d., Myric.

**Malignant:** Acon., *Ars.,* Crot-h., Lach., Merc., *Phos.*

**HYPOCHONDRIA, Pain in left side:** *Alum.,* Am-m., Arg-n., *Bapt-c.,* Carb-v., *Cean., Cimic.,* Con., Dig., Grind., Kali-c., Lyc., Nat-c., Nat-m., Nit-ac., *Ox-ac.,* Parth., Polym., *Puls.,* Querc., Sep., Squil., Urt-u. (See **Spleen**.)

**Pain in right side:** Aesc., *Aloe,* Aur., Bapt., *Berb.,* Bol-l., *Bry.,* Calc., Carb-v., *Chel., Chin.,* Con., *Dios.,* Gins., Jac-c., Jatr., *Kali-bi.,* Kali-c., Lim., *Lyc.,* Merc., *Nat-s.,* Nux-v., Ol-j., Phyt., *Podo., Ptel.,* Quas., Ran-s., Sulph., Wye. (See **Liver**.)

**LIVER, Abscess:** Ars., *Bell.,* Bold., Bry., Chinin-ar., *Hep.,* Lach., *Merc.,* Phos., Raph., Rhus-t., *Sil.,* Vip.

**Affections in general:** Abies-c., Aesc., *Aloe, Am-m.,* Ars-i., *Astac.,* Aur., *Aur-m-n.,* Barb., *Berb.,* Brass., *Bry.,* Calc., *Card-m., Cean., Cham., Chel.,* Chelo., Chen-a., *Chin., Chion.,* Chol., Cob., Con., Corn., Croc., Crot-h., Dios., Dol., *Eup-per.,* Euon., Fab., *Ferr-pic., Hep.,* Hydr., Iod., Iodof., *Iris, Kali-c.,* Kali-i., Lach., *Lept., Lyc., Mag-m.,* Mang-s., Marr., *Merc., Myric., Nat-s., Nux-v., Phos.,* Plb., *Podo., Ptel.,* Puls., Querc., Raph., Sel., *Sep.,* Stel., *Sulph., Tarax.,* Thlas., Uran-n., Vanad.

**Atrophy, acute, yellow:** Dig., *Phos.,* Podo.

**Atrophy (cirrhosis):** Abies-c., Apoc., Ars., *Ars-i.,* Aur., *Aur-m.,* Calc-ar., *Card-m.,* Cas-s., *Chin.,* Fel., Fl-ac., Graph., Hydr., *Iod.,* Kali-bi., Kali-i., *Lyc., Merc.,* Merc-d., *Nast.,* Nat-ch., Nit-ac., Nit-m-ac., Nux-v., *Phos.,* Plb., Podo., Quas., Senec.

**Cancer:** Ars., Chel., *Chol.,* Con., Hydr., Lach., Nit-ac., Phos.

**CONGESTION (hyperemia, fullness, torpidity):** Abies-c., *Aesc.,* Aesc-g., Agar., *Aloe,* Ars., *Berb.,* Berb-a., Brass., *Bry., Card-m.,* Cham., *Chel.,* Chelo., *Chin.,* Chinin-s., Croc., Dig., Eup-per., Euon., *Hep., Hydr., Iris,* Kali-bi., *Kali-m., Lach., Lept., Lyc., Mag-m., Merc., Merc-d.,* Muc-u., Nat-s., Nit-ac., Nit-m-ac., *Nux-v., Phos.,* Pic-ac., *Podo.,* Quas., Senn., *Sep.,* Stel., Still., *Sulph.,* Trom., *Vip.*

**Congestion, chronic:** Am-m., *Chel.,* Chin., *Chol.,* Con., *Hep.,* Hydr., Iod., *Kali-c.,* Lept., *Lyc.,* Mag-m., Merc., Merc-d., Nat-s., *Podo.,* Sel., *Sep., Sulph., Vip.*

**Enlargement (hypertrophy):** Aesc., Agar., *Ars.,* Calc-ar., Card-m., *Chel., Chin.,* Chinin-ar., *Chion.,* Coloc., Con., *Dig.,* Ferr-ar., Ferr-i., Glyc., Graph., Iod., Kali-c., Mag-m., Mang-act., *Merc., Merc-d.,* Nat-s., *Nux-v.,* Podo., Sec., *Sel.,* Stel., *Tarax.,* Vip., Zinc. (See **Congestion**.)

**Enlargements in drunkards:** Absin., Am-m., Ars., Fl-ac., Lach., Nux-v., Sulph.

**Fatty degeneration:** Aur., Chel., Kali-bi., Phlor., *Phos., Pic-ac.,* Vanad.

**Induration:** Abies-c., Ars., *Aur.,* Chin., *Con., Fl-ac., Graph.,* Lyc., Mag-m., Merc., Nux-v., Sil., *Tarax.,* Zinc. (See **Cirrhosis**.)

**Inflammation (perihepatitis, hepatitis):** Acon., Act-sp., Ars., Aur., *Bry.,* Cham., *Chel.,* Corn., *Hep.,* Iod., Kali-i., *Lach., Merc.,* Merc-d., Nat-s., *Phos.,* Psor., Sil., Stel., Sulph.

**PAIN (hepatalgia):** Acon., *Aesc.,* Aloe, Am-c., Am-m., Ars., Bell., Berb., Bold.,

*Bry.*, Calc-s., Carb-v., *Card-m., Cean., Chel.*, Chelo., *Chin.*, Chol., Cob., Con., Crot-h., *Dig., Dios.*, Jatr., Kali-c., Lach., *Lept., Lyc., Mag-m., Merc., Merc-d., Myric., Nux-v.*, Ol-j., Parth., *Podo., Ptel.*, Ran-b., *Ran-s.*, Sang., Sel., *Sep.*, Stann., Sulph., Tarax., Yuc.

**Pain dragging, on turning on left side:** Bry., Ptel.

**Pain, pressive:** Anac., Carb-an., Chin., *Kali-c.*, Lyc., Mag-m., Merc.

**Pain, stitching:** *Acon., Agar.*, Am-m., Bell., Benz-ac., *Berb., Bry.*, Carb-v., *Chel.*, Chin., Dios., Hep., Jug-c., Kali-bi., *Kali-c.*, Merc., Merc-c., Nat-m., Nat-s., *Nux-v.*, Ox-ac., Quas., Ran-b., Sep., Stel., Sulph.

**Pain, relieved by lying on painful side:** Bry., Ptel., Sep.

**Pain, relieved by rubbing and shaking liver region:** Podo.

**Pains worse lying on left side:** *Bry.*, Nat-s., *Ptel.*

**Pain worse lying on right side:** Chel., Dios., Kali-c., *Mag-m., Merc.*

**PIGMENTARY degeneration:** Arg-n.

**SENSITIVENESS to touch, pressure:** *Aesc., Aloe*, Bapt., *Bell., Berb., Bry.*, Calc., *Card-m.*, Chap., *Chel.*, Chelo., *Chin., Chion., Dig., Eup-per.*, Fl-ac., Graph., Hydr., Iod., *Iris, Kali-c., Lach.*, Lept., *Lyc., Mag-m.*, Merc., *Merc-d.*, Nat-s., *Nux-v.*, Nyct., Phos., *Podo., Ptel., Ran-b.*, Sanic., Senn., *Sep.*, Stel., Sulph., Tarax., Zinc.

**SYPHILIS:** Aur., Kali-i., Merc-i-r. (See **MALE SEXUAL SYSTEM.**)

**WAXY liver:** Calc., *Kali-i.*, Phos., Sil.

**PANCREAS: Affections:** Ars., *Atro.*, Bar-m., Bell., Calc-ar., Carb-an., Carb-v., Chion., *Iod., Iris*, Jab., Kali-i., *Merc.*, Nux-v., Pancr., *Phos.*, Pilo., Puls.

**PERINEUM:** Ars., Asaf., Bell., Bov., Cann-i., Carb-v., *Chim., Cycl.*, Kali-bi., Lyc., Mela., Merc., *Ol-an., Paeon., Sanic.*, Santal., Sel., Tell.

**PERITONITIS:** *Acon., Apis*, Arn., Ars., Atro., *Bell., Bry.*, Calc., *Canth.*, Carb-v., Cham., *Chin.*, Cimic., *Coloc., Crot-h.*, Ferr-p., Hep., Ip., Kali-chl., *Lach.*, Lyc., *Merc., Merc-c.*, Merc-d., *Rhus-t.*, Sangin-n., *Sin-n.*, Sol-n., Sulph., Ter., Verat-v., *Wye.*

**Chronic:** Apis, *Lyc.*, Merc-d., Sulph.

**Pseudo-peritonitis, hysterical:** Bell., Coloc., Verat.

**Tubercular:** *Abrot.*, Ars., Ars-i., Calc., Carb-v., *Chin.*, Iod., Psor., Sulph., *Tub.*

**PERITYPHILITIS:** *Ars.*, Bell., *Iris-t, Lach.*, Merc-c., Rhus-t.

**SPLEEN, Atrophy, induration:** Agn., Eucal., *Iod.*, Phos.

**Diseases, epidemic, in domestic animals:** Anthraci.

**Enlargement:** Agar., Agn., Aran., *Ars.*, Ars-i., Aur-m., Bell-p., *Calc-ar.*, Caps., Card-m., *Cean.*, Cedr., Chion., *Chin., Chinin-s.*, Ferr-act., *Ferr-ar.*, Ferr-i., Grin., *Helia.*, Iod., Mag-m., Malar., Merc-i-r., *Nat-m.*, Ph-ac.,

Phos., Polyg-h., *Polym., Querc.*, Succ., Sul-ac., Urt-u.

**Inflammation (splenitis):** Aran., Arn., *Cean., Chin., Chinin-s.,* Ferr-p., Iod., Plb-i., *Polym.,* Succ., Verat-v. (See **Enlargement**.)

**Pain:** *Agar.,* Agn., Am-m., Arn., *Ars.,* Ars-met., Caps., *Cean.,* Chin., Cimic., Cob., *Dios.,* Grin., *Helia., Helon.,* Ilx-a., Iod., *Kali-i., Lob-c., Nat-m.,* Parth., Plb., *Polym.,* Ptel., Quas., Quer., Ran-b., Rhus-t., Squil., Sulph., Urt-u.

**Pain, stitching:** Agar., Alst., Am-m., *Bell-p.,* Berb., Carb-v., *Cean.,* Chel., Chin., Con., Kali-bi., Nat-m., Ran-b., Rhod., Sulph., Tarax., *Ther.*

**TYPHILITIS, APPENDICITIS:** Acon., Arn., *Ars.,* Bapt., *Bell., Bry.,* Canth., Card-m., Colch., Coll., *Coloc.,* Crot-h., *Dios., Echi.,* Ferr-p., Gins., Hep., Iris-t., Kali-m., *Lach.,* Lyc., Merc., *Merc-c., Nux-v.,* Op., Plb., Rham-cal., *Rhus-t.,* Sil., Sulph., Verat.

**UMBILICUS, Navel, Bleeding from, in newborn:** Abrot., *Calc-p.*

**Bubbling sensation:** Berb.

**Burning:** Acon., Ars.

**Eczema:** Merc-pr-r.

**Pain, soreness about:** Aesc., *Aloe,* Anac., Benz-ac., *Bov.,* Bry., *Calc-p.,* Carb-v., Caust., *Cham.,* Chel., Chion., *Cina,* Cocc., *Coloc.,* Con., Crot-t., *Dulc.,* Euon., *Gamb., Gran.,* Hyper., *Ip.,* Lept., Lyc., *Nux-m.,* Nux-v., Olnd., Ox-ac., Paraf., *Ph ac.,* Plat., *Plb.,* Ran-s., Raph., *Rheum,* Senec., Sil., *Spig., Stann.,* Sulph., Tax., Verb., *Verat.,* Zinc.

**Retraction:** Calc-p., *Plb.,* Podo.

**Ulcer, above:** Ars.

**Urine, oozing from:** Hyos.

**WORMS: Remedies in general:** *Aesc., Ambro.,* Apoc-a., *Ars.,* Bapt., Bell., Calad., *Calc., Chelo.,* Cic., *Cina,* Cupr-act., Cupr-ox., *Ferr-m.,* Ferr-s., *Fil., Gran.,* Ign., Indg., Ip., Kali-m., Kuo., Lyc., Merc-c., *Naphtin., Nat-p.,* Passi., Puls., Quas., *Rat., Sabad., Santin.,* Sil., *Spig., Stann.,* Sulph., Sumb., Ter., *Teucr.,* Verat., *Viol-o.*

**Ascaris lubricoides:** *Abrot.,* Aesc., Ant-c., Calc., *Chelo., Cina,* Ferr., Gran., Helm., Ign., Indg., Kali-chl., Lyc., Merc-d., Naph., Pin-s., *Sabad., Santin., Spig.,* Stann., Sulph., Ter., *Teucr.,* Urt-u.

**Oxyuris vermicularis:** Ars., Bapt., *Chelo., Cina,* Ign., Indg., Lyc., *Merc., Merc-d.,* Nat-p., Rat., *Santin.,* Sil., Sin-n., Spig., *Teucr.,* Valer.

**Taenia:** Arge., Carb-v., Cuc-p., Cupr-act., Cupr-ox., *Fil., Gran.,* Graph., Kali-i., Kam., *Kuo.,* Mag-m., Merc., Pellin., Phos., Puls., Sabad., Sabin., Santin., Stann., Sulph., Ter., Valer.

**Trichnae:** Ars., Bapt., Cupr-ox.

# URINARY SYSTEM

**AFFECTIONS, in old men:** Alf., Aloe, Cop., Hep., Phos., *Pop-t.,* Staph., Sulph. (See **Weakness.**)

**Bladder: Atony:** *Ars.,* Dulc., Hep., Op., *Plb.,* Rhus-a., Rhus-t., Squil., Ter. (See **Paralysis.**)

**Cystocele:** Staph.

**ENURESIS, Incontinence, Remedies in general:** Acon., Agar., Apis, *Arg-n.,* Arn., Ars., Atro., *Bell., Benz-ac.,* Calc., Canth., *Caust.,* Cic., Cimic., *Cina,* Con., *Dulc., Equis-h.,* Ery-a., Eup-per., *Eup-pur.,* Ferr., *Ferr-p., Gels.,* Hydrang., Hyos., *Kali-br.,* Kali-n., Kali-p., *Kreos.,* Lina., *Lup.,* Lyc., Mag-p., Med., *Nux-v.,* Op., Petr., Ph-ac., Phys., Plan., *Puls., Rhus-a.,* Rhus-t., *Sabal,* Sanic., *Santin.,* Sec., Seneg., *Sep.,* Sil., Stram., *Sulph.,* Ter., *Thyr.,* Thuj., Tritic., Tub., *Uran-n., Verb.,* Zinc. (See **Flow.**)

**TYPE, OCCURRENCE, Diurnal:** Arg-n., Bell., Caust., Equis-h., *Ferr., Ferr-p.,* Sec.

**In old people:** Aloe, Am-be., *Arg-n., Benz-ac.,* Canth., *Dam.,* Equis-h., *Gels.,* Nit-ac., *Rhus-a.,* Sec., Seneg.

**Nocturnal:** Am-c., Arg-n., Arn., Ars., *Bell.,* Benz-ac., Calc., *Caust.,* Cina, Coca, *Equis-h.,* Eup-pur., Ferr-i., Ferr-p., Gels., Hep., Ign., Kali-br., Mag-p., *Med.,* Phys., *Plan., Puls.,* Quas., *Rhus-a.,* Santin., Sec., *Sil., Sulph.,* Thuj., *Thyr.,* Uran-n., Verb.

**CAUSE, Catheterization, after:** Mag-p.

**Digestive disturbances:** Benz-ac., *Nux-v.,* Puls.

**During first sleep, child aroused with difficulty:** Caust., Kreos., *Sep.*

**During full moon, intractable cases, eczematous history:** Psor.

**Habit, the only ascertainable cause:** Equis-h.

**History of sycosis:** Med.

**Hysteria:** Ign., Valer.

**Weak or paretic sphincter vesicae:** Apoc., *Bell., Caust.,* Con., Ferr-p., *Gels.,* Nux-v., Rhus-a., *Sabal,* Sec., *Stry.* (See **Paralysis.**)

**Worms:** Cina, *Santin.,* Sulph.

**FEELING, As if ball or plug, in bladder:** Anac., Kali-br., Lach., Santa.

**Feeling as if chill rising from, to back:** Sars.

**Feeling, as if distended:** Anth., *Apoc.,* Ars., Berb., *Con.,* Conv., Dig., *Equis-h.,* Eup-per., Gels., *Hyos.,* Mel-c-s., Pareir., *Puls.,* Ruta, Santin., *Sars.,* Sep., Staph., *Sulph.,* Uva.

**Hemorrhage:** *Amgd-p.,* Cact., Carb-v., Erig., *Ham.,* Mill., *Nit-ac.,* Rhus-a., *Sec., Thlas.* (See **Hematuria.**)

**Hypertrophy, concentric:** Fab.

**INFLAMMATION (cystitis), Acute:** Acon., Ant-t., Apis, Ars., Aspar., *Bell.*, Benz-ac., Berb., *Camph.*, Camph-ac., *Cann-s.*, *Canth.*, Caps., Chim., Con., *Cop.*, *Cub.*, Dig., *Dulc.*, Elat., *Equis-h.*, Erig., *Eucal.*, *Eup-pur.*, Fab., Ferr-act., *Ferr-p.*, *Gels.*, Hell., Hydrang., Hyos., Lach., *Merc-c.*, Methyl., Nit-ac., Nux-v., *Ol-sant.*, *Pareir.*, Petros., Pip-m., *Pop.*, Prun., *Puls.*, Sabal, *Sabin.*, Sars., *Saur.*, Sep., *Stigm.*, Sulph., *Ter.*, Tritic., Uva, Vesi.

**From abuse of cantharis:** Apis, Camph.

**From gonorrhea:** Bell., Benz-ac., *Canth.*, *Cop.*, Cub., Merc-c., Puls., Sabal.

**From operations, and in pregnancy:** Pop-t.

**With fever, strangury:** *Acon.*, Bell., *Canth.*, Gels., Hydrang., Stigm.

**Inflammation, chronic:** *Ars.*, Bals-p., *Baros.*, *Benz-ac.*, Berb., *Cann-s.*, *Canth.*, Carb-v., *Caust.*, *Chim.*, Coc-c., Coloc., *Cop.*, Cub., *Dulc.*, *Epig.*, Ery-a., Eucal., *Eup-pur.*, Fab., Grin., *Hydr.*, Iod., Juni-c., Lith-c., Lyc., *Merc-c.*, Nit-ac., *Pareir.*, Pip-m., *Pop.*, Prun., *Puls.*, Rhus-a., *Sabal,* Santin., Seneg., *Sep.*, Silphu., *Stigm.*, *Ter.*, Thlas., Thuj., Tritic., Tub., *Uva,* Vesi.

**IRRITABILITY: Bladder and neck:** *Acon.*, Alf., Aloe, *Apis,* Baros., *Bell.*, *Benz-ac.*, *Berb.*, Calc., *Camph.*, Cann-s., *Canth.*, Caps., Caust., *Cop.*, Cub., Dig., *Equis-h.*, Erig., Ery-a., *Eup-pur.*, Ferr-act., Ferr., *Ferr-p.*, Guaj., Hyos., Kali-br., Mit., Nit-m-ac., *Nux-v.*, Oxyt., Pareir., *Petros.*, Prun., Rhus-a., *Sabal,* *Senec.*, Seneg., *Sep.*, *Staph.*, *Stigm.*, *Ter.*, Thuja, *Tritic.*, Vesi.

**Irritability in women:** Berb., Cop., Cub., *Eup-pur.*, Gels., Hed., Kreos., Senec., *Sep.*, Staph.

**PAIN:** *Acon.*, Ambr., *Bell.*, *Berb.*, Camph., *Canth.*, Carb-v., Caul., *Caust.*, Coc.c., *Cop.*, Dig., *Dulc.*, *Equis-h.*, Erig., *Ery-a.*, Fab., Ign., Lach., *Lyc.*, Naph., Nit-ac., Op., *Pareir.*, Pilo., *Pop.*, Prun., Pulx., *Puls.*, *Rhus-a.*, *Staph.*, Stigm., Stry., *Ter.*, Thuj., Tritic., Uran-n., *Uva.* (See **Cystitis.**)

**TYPE, Aching:** Berb., Conv., *Equis,* Eup-pur., *Pop.*, Sep., Stict., Ter.

**Burning:** *Acon.*, Ars., Baros., *Berb.*, Camph., *Canth.*, *Cop.*, *Ferr-pic.*, Staph., *Ter.*, Thuj., *Uva.*

**Cramp-like constricting:** *Bell.*, *Berb.*, *Cact.*, Cann-s., Canth., *Caps.*, Lyc., Op., *Polyg-h.*, Prun., *Sars.*, Ter.

**Cutting, stitching:** *Acon.*, Aeth., *Bell.*, *Berb.*, *Canth.*, Coc-c., Con., *Lyc.*, *Ter.*

**Neuralgic, spasmodic:** *Bell.*, *Berb.*, Canth., Caul., Lith-c., *Lyc.*, Merc-c., *Pareir.*, Puls., *Staph.*, Uva.

**Pressing:** Aloe, Brach., *Cact.*, Carb-v., Coc-c., *Con.*, Dig., *Dulc.*, *Equis-h.*, Lach., Lil-t., Lyc., Mel-c-s., *Pop.*, Pulx., *Puls.*, Ruta, *Sep.*, *Staph.*, Sulph., Ter., Verb.

**Radiating to spermatic cord:** Clem., Lith-c., Puls., Spong.

**MODALITIES, AGGRAVATIONS, After urination:** *Canth.,* Caust., Epig., *Equis-h.,* Fab., Ruta. (See **Urination**.)

**From drinking water:** Canth.

**From lithotomy:** Staph.

**From walking:** Con., Prun.

**AMELIORATIONS, From rest:** Con.

**From urination:** Coc-c., Hed.

**From walking:** Ign., Ter.

**PARALYSIS:** Alum., Apoc., *Arn., Ars.,* Aur., Cact., Camph., Cann-i., *Canth., Caust.,* Con., Dig., Dulc., Eucal., *Equis-h., Ferr.,* Ferr-p., *Gels.,* Hell., *Hyos.,* Lach., Morph., *Nux-v., Op., Plb.,* Psor., Puls., *Sec.,* Stry., Thuj.

**Paralysis of sphincter:** Ars., *Bell., Caust.,* Cic., *Dulc., Hyos.,* Ign., Lach., Laur., Nat-m., Op., Sulph., Thuj., *Zinc.*

**POLYPI: Papilloma:** Ars., *Calc.,* Thuj.

**Prolapsus:** Hyos., Pyrus, Staph.

**Sensitiveness, tenderness of vesical region:** *Acon., Bell.,* Berb., *Canth.,* Coc-c., *Equis-h.,* Eup-pur., Merc-c., Sars., Stict., *Ter.* (See **Pain**.)

**Spasm (cystopasm):** Canth., Gels., *Hyos.,* Nux-v., Puls.

**Spasm following operations on orifice:** *Bell.,* Coloc., *Hyper.*

**TENESMUS VESICAE:** *Acon., Apis,* Arn., *Bell.,* Benz-ac., Camph., Cann-s., *Canth., Caps.,* Cham., Chim., Coc-c., *Coloc.,* Cop., Cub., Epig., *Equis-h.,* Ery-a., *Eup-pur.,* Fab., *Ferr-p.,* Hydrang., Hyos., Ip., *Lil-t.,* Lith-c., Lyc., Med., *Merc-c.,* Nit-ac., *Nux-v., Onis., Plb., Pop-t.,* Prun., *Puls.,* Rham-cal., Rhus-t., *Sabal,* Sars., *Senec.,* Staph., *Stigm., Ter.,* Vesi.

**WEAKNESS, Inability to retain urine, dribbling:** Aloe, Anan., *Apoc., Bell., Benz-ac.,* Brach., Camph., *Cann-i., Caust.,* Clem., *Con., Equis-h.,* Erig., Euphr., *Gels.,* Hep., Lycpr., *Nux-v.,* Petr., Pic-ac., Pulx., Puls., *Rhus- a.,* Santin., Sabal, *Sars.,* Sel., *Staph.,* Ter., Thymol., Trib., Uva, *Verb.,* Vesi., Xero.

**Weakness in old men:** Alum., *Benz-ac.,* Carb-ac., Clem., Con., *Pop-t.,* Sel., *Staph.* (See **Paralysis**.)

**KIDNEYS, Abscess (perinephritic):** Arn., Bell., *Hep.,* Merc., Verat-v.

**CALCULI, GRAVEL (nephrolithiasis), COLIC:** *Arg-n.,* Baros., *Bell.,* Benz-ac., *Berb.,* Calc., Calc-ren., *Canth.,* Cham., Chinin-s., *Coc-c.,* Coloc., *Dios., Epig.,* Erig., Ery-a., *Eup-pur., Fab.,* Hedeo., Hep., Hydrang., Ipom-p., *Lyc.,* Med., *Nit-ac., Nux-v., Oci.,* Onis., Op., Oxyd., *Pareir.,* Pipe., Polyg-h., *Sars.,* Sep., *Solid., Stigm., Tab.,* Thlas., Urt-u., Uva, Vesi.

**Colic, worse left side:** *Berb.,* Canth., Tab.

**Colic, worse right side:** *Lyc.,* Nux-v., Oci., Sars.

**Inter-paroxysmal treatment:** *Berb., Calc.,* Chinin-s., Hydrang., *Lyc.,* Nux-v., *Sep.,* Urt-u.

**CONGESTION, acute:** *Acon.,* Arg-n., Arn., Aur., *Bell.,* Benz-ac., *Berb.,* Bry., Camph., *Canth.,* Dig., *Dulc.,* Eucal., Ery-a., *Hell., Helon.,* Hydr-ac., *Juni-c.,* Kali-bi., Merc-c., *Ol-sant.,* Op., Rhus-t., Senec., Solid., *Ter.,* Verat-v. (See **Nephritis.**)

**Congestion, chronic (passive, from heart or kidney disease):** Acon., Arn., Bell., *Coffin., Conv., Dig.,* Glon., Phos., *Stroph-h.,* Stry., Verat-v. (See **Heart.**)

**DEGENERATION, acute, amyloid, fatty:** Apis, *Ars., Aur-m.,* Bell., Cic., *Cupr-act.,* Ferr-m., Hydr-ac., *Kali-i.,* Lyc., *Nit-ac., Ph-ac., Phos.,* Rhus-t., Ter. (See **Nephritis.**)

**FLOATING KIDNEY (nephroptosis) reflex symptoms:** *Bell.,* Cham., Coloc., Gels., *Ign.,* Lach., Puls., *Stry-ar.,* Sulph., Zinc.

**INFLAMMATION (nephritis): Bright's disease.**

**ACUTE AND SUBACUTE PARENCHYMATOUS NEPHRITIS:** *Acon.,* Ant-t., *Apis,* Apoc., *Ars., Aur-m., Bell., Berb., Cann-s., Canth.,* Chel., *Chim., Chinin-s.,* Colch., Conv., *Cupr-ar.,* Dig., Dulc., Eucal., Eup-per., *Fab.,* Ferr-i., Fuch., Glon., *Hell.,* Helon., *Hep.,* Hydrc., Irid-met., Juni-c., Kali-bi., *Kali-chl.,* Kali-cit., Kalm., Lach., *Merc., Methy.,* Nit-ac., *Ol-sant.,* Ph-ac., *Phos.,* Pic-ac., Plb-act., Polyg-h., Rhus-t., *Sabin., Samb.,* Sec., Senec., Ser-ang., *Squil., Ter., Tub-k., Verat., Verat-v.,* Zing.

**CAUSE: From cold, or wet exposure:** *Acon.,* Ant-t., *Apis,* Canth., *Dulc.,* Rhus-t., Ter.

**From influenza:** Eucal.

**From malaria:** *Ars.,* Eup-per., Ter.

**From pregnancy:** Apis, Apoc., *Cupr-ar.,* Helon., Kalm., *Merc-c.,* Sabin. (See **FEMALE SEXUAL SYSTEM.**)

**From scarlet fever, diphtheria:** Acon., *Apis, Ars.,* Bell., *Canth.,* Conv., Cop., Dig., Ferr-i., *Hell., Hep.,* Kalm., Lach., *Merc-c.,* Methyl., Nat-s., Nit-s-d., *Rhus-t.,* Sec., *Ter.*

**From suppurations:** Apoc., Chinin-s., *Hep.,* Phos., Plb-chr., *Sil.,* Ter.

**CONCOMITANTS: Dropsy:** Acon., Adon., Ant-t., *Apis, Apoc., Ars.,* Aur-m., Canth., Colch., Cop., *Dig., Hell.,* Merc-c., Pilo., *Samb.,* Senec., *Squil.,* Ter. (See **Dropsy, GENERALITIES.**)

**Heart failure:** Adon., Ars., *Coffin., Dig.,* Glon., *Saroth.,* Stroph-h., Verat-v.

**Pneumonia:** Chel., Phos.

**Uremic symptoms:** Aeth., Am-c., Ars., Bell., Cann-i., *Carb-ac.,* Cic., *Cupr-ar.,* Hell., Hyos., *Morph., Op.,* Pilo., Stram., Urea.

**ACUTE, SUPPURATIVE NEPHRITIS:** Acon., Arn., Bell., Camph., Calc-s., *Cann-s.,* Canth., *Chinin-s.,* Eucal., Hecla, *Hep.,* Kali-n., *Merc-c.,* Naphtin., Sil., Verat-v.

**CHRONIC, INTERSTITIAL NEPHRITIS:** Apis, *Ars., Aur-m.,* Aur-m-n., Cact., *Chinin-s., Colch.,* Conv., *Dig.,* Ferr., *Ferr-m., Glon., Iod.,* Kali-c., *Kali-i.,* Lith-ac., Lith-be., Lith-c., *Merc-c.,* Merc-d., *Nat-i., Nit-ac.,* Nux-v., Op., Ph-ac., Phos., *Plb., Plb-c., Plb-i.,* Sang., Tub-k., Zinc-pic. (See **Arteriosclerosis, CIRCULATORY SYSTEM.**)

**CHRONIC, PARENCHYMATOUS NEPHRITIS:** Am-be., *Apis, Ars., Aur-m.,* Aur-m-n., Benz-ac., Berb., *Brach.,* Calc-ar., Calc-p., Cann-i., *Canth.,* Chinin-ar., Conv., Dig., Eup-pur., *Euon., Ferr-ar.,* Ferr-cit., *Ferr-m.,* Ferr-p., Form-ac., Glon., *Helon.,* Hydr-ac., Juni-c., Kali-ar., *Kali-chl.,* Kali-cit., *Kali-i., Kali-m.,* Kalm., Lon-c., *Lyc., Merc-c.,* Nat-chor., *Nit-ac., Pilo., Plb.,* Saroth., Senec., *Solania., Solid., Ter.,* Tub-k., Urea., *Vesi.*

**SYMPTOMS, UREMIA, In general:** *Am-c.,* Apis, Apoc., Ars., Asc-c., *Bell.,* Cann-i., *Canth., Carb-ac.,* Cic., Cupr-act., *Cupr-ar., Glon., Hell.,* Hydr-ac., Hyos., Kali-br., *Morph., Op.,* Phos., *Pic-ac.,* Pilo., Queb., Ser-ang., Stram., *Ter.,* Urea, Urt-u., *Verat-v.*

**Coma:** *Am-c.,* Bell., Bry., *Carb-ac.,* Cupr-ar., *Hell.,* Merc-c., *Morph., Op.,* Verat-v.

**Convulsions:** Bell., Carb-ac., Chlol., Cic., Cupr-act., *Cupr-ar.,* Glon., *Hydr-ac.,* Kali-br., Merc-c., Op., Pilo., Plb., Verat-v. (See **Convulsions, NERVOUS SYSTEM.**)

**Headache:** Arn., Cann-i., Carb-ac., Cupr-ar., *Glon.,* Hyper., *Sang.,* Zinc-pic. (See **HEAD.**)

**Vomiting:** *Ars.,* Iod., Kreos., Nux-v. (See **STOMACH.**)

**PAIN IN RENAL REGION, Burning:** *Acon.,* Ars., Aur., *Berb.,* But-ac., *Canth.,* Hed., *Helon.,* Kali-i., Lach., *Lyc.,* Merc-c., *Phos.,* Sabin., *Sulph., Ter.* (See **Back.**)

**Cutting, digging, boring:** Arn., *Berb., Canth.,* Eup-pur., Ip., *Lyc.,* Rhus-t., Ter.

**Drawing, tensive:** *Berb.,* Cann-s., *Canth.,* Chel., Coc-c., *Colch.,* Dulc., Lach., *Lyc.,* Nit-ac., Solid., *Ter.*

**Neuralgic, radiating (nephralgia), tearing, lancinating:** *Arg-n.,* Arn., *Bell., Berb.,* Calc., *Canth.,* Chel., Chinin-s., *Coc.c., Cocc-s., Dios.,* Ery-a., Ferr-m., *Hed., Hydrang.,* Lach., *Lyc.,* Kali-i., Nit-ac., *Nux-v., Oci.,* Oxyt., Pereir., Phos., Sabin., *Sars.,* Scroph-n., *Solid., Tab.,* Ter., Thlas., Vesp. (See **Nephrolithiasis**.)

**Pressing:** Arg-n., *Arn.,* Aur-m., *Berb., Canth.,* Chinin-s., *Lyc.,* Nit-ac., *Oci.,* Petr., *Ph-ac., Sep., Ter.,* Uva, Xero.

**Stitching:** *Berb., Canth.,* Colch., *Kali-c.,* Pareir.

**Throbbing:** Act-sp., *Berb.,* Chim., Med., *Sabin.*

**Weariness, aching, lameness:** *Acon.,* Alum., Am-br., Apis, *Arg-n., Benz-ac., Berb.,* Cann-i., *Canth.,* Chel., Cina, Conv., Cop., *Eup-pur., Hed., Helon.,* Hydrang., Juni-c., Kali-bi., Lyc., Nat-chor., *Nux-v., Ol-sant., Phyt., Pic-ac.,* Pin-s., *Sabin., Sep.,* Solid., Stel., Ter., Ust., *Uva,* Vesp. (See **Back.**)

**MODALITIES, AGGRAVATIONS, At 2 P.M.:** Kalm.

**From lifting, sudden effort:** Calc-p.

**From lying down:** Conv.

**From motion:** *Berb., Canth.,* Chel., Kali-i.

**From pressure:** *Berb.,* Canth., Colch., *Solid.*

**From sitting:** *Berb.,* Ferr-m.

**From stooping, lying down:** Berb.

**From stretching legs:** Colch.

**From wine:** Benz-ac.

**On left side:** Aesc., Berb., *Hed.,* Hydrang., Tab., Uva.

**On right side:** Am-be., Cann-i., *Chel.,* Equis-h., Lith-c., *Lyc.,* Oci., Phyt., Pic-ac., *Sars., Ter.*

**AMELIORATIONS, From lying on back:** Cain.

**From lying on back, legs drawn up:** Colch.

**From standing:** Berb.

**From urination:** Lyc., Med.

**From walking:** Ferr-m.

**PERI-NEPHRITIS:** Acon., Bry., Chinin-s., Hep., Merc., Sil.

**PYELITIS, Inflammation of pelvis, Acute:** Acon., *Ars.,* Aur., *Bell., Benz-ac.,* Berb., Bry., *Cann-s., Canth.,* Chin., *Cop., Cupr-ar.,* Epig., *Ferr-m.,* Hecla, Hep., Kali-bi., *Merc-c.,* Nit-ac., *Puls., Rhus-t.,* Stigm., *Ter.,* Thuj., *Tritic., Uva, Verat-v.*

**Calculus:** Hep., *Hydrang.,* Lyc., *Pipe.,* Sil., Uva. (See **Nephrolithiasis.**)

**Chronic:** Ars., *Baros., Benz-ac.,* Berb., *Chim.,* Chin., Chinin-s., *Cop.,* Hep., Hydrin-m., Hydrin-s., *Juni-c., Kali-bi., Ol-sant.,* Pareir., Puls., Sep., Sil., Sulph., Stigm., *Uva.*

**SENSITIVENESS, tenderness:** *Acon.,* Apis, *Berb.,* Calc-ar., Cann-s., *Canth.,* Equis-h., *Helon.,* Phyt., *Solid., Ter.* (See **Pain.**)

**SYPHILIS:** Aur., Kali-i., Merc-c. (See **MALE SEXUAL SYSTEM.**)

**TRAUMATISMS:** Acon., *Arn.,* Bell., Verat-v.

**TUBERCULOSIS:** *Ars-i.,* Bac., Calc., Calc-hp., *Calc-i., Chinin-ar.,* Chinin-s., Hecla, Kali-i., Kreos. (See **Tuberculosis, RESPIRATORY SYSTEM.**)

**URETHRA, Burning, smarting, heat:** *Acon.,* Apis, *Arg-n., Berb.,* Cain., Calc., *Cann-i., Cann-s., Canth., Caps.,* Chim., *Clem.,* Con., Cop., Dig., Gels.,

*Hydrang., Merc., Merc-c.,* Mez., Nat-c., Nit-m-ac., Onis., Petr., *Petros.,* Phos., Sel., Staph., *Sulph., Ter., Thuj., Uran-n.,* Zing.

**Burning between acts of urination:** Berb., Cann-s., Staph.

**Caruncle:** Cann-s., *Eucal.,* Teucr., *Thuj.*

**Discharge, mucus:** Hep., Merc-c., Nat-m.

**Hemorrhage:** Calc., Lyc.

**Inflammation (urethritis):** *Acon.,* Apis, *Arg-n.,* Camph., *Cann-s., Canth.,* Caps., Caust., *Cop., Cub., Dor., Gels.,* Kali-bi., Kali-i., Merc-c., Nux-v., Petr., Sabin., Sulph., *Thuj.,* Yohim. (See **MALE SEXUAL SYSTEM.**)

**Itching:** Acon., Alum., Ambr., *Arg-n.,* Canth., Caust., Coloc., Ferr., *Ferr-i.,* Gins., Lyc., *Merc.,* Mez., *Nit-ac.,* Ol-an., Pareir., Petr., *Petros.,* Staph., *Sulph.,* Thuj., Tus-p.

**MEATUS: Burning:** *Acon.,* Ambr., Borx., Cann-s., *Canth., Caps.,* Clem., Gels., Menth., *Petros.,* Sel., *Sulph.,* Zing.

**Eruptions around:** Caps.

**Itching:** Alum., *Ambr.,* Caust., Coloc., Gins., *Petros.*

**Ulcers around:** Eucal.

**Swelling:** Acon., Arg-n., *Cann-s., Canth.,* Cop., Gels., *Merc., Ol-sant.,* Sulph. (See **Urethritis.**)

**Membranous-prostatic involvement:** Sabal.

**PAIN IN URETHRA: Constricting:** *Arg-n., Cann-s.,* Caps., *Clem.,* Ferr-i., Ol-sant., *Petros.*

**Cutting:** Alum., Ant-c., *Berb., Canth.,* Nat-m., Onis., *Petros.*

**Soreness, tenderness, irritation:** Agn., Anag., *Arg-n., Berb.,* Brach., *Cann-s., Canth.,* Caust., Clem., *Cop.,* Cub., Ferr-pic., Gels., Kali-i., Tus-p.

**Stitching, stinging:** Agar., *Apis, Arg-n.,* Aspar., *Berb.,* Cann-i., *Cann-s.,* Caps., Carb-v., *Clem.,* Merc., Merc-c., Nit-ac., Petros., *Thuj.*

**SENSIBILITY: Diminished:** Kali-br.

**STRICTURE, organic:** Acon., Arg-n., Arn., Calc-i., *Canth., Clem.,* Eucal., Lob., Phos., Puls., Sil., *Sul-i.*

**Stricture, spasmodic:** *Acon.,* Bell., *Camph.,* Canth., Ery-a., Hydrang., Nux-v., Petros.

**URINARY FLOW, DESIRE, Constant desire:** Absin., *Acon.,* Anan., *Bell.,* Berb., Cact., *Cann-s., Canth.,* Carb-v., Caust., Cean., Coc-c., *Cop.,* Dig., Dulc., Equis-h., *Eup-pur., Ferr-m.,* Gels., Guaj., Kreos., *Lil-t.,* Lyss., *Murx.,* Op., *Pareir.,* Ruta, *Sabal, Senec.,* Sep., *Staph.,* Sulfon., *Sulph., Thuj., Tritic.,* Zing. (See **Cystitis.**)

**Constant after labor:** Op., *Staph.*

**Constant at night:** Dig., *Sabal.*

**Constant from prolapsus uteri:** Lil-t.

**Constant, on seeing running water:** Canth., *Lyss.,* Sulph.

**DIABETES INSIPIDUS: Copious, profuse, polyuria, diuresis:** *Acet-ac.*, Acon., *Alf.*, All-c., Am-act., Apoc., *Arg-met.*, *Arg-mur.*, Ars., *Aur-m.*, *Bell.*, Bry., Cain., *Cann-i.*, Caust., Chinin-s., Chion., Cina, *Cod.*, Conv., Dulc., *Equis-h.*, *Eup-pur.*, *Ferr-m.*, Ferr-n., *Gels.*, Glyc., *Glon.*, Gnaph., Gua., *Hell.*, *Helon.*, *Ign.*, Indol., *Kali-c.*, Kali-i., *Kali-n.*, *Kreos.*, Lac-ac., Led., *Lil-t.*, *Lith-c.*, *Lyc.*, Mag-p., Merc-c., Mosch., *Murx.*, *Nat-m.*, Nicc-s., *Nit-ac.*, Nux-v., *Ol-an.*, *Oxyt.*, *Ph-ac.*, Phos., Phys., Pic-ac., Plat-m-n., Puls., Quas., *Rhus-a.*, *Samb.*, Sang., Santin., Sars., Saroth., *Sin-n.*, *Squil.*, Staph., *Stroph-h.*, *Sulph.*, Tarax., Ter., Thymol., Thyr., *Uran-n.*, Verb., Verat-v. (See **Diabetes.**)

**Copious at night:** Ambr., Kali-i., *Lyc.*, *Murx.*, Petr., *Ph-ac.*, Quas., *Squil.*

**DYSURIA, Difficult, slow, painful:** *Acon.*, *Alum.*, Ant-t., *Apis*, Apoc., *Arg-n.*, Arn., *Ars.*, *Bell.*, *Benz-ac.*, Camph., *Cann-i.*, *Cann-s.*, *Canth.*, Caps., Casc., *Caust.*, Chim., *Clem.*, Coc-c., *Con.*, Cop., Cuc-c., Dig., Dulc., *Epig.*, Equis-h., *Eup-pur.*, *Fab.*, Ferr-p., *Hep.*, Hydrang., Hyper., Hyos., Kreos., Lith c., *Lyc.*, Med., Merc-c., *Morph.*, Mur-ac., *Nat-m.*, Nit-ac., Nux-v., Oci., *Ol-sant.*, *Op.*, *Pareir.*, Petros., *Plb.*, Pop., Puls., Rhus-t., Ruta, *Sabal*, *Santin.*, *Sars.*, Sel., *Sep.*, *Solid.*, Staph., Stigm., Tax., Thlas., *Tritic.*, *Uva.*, Verb., Vib., Zinc. (See **Scanty**.)

**Difficult, in pregnancy, and after confinement:** Equis-h.

**Difficult, in presence of others:** Ambr., Hep., Mur-ac., *Nat-m.*

**Difficult, in young, married women:** Staph.

**Difficult, must lie down:** Kreos.

**Difficult, must sit bent backwards:** Zinc.

**Difficult, must stand with feet wide spart, body inclined forward:** Chim.

**Difficult, must strain:** *Acon.*, *Alum.*, Asim., Cann-i., *Chim.*, Equis-h., *Hyos.*, Kali-c., *Kreos.*, Lyc., *Mag-m.*, Nux-v., Op., *Pareir.*, *Prun.*, Sabal, Zinc. (See **Bladder**.)

**Difficult, with prolapsus ani:** Mur-ac.

**Difficult, with prostatic or uterine diseases:** Con., Staph.

**Divided stream:** Anag., Arg-n., Cann-s., Canth.

**Feeble stream:** Cham., Clem., Hell., Hep., Merc., Sars.

**FREQUENT desire:** *Acon.*, Agar., Agn., Alf., Aloe, *Alum.*, Ant-c., *Apis*, Arg-n., *Aspar.*, *Aur-m.*, Bar-c., *Bell.*, Benz-ac., *Berb.*, Bor-ac., Calc., Calc-ar., *Cann-s.*, *Canth.*, Caps., Carl., *Caust.*, *Chim.*, Clem., Coc-c., *Colch.*, Coloc., Conv., Cub., Dig., *Equis-h.*, Ferr-p., *Fer-pic.*, Form., *Gels.*, Glyc., Hell., *Helon.*, Hydrang., Ign., Indol., Jatr., *Kali-c.*, Kalm., *Kreos.*, Lac-ac., *Lil-t.*, Lith-be., *Lith-c.*, *Lyc.*, Merc., Merc-c., Nat-c., Nit-ac., *Nux-v.*, Oci., *Ol-sant.*, Ox-ac., *Ph-ac.*, Pilo., Plb., *Prun.*, Pulx., *Puls.*, Sabal, Sabin., *Samb.*, Santin., *Sars.*, Sec., *Sep.*, Sil., *Squil.*, *Staph.*, Sulph., Tritic., *Uva*, *Vesp.*, Zing.

**Frequent desire at night:** Alum., *Aur-m.,* Borx., Calc., Carb-ac., *Caust.,* Coc-c., *Con.,* Ferr., *Ferr-pic.,* Glyc., *Graph., Kali-c., Kreos.,* Lycpr., Murx., Nat-m., *Ph-ac.,* Phys., Pic-ac., *Puls.,* Sang., Sars., Sep., Squil., *Sulph.,* Ter., Thuj., Xero.

**Imperative, irresistible, sudden desire:** Acon., Agar., Aloe, *Apis,* Arg-n., Borx., Cann-s., *Canth.,* Carls., Equis-h., Hed., Ign., *Kreos.,* Lath., Merc., *Merc-c.,* Murx., Naphtin., Ol-an., *Pareir., Petros., Pop.,* Prun., Puls., Quas., Ruta, Santin., Scut., *Sulph.,* Thuj.

**Intermittent, interrupted flow:** Agar., Cann-i., Caps., *Clem., Con.,* Gels., *Hep.,* Mag-s., Pulx., Puls., *Sabal,* Sars., Sed-ac., Thuj., Zinc.

**INVOLUNTARY:** Alum., *Arg-n.,* Arn., Ars., *Bell.,* Calc., *Caust., Cina, Dulc.,* Echi., *Equis-h.,* Ferr., *Gels., Hyos.,* Kali-br., *Kreos.,* Lycpr., Op., Petr., *Puls., Rhus-a.,* Rhus-t., Ruta, *Sabal,* Sapin., Sars., *Sel.,* Seneg., *Sil.,* Sulph., *Uva,* Xero. (See **Bladder**.)

**Involuntary at night:** Ars., *Bell.,* Calc., *Caust., Cina,* Kali-br., *Kreos.,* Plan., *Puls.,* Rhus-t., Seneg., *Sep.,* Sil., *Sulph.,* Uva. (See **Enuresis**.)

**Involuntary during first sleep:** Kreos., Sep.

**Involuntary when coughing, sneezing, walking, laughing:** Bell., Calc., Canth., Caps., *Caust.,* Ferr., Ferr-m., *Ferr-p.,* Ign., Kali-c., *Nat-m., Puls.,* Sel., *Squil.,* Sulph., Vib., Xero., *Zinc.*

**Involuntary when dreaming of act:** Equis-h., Kreos.

**Involuntary without consciousness of:** Apoc., *Arg-n., Caust.,* Sars.

**RETENTION (Ischuria):** *Acon.,* Ap-g., Apis, *Arn., Ars., Bell., Camph.,* Cann-i., Cann-s., *Canth., Caust.,* Chim., Cic., Cop., Dulc., *Equis-h., Eup-pur., Hyos.,* Ign., Lyc., Merc-c., *Morph., Nux-v., Op., Plb.,* Puls., Rhus-t., Sars., *Stigm.,* Stry., Sulph., *Ter.,* Zinc.

**From atony of fundus:** Ter.

**From cold or wet exposure:** *Acon., Dulc.,* Gels., Rhus-t.

**From fever, acute illness:** Ferr-p., Op.

**From fright:** *Acon.,* Op.

**From hysteria:** Ign., Zinc.

**From inflammation:** *Acon.,* Cann-i., *Canth.,* Nux-v., Puls.

**From overexertion:** Arn.

**From paralysis:** *Caust.,* Dulc., Hyos., Nux-v., *Op., Plb.,* Stry.

**From post-partum:** Hyos., Op.

**From prostatic hypertrophy:** Chim., Dig., Morph., Zinc. (See **MALE SEXUAL SYSTEM.**)

**From spasmodic constriction of neck of bladder:** *Bell.,* Cact., Camph., Canth., *Hyos.,* Lyc., *Nux-v.,* Op., Puls., Rhus-t., Stram., Thlas.

**From suppressed discharges or eruptions:** Camph.

**From surgical operations:** Caust.

**SCANTY FLOW:** *Acon.,* Adon., *Alf.,* Apis, Apoc., *Arg-n., Ars.,* Aur-m., *Bell., Benz-ac., Berb.,* Bry., Camph., Cann-s., *Canth.,* Carb-ac., Carb-v., *Chim.,* Clem., *Colch.,* Coloc., Conv., Cupr-ar., *Dig.,* Dulc., Equis-h., Eup-pur., Fl-ac., Graph., *Hell., Juni-c.,* Kali-bi., Kali-chl., Kali-i., Kreos., Lach., Lec., Lil-t., Lith-c., Lyc., Lyss., Menth., *Merc-c.,* Merc-cy., *Nit-ac., Nux-v.,* Op., Phos., Pic-ac., *Pilo., Plb.,* Prun., Pulx., Puls., Ruta, *Sabin., Sars.,* Sel., Senec., Seneg., Sep., Ser-ang., *Solid., Stroph-h., Squil.,* Sul-ac., Sulfon., Sulph., *Ter., Uva,* Zing.

**Scanty, drop by drop:** *Acon.,* Aesc., *Apis,* Arn., *Bell.,* Borx., *Canth.,* Caps., Caust., Clem., Colch., *Cop.,* Dig., Equis-h., Inul., *Lyc.,* Merc., *Merc-c.,* Nux-v., Plb., *Puls.,* Rhus-t., *Sabal,* Staph., Sulph.

**STRANGURY:** *Acon.,* Ant-t., *Apis,* Apoc., *Ars., Bell., Camph., Cann-s., Canth., Caps.,* Coloc., Con., *Cop., Dulc.,* Ery-a., *Eup-pur.,* Hydrang., Junc-e., Juni-c., Juni-v., Lyc., *Merc-c.,* Morph., Nux-m., *Nux-v., Pareir., Petros.,* Prun., Puls., Sabin., Sars., Senn., Stigm., *Ter.,* Thlas., *Tritic., Urt-u.,* Verb., Zing.

**In children:** *Borx.,* Lyc., Sars.

**In females:** Apis, Caps., *Cop.,* Dig., *Eup-pur.,* Lil-t., *Sabin.,* Staph., Verat-v., Vib.

**Nervous type:** Apis, *Bell.,* Caps., *Ery-a.,* Morph., Petros.

**SUPPRESSION (anuria):** *Acon.,* Agar-ph., Alf., *Apis,* Apoc., *Ars.,* Ars-h., *Bell.,* Bry., *Camph., Canth.,* Coff., *Colch., Cupr-act., Dig.,* Form., *Hell.,* Juni-v., *Kali-bi., Kali-chl., Lyc., Merc-c.,* Merc-cy., Nit-ac., *Op., Oxyd.,* Petr., Phyt., Pic-ac., Puls., Sec., *Solid.* Stigma., *Stram., Ter.,* Verat., Zing.

**URINATION, COMPLAINTS BEFORE ACT, Anxiety, agony:** *Acon.,* Borx., *Canth.,* Ph-ac.

**Burning:** Ars., *Berb., Camph., Cann-s., Canth.,* Cochl., Cop. (See **Urethra.**)

**Leucorrhea, yellow:** Kreos.

**Pain:** *Acon., Berb., Borx., Canth.,* Cann-s., Erig., Kali-c., Lith-c., *Lyc.,* Pilo., *Rhus-a.,* Sanic., *Sars.,* Seneg., Sep. (See **Pain, Bladder, Kidneys, Urethra.**)

**COMPLAINTS DURING ACT: Burning, smarting:** *Acon.,* All-c., Ambr., Anac., Anag., *Apis,* Apoc., *Arg-n., Ars., Berb.,* Bor-ac., *Borx.,* Camph., Cann-i., *Cann-s., Canth.,* Caps., Carb-v., Chim., *Cop.,* Cub., Dig., Epig., *Equis-h.,* Erig., Ery-a., *Eup-pur.,* Gels., Glyc., Hell., *Kreos., Lyc.,* Merc., *Merc-c.,* Nit-ac., Nux-v., Oci., *Ol-sant.,* Ox-ac., *Pareir.,* Phos., Puls., Rhus-a., *Sep.,* Staph., *Sulph., Ter.,* Thuj., Uva, Verb., *Vesp.*

**Chill:** *Acon.,* Sars., Sep.

**Meatus, agglutination:** Anag., Cann-s.

**Meatus, burning (also prepuce):** Calad., Calc., *Cann-s.,* Gels., Menth., *Merc-c.,* Puls.

**Meatus, itching:** Ambr., Cop., Lyc., Nux-v.

**PAINS IN GENERAL:** *Acon., Apis, Arg-n., Berb.,* Berb-a., Blatta-a., Bor-ac., Camph., *Cann-s., Canth., Caps., Chim., Coloc.,* Dig., Dory., *Equis-h.,* Erig., Graph., Hed., *Lith-c., Lyc.,* Merc., Nit-ac., *Nux-v., Pareir., Petr.,* Phos., Puls., *Rhus-a.,* Sabal, *Sars., Sep.*

**Cutting, stinging, stitching:** *Acon.,* Ant-c., Apis, *Berb.,* Berb-a., Borx., Camph., *Cann-s., Canth.,* Cochl., Coloc., Con., Hydrang., Nux-v., *Pareir.,* Puls.

**Drawing, radiating to labia:** Eupi.

**Drawing, radiating to chest and shoulders:** Glyc.

**Drawing, radiating to perineum:** Lyc., Sep.

**Drawing, radiating to sacrum, coccyx:** Graph.

**Drawing, radiating to testicles:** *Berb.,* Cain., Erig.

**Drawing, radiating to thighs:** Berb., Pareir.

**Pressive:** Camph., Cop., Lyc., *Sep.*

**Pressive in heart:** Lith-c.

**Spasmodic, toward end of act:** *Arg-n.,* Bor-ac., Puls.

**Stool, involuntary:** Sulph.

**Sweating:** Merc-c.

**COMPLAINTS AFTER ACT, Burning, smarting:** *Acon.,* Anac., Apis, *Arg-n.,* Bell., *Berb.,* Camph., *Cann-s., Canth., Caps.,* Chim., Cochl., Cub., *Fab., Kreos.,* Lyc., Mag-s., *Merc-c.,* Nat-c., *Nat-m.,* Ph-ac., Puls., Rhus-t., Seneg., Staph., *Sulph., Thuj., Uva.*

**Dribbling:** *Arg-n.,* Benz-ac., Calc., Camph., Cann-i., Caust., *Clem.,* Con., Lyc., *Pareir., Sel.,* Thuj., Zing. (See **Bladder**.)

**Emissions, seminal:** Calad., Hep., Ph-ac.

**Exhaustion:** Ars., Berb.

**Hemorrhoids:** Bar-c.

**Meatus, and urethra, tingling:** Clem., Thuj.

**Meatus, burning:** Caps., Puls.

**PAINS, Aching, bruised:** *Berb.,* Equis-h., Sulph.

**Cutting, tearing, stitching:** *Berb.,* Bov., Camph., *Cann-s., Canth., Caps.,* Coch., *Cub.,* Guaj., Mag-s., Merc-act., *Nat-m.,* Nux-v., Petros., Prun., *Sars., Thuj.,* Uva.

**Pressive, in perineum:** Am-m., Lyc.

**Sensation as if urine remained behind:** Alum., *Berb.,* Dig., Eup-pur., Ery-a., Gels., *Hep., Kali-bi.,* Ruta, Sec., Sil., Staph., *Thuj.*

**Severe, at close, and after act:** Apis, *Berb.,* Canth., Echi., *Equis-h., Lith-c.,* Med., Merc-act., *Nat-m.,* Petros., Puls., Ruta, *Sars.,* Staph., *Thuj.*

**Spasmodic:** *Nat-m.,* Nux-v., Puls.

**Perspiration:** Merc-c.

**Tenesmus, urging, straining:** Arg-n., *Camph., Canth.,* Chim., Epig., *Equis-h.,* Ery-a., Fab., Lith-c., Nit-ac., *Pop-t., Puls.,* Ruta, Sabal, Sars., *Staph.,* Stigm., Sulph.

**URINE, TYPE, Acid:** Acon., *Benz-ac.,* Canth., Chinin-s., Euon., Lith-c., *Lyc., Merc-c.,* Mur-ac., *Nit-ac.,* Nit-m-ac., Nux-v., Oci., Puls., *Sars.,* Sep., *Sulph., Uva.* (See **Burning.**)

**Albuminuria, Albuminous:** Acetan., Adon., *Am-be.,* Ant-t., *Apis, Ars.,* Aur-m., Bell., *Berb., Calc-ar.,* Cann-s., *Canth.,* Carb-ac., Chinin-s., *Colch.,* Conv., Cop., Cupr-act., Cupr-ar., *Dig.,* Equis-h., *Euon., Eup-pur.,* Ferr-ar., *Ferr-m.,* Ferr-pic., Form., Fuch., Glon., *Hell.,* Helon., Kali-chl., *Kalm.,* Lach., Lec., Lith-c., Lyc., *Merc-c.,* Merc-cy., Methyl., Mur-ac., Nit-ac., Oci., Ol-sant., *Osm.,* Ph-ac., *Phos.,* Plb., *Plb-chr.,* Rad-met., Sabin., *Sec.,* Sil., *Solid.,* Squil., *Stroph-h., Ter.,* Thyr., Uran-n., Visc.

**Alkaline:** Am-c., Benz-ac., *Kali-act.,* Mag-p., Med., *Ph-ac.* (See **Nephritis.**)

**Bloody (hematuria):** *Acon.,* Ant-t., Apis, *Arn.,* Ars., Ars-h., *Bell., Berb.,* Cact., Camph., *Cann-s., Canth., Carb-ac.,* Chin., Chinin-s., Cina, *Coc-c., Colch., Cop., Crot-h.,* Dulc., Epig., *Equis-h., Erig.,* Eucal., Fab., Ferr-p., Fic-r., Gal-ac., Ger., *Ham.,* Hep., *Ip.,* Kali-chl., Kreos., *Lach., Lyc.,* Mangi., Merc., Merc-c., *Mill., Nit-ac., Nux-v.,* Oci., Ol-sant., *Pareir., Phos.,* Pic-ac., Plb., *Rhus-a.,* Sabin., Santin., *Sars.,* Sec., *Senec., Solid.,* Squil., Stigm., *Ter., Thlas., Uva.*

**Burning, scalding, hot:** *Acon.,* Apis, Bell., Benz-ac., *Borx.,* Camph., *Cann-s., Canth.,* Coc-c., Conv., Fab., Hep., Kali-bi., Kalm., *Lyc., Merc-c.,* Nit-ac., Phos., Pop., *Sars.,* Sulph. (See **Acid.**)

**Cold feeling:** Nit-ac.

**Heavy feeling:** Thlas.

**Oily pellicle:** Adon., *Crot-t.,* Hep., Lyc., *Iod.,* Petr., *Phos.,* Sumb.

**Viscid, gluey:** *Cot.,* Pareir., *Ph-ac.* (See **Deposit.**)

**COLOR, APPEARANCE, Black, inky:** *Apis,* Arn., *Benz-ac., Benz-d.,* Canth., *Carb-ac., Colch.,* Dig., *Hell.,* Kreos., Lach., Merc-c., Naphtin., Nit-ac., Pareir., *Ter.*

**Brown, dark:** *Apis,* Apoc., Arg-n., Arn., Ars., *Bell., Benz-ac., Bry., Canth.,* Carb-ac., Carb-v., *Chel.,* Chinin-s., Coc-c., *Colch.,* Crot-h., *Dig.,* Fl-ac., Hell., Kali-c., Kali-chl., Lach., *Lyc.,* Merc-c., Myric., Nat-c., Nat-chor., *Nit-ac., Nux-v.,* Ph-ac., Phos., Phyt., Pic-ac., Plb., Prun., *Rhus-t., Sep.,* Solid., Staph., Sulfon., *Ter.*

**Cloudy, turbid:** *Ambr.,* Am-c., Apoc., *Arg-met.,* Ars., *Aur-m., Bell., Benz-ac., Berb.,* Camph., *Cann-s., Canth.,* Card-m., Caust., Chel., *Chim., Chinin-s., Cina, Colch.,* Coloc., Con., *Cop.,* Crot-t., Daph., *Dig.,* Dulc., Graph., Hell., Helon., *Hep.,* Kali-c., Kreos., Lith-c., *Lyc.,* Lyss., Nit-ac., Nit-m-ac., *Oci.,* Petr., *Ph-ac., Phos., Plb., Puls.,* Raph., Rhus-t., *Sars., Sep.,* Solid., Sulph., *Ter.,* Thuj., Zing.

**Deep:** *Bell.,* Calc., Dig., Hell., Lach., *Lyc.,* Merc., Nit-ac., *Sep.*

**Frothy:** Apis, *Berb.,* Cop., Crot-t., Cub., *Lach.,* Myric., Raph., Sars.

**Greenish:** Ars., *Berb.,* Camph., Cann-i., *Carb-ac., Cean.,* Chim., Cop., Cyt-l., Mag-s., Ol-an., Ruta, *Santin.,* Uva.

**Milky:** Chel., *Cina,* Coloc., Con., Dulc., Eup-pur., Iod., Lil-t., Merc., *Ph-ac.,* Phos., Raph., Still., Uva, *Viol-o.*

**Pale, clear, limpid:** *Acet-ac.,* Berb., Caust., Crot-t., Equis-h., *Gels.,* Helon., *Ign.,* Kreos., Lycps-v., Mag-m., Mosch., *Nat-m.,* Nit-ac., Nux-v., *Ph-ac., Phos.,* Puls., Staph., *Sulph.* (See **Polyuria**.)

**Pink:** Sulfon.

**Red, dark:** *Acon., Apis,* Bell., Benz-ac., *Bry.,* Canth., Carb-v., Coc-c., Cupr-act., *Dig.,* Hep., *Kali-bi.,* Lob., Merc-c., Merc-d., Nux-v., Petr., Phyt., Sel., Solid., Squil.

**Red, fiery, high colored:** *Acon.,* All-c., Ant-c., *Apis,* Apoc., Arg-n., Ars., *Bell., Benz-ac., Berb., Bry.,* Camph., Cann-s., *Canth.,* Carb-ac., Chel., Chim., Cupr-act., *Equis-h.,* Euon., Glon., *Hell., Hep.,* Kali-bi., *Lith-c., Lyc.,* Merc-d., *Myric.,* Nit-ac., Oci., Phyt., Pic-ac., Puls., Rheum, *Rhus-t.,* Sabin., *Sars.,* Sel., Senec., Sulph., *Ter.,* Thuj., Uva, Verat-v.

**Smoky:** Am-be., *Benz-ac.,* Hell., *Ter.* (See **Bloody**.)

**Thick:** Am-be., Anan., *Benz-ac.,* Camph., Cina, Coc.c., *Coloc.,* Con., Daph., Dig., *Dulc., Hep.,* Iod., *Merc-c.,* Oci., *Phos.,* Still., Sep., Zing.

**Yellow:** Absin., Bell., Berb., *Card-m.,* Cean., Chin., Daph., Hydr., Ign., Kalm., Lac-ac., Oci., Op., Plb., Solid., Uva.

**Yellow, dark:** Bov., Bry., Camph., *Chel.,* Chen-a., Crot-t., *Iod., Kali-p.,* Myric., Petr., *Pic-ac.,* Podo.

**ODOR, Fetid, foul:** *Am-be.,* Am-c., Apis, Ars., *Aspar., Bapt., Benz-ac.,* Berb., *Calc.,* Camph., Carb-an., *Chim.,* Coloc., Conv., Cupr-ar., Daph., *Dulc., Graph.,* Hydr., Ind., Kali-bi., Kreos., Lach., *Lyc.,* Merc, Naphtin., *Nit-ac.,* Oci., Petr., *Phos.,* Phys., Pulx., *Sep., Solid.,* Stront-br., Sulph., Trop., Uran-n.

**Fish-like:** Uran-n.

**Garlicky:** Cupr-ar.

**Musk-like:** Oci.

**Pungent, ammoniacal:** *Borx.,* Cain., Cop., Dig., Naphtin., *Nit-ac., Pareir.,* Petr., Solid., Stigm.

**Sharp, intensely strong:** *Absin., Am-be.,* Arg-n., *Benz-ac., Borx., Calc.,* Carb-v., *Chinin-s.,* Erig., *Lyc.,* Pic-ac., Pin-s., *Sulph.,* Viol-o., Zing.

**Sharp, like cat's urine:** Caj., Viol-t.

**Sharp, like horse's urine:** Benz-ac., *Nit-ac.*

**Sour:** Calc., *Graph.,* Nat-c., Petr., Sep., Solid.

**Sweet, violaceous:** Arg-met., *Cop.,* Cub., Eucal., Ferr-i., Inul., *Juni-c.,* Phos., Prim-o., Salol., *Ter.,* Thyr.

**Valerian, like:** Murx.

**SEDIMENT, TYPE, acetone (azoturia):** Ars., Aur-m., *Calc-m.,* Carb-ac., *Caust.,* Colch., Cupr-ar., *Euon.,* Nat-sal., Phos., *Senn.*

**Bile:** Cean., Chion., *Chel.,* Kali-chl., Myric., Nat-s., Sep. (See **Liver**.)

**Blood:** Ars., *Berb.,* Cact., *Cann-s., Canth., Carb-ac.,* Colch., Dulc., *Ham.,* Hep., Lyc., *Nit-ac.,* Pareir., *Phos.,* Ter. (See **Bloody**.)

**Casts:** *Apis, Ars.,* Aur-m., Brach., *Canth., Carb-ac.,* Chel., Fab., Crot-h., Kali-chl., Merc-c., Nat-chl., *Phos.,* Pic-ac., *Plb.,* Rad-br., Sulfon., Ter. (See **Nephritis**.)

**Cells, debris:** Arg-n., *Ars., Berb.,* Brach., Cact., *Canth., Carb-ac.,* Chel., Crot-h., Hep., Kali-bi., *Merc-c., Phos.,* Pic-ac., Solid., Ter. (See **Nephritis**.)

**Chlorides, diminished:** Bar-m., Chel., Coloc.

**Chlorides, increased:** Chinin-s., Rad-br., Senn.

**Chyluria:** Coloc., Iod., *Kali-bi., Ph-ac.,* Uva. (See **Milky Urine**.)

**Coffee ground like:** Dig., *Hell.,* Ter.

**Flocculent, flaky:** *Berb.,* Caust., Phos., *Sars.*

**Gelatinous gluey, viscid:** Berb., *Cina, Coloc., Oci., Ph-ac.,* Puls. (See **Mucus**.)

**Grayish-white, granular:** Berb., Calc., Canth., *Graph.,* Sars., Sep.

**Hemato-porphyrinuria:** *Sulfon.,* Trion.

**Hemoglobinuria:** *Ars-h.,* Carb-ac., Chinin-ar., Chinin-s., Ferr-p., Kali-bi., *Kali-chl.,* Nat-n., Phos., Pic-ac., Santin.

**Indican:** Alf., Indol., Nux-m., Pic-ac.

**Lithic acid, uric acid, gravel, brick dust:** Arg-n., Arn., *Aspar.,* Baros., *Bar-m.,* Bell., *Benz-ac., Berb., Calc.,* Calc-ren., Cann-s., *Canth.,* Caust., Chel., *Chin., Chinin-s., Coc-c.,* Cocc-s., Coch., Colch., Coloc., Dig., Dios., *Epig., Eup-a., Eup-pur.,* Ery-a., Fab., Ferr-m., Gali., Graph., *Hed., Hydrang., Kali-c.,* Kali-i., Kreos., *Lith-be., Lith-c.,* Lob., *Lyc.,* Merc-c., Nat-m., Nat-s., *Nit-ac.,* Nit-m-ac., *Nux-v., Oci.,* Pareir., Pariet., Ph-ac., Phos., Phys., Pipe., Plb-i., Puls., *Sars.,* Sel., Senn., *Sep.,* Skook., *Solid.,* Stigm., *Thlas.,* Tritic., *Urt-u.,* Vesi. (See **Calculi**.)

**Mucus, slime:** Apoc., Ars., Aspar., Bals-p., *Baros., Benz-ac., Berb.,* Brach., Calc., *Cann-s., Canth., Chim.,* Chinin-s., Cina, *Cub., Dulc.,* Epig., *Equis-h.,* Eup-pur., Fab., *Hep.,* Hydrang., *Kali-bi.*, *Lyc.,* Menth., Merc-c., Nit-ac., Nux-v., *Pareir., Pop., Puls., Sars.,* Seneg., Sep., *Solid.,* Stigm., Sulph., *Tritic., Uva.* (See **Cystitis**.)

**Oxalates (oxaluria):** *Berb.,* Brach., *Kali-s.,* Lysd., Nat-p., Nit-ac., *Nit-m-ac.,* Ox-ac., Senn.

**Phosphates (phosphaturia):** *Alf.,* Arn., Aven., Bell., Benz-ac., Brach., Calc., *Calc-p.,* Cann-s., Chel., Chinin-s., Graph., Gua., Guaj., Helon., Hydrang., Kali-chl., Lec., Nit-ac., *Ph-ac., Pic-ac.,* Sang., Senn., *Solid.,* Thlas., Uran-n.

**Pus (pyuria):** *Ars.,* Aspar., *Baros., Benz-ac.,* Berb., Bry., Calc., *Cann-s., Canth., Chim.,* Cop., *Dulc., Epig.,* Eucal., Fab., *Hep.,* Hyos., *Kali-bi.,* Lith-c., *Lyc., Merc-c.,* Nit-ac., Nux-v., Oci., *Phos., Pop.,* Sars., Sep., Stigm., Sulph., Ter., Thlas., Tritic., *Uva.*

**Rose colored:** Am-ph.

**DIABETES: Sugar:** *Acet-ac., Adren.,* Am-act., *Arg-met.,* Arg-n., Arist-m., Arn., *Ars., Ars-br.,* Ars-i., *Aur.,* Aur-m., Bell., *Bor-ac.,* Bov., *Bry.,* Caps., Carb-ac., Cean., *Cham.,* Chel., *Chim., Chion., Coca, Cod.,* Colch., *Crot-h.,* Cupr-ar., *Cur.,* Eup-pur., Fel., Ferr-i., Ferr-m., Fl-ac., Glon., Glyc., Grin., *Hell., Helon.,* Iod., *Iris,* Kali-act., Kali-br., *Kreos., Lac-ac.,* Lach., Lec., Lyc., Lycps-v., Lyss., Morph., *Mosch.,* Murx., Nat-m., *Nat-s.,* Nit-ac., Nux-v., Op., *Pancr.,* Phase., *Ph-ac., Phos.,* Phlor., Pic-ac., Plb., Plb-i., Podo., *Rhus-a.,* Sec., *Sil.,* Squil., Stry-ar., Sulph., *Syzyg.,* Tarent., Tarax., Ter., *Uran-n.,* Urea., Vanad., Vince.

**Assimilative disorders:** Uran-n.

**Gastro-hepatic origin:** *Ars-i.,* Ars., Bry., Calc., Cham., Chel., Kreos., *Lac-ac.,* Lept., Lyc., *Nux-v., Uran-n.*

**Nervous origin:** Ars., Aur-m., Calc., *Ign., Ph-ac.,* Stry-ar.

**Pancreatic origin:** Iris, Pancr., Phos.

**With debility:** Acet-ac., Op.

**With gangrene, boils, carbuncles, diarrhea:** Ars.

**With gouty symptoms:** *Lac-ac., Nat-s.*

**With impotency:** Coca, Mosch.

**With melancholia, emaciation, thirst, restlessness:** Helon.

**With motor paralysis:** Cur.

**With rapid course:** Cur., Morph.

**With ulceration:** Syzyg.

■

# MALE SEXUAL SYSTEM

**BUBO:** Acon., Ang., Apis, Aur-m., Bad., *Bell.,* Calen., *Carb-an.,* Carb-v., Caust., *Cinnb., Hep.,* Jac-c., *Kali-i., Merc., Merc-i-r.,* Merc-p-r., *Nit-ac.,* Ph-ac., *Phyt.,* Sil., Sulph., Syph., Tarent-c.

**Bubo, chancroidal:** Ars-i., *Merc.,* Merc-c., *Merc-i-r.,* Sil.

**Bubo, indurated:** Alum., Bad., *Carb-an.,* Merc.

**Bubo, phagedenic:** *Ars.,* Graph., Hydr., *Kali-i.,* Lach., *Merc., Merc-i-r., Nit-ac.,* Sil., Sulph.

**CHANCROID:** Cor-r., *Jac-c.,* Kali-bi., *Merc.,* Merc-p-r., *Nit-ac.,* Thuj.

**Chancroid, complications:** *Ars.,* Hecla, *Hep.,* Lach., *Sil.,* Sulph., Thuj.

**COITUS, Aversion to:** Arn., Graph., Lyc. (See **Desire**.)

**Coitus, followed by backache:** *Cann-i.,* Kali-c.

**Coitus, followed by irritability:** Sel.

**Coitus, followed by nausea, vomiting:** Mosch.

**Coitus, followed by pain in perineum:** Alum.

**Coitus, followed by pain in urethra:** Canth.

**Coitus, followed by prostration:** Agar., Calc., *Chin.,* Con., Dig., *Kali-c.,* Kali-p., Nat-c., Sel., Ziz. (See **Impotence**.)

**Coitus, followed by pollution, increased desire:** Nat-m., Ph-ac.

**Coitus, followed by toothache:** Daph.

**Coitus, followed by urging to urinate:** Staph.

**Coitus, followed by vertigo:** Bov., Sep.

**Coitus, followed by vomiting:** Mosch.

**Coitus, followed by weak vision:** Kali-c.

**Coitus, painful:** Arg n., Calc., Sabal. (See **Impotence**.)

**CONDYLOMATA:** Aur-m., *Cinnb.,* Euphr., Kali-i., *Lyc., Merc.,* Nat-s., *Nit-ac., Sabin.,* Staph., *Thuj.* (See **Syphilis**.)

**CONTUSIONS, of genitals:** Arn., Con.

**DESIRE, Diminished, lost:** *Agn., Arg-n.,* Bar-c., Berb., *Calc.,* Caps., *Con.,* Hep., Ign., Iod., Kali-br., *Kali-c.,* Lec., *Lyc.,* Nit-ac., Nuph., Onos., Oxyt., Ph-ac., *Sabal, Sel.,* Sil., Sulph., X-ray. (See **Impotence**.)

**Desire increased (erethism, satyriasis):** Alum., Anac., Bov., Calad., *Camph., Cann-i.,* Cann-s., *Canth., Dulc.,* Fl-ac., *Gins.,* Graph., Hipp., *Hyos.,* Ign., *Kali-br.,* Lach., Lyc., Lyss., *Mosch.,* Nat-m., *Nux-v.,* Ol-an., Onos., *Orig., Phos., Pic-ac., Plat.,* Sabin., *Sal-n.,* Stram., *Tarent.,* Thymol., Upa., Verat., *Zinc-p.,* Ziz.

**Desire increased in old men but impotent:** Lyc., Sel.

**Desire perverted:** Agn., Nux-v., Plat., Staph.

**Desire suppressed, ill effect from:** Con.

**GENITALS, Burning, heat,** Spong., Sil. (See **Gonorrhea**.)

**Genitals, itching (pruritus):** Agar., *Ambr.,* Anac., *Calad.,* Crot-t., *Fago.,* Rhus-d., *Rhus-t.,* Sep., Sulph., Tarent-c. (See **SKIN.**)

**Genitals, relaxed, flabby, cold, weak:** Absin., *Agn., Calad.,* Caps., *Chin., Con., Dios., Gels.,* Ham., *Lyc.,* Nuph., *Ph- ac.,* Phos., *Sel.,* Sep., Staph., Sulph., Uran-n. (See **Impotence.**)

**GONORRHEA (specific urethritis) Remedies in general:** *Acon.,* Agn., Apis, *Arg-n., Baros.,* Benz-ac., *Camph., Cann-s., Canth., Caps., Clem., Cop., Cub.,* Dig., *Dor.,* Echi., Equis-h., Erig., Eucal., Euph-pi., Fab., Ferr., *Gels.,* Hep., *Hydr.,* Ichth., Jac-c., *Kali-bi.,* Kali-s., Kreos., Med., *Merc., Merc-c.,* Merc-pr-r., Methyl., Naphtin., Nat-s., *Nit-ac.,* Nux-v., *Ol-sant.,* Pareir., *Petros.,* Pin-c., *Puls.,* Sabal, Sabin., Sal-n., *Sep.,* Sil., Stigm., *Sulph.,* Ter., *Thuj.,* Tritic., *Tus-p.,* Zing.

**Acute, inflammatory stage:** *Acon.,* Arg-n., Atrop., *Cann-s., Canth.,* Caps., *Gels.,* Petros.

**Adenitis, tymphangitis:** Acon., Apis, *Bell.,* Hep., *Merc.*

**Chordee:** Acon., *Agav-a., Anac.,* Arg-n., Bell., Berb., *Camph-mbr., Cann-i.,* Cann-s., *Canth.,* Caps., Clem., Cop., Gels., Hyos., Jac-c., *Kali-br., Lup.,* Merc., Oena., Ol-sant., Phos., *Pic-ac.,* Pip-m., Sal-n., Ter., Tus-p., Yohim., Zinc-pic.

**Chronic, subacute stage:** Arg-n., Cann-s., *Cop., Cub.,* Erig., *Hep.,* Hydr., *Kali-s.,* Merc., Merc-c., Merc-i-r., Naphtin., *Nat-s., Ol-sant.,* Pin-c., Psor., *Puls.,* Rhod., *Sabal,* Sep., Sil., Stigm., *Sulph., Thuj.* (See **Gleet.**)

**Cowperitis:** Acon., *Cann-s.,* Gels., Fab., *Hep.,* Merc-c., Petros., *Sabal,* Sil. (See **Bladder**.)

**DISCHARGE: Acrid, corroding:** Cop., Gels., *Hydr., Merc-c.,* Thuj.

**Bloody:** Arg-n., *Canth.,* Cub., *Merc-c.,* Mill.

**Milky, glairy, mucus:** Cann-i., *Cann-s.,* Cop., Cupr-ar., Graph., *Hydr., Kali-bi., Nat-m., Petros.,* Puls., Sep. (See **Gleet**.)

**Muco-purulent, yellowish-green:** Agn., Alum., *Arg-n.,* Baros., *Cann-s.,* Canth., Caps., Cob., *Cop., Cub.,* Dig., *Hep., Hydr.,* Jac-c., Kali-i., *Kali-s., Merc., Merc-c.,* Nat-m., *Nat-s.,* Ol-sant., *Puls.,* Sabin., Sep., Sil., Sulph., *Thuj.,* Tus-p., Zing. (See **Gleet**.)

**Watery:** *Cann-s.,* Fl-ac., Mez., Mill., *Nat-m.,* Sep., Sulph., Thuj.

**Folliculitis:** Caps., Hep., Merc., Sep., Sil.

**GLEET:** Abies-c., *Agn.,* Arg-n., Calad., Calc-p., *Cann-s., Canth.,* Caps., Chim., *Cinnb.,* Clem., *Cub.,* Dor., Erig., Graph., *Hydr.,* Kali-bi., Kali-i., *Kali-s.,* Mati., Med., Merc., *Naphtin., Nat-m.,* Nat-s., *Nit-ac.,* Nux-v., *Ol-sant.,* Petros., Pip-m., Pop., *Puls., Sabal,* Sel., *Sep.,* Sil., *Thuj.,* Zinc-m.

**Ophthalmia:** *Acon.,* Apis, Arg-n., *Bell.,* Ip., Merc-c.

**Orchitis, epididymitis:** Aur., Clem., Gels., Ham., Puls., Rhod., *Spong.*

**Prostatic involvement:** Caps., Cub., Pareir., *Thuj.* (See **Prostatitis.**)

**Rheumatism:** *Acon.,* Arg-n., Clem., Cop., *Daph.,* Gels., Guaj., Iod., *Irisin,* Kali-i., *Med., Merc.,* Nat-s., *Phyt., Puls., Sars.,* Sulph., *Thuj.*

**Stricture, organic:** Acon., *Arg-n.,* Calc-i., Canth., Caps., *Clem.,* Cop., *Fl-ac.,* Iod., *Kali-i., Merc.,* Merc-pr-r., Nux-v., Ol-sant., Pareir, Petros., Puls., Sep., *Sil.,* Sul-i., Sulph., *Thiosin., Thuj.*

**Suppression ill effects:** *Agn.,* Ant-t., Benz-ac., *Clem.,* Kali-i., *Med.,* Nat-s., *Puls.,* Sars., *Thuj.,* X-ray.

**IMPOTENCE:** *Agn.,* Anac., Ant-c., *Arg-n.,* Arn., Ars., Aven, Bar-c., Berb., *Calad.,* Calc., Camph., Carbn-s., *Chin.,* Chinin-s., *Cob., Con.,* Dam., Dig., *Dios., Gels.,* Glyc., Graph., Hyper., Ign., Iod., Kali-br., Kali-i., Lec., *Lyc.,* Nat-m., Nit-ac., Nuph., *Nux-v.,* Onos., *Ph-ac., Phos., Pic-ac.,* Plb., *Sabal, Sal-n., Sel.,* Sep., Sil., Staph., *Stry.,* Sulph., Thuj., Trib., *Yohim.,* Zinc., Zinc-p. (See **Spermatorrhea.**)

**MASTURBATION, Ill effects:** Agn., *Anac.,* Apis, Arg-met., Bell-p., *Calad., Calc., Calc-p., Chin., Con., Dios., Gels.,* Graph., Grat., *Kali-br., Lyc.,* Nat-m., *Nux-v., Ph-ac., Pic-ac.,* Plat., *Sal-n., Staph.,* Still., *Sulph.,* Tab., Thuj., Trib., Ust., Zinc., Zinc-o.

**PENIS, Atrophy:** Ant-c., Arg-met., Staph.

**Glans, Epithelioma:** Arg-n., *Ars.,* Con., Thuj.

**Gangrene:** Canth., Lach.

**Itching:** *Acon.,* Ars., Bell., *Calad., Canth.,* Caps., Chin., Cinnb., Coc-c., *Con.,* Cop., Cor-r., *Crot-t.,* Graph., Ham., *Hep.,* Ign., Kali-bi., Lyc., *Merc.,* Nat-m., Nux-v., *Puls.,* Sel., Sep., Staph., *Sulph.,* Thuj., *Viol-t.*

**PAINS, Burning, sore:** Anac., *Ars.,* Bell., *Cann-s., Canth., Caps.,* Chin., *Cinnb.,* Con., Cop., Cor-r., Crot-t., *Gels.,* Ign., Lyc., *Merc-c.,* Mez., *Nit-ac.,* Nuph., Nux-v., Puls., Rhus-t., Sep., *Sulph., Thuj.,* Viol-t.

**Cutting, stitching, tearing:** *Acon.,* Apis, *Arg-n.,* Asim., Calad., *Cann-s., Canth., Caps.,* Con., *Hep., Lyc.,* Naphtin., Nat-m., *Nit-ac., Pareir.,* Petr., Ph-ac., *Phyt.,* Prun., *Sars.,* Staph., Sulph.

**Pressing, pinching:** *Canth.,* Caps., Graph., Kali-bi., *Nit-ac.,* Puls., *Rhod.*

**Throbbing:** Coc-c., Ham., Lith-c., Nat-m., *Nit-ac.*

**PRIAPISM:** (See **Chordee.**)

**PUSTULES:** *Ars-h.,* Coc-c., *Hep., Kali-bi.,* Merc.

**RASH AND SPOTS:** Antip., *Bell.,* Bry., Calad., Cann-s., Caust., *Cinnb.,* Gels., Lach., *Merc.,* Nat-m., Petr., *Rhus-t.,* Sep., *Sulph.,* Thuj.

**SWOLLEN, inflamed glans:** *Acon.,* Antip., *Apis, Arg-n.,* Arn., Ars., Calad., *Cann-s., Canth., Cop.,* Cor-r., *Cub.,* Dig., *Gels.,* Ham., Merc., *Merc-c., Nit-ac.,* Ph-ac., *Rhus-t.,* Sars., *Thuj.* (See **Gonorrhea.**)

**ULCERS, excoriations:** *Ars., *Cann-s., *Caust.,* Cop., *Cor-r.,* Crot-t., *Hep., Merc., Merc-c.,* Mez., *Nit-ac.,* Osm., Sep., *Thuj.*

**PREPUCE, Constriction (Paraphimosis, phimosis):** Acon., *Apis,* Arn., Bell., Cann-s., *Canth.,* Caps., Dig., Euphr., Ham., *Merc., Merc-c., Nit-ac.,* Ol-sant., Ph-ac., *Rhus-t.,* Sabin., Sulph., *Thuj.*

**Herpes:** Ars., Carb-v., Caust., *Crot-t.,* Graph., *Hep.,* Jug-r., *Merc.,* Mez., *Nit-ac.,* Petr., Ph-ac., *Rhus-t.,* Sars., *Thuj.*

**Inflammation (balanitis, balano-postitis):** *Acon.,* Apis, Calad., *Cann-s., Canth., Cinnb.,* Coc-c., Con., Crot-t., Dig., *Gels., Jac-c.,* Lyc., *Merc.,* Merc-c., *Nit-ac.,* Ol-sant., *Rhus-t.,* Sulph., *Thuj.,* Viol-t.

**Itching:** Ars., *Canth., Caps.,* Cinnb., *Con.,* Graph., Ign., Lyc., *Merc.,* Nit-ac., Nux-v., Puls., *Rhus-t.,* Sil., *Sulph.,* Thuj., Zing.

**Pains:** *Acon.,* Bell., *Berb.,* Calad., *Cann-s., Canth.,* Cinnb., Coc-c, Con., *Cop.,* Cor-r., Ign., *Merc.,* Merc-c., *Nit-ac.,* Nux-v., *Rhus-t.,* Sep., Sulph., *Thuj.*

**Ulcers, excoriations:** *Ars.,* Cann-s., *Caust.,* Cop., *Cor-r., Hep.,* Ign., *Merc., Nit-ac.,* Nux-v., Ph-ac., Phyt., Sep., *Sil., Thuj.*

**Varices:** Ham., Lach.

**Warts, condylomata:** Apis, *Cinnb.,* Hep., Kreos., Lyc., Nat-m., *Nit-ac.,* Ph-ac., *Sabin.,* Sep., Staph., *Thuj.*

**PROSTATE GLAND, Affections in general:** Aesc., Aloe, Baros., Caust., Dam., Fab., *Ferr-pic.,* Hep., *Hydrang., Iod.,* Kali-i., *Mela.,* Merc., Pareir., Phyt., Pic-ac., Pop., *Sabal, Solid.,* Staph., Sul-i., *Thuj.*

**Congestion:** *Acon., Aloe,* Arn., Bell., *Canth.,* Con., Cop., Cub., Ferr-p., Gels., Kali-br., Kali-i., Lith-c., *Ol-sant.,* Puls., *Sabal,* Thuj.

**Hypertrophy:** Alf., *Aloe,* Am-m., *Arg-n., Bar-c.,* Benz-ac., Calc-f., Calc-i., *Chim.,* Chr-s., *Cimic.,* Con., Eup-pur., *Ferr-pic., Gels.,* Graph., Hep., *Hydrang.,* Iod., Kali-bi., Kali-br., Lyc., Med., Ol-sant., Oxyd., Pareir., Pic-ac., Pip-m., *Pop.,* Puls., Rhus-a., *Sabal,* Sars., *Senec., Solid.,* Staph., *Sulph., Thiosin., Thuj.,* Thyr., Trib., Tritic.

**Inflammation (prostatitis), Acute:** Acon., *Aesc.,* Aloe, Apis, *Bell.,* Bry., Canth., *Chim.,* Colch., *Cop.,* Cub., Dig., *Fab.,* Ferr-p., *Gels., Hep., Iod.,* Kali-br., Kali-i., Kali-n., Merc-c., *Merc-d., Nit-ac.,* Ol-sant., Pic-ac., *Puls.,* Sabad., *Sabal,* Sal-n., Sel., *Sil.,* Solid., *Staph., Thuj.,* Tritic., *Verat-v.,* Vesi.

**Inflammation, chronic:** Alum., *Aur.,* Bar-c., Brach., Calad., Carbn-s., Caust., Clem., *Con., Ferr-pic.,* Graph., Hep., Hydrc., Iod., *Lyc., Merc., Merc-c., Nit-ac.,* Nux-v., Phyt., *Puls.,* Sabad., *Sabal, Sel., Sep.,* Sil., Solid., *Staph.,* Sulph., *Thuj., Trib.* (See **Prostatitis.**)

**Weakness (prostatorrhea), discharge during stool, urination, straining:** Acet-ac., Aesc., *Agn., Alum.,* Anac., *Arg-n., Cann-s.,* Caust., *Chim.,* Con.,

Cub., *Dam.,* Ery-a., Hep., Juni-c., Kali-bi., Lyc., Nit-ac., Nuph., Nux-v., Petr., *Ph-ac.,* Phos., Puls., Sabal, *Sel.,* Sil., *Sulph.,* Ter., Thuj., Thymol., Zinc.

**PUBIC HAIR, Loss:** Merc., Nit-ac., Sel., Zinc.

**SCROTUM: Cancer, epithelioma:** Ars., Fuli., Thuj.

**Cold, relaxed:** *Agn., Calad.,* Calc., *Caps.,* Gels., Lyc., Merc., *Ph-ac.,* Sep., Staph., Sulph. (See **Impotence.**)

**Eczema:** Alumn, Ant-c., Canth., *Crot-t., Graph.,* Hep., Olnd., Petr., Ph-ac., *Rhus-t.,* Sanic., Sulph.

**Hydrocele: Edema:** Abrot., Ampe-tr., *Apis,* Ars., *Aur.,* Bry., Calad., *Calc.,* Calc-f., Calc-p., Canth., Chel., Chin., *Con.,* Dig., Dulc., *Fl-ac., Graph.,* Hell., *Iod., Kali-i.,* Merc., *Puls., Rhod.,* Rhus-t., Samb., *Sel., Sil., Spong.,* Squil., Sulph.

**Induration:** Calad., Rhus-t.

**Inflammation:** *Apis,* Ars., Crot-t., Euph-l., *Ham.,* Rhus-t., Verat-v.

**Itching:** *Ambr,* Carb-v., Caust., *Crot-t.,* Euph-l., *Graph., Hep.,* Nit-ac., Nux-v., Petr., Ph-ac., Rhus-t., *Sars.,* Sel., Thuj., Urt-u. (See **SKIN.**)

**Hematocele, acute:** Acon., *Arn.,* Con., Erig., *Ham.,* Nux-v., *Puls., Sulph.*

**Hematocele, chronic:** Iod., *Kali-i.,* Sulph.

**Nodules, hard, suppurating:** Nit-ac. (See **SKIN.**)

**Numbness:** *Ambr,* Am-c., Sep. (See **Itching.**)

**Pain:** Am-c., Berb., *Clem.,* Iod., Kali-c., *Merc.,* Nux-v., *Thuj.* (See **Inflammation.**)

**Prurigo:** *Ant-c.,* Aur., *Graph.,* Mur-ac., Nat-s., *Nit-ac.,* Nux-v., *Rhus-t.,* Staph.

**Retraction:** Plb.

**Spots, brown:** Con.

**Sweat:** Bell., *Calad.,* Calc., Cor-r., Cupr-ar., *Dios.,* Fago., Nat-m., *Petr.,* Sep., *Sil., Sulph.,* Thuj., Uran-n.

**Swelling:** *Apis, Ars., Bell.,* Brom., *Canth., Clem.,* Con., Ign., Nit-ac., *Puls.,* Rhus-d., *Rhus-t.,* Sep. (See **Inflammation.**)

**Tubercles:** Con., *Iod.,* Sil., Sulph., Teucr.

**Varicocele:** Acon., Arn., *Ferr-p., Ham.,* Lach., Nux-v., Plb., *Puls.,* Ruta, Sulph.

**SEMINAL VESICULITIS, Acute:** *Acon.,* Aesc., Aloe, *Bell.,* Canth., Cub., *Ferr-p.,* Hep., Kali-br., *Merc.,* Phyt., *Puls.,* Sel., Sil., Verat-v.

**Chronic:** *Agn., Arg-n.,* Aur., Bar-c., Calad., *Cann-s.,* Chin., Clem., *Con., Cub.,* Ferr-pic., Graph., *Hep., Iod.,* Kali-br., *Lyc.,* Merc., *Nux-v., Ox-ac., Ph-ac.,* Phyt., *Puls., Sel.,* Sep., *Sil.,* Staph., Sulph., Trib., Zinc. (See **Prostatitis.**)

**SEXUAL EXCESSES, Ill effects:** Agar., *Agn., Anac.,* Aven., Calad., Calc.,

*Chin.*, Con., Digin., *Gels.*, Graph., Kali-br., Kali-p., Lyc., Lyss., Nat-m., *Nux-v.*, *Ph-ac.*, Phos., Samb., Sel., Sil., Staph., Trib. (See **Impotence, Spermatorrhea.**)

**SPERMATIC CORD, Pain in general:** Anth., *Arg-n.*, Arund., Aur., *Bell.*, *Berb.*, Calc., Cain., *Cann-s.*, Caps., Chin., *Clem.*, Con., *Dios.*, *Ham.*, Ind., Kali-c., Lith-c., *Merc-i-r.*, Morph., *Nit-ac.*, Nux-v., Ol-an., Osm., *Ox-ac.*, Oxyt., *Phyt.*, Pic-ac., *Puls.*, Sars., *Senec.*, Sil., *Spong.*, Staph., Sulph., *Thlas.*, *Thuj.*, Tus-p., Verat-v.

**Drawing:** *Cain.*, Calc., *Clem.*, Con., *Ham.*, Ind., Ol-an., *Puls.*, Rhod., Senec., *Staph.*, Zinc.

**Neuralgic:** *Arg-n.*, Aur., *Bell.*, *Berb.*, Clem., Ham., Mentho., Nit-ac., Nux-v., *Ox-ac.*, Phyt., *Spong.*

**Swelling:** Anth., *Cann-s.*, Chin., *Ham.*, Kali-c., *Puls.*, *Spong.*

**Tenderness:** *Bell.*, *Clem.*, Ham., Merc-i-r., *Ox-ac.*, Phyt., Rhod., *Spong.*, Tus-p.

**SPERMATORRHEA, (Sexual debility, deficient physical power, nocturnal pollutions):** Absin., *Agn.*, *Anac.*, Arg-met., *Arg-n.*, Arn., Ars., Aur., *Aven.*, *Bar-c.*, *Calad.*, *Calc.*, *Calc-p.*, Camph-mbr., Cann-i., *Canth.*, Carb-v., Carbn-s., *Chin.*, Chlor., Cimic., *Cob.*, Coca, Cocc., *Con.*, Cupr., Dam., *Dig.*, *Digin*, *Dios.*, Ery-a., *Ferr-br.*, Form., *Gels.*, *Gins.*, *Graph.*, Hyper., Iod., Iris, *Kali-br.*, *Kali-c.*, *Kali-p.*, *Lyc.*, Lyss., *Lup.*, *Med.*, Mosch., *Nat-m.*, Nit-ac., *Nuph.*, *Nux-v.*, *Onos.*, Orch., *Ph-ac.*, *Phos.*, *Pic-ac.*, Plb-p., *Sabal*, *Sal-n.*, Scut., *Sel.*, *Sep.*, *Sil.*, *Staph.*, *Stry.*, Sul-ac., *Sulph.*, Sumb., Thuj., *Thymol.*, Titan., Trib., Upa., Ust., Viol-t., *Yohim.*, *Zinc-pic.*

**With brain fag, mental torpidity:** Ph-ac.

**With debility, backache, weak legs:** Aur., Calc., Calc-p., *Chin.*, *Cob.*, Con., Cupr., Dam., Dig., *Dios.*, Ery-a., Form., Gels., *Kali-c.*, Lyc., Med., Nat-p., *Nux-v.*, *Ph-ac.*, *Pic-ac.*, Sars., Sel., *Staph.*, *Sulph.*, Zinc.

**With dreams absent:** Anac., *Arg-n.*, Dig., Gels., Hep., Nat-p., *Pic-ac.* (See **Sleep.**)

**With dreams amorous:** Ambr., *Calad.*, Cann-i., Cob., Con., Dios., Lyc., *Nux-v.*, *Phos.*, Sars., Sel., Senec., Staph., Thymol., Ust., Viol-t. (See **Sleep.**)

**With emission and orgasm absent:** Calad., Calc., Sel.

**With emissions, bloody:** Ambr., *Canth.*, Led., *Merc.*, Petr., Sars.

**With emissions, diurnal, straining at stool:** *Alum.*, Canth., *Chin.*, Cimic., Digin., Gels., Kali-br., *Nuph.*, *Ph-ac.*, Phos., Pic-ac., *Sel.*, Trib. (See **Prostatorrhea.**)

**With emissions, premature:** *Agn.*, Bar-c., *Calad.*, *Calc.*, Carb-v., *Chin.*, *Cob.*, Con., *Graph.*, *Lyc.*, Ol-an., Onos., *Ph-ac.*, Phos., *Sel.*, Sep., Sulph., Titan., Zinc.

**With emissions profuse, frequent, after coitus:** Ph-ac.

**With emissions too slow:** Calc., Lyc., Nat-m., Zinc.

**With erections deficient:** Agar., *Agn.,* Arg-met., Arg-n., Calad., *Calc.,* Caust., *Con.,* Graph., Hep., Kali-c., *Lyc.,* Mag-c., Nit-ac., Nuph., *Ph-ac.,* Phos., *Sel.,* Sulph., Zinc.

**With erections painful:** Cann-i., *Canth.,* Ign., Merc., Mosch., *Nit-ac.,* Nux-v., Pic-ac., Puls., Sabad., Thuj.

**With irritability, despondency:** *Aur., Calc.,* Calad., *Chin., Cimic.,* Con., Dios., Kali-br., *Nux-v.,* Ph-ac., Phos., *Sel., Staph.*

**With masturbatic tendency:** Ust.

**With rheumatic pains:** Gins.

**With vision weak:** Kali-c.

**With wasting of testes:** *Iod.,* Sabal.

**SYPHILIS, Remedies in general:** *Aeth-m.,* Aln., Anac., Ant-c., Arg-i., *Ars.,* Ars-br., Ars-i., *Ars-met.,* Ars-s-f., Asaf., *Aur., Aur-ar.,* Aur-i., Aur-m., Aur-m-n., Bad., Bapt., *Berb-a.,* Calc-f., *Calo., Carb an.,* Carb-v., Caust., Chinin-ar., *Cinnb., Cory.,* Cund., Echi., *Fl-ac.,* Franc., Gels., Graph., *Gua,* Guaj., Hecla, *Hep.,* Hippoz., Hydrc., *Iod., Jac-c., Kali-bi., Kali-i.,* Kali-m., *Kreos., Lach.,* Lon-x., Lyc., *Merc., Merc-aur.,* Merc-br., *Merc-c.,* Merc-d., *Merc-i-f., Merc-i-r., Merc-n., Merc-pr-r.,* Merc-tn., *Mez., Nit-ac.,* Osm., Ph-ac., Phos., *Phyt.,* Plat., *Plat-m.,* Psor., Rhus-g., Sars., Staph., *Still.,* Sulph., *Syph., Thuj.*

**Abuse of mercury:** Ang., *Aur.,* Calo., Carb-an., Fl-ac., *Hep.,* Kali-i., *Nit-ac.,* Rhus-g., Sulph.

**Adenopathy:** *Bad.,* Carb-an., Graph., *Hep.,* Iod., Merc., *Merc-i-f., Merc-i-r.,* Phyt. (See **Glands, GENERALITIES.**)

**Alopecia:** *Ars.,* Aur., Carb-v., Cinnb., *Fl-ac.,* Graph., *Hep.,* Kali-i., *Lyc.,* Merc., Merc-i-f., *Nit-ac., Phos.,* Sulph. (See **Scalp, HEAD.**)

**Bone and cartilage lesions:** Arg-met., *Asaf., Aur.,* Aur-m., Calc-f., Carb-v., *Fl-ac.,* Hep., *Kali-bi., Kali-i.,* Lach., *Merc., Mez., Nit-ac.,* Ph-ac., *Phos.,* Phyt., Sars., *Sil.,* Staph, Still., Sulph. (See **Bones, GENERALITIES.**)

**Cachexia, anemia, emaciation:** *Ars., Aur.,* Calo., Carb-an., Carb-v., Ferr-i., Ferr-lac., *Iod.,* Merc., Sars.

**Chancre and primary lesions:** Anan., Apis, Arg-n., Ars., Asaf., *Cinnb.,* Cor-r., Hep., *Jac-c.,* Kali-bi., *Kali-i.,* Lyc., *Merc., Merc-c., Merc-i-f., Merc-i-r., Nit-ac.,* Ph-ac., Phos., Plat., Plat-m., Sil., Sulph.

**Chancre, gangrenous:** Ars., Lach.

**Chancre, hard:** Carb-an., Kali-i., Merc., Merc-i-f., *Merc-i-r.*

**Chancre, indurated, with lardaceous base, deep, round, penetrating, painful, bleeding, raw, everted edges:** Merc.

**Chancre, phagedenic:** *Ars., Cinnb.,* Hydr., Lach., *Merc-c., Nit-ac.,* Sil.
**Chancre, soft:** Cor-r., Merc., Nit-ac., Thuj.
**Condylomata:** Aur-m., *Cinnb.,* Euphr., Kali-i., Mercuries, Plat-m., Nat-s., *Nit-ac., Sabin.,* Staph., *Thuj.*
**Congenital, infantile:** *Aethi-m.,* Ars-i., Ars-met., *Aur.,* Calc-f., *Calc-i.,* Cor-r., Kali-i., *Kreos., Merc., Merc-d., Nit-ac.,* Psor., Syph.
**Exotoses:** *Calc-f.,* Fl-ac., *Hecla,* Merc-p., Phos. (See **Bones, GENERALITIES**.)
**Fever:** *Bapt.,* Chin., *Chinin-s.,* Gels., *Merc.,* Phyt.
**Gummata, nodes:** Asaf., *Aur.,* Berb-a., *Calc-f.,* Carb-an., *Cory.,* Cund., *Fl-ac.,* Iod., *Kali-bi., Kali-i.,* Merc., Mez., Nit-ac., *Phyt.,* Sil., Staph., *Still.,* Sulph., Thuj.
**Headache:** *Kali-i.,* Merc., Sars., Still., *Syph.* (See **HEAD**.)
**Mucus patches:** *Asaf.,* Aur., Calc-f., Calo., *Cinnb., Cund.,* Fl-ac., *Hep.,* Iod., *Kali-bi.,* Kali-i., Kali-m., *Merc., Merc-c.,* Merc-d., *Merc-n., Merc-pr-r., Nit-ac.,* Phyt., Sang., Staph., Still., *Thuj.*
**Onychia, paronychia:** *Ant-c.,* Ars., Graph., Kali-i., *Mercuries.* (See **Whitlow, SKIN**.)
**Ozena:** *Aur.,* Kali-bi., Still. (See **NOSE**.)
**Nervous lesions:** *Anac.,* Asaf., *Aur.,* Iod., *Kali-i.,* Lyc., Merc-n., *Merc-p.,* Mez., *Phos.*
**Nocturnal pains (osteocopic):** Asaf., *Aur.,* Calc-f., Cinnb., *Cory., Eup-per.,* Fl-ac., Hep., *Kali-bi., Kali-i.,* Lach., Lyc., *Merc., Mez.,* Phos., *Phyt.,* Sars., Still.
**Rheumatism:** *Guaj.,* Hecla, Hep., *Kali-bi.,* Kali-i., *Merc.,* Nit-m-ac., *Phyt.,* Still. (See **LOCOMOTOR SYSTEM**.)
**Secondary stage:** *Aur.,* Berb-a., Calo., *Cinnb.,* Fl-ac., *Graph.,* Guaj., Iod., *Kali-bi., Kali-i.,* Lyc., *Merc.,* Merc-br., Merc-c., *Merc-i-f., Merc-i-r., Nit ac.,* Osm., Phos., Phyt., Rhus-g., Sars., *Still.,* Thuj.
**Stomatitis, mercurial:** Nit-ac.

**SYPHILIDES, Bullae:** Kali-i., Syph.
**Eczematous:** *Ars., Graph.,* Kreos., Merc., Petr., Phyt., *Sars.* (See **SKIN**.)
**Papular:** *Calo.,* Kali-i., Lach., Merc., Merc-c., *Merc-i-r.*
**Pigmentary:** Calc-s., Nit-ac.
**Psoriasis:** Asaf., *Graph., Kali-bi.,* Nit-ac., Phos.
**Pustular:** *Ant-t.,* Asaf., *Calo.,* Fl-ac., *Hep.,* Ign., *Kali-bi.,* Kali-i., Lach., *Merc-n.,* Mez., *Nit-ac.*
**Roseolae:** Kali-i., *Merc.,* Merc-c., Merc-i-r., Phos., Phyt.
**Rupia:** Ars., *Berb-a.,* Kali-i., *Merc., Nit-ac.,* Phyt., Syph.
**Spots, copper colored:** *Carb-an.,* Carb-v., *Cor-r.,* Kali-i., Lyc., Merc., Nit-ac., Sulph.

**Squamous:** *Ars.*, Ars-i., *Ars-s-f.*, Borx., *Cinnb.*, Fl-ac., Kali-i., Merc., Merc-c., Merc-i-f., Merc-n., *Merc-pr-r.*, Merc-tn., *Nit-ac.*, *Phos.*, Phyt., *Sars.*, Sulph.

**Tubercular:** *Ars.*, Aur., *Carb-an.*, Fl-ac., Hydrc., *Kali-i.*, Merc-i-r., Still., Thuj.

**Ulcerations:** Ars., *Asaf.*, *Aur.*, *Aur-m.*, Carb-v., *Cinnb.*, Cist., *Cund.*, *Cor-r.*, *Fl-ac.*, Graph., *Hep.*, lod., *Kali-bi.*, Kali-i., Lach., Lyc., Merc., *Merc-c.*, Merc-cy., Merc-d., *Merc-pr-r.*, Mez., *Nit-ac.*, *Phyt.*, Sil., Staph., Still., Sulph., *Thuj.* (See **Mucus patches**.)

**Vesicular:** *Cinnb.*, Merc-c., *Merc-i-r.*, Thuj.

**Tertiary stage:** Ars-i., *Aur.*, Aur-m., Calcareas., Carb-v., Cinnb., *Fl-ac.*, Graph., Guaj., Iod., *Kali-bi.*, *Kali-i.*, Lyc., *Mercuries*, *Mez.*, *Nit-ac.*, Ph-ac., *Phos.*, *Phyt.*, Psor., Staph., Strych-g., Sulph., Thuj.

**Throat symptoms:** Borx., Calc-f., *Cinnb.*, Fl-ac., Kali-bi., Lyc., Merc., *Merc-c.*, Merc-d., Merc-i-f., Merc-i-r., *Nit-ac.*, *Phyt.*, Still.

**Visceral symptoms:** *Ars.*, Ars-i., Aur., Cean., Hep., *Kali-bi.*, Kali-i., Merc., Merc-aur., *Merc-c.*, Merc-i-r., Merc-tn., *Nux-v.*

**TESTICLES: Abscess:** Hep., Merc., Still.

**Atrophy:** Agn., Ant-c., *Arg-n.*, *Aur.*, Caps., Carbn-s., Cere-s., *Iod.*, Kali-br., Lyss., *Rhod.*, *Sabal.*

**Coldness:** *Agn.*, Berb., *Dios.*, Merc., Sil. (See **Impotence**.)

**Cysts:** *Apis,* Con., *Graph.*, Sep., Sulph.

**Hernia:** Ars., *Bar-c.*, Calc., Carb-v., Hep., *Merc.*, Nit-ac., *Sil.*, Thuj.

**Hypertrophy:** Bar-c., *Berb.*, Cinnb., Con., *Ham.*, *Iod.*, *Merc.*, Merc-i-r., Puls., Stigm. (See **Inflammatory**.)

**Induration, hard:** Acon., *Agn.*, Arg-n., Arn., *Aur.*, *Bar-c.*, Bell., *Brom.*, *Calc-f.*, Carb-v., *Clem.*, *Con.*, Cop., *Iod.*, Kali-c., Merc., Ox-ac., *Phyt.*, Plb., *Rhod.*, *Sil.*, *Spong.*, Sulph. (See **Inflammation**.)

**Inflammation of epididymis (epididymitis):** *Acon.*, Apis, Arg-n., *Bell.*, Cann-s., Chin., *Clem.*, *Gels.*, *Ham.*, *Merc.*, Phyt., *Puls.*, *Rhod.*, *Sabal*, *Spong.*, Sulph., Teucr-s., Thuj.

**Inflammation of testes (orchitis): Acute:** *Acon.*, Ant-t., Arg-met., Arg-n., *Bell.*, Brom., Cham., Chin., Chinin-s., *Clem.*, Cub., Gels., *Ham.*, Kali-s., *Merc.*, Nit-ac., Nux-v., Phyt., Polyg-s., *Puls.*, *Rhod.*, *Spong.*, Teucr-s., Verat-v.

**Inflammation, chronic:** Agn., *Aur.*, Bar-c., *Calc-i.*, Chin., *Clem.*, *Con.*, Gels., *Hep.*, Hyper., Iod., *Kali-i.*, Lyc., Merc., Nit-ac., Phyt., *Puls.*, Rhod., *Rhus-t.*, *Spong.*, Sulph.

**Inflammation, metastatic:** *Puls.*, Staph.

**Inflammation, syphilitic:** Aur., *Kali-i.*, Merc-i-r.

**PAINS, In general:** *Acon.,* Agn., *Apis,* Arg-met., *Arg-n.,* Asim., *Aur., Bell.,* Berb., *Brom.,* Cain., *Cann-s.,* Caps., Cere-b., Cham., *Clem., Con.,* Erio., Gins., *Ham.,* Hydr., Ign., Iod., Kali-c., Lyc., *Lycps-v.,* Merc., Merc-i-r., Nit-ac., Nux-v., *Ox-ac., Oxyt.,* Ph-ac., Pic-ac., *Puls., Rhod.,* Sal-n., Sep., *Spong.,* Staph., Sulph., *Thuj.*

**Aching, dragging, relaxed:** Apis, *Aur.,* Cann-s., *Clem., Con.,* Iod., Nit-ac., Nux-v., Ph-ac., *Puls., Spong.,* Staph., Sulph., *Thuj.*

**Bruised, crushed, squeezed, contractive pain:** *Acon., Arg-met., Arg-n., Aur.,* Cham., Carb-v., *Clem., Con.,* Gins., *Ham.,* Kali-c., Nit-ac., *Ol-an.,* Ox-ac., *Puls., Rhod.,* Sep., *Spong.,* Staph.

**Neuralgic (testalgia):** Arg-n., *Aur.,* Bell., *Berb., Clem., Coloc.,* Con., Euphr., *Ham.,* Ign., *Mag-p.,* Merc., Nux-v., Ol-an., *Ox-ac.,* Oxyt., *Puls.,* Spong., Verat-v., Zinc.

**Sensitive, sore, tender:** *Acon.,* Apis, *Bell.,* Berb., Brom., *Clem., Con.,* Cop., *Ham.,* Ind., Merc-i-r., *Ph-ac., Puls., Rhod.,* Sep., *Spong.,* Staph.

**RETRACTION:** Arg-n., *Aur.,* Bell., Brom., Camph., Chin., *Clem.,* Coloc., Euphr., Nit-ac., *Ol-an.,* Puls., *Rhod.,* Zinc.

**SWELLING:** *Acon.,* Agn., *Apis,* Arg-met., *Arg-n.,* Arn., Ars., *Aur.,* Aur-m-n., *Bell., Brom.,* Calc-p., Carb-v., *Clem., Con.,* Cop., Dig., Graph., *Ham., Iod., Kali-c.,* Lyc., Merc., *Merc-c.,* Mill., Oci., Ph-ac., *Puls., Rhod., Spong.,* Staph., Tus-p., *Verat-v.,* Zinc. (See **Inflammation**.)

**TUBERCULOSIS:** *Aur.,* Bac-t., *Merc.,* Scroph-n., Spong., *Teucr-s.*

**Tuberculosis, pseudo:** *Aur.,* Calc., Hep., *Merc-i-r., Sil.,* Spong., Sulph.

**TUMORS (sarcocele):** *Aur., Calc.,* Clem., Merc-i-r., Puls., *Rhod.,* Sil., *Spong.,* Tub. (See **Hypertrophy**.)

**UNDESCENDED testicle in boys:** Thyr.

■

# FEMALE SEXUAL SYSTEM

**COITION, Fainting during:** Murx., Orig., *Plat.*

**Coition, hemorrhage after:** Arg-n., Kreos., Nit-ac., Sep.

**Coition, painful:** Apis, Arg-n., Bell., *Berb.,* Ferr., Kreos., Lyc., Lyss., Plat., Sep., *Staph.,* Thuj. (See **Vaginismus.**)

**CONCEPTION, difficult (sterility):** *Agn.,* Alet., Am-c., Aur., *Bar-m., Borx.,* Calc., Cann-i., Caul., *Con.,* Eup-pur., Goss., *Graph.,* Helon., *Iod.,* Lec., *Med.,* Nat-c., *Nat-m.,* Nat-p., Phos., *Plat., Sabal.*

**Conception, easy:** Merc., Nat-m.

**DESIRE, diminished or lost:** *Agn.,* Am-c., Berb., Caust., Ferr-m., Graph., *Helon., Ign.,* Nat-m., *Onos.,* Plb., *Sep.*

**Desire, increased (nymphomania):** Ambr., *Aster.,* Arund., *Bufo,* Calc., *Calc-p.,* Camph., *Canth.,* Chin., Cimic., Coca, Dulc., *Ferul., Grat., Hyos.,* Kali-br., Kali-p., Kreos., Lach., Mosch., *Murx.,* Nux-v., *Orig.,* Phos., Pic-ac., *Plat.,* Raph., *Rob.,* Sabin., Sil., *Stram.,* Stry., *Tarent., Verat., Xero.,* Zinc.

**Desire, increased, must keep busy to repress it:** Lil-t.

**Desire, suppressed, ill effects:** *Con.,* Sabal.

**GONORRHEA:** Acon., Alumn., Apis, Arg-n., *Cann-s., Canth., Cop., Cub.,* Jac-c., Kreos., Med., *Merc.,* Merc-c., *Ol-sant.,* Petros., *Puls., Sep.,* Sulph., *Thuj.* (See **Leucorrhea, Vaginitis, Vulvitis.**)

**LEUCORRHEA, Remedies in general:** Agar., *Agn.,* Alet., Aln., *Alum.,* Am-c., *Am-m., Ambr.,* Arg-n., *Ars.,* Asaf., Aur-m., *Aur-m-n.,* Baros., Bar-m., Bell., *Borx., Bov., Calc.,* Calc-p., *Canth.,* Carb-v., *Caul.,* Caust., Cham., *Chin.,* Cimic., *Cocc., Con., Cop., Dict., Eucal.,* Eupi., Ferr-i., *Frax.,* Gels., *Graph.,* Hedeo., *Helon.,* Helin., Hep., *Hydr.,* Hydrc., Ign., Iod., Jac-c., Joan., *Kali-bi., Kali-c.,* Kali-m., *Kali-s., Kreos., Lil-t., Lyc.,* Mag-c., *Mag-m., Merc.,* Merc-pr-r., Mez., Murx., Naja, *Nat-m., Nat-s., Nit-ac.,* Nux-v., Orig., *Ovi-p.,* Pall., Pic-ac., *Psor.,* Pulx., *Puls., Sabin., Sec.,* Sil., Spira., *Stann.,* Sul-ac., Sulph., Thlas., *Thuj.,* Til., Tril-p., Vib., *Xan.,* Zinc.

**TYPE, Acrid, corroding, burning:** Aesc., *Alum., Am-c.,* Aral., *Ars.,* Ars-i., Aur., Aur-m., *Borx., Bov., Calc.,* Calc-i., Carb-ac., Carb an., Carb-v., Caul., *Cham., Con.,* Cop., Eucal., Ferr-br., *Graph., Gua.,* Helin., Hep., *Hydr.,* Ign., *Iod., Kreos.,* Lach., *Lit-t.,* Lyc., Med., *Merc., Nat-m., Nit-ac.,* Phos., Puls., Sabin., *Sep., Sil.,* Sul-ac., *Sulph.,* Ziz.

**Albuminous, slimy, mucus:** Agn., *Alum., Am-m., Ambr.,* Berb., *Borx.,* Bov., *Calc., Calc-p.,* Ferr-i., Graph., Haem., Hydr., Inul., Iod., Kali- m., *Kali-s.,* Kreos., Mag-c., Mez., Plat., *Puls.,* Sul-ac., *Thuj.,* Til.

**Blackish:** *Chin.,* Thlas.

**Bland:** Borx., Calc-p., Eupi., *Frax.,* Kali-m., Puls., Stann.

**Bloody:** Arg-n., Ars., Bufo, Calc-ars., Carb-v., *Chin.,* Cocc., Con., *Kreos., Merc., Merc-c.,* Murx., Nit-ac., Nux-m., *Sep., Spira.,* Sul-ac., *Thlas.*

**Brown:** *Aesc.,* Am-m., Kreos., *Lil-t.,* Nit-ac., *Sec., Sep.*

**Flesh colored, like washing of meat, non-offensive:** *Nit-ac.*

**Greenish:** *Bov.,* Carb-ac., Carb-v., *Kali-s.,* Lach., *Merc., Murx.,* Nat-s., Nit-ac., Phos., Pulx., *Puls.,* Sec., *Sep.,* Sulph., Thuj.

**Gushing:** Cocc., *Eupi., Graph., Sep.* (See **Profuse.**)

**Intermittent:** Con., Sulph.

**Itching:** *Ambr.,* Anac., Calc., *Calc-i.,* Carb-ac., *Chin.,* Hedeo., Helin., Hydr., *Kreos., Merc., Sep.* (See **Pruritus.**)

**Lumpy:** Ant-c., Hydr., Psor.

**Milky, white:** Aur., Bell., *Borx., Calc., Calc-i.,* Calc-p., Canth., Carb-v., *Con., Cop.,* Ferr., *Graph.,* Haem., Iod., *Kali-m.,* Naja, *Ovi-p.,* Paraf., *Puls., Sep., Sil., Stann.,* Sulph.

**Offensive:** Aral., Ars., Bufo, *Carb-ac.,* Chin., Eucal., Guaj., *Helon., Hep., Kreos., Merc.,* Med., Nat-c., Nit-ac., Nux-v., *Psor.,* Pulx., Rob., Sabin., Sang., *Sanic., Sec., Sep.,* Thlas., Ust.

**Painful:** Mag-m., Sil., Sulph. (See **Concomitants.**)

**Painless:** Am-m., Puls.

**Profuse:** *Alum.,* Ambr., Am-c., *Arg-n., Ars.,* Aur., Borx., *Calc.,* Calc-p., Carb-ac., *Caul.,* Caust., Con., Fl-ac., Graph., Gua., Helin., *Hydr.,* Hydrc., Iod., Kreos., *Lach.,* Lil-t., Mag-s., *Merc., Nat-m., Ovi-p.,* Phos., Pulx., *Puls., Sep.,* Sil., *Stann., Syph., Thuj.,* Til., Tril-p., Ziz.

**Purulent, staining, yellow:** Aesc., *Agn.,* Alumn., Arg-n., *Ars.,* Aur-m., *Bov.,* Calc., Cann-s., Carb-an., Cean., Cham., *Chin.,* Eupi., *Fago.,* Helin., *Hydr.,* Ign., Iod., *Kali-bi., Kali-s., Kreos.,* Lach., Lil-t., Lyc., *Merc.,* Merc-i-f., Nat-s., Pulx., *Puls., Sep., Stann.,* Sulph., Tril-p., Ust.

**Thick:** Aesc., Aur., *Bov.,* Canth., Carb-v., Con., Helin., *Hydr., Iod.,* Kali- m., Kreos., Mag-s., Merc., Murx., Nit-ac., *Puls.,* Sabin., *Sep.,* Thuj.

**Thin, watery:** *Am-c.,* Ars., Bell., Bufo, Cham., Frax., *Graph., Kali-s.,* Kreos., Lil-t., Merc., *Merc-c.,* Naja, Nat-m., *Nit-ac.,* Plat., Puls., *Sep., Syph.,* Sulph.

**Viscid, stringy, tough:** *Aesc., Alum.,* Asar., *Bov.,* Dict., Ferr-br., Graph., *Hydr.,* Iris, *Kali-bi., Kali-m.,* Nit-ac., *Pall.,* Phyt., Sabin., Tril-p.

**OCCURRENCE, MODALITIES, After coitus:** Nat-c.

**After menses and between periods:** Aesc., *Alum.,* Borx., *Bov., Calc., Cocc.,* Con., *Eupi., Graph.,* Hydr., *Iod.,* Kalm., *Kreos., Nit-ac.,* Ph-ac., *Puls.,* Sabin., *Sep.,* Thlas., *Xan.*

**After stool:** Mag-m.
**After urination:** *Am-m.,* Con., *Kreos.,* Mag-m., Nicc., Plat., *Sep.,* Sil.
**At climaxis:** Psor., Sang.
**At night:** Ambr., Caust., *Merc.,* Nit-ac.
**Before menses:** *Alum.,* Bar-c., Borx., *Bov., Calc.,* Calc-p., Carb-v., Con., *Graph.,* Kreos., Pic-ac., *Puls.,* Sep., Thlas.
**Better from washing with cold water:** Alum.
**From motion, walking:** *Bov.,* Carb-an., Euph-pi., Graph., Helin., *Mag-m.,* Til.
**From rest:** Fago.
**From sitting, relieved by walking:** Cact., *Cocc.,* Cycl.
**From urine, contact of:** Kreos., *Merc.,* Sulph.
**In daytime:** Alum., Plat.
**In infants, little girls:** *Asper., Calc.,* Cann-s., Carb-ac., *Caul., Cina, Cub.,* Hydr., Merc., Merc-i-f., *Mill., Puls., Sep.,* Syph.
**In old, weak women:** Ars., *Helon.,* Nit-ac., Sec.
**In pregnant women:** Cocc., Kali-c., Sep.
**Instead of menses:** *Cocc.,* Graph., *Iod., Nux-m.,* Phos., Puls., Senec., *Sep.,* Xan.

**CONCOMITANTS, Abdominal pain, colic preceding and attending:** *Am-m.,* Aral., *Ars.,* Bell., Calc., *Con.,* Graph., Ham., Haem., Ign., Lyc., *Mag-m.,* Nat-c., *Sep.,* Sil., *Sulph.,* Syph.
**Backache and weak feeling, preceding and attending:** *Aesc., Eupi,* Graph., *Helon.,* Kali-bi., Kreos., Mag-s., *Murx.,* Nat-chor., *or Nat-hchls., Nat-m.,* Ovi-p., Psor., *Stann.*
**Cervical erosion, bleeding easily:** Alum., *Aln.,* Arg-n., Dict., *Hydr.,* Hydrc., *Kali-bi.*
**Debility, weakness:** *Alet., Alum.,* Calc., Carb-an., Caul., Caust., Chin., *Cocc.,* Con., Guaj., *Helon.,* Helin., Hydr., *Kreos.,* Onos., Phos., *Psor.,* Puls., Sep., *Stann.*
**Diarrhea:** Puls.
**Feeling, as if warm water running:** Borx.
**Feeling of fullness, heat, relieved by cold water:** Acon.
**Hemorrhage, obstinate, intermittent:** Kreos.
**Hepatic derangement, costiveness:** Hydr.
**History of abortion:** Alet., Caul., *Sabin.,* Sep.
**Hysterical spasm in uterus and abdomen:** Mag-m.
**Mental symptoms:** Murx.
**Moth spots on forehead:** Caul., Sep.
**Metorrhagia following:** Mag-m.

**Pruritus vulvae:** Agar., Alum., *Ambr., Anac.,* Calc., *Fago., Helon.,* Hydr., Kreos., Merc., *Sep.,* Sulph.

**Relaxation of genitals:** Agn., *Caul.,* Sec., Sep.

**Spasmodic contraction of vagina:** Aur-m-n.

**Urinary irritation:** Berb., *Erig.,* Kreos., Sep.

**MAMMAE, Abscess:** Bry., Crot-t., Graph., *Hep., Phos.,* Phyt., *Sil.,* Sulph. (See **Mastitis.**)

**Atrophy:** Chim., *Con., Iod.,* Kali-i., Nit-ac., Onos., *Sabal.*

**Cancer:** *Arg-n., Ars.,* Ars-i., *Aster.,* Bad., Bapt., Bar-i., Brom., Bry., Calc-i., *Carb-an.,* Carc., Cic., Clem., *Con., Cund., Gali.,* Graph., Hep., *Hydr., Kali-i.,* Kreos., Lach., Phos., *Plb-i.,* Psor., Sang., *Scir.,* Semp., Sil., Strych-g., Sulph., Tarent., *Thuj.* (See **Tumors.**)

**Cancer, bleeding:** Kreos., Lach., *Phos.,* Sang., Strych-g., Thuj.

**Cancer, scirrhus:** Ars., Carb an., *Con.,* Cund., Hydr., Kreos., Lap-a., Phyt., *Scir., Sil.*

**Induration, hardness:** Alumn., Anan., *Aster.,* Bar-i., Bell., *Bry.,* Bufo, *Calc-f., Carb-an.,* Carb-v., Cham., Cist., Clem., *Con., Graph., Iod.,* Kreos., Lac-c., *Lap-a.,* Merc., Nit-ac., *Phyt., Plb., Plb-i.*

**Inflammation (mastitis):** *Acon.,* Ant-t., Apis, Arn., Ars., *Bell., Bry.,* Calc., *Cham.,* Cist., *Con., Crot-t.,* Ferr-p., Galeg., Graph., *Hep., Lac-c.,* Lach., *Merc., Phel., Phos., Phyt.,* Plan., *Puls.,* Sabad., *Sil.,* Sulph. (See **Pain, Swelling.**)

**NIPPLES, burning, itching:** *Agar.,* Arund., *Ars.,* Castm., *Crot-t.,* Lyc., Onos., Orig., Petr., Puls., Sil., *Sulph.*

**Cracks, fissures, ulcerations:** Anan., *Arn.,* Ars., *Aur-s.,* Calc-ox., Calen., Carb-v., *Castm.,* Caust., Cham., *Con., Crot-t., Cund., Eup-a.,* Gali., Ger., *Graph.,* Ham., Hep., Hipp., Merc., Nit-ac., *Paeon., Phel.,* Phos., *Phyt., Rat.,* Sep., *Sil.,* Sulph. (See **Soreness.**)

**Inflamed, tender to touch:** *Cham.,* Helon., Phyt.

**Retraction:** Carb-an., Hydr., Lap-a., Nux-m., *Sars.,* Sil.

**Soreness, tenderness:** Ap-g., *Arn.,* Borx., Calen., *Castm., Cham.,* Cist, *Con., Crot-t., Eup-a., Graph.,* Ham., Helon., *Hep.,* Hydr., Lac-c., Med., Oci., Orig., Paraf., *Phel.,* Phos., *Phyt., Rat.,* Sang., Sil., Sulph., Zinc.

**PAIN IN BREASTS (mastodynia):** Acon., All-s., Apis, Arg-n., *Aster.,* Aur-s., *Bell.,* Brom., *Bry., Calc.,* Carb-an., Cham., *Chim., Cimic., Con.,* Cot., Croc., *Crot-t., Hep.,* Hydr., Hyper., *Lac-ac.,* Lac-c., Lach., *Lap-a.,* Lepi., Med., *Merc.,* Merl., *Murx.,* Nat-m., Onos., Pall., *Phel., Phos., Phyt.,* Plb., *Plb-i.,* Poly-h., Prun., Psor., Puls., *Sang.,* Sil., Sumb., Zinc.

**Pain, inframammary:** *Cimic.,* Puls., *Ran-b.,* Raph., Sumb., Ust., Zinc.

**Pain relieved by supporting heavy mammae:** *Bry., Lac-c.,* Phyt.

**Pain worse from jar, toward evening:** Lac-c.

**SWELLING:** All-s., Anan., *Asaf., Aster.,* Aur-s., *Bell.,* Bell-p., *Bry.,* Castm., Dulc., *Graph.,* Helon., Lac-c., *Merc.,* Merl., Onos., Phos., *Phyt.,* Psor., Puls., Sol-o., Urt-u. (See **Mastitis.**)

**Tenderness, soreness:** Arg-n., *Aster., Bell., Bry.,* Calc., Carb-an., *Cham.,* Clem., *Con.,* Dulc., *Helon., Hep.,* Iod., Kali-m., *Lac-c.,* Lach., *Med.,* Merc., Onos., *Phyt.,* Plb., Rad-br., Sabal, Syph. (See **Pain.**)

**TUMORS, nodosities:** Ars-i., *Aster., Bell.,* Berb-a., *Brom.,* Bry., Calen., Calc., *Calc-f., Calc-i.,* Carb-an., Cham., *Chim.,* Clem., *Con.,* Cund., Ferr-i., Gnaph., *Graph.,* Hecla, *Hydr., Iod.,* Lach., Lap-a., Lyc., *Merc-i-f.,* Murx., Nit-ac., *Phos., Phyt., Plb-i.,* Psor., *Puls.,* Sabin., Sang., *Scir., Scoph-n., Sil.,* Thuj., *Thyr.,* Tub. (See **Cancer, Swelling, Inflammation.**)

**ULCERATION:** Aster., Calen., Clem., *Hep., Merc.,* Paeon., Phos., *Phyt., Sil.*

**MASTURBATION, In children, due to pruritus vulvae:** *Calad., Orig.,* Zinc.

**MENOPAUSE, Climacteric period, change of life, Remedies in general:** Acon., Agar., Alet., *Aml-ns.,* Aqui., Arg-n., *Bell., Bell-p.,* Bor-ac., *Cact.,* Calc., Calc-ar., Caps., Carb-v., *Caul., Cimic.,* Cocc., Coff., *Con.,* Cycl., Ferr., *Gels., Glon.,* Graph., Helon., *Ign., Jab.,* Kali-br., *Kali-c., Kreos., Lach.,* Mag-c., *Manc., Murx., Nux-m., Nux-v., Ov.,* Plb., *Puls., Sang.,* Semp., *Sep.,* Sul-ac., *Sulph.,* Ther., *Ust.,* Valer., Vip., Visc., *Zinc-val.*

**Anxiety:** Acon., *Aml-ns.,* Sep.

**Breasts enlarged, painful:** Sang.

**Burning in vertex:** *Lach.,* Nux-v., Sang., *Sulph.*

**Burning of palms and soles:** Sang., *Sulph.*

**Congestions:** Acon., *Aml-ns.,* Calc., *Glon.,* Lach., Sang., Sep., *Sulph., Ust.*

**Cough, burning in chest, periodical neuralgia:** Sang.

**Earache:** Sang.

**Fainting spells:** Cimic., Crot-h., Ferr., *Glon., Lach.,* Nux-m., Sep., *Sulph.,* Tril-p.

**Falling of hair:** Sep.

**Fatigue, persistent tiredness, fagged womb:** Bell-p.

**Fatigue without cause, muscular weakness, chilliness:** Calc.

**Flooding:** Aloe, Aml-ns., Apoc., *Arg-met.,* Arg-n., Aur-m., Calc., Caps., Chin., *Cimic.,* Ferr., Hydrtinin-m., Kali-br., Lach., Med., Nit-ac., *Plb.,* Sabin., Sanguiso., *Sed-ac,* Sep., Thlas., *Tril-p., Ust.,* Vinc. (See **Metrorrhagia.**)

**Flushings:** *Acon., Aml-ns.,* Bell., Bor-ac., Calc-p., *Cimic.,* Crot-h., Dig., Ferr., *Glon., Ign., Jab.,* Kali-br., Kali-c., *Lach., Mang-act.,* Nicc-s., Nux-v., Ov., Ph-ac., Pilo., *Sang.,* Sed-ac, Sep., Stront-c., Sul-ac., *Sulph., Sumb.,* Tub., *Ust.,* Valer., Verat-v., Vesp., Vinc., Zinc-val.

**Globus hystericus:** Aml-ns., *Lach.,* Valer., Zinc-val.

**Headache:** *Aml-ns.,* Cact., *Chin., Cimic.,* Croc., *Cypr.,* Ferr., *Glon.,* Ign., Lach., *Sang., Sep.,* Stront-c.

**Hysterical tendencies:** Ign., Valer., Zinc-val.

**Inframammary pains:** Cimic.

**Liver disorders:** Card-m.

**Mental depression or irritability:** *Cimic.,* Ign., Kali-br., *Lach.,* Manc., Psor., Valer., Zinc-val.

**Nervous erethism:** Absin., Arg-n., Cimic., Coff., Dig., *Ign.,* Kali-br., *Lach.,* Ov., *Ther.,* Valer., *Zinc-val.*

**Pains in uterus:** Agar., *Cimic.,* Cocc., Lach., Puls., *Sep.*

**Palpitation:** *Aml-ns., Calc-ar.,* Ferr., Glon., Kali-br., *Lach.,* Sep., Tril-p., Valer.

**Perspiration, profuse:** Aml-ns., Bell., Crot-h., Hep., *Jab.,* Lach., Nux-v., *Sep.,* Til., Valer.

**Pruritus:** Calad.

**Salivation:** Jab.

**Sexual excitement:** Manc., *Murx.*

**Sinking at stomach:** Cimic., Crot-h., Dig., Hydr-ac., *Ign., Sep.,* Tril-p.

**Ulcers, superficial, sores, on lower limbs:** Polyg-h.

**Vertigo, tinnitus:** Glon., Lach., Tril-p., Ust.

**Weakness:** Dig., Helon., Lach., *Sep.*

**MENSTRUATION; TYPE, AMENORRHEA, Remedies in general:** *Acon.,* Alet., Aln., *Apis,* Apoc., Ars., Aven., Bell., Bry., *Calc.,* Cann-s., *Caul.,* Caust., *Cimic.,* Con., *Cycl.,* Dulc., *Euphr., Ferr., Ferr-ar., Ferr-r.,* Gels., *Glon., Graph.,* Hedeo., *Hell., Helon.,* Joan., *Kali-c., Kali-perm.,* Lil-t., Mang-act., *Merl., Nat-m.,* Nux-v., Op., Parth., Ph-ac., Pin-l., *Plat.,* Plb., *Polyg-h., Puls.,* Sec., *Seneg., Sep.,* Spong., *Sulph.,* Tanac., Thyr., Ust., *Xan.*

**Before the proper age:** *Calc.,* Calc-p., Carb-v., Chin., Cocc., *Sabin.,* Sil., Verat.

**Delayed, first menses:** Calc., Calc-p., Dam., Ferr., *Graph., Kali-c.,* Kali-perm., Polyg-h., *Puls., Senec.,* Sep.

**Delayed, tardy flow:** Acon., Alet., *Caust., Cimic.,* Con., Cupr., Dulc., Euphr., *Gels.,* Glon., Goss., *Graph.,* Hell., Iod., Joan., *Kali- c.,* Kali-m., *Kali-p.,* Kali-s., Lac-d., *Mag-c., Nat-m.,* Nux-m., Phos., Pulx., *Puls.,* Rad-br., Sabad., *Senec., Sep., Stry-af-cit., Sulph.,* Valer., *Vib.,* Zinc., Ziz.

**Intermittent:** Coc-c., Ferr., *Kreos., Lac-c.,* Mag-s., *Meli.,* Murx., Nux-v., Phos., *Puls., Sabad., Sep.,* Sulph., Xan.

**Irregular:** Ambr., Caul., *Cimic., Cocc., Cycl., Graph.,* Iod., Joan., Lil-t., *Nux-m., Nux-v.,* Phos., Pisc., *Puls.,* Rad-br., Sec., Senec., *Sep.,* Sulph.

**Protracted:** Acon., Calc-s., Caust., *Con.,* Crot-h., *Cupr.,* Ferr., Graph., Iod., Kreos., *Lyc.,* Nat-m., Nux-m., Nux-v., *Phos.,* Rhus-t.

**Scanty flow:** Alet., *Alum.*, Apis, Berb., *Borx.*, Canth., *Caul.*, Caust., *Cimic.*, *Cocc.*, *Con.*, Cycl., Dulc., *Euphr.*, *Gels.*, *Graph.*, Ign., *Kali- c.*, *Kali-p.*, Kali-s., Lach., Lam., Lil-t., *Mag-c.*, Mang-act., *Meli.*, Merl., *Nat-m.*, Nux-v., *Ol-an.*, *Phos.*, Plat., *Puls.*, Sang., *Senec.*, *Sep.*, Sil., *Stry-af-cit.*, *Sulph.*, Valer., *Vib.*, Xan. (See **Dysmenorrhea**.)

**Suppressed:** *Acon.*, Apis, Bell., *Bry.*, Calc., Cean., Cham., Chion., *Cimic.*, *Con.*, Croc., Cupr., *Cycl.*, *Dulc.*, Ferr., Gels., *Glon.*, Graph., Helon., Ign., Kali-c., *Kali-m.*, Lach., Leon., Nat-m., Nux-m., *Op.*, Podo., *Puls.*, *Puls-n.*, *Senec.*, Sep., Sulph., *Tanac.*, Tax., Tub., *Verat-v.*, Zinc.

**Suppressed from anemic conditions:** Ars., Ars-i., Caust., Ferr-ar., Ferr-r., Graph., *Kali-c.*, Kali-p., Kali-perm., Mag-act., Nat-m., Ovi-p., *Puls.*, *Senec.*, *Stry-af-cit.*

**Suppressed from anger with indignation:** Cham., Coloc., Staph.

**Suppressed from cold water, exposure, chilling:** *Acon.*, *Ant-c.*, Bell., Calc., Cham., Cimic., *Con.*, *Dulc.*, Graph., Lac-c., *Lac-d.*, Phos., *Puls.*, *Rhus-t.*, Sulph., Verat-v., Xan.

**Suppressed from disappointed love:** Hell.

**Suppressed from fright, vexation:** Act-sp., Acon., Cimic., Coloc., Lyc., Op., Verat.

**Suppressed from transient, localilzed, uterine congestion, followed by chronic anemic state:** Sabal.

**Suppressed in emigrants:** Bry., Plat.

**Suppressed with asthma:** Spong.

**Suppressed with cerebral congestion:** *Acon.*, Apis, *Bell.*, Bry., Calc., Cimic., *Gels.*, *Glon.*, Lach., Psor., Sep., Sulph., *Verat-v.*

**Suppressed with congestion to chest:** Acon., Calc., Sep.

**Suppressed with cramps to chest:** Cupr.

**Suppressed with delirium, mania:** Stram.

**Suppressed with dropsy:** Apis, Apoc., Kali-c.

**Suppressed with fainting spells, drowsiness:** Kali-c., *Nux-m.*, Op.

**Suppressed with gastralgia or spasms:** Cocc.

**Suppressed with jaundice:** Chion.

**Suppressed with neuralgic pains about head, face:** *Gels.*

**Suppressed with ophthalmia:** Puls.

**Suppressed with ovaritis:** *Acon.*, Cimic.

**Suppressed with pelvic pressure, ovarian tenderness:** Ant-c., Bell.

**Suppressed with pelvic tenesmus:** Podo.

**Suppressed with rheumatic pains:** Bry., Cimic., Rhus-t.

**Suppressed with vicarious bleeding:** *Bry.*, Crot-h., Dig., Erig., Eupi., *Ferr.*, *Ham.*, Ip., Kali-c., Lach., Mill., Nat-s., *Phos.*, *Puls.*, Sabad., Sang., *Senec.*, Sil., Sulph., Tril-p., Ust.

**DYSMENORRHEA, Remedies in general:** Acetan., Acon., Am-act., Ap- g., *Apiol.*, Apis, Aqui., Atrop., Aven., *Bell., Borx.,* Bov., Brom., Bry., *Cact.,* Calc., Canth., Castm., *Caul., Cham., Cimic., Cocc., Coff.,* Coll., *Coloc.,* Croc., Cupr., Dulc., Epiph., Ferr., Ferr-p., *Gels.,* Glon., *Gnaph.,* Goss., Graph., *Guaj., Ham.,* Helon., Hyos., Ign., *Kali-perm.,* Lach., Lil-t., *Macrot., Mag-c.,* Mag-m., *Mag-p.,* Merc., Mill., Morph., Nux- m., Nux-v., Op., Plat., *Puls.,* Rhus-t., Sabin., Sang., Santin., *Sec., Senec.,* Sep., Stram., Thyr., Tub., Ust., *Verat.,* Verat-v., *Vib.,* Vib-p., *Xan., Zinc.*

**TYPE, Irregular, every two weeks, or so:** Borx., *Bov., Calc.,* Calc-p., Croc., Ferr-p., *Helon.,* Ign., Mag-s., Mez., Murx., Nit-ac., Nux-v., Ph-ac., *Phos.,* Phyt., Sabin., Sec., Thlas., *Tril-p.,* Ust.

**Irregular:** Am-c., *Bell.,* Bry., *Calc.,* Caul., *Cimic.,* Cocc., *Cycl.,* Guaj., Inul., Mag-s., Murx., *Nat-m., Nux-v.,* Phys., *Puls.,* Sec., *Senec., Sep.* (See **Amenorrhea.**)

**Membranous:** *Ars.,* Bell., *Borx., Brom.,* Bry., Calc., *Calc-act.,* Cham., Coll., Con., Cycl., Guaj., Helio., Lac-c., *Mag-p.,* Merc., Rhus-t., *Sulph.,* Ust., *Vib.*

**Non-obstructive, from ovarian irritation:** *Apis,* Bell., Ham., Xan.

**Non-obstructive, from uterine irritation:** *Cham.,* Coff., Nit-ac., Xan.

**Premature:** Am-c., *Calc.,* Caust., Cocc., Con., Cycl., Ign., *Kali-c.,* Lam., Lil-t., *Mag-p.,* Nat-m., *Nux-v.,* Ol-an., Phos., Sabin., Sep., Sin-n., Sil., *Sulph., Xan.* (See **Irregular**.)

**Rheumatic:** Caul., Caust., *Cimic.,* Cocc., Guaj., Rham-cal.

**Spasmodic, neuralgic:** Acon., Agar., *Bell., Caul.,* Cham., *Cimic.,* Coff., Coll., *Gels.,* Glon., Gnaph., Mag-m., *Mag-p., Nux-v., Puls.,* Sabin., Santin., *Sec.,* Senec., Sep., Verat-v., *Vib., Xan.*

**Spasmodic, with uterine congestion:** Acon., *Bell.,* Cimic., Coll., Gels., Puls., *Sabin.,* Sep., Verat-v.

**MENORRHAGIA, (profuse, premature flow), Remedies in general:** Achil-m., Agar., *Alet.,* Aloe, *Am-c.,* Ambr., Apoc., *Aran., Arn., Ars., Bell., Borx.,* Bov., Bry., *Cact., Calc.,* Calc-p., *Cann-i., Canth.,* Carb-v., Caul., Cean., *Cham., Chinin-s.,* Cimic., *Cinnm.,* Coll., Coloc., *Croc., Cycl.,* Dig., *Erig.,* Ferr., *Ferr-p.,* Ferr-r., Fic-r., *Ger.,* Glyc., *Ham., Helon.,* Hydr., Ign., Joan., *Kali-c., Kali-m., Kreos.,* Lac-c., Lach., Led., Lil-t., Mag-c., Mez., *Mill.,* Murx., *Nit-ac., Nux-v.,* Pall., Paraf., Ph-ac., *Phos.,* Phyt., *Plat., Plb.,* Ruta, *Sabin., Sec.,* Sed-ac., *Sep.,* Sil., *Stann.,* Sul-ac., Sulph., Thlas., *Tril-p.,* Ust., Vinc., *Xan.*

**After miscarriage, parturition:** Apis, Chin., *Cimic.,* Helon., Kali-c., *Nit-ac., Sabin.,* Sep., Sulph., Thlas., *Ust.,* Vib.

**Every alternate period, profuse:** Thlas.

**Protracted, premature, profuse:** *Aloe,* Asar., *Bell., Calc.,* Calc-i., Carb-an., *Cinnm.,* Coff., Ferr., Ferr-act., Fl-ac., Glyc., Grat., Ign., Kreos., *Mill.,* Murx., *Nux-v.,* Onos., *Plat.,* Raph., Rhus-t., *Sabin.,* Sanguiso., *Sec.,* Sulph., *Thlas., Tril-p.,* Tub., Xan.

**TYPE OF MENSTRUAL BLOOD, Acrid, corroding:** Am-c., Kali-c., Lach., Mag-c., Nat-s., Nit-ac., *Rhus-t.,* Sabin., Sil., *Sulph.*

**Bright red:** Acon., *Bell.,* Brom., Calc-p., *Cinnm., Erig.,* Glyc., Ferr-p., *Ip.,* Lac-c., *Mill., Sabin.,* Sang., *Tril-p.,* Ust.

**Changeable:** Puls.

**Coagulated:** Am-m., *Bell.,* Bov., *Cham., Chin.,* Cimic., *Coc-c.,* Cocc., Coff., *Croc., Cycl.,* Glyc., Helon., Jug-r., *Kali-m., Lil-t.,* Mag-m., Med., Murx., Nux-v., *Plat.,* Plb., *Puls., Sabin.,* Sang., Sulph., *Thlas.,* Tril-p., Ust.

**Dark, blackish:** Apis, *Asar.,* Bov., Calc-p., Canth., Caul., Cham., *Chin.,* Cimic., *Coc-c.,* Cocc., Coff., *Croc., Cycl.,* •Elaps, *Ham.,* Helon., *Ign., Kali-m., Kali-n.,* Kreos., Lach., *Lil-t.,* Mag-c., Mag-m., Mag-p., Med., Nit-ac., Nux-v., *Plat.,* Plb., *Puls.,* Sabin., Sec., Sep., *Thlas.,* Tril-p., *Ust., Xan.*

**Hot:** Bell.

**Membranous, shreddy, like meat washings:** Brom., *Cycl.,* Ferr., Nat-c., *Nit-ac.* (See **Coagulated**.)

**Offensive:** *Bell.,* Carb-v., Cimic., Cop., Helon., *Kali-c.,* Kali-p., *Lil-t.,* Mag-c., *Med.,* Plat., *Psor.,* Pyrog., *Sabin.,* Sang., *Sec.,* Sulph., Vib.

**Pale:** *Alum.,* Ars., *Carb-v., Ferr., Graph., Kali-c.,* Nat-p., *Puls.,* Sulph. (See **Watery**.)

**Partly fluid, partly clotted:** *Ferr.,* Ham., Plb., *Sabin., Sec.*

**Pitch-like:** Cact., Cocc., *Croc.,* Kali-m., *Mag-c.,* Med., *Plat.*

**Stringy, glairy, viscid, thick:** Arg-n., Coc-c., *Croc., Kali-m.,* Kreos., Lac-c., Mag-c., Mag-p., *Nit-ac.,* Nux-m., *Plat.,* Puls., Sulph., *Tril-p., Ust., Xan.*

**Watery, thin:** Aeth., Alumn., Eupi, Ferr-act., *Ferr-m.,* Goss., Kali-p., Nat-p., Phos., *Sabin., Sec.*

**COMPLAINTS, PRECEDING AND ATTENDING FLOW, Abdomen distended:** Apoc., Aran., Cham., *Chin., Cocc.,* Kali-c., Kreos., Nux-v. (See **ABDOMEN**.)

**Abdomen sore:** Ham., Sep. (See **ABDOMEN.**)

**Abdomen, weight:** Aloe, Bell., Glyc., Kali-s., Puls., *Sep.*

**Anus, sore:** Ars., *Mur-ac.* (See **Anus.**)

**Aphonia:** *Gels.,* Graph.

**Asthmatic seizures awaken her from sleep:** Cupr., *Iod., Lach.,* Spong.

**Axillae, itching:** Sang.

**Backache, general bad feelings:** Kali-c.

**Blindness:** Cycl., Puls.

**Breasts, icy cold:** Med.

**Breasts, milk in them, in place of menses:** Merc.

**Breasts, tender, swollen:** Bry., Calc., Canth., *Con.,* Graph., *Helon.,* Kali-c., *Lac-c.,* Mag-c., Merc., *Murx., Phyt., Puls.,* Sang.

**Burning in hands and soles:** Carb-v.

**Catalepsy:** Mosch.

**Chilliness, coldness:** Am-c., Apis, Calc., Cham., Glyc., Graph., Nux-v., Plat., *Puls.,* Sec., Sep., *Sil., Sulph., Verat.*

**Cholera-like symptoms:** Am-c., Bov., Verat.

**Colds:** Mag-c., Sep.

**Constipation:** Am-c., Coll., *Graph., Nat-m.,* Nux-v., Plat., *Plb.,* Sep., *Sil.,* Sulph.

**Cough:** *Graph.,* Lac-c., *Sulph.*

**Deafness, tinnitus:** Kreos.

**Diarrhea:** *Am-c.,* Am-m., Ars., *Bov.,* Cham., Kreos., Phos., *Puls., Verat.*

**Epistaxis:** Acon., *Bry.,* Dig., Gels., Nat-s., Sep., Sulph.

**Eruptions:** All-s., *Bell.,* Bell-p., Calc., *Cimic.,* Con., *Dulc.,* Eug., *Graph., Kali-ar.,* Kali-c., Mag-m., Mang-act., *Med.,* Psor., Sang., *Sars.,* Sil., Thuj., Verat.

**Eyes, blindness or fiery spots:** Cycl., Sep.

**Eyes, burning:** Nicc.

**Eyes, diplopia:** Gels.

**Eyes, ophthalmia:** Puls.

**Face flushed:** *Bell.,* Calc-p., Ferr., *Ferr-p.,* Gels., *Sang.*

**Face pale, eyes sunken:** Cycl., Ip., Verat.

**Feet and cheeks swollen:** Apis, Graph.

**Feet, cold damp:** Calc.

**Feet, pain in:** Am-m.

**Feet, swollen:** Graph., Lyc., Puls.

**Flushes of heat:** Ferr., Glon., *Lach., Sang.,* Sulph.

**Frenzy:** Acon.

**Genitals, sensitive:** Am-c., Cocc., *Lach.,* Kali-c., *Plat.* (See **Vaginismus.**)

**Headache, congestive symptoms:** Aster., *Bell.,* Bry., Cimic., Cocc., Croc., *Cycl.,* Ferr-m., Ferr-p., *Gels., Glon.,* Graph., Kali-p., Kreos., Lac-c., Lach., Nat-c., *Nat-m., Nux-v.,* Puls., *Sang., Sep., Sulph., Ust.,* Verat-v., Xan.

**Heart, pain, palpitation, etc.:** *Cact.,* Crot-h., Eupi., Lach., *Lith-c.,* Sep., Spong.

**Hoarseness, coryza, sweats:** Graph.

**Hunger:** Spong.

**Hysterical symptoms:** Caul., *Cimic.*, Gels., *Ign.*, *Mag.-m.*, Nux-v., Plat., Puls., Senec., Vib.

**Inflammation of throat, chest, bladder:** Senec.

**Insomnia:** Agar., Senec.

**Irritability:** *Cham.*, Cocc., Eupi., Kreos., Lil-t., Lyc., Mag-m., *Nux-v.*

**Joint pains:** Caul., Sabin.

**Labia burning:** Calc.

**Lachrymation, catarrhal state of eyes, nose:** Euphr.

**Leucorrhea:** Bar-c., Borx., *Calc.*, Carb-v., Caust., Graph., Iod., *Nat-m.*, Puls.

**Leucorrhea, acrid:** Lach., Sep.

**Mania, chorea:** Cimic.

**Mania, sexual:** Cann-i., *Dulc.*, Plat., Stram., Verat.

**Morning sickness, nausea, vomiting:** *Am-m.*, Borx., *Cocc.*, *Cycl.*, Graph., Ichth., *Ip.*, Kreos., Meli., Nat-m., *Nux-v.*, Puls., *Sep.*, Thlas., Verat.

**Mouth sore, swelling of gums, cheeks, bleeding ulcer:** Phos.

**Mouth, tongue, throat dry, especially during sleep:** Nux-m., Tarent.

**Nervous disturbance, restlessness:** *Acon.*, *Cham.*, Caul., *Cimic.*, Ign., Kreos., *Lach.*, Mag-m., *Mag-p.*, Nit-ac., Puls., *Sal-n.*, Senec., Sep., Tril-p., Vib., Xan.

**Nipples and breasts icy cold:** Med.

**Old symptoms aggravated:** Nux-v.

**Pain, burning in left ovarian region, on motion:** Croc., *Thuj.*, Ust.

**Pain, colicky, labor-like, spasmodic:** *Alet.*, Aloe, *Am-c.*, Am-m., Apis, *Bell.*, Borx., *Bov.*, Brom., Calc., *Caul.*, *Cham.*, Chin., *Cimic.*, *Cocc.*, *Coff.*, *Coloc.*, Cupr., *Cycl.*, Ferr., Ferr-p., *Gels.*, *Graph.*, *Haem.*, Helon., Ign., Joan., *Kali-c.*, Kreos., Lil-t., *Mag-c.*, *Mag-m.*, *Mag-p.*, Med., Meli., Nat-m., Nit-ac., Nux-m., *Nux-v.*, Plat., *Puls.*, *Sabin.*, *Sec.*, Sep., Stann., Thlas., *Verat.*, Verat-v., Vesp., *Vib.*, *Xan.*

**Pain, extending around pelvis, from sacrum to groin:** Plat., Puls., Sep., Vib.

**Pain extending down hips, thighs, legs:** *Am-m.*, Berb., Bry., Castm., *Caul.*, Cham., *Cimic.*, Coff., Coloc., Con., *Gels.*, Graph., Lil-t., Mag-c., Mag-m., Nit-ac., Plat., *Sep.*, Tril-p., *Vib.*, Xan.

**Pain, extending through pelvis antero-posteriorly or lateraly:** Bell.

**Pain, extending to back (sacrum, coccyx):** *Am-c.*, Am-m., Asar., Bell., *Borx.*, Calc., *Calc-p.*, Caust., *Cham.*, Cic., *Cimic.*, Cupr., Cycl., *Gels.*, Graph., *Helon.*, *Kali-c.*, Kreos., Mag-m., Nit-ac., *Nux-v.*, Phos., Plat., Podo., *Puls.*, Rad-br., Sabin., *Senec.*, *Sep.*, Spong., Vib., *Xan.*

**Pain, extending to chest:** Caul., Cham., Cimic., *Cupr.*

**Pain, extending to groins:** Borx., *Caul.,* Kali-c., Lil-t., Plat., Tanac., *Ust.*
**Pain, extending to liver:** Ph-ac.
**Pain, extending to pubes:** Aln., Bov., Coloc., Cycl., Rad-br., *Sabin.,* Sep., Vib.
**Pain, extending to rectum:** *Aloe,* Xero.
**Pain, in feet:** Am-m.
**Pain, in malar bones:** Stann.
**Pain, in ovaries:** *Apis,* Bell., Bry., Cact., Canth., Cimic., Coloc., Ham., Iod., Joan., Kali-n., *Lach., Lil-t.,* Pic-ac., Sal-n., Tarent., *Thuj.,* Vib.
**Pruritus:** Calc., *Graph.,* Hep., Inul., Kali-c., *Sil.,* Sulph.
**Rectal and vesical irritation:** Sabin.
**Sadness:** Am-c., Aur., Brom., Caust., *Cimic.,* Cocc., Ferr., Hell., Helon., *Ign.,* Lyc., Nat-c., *Nat-m.,* Nit-ac., Phos., Plat., *Puls., Sep.,* Stann., Vesp.
**Salivation:** Pulx.
**Sexual excitement:** Plat.
**Sore throat:** Canth., *Lac-c., Mag-c.*
**Spasms:** Art-v., *Bufo,* Calc-s., Caul., *Cimic.,* Cupr., Gels., *Hyos., Ign.,* Kali-br., Lach., Mag-m., Oena., *Plat.,* Tarent.
**Stomach disturbances:** Arg-n., Ars., *Bry.,* Kali-c., Lach., *Lyc.,* Nux-m., *Nux-v., Puls.,* Sep., Sulph.
**Stretching, yawning:** Am-c., Puls.
**Syncope:** Ars., Chin., Ign., *Mosch.,* Nux-m., *Nux-v.,* Verat.
**Tinnitus:** *Ferr.,* Kreos.
**Toothache:** Am-c., Calc., Cham., Mag-c., *Puls.,* Sep.
**Urinary symptoms:** Calc-p., *Canth.,* Coc-c., *Gels.,* Hyos., Mag-p., Med., Nux-v., Plat., Pulx., Puls., *Senec.,* Sep., Verat-v., Vib.
**Vertigo:** Calc., Cycl., Nux-v.
**Weakness:** *Alum., Am-c.,* Carb-an., *Chin., Cocc.,* Ferr., Glyc., Graph., *Helon., Haem.,* Ign., Iod., Nicc., Puls., *Verat.*

**COMPLAINTS FOLLOWING MENSES, Diarrhea:** Graph., Puls.
**Erethism, neuralgic pains, inframammary pains, insomnia:** Cimic.
**Eruption:** Kreos.
**Headache:** Croc., Lach., Lil-t., Puls., Sep.
**Headache, throbbing, with sore eyes:** Nat-m.
**Hemorrhoids:** Cocc.
**Hysterical symptoms:** Ferr.
**Leucorrhea:** Aesc., Alum., Graph., *Kreos.,* Nit-ac. (See **Leucorrhea.**)
**Mammae swollen, milky secretion:** Cycl.
**Old symptoms aggravated:** Nux-v.
**Ovarian pain:** Zinc.

**Pains (intermenstrual):** *Bry.,* Ham., Iod., Kreos., *Sep.*

**Pruritus:** Con., Lyc., *Tarent.*

**Show occasional, every few days:** Borx., Bov.

**Vomiting:** Crot-h.

**Weakness, profound:** *Alum.,* Am-c., Am-m., *Ars.,* Calc., *Carb-an.,* Carb-v., *Chin.,* Cimic., *Cocc.,* Ferr., Glyc., Graph., Iod., Ip., Kali-c., Mag-c., Phos., Thlas., *Tril-p., Verat.,* Vinc.

**MODALITIES, AGGRAVATION, At night:** Am-c., *Am-m., Borx., Bov.,* Coc-c., *Mag-c.,* Mag-m., Zinc.

**During flow:** *Cimic.,* Ham., Kreos., *Puls., Tub.*

**From excitement:** *Calc., Sulph.,* Tub.

**From lying down, rest:** *Am-c.,* Am-m., *Bov., Cycl., Kreos., Mag-c., Zinc.*

**From motion:** Bov., Bry., Canth., Caust., Erig., *Lil-t.,* Mag-p., *Sabin., Sec.,* Thlas., *Tril-p.*

**From sleep:** Mag-c.

**In morning, daytime:** Borx., Cact., Carb-an., *Caust.,* Cycl., *Lil-t., Puls., Sep.*

**AMELIORATION, From establishment of flow:** Aster., Cer-ox., *Cycl.,* Eupi., *Lach., Mag-p., Senec., Zinc.*

**From cold drinks:** Kreos.

**From hot applications:** Mag-p.

**From lying down:** Bov., Cact., Caust., Lil-t.

**From motion:** Am-m., *Cycl.,* Kreos., *Mag-c., Sabin.*

**NYMPHOMANIA:** Ambr., Aster., Bar-m., Calc-p., Camph., *Canth.,* Coca, Dulc., *Ferul.,* Fl-ac., *Grat., Hyos.,* Kali-br., Lach., *Lil-t., Murx.,* Orig., *Phos., Plat.,* Raph., *Rob., Sal-n.,* Stram., Stry., *Tarent.,* Valer., *Verat.*

**OVARIES, Abscess:** Chin., *Hep.,* Lach., *Merc.,* Ph-ac., Pyrog., *Sil.*

**Atrophy:** *Iod.,* Ov., Orch.

**Complaints attending, or following, ovariotomy:** Ars., *Bell., Bry.,* Chin., Coff., *Coloc.,* Hyper., Ip., Lyc., Naja, Nux-v., *Ov.,* Orch., *Staph.*

**Congestion:** *Acon.,* Aesc., Aloe., Am-br., *Apis,* Arg-n., *Bell., Bry.,* Canth., *Cimic.,* Coloc., Con., *Gels., Ham.,* Iod., *Lil-t.,* Merc., Naja, *Nat-chor.,* Sep., Tarent., Ust., *Vib.* (See **Inflammation.**)

**CYSTS, DROPSY:** *Apis,* Apoc., Arn, Ars., *Aur-i.,* Aur-m-n., Bell., Bov., Bry., Chin., *Coloc.,* Con., Ferr-i., Graph., *Iod.,* Kali-br., Lach., Lil-t., *Lyc.,* Med., *Ov.,* Rhod., Sabin., Ter., Zinc.

**Induration:** Aur., Aur-m-n., Carb-an., *Con.,* Graph., *Iod.,* Lach., Pall., Plat., Ust.

**Inflammation (ovaritis): Acute:** *Acon.,* Am-br., *Apis, Bell., Bry.,* Cact., *Canth., Cimic., Coloc.,* Con., Ferr-p., Guaj., *Ham., Iod., Lach.,* Lil-t., Merc., *Merc-c.,* Ph-ac., Plat., *Puls.,* Sabin., Thuj., Visc.

**Acute, with peritoneal involvement:** *Acon.,* Apis, Ars., *Bell.,* Bry., Canth., Chin., Chinin-s., Coloc., *Hep., Merc-c.,* Sil.

**Inflammation, chronic, with induration:** *Con.,* Graph., *Iod.,* Lach., Pall., Plat., Sabal, Sep., *Thuj.*

**PAIN, Boring:** *Coloc.,* Zinc.

**Burning:** *Apis, Ars.,* Bufo, *Canth.,* Con., Eupi., *Fago.,* Kali-n., Lil-t., Plat., Thuj., *Ust.,* Zinc-val.

**Crampy, constrictive:** *Cact.,* Coloc., Naja.

**Cutting, darting, tearing:** Absin., Acon., *Bell.,* Bry., Caps., *Coloc.,* Con., Croc., *Lil-t.,* Naja, Puls.

**Cutting, extending to thighs, legs:** Bry., *Cimic.,* Croc., Lil-t., Phos., Podo., Wye., *Xan.,* Zinc-val.

**Dull, constant:** Aur-br., Hydrc., Nicc., Sep.

**Dull, numb, aching:** Podo.

**Dull, wedge like in uterus:** Iod.

**Neuralgic (ovaralgia):** Am-br., Ap-g., *Apis, Atrop., Bell.,* Berb., Bry., *Cact.,* Canth., *Caul., Cimic., Coloc., Con.,* Ferr., Ferr-p., *Gels.,* Goss., Graph., Ham., Hyper., Kali-br., *Lach., Lil-t., Mag-p.,* Meli., Merc., Merc-c., *Naja,* Phyt., *Plat.,* Podo., Puls., *Sabal,* Sal-n., Sumb., *Staph.,* Thea, *Ust., Vib., Xan., Zinc-val.*

**Neuralgic, intermittent:** *Goss.,* Ziz.

**Stinging:** *Apis,* Canth., Con., Lil-t., Merc.

**Throbbing:** Bell., Brach., Bran., *Cact.,* Hep.

**Pain, in left ovary:** Am-br., Ap-g., Apis, *Arg-met.,* Caps., Carb-ac., *Cimic., Coloc.,* Erig., Eup-pur., Frax., Graph., Iod., *Lach., Lil-t.,* Med., Murx., *Naja,* Ovi-p., Phos., Pic-ac., Thea, *Thuj.,* Ust., *Vesp.,* Wye., *Xan.,* Zinc., Ziz.

**Pain, in right ovary:** Absin., *Apis,* Ars., *Bell.,* Bran., *Bry.,* Coloc., Eupi., Fago., Graph., Iod., Lach., Lil-t., *Lyc., Pall.,* Phyt., *Podo.,* Ust.

**Pain, with aggravation, from deep breathing:** Bry.

**Pain, with aggravation, from walking, riding, relieved by lying down:** Carb-ac., Podo., Sep., *Thuj.,* Ust.

**Pain, with frequent urination:** Vesp.

**Pain, with numbness, shifting gases in ascending colon:** Podo.

**Pain, with relief, by drawing up leg:** Ap-g., Coloc.

**Pain, with relief by flow:** Lach., Zinc.

**Pain, with relief from pressure, tight bandage:** Coloc.

**Pain, with restlessness, can't keep still:** Kali-br., Vib., *Zinc.*

**Pain, with sympathetic heart symptoms:** Cimic., *Lil-t.,* Naja.

**Swelling:** *Am-br., Apis, Bell.,* Brom., Graph., Ham., *Lach.,* Pall., *Tarent.,* Ust. (See **Congestion, Inflammation.**)

**Tenderness, to touch, motion:** Ant-c., *Apis, Bell., Bry.,* Canth., Carb-an., *Cimic., Ham.,* Hep., Iod., *Lach.,* Lil-t., *Plat.,* Sabal, *Tarent.,* Thea, Thuj., Ust., Zinc-val.

**Traumatic conditions:** Arn., *Ham.,* Psor.

**Tumors:** *Apis,* Aur-m-n., Bov., *Coloc.,* Con., Graph., *Iod., Kali-br.,* Lach., Ov., Podo., Sec. (See **Cysts.**)

**PELVIC, Abscess:** Apis, Calc., *Hep.,* Merc-c., Pall., *Sil.*

**Pelvic cellulitis:** Acon., *Apis,* Ars., Bell., *Bry.,* Calc., Canth., *Cimic.,* Hep., Med., Merc., *Merc-i-r.,* Pyrog., *Rhus-t.,* Sil., Ter., Til., *Verat-v.*

**Pelvic hematocele:** Acon., Apis, *Arn.,* Ars., Bell., Canth., Chin., Coloc., Dig., *Ferr., Ham.,* Ip., *Kali-i.,* Lach., *Merc.,* Mill., Nit-ac., Phos., Sabin., *Sec., Sulph.,* Ter., Thlas.

**Pelvic peritonitis:** *Acon., Apis,* Arn., Ars., *Bell., Bry., Canth.,* Chin., Chinin-s., Cimic., *Coloc.,* Gels., *Hep.,* Hyos., *Lach., Merc-c.,* Op., Pall., Rhus-t., Sabin., Sec., *Sil.,* Ter., Verat-v. (See **Cellulitis, Metritis.**)

**Pelvic peritonitis, with menorrhagia:** Ars., Ham., Sabin., Thlas.

**PREGNANCY AND LABOR, ABORTION, Remedies in general:** Acon., *Alet.,* Arn., Bell., Calc-f., *Caul.,* Cham., Chin., *Cimic.,* Cinnm., Coff., Croc., Goss., *Helon.,* Hyos., Ip., *Kali-c.,* Mill., Nit-ac., Nux-v., Op., *Pin-l.,* Pyrog., Rhus-t., *Sabin., Sec., Sep.,* Tanac., Thlas., Tril-p., *Vib.*

**Abortion: From debility:** *Alet.,* Caul., Chin., Chinin-s., *Helon.,* Sec.

**From fatty degeneration of placenta:** Phos.

**From fright, emotions:** *Acon.,* Cham., Cimic., Op.

**From mental depression, shock, watching, low fever:** Bapt.

**From ovarian disease:** Apis.

**From syphilitic taint:** Aur., Kali-i., *Merc-c.*

**From traumatism:** Arn., Cinnm.

**With blood dark, fluid, formication:** Sec.

**With blood intermittent, pains spasmodic, excites suffocation, fainting, craves fresh air:** Puls.

**With blood light, fluid, painless:** Mill.

**With hemorrhage persisting:** Nit-ac., Thlas.

**With pains, frequent, labor-like, no discharge:** Sec.

**With pains, from small of back, around to abdomen, ending in crampy, squeezing, bearing down, tearing down thighs:** Vib.

**With pains, from samll of back, to pubes, worse from motion, blood partly clotted:** Sabin.

**With pains from small of back to thighs, weak back, pains worse from motion;also subsequent debility and sweat:** Kali-c.

**With pains, flying across abdomen, doubling her up, chills, pricking in breasts, pains in loins:** Cimic.

**With pains, irregular, feeble, tormenting, scanty flow, or long continued, passive oozing, backache, weakness, internal trembling:** Caul.

**With retained secundines:** Chin., Pyrog.

**With septicemia:** Pyrog.

**With sequelae:** Kali-c., Sabin., Sulph.

**Tendency to abort:** *Alet.,* Apis, Aur., Bac., Calc., *Caul., Cimic., Helon.,* Kali-c., Kali-i., Merc., Merc-c., Plb., Puls., *Sabin., Sec., Sep.,* Sil., Sulph., Syph., *Vib., Vib-p.,* Zinc.

**Tendency to abort at second or third month:** *Cimic.,* Kali-c., *Sabin., Sec.,* Vib.

**Threatened:** *Acon.,* Arn., *Bapt.,* Bell., *Caul., Cham.,* Chin., Cimic., Coff., Croc., Eup-pur., Ferr., *Helon.,* Mill., Plb., Puls., *Sabin., Sec.,* Tril-p., *Vib.,* Vib-p.

**COMPLAINTS DURING, Abdomen, must lie on, during early months:** Acet-ac., Podo.

**Acne:** *Bell.,* Sabin., Sep. (See **SKIN.**)

**Albuminuria:** *Apis, Ars.,* Aur-m., Cupr-ar., Gels., Glon., *Helon.,* Ind., *Kali-chl.,* Kalm., *Merc-c., Phos.,* Sabin., Thlas., Thyr., *Verat-v.* (See **Kidneys, URINARY SYSTEM.**)

**Arms hot, sore, painful:** Zing.

**Backache:** *Aesc.,* Kali-c. (See **LOCOMOTOR SYSTEM.**)

**Bilious complications:** Chel.

**Bladder disturbances, tenesmus:** *Bell., Canth., Caust.,* Equis-h., Ferr., Nux-v., Pop., *Puls.,* Staph.

**Breasts, painful, inflammatory:** *Bell., Bry.*

**Breasts, painful, neuralgic:** *Con.,* Puls.

**Congestion of brain:** *Glon.* (See **HEAD.**)

**Constipation:** Alum., *Coll.,* Lyc., Nux-v., Op., *Plat.,* Plb., *Sep.* (See **ABDOMEN.**)

**Convulsions, spasms:** Aml-ns., Cupr., *Glon.,* Hyos., Lyss., *Oena.* (See **NERVOUS SYSTEM.**)

**Cough:** Acon., *Apoc., Bell.,* Bry., *Cham.,* Caust., *Con.,* Cor-r., *Dros.,* Glon., *Hyos., Kali-br.,* Ip., Nux-v., Vib.

**Cramps, in calves:** Cham., *Cupr.,* Mag-p., Nux-v., *Verat.*

**Cravings, abnormal:** *Alum.,* Calc., Carb-v., *Sep.* (See **STOMACH.**)

**Diarrhea:** Ferr., Hell., Nux-m., Petr., Ph-ac., *Puls.,* Sec., *Sulph.*

**Discharge, bloody:** Erig., Kali-c., Phos., Rhus-t. (See **Abortion.**)

**Dyspepsia (heartburn, acidity):** Acet-ac., Anac., Calc., Canth., Caps., Dios., *Nux-v., Puls.* (See **STOMACH.**)

**Dyspnea:** Apoc., Lyc., Nux-v., Puls., *Viol-o.* (See **RESPIRATORY SYSTEM.**)

**False pregnancy:** *Caul.,* Croc., Nux-v., *Thuj.*
**Gastralgia:** Petr.
**Goitre:** Hydr.
**Hemorrhoids:** Coll., Podo., Sulph. (See **ABDOMEN.**)
**Herpes:** Sep.
**Hiccough,** Cycl. (See **STOMACH.**)
**Insanity:** Hyos. (See **MIND.**)
**Mental symptoms:** Acon., Cham., *Cimic.,* Puls. (See **MIND.**)
**Metrorrhagia:** Chin., Cinnm., Ip., Nit-ac., Sec., Tril-p. (See **Uterus.**)
**Morning sickness (nausea, vomiting):** Acet-ac., Acon., Alet., *Amgd-p.,* Anac., Ant-t., *Apom.,* Arg-n., *Ars.,* Bry., Carb-ac., *Cer-ox., Cimic., Cocc.,* Colch., *Cuc-p.,* Cupr-act., Cycl., Gnaph., *Goss.,* Ing., *Ip.,* Iris, Kali-m., *Kreos.,* Lac-ac., Lac-d., *Lob.,* Mag-c., Merc., Nat-p., Nux-m., *Nux-v.,* Petr., Phos., Pilo., Psor., *Puls., Sep.,* Staph., *Sym-r.,* Tab., Ther., *Thyr.* (See **STOMACH.**)
**Mouth, sore:** Hydr., Sin-a. (See **MOUTH.**)
**Nervous sensitiveness, extreme:** Acon., Asar., Cimic., *Ther.*
**Pain, false labor:** *Caul., Cham., Cimic.,* Gels., *Puls., Sec.*
**Pain in abdomen, as if strained, left side:** Am-m.
**Pain, in lumbar region, dragging, distressful:** Arn., *Bell., Kali-c.,* Nux-v., Puls., Rhus-t.
**Pain, rheumatic:** Acon., Alet., *Cimic.,* Op., Rhus-t.
**Plethora:** Acon.
**Pruritus, vulvae et vaginae:** Acon., *Ambr.,* Ant-c., Borx., *Calad., Coll.,* Ichth., *Sep.,* Tab. (See **Vulva.**)
**Retinitis:** Gels.
**Salivation:** Acet-ac., Ars., *Iod., Jab.,* Kreos., Lac-ac., *Merc.,* Nat-m., *Pilo.,* Sulph.
**Sexual excitement:** Plat. (See **Nymphomania.**)
**Sleeplessness:** Acon., Cimic., *Coff.,* Nux-v., Puls., Sulph.
**Toothache:** Acon., Bell., *Calc-f., Cham.,* Coff., *Kreos., Mag-c.,* Nux-v., Rat., Sep., *Staph.,* Tab.
**Toxemic conditions:** Kali-chl.
**Uterine and abdominal soreness:** Ham., Puls.
**Varicose veins:** Arn., Bell-p., Calc., Carb-v., Ham., Lyc., Mill., Sulph., Zinc.
**Vertigo:** Bell., Cocc., Nux-v.
**Weariness in limbs, cannot walk:** Bell-p.

**PARTURITION, LABOR, CONVULSIONS (eclampsia):** *Acon.,* Aeth., Aml-ns., Arn., *Bell.,* Canth., Cham., *Chlol., Cic.,* Cimic., Coff., Cupr., *Cupr-ar.,* Gels., Glon., *Hydr-ac., Hyos.,* Ign., Ip., Kali-br., Merc-c., Merc-d., *Oena.,* Op., Pilo., Plat., Sol-n., Spira., Stram., *Verat-v., Zinc.*

**PAINS, Backache violent, wants it pressed:** Caust., *Kali-c.*

**Excessive:** *Bell.,* Coff.

**False labor pains:** Bell., Cham., *Caul., Cimic.,* Gels., Nux-v., *Puls.,* Sec., Vib.

**Hour glass contraction:** Bell., Sec.

**Labor delayed:** Kali-p., Pituin.

**Labor premature:** Sabin.

**Needle-like prickings in cervix:** Caul.

**Shifting, across abdomen, doubling her up, pricking in mammae, shivers during first stage:** Cimic.

**Shifting, all over, exhaustion, fretful, shivering:** Caul.

**Shifting, from back to rectum, with urging to stool, or urination:** Nux-v.

**Shifting from loins down legs:** Aloe, *Bufo,* Carb-v., Caul., Cham., *Nux-v.*

**Shifting upwards:** *Cham.,* Gels.

**Spasmodic, irregular, intermittent, ineffectual, fleeting:** Arn., Art-v., *Bell.,* Borx., *Caul.,* Caust., *Cham., Chin.,* Chlol., *Cimic.,* Cinnm., Coff., *Gels.,* Kali-c., Kali-p., Nat-m., *Nux-v.,* Op., Pituin., *Puls.,* Sacch., *Sec.*

**With dyspnea from constriction of middle of chest arresting pains:** Lob.

**With hypersensitiveness to pain:** *Acon.,* Bell., *Caul.,* Caust., *Cham.,* Chin., *Cimic., Coff., Gels.,* Hyos., Ign., *Nux-v.,* Puls.

**With relief from pressure in back:** Caust., *Kali-c.*

**With syncope:** Cimic., Nux-v., Puls., Sec.

**PLACENTA, Retained:** *Arn.,* Canth., Caul., Chin., Cimic., Ergot., Goss., *Hydr., Ign., Puls., Sabin., Sec.,* Visc.

**RIGID OS:** Acon., *Bell., Caul.,* Cham., Cimic., *Gels.,* Lob., *Verat-v.*

**PUERPERIUM (Lying in period): After-pains:** *Acon.,* Aml-ns., *Arn., Bell.,* Calc., *Caul.,* Carb-v., *Cham., Cimic.,* Cocc., *Coff., Cupr.,* Cupr-ar., *Gels.,* Ign., Kali-c., Lach., Nux-v., *Puls.,* Pyrog., Rhus-t., *Sabin., Sec.,* Sep., Vib., *Vib-p., Xan.*

**After pains, across lower abdomen, into groins:** Caul., Cimic.

**After pains, extending into shins:** Carb-v., Cocc.

**After pains severe, distressing, in calves and soles:** Cupr.

**Backache, debility, sweat:** Kali-c.

**Complications prevented:** *Arn.,* Calen.

**Constipation:** *Bry., Coll.,* Nux-v., Verat., Zinc.

**Diarhea:** *Cham.,* Hyos., Puls.

**Hemorrhage (flooding, post partum):** *Acet-ac.,* Am-m., Aml-ns., Arn., Ars., *Bell.,* Caul., Cham., *Chin., Cinnm., Croc.,* Cycl., Ferr., Ger., *Ham.,* Hyos., Ign., *Ip.,* Kali-c., *Mill.,* Nit-ac., Puls., *Sabin., Sec.,* Tril-p., Ust.

**With bright red fluid, painless flow:** Mill.
**With bright red, hot, profuse flow in gushes:** Bell.
**With bright red, hot, profuse flow, collapsic symptoms:** Ip.
**With colicky, bearing down pains, relieved by gush of blood:** Cycl.
**With dark, thick, paroxysmal flow, debility:** Chin.
**With habitual tendency, profuse, dark, clotted:** Tril-p.
**With pain from back to pubes, dark, clotted, painless flow:** Sabin.
**With passive, dark, fluid blood, worse from motion, thin females, relaxed uterus, formication:** Sec.
**With uterine inertia:** Am-m., Caul., Puls., Sec.
**Hemorrhoids:** Acon., *Aloe.,* Bell., Ign., Puls.

**LOCHIA, Acrid:** Bapt., Kreos., *Nit-ac.,* Pyrog.
**Lochia, bloody:** Chr-ac., *Tril-p.*
**Lochia, bloody, dark:** Caul., Cham., Kreos., Nit-ac., Pyrog., *Sec.*
**Lochia, bloody, in gushes, worse from motion:** Erig.
**Lochia, hot, scanty:** Bell.
**Lochia, intermittent:** Con., *Kreos.,* Pyrog., Rhus-t., Sulph.
**Lochia, offensive:** Bapt., *Bell.,* Carb-ac., *Carb an.,* Carb-v., Chr-ac., Crot-t., Erig., *Kreos.,* Nit-ac., Pyrog., Rhus-t., *Sec.,* Sep., Sulph.
**Lochia, prolonged:** Calc., *Caul.,* Chin., Helon., Mill., *Rhus-t.,* Sabin., *Sec.,* Tril-p., *Ust.*
**Lochia, scanty:** Bell., Cham., Puls.
**Lochia, suppressed:** *Acon.,* Aral., Bell., *Bry.,* Cham., Echi., Hyos., Leon., Op., *Puls.,* Pyrog., *Sec., Sulph.,* Zinc.
**Nymphomania:** Chin., *Plat.,* Verat.
**Panaritium:** All-c.
**Prolapsus recti:** Ruta. (Sec **ABDOMEN.**)
**Puerperal cellulitis:** Hep., *Rhus-t.,* Verat-v.
**Puerperal fever (milk fever):** Acon., *Bry., Calc.,* Cham.
**Puerperal fever, septic (septicemia):** *Acon.,* Ail., Arn., *Ars., Bapt., Bell.,* Bry., Calc., *Carb-ac.,* Canth., Cham., *Chinin-s.,* Cimic., Crot-h., *Echi., Hydrc-ac.,* Hyos., Kali-c., Kali-p., Lach., Lyc., Merc., *Merc-c.,* Nux-v., *Puls., Pyrog., Rhus-t.,* Sec., Sep., Ter., *Verat-v.* (See **Pyemia, GENERALITIES.**)
**Puerperal mania:** Bell., *Cann-i.,* Cimic., *Hyos.,* Plat., Senec., *Stram.,* Verat-v., Zinc. (See **MIND.**)
**Puerperal melancholia:** *Agn.,* Aur., *Cimic.,* Plat., Puls. (See **MIND.**)
**Puerperal metritis:** Bell., *Canth.,* Lach., Nux-v., Til. (See **Uterus.**)
**Puerperal peritonitis:** Acon., *Bell.,* Bry., *Merc-c.,* Pyrog., Sulph., Ter. (See **ABDOMEN.**)

**Puerperal phlebitis after forceps delivery:** All-c.
**Puerperal tympany:** Ter.
**Sweating:** Cham., Samb., Stram.
**Urinary incontinence:** Arn., Bell., Caust., Hyos., Tril-p.
**Urinary retention, suppression:** Acon., *Arn., Bell.,* Equis-h., *Hyos., Op.,* Staph., Stram.

**COMPLAINTS AFTER PUERPERIUM, Acne on chin:** Sep.
**Constipation:** Lil-t., *Lyc.,* Mez., Verat. (See **ABDOMEN.**)
**Hair falls out:** Carb-v., Nat-m., *Sep.*
**Hemorrhoids:** Ham. (See **ABDOMEN.**)

**LACTATION, Discharge from vagina, bloody during nursing:** Sil.
**Excitement, sexual, during nursing:** Calc-p.
**Menses during:** Calc., Pall.
**Milk, absent, or scanty, tardy (agalactea):** Acon., *Agn., Asaf.,* Bry., *Calc.,* Caust., Cham., Chel., Form., Frag., *Lac-c.,* Lac-d., *Ph-ac.,* Phos., Phyt., Pilo., *Puls., Ric.,* Sec., *Sil.,* Stict., *Thyr.,* Urt-u., X-ray.
**Milk, bloody:** Bufo.
**Milk, bluish, transparent, sour, impoverished, or faulty, so child rejects it:** *Acet-ac.,* Calc., *Calc-p.,* Merc., *Ph-ac.,* Sabal, *Sil.,* Sulph.
**Milk suppressed:** *Acon.,* Agn., Bell., *Bry.,* Camph-mbr., Cham., Phyt., *Puls.,* Sec., Zinc.
**Milk, too profuse (galactorrhea):** Bell., *Borx., Calc.,* Cham., Chim., *Con.,* Erig., Iod., Lac-c., Lact., *Medus.,* Parth., Phos., Phyt., Pip-m., Rheum, Ric., Sabal, *Salv.,* Sec., *Sol-o.,* Spira., Ust.
**Milk, too profuse (to dry up during weaning):** Asaf., Bry., *Calc.,* Con., *Lac-c., Puls.,* Urt-u.
**Pain, drawing from nipple, all over body, during nursing:** Phyt., Puls., Sil.
**Pain, drawing from nipple through to back, during nursing, nipple very sore:** Crot-t.
**Pain, intolerable, between nursings:** Phel.
**Pain, in opposite breast:** Borx.
**Prolonged nursing, with anemia, debility:** *Acet-ac.,* Calc-p., Carb-an., *Chin.,* Ph-ac.
**Menorrhagia:** *Calc.,* Phos., *Sil.*
**Milk leg (phlegmasia alba dolens):** Acon., Apis, *Ars.,* Bell., Bism., Bry., *Bufo,* Crot-h., *Ham.,* Lach., *Puls., Rhus-t.,* Sulph., Urt-u.
**Nipples fissured from nursing:** Graph., Rat., Sep.
**Prolapsus uteri:** Podo. (See **Uterus.**)
**Sore mouth:** Hydr., Sin-a.

**Sub-involution:** *Aur-m-n.,* Calc., Caul., Cimic., Croc., *Epip.,* Ferr-i., *Frax., Helon.,* Hydr., *Kali-br., Lil-t.,* Mel-c-s., Nat-hchls., Podo., *Sec., Sep.,* Ust.

**Weakness:** Chin., Chinin-s., Kali-c.

**Weaning, ill effects:** Bry., Cycl., Frag., Puls.

**PUBIC HAIR, Falls out:** Nat-m., Nit-ac., Zinc.

**TUBES, FALLOPIAN, Inflammation (salpingitis):** Acon., Apis, *Ars.,* Bry., Canth., Chinin-s., *Coloc.,* Eupi., Hep., *Merc-c.,* Sabal. (See **Metritis, Peritonitis.**)

**UTERUS, Atony, weakness, relaxation:** Abies-c., *Alet.,* Aloe, Alst., Alum., Bell-p., *Caul., Chin.,* Ferr-i., *Helon.,* Lappa, *Lil-t.,* Puls., Rhus-a., *Sabin., Sec., Sep., Tril-p.,* Ust. (See **Displacements.**)

**CERVIX, Induration of, and os:** Alumn., *Aur., Aur-m.,* Aur-m-n., Carb-an., Con., Helon., *Kali-cy., Iod.,* Kalm., Mag-m., Nat-c., *Plat.,* Sep.

**Cervix, inflammation (endocervicitis):** Ant-t., Arg-n., *Ars., Bell.,* Calen., Hydr., Lyc., Merc., *Merc-c.,* Nit-ac., Sep. (See **Ulceration.**)

**Cervix, redness:** Hydrc., Mit.

**Cervix, swelling, scirrhus-like:** Anan.

**Cervix, swelling, with urinary symptoms:** Canth.

**Cervix, tenesmus:** Bell., Ferr.

**Cervix, tumors, cancerous:** Carb-an., Iod., Kreos., Thuj.

**Cervix, ulceration:** Aln., *Arg-met.,* Arg-n., *Ars., Aur-m-n.,* Bufo, *Carb-ac.,* Carb-an., Fl-ac., *Hydr., Hydrc.,* Kali-ar., *Kreos.,* Lyc., *Merc., Merc-c.,* Murx., Phyt., *Sep.,* Sul-ac., Thuj., *Ust., Vesp.*

**Cervix, ulceration bleeding easily:** Aln., Arg-n., Carb-an., Kreos.

**Cervix, ulceration, deep:** Merc-c.

**Cervix, ulceration, in aged:** Sul-ac.

**Cervix, ulceration, spongy:** Arg-n., Kreos.

**Cervix, ulceration, superficial:** *Hydr.,* Merc.

**Cervix, ulceration, with fetid, acrid discharge:** Ars., Carb-ac.

**Cervix, ulceration, with fetid, ichorous, bloody discharge:** Carb-an., Kreos.

**CONGESTION:** Acon., *Aloe,* Aur., *Bell.,* Bell-p., *Caul.,* Cimic., *Coll.,* Croc., *Frax.,* Gels., Iod., *Lit-t.,* Mag-p., Mit., Murx., Puls., Sabal, Sabin., *Sep.,* Stroph-h., Sulph., Tarent., *Verat-v.* (See **Inflammation.**)

**Congestion, chronic or passive:** Aesc., *Aur.,* Calc., Cimic., *Coll., Helon.,* Lach., *Polym.,* Sep., Stann., Sulph., *Ust.*

**Consciousness of a womb, very tender to jars:** *Helon.,* Lyc., Lyss., *Med.,* Murx.

**Disorders, with reflex heart symptoms:** Cimic., Lil-t.

**Disorders, with toothache, headache, salivation, neuralgia:** Sep.

**DISPLACEMENTS (flexions, versions):** *Abies-c.,* Aesc., *Bell.,* Carb-ac., *Eupi.,* Ferr., *Ferr-i., Frax.,* Helio., *Helon.,* Lappa, *Lil-t.,* Mel-c-s., Murx., Pall., *Puls.,* Sabal, Sec., Senec., *Sep., Stann.*

**Displacements, prolapsus:** Abies-c., Aesc., Agar., *Alet.,* Aloe, Arg-met., Asper., *Aur-m-n., Bell.,* Benz-ac., *Calc.,* Calc-p., Calc-sil., Caul., *Coll.,* Con., Ferr., Ferr-br., *Ferr-i., Frax.,* Graph., *Helon.,* Ign., Kali-bi., Kreos., Lach., *Lil-t.,* Lyss., *Mel-c-s., Murx.,* Nat-chor., Nat-m., Nux-m., *Nux-v.,* Onos., Pall., Plat., *Podo., Puls., Rhus-t.,* Sec., Senec., *Sep., Stann.,* Staph., Til., Tril-p., Zinc-val.

**HEMORRHAGE (Metrorrhagia), Remedies in general:** Acet-ac., Achil., Agar., *Ambr.,* Apis., Arg-n., Arg-ox., *Arn., Ars.,* Aur-m-k., *Bell., Bov.,* Bry., *Cact., Calc.,* Canth., *Caul., Cham., Chin.,* Cimic., Cina, *Cinnm.,* Coll., *Croc.,* Crot-c., Crot-h., Dict., Elaps, *Erig.,* Ferr., *Ferr-act., Ferr-p.,* Fuli., *Ham.,* Helon., Hydr., Iod., *Ip.,* Joan., Jun-v., *Kali-n.,* Kreos., *Lach.,* Lil-t., Mag-m., Mangi-h., Mill., Mit., Nat-chor., *Nit-ac.,* Nux-v., *Phos.,* Plat., Plb., Puls., *Pyrog., Rhus-a.,* Rob., *Sabin., Sec., Sep.,* Sul-ac., Sulph., *Stram.,* Ter., *Thlas., Tril-p.,* Ust., *Vinc.,* Visc., Xan.

**From chlorosis, climacteric, cancer uteri:** Med., Phos., Thlas., Ust.

**From currettage:** Nit-ac.

**From fibroids:** Calc., Nit-ac., *Phos.,* Sabin., Sec., Sul-ac., *Thlas., Tril-p.,* Vinc.

**From mechanical injury, straining, undue exertion:** *Ambr.,* Arn., *Cinnm.,* Ham.

**From parturition, abortion:** Caul., Cham., Chin., Croc., Ip., Mill., Nit-ac., *Sabin., Sec.,* Thlas. (See **Pregnancy**.)

**From retained placenta:** Sabin., Sec., Stram.

**From uterine atony, malarial cases:** Chin.

**Inter-menstrual:** *Ambr.,* Arg-n., *Bov., Calc.,* Cham., Elaps, *Ham., Ip.,* Mag-s., *Phos.,* Rhus-t., Rob., *Sabin.,* Vinc.

**With backache, relieved by pressure, sitting:** Kali-c.

**With blood, black:** Caul., *Croc.,* Elaps, Mag-c., *Plat.*

**With blood, bright red, profuse, gushing, from least motion:** Acal., *Bell.,* Bov., Cham., Erig., *Ip.,* Med., *Mill.,* Mit., Phos., *Sabin., Sec., Tril-p.,* Ust., Visc.

**With blood, clotted or partly clotted:** Acal., *Bell.,* Cham., *Chin.,* Cocc., *Croc.,* Cycl., Erig., *Ip.,* Kali-c., Lach., *Plat., Plb.,* Puls., Rhus-t., *Sabin.,* Thlas., Tril-p., Ust., Visc.

**With blood clotted or fluid, paroxysmal or continual flow, nausea, vomiting, palpitation, pulse quick, feeble when moved, vital depression, fainting on raising head from pillow:** Apoc.

**With blood dark fluid, offensive:** Crot-h.

**With blood, profuse, painless:** Mill., Nit-ac.
**With blood, profuse, painless, dark, venous:** *Ham.,* Mang.
**With blood profuse, passive, obstinate:** Caul., Cinnm.
**With blood, profuse, passive, thin, fetid, in cachetic females:** Sec.
**With blood, profuse, very dark, thick, tarry, dragging, downward, pressing in pelvis and groins, followed by sacral pain, unnatural genital sensibility and irritability:** Plat.
**With blood thin, painless flow:** Carb-an., Chin., Sec.
**With congestive headache:** Bell., Glon.
**With fainting:** Apis, *Chin.,* Ferr., *Tril-p.*
**With faintness in stomach:** Crot-h., Tril-p.
**With feeling, as if back and hips were falling to pieces, relieved by bandaging, fainting:** Tril-p.
**With feeling of enlarged head:** Bad.
**With flow in paroxysms, bright red, joint pains:** Sabin.
**With flow in paroxysms, thin, light blood, firm coagula, severe labor-like pains:** Cham.
**With heavy abdomen, faintness, stinging pains:** Apis.
**With hysteria:** Caul., Cimic., Mag-m.
**With labor like pains:** *Caul., Cham., Cimic.,* Ham., Sabin., Sec., Thlas., Visc.
**With nausea:** Apoc., Caps., *Ip.*
**With nervous erethism at menopause:** Arg-n., *Lach.*
**With painful micturition, pallor, violent irritation of rectum, bladder, prolapsus:** Erig.
**With pain extending to navel, dyspnea:** Ip.
**With pain passing around pelvis, from sacrum to groin:** Puls., Sep.
**With pain passing from sacrum to pubes:** Sabin.
**With pain passing through pelvis, antero-posteriorly or laterally:** Bell.
**With septic fever:** Pyrog.
**With sexual excitement:** Ambr., Plat., Sabin.
**With uterine congestion, inflammation:** Sabin.
**With weak heart:** Am-m., Dig.

**HYDROMETRA:** Nat-hchls., Sep.
**Induration:** Aur., Aur-m-k., *Aur-m-n.,* Carb-an., *Con.,* Graph., *Iod.,* Kalm., Kreos., Mag-m., Plat., *Sep.*

**INFLAMMATION (endometritis, metritis): Acute:** *Acon.,* Ant-i., *Apis,* Arn., *Ars., Bell., Bry.,* Canth., Cham., Chin., *Cimic.,* Con., *Gels.,* Hep., Hyos., *Iod.,* Kali-c., Kali-i., Lach., Lil-t., *Mel-c-s., Merc-c.,* Nux-v., Op., Ph-ac., Plat., *Puls.,* Rhus-t., *Sabin., Sec., Sep., Sil.,* Stram., Sulph., Ter., Til., *Verat-v.*

**Inflammation, chronic:** Alet., Aloe, *Ars., Aur., Aur-m-n.,* Borx., *Calc., Carb-ac.,* Caul., Chinin-ar., *Cimic., Con.,* Graph., *Helon., Hydr.,* Hydrc., Inul., *Iod., Kali-bi.,* Kali-c., Kali-s., Kreos., Lach., *Mag-m., Mel-c-s.,* Merc., *Murx.,* Nat-m., Nit-ac., *Nux-v., Ph-ac.,* Phos., Plb., *Puls.,* Rhus-t., *Sabin., Sec., Sep.,* Sil., Stram., *Sulph.*

**Inflammation, chronic, follicular:** *Hydr.,* Hydrc., Iod., Merc.

**Inflammation, chronic, with arterial congestion:** Bell., Lil-t., *Sabin.*

**Inflammation, chronic, with venous congestion:** Aloe, *Coll.,* Mag-m., Murx., *Sep.*

**Inflammation, hemorrhagic cases:** Ars., Ham., Led., Phos., *Sec., Thlas.*

**Inflammation, peri or para metritis:** Acon., *Bell.,* Canth., Coloc., Hep., *Merc-c.,* Sil.

**IRRITABLE uterus (hysteralgia):** Bell., Caul., *Cimic.,* Ign., *Lil-t., Mag-m.,* Murx., Tarent. (See **Pain.**)

**MOLES, foreign bodies, promote expulsion:** Canth., Sabin.

**PAIN: Bruised, broken feeling, of pelvic bones:** *Aesc.,* Arn., Bell-p., Lappa, *Tril-p.*

**Burning:** Acon., *Ars., Bell.,* Bufo, Calc-ar., *Canth.,* Carb-an., Con., Hep., Kreos., Lap-a., Murx., Pall., *Sec., Ter.,* Xan.

**Colicky, cramps, labor-like, bearing down:** *Agar.,* Apis, Arg-met., Calad., Calc., Cann-i., *Caul.,* Caust., Cham., *Cimic., Cocc., Coloc.,* Con., *Cupr.,* Dios., Ferr., Ferr-i., *Gels., Goss.,* Hedeo., *Ign.,* Inul., *Ip., Lach.,* Mag-p., Nat-m., *Nux-v.,* Onos., Op., Plat., *Puls., Sabin., Sec.,* Sil., Thlas., Til, *Vib.,* Xan. (See **Labor.**)

**Constricting, squeezing:** *Bell-p., Cact.,* Cham., Chin., *Gels., Mag-p.,* Nux-v., Polyg-h., *Sep.,* Ust.

**Neuralgic, lancinating, spasmodic, tearing, shooting, cutting, stitching:** Acon., *Agar.,* Apis, *Aran., Bell.,* Bry., Bufo, Calc., Chin., *Cimic., Coloc., Con.,* Crot-c., Cupr-ar., *Dios.,* Ferr., Graph., Kali-p., Lach., *Lil-t.,* Mag-m., *Mag-p.,* Merc., *Murx.,* Op., *Plat.,* Puls., Sec., Tarent., *Vib.,* Visc. (See **Dysmenorrhea.**)

**Neuralgic, from back, circumferentially:** Plat., Sep.

**Neuralgic, from back to abdomen:** Sep., Visc.

**Neuralgic, from back to pubes:** Bell., Sabin.

**Neuralgic, from back to thighs, legs:** Bufo, Carb-ac., Cham., *Cimic.,* Puls., *Sabin.*

**Neuralgic, from hip to hip:** *Bell.,* Calc., Chin., *Cimic., Coloc.,* Pall.

**Neuralgic, from navel to uterus:** Ip.

**Neuralgic, radiating to chest:** Lach., Murx., Vesp.

**Neuralgic, right side, upward across body, thence to left mamma:** Murx.

**Pressing, as if viscera would protrude from vagina:** *Agar., Bell.,* Calc-o-t., Cimic., Cinnm., Crot-h., Ferr., *Ferr-i., Frax.,* Goss., Helio., Kali- fcy., *Kreos., Lac-c., Lil-t.,* Lyc., Mosch., *Murx., Nat-c.,* Nat-chor., Nat-m., *Nux-v.,* Onos., Pall., *Podo., Puls., Sanic., Sep., Stann., Sulph., Til.,* Tril-p., Vib., *Xan.,* Xero.

**Pressing, heaviness, fullness, dragging in pelvis:** Agar., Alet., *Aloe,* Ant-c., *Aur-m-n., Bell.,* Calc., Calen., Carb-ac., Chin., *Cimic., Cocc., Coll.,* Con., Ferr-br., Frax., Glyc., Gnaph., *Goss., Helon.,* Kali-bi., Lappa, *Lil-t.,* Mag-c., *Mag-m.,* Merc., Murx., Nat-c., Nat-chor., *Nux-v., Plat.,* Plb., *Podo.,* Polyg-h., *Sep.,* Sulph., Tril-p., Wye., Zinc val.

**Pressing in back:** Agar., *Bell.,* Carb-ac., Cham., *Cimic., Gels.,* Goss., Hedeo., *Helon.,* Inul., *Kali-c.,* Kreos., Nat-m., Onos., Tril-p., Vesp., Vib.

**Pulsating, throbbing:** *Aesc.,* Bell., *Cact.,* Hep., Murx.

**Splinter-like when walking or riding:** Arg-n.

**Ulcerative, between anus and perineum, when walking or sitting:** Cycl.

**PHYSOMETRA:** Bell., Bry., *Brom.,* Lac-c., *Lyc.,* Nux-v., Ph-ac., Sang.

**Soreness, tenderness of uterus:** Abies-c., Acon., *Apis,* Arg-met., Arn., *Bell., Bell-p., Bry., Cimic.,* Conv., *Helon.,* Kreos., *Lach.,* Lappa, *Lil-t.,* Lyss., Mag-m., *Mel-c-s.,* Merc., *Murx.,* Plat., Sanic., *Sep., Thlas., Til.*

**TUMORS; Cancer, malignant disease:** *Arg-met., Ars., Ars-i., Aur-m-n.,* Bell., Bov., Calc-ar., Calc-o-t., Calc-s., *Calth., Carb-an.,* Carc., Cham., Chin., *Con., Graph., Hydr.,* Iod., Irid-met., *Kali-bi.,* Kali-p., Kali-s., *Kreos.,* Lach., *Lap-a.,* Mag-p., Med., Murx., *Phos.,* Phyt., Rhus-t., *Sec.,* Sep., *Sil.,* Staph., Sulph., Tarent., Thlas., *Thuj.,* Tril-p., Zinc.

**Cancer, hemorrhage:** Bell., Crot-h., Kreos., Lach., Sabin., *Thlas.,* Ust.

**Fibroids, polypi, myo-fibromata:** *Aur-i., Aur-m.,* Bell., *Calc., Calc-i.,* Calc-p., *Calen.,* Chin., *Con.,* Erod., Ferr., *Frax.,* Ham., Hydr., *Hydrc., Iod.,* Ip., *Kali-i., Lach.,* Led., Lyc., Merc-c., *Merc-i-r., Nit-ac., Phos.,* Plat., Plb., Puls., Sabal, *Sabin.,* Sang., Sec., Sep., Sil., Solid., Staph., Sulph., *Thlas., Thuj., Thyr.,* Tril-p.

**VAGINA: Apthous patches, ulcers, erosions:** Alumn., *Arg-n.,* Carb-v., *Caul., Graph., Helon., Hydr.,* Ign., Kreos., Lyc., Lyss., Merc., Nat-m., *Nit-ac.,* Rhus-t., Rob., *Sep.,* Thuj.

**Burning, heat:** *Acon.,* Alum., Antip., Aur-m., *Bell., Berb.,* Bov., *Canth.,* Carb-an., Carb-v., Ferr-p., *Hydrc.,* Kali-bi., Kali-c., *Kreos.,* Lyc., Lyss., Merc., *Merc-c.,* Nat-m., *Nit-ac.,* Pop-c., Pulx., *Sep.,* Spira., *Sulph.*

**Burning, heat, after coitus:** Lyc., Lyss.

**Coldness:** Bor-ac.

**Cysts:** Lyc., Puls., *Rhod.,* Sil.

**Dryness:** Acon., Apis, *Bell.,* Ferr-p., *Lyc.,* Lyss., *Nat-m.,* Spira. (See **Inflammation.**)

**Flatus, emission:** *Brom.,* Lac-c., *Lyc.,* Nux-m., Sang.

**Inflammmation (vaginitis): Acute:** *Acon., Apis,* Arn., Ars., *Bell.,* Cann-s., *Canth.,* Cimic., Con., *Crot-t.,* Gels., *Helon., Hydr.,* Kali-c., Kali-m., *Kreos., Merc-c.,* Rhus-t., *Sep.,* Sulph., Thuj.

**Inflammation, chronic:** Ars., Borx., *Calc.,* Grin., Hydr., Iod., *Kreos.,* Kali-m., *Merc.,* Nit-ac., *Puls., Sep.,* Sulph. (See **Vulvitis.**)

**Itching:** Antip., Arund., Aur-m., *Calad., Canth., Con., Helon.,* Hydr., Hydrc., *Kreos.,* Merc., Scroph-n., *Sep.,* Sil., Sulph. (See **Pruritus Vulvae**.)

**Pain, pressing:** *Bell.,* Calc., Chim., Cinnb., *Ferr-i.,* Stann.

**Pain, stinging, stitching, shooting, tearing:** *Apis,* Cimx., Cimic., Coloc., Kreos., *Rhus-t.,* Sabin., *Sep.*

**Pain, throbbing:** Bell.

**Prolapsus vaginae:** Alum., *Bell.,* Ferr., Gran., Kreos., Lach., *Lappa,* Nux-m., Nux-v., Oci., *Sep., Stann.,* Staph., Sul-ac.

**Sensitiveness (vaginismus):** Acon., Aur., *Bell., Berb., Cact., Caul.,* Caust., Carb-v., *Cimic., Cocc., Coff.,* Con., Ferr., Ferr-i., Ferr-p., *Gels.,* Ham., *Ign.,* Kreos., Lac-c., Lyss., *Mag-p., Murx.,* Mur-ac., Nit-ac., Nux-v., Orig., *Plat., Plb.,* Sil., *Staph.,* Tarent., *Thuj.*

**VULVA-LABIA: Abscess (vulvo-vaginal):** *Apis, Bell.,* Borx., *Hep.,* Kreos., Iod., Lach., *Merc.,* Puls., Rhus-t., Sep., *Sil.,* Sulph.

**Burning:** Acon., Am-c., Aur., Bov., *Canth.,* Carb-v., Graph., Helon., *Kreos.,* Lyc., *Merc.,* Puls., *Rhus-t.,* Sep., Sil., *Sulph.,* Thuj. (See **Pain**.)

**Cancer:** *Ars.,* Con., Thuj.

**Dryness:** *Acon., Bell.,* Calc., Lyc., Tarent. (See **Vulvitis**.)

**Eczema:** Rhus-t.

**Erysipelas, with edema:** *Apis.*

**Hair falling out:** Merc., Nit-ac.

**Hyperesthesia, soreness:** Acon., *Bell., Cimic.,* Cocc., *Coff.,* Ferr-i., *Gels.,* Hep., *Ign.,* Kali-br., *Kreos.,* Mag-p., *Merc., Murx., Nit-ac.,* Nux-v., Petr., *Plat., Sep.,* Sulph., *Thuj.,* Til., Zinc.

**Inflammation (vulvitis):** *Acon.,* Ambr., *Apis,* Ars., *Bell.,* Brom., *Calc., Canth., Carb-v.,* Chim., Coc-c., Coll., *Cop.,* Eupi., Goss., *Graph.,* Ham., *Helon., Hydr., Kreos.,* Lyc., Mag-p., *Merc., Merc-c.,* Oci., Plat., Puls., Rhus-d., *Rhus-t., Sep.,* Sil., Sulph., *Thuj.*

**Vulvitis, follicular, herpetic:** Ars., Crot-t., *Dulc.,* Merc., Nat-m., Rob., *Sep.,* Spira., Thuj., *Xero.*

**Itching (pruritus):** Agar., *Ambr.,* Apis, *Ars.,* Arund., Berb., Bov., *Calad., Calc., Canth.,* Carb-ac., *Carb-v.,* Caust., Coff., *Coll., Con.,* Conv., Cop., Crot-t., Dulc., *Fago.,* Ferr-i., *Graph.,* Grin., Guaj., *Helon.,* Hydr., Kali-bi., Kali-br., Kali-c., *Kreos.,* Lil-t., *Lyc., Merc.,* Mez., Nat-m., Nit-ac., *Orig.,* Petr., Pic-ac., *Plat., Rad-br.,* Rhus-d., *Rhus-t.,* Rhus-v., Scroph-n., *Sep.,* Spira., Staph., *Sulph., Tarent.,* Tarent-c., Thuj., *Urt-u.,* Xero., Zinc.

**Pain:** Apis, Ars., *Bell., Berb., Calc-c., Cann-s.*, Con., Ferr., Kali-c., *Kreos.*, Lyc., Meli., *Merc-c., Phos.*, Plat., Sabin., *Sep.*, Sulph. (See **Vulvitis.**)

**Papules, pustules:** *Carb-ac.*, Graph., *Sep.*, Sulph.

**Polypi:** Bell., Calc., *Phos.*, Teucr., *Thuj.*

**Sensation, as if wet:** Eup-pur., Petr.

**Soreness, tenderness:** *Acon.*, Ambr., *Bell.*, Caust., Conv., *Graph., Helon.*, Hep., *Kreos.*, Ovi-p., *Plat., Sep.*, Sulph., Tarent., Urt.

**Soreness, with ulcers:** Arg-n., *Hep.*, Merc., *Nit-ac.*, Thuj.

**Sweat, offensive:** *Calc.*, Fago., Lyc., *Merc.*, Petr., *Sulph.*, Thuj.

**Ulcers:** *Ars., Aur-m-n.*, Graph., Mur-ac., *Nit-ac.*, Sep., Syph.

**Varices:** Calc., Carb-v., Lyc.

**Warts:** Aur-m., Med., Thuj.

■

# RESPIRATORY SYSTEM

**BRONCHIAL TUBES, ASTHMA, Remedies in general:** *Acon.,* Alumn., Ambro., Aml-ns., Anis., Ant-ar., *Ant-t.,* Apis, *Aral., Ars.,* Ars-i., Atrop., *Bac.,* Bell., *Blatta-o.,* Brom., Bry., *Carb-v.,* Chin., Chinin-ar., Chlor., Cic., *Coca,* Cocain., Coff., *Crot-t., Cupr-act.,* Cupr-ar., *Dros.,* Dulc., Egg vaccine, Glon., *Grin.,* Hep., *Hydr-ac., Ictod.,* Iod., *Ip., Kali-bi., Kali-c.,* Kali-chl., *Kali-i., Kali-n.,* Kali-p., *Kola,* Lach., Led., *Lob.,* Lyc., Magn-gr., Meph., Morph., Naja, *Naphtin., Nat-s., Nux-v., Passi.,* Psor., *Ptel.,* Puls., Queb., Sabad., *Samb.,* Sang., Scroph-n., Silphu., Squil., Stram., Stry., *Sulph.,* Syph., Tab., Tela, *Thuj.,* Tub., Verat., Verat-v., *Visc.,* Zinc., *Zing.*

**TYPE, OCCURRENCE, Alternates with eruptions:** Calad., Caust., Rhus-t., *Sulph.*

**Alternates, with itching rash:** Calad.

**Alternates, with spasmodic vomiting:** Cupr., Ip.

**Anger, from:** Cham., Nux-v.

**Cardiac:** Cact., Digin., Grin., Stroph-h. (See **Heart**.)

**Epiglottis, spasm or weakness:** Med.

**Eruptions, suppressed, from:** Ars., Hep., Psor., *Sulph.*

**Foot sweat, suppressed, from:** Ol-an

**Hay asthma:** Aral., *Ars.,* Ars-i., Chinin-ar., *Ip., Lob.,* Naphtin., Nat-s., Nux-v., *Sabad.,* Sang., Stict., Sul-i. (See **Rhinitis, NOSE**.).

**Hebdomadal:** Chin., Ign.

**Humid:** Acon., *Ant-i.,* Ars., *Bac.,* Bry., *Cann-i.,* Coch., Cupr., *Dulc.,* Eucal., Euph-pi., Grin., Hyper., Iod., *Kali-bi., Nat-s.,* Pulm-v., Sabal, *Seneg,* Stann., *Sulph.,* Thuj.

**Humid, in children:** *Nat-s.,* Samb., Thuj.

**Millar's:** Arum-d., *Arund.,* Cor-r., Cupr., Guar., Hep., Ip., Lach., Lob., Mosch., *Samb.* (See **Laryngismus stridulus**.)

**Miner's:** Card-m., Nat-ar.

**Nervous:** Acon., Ambr., Aml-ns., *Asaf.,* Chinin-s., Cina, Coff., *Cupr.,* Grin., *Hydr-ac., Ip.,* Kali-p., Lob., *Mosch.,* Nux-m., *Nux-v.,* Sumb., Tela, Thymu., *Valer.,* Verat.

**Periodical:** *Ars., Chin.,* Chinin-ar., Ip.

**Preceded by coryza:** Aral., Naja, Nux-v.

**Preceded by formication:** Cist., Lob.

**Preceded by nose cold:** Sang.

**Recent, uncomplicated cases:** Hydr-ac.

**Sailors on shore:** Brom.

**Senile cases:** Bar-m.

**Tetter recedes with attack:** Sulph.

**CONCOMITANTS, With bronchial catarrh:** Acon., *Ant-t., Ars.,* Blatta-a., *Bry.,* Cupr-act., *Erio.,* Eucal., *Grin., Ip.,* Kali-i., Lob., Nat-s., Onis., Sabal, Sulph. (See **Humid.**)

**With burning in throat and chest:** Aral.

**With constriction of throat:** Cham., Dros., *Hydr-ac.,* Lob, *Mosch.*

**With cramp, muscular spasm of various parts:** Cupr.

**With cyanosis:** Ars., Cupr., Samb.

**With despondency, thinks he will die:** *Ars.,* Psor.

**With diarrhea following:** Nat-s.

**With dysuria, nocturnal:** Solid.

**With every fresh cold:** Nat-s.

**With gastric derangement:** Arg-n., *Bry.,* Carb-v., Ip., Kali-m., *Lob.,* Lyc., *Nux-v.,* Puls., Sang., Verat-v., Zing.

**With gout, rheumatism:** Led., Sulph., *Visc.*

**With hemorrhoids:** Junc-e., Nux-v.

**With hydrothorax:** Colch.

**With insomnia:** Chlol., Tela.

**With nausea, cardiac weakness, vertigo, vomiting, weak stomach, cold knees:** Lob.

**With palpitation:** Ars., Cact., Eucal., Puls.

**With thirst, nausea, stitches, burning in chest:** Kali-n.

**With urine, supersaturated with solids:** Nat-n.

**MODALITIES, AGGRAVATION, After sleep:** Aral., Grin., *Lach.,* Samb.

**At night, lying down:** *Aral.,* Ars., Cist., Con., Ferr-act., *Grin.,* Lach., Merc-pr-r., Naja, Puls., *Samb.,* Sulph.

**From cold, damp weather:** Ars., *Dulc., Nat-s.* (See **Humid.**)

**From cold, dry weather:** Acon., Caust., Hep.

**From falling asleep:** Am-c., *Grin.,* Lac c., *Lach., Merc-pr-r.,* Op.

**From food**: Kali-p., *Nux-v.,* Puls.

**From inhaling dust:** Ictod., *Ip.,* Kali-c.

**From odors:** Sang.

**From sitting up:** Ferr-act., Laur., Psor.

**From talking:** Dros., Meph.

**In early A.M.:** Am-c., Ant-t., *Ars.,* Grin., Kali-bi., *Kali-c.,* Nat-s., Nux-v., Zing.

**In spring:** Aral.
**In summer:** Syph.

**AMELIORATION, At sea:** Brom.
**From bending forward, rocking:** Kali-c.
**From eructation:** *Carb-v.,* Nux-v.
**From expectoration:** Aral., *Erio.,* Grin., Hyper., *Ip.,* Kali-bi., Zinc.
**From lying down, keeping arms spread apart:** Psor.
**From lying on face, protruding tongue:** Med.
**From motion:** Ferr., Lob.
**From sitting up:** Ars., Kali c., Merc-pr-r., Nux-v., *Puls.*
**From sitting up, with head bent backward:** Hep.
**From stool:** Ictod.
**From vomiting:** Cupr.
**In damp weather:** Caust., Hep.
**In open air:** Naphtin.

**BRONCHIECTASIS, BRONCHORRHEA, Dilatation, with profuse, fetid, purulent sputum:** Acet-ac., All-s., Alumn., Ant-t., *Bac., Bals-p.,* Benz-ac., *Calc.,* Eucal., Ferr-i., Grin., *Hep.,* Ichth., *Kali-bi., Kali-c.,* Kreos., *Lyc.,* Myos-a., Myrt-ch., *Puls.,* Sang., *Sil., Stann.,* Sulph., Tub. (See **Chronic Bronchitis.**)

**BRONCHITIS, Inflammation, acute:** *Acon.,* Am-c., Am-i., Am-p., Ant-ar., Ant-i., *Ant-t.,* Ars., Ars-i., Asc-t., *Bell.,* Blatta-o., *Brom., Bry., Caust.,* Cham., Chin., Colch., Cop., *Dulc.,* Eup-per., Euphr., *Ferr-p.,* Gels., Grin., *Hep.,* Hyos., *Ip., Kali-bi.,* Lob, Mang-act., *Merc.,* Naphtin., Nat-ar., Nit-ac., *Phos.,* Pilo., *Puls.,* Rhus-t., *Rumx., Sang., Sang-n.,* Solid., Spong., *Squil., Stict.,* Sul-ac., *Sulph.,* Thuj., Tub., Tub-a., Verat., Verat-v., Zinc.

**Capillary:** *Alum-sil.,* Am-c., Am-i., Ant-ar., *Ant-t.,* Ars., Bac., *Bell.,* Bry., Calc., Camph., *Carb-v.,* Chel., Cupr-act., *Ferr-p., Ip.,* Kali-c., Kali-i., Nit-ac., Ph-ac., Phos., *Seneg., Solin.,* Sulph., *Ter.,* Verat.

**Chronic (winter catarrhs):** Alum., Alumn., *Am-c.,* Am-caust., Am-i., Am-m., *Ammc.,* Ant-ar., Ant-i., *Ant-s-aur., Ant-t., Ars., Ars-i.,* Bac., *Bals-p.,* Bar-c., *Bar-m., Calc.,* Calc-i., Calc-sil., Canth., Carb an., *Carb-v.,* Cean., Chel., *Chin.,* Coc-c., Con., *Cop.,* Cub., Dig., Dros., *Dulc.,* Erio., Eucal., Grin., *Hep.,* Hydr., Hyos., Ichth., Iod., *Ip., Kali-bi.,* Kali-c., Kali-hp., *Kali-i.,* Kali-s., Kreos., Lach., *Lyc., Merc.,* Myos-s., Myrt-ch., Nat-m., Nat-s., *Nit-ac.,* Nux-v., Phos., Pix, *Puls.,* Rumx., Sabal, Sang., Sec., *Seneg,* Sep., *Sil.,* Silphu., Spong., *Squil., Stann.,* Stry., *Sulph.,* Tax., Ter., Tub., Verat.

**Fibrinous:** *Calc-act.,* Bry., Brom., *Kali-bi.,* Phos.

**Toxemic:** Am-c., Ant-t., Bry., Colch., Diphtox., *Merc-c.*

**Irritation of tubes:** Acet-ac., *Acon.,* Alumn, Ambro., Brom., *Bry.,* Chlor., Ferr-p., *Hep., Phos.,* Pilo., *Rumx.,* Sang-n., Spong. (See **Bronchitis.**)

**Sensitiveness, to cold air:** All-s., *Aral.,* Bac., Calc-sil., *Cham.,* Chin., *Cor-r., Dulc., Hep.,* Iod., Kali-c., Mang-act., *Merc.,* Naja, *Psor., Sil., Tub.*

**CHEST, Affections, after brain fag:** Ph-ac.

**Affections, after operations, for fistulae:** Berb., Calc-p., Sil.

**Affection, after operation, for hydrothorax, empyema:** Abrot.

**Affection, after suppressed skin eruptions:** Hep.

**Affections, in circumscribed spots, persistent after inflammation:** Seneg.

**Affections, in stone cutters with adynamia:** Sil.

**Burning:** Acet-ac., *Acon.,* Am-c., Am-m., Ant-t., Apis, Aral., *Ars.,* Bell., *Brom.,* Bry., *Calc., Carb-v.,* Cic., Euph., Kreos., Lyc., Mag-m., Mang-act., *Merc.,* Merc-sul., Mez., Myrt-c., Ol-j., Op., *Phos.,* Prim-v., Ran-s., *Sang.,* Sangin-n., *Spong., Sulph.,* Wye., Zinc.

**Coldness:** Abies-c., *Am-m., Brom.,* Carb-an., Cist., *Cor-r., Elaps,* Helo., *Kali-c.,* Lith-c.

**Eruptions on:** Arund., Jug-c., Kali-br., Lyc., Petr.

**Inability to lie down (orthopnea):** Acon-f., *Ars., Conv.,* Dig., Grin., Lach., Mag-p., Puls., Visc. (See **Respiration.**)

**Inability, to lie on left side:** *Phos.,* Puls.

**Inability, to lie on right side:** Merc.

**Injury followed by phthisis:** Mill., Ruta.

**Itching, extending to nares:** Coc-c., Con., Iod., *Ip.,* Puls.

**Lightness, emptiness, eviscerated feeling:** Cocc., Nat-s., *Phos., Stann.*

**PAINS, In general:** Abrot., Acal., *Acon., Apis,* Arg-n., *Arn.,* Ars., *Bell.,* Borx., Brom., Bry., *Cact.,* Calc., Caul., *Caust.,* Chel., *Cimic.,* Coll., Com., Crot-t., Dig., Elaps, Erio., Gad., *Hydr-ac.,* Ictod., Jug-c., *Kali-c.,* Kali- n., *Kreos.,* Lycpr., Med., Morph., Myrt-c., *Ox-ac., Phos.,* Psor., Puls., *Ran-b., Rumx., Sang.,* Stict., Stry-p., Succ., Sulph.

**Bruised, ulcerative:** Ampe-qu., *Arn.,* Calc., Eup-per., Kreos., Lyc., Phase., *Psor., Puls.,* Ran-b., Ran-s., Sang.

**Constriction, must frequently breathe deeply to expand lungs:** Adon., Asaf., *Bry., Dig.,* Ign., Iod., Lach., Meli., Mill., *Mosch.,* Nat-s., *Phos.,* Squil., Xan.

**Constriction, spasmodic, tightness, fullness, oppression:** Abies-n., *Acon.,* Adren., Ambro., Am-c., *Ant-t., Ap-g.,* Apis, *Apoc., Aral.,* Arg-n., *Ars.,* Asaf., *Bac.,* Bell., Brom., *Bry., Cact., Calc.,* Calc-ar., Caps., Carb-v., Cham., *Chlor.,* Cic., Coca, Cocc., Coff., Cupr., *Cupr-act., Dig.,* Dios., Dulc., *Ferr.,* Ferr-p., Glon., Glyc., *Grin.,* Haem., Hep., *Hydr-ac., Ip., Just.,* Kali-bi., *Kali-c., Kali-n., Kreos.,* Lach., Lact., Laur., *Lob.,* Lyc.,

Magn-gr., Med., Morph., *Mosch.,* Naja, Naphtin., *Nat-ar., Nat-s., Nit-sp-d., Nux-v.,* Orni., Ox-ac., *Phos., Puls.,* Ran-b., Ruta, *Samb.,* Sang., Seneg., Sep., Sil., Silphu., Sol-n., Spig., Spong., Stram., Stry., Sul-ac., *Sulph.,* Verat-v.

**Cutting:** *Bry.,* Kali-c., Kali-n., Sulph., Zinc.

**Pressing, heaviness, weight:** *Abies-n.,* Abrot., Acon., Am-c., *Anac.,* Arg-n., Arn., *Ars.,* Aur., Bry., *Cact., Calc.,* Cham., Chel., Ferr-i., Haem., Ip., Kali-n., *Kreos., Lil-t., Lob.,* Lyc., Ph-ac., *Phos.,* Prun-p., Ptel., *Puls.,* Ran-b., Ruta, Samb., Sangin-n., Seneg., Sil., *Spong., Sulph.,* Verat-v.

**Stitching, tearing, darting, shooting:** *Acon.,* Agar., All-s., Am-c., Ant-t., Ap-g., Ars., *Asc-t.,* Bell., Berb., *Borx.,* Brom., *Bry.,* Calc., Canth., Caps., *Carb-an.,* Carb-v., *Caust., Chel., Chin.,* Cimic., Coc-c., Colch., Crot-t., *Elaps,* Form., *Guaj.,* Haem., Inul., *Kali-c.,* Kali-i., Kalm., *Lob-c.,* Lyc., Mentho., Merc., Merc-c., Myrt-c., *Nat-s.,* Nit-ac., Nux-v., *Ol-an.,* Ol-j., Paeon., Phel., *Phos., Ran-b.,* Rhod., Rhus-r., Rhus-t., Rumx., Sang., Sep., *Sil.,* Spig., *Squil.,* Stann., *Stict., Sulph., Ther.,* Thuj., Tril-p., Zing.

**LOCATION, Cartilages, costal, Perichondritis:** Arg-met., Bell., Cham., *Cimic.,* Guaj., Olnd., Plb., *Ruta.*

**Infra-mammary:** *Cimic.,* Puls., Ran-b., Ust. (See **FEMALE SEXUAL SYSTEM.**)

**Intercostal (pleurodynia):** *Acon., Am-c.,* Arist-m., *Arn.,* Ars., *Asc-t.,* Aza., Borx., *Bry.,* Caust., Chel., *Cimic., Colch.,* Echi., Gaul., Guaj., *Kali-c., Nux-v.,* Ox-ac., *Phos., Puls., Ran-b.,* Rham-cal., Rhod., Rhus-r., *Rhus-t.,* Rumx., Seneg., Sin-n., Sul-ac.

**Lung, left: Apex and middle portion:** Acon., Am-c., *Anis.,* Ant-s-aur., Crot-t., *Lob-c., Myrt-c.,* Paeon., Phos., *Pix,* Puls., *Ran-b.,* Rumx., Sil., Spig., Stann., Stict., *Sulph., Ther.,* Tub., Ust.

**Lower portion:** Agar., Ampe-qu., Asc-t., Calc-p., Cimic., *Lob-s.,* Lyc., Myos-s., *Nat-s., Ox-ac., Rumx.,* Squil., Sil.

**Lung, right: Apex and middle portion:** Abies-c., *Anis., Ars.,* Borx., *Calc.,* Com., Crot-t., *Elaps,* Erio., Iodof., *Phel.,* Sang., Upa.

**Lower portion:** Am-m., Berb., Bry., Cact., Card-m., *Chel.,* Dios., Kali-c., Lyc., *Merc.*

**Substernal:** Ap-g., Ars., *Asc-t.,* Aster., Aur., Aza., *Bry.,* Card-m., *Caust.,* Chel., Con., *Dios.,* Jug-r., Kali-n., Kalm., *Kreos.,* Lact., Morph., Nit-ac., Nit-s-d., Osm., Ph-ac., Phel., Phos., Psor., Puls., *Ran-b.,* Ran-s., *Rumx.,* Ruta, Samb., *Sang.,* Sang-n., Sep., Sil., Spig., Sulph., Tril-p.

**MODALITIES, AGGRAVATIONS, From ascending:** Ars., Sep.

**From bending forward:** Sulph.

**From breathing, coughing:** Am-m., Arn., *Bry.,* Colch., Mentho., Nat-m., Phos., *Ran-b.,* Seneg., Sep., Sil., Sulph.

**From cold drinks:** Thuj.

**From cold weather:** Petr., Phos.

**From damp weather:** Ran-b., Rhus-t., Spig.

**From lying down, at night:** Calc., Sep.

**From lying on affected side:** Nux-v., Phos., Stann.

**From lying on left side:** Phos.

**From lying on right side:** Kali-c., *Merc.*

**From motion:** Arn., Ars., *Bry.,* Calc., Card-m., Jug-r., Kali-c., Mag-c., Phos., *Ran-b.,* Seneg., Sep., Spig., Sulph.

**From pressure:** Arn., Ars., *Bry.,* Colch., Nux-v., *Phos., Ran-b.*

**From spinal irritation:** Agar., Ran-b.

**From talking:** Alum., Hep., *Stann.*

**From working:** Am-m., Lyc., Sep.

**AMELIORATIONS, From bending forward:** Asc-t., Hyos.

**From eructation:** Bar-c.

**From lying down:** Psor.

**From lying on affected side:** Bry., Puls.

**From motion:** Ign., Puls.

**From rapid walking:** Lob.

**From rest:** Bry.

**In open air:** Anac., Puls.

**SENSITIVENESS, tenderness, rawness of chest:** *Alum-sil.,* Ant-t., Aral., *Arn.,* Ars., *Asc-t., Bry., Calc.,* Calc-p., Calc-sil., *Carb-v., Caust.,* Cimic., Cur., *Eup-per.,* Ferr-p., Ham., *Iod.,* Kali-c., *Merc.,* Naphtin., *Nat-s.,* Nit-ac., *Ol-j., Phos.,* Pop-c., Puls., *Ran-b., Ran-s., Rumx., Sang., Seneg.,* Sep., Spong., Stann., Sulph.

**SPOTS on, brown:** Sep.

**Spots on, yellow:** Phos.

**WEAKNESS, from least exertion, even talking, laughing, singing:** Alumn., Am-c., *Arg-met., Calc.,* Canth., *Carb-v.,* Cocc., *Dig.,* Iod., Kali-c., Lob., *Ph-ac.,* Phos., Psor., Ran-s., Rhus-t., Ruta, Spong., *Stann., Sulph.*

**COUGH, Remedies in genereal:** *Acal., Acet-ac., Acon., All-c., All-s., Alum.,* Am-br., *Am-c.,* Am-caust., Am-m., *Ambr.,* Ant-ar., Ant-s-aur., *Ant-t.,* Aral., Arn., *Ars., Ars-i.,* Asc-t., Bals-p., *Bell., Bism., Brom., Bry., Calc.,* Canth., *Caps.,* Carb-ac., *Carb-v.,* Caust., Cham., Chel., *Cimic., Cina, Coc-c., Cod., Con., Cor-r., Crot-h.,* Cupr., Cupr-act., *Dros.,* Dulc., *Eup-per.,* Euphr., *Ferr-p., Hep.,* Hydr-ac., *Hyos.,* Hyosin-hbr., Ign., *Iod., Ip., Kali-bi., Kali-c.,* Kali-chl., *Lach., Lact., Laur., Lob, Lyc., Mag-p.,* Mang-act., *Menth.,* Meph., *Merc.,* Myrt-c., *Naja,* Nat-m., *Nit-ac., Nux-v.,* Op., *Osm.,* Phel., *Phos.,* Pop-c., *Puls.,* Rhus-t., *Rumx., Samb., Sang., Santin., Seneg.,*

Sil., *Spong., Squil.,* Stann., *Stann-i., Stict., Sulph.,* Trif-p., Tub., *Verb., Viol-o.,* Wye.

**CAUSE, OCCURRENCE, AGGRAVATION, Abdomen, irritation from:** Sep.

**After anger in children:** Anac., Ant-t.

**After anger, vexation, cleaning teeth:** Staph.

**After diarrhea:** Abrot.

**After falling asleep, especially, in children, constant tickling cough without waking:** *Acon.,* Agar., *Aral., Cham.,* Cycl., Lach., Nit-ac., Sulph., Tub., Verb. (See **Evening.**)

**After sleep:** Brom., Lach., Spong.

**Afternoon, in:** Am-m., Lyc., Thuj.

**Air, hot:** Kali-s.

**Arsenical wall paper:** Calc.

**Ascending:** Am-c.

**Bathing:** Nux-m.

**Catarrh:** Am-m., Caust., *Ip.,* Kreos., *Squil.,* Stict.

**Catarrh, post-nasal, in children and adults:** Hydr., Pop-c., Spig.

**Chest, feeling as if lump in:** Abies-n.

**Cold air:** *Acon., All-c.,* Alum., Am-c., Ars., Bar-c., Brom., Calc-sil., *Carb-v., Hep.,* Lach., *Menth.,* Nit-ac., *Phos.,* Rhus-t., *Rumx.,* Seneg., *Spong.,* Squil., Trif-p.

**Cold air, to warm:** Ant-c., *Bry.,* Ip., *Nat-c.,* Squil., Verat.

**Condiments, vinegar, wine:** Alum.

**Dampness:** Ant-t., Calc., *Dulc., Nat-s.,* Nux-m.

**Daytime only:** *Euphr., Ferr.,* Nat-m., Stann., Staph., Viol-o.

**Drinking:** Ars., *Bry., Carb-v.,* Dros., Hyos., Lyc., Phos., Staph.

**Drinking, cold:** *Carb-v., Hep.,* Merc., Rhus-t., Sil., *Spong.,* Squil., Verat.

**Eating:** Anac., Ant-ar., Ant-t., *Bry., Calc., Carb-v., Chin.,* Hyos., Kali-bi., *Lach., Mez.,* Myos., *Nux-v., Phos.,* Staph., Tax., Zinc.

**Eczema or itch suppressed:** Psor.

**Entering, warm room:** Acon., *Ant-c.,* Anth., *Bry., Caust.,* Cham., Merc., *Nat-c., Puls.,* Ran-b., Verat.

**Evening, night:** Acal., *Acon., Am-br.,* Am-c., Ant-t., Arn., *Ars., Bell., Bry., Calc.,* Caps., *Carb-v., Caust., Cimic., Cod., Colch., Con., Dros., Eup-per., Hep.,* Hydr-ac., *Hyos.,* Kali-br., Ign., Laur., Lyc., Menth., Meph., *Merc., Nit-ac.,* Op., Passi., *Phos., Prun-v., Psor., Puls., Rhus-t., Rumx., Samb.,* Sang., *Sanic.,* Santin., Sep., *Sil., Spong., Stann., Stict., Sulph.,* Tub., *Verb.*

**Before midnight:** Aral., *Bell.,* Carb-v., Mag-m., *Phos.,* Samb., *Spong.,* Stann.

**After midnight, early A.M.:** *Acon.,* Am-br., Am-c., *Ars.,* Cupr., *Dros., Hep., Kali-c., Nux-v.,* Phel., Rhus-t.

**Constriction in larynx, trachea:** Ign.

**Excitement:** Ambr., Cor-r., Ign., Spong., Tarent. (See **Nervous.**)

**Expiration:** *Acon., Caust., Nux-v.*

**Exposure even of hand from under cover:** Bar-c., Hep., Rhus-t.

**Heart disease:** Arn., Hydr-ac., Lach., Laur., Lycps-v., *Naja, Spong.*

**Influenza:** All-c., *Erio.,* Hyos., *Kali-bi.,* Kali-s., *Kreos., Pix, Sang.,* Seneg., Stann., Stry.

**Injuries:** Arn., Mill.

**Inspiration:** *Acet-ac.,* Acon., *Bell., Brom.,* Bry., Cina, Iod., *Ip.,* Kali-bi., Lach., Menth., Nat-m., *Phos., Rumx., Spong.,* Squil., *Stict.*

**Intermittent, suppressed:** Eup-per.

**Liver affections:** Am-m.

**Lying down:** Ant-ar., *Aral.,* Ars., *Bell.,* Bry., *Caust.,* Coch., *Con.,* Croc., Crot-t., *Dros.,* Dulc., *Hyos.,* Ign., Inul., Lith-c., Meph., Nit-ac., Nux-v., Petr., *Phos., Prun-v.,* Psor., *Puls., Rumx.,* Sabad., *Sang., Sil.,* Stict., Tub., Verb.

**Lying on back:** Am-m., Ars., Iod., *Nux-v.,* Phos.

**Lying on left side:** Dros., *Phos.,* Ptel., Rumx., Stann.

**Lying on right side:** Am-m., Benz-ac., *Merc.*

**Lying with head low:** Am-m., *Spong.*

**Measles:** Dros., Dulc., Eup-per., Euphr., Ip., Kali-bi., *Puls.,* Sang., Squil., *Stict.* (See **FEVER.**)

**Menses, or piles, suppressed:** Mill.

**Mental exertion:** Nux-v.

**Morning:** Acal., All-s., *Alum.,* Ambr., Calc., Cina, *Coc-c., Hep., Iod.,* Kali-bi., Kali-i., Kali-n., Lyc., Nat-m., *Nit-ac., Puls.,* Rhus-t., Sel., Sep., Stict., Sil., Tab.

**Morning, early:** *Am-br., Am-c., Ars.,* Caust., Cupr., Hep., *Kali-c., Nux-v.,* Phel., Puls., Sulph.

**Morning, on waking:** Alum., Ambr., *Bry., Coc-c.,* Kali-bi., Psor., Rhus-t.

**Motion:** Ars., Bell., *Bry., Cina,* Hep., Iod., *Ip.,* Nux-v., Puls., Seneg., Spong., Verat.

**Odors strong, presence of strangers:** Phos.

**Old people:** Ant-i., Ant-t., Bar-c., Bar-m., *Carb-v., Hyos.,* Kreos., Myrt-c., Rhus-t., *Seneg.,* Sil., Stict.

**Operations for fistulae, after:** Berb., Calc-p., Sil.

**Periodic, recurring in spring, autumn:** Cina.

**Pertussis after, from least cold:** Caust., Sang.

**Physical exhaustion:** Squil., *Stict.*

**Pregnancy:** *Apoc.,* Bry., Caust., *Con., Kali-br.,* Nux-m., Vib-od.

**Reading, laughing, singing, talking:** Alum., *Ambr.,* Anac., *Arg-met., Arg-n.,* Arum-t., Carb-v., *Caust.,* Cimic., Coll., *Con., Dros., Hep., Hyos.,* Irid-met., Lach., *Mang-act.,* Menth., Nux-v., *Phos., Rumx.,* Sil., Spong., *Stann.,* Sulph.

**Reflex:** Ambr., Apis, Phos.

**Sciatica in summer, alternating:** Staph.

**Standing still during a walk:** Astac., Ign.

**Stomach, irritation, from:** Bism., *Bry.,* Calad., Cer-ox., Kali-m., *Lob,* Nat-m., Nit-ac., Nux-v., Phos., *Sang., Sep.,* Sulph., Verat.

**Swallowing, from:** Spong.

**Sweets:** Med., *Spong.,* Zinc.

**Tickling, as from dust, feather:** Am-c., Ars., *Bell., Calc.,* Caps., Caust., *Carb-v.,* Cina, *Dros.,* Euph-l., *Ign.,* Lac-c., Lach., *Lact.,* Nat-m., Nux-v., Par., *Phos., Rumx.,* Sep.

**Tickling, in chest (substernal, suprasternal fossa):** Am-br., *Ambr., Ant-c.,* Apis, Arn., Ars., Brom., *Bry., Calc.,* Caps., *Carb-v., Caust.,* Cham., Coc-c., *Con.,* Ferr-act., *Ign., Iod.,* Ip., Kali-bi., Kreos., *Lach., Menth.,* Myrt-c., *Nux-v., Osm.,* Par., Ph-ac., *Phos.,* Puls., Rad-br., Rhus-t., *Rumx.,* Sang., Sep., *Sil.,* Spong., *Stann.,* Sulph., Verat.

**Tickling, in larynx:** *All-c.,* Alum., *Arg-met., Bell.,* Brom., *Calc.,* Caps., *Carb-v.,* Caust., Coch., *Coc-c., Con.,* Crot-h., *Dros.,* Dulc., Ery-a., Hep., *Ign.,* Iod., Ip., Kreos., *Lach.,* Menth., Nit-ac., *Phos.,* Puls., *Rumx.,* Sang., *Sil.,* Spong., *Sulph.*

**Tickling, in throat:** Alum., Am-br., Ambr., Am-c., *Aral., Arg-n.,* Bell., *Calc., Caps.,* Cham., Cimic., Cina, *Con., Dros., Hep.,* Hepat., *Hyos., Ign., Iod.,* Kali-c., Lact., *Lob,* Meli., Menth., Nux-v., *Phos.,* Rumx., Stann-i., Sulph., Wye.

**Tobacco smoke:** Menth., Merc., Spong., *Staph.*

**Tonsils, enlarged:** Bar-c., Lach.

**Touch, pressure:** Lach., *Rumx.*

**Undressing, or uncovering body:** Bar-c., *Hep.,* Kali-bi., *Rhus-t., Rumx.*

**Uvula, relaxed:** Bar-c., *Hyos.,* Kali c., Merc-i-r.

**Warmth:** *Ant-c., Bry.,* Caust., Dros., Dulc., Ip., *Merc.,* Nat-c., Nux-m., Puls., Squil.

**Weeping:** Arn.

**Winter:** Aloe, *Ant-s-aur.,* Bry., Cham., Ip., Kreos., Lip., Psor. (See **Chronic Bronchitis**.)

**Worms:** Cina, Ter.

**Young, phthisical persons with constant, distressing night cough:** Dros.

**TYPE, Barking:** *Acon.*, Ambr., *Bell.*, Cor-r., *Dros.*, Hep., Iod., *Kali-bi.*, Phos., Samb., Sin-n., *Spong.*, Verat. (See **Dry, hoarse, spasmodic.**)

**Chronic (phthisical):** *All-s.*, *Ant-t.*, Ars-i., Bar-c., Bry., Calc-i., Calc-p., Cham., *Cod.*, Crot-h., *Dros.*, Dulc., Eup-per., Hyosin-hbr., Kreos., Laur., Lob., Lyc., Mang-act., Merc., Naja, *Nit-ac.*, Phel., *Phos.*, Psor., Puls., Rumx., *Sang.*, Sil., *Spong.*, Squil., Stict., Sulph. (See **Tuberculosis.**)

**Croupy:** *Acon.*, Brom., Gels., *Hep.*, Iod., *Kali-bi.*, Nit-ac., Phos., *Spong.*, Staph. (See **Croup.**)

**Dry, hard, racking, hacking, short, tight, tickling:** *Acal.*, *Acon.*, *All-c.*, *Alum.*, Alumn., *Am-br.*, Am-c., Ant-s-aur., *Ars.*, Ars-i., *Arum-t.*, Asc-t., *Bell.*, *Brom.*, *Bry.*, *Calc.*, Calc-i., Canth., *Caps.*, Carb-ac., Carb-v., *Caust.*, *Cham.*, Cimic., *Cina*, Coch., *Cod.*, Coff., *Con.*, *Cor-r.*, Dig., Dros., Euphr., Ferr-p., Glyc., *Hep.*, *Hydr-ac.*, *Hyos.*, Hyosin-hbr., *Ign.*, *Iod.*, Just., *Kali-bi.*, *Kali-br.*, *Kali-c.*, Kali-m., Kreos., *Lach.*, *Laur.*, *Lob.*, Lyc., Lycpr., Lycps-v., Mang-act., Med., *Menth.*, Mentho., Merc., *Morph.*, *Naja*, Nat-m., *Nit-ac.*, *Nux-v.*, Ol-j., *Onos.*, Op., *Osm.*, Petr., *Phos.*, *Puls.*, *Rhus-t.*, *Rumx.*, Salv., Samb., Sang., *Sang-n.*, *Seneg.*, *Sep.*, *Sil.*, *Spong.*, Squil., Stann., *Stict.*, Sul-ac., Sulph., Tela, Tub., Tub-a., Vanad., Verat., *Verb.*, Wye.

**Explosive, noisy:** *Caps.*, Dros., *Osm.*, Lycpr., Stry. (See **Spasmodic.**)

**Fatiguing, exhausting, irritating:** *Acon.*, Am-c., Ant-i., *Ars.*, *Arum-t.*, Bals-p., *Bell.*, Bry., Calc., *Caust.*, Cham., Chel., *Cod.*, Coll., Con., *Cor-r.*, *Dros.*, Eucal., Hep., *Hyos.*, Hydr-ac., *Ign.*, Iod., *Ip.*, Kali-br., Kreos., Lact., Laur., *Lob*, Lyc., *Menth.*, Mentho., Merc., Myrt-c., *Naja*, Nit-ac., Op., Phel., *Phos.*, Psor., Rumx., Rumx-act., Sang., *Seneg.*, *Sep.*, *Sil.*, Silphu., *Squil.*, *Stict*, Stry., Tela, Tub-a. (See **Spasmodic.**)

**Hoarse, hollow, deep, metallic:** *Acon.*, Am-p., *Ambr.*, Ant-t., Apoc., Ars-i., *Arum-t.*, Bell., Brom., Bry., *Carb-v.*, *Caust.*, *Cina*, *Dros.*, Dulc., Euph., Euphr., *Hep.*, Ign., Iod., Irid-met., *Kali-bi.*, Lip., Lyc., Mang-act., Med., Meph., Myrt-c., Nit-ac., *Phos.*, Samb., *Spong.*, Stann., Verat., *Verb.* (See **Spasmodic.**)

**Laryngeal, nervous:** Acon., *Ambr.*, Asar., *Bell.*, *Brom.*, Caps., Carb-v., *Caust.*, Cina, *Cor-r.*, *Cupr.*, *Dros.*, Gels., *Hep.*, Hydr-ac., *Hyos.*, *Ign.*, Ip., Kali-br., Kali-m., Lach., Med., Merc., *Nit.*, *ac.*, Nux-v., *Phos.*, Puls., *Rumx.*, *Santin.*, *Spong.*, Sulph., Tarent., Ter., Verat., Viol-o.

**Loose, rattling, gagging, choking, strangling:** Am-br., Am-m., Ant-s-aur., *Ant-t.*, Ars., Asc-t., Bals-p., *Brom.*, *Calc.*, *Calc-act.*, *Chel.*, Cina, Coc-c., Cupr., Dros., *Dulc.*, Eup-per., *Hep.*, *Ip.*, Kali-bi., Kali-c., Kali-m., Kali-s., Lyc., *Merc.*, *Nat-s.*, Nit-ac., Phos., *Puls.*, Rhus-t., Samb., Sang., *Senec.*, Seneg., Sep., Sil., Squil., *Stann.*, Stict., *Sulph.*, Ter., Verat.

**Spasmodic, paroxysmal, nervous, violent, suffocative:** *Acon.*, Agar., *Ambr., Ambr.*, Ant-ar., Ant-t., Aral., *Arn., Ars.*, Asar., *Bell., Brom., Bry.*, Caps., Carb-ac., *Carb-v., Caust.*, Cham., *Chel., Cina,* Coc-c., *Con., Cor-r.*, Crot-t., *Cupr., Cupr-act., Dros.*, Dulc., Gels., Glyc., *Hep., Hydr-ac., Hyos., Ign.*, Iod., *Ip., Just., Kali-br., Kali-c., Kreos., Lach., Lact-v.*, Laur., Led., Lyc., *Mag-p., Meph., Merc.*, Naphtin., *Nat-m., Nit-ac.*, Nux-m., *Nux-v.*, Op., *Osm.*, Pert., *Phos.*, Rad-br., *Rumx., Samb.*, Sang., Santin., Sep., *Sil., Spong., Squil., Stann.*, Stict., Sulph., Trif-p., Verat., *Viol-o.*

**Successive, in two paroxysms:** Merc., Puls.

**Successive, in three paroxysms:** Cupr., Stann.

**Wheezing, asthmatic:** Ambro., Ant-t., *Ars.*, Benz-ac., Croc., Hep., Iod., *Ip.*, Kali-bi., *Lob.*, Meph., Nit-ac., Rhod., Samb., *Sang.*, Seneg., *Spong.* (See **Spasmodic**.)

**WHOOPING (pertussis):** *Acon.*, Alumn., Am-br., Am-m., Am-pic., Ambr., *Ambro.*, Ant-c., *Ant-t., Arn.*, Bad., *Bell.*, Bry., Brom., Caps., Carb-ac., Carb-v., Caust., *Castn-v.*, Cer-ox., *Chel.*, Chin., *Cina,* Cocain., *Coc-c.*, Con., *Cor-r., Cupr., Cupr-act., Dros., Dulc.*, Eucal., Euph-l., Euphr., *Form.*, Grin., *Hep., Hydr-ac., Hyos., Ip., Just., Kali-bi.*, Kali-br., *Kali-c., Kali-m.*, Kali-p., Kali-s., Led., *Lob.*, Lob-m., *Mag-p., Meph., Merc., Naphtin.*, Nit-ac., Ol-j., Op., Passi., Pert., Phos., Podo., *Puls.*, Samb., Sangin-n., *Sep.*, Sil., Sol-c., Stict., Sulph., Thymu., Tong., *Trif-p., Verat.*, Viol-o. (See **Spasmodic**.)

**Whooping at night, "minute gun" during day:** Cor-r.

**Whooping, convulsions:** *Bell.*, Cina, Cupr., *Cupr-act.*, Hydr-ac., Hyos., Kali-br., Mag-p., Narc-po., *Sol-c.*

**Whooping, early stage (spasmodic):** *Acon., Bell.*, Carb-ac., Carb-v., *Castn-v.*, Chel., *Cina,* Coc-c., Cor-r., Cupr., *Dros.*, Hyos., Ip., Mag-p., Meph., Naphtin., Narc-po., Samb., Stann., Thymu.

**Whooping, hemorrhage:** *Arn., Cer-ox.*, Cor-r., Cupr., *Dros.*, Ind., *Ip.*, Merc.

**Whooping, later stages (catarrhal):** *Ant-t.*, Chin., Hep., *Ip.*, Puls.

**Whooping, vomiting:** Ant-t., Bell., Carb-v., *Cer-ox., Coc-c., Cupr., Dros., Ip.*, Lob, Verat.

**CONCOMITANTS, Body stiff, rigid, cyanosis:** Am-c., *Ant-t.*, Carb-v., Cina, Cor-r., *Cupr., Cupr-act.*, Iod., *Ip.*, Mag-p., Meph., Op., Samb., *Verat.*

**Coryza:** Alum., Lyc., Nat-c.

**Crowing inspiration absent:** Ambr.

**Crying:** *Arn.*, Bry., *Caps.*, Samb.

**Diarrhea:** Ant-t., *Cupr-ar.*, Euph-l., Ip., *Rumx.*, Verat.

**Dyspnea:** Ambr, Am-c., *Ant-t.*, Bell., Brom., *Carb-v.*, Cina, Cor-r., *Cupr., Dros.*, Euph., Hep., Hipp., Iod., *Ip.*, Kali-bi., *Lob., Meph.*, Naphtin., Op., *Samb.*, Senec., *Verat., Viol-o.* (See **Respiration**.)

**Epistaxis, bleedings:** *Arn.,* Bell., Cer- ox., Cor-r., *Cupr., Dros., Ind., Iod.,* Ip., Merc.

**Paroxysms follow each other rapidy and violently:** Dros.

**Paroxysms wakes child at 6-7 A.M., vomiting of ropy mucus:** Coc-c.

**Paroxysms with flow of tears:** Nat-m.

**Spasm of glottis:** Cupr., Meph., Mosch.

**Sublingual ulcer:** Nit-ac.

**Vomiting of solid food after regaining consciousness:** Cupr.

**With every cold, severe cough returns:** Sang.

**EXPECTORATION, TYPE: Acid:** Carb-an., Nit-ac., Puls.

**Albuminous, clear, white:** *Arg-met.,* Ars., Bry., Coc-c., Eucal., Kali-m., *Sel.,* Squil., Sulph.

**Bitter:** Bry., Calc., Cham., Dros., Kali-n., Nit-ac., *Puls.*

**Bloody, blood streaked:** *Acon.,* Arg-n., *Arn., Ars., Bell., Bry.,* Calc., Cann-s., Canth., *Cetr.,* Cor-r., Crot-h., *Dig.,* Dros., Dulc., *Elaps, Ferr-p., Hep.,* Hyos., Iod., Ip., Kali-c., *Kali-n., Laur., Led.,* Lyc., Merc., Merc-c., *Mill.,* Nit-ac., Nux-v., Op., *Phos.,* Puls., *Rhus-t.,* Sel., Sil., Sulph., *Tril-p.*

**Casts:** *Calc-act.,* Kali-bi.

**Daytime:** Ambr., Bry., Calc., Hyos., Stann.

**Easy, raising:** *Arg-met.,* Carb-v., Dulc., Erio., Kali-s., *Nat-s.,* Puls., Squil, *Stann.,* Tub.

**Fetid, offensive:** Ars., Borx., *Calc., Caps.,* Carb-v., Cop., Euphr., Kali-c., *Kali-hp.,* Lyc., Nit-ac., Ph-ac., *Phel., Pix,* Psor., *Sang.,* Sep., *Sil., Stann.,* Sulph.

**Globular, lumpy:** *Agar.,* Arg-met., Am-m., Ant-t., *Bad.,* Calc., Calc-f., *Chel., Kali-c.,* Mang-act., Nat-sel., Rhus-t., *Sil.*

**Gray, greenish, mucus:** Alum-sil., Am-p., Ant-s-aur., Ars., *Benz-ac.,* Calc., Calc-i., Calc-p., Calen., Cann-s., *Carb-v., Cop.,* Dros., Dulc., Ferr-act., *Kali-i.,* Kali-m., Kali-s., *Lyc.,* Nat-c., *Nat-s., Par.,* Phos., Psor., *Puls.,* Seneg., Sep., Silphu., Spong., *Stann.,* Sulph., Thuj.

**Herby taste:** Borx.

**Liver colored:** Graph., Lyc., Puls., Sep., Stann.

**Profuse:** All-s., *Am-m., Ammc.,* Ant-ar., *Ant-i.,* Ant-t., Arg-met., *Ars-i.,* Asc-t., *Bals-p.,* Calc., Calc-sil., Canth., *Carb-v.,* Cean., Chel., Chin., *Coc-c.,* Cop., Dros., *Dulc.,* Eucal., Grin., *Hep.,* Hepat., Hydr., *Ip., Kali-bi.,* Kali-c., Kali-i., *Kreos., Laur., Lyc.,* Merc., Myos., Myrt-ch., Nat-ar., Nat-s., Ph-ac., Phel., Pilo., *Puls.,* Ruta, Sang., *Seneg, Sep., Sil.,* Silphu., *Squil., Stann., Sulph.,* Ter., Tril-p., Zing.

**Purulent, muco-purulent:** Ammc., Ant-i., Ars-i., Asc-t., *Bac., Bals-p., Calc.,* Calc-p., Calc-s., Calc-sil., *Carb-v.,* Chin., Cop., Dros., Eucal., *Eryn., Hep.,*

Hepat., *Hydr.,* Iod., *Kali-bi.,* Kali-c., Kali-i., *Kali-p.,* Kali- s., *Kreos.,* Laur., *Lyc.,* Merc., *Myos.,* Myrt-c., Myrt-ch., Nat-c., Nit-ac., Ph-ac., *Phos., Pix,* Psor., Ruta, Sang., Sangin-n., Sep., *Sil.,* Sol-n., Squil., *Stann., Sulph.,* Ter., *Teucr-s.,* Tril-p.

**Rust colored:** *Bry.,* Ferr-p., *Phos.,* Rhus-t., *Sang.*

**Salty:** Ambr, Ars., Calc., *Kali-i., Lyc., Mag-c.,* Nat-c., Nat-m., Ph-ac., Phos., Psor., Puls., *Sep.,* Sil., Squil., Stann.

**Scanty:** Alum., Am-m., *Ant-t., Ars.,* Asc-t., Brom., Bry., *Caust.,* Cimic., Kali-c., Kali-hp., Ign., Lach., Morph., Nit-ac., *Nux-v.,* Op., *Phos.,* Rumx., Sang., Spong., Squil., Zinc. (See **Viscid**.)

**Serous, frothy, watery:** *Acon.,* Am-c., *Ant-ar., Ars.,* Bry., Carb-v., Croc., Ferr-p., Grin., *Kali-i.,* Lach., Merc., Nat-m., Oena., Phos., Pilo., Silphu., Tanac.

**Slips back, or must be swallowed:** Arn., *Caust.,* Con., Iod., *Kali-c.,* Lach., Nux-m., Spong.

**Soapy:** Caust.

**Sour:** Calc., Iris, Lach., Nit-ac., Nux-v., Ph-ac., Phos., Stann., Zinc.

**Sweetish:** Hepat., Phos., Sangin-n., *Stann.,* Sulph.

**Viscid, tenacious, difficulty on raising:** All-s., *Alum., Am-c., Am-m.,* Ammc., Ant-i., Ant-s-aur., *Ant-t.,* Aral., *Ars.,* Asc-t., Bals-p., Bar-c., Bar-m., Bell., Bov., *Bry.,* Calc., Cann-s., *Canth., Carb-v., Caust.,* Chel., Chin., *Coc-c.,* Cupr., Dulc., Eucal., Grin., *Hydr., Ip., Kali-bi.,* Kali-c., *Kali-hp.,* Kali-m., *Lach.,* Laur., Lyc., Mang-act., Merc., Morph., Myrt-c., Naphtin., Nat-s., Nux-v., Osm., *Par.,* Phos., Psor., Quill., Rumx., *Sang.,* Sangin-n., *Seneg., Sep., Sil.,* Silphu., Squil., Stann., Sulph.

**EMPTY FEELING IN CHEST:** Ph-ac., *Stann.*

**ERUCTATIONS:** Ambr., Caps.

**FAINTNESS:** Sep.

**GAPING, alternates with cough:** Ant-t.

**GRASPS genitals:** Zinc.

**GRASPS throat:** Acon., *All-c., Iod.,* Lob.

**GURGLING, from throat to stomach:** Cina.

**HERPES facialis:** Arn. (See **SKIN.**)

**HICCOUGH:** Tab.

**HOARSENESS:** Am-c., Ambr., *Brom.,* Calc., Calen., Carb-v., *Caust., Dros., Eup-per., Hep.,* Iod., Lach., Meph., *Merc., Phos.,* Sil., *Spong.,* Sulph.

**HYPERESTHESIA of mucosa:** *Bell.,* Con., *Hyos.,* Lach., Phos., *Rumx.,* Stict.

**LACHRYMATION:** *All-c.,* Caps., Cina, *Euphr.,* Nat-m., *Squil.*

**LEFT BREAST, feels cold:** Nat-c.

**PAIN, Chest:** Abies-n., Ars., *Bell.,* Brom., *Bry.,* Caps., Carb-v., *Caust.,* Chel.,

Chin., Cina, Com., *Dros.*, Dulc., Elaps, *Eup-per.*, Euph., Ign., *Iod.*, Just., Kali-bi., *Kali-c.*, Kali-i., Kali-n., *Kreos.*, *Lact.*, Lyc., Meph., *Merc.*, Myrt-c., Nat-c., *Nat-s.*, *Nicc.*, Nux-v., Phel., *Phos.*, Phyt., *Rumx.*, Seneg., Sil., Spong., *Stict.*, *Sulph.*, Ziz.

**Distant parts:** Agar., Am-c., Bell., *Bry.*, *Caps.*, *Caust.*, Chel., Lach., Nat-m., Seneg.

**Head:** Aeth., Anac., Asc-t., Bell., *Bry.*, Carb-v., Eup-per., Ferr., Form, Lyc., *Nat-m.*, *Nux-v.*, Sep., Sulph.

**Head, he places hands to it:** *Bry.*, Caps., Nat-m., Nat-s.

**Larynx:** *Acon.*, *All-c.*, Ant-t., Arg-met., Arum-t., Asc-t., *Bell.*, Caust., Hep., Inul., *Iod.*, Nit-ac., *Phos.*, Rumx., *Spong.*

**Stomach, abdomen:** Asc-t., *Bry.*, Calc., *Nux-v.*, Puls., Sep., Sil., Sulph., Thuj.

**Throat:** *Bell.*, *Lach.*, Merc-i-r., Sil.

**POLYURIA:** Squil.

**PROSTRATION:** Am-c., *Ant-t.*, *Ars.*, Cor-r., *Cupr.*, Cur., Hep., Iod., *Ip.*, Meph., Nit-ac., Ph-ac., Rumx., *Verat.*

**RAWNESS, soreness of chest:** Amyg., Ant-s-aur., Ars., *Bry.*, Calc., Carb-v., *Caust.*, Cor-r., Dig., *Eup-per.*, Ferr-p., Gels., Graph., Mag-m., Meph., *Merc.*, *Phos.*, Rhus-t., *Rumx.*, Sel., Seneg., *Stann.*

**RUBS face, with fists:** Squil.

**SLEEPINESS, between attacks:** Euph-l.

**SNEEZING, at end:** Agar., Bell., Cina, Dros., *Just*, *Squil.*, Seneg.

**SPASMS:** *Bell.*, Cina, *Cupr.*, *Cupr-act.*, Hydr-ac., Oena., *Sol-c.*

**SPASM of chest:** Samb.

**TINGLING, in chest:** Acon.

**URINE, involuntary, spurting:** Alum., *Anemps.*, Caps., *Caust.*, Colch., *Ferr.*, *Ferr-m.*, Ferr-p., Nat-m., *Puls.*, Rumx., *Squil.*, Verat., Verb., Zinc.

**VOMITING, retching, gagging:** Alumn., Anac., *Ant-t.*, *Bry.*, Carb-v., Coc-c., Cupr., *Cupr-act.*, Cupr-ar., Cur., *Dros.*, Euph-l., Euphr., *Ferr.*, *Hep.*, *Ip.*, *Kali-c.*, Kreos., Meph., Myos., Nit-ac., *Nux-v.*, Phos., Puls., Sep., *Sil.*, Verat.

**AMELIORATIONS: From drinking, cold things:** *Caust.*, *Cupr.*, Phos., Tab.

**From drinking, warm things:** Spong.

**From eating:** Anac., Bism., Ferr., *Spong.*

**From eructations:** Ambr., Ang., Sang.

**From expectoration:** Zinc.

**From lying down:** Calc-p., Ferr., *Mang-act.*, Sin-n.

**From lying on right side:** Ant-t.

**From lying on stomach:** Med.

**From placing hands, on chest:** *Bry.,* Caps., Cina, Dros., *Eup-per.,* Lact., *Nat-s.*

**From resolute suppression of cough:** Ign.

**From resting, on hands and feet:** Eup-per.

**From resting, with hands on thighs:** Nicc.

**From sitting up:** *Bry.,* Crot-t., *Dros.,* Hep., *Hyos.,* Nat-s., Phel., *Puls.,* Sang.

**From warming air by covering head with bedclothes:** Hep., Rhus-t., *Rumx.*

**From warmth:** Bad.

**LARYNX, Anesthesia:** Kali-br.

**Burning:** Am-caust., Am-m., Arg-met., *Ars.,* Canth., Mang-act., *Merc.,* Mez., *Par.,* Phos., *Rumx., Sang., Spong.,* Zing. (See **Pain**.)

**Cancer:** Nit-ac., Thuj.

**Coldness:** *Brom.,* Rhus-t., Sulph.

**Constricted feeling:** Acon., *Bell.,* Brom., Calad., *Chlor., Cupr.,* Dros., Guaj., Hydr-ac., *Iod.,* Mang-act., Med., *Mosch.,* Naja, Ox-ac., Phos., *Spong.,* Still., Verat. (See **Spasms**.)

**Dryness:** Ars., *Bell.,* Carb-v., Caust., Dros., Dub., Hep., Iod., Kali-bi., Kali-i., Lem-m., *Mang-act.,* Mez., *Phos.,* Pop-c., *Sang.,* Seneg., *Spong.* (See **Inflammation**.)

**Edema of glottis:** *Apis, Ars.,* Bell., Chinin-ar., Chlor., *Kali-i.,* Lach., Merc., Pilo., *Sang.,* Stram., *Vip.*

**Epiglottis, affections:** All-c., Chlor., Hepat., Wye.

**INFLAMMATION, LARYNGITIS, Acute, catarrhal:** *Acon.,* Aesc., *All-c.,* Ant-t., Apis, Arg-met., Ars-i., *Arum-t., Bell.,* Brom., Bry., Canth., Carb-v., *Caust.,* Cub., Dros., *Dulc.,* Eup-per., *Ferr-p.,* Guaj., *Hep.,* Iod., Ip., *Kali-bi.,* Kali-i., *Merc.,* Mentho., Osm., *Phos., Rhus-t., Rumx., Samb.,* Sang., *Spong.,* Stict., Sulph.

**Inflammation, atrophic:** Am-m., *Kali-bi.,* Kali-i., Lach., Mang-act., Phos., Sang.

**Inflammation, chronic, catarrhal:** Am-br., Am-i., Ant-s-aur., Ant-t., *Arg-met., Arg-n.,* Bar-c., Bar-m., Calc., Calc-i., *Carb-v., Caust., Coc-c.,* Cot., *Dros., Hep.,* Iod., Irid-met., *Kali-bi.,* Kali-c., *Kali-i., Lach., Mang-act., Merc.,* Merc-c., Nat-m., Nat-sel., Nit-ac., *Nux-v., Par., Phos., Puls.,* Rhus-t., Sang-n., *Sel., Seneg., Stann.,* Still., *Sulph.,* Thuj.

**Inflammation, follicular:** Arg-n., Hep., *Iod.,* Kali-i., Sel., *Sulph.*

**Inflammation, membranous exudate, MEMBRANOUS CROUP:** *Acet-ac.,* Acon., *Alum-sil., Am-caust.,* Ammc., Ant-t., Ars., Ars-i., Bell., *Brom.,* Calc-i., Con., Dros., Ferr-p., Hep., *Iod., Kali-bi.,* Kali-chl., *Kali-m.,* Kali-n., Lach., *Merc.,* Merc-cy., Phos., Samb., *Sang., Spong.,* (See **Diphtheria, THROAT**.)

**Inflammation, SPASMODIC CROUP:** *Acon.,* Alum-sil., Ant-t., Ars., Bell., Benzo., *Brom.,* Bry., *Calc-f.,* Calc-i., *Chlor.,* Cupr., Euph., Ferr-p., *Hep.,* Ictod., Ign., *Iod.,* Ip., *Kali-bi.,* Kali-br., *Kali-n.,* Lach., Meph., Merc-i-f., Mosch., Naja, Petr., *Phos.,* Samb., Sang., *Spong., Verat-v.*

**Inflammation, syphilitic, associated with, secondary symptoms:** Merc., Merc-c., Nit-ac.

**Inflammation, syphilitic, associated with, tertiary symptoms:** *Aur.,* Cinnb., Iod., *Kali-bi., Kali-i.,* Lach., *Merc-c.,* Merc-i-f., Merc-i-r., Mez., *Nit-ac.,* Sang., Thuj. (See **Syphilis, MALE SEXUAL SYSTEM**.)

**Inflammation, syphilitic, hereditary:** *Aur.,* Fl-ac., *Hep.,* Kreos., Merc., Merc-i-f., *Merc-i-r., Nit-ac., Phyt.,* Sulph., Thuj.

**Inflammation, tuberculous:** *Arg-n.,* Ars., *Ars-i.,* Atrop., Bapt., Brom., *Calc.,* Calc-p., Canth., Carb-v., *Caust.,* Chr-o., Cist., *Dros.,* Ferr-p., Hep., *Iod.,* Ip., Jab., Kali-c., Kali-m., Kreos., Lyc., *Mang-act.,* Merc-n., Naja, *Nat-sel.,* Nit-ac., *Phos., Sel.,* Spong., *Stann.,* Sulph.

**Irritation:** *Arg-met.,* Bar-c., Caust., Chlor., *Hep.,* Kali-bi., Kali-i., Kali-perm., *Lach.,* Mang-act., Nux-v., *Phos.* (See **Rawness**.)

**Motion, up and down, violent:** *Sul-ac.*

**Mucus:** Ant-t., *Arg-met.,* Arg-n., *Brom., Bry.,* Canth., Dros., *Hep., Kali-bi.,* Kali-c., Lach., *Mang-act.,* Ox-ac., Par., Phos., Rumx., *Samb.,* Sang., Sel., Seneg, Stann. (See **Inflammation**.)

**Pains:** Acon., *All-c.,* Alum., Arg-n., Arum-t., *Bell.,* Bry., *Hep., Iod.,* Just., Kreos., Lach., *Mang-act.,* Med., Merc-c., Nit-ac., *Osm., Phos.,* Sang., *Spong.* (See **Inflammation**.)

**Polypus:** Berb., Psor., Sang., *Sang-n., Teucr.,* Thuj.

**Rawness, roughness, soreness, sensitiveness:** Acon., Alum., Alum-sil., Am-caust., *Arg-met.,* Arn., *Arum-t., Bar.c., Bell.,* Benzo., Brom., Bry., *Caust., Cham.,* Cist., Dros., Eup-per., *Hep.,* Iod., Kali-bi., *Kali-i.,* Kali- perm., *Lach.,* Lyc., *Mag-p., Mang-act.,* Med., *Merc.,* Nux-v., Osm., Ph-ac., *Phos.,* Puls., Rhus-t., *Rumx.,* Sang., *Spong., Sulph.,* Zinc.

**Spasm (laryngismus stridulus):** *Acon.,* Agar., Am-caust., Ars-i., Arum-t., *Bell.,* Brom., *Calc.,* Calc-i., Calc-p., Chel., Chin., Chlol., *Chlor.,* Cic., *Cor-r., Cupr., Cupr-act., Form., Gels.,* Gran., Ign., *Iod., Ip.,* Kali-br., *Lach.,* Meph., *Mosch.,* Phos., *Samb.,* Spong., Stram., *Stry.,* Vesp., Zinc.

**Suffocative catarrh:** Ambr., Ars., Calc., Coff., Sang., Spong.

**Tickling:** All-c., Alum., *Ambr.,* Ant-s-aur., *Bell.,* Calc., Caps., Carb-v., *Coc-c.,* Cop., Dros., Dulc., *Iod.,* Kali-bi., *Phos.* (See **Cough**.)

**Tumors, benign:** Caust., Kali-bi., Sang., Thuj.

**Tumors, malignant:** *Ars.,* Ars-i., Bell., Carb-an., Clem., *Con.,* Hydr., Iod., Kreos., Lach., Morph., *Phyt.,* Sang., Thuj.

**Vocal cords, ulceration:** Aur-i., Iod., Lyc., Merc-n.

**Vocal cords, weak:** *Carb-v., Caust.,* Coca, Dros., Graph., Pen., Phos. (See Voice.)

**VOICE, Deep, bass:** Brom., Camph., Carb-v., *Caust., Dros.,* Phos., Pop-c., Sangin-n., Stann., Sulph., *Verb.*

**High, piping:** *Bell.*

**Hoarse, aphonia:** *Acon.,* Alum., Alumn., Am-c., *Am-caust., Am-m.,* Ant-c., Antip., Arg-i., *Arg-met., Arg-n.,* Arn., Ars-i., *Arum-t.,* Asc-t., Bar-c., *Bell.,* Benzo., *Brom., Bry., Calc.,* Calc-caust., Camph., *Carb-v., Caust.,* Cham., Chlor., Cina, *Coca,* Coc-c., Coch., Cub., *Dros.,* Dub., *Dulc., Eup-per.,* Ferr-p., Gels., Graph., *Hep.,* Hyos., Ign., Iod., *Ip.,* Just., *Kali-bi., Kali-c.,* Kali-chr., Kreos., Mag-p., *Mang-act., Merc., Nit-ac.,* Nux- m., *Nux-v.,* Op., Osm., *Ox-ac.,* Par., Pen., Petr., *Phos.,* Plat., *Pop-c., Puls., Rhus-t., Rumx., Samb.,* Sang., Sangin-n., *Sel.,* Seneg, Sep., Sil., *Spong.,* Stann., Stict., *Still., Sulph.,* Thuj., Verat-v., *Verb.,* Viol-o.

**Hoarseness, capricious:** Hep., Puls.

**Hoarseness, chronic:** Ampe-qu., *Arg-n.,* Bar-c., Calc., *Carb-v., Caust.,* Graph., *Mang-act., Phos., Sulph.*

**Hoarseness, croupy:** Acon., Ail., All-c., Brom., Caust., *Hep.,* Kali-s., *Spong.*

**Hoarseness, from cold weather:** Carb-v., Caust., Rumx., Sulph.

**Hoarseness, from overheating:** Ant-c., Ant-t., Brom.

**Hoarseness, from overusing voice, especially public speakers, professional singers:** Alum., *Arg-met., Arg-n.,* Arn., *Arum-t.,* Carb-v., *Caust., Coca,* Ferr-p., Ferr-pic., *Hep.,* Iod., Mang-act., Med., Merc., Merc-cy., Nat-sel., Phos., *Rhus-t., Sel.,* Spong., Stil., Sulph., Tab., Ter.

**Hoarseness, hysterical:** Cocc., *Gels., Ign.,* Nux-m., Plat.

**Hoarseness, painless:** Bell., *Calc.,* Carb-v., Par.

**Hoarseness, paretic:** Am-caust., Bell., *Caust., Gels.,* Lach., *Ox-ac.,* Phos., Rumx., Sil.

**Hoarseness, relieved temporarily by coughing or expectoration:** Stann.

**Hoarseness, worse, at end of cold:** Ip.

**Hoarseness, worse, in A.M.:** *Arum-t.,* Benz-ac., Calc., *Caust.,* Eup-per., Hep., *Mang-act.,* Nit-ac., *Nux-v.,* Sulph.

**Hoarseness, worse, in P.M.:** *Carb-v.,* Kali-bi., Phos., *Rumx.*

**Hoarseness, worse, in damp weather:** Carb-v.

**Hoarseness, worse, talking, singing, swallowing:** Spong.

**Hoarseness, worse, walking against wind:** Acon., Arum-t., *Euphr.,* Hep., *Nux-m.*

**Hoarseness, worse when crying:** Acon., *Bell.,* Phos., Spong.

**Menstrual:** Gels.

**Nervous aphonia with cardiac disorder:** Coca, Hydr-ac., Nux-m., Ox-ac.

**Timbre, varies continually:** Ant-c., Arg-met., *Arum-t.*, Bell., Carb-v., Caust., Dros., Lach., Rumx.

**Voice producer, instantaneous:** Arum-t., Caust., *Coca,* Ferr-p., *Pop-c.*

**Voice, low, monotonous, economical speech:** Mang-act., Mang-o.

**Whispering, weak voice:** Arg-met., Camph., Canth., Carb-v., *Caust.,* Dub., *Phos., Pop-c.,* Prim-v., Puls., Verat.

**LUNGS, Abscess:** Acon., *Ars-i.,* Bell., Caps., *Chin.,* Chinin-ar., *Hep.,* Iod., Kali-c., Merc., *Sil.*

**Congestion:** *Acon.,* Adren., Ars-i., *Bell.,* Both., *Cact.,* Conv., *Ferr-p.,* Iod., Kali-n., Lyc., Nux-v., Op., Phos., Stroph-h., Sulfon., Upa., *Verat-v.* (See **Inflammation**.)

**Congestion, passive:** Carb-v., *Dig.,* Ferr., Hydr-ac., Nux-v., Phos., *Sulph.*

**Dilation of cells (emphysema):** *Am-c., Ant-ar.,* Ant-t., *Ars., Aur-m.,* Bell., Bry., Calc., *Calc-p.,* Carb-v., Chin., Chinin-ar., Dig., *Dros.,* Eucal., Glon., Grin., Hep., Ip., Kali-c., *Lob, Lyc.,* Myrt-c., Naphtin., Nux-v., Phel., *Phos.,* Puls., Sep., Spong., *Stry.,* Sulph. (See **Asthma**.)

**Distended feeling:** Ter.

**Edema:** *Am-c.,* Am-i., *Ant-t., Apis, Ars.,* Coch., *Kali-c.,* Kali-i., Lach., *Phos.,* Pilo., Pulm-v., *Sang.,* Senec., Stroph-h., Tub.

**Gangrene:** Arn., *Ars., Caps.,* Carb-an., *Carb-v., Crot-h.,* Eucal., Dulc., Hep., Kreos., *Lach.,* Lyc., *Sec.,* Sil.

**HEMORRHAGE (hemoptysis):** *Acal.,* Acet-ac., *Achil., Acon., All-s., Arn., Cact.,* Carb-v., *Chin.,* Chinin-ar., Cinnm., Dig., Erech., Ergot., *Erig., Ferr-act.,* Ferr., *Ferr-p.,* Gelin., *Ger., Ham.,* Helx., *Hydrin-m., Ip.,* Kali- c., Kreos., *Lam., Led.,* Mangi., Meli., *Mill.,* Nat-n., *Phos.,* Rhus-t., Sang., Stroph-h., *Sul-ac.,* Ter., *Tril-p., Verat-v.*

**Hemorrhage, bright red, blood:** Acal., *Acon.,* Aran., Cact., Ferr-act., *Ferr-p.,* Ger., Led., *Mill.,* Nit-ac., Rhus-t., Tril-p.

**Hemorrhage, dark, clotted blood:** Arn., Crot-h., *Elaps,* Ferr-m., *Ham.,* Sul-ac.

**Hemorrhage, during menopause:** Lach.

**Hemorrhage, hemorrhoidal:** Mez., Nux-v.

**Haemorrhage, in drunkards:** Hyos., *Led.,* Nux-v., *Op.*

**Hemorrhage, in periodical attacks:** Kreos.

**Hemorrhage, in puerperal fevers:** Ham.

**Hemorrhage, traumatic:** Mill.

**Hemorrhage, tubercular:** Acal., Ferr-p., Mill., Nux-v., Tril-p.

**Hemorrhage, vicarious:** Bry., Ham., Phos.

**Hemorrhage, with cough:** *Acon.,* Acal., *Ferr-act.,* Ferr-p., *Ip., Led.,* Phos. (See **Cough**.)

**Hemorrhage, without cough, or effort:** *Acon., Ham.,* Mill., Sul-ac.

**Hemorrhage with valvular disease:** Cact., Lycps-v.

**Hot feeling:** Acon. (See **Congestion**.)

**INFLAMMATION, BRONCHO-PNEUMONIA:** *Acon.,* Am-i., Ant-ar., *Ant-t.,* Ars., *Ars-i.,* Bell., Bry., *Chel.,* Ferr-p., Glyc., Iod., *Ip.,* Kali-c., *Phos.,* Puls., Solin., *Squil., Tub., Tub-k.*

**Inflammation, CROUPOUS PNEUMONIA:** *Acon.,* Agar., Am-i., Ant-ars., Ant-i., Ant-s-aur., *Ant-t.,* Apom., Arn., Ars., *Bell., Brom., Bry.,* Camph., Carb-ac., Carb-v., *Chel.,* Chin., Coffin., Dig., *Ferr-p.,* Gels., Hep., *Iod.,* Ip., Kali-bi., *Kaii-c.,* Kali-i., Lach., *Lyc., Merc.,* Mill., Nat-s., Nit-ac., Op., Ox-ac., *Phos.,* Pneu., Pneumotox., Pyrog., Ran-b., Rhus-t., *Sang.,* Seneg, Squil., Stry., *Sulph.,* Tub., Verat., *Verat*-v.

**Stages of pneumonia: Congestive:** *Acon.,* Aesc., Bell., Bry., *Ferr-p., Iod.,* Sang., *Verat-v.*

**Consolidation:** Ant-t., *Bry., Iod.,* Kali-i., Kali-m., *Phos.,* Sang., Sulph.

**Resolution:** *Ant-t.,* Ant-s-aur., Ars., Ars-i., Carb-v., *Hep.,* Iod., *Kali-i.,* Kali-s., *Lyc.,* Nat-s., *Phos., Sang.,* Sil., Stann-i., *Sulph.*

**Type, Bilious:** Ant-t., *Chel.,* Lept., Merc., Phos., Podo.

**Latent:** Chel., Phos., *Sulph.*

**Neglected, lingering, cases:** Am-c., Ant-i., Ant-s-aur., *Ant-t.,* Ars-i., Bry., *Carb-v.,* Chin., Hep., Kali-i., Lach., *Lyc.,* Phos., Plb., Sulph.

**Secondary:** Ant-ar., *Ant-t., Ferr-p.,* Phos.

**Senile:** Ant-ar., *Ant-t.,* Dig., Ferr-p.

**Sycotic:** Nat-s.

**Typhoid:** *Hyos.,* Lach., Laur., Merc-cy., Op., *Phos., Rhus-t.,* Sang., Sulph.

**PARALYSIS of lungs:** Am-c., *Ant-ar., Ant-t.,* Arn., Bac., Carb-v., Cur., Diphtox., Dulc., *Grin.,* Hydr-ac., Ip., Lach., *Laur., Lob-p.,* Lyc., Merc-cy., Morph., Mosch., Phos., *Solania.*

**Tired feeling:** Ail., Arum-t.

**TUBERCULOSIS (phthisis pulmonalis):** Acal., Acon., Agarin., *All-s.,* Ant-ar., *Ant-i., Ars., Ars-i.,* Aur-ar., Atrop., *Bac.,* Bals-p., *Bapt.,* Bell., Blatta-o., *Bry., Calc.,* Calc-ar., Calc-chln., Calc-hp., *Calc-i., Calc-p.,* Calo., Cann-s., *Cetr., Chinin-ar.,* Cimic., Coc-c., Cod., *Crot-h.,* Cupr-ar., *Dros.,* Dulc., Erio., Ferr., Ferr-act., *Ferr-ar.,* Ferr-i., *Ferr-p.,* Form., Form-ac., *Gal-ac.,* Guaj., *Guajol.,* Ham., Hep., Helx., Hippoz., Hydr., Hyos-hbr., Hysterion, Ichth., *Iod.,* Iodof., Ip., Kalag., Kali-bi., *Kali-c.,* Kali- n., *Kreos.,* Lac-ac., Lach., *Lachn.,* Laur., Lec., *Lyc.,* Mang-act., Med., Mill., *Myos.,* Myrt-c., Naphtin., *Nat-cac., Nat-sel.,* Nat-s., *Nit-ac.,* Nux-v., Ox-ac., Ph-ac., *Phel., Phos.,* Pilo., Pineal., *Polyg-a.,* Puls., Rumx., Ruta, Salv., *Sang.,* Sep., *Sil.,* Silpho., *Spong., Stann.,* Stann-i., Stict., Succ., *Sulph.,* Teucr-s., Thea, Ther., *Tub.,* Tub-a., Urea., Vanad.

**Acute (phthisis florida):** Ant-t., *Ars.,* Calc., Calc-i., Ferr., Ferr-act., Ferr-m., *Iod., Phos.,* Pilo-m., *Sang.,* Ther., Tub.

**Cough:** All-s., Ars., *Ars-i.,* Bapt., *Bell.,* Calc., Caust., Chin., *Cod.,* Con., *Cor-r.,* Crot-h., *Dros.,* Ferr-ac., *Hep., Hyos.,* Ip., *Kali-c.,* Lach., Laur., Lob., Myos., *Nit-ac., Phos.,* Rumx., Sang., *Sil.,* Silpho., Spong., *Stann.,* Stict., Tub-a.

**Debility:** Acal., Ars., *Ars-i., Chinin-ar.,* Phos., Sil., Tub-a. (See **NERVOUS SYSTEM.**)

**Diarrhea:** Acet-ac., Arg-n., Arn., *Ars.,* Ars-i., Calc., *Chin., Coto,* Iod., Iodof., *Ph-ac., Phos.,* Sil. (See **ABDOMEN.**)

**Digestive disorders:** Ars., Calc., Carb-v., *Cupr-ar.,* Ferr-act., Ferr-ar., Gal-ac., *Hydr.,* Kreos., *Nux-v.,* Strych., Tub-a. (See **STOMACH.**)

**Dyspnea:** Carb-v., Ip., Phos.

**Emaciation:** All-s., Ars., *Ars-i.,* Calc-p., Erio., *Iod.,* Myos., Phos., Sil., Silpho., *Tub.* (See **GENERALITIES.**)

**Fever:** Acon., All-s., Ars., Ars-i., *Bapt.,* Calc-i., Chin., *Chinin-ar., Ferr-p.,* Iod., Lyc., Nit-ac., Phos., Sang., Sil., Stann.

**Fibroid:** Bry., Calc., Sang., *Sil.*

**Haemoptysis:** Acal., *Achil., Acon.,* Calc-ar., Ferr., *Ferr-act., Ferr-p., Ham., Ip.,* Mill., Nit-ac., *Phos.,* Pilo-m., *Tril-p.* (See **Hemoptysis.**)

**Incipient:** Acal., Agar., *Ars-i., Calc.,* Calc-i., Calc-p., *Dros., Ferr-p.,* Iod., Kali-c., Kali-i., Lachn., Mang-act., Med., Myrt-c., Ol-j., *Phos.,* Polyg-a., Puls., Sang., Sec., Succ., Sulph., Tril-p., *Tub.,* Vanad.

**Insomnia:** All-s., *Coff.,* Dig., Sil. (See **NERVOUS SYSTEM.**)

**Liver disturbance:** Chel.

**Mechanical injury, after:** Mill., Ruta.

**Night sweats:** *Acet-ac., Agarcin., Ars.,* Ars-i., Atrop., *Chin.,* Erio., Gal-ac., Hep., *Jab.,* Kali-i., Lyc., Myos., *Ph-ac., Phos.,* Pilo., Pilo-m., Salv., Samb., Sec., *Sil.,* Silpho., Stann. (See **FEVER.**)

**Pains in chest:** Acon., *Bry.,* Calc., Cimic., Guaj., *Kali-c.,* Myrt-c., Phos., Pix. (See **Chest.**)

**Sore mouth:** Lach.

**PLEURAE, EMPYEMA:** Arn., *Ars.,* Calc., *Calc-s., Chin.,* Echi., Ferr., *Hep.,* Ip., Kali-c., *Merc.,* Nat-s., Phos., *Sil.*

**Hydrothorax:** *Adon.,* Ant-t., *Apis,* Apoc., *Ars., Ars-i.,* Canth., Carb-v., Chin., Colch., *Dig.,* Fl-ac., Hell., *Iod., Kali-c.,* Kali-i., *Lact.,* Lyc., *Merc-sul.,* Phase., Phos., Pilo., *Ran-b., Seneg.,* Squil., *Sulph.*

**PLEURISY:** Abrot., *Acon.,* Ant-ar., Ant-t., *Apis,* Arn., *Ars., Asc-t.,* Bell., Borx., *Bry., Canth.,* Carb-an., Chin., *Dig.,* Erio., Ferr-m., *Ferr-p.,* Form., *Guaj.,* Hep., *Iod., Kali-c.,* Kali-i., Led., Lob-c., *Merc.,* Nat-s., Op., Phos., Ran-b., Rhus-t., Sabad., *Seneg,* Sep., Sil., Spig., *Squil., Sulph.,* Tub.

**Adhesions:** Abrot., Carb-an., Hep., Ran-b., Sulph.

**Chronic:** Ars-i., *Hep., Iod.,* Kali-i., Squil., *Sulph.*

**Diaphragmatic:** Acon., *Bry.,* Cact., Cupr., Mosch., *Ran-b.*

**Rheumatic:** Acon., Arn., *Bry.,* Ran-b., Rhod., Rhus-t.

**Tuberculosis:** Ars-i., Bry., Hep., *Iod.,* Iodof., Kali-c.

**With Bright's disease:** Ars., *Merc-c.* (See **URINARY SYSTEM.**)

**RESPIRATION, Arrested (apnea):** Ars., Bov., Camph., Hydr-ac., *Lat-m.,* Lyss., Upa.

**Arrested, on falling asleep:** *Am-c.,* Dig., *Grin.,* Lac-c., *Lach.,* Merc-p-r., *Op., Samb.*

**Cheyne-Stokes:** *Acon-f.,* Antip., Atrop., Bell., Carb-v., Cocain., *Grin.,* Kali-cy., *Morph.,* Op., Parth., *Saroth.*

**DYSPNEA (difficult, embarrassed, oppressed, anxious):** *Acet-ac., Acon., Acon-f.,* Adren., *All-c., Am-c.,* Aml-ns., *Ant-ar.,* Ant-i., *Ant-t., Apis,* Apoc., *Aral., Ars.,* Ars-i., Aur., *Bac.,* Bell., *Blatta-o, Brom., Bry., Cact.,* Caj., *Calc., Calc-ar.,* Canth., Caps., *Carb-v.,* Caust., Cham., Chel., Chin., *Chlor., Coca,* Coll., *Conv., Crat.,* Cupr., *Cupr-act., Cur., Dig.,* Dios., Dros., *Ferr.,* Ferr-p., Fl-ac., *Formal.,* Glon., *Grin., Hep.,* Hydr-ac., Ictod., Ign., Iod., *Ip., Just., Kali-bi., Kali-c., Kali-n., Lach., Laur., Lob., Lyc.,* Merc-c., *Merc-sul.,* Mosch., *Naphtin., Nat-ar., Nat-s., Nux-v.,* Op., *Phos.,* Phyt., *Puls.,* Pulm-v., *Queb.,* Ran-b., Ruta, *Samb., Sang.,* Senec., *Seneg,* Ser-ang., *Sil., Spig., Spong., Squil.,* Stann., *Stroph-h.,* Stry., *Sulph.,* Tab., Verat., Verat-v, *Viol-o., Zinc.* (See **Asthma**).

**Dyspnea, aggavated at P.M.:** Act-sp., *Ars.,* Aur., Cain., Calc., Carb-v., *Dig.,* Phos., Puls., *Samb.,* Sep., *Sulph.,* Trif-p.

**Dyspnea, aggravated during damp, cloudy weather:** Nat-s.

**Dyspnea, aggravated from ascending stairs:** Am-c., Ars., Borx., Calc., Chinin-ar., Iod., Ip., Lob, Nat-m., Sep.

**Dyspnea, aggravated from exposure to cold air:** Act-sp., Lob.

**Dyspnea, aggravated from foreign bodies:** Ant-t., Sil.

**Dyspnea, aggravated from least thing coming near mouth or nose:** Lach.

**Dyspnea, aggravated from lying down:** Abies-n., Act-sp., Aral., *Ars.,* Cain., Dig., Grin., Lach., Merc-sul., Puls., Sep., Stry-ar., Sulph.

**Dyspnea, aggravated from lying on left side:** Naja, Spig., Tab., Visc.

**Dyspnea, aggravated form lying on right side:** Visc.

**Dyspnea, aggravated from lying with head low:** Chin., Kali-n., Spong.

**Dyspnea, aggravated from myocardial disease:** Sarcol-ac.

**Dyspnea, aggravated from nervous causes:** Ambr., Arg-n., Ars., Asaf., *Caj., Mosch.,* Nux-m., Puls., *Valer.,* Viol-o.

**Dyspnea, aggravated from rest:** Sil.

**Dyspnea, aggravated from sinking sensation in abdomen:** Acet-ac.
**Dyspnea, aggravated from sitting up:** Carb-v., Laur., Psor., Sep.
**Dyspnea, aggravated from sleep:** Dig., *Lach., Samb.,* Sep., Spong.
**Dyspnea, aggravated from sleep; sitting indoors, relieved by rapid motion:** Sep.
**Dyspnea, aggravated from stooping:** Calc., Sil.
**Dyspnea, aggravated from walking:** *Acon.,* Am-c., Carb-v., Con., *Ip.,* Kali-c., Nat-m., Sep., Sil.
**Dyspnea, aggravated from working:** Am-m., Calc., Lyc., Nat-m., Nit-ac., Sep., Sil., Sumb.
**Dyspnea, aggravated in aged, alcoholics, athletics:** Coca.
**Dyspnea, aggravated in children:** Lyc., Samb.
**Dyspnea, aggravated in lower chest:** Lob-s., Nux-v.
**Dyspnea, aggravated in morning:** Ant-t., Con., Kali-bi., Kali-c., Nat-s.
**Dyspnea, aggravated in warm room:** Am-c., Puls., Sep.
**Dyspnea, relieved from bending forward:** Ars., Kali-c.
**Dyspnea, relieved from bending shoulders backwards:** Calc.
**Dyspnea, relieved from eructating:** Ambr., Ant-t.
**Dyspnea, relieved form expectoration:** *Ant-t.,* Ars., Kali-bi., Zinc.
**Dyspnea, relieved from fanning rapidly:** Carb-v.
**Dyspnea, relieved from fanning slowly and at a distance:** Lach.
**Dyspnea, relieved from lying down:** Kali-bi., *Psor.*
**Dyspnea, relieved from lying on right side:** Ant-t.
**Dyspnea, relieved from lying on right side, head high:** Cact., Spig., Spong.
**Dyspnea, relieved from motion:** Lob, Sep.
**Dyspnea, relieved from sitting up:** Acon-f., Ant-t., *Ars.,* Dig., Laur., Merc-sul., Nat-s., *Samb.,* Sulph., Ter.
**Dyspnea, relieved from standing up:** Cann-s.
**Dyspnea, relieved from stretching arms apart:** Psor.
**Dyspnea, relieved in open air:** Calc., Lach., *Sulph.*
**Gasping:** Brom., Hydr-ac., *Ip.,* Phos., Samb.
**Hoarse, hissing:** Acet-ac.
**Inspiration difficult:** Brom., Cact., Chel., Iod., Nicot., *Ox-ac.* (See **Dyspnea.**)
**Inspiration free, expiration impeded:** *Chlor.,* Med., Meph., *Samb.*
**Irregular:** Ail., *Ant-t.,* Bell., Crat., *Dig.,* Hell., Hippoz., *Hydr-ac.,* Op., Tril-p.
**Rapid, short, superficial:** Acon., *Acon-f.,* Am-c., *Ant-t.,* Apis, *Apoc.,* Aral., *Ars.,* Bell., *Bry.,* Calc., Carb-v., Cupr., Cupr-act., Cur., *Ferr-p.,* Hippoz., Kali-bi., Lach., Lob-p., Lyc., Mag-p., Merc-cy., Merc-sul., Nat-s., *Nux-v.,* Ox-ac., Ph-ac., *Phos.,* Prun., Seneg, Sil., *Spong.,* Stann., Sul-ac.

**Rattling:** All-s., Am-c., Am-caust., Am-m., *Ammc., Ant-ar., Ant-t.,* Bals-p., Bar-c., Bar-m., *Brom.,* Calc., Calc-act., Cann-s., Carb-v., Cham., *Chel., Chin.,* Chlor., Cupr., Dulc., Ferr-p., Grin., *Hep., Ip.,* Kali-bi., Kali-c., Kali-m., Kali-n., *Kali-s.,* Lyc., Meph., *Nat-s.,* Oena., *Op.,* Phos., Pix, *Puls., Seneg,* Sil., Squil., *Stann., Sulph.,* Verat.

**Sawing:** Brom., Iod., Samb., *Spong.*

**Sighing:** Ail., Apoc., Cact., *Calc-p.,* Carb-ac., Cere-b., *Dig.,* Gels., Gran., Hell., *Ign., Lach.,* Led., Naphtin., Nat-p., *Op.,* Phase., Pilo., Samb., Sec., Sulfon.

**Slow, deep:** Am-c., Aur., Ben-d., Cact., Cann-i., Chin., Dig., Gad., Gels., *Hell., Hydr-ac.,* Laur., Lob-p., *Op.,* Phase., Pilo., *Verat*-v.

**Stertorous:** Acon., Am-c., Arn., Bell., Bry., Cann-i., *Chin.,* Euph-l., *Hell.,* Hippoz., *Hydr-ac.,* Lob-p., Naja, Nat-sal., *Oena., Op.,* Phase., Phos., Pilo., Sec., *Sulfon.,* Tanac., Trion., Verat-v., Visc.

**Suffocative:** *Acon-f., Ant-t., Apis, Ars.,* Bell., Brom., Cact., *Calc.,* Camph., *Chin., Chlor.,* Cor-r., Cupr., *Dig.,* Graph., *Grin., Guaj.,* Hep., Hydr-ac., Iod., *Ip.,* Kali-bi., Kali-i., *Lach., Lat-m.,* Led., Lil-t., Lob, Lyc., Meli., Meph., Merc-cy., *Merc-p-r.,* Morph., *Mosch.,* Naja, Puls., *Samb., Spong., Sulph.,* Tub., Trif-p., Verat., Visc.

**Wheezing:** Alum., Am-c., Ant-i., *Ant-t.,* Aral., *Ars.,* Cann-s., Carb-v., Card-m., Erio., *Grin., Hep.,* Iod., Iodof., *Ip.,* Just., Kali-bi., *Kali-c.,* Lob, Lycps-v., Nux-v., Prun., *Samb.,* Seneg., *Spong.* (See **Asthma**.)

**Whistling:** Ars., Ip., Samb.

**TRACHEA, Burning:** *Ars.,* Kali-bi., Sang. (See **Irritation**.)

**Catarrh:** Alum., Anis., *Ant-t.,* Arg-n., Ars., *Bry.,* Calc., Cann-s., Carb-v., *Caust.,* Coc-c., Conv., Cot., Ferr-i., Hep., Iber., *Kali-bi.,* Mang-act., *Merc.,* Naphtin., Nat-m., Nux-v., Par., *Rumx.,* Sil., *Stann.,* Stict., Sulph., Tab.

**Constricted feeling:** Brom., Cist., Gua., *Mosch., Nux-v.,* Xero.

**Dryness:** Ars., Bell., Carb-v., *Rumx.,* Sang., Spong. (See **Irritation**.)

**Irritation, rawness, hypersensitiveness:** Acet-ac., *Aesc.,* Alum-sil., Ambro., Apis, Arg-met., *Arg-n.,* Ars., *Bell.,* Brom., *Bry.,* Cann-s., Carb-an., Carb-v., *Caust.,* Ferr-p., *Hyos.,* Kali-bi., *Lach.,* Menth., *Osm., Phos., Rumx., Sang.,* Stann., Still., Sulph., Syph., Xero.

**Tickling:** Ambro., Brom., Calc., Caps., *Carb-v.,* Cop., Ip., *Lach.,* Nux-v., *Phos., Rumx.* (See **Cough**.)

■

# CIRCULATORY SYSTEM

**ARTERIES, AORTA, Inflamed, acute (aortitis):** Acon., Apis, Glon., Tub.

**Aorta, inflamed, chronically (aortitis chronica):** Adon., *Adren., Ant-ar., Ars-i.,* Aur., Aur-ar., *Cact.,* Chinin-s., Crat., Cupr., Glon., Kali-i., Lyc., *Nat-i.,* Spig., Stroph-h.

**Aortitis, ulcerative:** Acon., Ars., Chinin-s.

**Aorta, pain:** Adren., Strych. (See **Angina Pectoris.**)

**Arteritis:** Ars., Carb-v., Echi., *Kali-i.,* Lach., *Nat-i.,* Sec.

**Atheroma of arteries (arteriosclerosis):** Adren., *Am-i.,* Am-van., Ant-ar., Arn., Ars., *Ars-i.,* Aur., *Aur-i.,* Aur-m-n., *Bar-c.,* Bar-m., Cact, Calc-f., Chinin-s., Con., Crat., Ergot., *Glon., Kali-i.,* Kali-sal., Lach., Lith-c., *Nat-i.,* Phos., Plb., *Plb-i., Polyg-a.,* Sec., Stront-c., *Stront-i.,* Stroph-h., Sumb., Thyr., *Vanad.* (See **Interstitial Nephritis.**)

**Carotids, pulsate:** *Acon.,* Aml-ns., *Bell., Cact.,* Chin., Fago., *Glon.,* Lil-t., Sabin., *Verat-v.* (See **Pulse.**)

**Circulation, sluggish:** Aeth., Calc., *Calc-p.,* Carb-an., *Carb-v.,* Cimic., Cinnm., Ferr-p., *Gels.,* Led., Nat-m., *Rhus-t., Sil.* (See **Heart.**)

**Congestion of blood (local):** *Acon.,* Aesc., Ambr., *Aml-ns.,* Aur., *Bell., Cact.,* Calc., Cent., Cupr., Ferr., *Ferr-p.,* Gad., *Glon.,* Kali-i., Lil-t., Lon-c., *Meli.,* Mill., Phos., *Sang., Sep.,* Sil., Spong., Stel., *Sulph., Verat-v.*

**Degeneration, fatty:** Phos. (See **Heart.**)

**Dilatation: Aneurism:** Acon., Ars-i., *Bar-c., Bar-m.,* Cact., Calc-f., Calc-p., Glon., Iod., *Kali-i.,* Kalm., Lach., Lith-c., *Lyc.,* Lycps-v., Morph., *Nat-i.,* Plb., Puls., Spig., Spong., *Verat-v.*

**Aneurism, capillary:** *Calc-f.,* Fl-ac., Tub.

**Aneurism, pain:** Cact. (See **Angina Pectoris.**)

**RUPTURE of artery (apoplexy):** *Acon.,* Apis, *Arn.,* Aster., Bar-c., *Bell.,* Cact., Camph., Caust., Chen-a., Chin., Croc., Crot-h., Cupr., Form., *Glon.,* Hydr-ac., Hyos., Juni-v., Kali-br., Kali-i., *Lach., Laur., Nux-v., Op., Phos.,* Sep., Stram., Sulph., Verat., *Verat-v.*

**Rupture of artery, post-hemiplegia:** *Arn.,* Ars., *Bar-c.,* Bell., Both., *Caust., Cocc.,* Cupr., Cur., Lach., Nux-v., Phos., *Plb.,* Rhus-t., Vip., Zinc.

**Rupture of artery, predisposition to, or threatened:** *Acon.,* Arn., Ars., Bar-c., *Bell.,* Calc-f., *Gels., Glon.,* Guaj., Hyos., *Lach.,* Laur., *Nux-v., Op., Phos.,* Stront-c.

**HEART, Action tumultuous, violent, labored:** Abies-c., Absin., *Acon.,* Aesc., *Agar., Aml-ns.,* Ammc., Ars., *Aur., Bell.,* Bry., *Cact.,* Carb-ac., Cimic., Colch., Conv., Ephe., Gels., *Glon.,* Helo., Iber., Kalm., *Lil-t., Lycps-v., Nat-m.,* Phys., Prun., Pyrog., *Spig.,* Spong., *Verat-v.* (See **Pulse.**)

**AFFECTIONS in general:** *Acon., Adon.,* Am-c., Am-m., *Aml-ns.,* Apoc., Arn., *Ars., Ars-i.,* Aur., Aur-m., Bar-c., Bell., Benz-ac., *Bry., Cact., Calc-ar.,* Calc-f., Carb-v., Chin., Cimic., Coca, Colch., *Coll., Conv.,* Coron-v., *Crat., Crot-h., Dig., Digin.,* Ferr., Ferr-p., Gels., *Glon.,* Grin., *Hydr-ac., Iber.,* Ign., Iod., Kali-c., *Kali-chl., Kalm., Lach.,* Laur., Lepi., *Lil-t.,* Lith-c., *Lycps-v.,* Merc-c., Mosch., *Naja,* Nat-i., Nat-m., Nux-v., *Ox-ac., Phase., Phos.,* Pilo., *Saroth., Spig., Spong.,* Squil., *Stroph-h., Strych.,* Sumb., Thyr., Valer., Verat-v. (See Separate **Diseases of Heart**.)

**Affections, rheumatic:** Acon., Aur., Benz-ac., *Bry.,* Cact., Caust., Cimic., *Colch.,* Ign., Kalm., Led., Lith-c., Lycps-v., Naja, Phyt., *Rhus-t., Spig.,* Verat-v.

**Affections, with hemorrhoids:** Cact., *Coll.,* Dig.

**CYANOSIS:** Acetan., Am-c., *Ant-ar., Ant-t., Ars.,* Ben-n., Carb-an., *Carb-v.,* Crot-h., Cupr., *Dig.,* Hydr-ac., Lach., *Laur.,* Lycps-v., Merc-cy., Nat-n., Phos., Pilo., Psor., *Rhus-t.,* Samb., Tab., Zinc.

**DEBILITY, weakness:** Acetan., Acet-ac., *Adon.,* Adren., *Am-c., Am-m.,* Ant-ar., *Ars., Ars-i.,* Aur., *Cact., Calc-ar.,* Camph., Carb-ac., *Carb-v.,* Chin., Chinin-ar., *Conv., Crat., Dig.,* Dios., Euph., Ferr., Grin., Helo., *Hydr-ac., Iber.,* Kali-c., Kalm., Lach., Lil-t., Lycps-v., Morph., Mosch., Nit-ac., Nux-m., Olnd., Phase., Plb., Prun., Psor., Pyrog., Sarcol-ac., *Saroth.,* Ser-ang., Spig., Squil., *Stroph-h.,* Tab., Thyr., *Verat.*

**Debility, weakness, muscular, "heart failure":** Adon., Adren., Aether., Agarin., *Alco.,* Aml-ns., Ant-t., Atrop., *Coffin.,* Camphorated oil, Cocain., Conv., Crat., *Dig., Digit., Glon.,* Oxygen inhalation, Sacch., Saline infusion, Saroth., Ser-ang., *Stroph-h., Stry-s.,* Verat.

**Debility, weakness, nervous:** Adren., Cact., *Iber.,* Ign., *Lil-t.,* Lith-c., *Mosch., Naja,* Pilo., Prun., Saroth., *Spig.,* Tab., *Valer.*

**Debility, weakness, with dropsy:** *Acetan., Adon., Apoc., Ars.,* Ars-i., Asc-c., Cact., *Coffin.,* Coll., *Conv., Dig.,* Iber., Lach., Lycps-v., Olnd., Saroth., Squil., *Stroph-h.* (See **GENERALITIES**.)

**DEGENERATION, fatty:** Adon., Adon-ae., Arn., *Ars.,* Ars-i., *Aur., Bar-c.,* Cimic., Crat., Cupr-act., Fuc., *Kali-c.,* Kali-fcy., Kalm., Ph-ac., *Phos.,* Phys., *Phyt.,* Sacch., Stroph-h., Stry-ar., Stry-p., *Vanad.*

**DILATATION:** Adon., Am-c., *Ars.,* Ars-i., *Bar-c., Cact.,* Cimic., Conv., *Crat., Dig.,* Gels., Iber., *Naja, Phase.,* Phos., Phys., Prun., Saroth., *Spig.,* Stroph-h., Tab., Verat-v. (See **Debility, muscular**.)

**DYSPNEA (Cardiac):** Acon., *Acon-f.,* Adon., *Adren.,* Am-c., Apis, Arn., Ars., Ars-i., Aur., *Cact., Calc-ar.,* Carb-v., *Chinin-ar.,* Cimic., Coll., Conv., *Dig., Glon., Iber.,* Kali-n., Kalm., Lach., Laur., Lycps-v., Magn-gr., Naja, Ox-ac., Op., *Queb.,* Spig., Spong., Stroph-h., Stry-ar., Sumb., Visc. (See **RESPIRATORY SYSTEM**.)

**Hydropericardium:** Apis, Apoc., Ant-ar., Ars., Iod., Lach.

**HYPERTROPHY:** *Acon., Arn.,* Ars., Aur., Bell., *Brom., Cact.,* Coffin., *Caust.,* Cere-b., *Conv., Crat., Dig.,* Glon., *Iber.,* Iod., Kalm., Lil-t., Lycps-v., *Naja,* Phos., Phyt., *Rhus-t.,* Spig., *Spong.,* Stroph-h., Stry-ar., *Verat-v.,* Visc.

**Hypertrophy uncomplicated, of athletes:** Arn., Brom., Caust., *Rhus-t.*

**INFLAMMATION (ENDOCARDITIS): Acute:** *Acon.,* Ars., Bell., *Cact., Colch.,* Conv., Dig., *Lach.,* Magn-gr., *Naja,* Phos., *Spig.,* Spong., Tab., Verat-v. (See **Pericarditis.**)

**Endocarditis, malignant:** Acon., Ars., *Chinin-s.,* Crot-h., Lach., Vip.

**Endocarditis, rheumatic:** Acon., Adon., Bell., *Bry., Colch.,* Kali-c., Kalm., Rhus-t., *Spig.*

**MYOCARDITIS:** Acon., Adon., *Ars-i.,* Aur-m., Cact., Chinin-ar., Crat., *Dig.,* Gala., Iod., Lach., Phos., Stroph-h., *Vip.* (See **Weakness, Degeneration.**)

**PERICARDITIS, acute:** *Acon.,* Adon., Ant-ar., *Apis, Ars.,* Asc-t., Bell., *Bry.,* Cact., Cann-s., *Canth., Colch.,* Dig., Iod., Kali-c., *Kali-i.,* Kalm., Magn-gr., *Merc.,* Merc-c., Naja, Nat-m., Phase., *Spig., Spong.,* Squil., Sulph., Verat., Verat-v.

**Pericarditis, chronic:** Apis, *Aur-i.,* Calc-f., Kali-c., Spig., Squil., Sulph.

**Pericarditis, rheumatic:** Acon., Anac., Bry., Colch., *Colchin.,* Crat., Kalm., Rhus-t., *Spig.*

**NEUROSES:** *Acon.,* Adren., Cact., Cham., Chin., *Coff.,* Ferr., *Gels., Iber., Ign.,* Lach., *Lil-t.,* Lycps-v., *Mosch., Nux-v.,* Prun-v., Scut., Sep., *Spig., Tab.,* Verat., Zinc.

**Neuroses, irritable from influenza:** Iber., Saroth.

**Neuroses, irritable from tea, coffee:** Agarin.

**Neuroses, irritable from tobacco:** *Agarin.,* Agn., Ars., Calad., *Conv.,* Dig., *Kalm.,* Lycps-v., Nux-v., *Phos., Spig.,* Staph., *Stroph-h.,* Tab., Verat.

**Neuroses, irritable from suppressed hemorrhoids:** Coll.

**Neuroses, irritable from utero-ovarian disease:** Cimic., Lil-t.

**Neuroses, irritable tremulousness, from scarlet fever:** Lach.

**PAIN:** Abies-n., *Acon., Adon., Aml-ns.,* Apis, Arn., *Ars.,* Aster., *Bry., Cact.,* Calc-f., Canth., Cere-b., Cere-s., *Cimic.,* Coff., *Colch.,* Conv., Crat., Daph., *Dig.,* Dios., *Ferr-t., Haem., Hydr-ac.,* Iber, *Kalm.,* Lach., *Lat-m.,* Lepi., *Lil-t., Lith-c.,* Lob., Lycps-v., Magn-gr., Med., *Naja,* Onos., *Ox-ac.,* Ovi-p, *Paeon.,* Pip-n., Ptel., *Spig., Spong., Stroph-h.,* Syph., Tab., *Ther.,* Thyr., *Verat-v.,* Zinc-val.

**Pain at apex:** Lil-t.

**Pain at base:** Lob.

**Pain constricting, as if squeezed in vise:** *Acon.,* Adon., Aml-ns., Arn., Ars., *Cact.,* Cadm-s., Calc-ar., Coc-c., Colch., *Iod.,* Iodof., Kali-c., Lach., Laur., *Lil-t.,* Lycps-v., Mag-p., Magn-gr., Nux-m., Ptel., Spong., *Thyr.*

**Neuralgic, ANGINA PECTORIS:** *Acon., Adren., Aml-ns.,* Arg-cy., Arg-n., *Arn., Ars.,* Ars-i., Aur-m., Bism., *Cact.,* Camph., Cere-b., Chinin-ar., *Cimic., Cocain.,* Conv., *Crat.,* Crot-h., *Cupr., Cupr-act.,* Dig., Dios., *Glon., Haem., Hydr-ac.,* Kali-c., Kali-i., Kalm., *Lat-m.,* Lil-t., Lith-c., Lob., *Mag-p.,* Magn-gr., Morph., *Naja, Nat-i.,* Nat-n., *Nux-v.,* Olnd., *Ox-ac.,* Phos., Phyt., Pip-n., Prun., Samb., Saroth., *Spig., Spong.,* Staph., Stront-c., Stront-i., *Tab.,* Thyr., Verat-v., Zinc-val.

**From abuse of coffee:** Coff.

**From abuse stimulants:** Nux-v., Spig.

**From muscular origin:** Cupr., Hydr-ac.

**From organic heart disease:** *Ars-i., Cact.,* Calc-f., Crat., Kalm., Nat-i., Stront-i., Tab.

**From rheumatism:** Cimic., Lith-c.

**From straining, overlifting:** *Arn.,* Carb-an., Caust.

**From tobacco:** Kalm., Lil-t., Nux-v., Spig., Staph., Tab.

**Pseudo-angina pectoris:** Aconin., Cact., *Lil-t., Mosch.,* Nux-v., Tarent. (See **Pain.**)

**Precordial oppression, anxiety, heaviness:** *Acon., Adon., Adren.,* Aesc., Agar., Am-c., Aml-ns., Apis, *Ars., Ars-i.,* Aspar., Aur., Brom., Bry., *Cact.,* Calc., Calc-ar., *Camph.,* Carb-v., Cere-b., Cimic., *Colch.,* Coll., Cot., *Crat.,* Cupr., *Dig.,* Dios., Ferr., Glon., Haem., *Hydr-ac., Iber.,* Ign., *Iod.,* Ip., Kalm., *Lach., Lat-m.,* Laur., *Lil-t.,* Lith-c., *Lycps-v.,* Magn-gr., Meny., *Naja,* Nat-ar., Prim-v., *Puls.,* Sapo., *Spig., Spong.,* Tab., *Thea,* Thyr., Vanad., Verat-v.

**Shooting, down left shoulder, arm to fingers:** *Acon.,* Arn., Asper., Bism., *Cact.,* Cimic., Crot-h., *Kalm., Lat-m.,* Lepi., Naja, *Ox-ac., Rhus-t., Spig.,* Tab.

**Shooting, from apex to base:** Med.

**Shooting, from base to apex at night:** Syph.

**Shooting from back to clavicle, shoulder:** Spig.

**Shooting, lancincating, tearing:** Ars., Bell., *Cact.,* Cere-b., Cimic., Colch., Daph.., Glon., *Iber., Kalm., Lat-m.,* Lil-t., Lith-c., Magn-gr., Mentho., *Ox-ac.,* Paeon., Phyt., *Spig.,* Syph., Tab. (See **Neuralgia**.)

**Stitching, cutting:** *Abies-n., Acon.,* Anac., Ars., Asc-t., *Bry., Cact.,* Cann-i., Caust., Cere-b., Dig., Iber., *Kali-c.,* Kali-n., Lith-c., Naja, *Spig.*

**PALPITATION:** *Abies-c., Acon., Adon., Agar.,* Agarin., Aml-ns., Apis, *Arg-n., Ars.,* Asaf., *Aur.,* Aur-m., Bar-c., *Bell., Cact.,* Calc., *Calc-ar.,* Camph., Canth., Cann-i., Carb-v., Chin., Chinin-ar., *Cimic., Coca, Cocc., Coff.,* Colch., Con., *Conv.,* Crat., Cupr., *Dig.,* Digin., Fago., Ferr., Ferr-p., *Gels., Glon.,* Hydr., *Hydr-ac., Iber., Ign., Iod., Kali-c.,* Kali-fcy., *Kalm., Lach.,* Laur., *Lil-t.,* Lob., *Lycps-v., Mosch.,* Naja, *Nat-m.,* Nux-m., *Nux-v.,* Ol-j.,

Olnd., Ox-ac., Ph-ac., *Phase.*, *Phos.*, Plat., *Puls.*, *Pyrog.*, Sec., Sep., *Spig.*, *Spong.*, *Sulph.*, *Sumb.*, *Tab.*, Thea, *Thyr.*, Valer., Verat-v., Zinc.

**CAUSE, Anemia, vital drains:** Ars., *Chin.*, Dig., *Ferr-r.*, Kali-c., Kali-fcy., Nat-m., *Ph-ac.*, Phos., *Puls.*, Spig., Verat.

**Children, growing too fast:** Ph-ac.

**Dyspepsia:** Abies-c., *Abies-n.*, Arg-n., Cact., *Carb-v.*, *Chin.*, Coca, Coff., Coll., Dios., Hydr-ac., Lyc., *Nux-v.*, Puls., Prun-v., Sep., Spig., Tab.

**Emotional causes:** *Acon.*, Ambr., Am-val., Anac., Cact., *Calc-ar.*, Cham., *Coff.*, Gels., Hydr-ac., *Ign.*, Iod., Lach., Lith-c., *Mosch.*, Nux-m., Nux-v., Op., Plat., Sep., Tarent.

**Eruption suppressed:** Calc.

**Exertion, even slightest:** Bell., Brom., Cimic., Coca, Conv., *Dig.*, *Iber.*, *Iod.*, Nat-m., Sarcol-ac., *Thyr.*

**Grief:** *Ign.*, Ph-ac.

**Heart strain:** *Arn.*, Borx., *Caust.*, Coca.

**Nervous irritaion:** Atrop., Cact., *Coff.*, *Glon.*, Hydr-ac., Hyos., Ign., Kali-c., Kali-p., Lil-t., *Lycps-v.*, Mag-p., *Mosch.*, *Naja*, Sep., Spig., *Sumb.*

**Prolonged brain work, sexual excesses:** Coca.

**Tea drinking:** Chin.

**Tobacco:** Agar., Ars., Cact., *Gels.*, Nux-v., Stroph-h.

**Uterine disease:** Conv., Lil-t.

**Worms:** Spig.

**CONCOMITANTS, With anguish, restlessness:** *Acon.*, Aeth., Ars., Calc., Coff., Ign., Lach., Nat-m., Phase., *Phos.*, *Puls.*, Sapo., Spig., *Spong.*, Verat., Zinc.

**With burning at heart:** Kali-c.

**With choking in throat:** Iber., Lach., Naja.

**With dim vision:** Puls.

**With dyspnea:** Am-c., *Cact.*, Dig., *Glon.*, Glyc., Lach., Olnd., Naja, Ox-ac., *Phos.*, Spig., *Spong.*, Verat., Zinc.

**With face red:** Agar., Aur., Bell., Glon.

**With fainting:** Acon., *Cham.*, *Lach.*, Nat-m., *Nux-m.*, Petr., *Tab.*

**With fetor oris:** Spig.

**With flatulence:** *Arg-n.*, Cact., Carb-v., *Nux-v.*

**With headache:** Aeth., Bell., Lith-c.

**With heart labored, reverberates in head:** Aur., Bell., *Glon.*, Spig., Spong.

**With heart weak:** Coca, Dig.

**With hot feeling, uncomfortable:** Ant-t., Calc., Kali-c., Petr.

**With pain, precordial:** *Acon.*, Ars., *Cact.*, Cham., Caust., *Coff.*, *Hydr-ac.*, Laur., Mag-m., Naja, *Spig.*, Spong.

**With piles or suppressed menses, alternating:** Coll.
**With sleeplessness:** Cimic., Coca, *Ign.,* Spig.
**With stomach, heavy feeling in:** Upa.
**With stomach, sinking in:** Cimic.
**With tinnitus, mental depression, anorexia, chest oppression:** Coca.
**With trembling:** Asaf., Lach., Rhus-t., *Sul-ac.*
**With urination, copious:** Coff.
**With uterine soreness:** Conv.
**With vertigo:** Adon., Aeth., Cact., Coron-v., *Iber.,* Spig.
**With weakness, empty feeling in chest:** Olnd.

**AGGRAVATION, After eating:** Calc., Lil-t., Lyc., Nat-m., *Nux-v.,* Puls.
**At approach of menses:** *Cact.,* Crot-h., Spong.
**At night:** *Ars.,* Cact., Calc., Iber., Ign., Lil-t., Lyc., Nat-m., Phos., Tab.
**During sleep:** Alst., Am-c., *Cann-i.,* Iber., Ph-ac., Spong.
**From least motion:** Acon., Bell., *Cact., Calc-ar.,* Cimic., *Dig.,* Ferr., Iber., *Lil-t.,* Nat-m., *Spig.*
**From lying down:** *Ars.,* Kali-c., Lach., Lil-t., Nat-m., Nux-v., Sep., Spig., Thyr.
**From lying on left side:** Bar-c., *Cact.,* Lac-c., *Lach.,* Lyc., Nat-m., *Phos.,* Puls., *Tab.,* Thea.
**From lying on right side:** *Alumn.,* Arg-n.
**From mental exertion:** Calc-ar.
**From rising:** Cact.
**From sitting:** Mag-m., Phos., Rhus-t.
**From sitting bent forward:** Kalm.
**From stooping forward:** Spig.
**From thinking of it:** Bar-c., Gels., *Ox-ac.*
**In morning on waking:** Kali-c., Nux-v.

**AMELIORATION, Lying on right side:** Lac-c., Tab.
**Motion:** Ferr., Gels., *Mag-m.*

**PULSE, Full, round, bounding, strong, felt all over:** *Acon.,* Aesc., Am-m., *Aml-ns.,* Antip., Arn., *Aur.,* Bar-c., *Bell.,* Bry., *Cact.,* Calc., Canth., Coff., Cupr., Fago., Ferr., *Glon.,* Ictod., *Iod., Lil-t.,* Lycps-v., Onos., *Op., Phys.,* Pilo., Puls., *Sabin.,* Spig., Spong., *Verat-v.*
**Intermittent:** Acon., *Apoc.,* Bapt., *Cact., Carb-v.,* Chin., Colch., Conv., *Crat., Dig.,* Ferr-m., *Iber.,* Ign., *Kali-c.,* Kalm., Lil-t., *Lycps-v.,* Merc-c., Merc-cy., *Nat-m.,* Nux-m., Ph-ac., Pip-n., Rhus-t., Sec., *Sep., Spig., Stroph-h.,* Tab., Ter., Thea, Verat., *Verat-v.,* Zinc.
**Intermittent, every third to seventh beat:** Dig., *Mur-ac.*
**Irregular:** Acetan., Acon., Adon., Adren., *Agarin.,* Antip., Apoc., Arn., *Ars., Ars-i., Aur.,* Bell., *Cact.,* Coffin., Camph., *Chin.,* Cimic., *Conv., Crat.,*

*Dig.*, Ferr., Gels., *Glon.*, *Hydr-ac.*, *Iber.*, Ign., Kali-c., Kalm., *Lach.*, Laur., *Lil-t.*, *Lycps-v.*, Mur-ac., *Naja*, *Nat-m.*, Nux-m., *Ph-ac.*, *Phase.*, Pilo., Puls., Rhus-t., Sang., Sec., Ser-ang., *Saroth.*, Spig., Stroph-h., Stry-ar., Stry-p., Sumb., *Tab.*, Thea, Verat., *Verat-v.*, Zinc.

**Rapid (tachycardia):** *Abies n.*, *Acon.*, Adon., Adren., *Agn.*, Am-val., Ant-ar., Ant-c., *Ant-t.*, Antip., Apoc., Arn., Ars-i., *Bell.*, Bry., *Cact.*, Canth., Carb-v., Coff., Colch., Coll., *Conv.*, *Crat.*, *Dig.*, Diph., Ferr-p., *Gels.*, Glon., *Iber.*, Kalm., Kali-chl., Lach., Lat-m., Led., *Lil-t.*, *Lycps-v.*, Merc-c., *Morph.*, Mur-ac., *Naja*, Nat-m., Phase., *Phos.*, Phyt., Pilo., Pyrog., Rhod., Rhus-t., Sec., Sep., Ser-ang., Spong., Stroph-h., Stry-p., Tab., Ter., Thea., *Thyr.*, Verat., Verat-v. (See **Weak.**)

**Rapid in morning:** Ars., Sulph.

**Rapid, out of all proportion to temperature:** Lil-t., *Pyrog.*

**Slow (bradycardia):** *Abies-n.*, Adon., Adren., Aesc., *Apoc.*, Cact., *Camph.*, *Cann-i.*, Canth., Caust., Colch., Cupr., *Dig.*, Esin., *Gels.*, Helo., Hell., *Kalm.*, Lat-m., *Lup.*, Lycpr., *Morph.*, Myric., Naja, *Op.*, Pip-n., Rhus-t., Spig., Tab., Verat., *Verat-v.* (See **Weak.**)

**Slow, alternating with rapid:** Chin., Dig., *Gels.*, Iod., Morph.

**Soft, compressible:** Acal., *Ars.*, Bapt., *Coffin.*, Conv., Ferr., *Ferr-p.*, *Gels.*, Kali-c., *Phos.*, Plb., Verat., *Verat-v.* (See **Weak.**)

**Weak, fluttering, almost imperceptible:** Acetan., *Acon.*, *Adon.*, Adren., Aeth., *Agarin.*, Ail., Am-m., Ant-ar., Ant-t., Apis, Arn., *Ars.*, *Ars-i.*, *Aur.*, Aspar., Bar-m., *Cact.*, *Coffin.*, *Camph.*, Carb-ac., Carb-v., Cimic., Colch., Coll., *Conv.*, Crat., Crot-h., *Dig.*, Diph., *Ferr.*, *Gels.*, *Hydr-ac.*, Hyosin-hbr., Iod., *Kali-c.*, Kali-chl., *Kali-n.*, Kalm., *Lach.*, *Lat-m.*, *Laur.*, Lycps-v., Merc-c., *Merc-cy.*, Morph., *Mur-ac.*, Naja, Op., Ox-ac., *Ph-ac.*, *Phase.*, *Phos.*, Phys., Plb., Rhus-t., Sang., *Sapo.*, *Saroth.*, Sec., Ser-ang., *Spig.*, Sulph., *Tab.*, Ter., *Thyr.*, *Verat.*, *Verat-v.*, Visc., Zinc.

**SENSATIONS, As if drops were falling from heart:** Cann-s.

**As if heart were burning:** Kali-c., Op., Tarent.

**As if heart were ceasing its beat:** Antip., Chinin-ar., Cimic., Crat., *Dig.*, Lob., *Phase.*, Trif-p.

**As if heart were ceasing its beat, then started suddenly:** *Aur.*, Conv., Lil-t., Sep.

**As if heart were ceasing its beat when moving about, must keep still:** Cocain., *Dig.*

**As if heart were ceasing its beat when resting, must move about:** Gels., Trif-p.

**As if heart were cold:** Calc., *Carb-an.*, Graph., *Helo.*, Kali-bi., *Kali-m.*, Kali-n., Lil-t., *Nat-m.*, Petr.

**As if heart were fluttering:** Absin., *Acon.*, Aml-ns., Apoc., Asaf., *Cact.*,

*Cimic.*, Conv., Crot-h., Ferr., Glon., *Iber.*, *Kalm.*, Lach., *Lil-t.*, Lith-c., *Mosch.*, Naja, *Nat-m.*, Nux-m., Ph-ac., *Phase.*, *Phys.*, Pyrog., *Spig.*, Sul-ac., Thea. (See **Palpitation**.)

**As if heart were purring:** Pyrog., Spig.

**As if heart were squeezed by iron hand:** Arn., *Cact.*, Iod., *Lil-t.*, Sulph., Vanad., Visc.

**As if heart were suspended by thread:** Kali-c., Lach.

**As if heart were too full, bursting:** *Aesc.*, Aml-ns., Aur-m., *Bell.*, Bufo, *Cact.*, Cench., Coll., Conv., *Glon.*, Glyc., Iber., Lact., *Lil-t.*, Pyrog., *Spig.*, Stroph-h., *Sulph.*, Vanad.

**As if heart were tired:** Pyrog.

**As if heart were twisted:** *Lach.*, Tarent.

**Soreness, tenderness of heart:** *Arn.*, *Cact.*, Camph., Gels., Haem., Lith-c., Lycps-v., *Naja*, Sec., *Spig.*

**SYNCOPE, (fainting):** Acetan., Acet-ac., *Acon.*, Alet., Aml-ns., Apis, *Ars.*, Cact., *Canth.*, Carb-v., Cham., *Chin.*, Cimic., Coll., Croc., Cupr., *Dig.*, Ferr., Glon., *Ign.*, Ip., Lach., Lil-t., *Lina.*, Mag-m., Magn-gr., *Mosch.*, *Nux-m.*, Nux-v., Op., Ph ac., Phase., Phos., Puls., Sep., *Spig.*, Spong., *Sulph.*, *Sumb.*, Tab., Thyr., Tril-p., *Verat.*, Zinc.

**Syncope from odors, in morning, after eating:** Nux-v.

**Syncope, lipothymia, hysterical:** *Acon.*, Apisin., Asaf., Cham., Cocc., Cupr., *Ign.*, Lach., *Mosch.*, Nux-m.

**VALVULAR DISEASE:** Acon., *Adon.*, Apoc., *Ars.*, *Ars-i.*, Aur., Aur-br., Aur-i., *Cact.*, Calc-f., Camph, *Conv.*, *Crat.*, *Dig.*, Ferr., Galan., *Glon.*, Iod., Kalm., Lach., Laur., Lith-c., *Lycps-v.*, *Naja*, Ox-ac., Phos., Plb., Rhus-t., Sang., Ser-ang., *Spig.*, *Spong.*, Stigm., Stroph-h., Thyr., Visc.

**VEINS, Engorged, distended (plethora):** Adon., *Aesc.*, *Aloe*, Arn., Ars., Aur., Bell-p., Calc., Calc-hp., Camph., *Carb an.*, *Carb-v.*, Chinin-s., *Coll.*, Conv., *Dig.*, Fl-ac., *Ham.*, Lept., Lyc., *Nux-v.*, Op., Plb., *Podo.*, *Puls.*, *Sep.*, Spong., Stel., *Sulph.*, Verb.

**Veins engorged (pelvic):** *Aloe*, Coll., *Sep.*, Sulph.

**Veins engorged (portal):** Aesc., *Aloe*, *Coll.*, Lept., Lyc., *Nux-v.*, *Sulph.*

**Veins inflamed (phlebitis):** Acon., Agar., *Apis*, Arn., *Ars.*, Bell., Crot-h., *Ham.*, Kali-c., *Lach.*, Lyc., Merc., Phos., *Puls.*, Stront-c., Vip.

**Veins inflamed, chronic:** Arn., Merc., *Puls.*, Ruta.

**Veins varicosed:** Acet-ac., Aesc., Alumn., Apis, Ars., Bell-p., Calc., *Calc-f.*, *Calc-i.*, Carb-v., *Card-m.*, Caust., Coll., Ferr-p., *Fl-ac.*, Graph., *Ham.*, Kali-ar., Lach., *Lyc.*, Magn-gr., Mur-ac., Nat-m., Paeon., Plb., Polyg-h., *Puls.*, Ran-s., Ruta, Scir., Sep., *Staph.*, Stront-c., Sul-ac., Sulph., *Vip.*, *Zinc.*

■

# LOCOMOTOR SYSTEM

**AXILLAE, Abscess:** *Hep.,* Irid-met., Jug-r.

**Acne:** Carb-v.

**Eczema:** Elaps, Nat-m.

**Herpes:** Carb an.

**Pain, in muscles, right side:** Prim-v.

**Pain, with, or without swelling:** Jug-c.

**Sweat, profuse, offensive:** Bov., *Calc.,* Hep., *Kali-c.,* Lyc., *Nit-ac.,* Osm., Petr., Sep., Sil., *Stry-p.,* Sulph., *Tell.,* Thuj.

**BACK Bent, arch-like, opisthotonos:** Ang., *Cic.,* Nat-s., *Nicot.,* Op., Phyt., *Stry.* (See **Convulsions, NERVOUS SYSTEM.**)

**Burning between scapulae:** Glon., *Lyc., Phos.,* Sulph.

**Burning:** *Alum., Ars.,* Aur-m., Berb., Calc-f., Carb-an., Helo., *Helon.,* Kali-p., Lyc., Med., Nit-ac., *Phos., Pic-ac.,* Sep., Ter., Ust., Xero.

**Burning in small spots:** Agar., *Phos.,* Ran-b., Sulph.

**Coldness between scapulae:** *Abies-c., Am-m.,* Helo., *Lachn.,* Sep.

**Coldness:** *Abies-c.,* Acon., Ars., Benz-ac., *Gels.,* Gins., Quas., Raph., Sep., *Stry.,* Verat.

**Curvature (scoliosis):** Bar-c., *Calc.,* Ph-ac., Phos., *Sil.,* Sulph.

**Eruption:** Sep.

**Lameness, stiffness:** Abrot., Acon., Aesc., Agar., Am-m., Bell., *Berb., Bry.,* Calc., Camph-mbr., *Caust., Cimic., Cupr-ar.,* Dios., Dulc., Get., Gins., *Helon.,* Hyper., *Kali-c.,* Kali-p., Kalm., Lachn., Led., Lyc., Nicot., Phys., *Phyt.,* Rhus-t., Ruta, Sarcol-ac., *Sep.,* Spong., Staph., *Stry.,* Sul-ac., *Sulph.,* Zing.

**Numbness:** *Acon., Berb.,* Calc-p., *Ox-ac.,* Oxyt., Sec., Sil.

**PAIN in general:** Abrot., *Acon., Aesc., Agar.,* Alum., Am-c., Ang., *Ant-t.,* Apis, Arg-met., Arg-n., *Arn.,* Bar-c., Bell., *Berb., Bry., Calc.,* Calc-p., *Cann-i.,* Carb-ac., Caul., *Caust.,* Cham., Chin., Chinin-s., Cic., *Cimic., Cob., Cocc.,* Colch., Coloc., Dulc., *Eup-p.,* Graph., *Gua.,* Ham., *Helon.,* Hom., Kali-bi., *Kali-c.,* Kali-m., Lach., Lil-t., Lyc., Mag-m., Mag-s., Med., *Merc.,* Mez., Mom-b., Nat-c., *Nat-m.,* Nit-ac., *Nux-v.,* Ox-ac., Paraf., Petr., Ph-ac., *Pic-ac.,* Puls., *Rad-br.,* Ran-a., Rhod., *Rhus-t.,* Ruta, *Sabin.,* Sang., Sarr., Scol., Sec., Sel., *Sep.,* Sil., Staph., *Stel.,* Stry., *Sulph.,* Tarent., *Tell.,* Ther., Trios., *Upa., Vario.,* Wye., Xero., *Zinc.*

**Aching, as if it would break and give out:** *Aesc.,* Aeth., Am-m., *Bell.,* Calc-o-t., Cann-i., Cham., *Chel.,* Dulc., *Eup-per.,* Eupi., Graph., *Ham.,*

Kali-bi., *Kalm.,* Kreos., *Nat-m.,* Ol-an., *Phos.,* Plat., *Puls., Rhus-t., Sarcol-ac.,* Sanic., Seneg., Sil., *Tril-p.*

**Aching, dull, constant (backache):** Abies-n., *Aesc., Agar.,* Aloe, Am-m., *Ant-t.,* Apoc., Arg-met., Arg-n., *Arn.,* Bapt., Bell-p., *Berb.,* But-ac., *Calc., Calc-f.,* Canth., *Cimic., Cob., Cocc.,* Cocc-s., Colch., Con., Conv., Cupr-ar., *Dulc.,* Euon., Eupi., Ferr-p., Gels., Glyc., *Helon.,* Hyper., Inul., Ipom., *Kali-c.,* Kali-i., *Kalm.,* Kreos., Lach., Lith-be., *Lyc.,* Lycpr., Morph., *Nat-m, Nux-v.,* Ol-an., *Ol-j., Ox-ac.,* Pall., Petr., Ph-ac., *Phyt.,* Pic-ac., Pisc., *Pulx., Puls., Rad-br., Rhus-t.,* Ruta, *Sabal,* Sabin., Senec., *Sep.,* Solid., *Staph., Still., Sulph.,* Symph., *Ter.,* Upa., *Vib.,* Visc., Zinc.

**Between scapulae:** *Acon.,* Apom., Asc-t., Bar-c., *Calc.,* Cann-i., Con., Gua., Guaj., Jug-c., Kali-c., Med., *Podo.,* Rad-br., *Rhus-t.,* Sep., Sulph., Zinc.

**Bruised:** *Acon.,* Aesc., Agar., Ant-t., *Arn.,* Bar-c., *Berb.,* Bry., Cina, *Dulc.,* Gins., Graph.., *Ham.,* Mag-s., *Merc.,* Nat-m., *Nux-v.,* Ph-ac., Phyt., *Rhus-t.,* Ruta, Sil., Sulph., Tell.

**Crampy:** *Bell.,* Calc-o-t., Chin., Cimic., *Coloc.,* Graph., Iris, Mag-p., Sep.

**Digging, cutting:** Sep.

**Drawing:** Anac., Carb-v., *Caust., Kali-c.,* Lyc., Nux-v., Rhus-t., *Sabin.,* Sulph.

**Falling apart sensation, involving small of back, sacro-iliac synchondroses, relieved by bandaging tightly:** Tril-p.

**Heaviness, dragging, weight:** *Aesc., Aloe, Am-m.,* Anac., Ant-c., Benz-ac., *Berb.,* Bov., Colch., *Eup-pur., Helon.,* Hydr., Kali-c., *Kreos., Lil-t.,* Nat-s., Pic-ac., *Sep.* (See **FEMALE SEXUAL SYSTEM.**)

**Lancinating, drawing, tearing:** Alum., Asc-t., *Berb.,* Colch., Coloc., Kali-m., Lyc., Mim-h., Nux-v., *Scol.,* Sep., Sil., Stel., *Stry.*

**Lancinating, extends down thighs, legs:** *Aesc.,* Aur-m., Bapt., *Berb.,* Carb-ac., Cocc., *Coloc.,* Cur., Ham., *Helon.,* Kali-c., Kali-m., Lac-c., *Ox-ac.,* Phyt., *Scol., Stel.,* Tell., Xero.

**Lancinating, extends to pelvis:** *Arg-n.,* Aur-m., Berb., Cham., *Cimic.,* Eupi., Ham., Sil., *Vario.,* Visc.

**Lancinating, extends to pubes:** *Sabin.,* Vib., Xan.

**Lancinating, extends upwards:** Aspar., *Gels.*

**Paralytic:** Cocc., Kali-p., Nat-m., Sil.

**Pressing, plug-like:** *Aesc., Agar., Anac.,* Aur-m., Benz-ac., *Berb.,* Colch., Hyper., Nat-m., *Nux-v.,* Sep., Tell.

**Sensitiveness extreme of sacrum:** Lob.

**Stitching, piercing, pricking:** Agar., Aloe, Alum., Apis, *Berb., Bry.,* Guaj., Hyper., *Kali-c., Merc.,* Nat-s., Sulph., Tell., Ther.

**MODALITIES, AGGRAVATION, After emission:** Cob.

**After masturbation:** Nux-v., Ph-ac., Staph.

**At night:** Aloe, Calc., Lyc., *Merc.,* Mez., Nat-m., *Staph.,* Visc.
**From cold exposure:** Acon., *Bry., Rhod.,* Sulph.
**From damp exposure:** Dulc., Phyt., *Rhus-t.*
**From eating:** Kali-c.
**From exertion:** Agar., *Berb.,* Cocc., Hyper., Kali-c., Kali-p., Ox-ac., Sulph. (See **Motion.**)
**From jar, touch:** *Acon.,* Berb., *Bry.,* Kali-bi., *Lob.,* Mez., Sil., *Tell.*
**From lying down:** Bell., *Berb.,* Nicc-s., Nux-v., Rhus-t.
**From motion, beginning:** Lac-c., *Rhus-t.*
**From motion, walking:** *Aesc.,* Aloe, *Ant-t.,* Bell., *Bry., Caust.,* Chel., Chin., *Colch.,* Kali-bi., *Kali-c.,* Mez., *Nux-v.,* Ox-ac., Paraf., Petr., Phyt., Ran-a., Sep., *Sulph.*
**From resting, sitting:** *Agar.,* Alum., Ant-t., *Bell., Berb.,* Cann-i., Cob., Ferr-m., Kali-p., Kreos., *Lac-c.,* Merc., Nux-v., Puls., *Rhus-t.,* Sep., Sulph., *Zinc.*
**From standing:** *Aesc.,* Bell., Nux-v., Sarcol-ac., Sep.
**From stooping:** *Aesc.,* Berb., Dios., Gua., Tell.
**From warmth:** *Kali-s.,* Puls., Sulph.
**In morning:** Agar., *Berb.,* Bry., Conv., Kali-c., Nat-m., Nux-v., Petr., Phyt., Ruta, Sel., *Staph.*
**When rising from seat:** Aesc., Arg-n., *Berb., Caust.,* Kali-p., *Lach.,* Sil., Sulph., Tell.

**AMELIORATON, After rising:** Kali-c., Ruta, Staph
**From bending backward:** Rhus-t.
**From bending forward:** Lob.
**From emission:** Zinc.
**From lying on abdomen:** Acet-ac.
**From lying on back:** Aesc., *Cob.,* Gnaph., Nat-m., Rhus-t., Ruta.
**From lying on something hard, or firm support:** Eupi, *Nat-m., Rhus-t.,* Sep.
**From lying, sitting:** Sep.
**From motion, walking:** Arg-n., Bell., Caust., *Cob.,* Ferr-m., *Helon.,* Kali-m., Kreos., Merc., *Puls.,* Rad-br., *Rhus-t.,* Sep., Staph., *Sulph., Zinc.*
**From rest:** *Aesc.,* Colch., Nux-v., Sil.
**From sitting:** Bell.
**From standing:** Arg-n., Caust., Sulph.
**From urination:** *Lyc.,* Med.

**WEAKNESS, of back:** Abrot., *Aesc., Aesc-g.,* Alum., Ant-t., Arn., Berb., But-ac., Calc., *Calc-p., Chin., Cocc.,* Glyc., Graph., Gua., *Helon.,* Ign., Irid-met., Jac-c., *Kali-c.,* Merc., Nat-m., Nux-v., Ox-ac., Petr., Ph-ac., Phos., *Pic-ac.,* Podo., *Sarr., Sep., Sil.,* Staph., *Zinc.*

**BODY, Bruised, sore feeling, all over:** Abrot., Ampe-qu., Apis, *Arn., Bapt., Bell-p,* Caust., *Chin.,* Cic., Cimic., *Eup-per., Gels.,* Ham., Hep., Iber., Lil-t., Lycpr., *Mang-act.,* Med., Morph., Nux-m., *Phyt.,* Psor., *Pyrog., Rad-br., Rhus-t., Ruta,* Staph., Tell., *Thuj.,* Wye.

**Burning, in various parts:** Acon., *Agar.,* Apis, *Ars., Canth.,* Caps., *Carb-an.,* Ph-ac., *Phos.,* Sulph.

**Coldness:** Acon., *Aeth.,* Ant-t., Ars., Atha., *Bar-m., Bor-ac.,* Cadm-s., *Camph.,* Camph-mbr., *Chlol.,* Cupr., *Helo., Jatr.,* Lachn., Luf-op, *Sec.,* Tab., *Verat.,* Zinc.

**Constriction, as if caged:** Cact., Med.

**Numbness:** *Acon.,* Ars., Cic., Con., *Ox-ac., Phos.,* Plb., *Sec.*

**Swelling:** *Apis,* Dory., Frag. (See **Dropsy, GENERALITIES.**)

**Trembling:** *Agar.,* Cod., *Con., Gels.,* Hyos., Iber., Lon-x., *Mygal.,* Phos., Sarcol-ac.

**COCCYX: Burning on touch:** Carb-an.

**Itching:** Bov., Graph.

**Neuralgia, worse rising from sitting posture:** Lach.

**Numbness:** Plat.

**Pain (coccygodynia):** Ant-t., Arn., *Bell., Bry., Calc-caust.,* Castm., *Caust., Cic., Cimic.,* Cist., Con., *Ferr-p.,* Fl-ac., *Graph., Hyper.,* Kali-bi., Kali-c., Kali-i., *Kreos.,* Lac-c., *Lach.,* Lob., Mag-c., *Mag-p., Merc., Par.,* Petr., Phos., *Rhus-t.,* Sil., *Tarent.,* Tet., Xan., Zinc-

**Bruised:** Am-m., *Arn.,* Caust., Ruta, Sulph.

**Bruised from injury:** Hyper.

**Dragging, drawing:** *Ant-t., Caust.,* Graph., Kreos.

**Tearing, lancinating:** *Bell.,* Canth., *Cic.,* Kali-bi., *Mag-p.,* Merc.

**Ulcer:** Paeon.

**EXTREMITIES: Coldness:** Acon., Agar., *Agar-ph., Bell., Calc.,* Calc-hp., *Calc-p., Camph., Cocc-s.,* Crat., Dulc., *Ferr.,* Hed, *Helo., Hydr-ac.,* Ign-Kalm., Lol., Lon-x., Meli., Merc., *Mur-ac.,* Nat-m., Nux-m., Olnd., Op., *Phyt.,* Quas., Sang., *Sec.,* Sulfon., Tril-p., *Verat.,* Zinc.

**Itching:** *Arund.,* Kali-c., Lyc., Pall., *Phos.,* Prun-v., Valer.

**Lameness, stiffness:** *Agar.,* Agarin., Aloe, *Calc-p.,* Carb-v., *Cocc., Eucal.,* Gins., Ip., Kali-p., *Lith-c., Rhus-t.,* Trios., Xero., Zinc.

**Numbness, tingling, fall asleep:** Absin., *Acon.,* Alum., Aran., *Arg-n.,* Aven., Bar-c., Calc., *Calc-p.,* Camph., *Carb-v., Caust.,* Cham., Chin., Cic., *Cocc., Gels.,* Helo., *Kali-c.,* Kalm., *Lon-x.,* Lycpr., *Morph.,* Nat-m., *Onos., Op., Ox-ac., Phos., Pic-ac., Plat.,* Plb., *Sec., Sil.,* Sulph., *Thal.,* Verat., *Zinc.*

**PAIN, Aching:** Aesc., All-c., Apis, *Arn.,* Ars., Aza., *Bry.,* Calc., Carb-v., Caust., Chin., *Cimic., Con.,* Cur., Cycl., Echi., Eucal., *Gels.,* Hedeo., *Kalm.,*

*Merc.*, Myric., *Pyrog.*, Quas., *Rad-br.*, Ran-s., *Rhod.*, *Rhus-t.*, Sec., Sil., Staph., *Stel.*, Stry., Thyr.

**Bone pains:** Aran., Aur., Calc-p., *Eup-per.*, *Gels.*, *Kali-bi.*, Kali-i., Mag-m., Mang-act., *Merc.*, *Mez.*, *Ph-ac.*, *Ran-s.*, Rhus-v., Ruta, *Sang.*, Sars., *Still.*, Stront-c., Trios.

**Cramp-like, constricting:** Abrot., Alumn., Ant-t., Antip., *Asaf.*, Calc., Canth., Carbn-s., *Cocc.*, *Coloc.*, Croc., *Cupr.*, Gins., Mag-p., Meny., *Plat.*, Sec., Sil., *Stry.*, Verat.

**Drawing:** Camph., Caust., Graph., Hep., Kali-c., Lyc., Nat-m., Rhus-t.

**Erratic, fly about:** *Caul.*, Iris, Kali-bi., *Kali-s.*, Kalm., *Lac-c.*, Magn-gr., *Mang-act.*, Phyt., *Puls.*, Rhod., Sal-ac., *Stel.*

**Growing pains:** Ap-g., Calc-p., *Guaj.*, Hipp., Ph-ac. (See **Bones, GENERALITIES.**)

**Hysterical contractures:** Bell., *Cocc.*, *Cupr.*, Hyos., *Ign.*, Lyc., Merc., Nux-v., Stram., Zinc.

**Neuralgic, lancinating, tearing, shooting:** Absin., *Acon.*, Alum., *Bell.*, Bran., *Carbn-s.*, Caul., *Cham.*, Daph., Elat., Eucal., Gels., Guaj., Kali-c., Kalm., Lyc., *Mag-p.*, Magn-gr., *Mim-p.*, Nit-ac., *Ox-ac.*, Phos., Phyt., *Rhod.*, Rhus-t., Sars., Sil., Stry.

**Rheumatico-gouty:** *Acon.*, Anag., Ant-t., Apis, *Arn.*, Aspar., Bell., Bran., *Bry.*, Calc., *Calc-p.*, Caul., Caust., Cham., *Colch.*, Dulc., Eucal., Guaj., Iod., Kali-c., *Kalm.*, Lac-c., Lyc., *Merc.*, Prun-v., *Rad-br.*, *Rhod.*, *Rhus-t.*, Sang., *Stel.*, Stict.

**Shock-like, paralytic:** Cina, Colch., *Phyt.*, *Thal.*, Verat-v., Verin., Xan.

**Sprained, dislocated feeling:** *Arn.*, Bell-p, Calc., Carb-v., *Chin.*, Rhus-t., *Ruta.* (See **Joints.**)

**Paralysis:** *Acon.*, Alum., *Bar-act.*, *Caust.*, *Cocc.*, *Con.*, Cur., Dub., *Dulc.*, Hedeo., Kalm., *Lol.*, Nux-v., Olnd., Op., *Phos.*, Pic-ac., Rhus-t., Sec., Sil. (See **NERVOUS SYSTEM.**)

**Sprains, chronic:** Graph., Petr., *Stront-c.* (See **GENERALITIES.**)

**Stretching continually:** Alum., Aml-ns., Ang., *Ars.*, Chin., Quas., Sep.

**Trembling, twitching, jerking:** Acon., *Agar.*, Alum., Apis, *Arg-n.*, Ars., Bell., Calc-p., Carb-v., Caust., Chin., *Cimic.*, *Cina*, *Cocc.*, *Con.*, *Cupr.*, Cupr-ar., *Gels.*, Helo., *Hyper.*, *Hyos.*, *Ign.*, Kali-c., *Lach.*, *Lol.*, Lon-x., Lyc., Mag-p., *Merc.*, *Morph.*, *Mygal.*, *Op.*, Ph-ac., *Phos.*, Phys., Rhus-t., *Sec.*, Sep., Sil., Stram., *Stry.*, Sulfon., Sulph., *Tarent.*, Thal., *Valer.*, Viol-o., Xero., *Zinc.*, Zinc-s. (See **Weakness.**)

**Weakness, debility:** Aeth., Agar., *Alum.*, *Am-caust.*, Am-m., Anac., Apis, Arg-n., *Ars.*, Asar., Bell-p., Bism., *Calc.*, *Caust.*, *Chin.*, *Cocc.*, *Con.*, Cupr., Cur., Cypr., Dig., Eucal., *Gels.*, Gins., Helon., Hipp., *Kali-bi.*, Kalm., Lec., Lyc., Mag-p., Med., Merc., *Mur-ac.*, Myric., Nat-c., Nat- m., Nicc-s., Nux-v., *Onos.,* Ox-ac., *Ph-ac., Phos., Pic-ac., Plat.,* Prim-v., Puls., *Sarcol-ac.,* Scut., Sel., Sep., Sil., *Stann.,* Stry-p., Sulfon., *Thal.,* Thuj., Verat., *Zinc.* (See **Neurasthenia, NERVOUS SYSTEM.**)

**UPPER EXTREMITIES, ARM:** (See **Extremities in general.**)

**Coldness:** Apis, Carb-v., Raph., Verat.

**Eruptions:** Arund., Caust., Ph-ac., Sulph.

**Gangrenous ulceration:** Ran-fl.

**Heaviness:** *Acon., Alum.,* Cann-i., Cimic., *Cur.,* Ham., Hep., *Lat-m.,* Lyc., Nat-m., Verat.

**Intolerant of band around:** Ovi-p.

**Itching:** Fago.

**Jerking, involuntary motion:** *Agar.,* Ant-c., *Cic., Cina,* Cocc., *Ip.,* Lact., Lyc., Op., Tarent., *Thlas.*

**Jerking, or involuntary motion, of one arm, and leg:** Apoc., *Bry., Hell.,* Mygal., Zinc.

**Lameness, stiffness:** *Acon.,* Am-c., Bapt., Cann-i., *Caust.,* Par., *Rhus-v.,* Verat., Ziz.

**Nodules:** Hippoz.

**Numbness, fall asleep:** *Acon.,* Ambr., Aran., Aster., Bar-c., *Cact.,* Cham., Cimic., *Cocc.,* Dig., *Graph.,* Iber., Ign., Kali-c., *Lat-m.,* Lil-t., Lyc., *Mag-m.,* Magn-gr., *Nux-v.,* Par., Phos., *Rhus-t.,* Sep., Sil., Xan.

**Numbness, left arm:** Acon., Dig., Kalm., Puls., *Rhus-t.,* Sumb.

**Numbness, right arm:** Phyt.

**PAINS:** Aesc., All-c., *Alum., Anag.,* Calc., *Caust.,* Cic., Cinnb., *Eup-per.,* Ferr-pic., Gels., Gua., *Guaj.,* Ind., Lycpr., Mag-m., Nat-m., Phos., *Phyt., Rhus-t., Sang., Stel.,* Stict., *Sulph.,* Wye., *Zinc.*

**Pain in left arm:** Acon., Agar., Aster., *Cact., Cimic.,* Colch., Crot-h., Iber., Kalm., *Lat-m.,* Mag-s., Magn-gr., *Rhus-t., Spig.,* Tab., Xan.

**Pain in right arm:** *Ferr-m.,* Ferr-pic., Lycpr., Pip-m., Rhus-v., *Sang.,* Viol-o., Wye.

**Aching:** Bapt., Berb., *Caust.,* Gels., Jal., Lith-c., Nat-ar., Ol-j., Sarr.

**Aching, weakness, when singing, using voice:** Stann.

**Bruised, cramp-like:** Acon., Arg-n., *Cocc.,* Cupr., Olnd., *Ph-ac.,* Sec., Sul-ac., Verat-v., *Zinc-s.*

**Drawing:** Calc., *Caust.,* Lyc., *Mag-m.,* Mur-ac., Olnd., Sep., Sil., Zinc.

**Neuralgic (brachalgia):** *Acon.,* Alum., Bry., *Hyper.,* Kali-c., *Kalm.,* Lyc., Merc., *Nux-v.,* Pip-m., *Puls., Rhus-t.,* Scut., Sulph., Teucr., Verat., Visc.

**Paralysis:** Cocc., Ferr., Gels., Nux-v., Rhus-t.

**Sensibility, diminished:** Carbn-s., Phos.

**Tearing, stitching:** Calc., Ferr., Hep., Phos., Sep., Sil.

**Trembling:** Cod., Cocc., *Gels.*, Kali-br., *Phos.*, Sil. (See **Weakness.**)

**Weakness:** *Alumn.*, Anac., *Cur.*, Dig., Iod., Kali-c., Lach., Lyc., Mag-p., Med., *Nat-m.*, *Sarcol-ac.*, Sep., *Sil.*, *Stann.*, Sulph.

**FOREARM** (See **Extremities.**).

**Coldness:** Arn., Brom., Med.

**Pain:** Anac., Cinnb., *Eup-per.*, Ferr-m., Ferr-pic., Gels., Gua., *Hyper.*, Kali-c., *Kalm.*, Phyt., *Rhus-t.*, Sep., Stann.

**Paralysis:** Arg-n., Nux-v., Plb., Sil. (See **NERVOUS SYSTEM.**)

**Soreness of flexor carpi ulnaris:** Brach.

**Unsteadiness of muscles of forearm, hands:** Caust.

**HAND, Automatic motion of hand and head:** Apoc., Bry., Hell., Zinc.

**Blueness, distended veins:** Am-c., Aml-ns., *Ant-t.*, *Carb-an.*, Dig., Elaps, Laur., *Nit-ac.*, Olnd., Samb., Stront-c., *Verat.* (See **Cyanosis, CIRCULATORY SYSTEM.**)

**Burning, heat:** *Acon.*, Agar., Carb-v., Cocc., *Lach.*, Lyc., *Med.*, Ol-j., *Phos.*, Sang., Sil.

**Chapping:** Alum., *Calc.*, Castor-eq., Cist., *Graph.*, Lyc., Mag-c., Nat-ar., *Nat-c.*, *Petr.*, Sars., Sulo-ac.

**Coldness:** Abies-c., Acon., *Ant-t.*, Apis, *Ars.*, Cact., Calc., *Camph.*, *Carbn-o.*, *Chin.*, Cic., Con., *Cupr.*, *Dig.*, Iod., *Meny.*, Nat-m., Nit-ac., Squil, *Tab.*, Thuj., Trif-p., *Verat.*

**Coldness of one, warmth of the other:** Chin., Dig., Ip., Puls.

**Cramps:** Bell., Calc., *Sec.*, Sil.

**Cramps (writer's), piano or violin players, typists:** Ambr., *Arg-met.*, *Arg-n.*, Brach., *Caust.*, *Cimic.*, Cupr., Cycl., *Gels.*, Graph., Hep., *Mag-p.*, Ruta, *Stann.*, Sul-ac., Sulph. (See **NERVOUS SYSTEM.**)

**Dryness:** Lyc., Zinc.

**Enlarged feeling:** *Aran.*, Caust., *Cocc.*, Gins., Kali-n.

**Eruption:** Borx., Cist., Ped., *Pix.* (See **SKIN.**)

**Fidgety:** *Kali br.*, *Mygal.*, Tarent., Zinc.

**Hypothenar eminences bright red:** Acon.

**Itching:** Agar., Tell.

**Nodosities, gouty, on dorsum:** *Am-p.*, Eucal., Med. (See **Fingers.**)

**Numbness, go asleep:** *Acon.*, Arg-n., Ars., Borx., Cann-i., *Caust.*, *Cocc.*, Cod., *Colch.*, Cyt-l., Graph., *Hyper.*, Iber., Lil-t., Lyc., Mag-p., Nat-c., Nux-v., *Phos.*, Phys., Pyrog., Raph., Sec., Tela.

**Pains: Bruised:** *Ruta*, Verat.

**Lancinating:** *All-c*, Lappa, Sel., Sulph.

**Paralysis:** Cyt-l., Ferr., Merc., Plb-act., Ruta, Sil.

**Rheumatic:** Ambr., Berb., *Caul.*, *Caust.*, Chel., Guaj., Led., Lycpr., *Puls.*, *Rhus-t.*, *Ruta*, Sang.

**PALMS, Blisters:** Bufo.

**Burning:** *Aza.,* Bol-la., Ferr., Ferr-p., Gad, *Lach.,* Lachn., Lim., Nat-m., Ol-j., Petr., *Phos.,* Prim-v., Puls-n., *Sang.,* Sep., *Sulph.*

**Chapping, fissuring:** Calc-f., *Ran-b.*

**Cramps:** *Cupr.,* Scroph-n., Zing.

**Desquamation:** Elaps.

**Eruption, dry, bran-like, itching:** Anag., *Ars.,* X-ray.

**Injary with intolerable pain:** Hyper.

**Itching:** Ant-s-aur., *Fago., Gran.,* Lim., Ran-b., Tub.

**Pains:** Aza., Trif-p.

**Stiffness of hands while writing:** Kali-m.

**Sweating:** *Calc.,* Cocc., Con., Dulc., Fago., *Fl-ac.,* Nat-m., Pic-ac., Sep., *Sil., Stry-p., Sulph.,* Wye.

**Swelling:** Aesc., Agar., *Apis,* Arg-n., Ars., Arund., Bry., *Cact.,* Calc., Crot-h., Elaps, Ferr-p., Nat-chor., *Rhus-d.* (See **Dropsy, GENERALITIES**.)

**Twitching, trembling, weakness:** Act-sp., Anac., Ant-c., Ant-t., *Arg-n.,* Arn., Aven., Calc., *Cic., Cina, Cocc., Con., Cur., Gels.,* Hipp., Lach., Lact., Lol., *Mag-p., Merc., Phos.,* Sars., *Sarcol-ac.,* Sil., *Stann., Stram.,* Sulph., Tab., *Zinc.*

**Warts:** *Anac.,* Ant-c., Calc., *Dulc.,* Ferr-ma., *Ferr-pic.,* Nat c., Nat-m., *Ruta.*

**Yellow color:** Chel., Sep. (See **SKIN.**)

**FINGERS: Blueness, coldness:** Chel., Crat., Cupr., Verat. (See **Hands**.)

**Blue, numb, shrivelled, spread apart, or bent backward:** Sec.

**Burning:** *Aza.,* Gins., Olnd., Sars., *Sulph.*

**Chapped tips cracks, fissures:** Alum., *Graph.,* Nat-m., *Petr., Ran-b., Sanic.,* Sars.

**Cramp-like, contracted, clenching:** *Aeth.,* Ambr., Anag., *Arg-n.,* Bism., *Brach.,* Cann-s., Caust., *Cic., Cina,* Cocc., Colchin., *Cupr., Cupr-act.,* Cycl., Dios., *Hell.,* Kali-bi., Laur., Lyc., Par., Ruta, *Sec.,* Sol-t., Stann., *Sul-ac.*

**Crooked:** Kali-c., Lyc.

**Crushed, mashed tips:** Hyper.

**Eruptions:** Aln., Anac., *Barbit., Bov., Graph.,* Lim., *Lob-e.,* Nat-c., Nit-ac., *Petr.,* Prim-f., *Rhus-t.,* Sars., Sel. (See **SKIN.**)

**Exostoses:** Calc-f., *Hecla.*

**Fidgety, must move constantly:** Kali-br.

**Hypertrophy:** Aur-m.

**Impression deep, from scissors:** Bov.

**Itching between:** Ph-ac. (See **SKIN.**)

**Jerking, when holding pen:** *Caust.,* Cina, Cycl., Kali-c., *Stann.,* Sul-ac.

**Joints, inflamed, painful:** *Benz-ac.,* Berb., *Bry.,* Fl-ac., Lyc., Med., *Nat-p.,* Pip-m., Prim-o., Puls., *Rhus-t.,* Staph., *Stel.* (See **Rheumatism**.)

**Joints, nodosities on:** *Am-p.,* Ben., *Benz-ac.,* Calc., Calc-f., *Caul., Colch.,* Graph., Led., Lith-c., *Lyc., Med.,* Staph., Stel. (See **Joints**.)

**Joints, pain in:** Bry., Graph., Led., Lyc., Sil., Sulph.

**Joints, stiff:** Carb-v., *Caul.,* Lyc., Prim-o., Puls. (See **Joints**.)

**Numbness, tingling of fingers:** *Acon.,* Aesc., Ambr., Apis, Ars., Aster., Bar-c., Calc., *Cocain.,* Con., *Dig.,* Lath., Lyc., Mag-p., Mag-s., Nat-m., Nit-ac., *Ox-ac., Par.,* Phos., Prop., Sarcol-ac., *Sec., Sil., Thal.,* Thuj., Upa., Verb., Zinc.

**Pains, at root of nails:** *All-c.,* Berb., Bism., Myris.

**Pains in general:** Abrot., Aza., Lil-t., Sec.

**Pains in tips:** Am-m., Borx., Chel., *Hyper.,* Kali-c., *Sec.,* Sil., Teucr.

**Pains, rheumatic:** *Act-sp., Ant-c.,* Berb., *Caul.,* Colch., Fago., Gran., Graph., Gua., Hyper., Lappa, *Led.,* Lith-c., Lyc., Med., Paeon., Puls., Ran-s., *Rhus-t.* (See **Rheumatism**.)

**Pains, tearing:** *Act-sp.,* Am-m., *Caul.,* Caust., Cedr., Led., Lyc., *Puls.,* Rhus-t.

**Pains, throbbing:** Aml-ns., Borx.

**Panaritium:** Alum., Am-c., Dios., Myris., Sil.

**Sensibililty, diminished:** *Carbn-s.,* Pop-c., Sec.

**Sensitive to cold:** *Cist.,* Hep.

**Skin, dry, shrivelled:** Aeth. (See **SKIN.**)

**Skin peels off:** Elaps. (See **SKIN.**)

**Soreness between:** Nat-ar. (See **SKIN.**)

**Stiffness, rigidity:** Am-c., Carbn-s., *Caul.,* Cocc., Lyc., Olnd., Puls., Sil. (See **Joints**.)

**Swelling:** *Am-c.,* Bry., Carbn-s., Cinnm., Hep., Kali-m., *Lith-c.,* Mang-act., Olnd., *Puls., Thuj.*

**Thick, horny tips:** *Ant-c.,* Pop-c.

**Trembling:** Bry., Iod., Kali-br., Lol., Merc., Olnd., Rhus-t., Zinc.

**Ulcers:** Alum., Arund., Ars., Borx., Sep.

**Weariness:** Bov., Calc., *Cur., Gels.,* Hipp., Phos., Sil. (See **Hand.**)

**LOWER EXTREMITIES, BUTTOCKS (glutel), Cold feeling:** Daph.

**Cold feeling, fall asleep:** Calc-p.

**Cramp:** Graph.

**Emaciation:** Lath.

**Pain to hips, small of back:** Staph.

**Pricking:** Guaj.

**Swelling:** Ph-ac.

**LOINS, LUMBAGO:** *Acon.,* Act-sp., *Aesc.,* Agar., *Aloe, Ant-t., Arn.,* Bell., *Berb., Bry., Calc-f., Calc-p., Carb-ac.,* Carbn-s., *Caul., Cham.,* Chel., *Cimic.,* Cina, Colch., Coloc., Dios., *Dulc., Eup-per.,* Ferr., *Gins., Gnaph.,* Guaj., Hydr., *Hymos.,* Ipom., Kali-bi., *Kali-c.,* Kali-i., Kali-o., Lath., Led., Lith-be., Lyc., *Macro.,* Merc., Nat-m., *Nux-v.,* Pimp., Pic-ac., Phyt., Puls., Rad-br., Rham-cal., Rhod., *Rhus-t.,* Ruta, *Sabal,* Senec., Sep., Spira., *Sulph.,* Ter., Vib.

**Alternates, with headache, piles:** Aloe.

**With aggravation in open air:** Agar.

**With aggravation on beginning to move:** Anac., Con., Glyc., *Rhus-t.*

**With aggravation, on beginning to move, relieved by continued motion:** Calc-f., *Rhus-t.*

**With aggravation on exertion, during day, while sitting:** Agar.

**With aggravation on lying down:** Bell., Murx.

**With chronic tendancy:** Aesc., Berb., *Calc-f., Rhus-t.,* Sil.

**With masturbatic origin, sexual weakness:** Nux-v.

**With numbness, in lower part of back, weight in pelvis:** Gnaph.

**With relief, from lying down:** Euon., Sep.

**With relief, from slow walking:** Ferr.

**With retching, cold, clammy sweat, from least motion:** Lath.

**With sciatica:** *Rhus-t.*

**THIGHS-LEGS, Blue, painful, swollen, if hanging down:** Lath.

**Burning:** *Ars.,* Arund., Bar-c., Kali-c., Led., Lyc., Mez., Still.

**Coldness:** Acon., Alum., Berb., Bism., *Calc.,* Calc-p., *Carb-an., Carb-v.,* Colch., Crot-h., Lac-ac., Lact., *Laur.,* Lyc., Merc., Mez., *Nat-m.,* Nit-ac., Ox-ac., Oxyt., Sep., Sil., *Tab., Verat.,* Zinc.

**Contractions of hamstrings, tendons:** *Am-m., Caust.,* Cimx., Coloc., Graph., Guaj., Lach., Med., Nat-m., Ruta, Sulph.

**Curved limbs, cannot be straightened, and vice versa:** Cic.

**Emaciation:** *Abrot.,* Acet-ac., Kali-i., *Lath.,* Pin-s.

**Enlargement of femur, in rachitic infants:** Calc-f.

**Eruptions:** Calc., Chrysar., Gins., *Graph.,* Mag-c., *Petr.,* Sulph. (See **SKIN.**)

**Erysipelas:** Sulph. (See **SKIN.**)

**Excoriation, itching over tibia:** Bism.

**Heaviness:** *Alum.,* Bry., Calc., Cann-i., Cimic., *Con.,* Gins., *Gua.,* Hell., Med., Nux-v., Pall., *Pic-ac.,* Sep., Sulfon., *Sulph.,* Verb., Vib-o.

**Itching:** Bell-p., Bov., *Fago.,* Nit-ac., *Rumx.,* Stel.

**Motion involuntary:** Bry., Hell., Lyc., *Mygal.,* Tarent. (See **Trembling**.)

**Numbness, formication "going asleep":** *Agar., Alum.,* Aran., Calc., *Calc-p., Caust.,* Carbn-s., *Cocc.,* Coloc., Crot-h., *Gnaph.,* Graph., Kali-c., Kali-i., Lact., Mez., *Nux-v.,* Onos., *Phos., Rhus-t.,* Sarcol-ac., *Sec.,* Sep., *Sulph.,* Tarent., Tela, *Trios.,* Zinc.

**PAINS, In general:** Agar., Anis., Aran., Cann-i., *Caps.,* Carb-an., *Carbn-s.,* Chel., Cic., *Dios.,* Euph., Ferr., *Gels., Gnaph.,* Helo., Indg., Iod., Irid-met., *Kali-c., Kalm.,* Lach., Mag-m., Mang-act., Mang-o., Menis., Murx., Nat-s., Nit-ac., Ph-ac., *Phos.,* Pic-ac., *Plb.,* Puls., *Rhus-t.,* Sabin., Sil., Tong., Trif-p., Vib., *Vip.*

**Aching, bruised:** Arg-n., *Arn., Bapt.,* Calc., Cimic., Cocc., *Colch.,* Dios., *Eup-per., Gels.,* Guaj., Laur., Lil-t., Lycpr., Mag-c., Med., *Ph-ac., Pyrog.,* Sabin., Sarcol-ac., Sep., Staph., Ulm-c., *Vario.*

**Cramps, contractions:** Abrot., Aesc-g., Agar., Am-br., *Am-m.,* Ambr., Anac., *Arn.,* Bapt., Bar-c., *Calc., Camph.,* Carb-ac., Carb an., Carb-v., *Caust.,* Chin., Cho., Cimic., *Cimx., Cocc.,* Colch., *Coloc.,* Con., *Cupr., Cupr-ar.,* Eupi., Ferr., *Gels.,* Hyper., Hyos., Irid-met., Jatr., Lath., Lol., *Lyc., Mag-p.,* Med., Nit-ac., *Nux-v.,* Ox-ac., Pin-s., Plb., Puls., *Rhus-t.,* Sarcol-ac., *Sec.,* Sep., *Sil.,* Sol-t., *Sulph.,* Ust., *Verat.,* Vip., Zinc-s.

**Cramps (tailor's):** Anac., Anag., Mag-p.

**Pains in tibia:** Ars., Bad., Carb-an., *Dulc.,* Ferr., *Kali-bi., Lach.,* Mang-o., *Mez., Phos.,* Sep.

**Paralysis:** *Agar.,* Alum., Bry., *Cann-i.,* Chel., *Cocc., Crot-h.,* Dulc., Gels., *Gua.,* Kali-i., Kali-t., *Lath.,* Nux-v., Olnd., *Plb., Rhus-t.,* Sec., Sulfon., Tab., *Thal.,* Verat., Zinc. (See **NERVOUS SYSTEM.**)

**Rending, tearing, lancinating:** *Am-m.,* Ars., Bapt., Bar-act., *Bell.,* Bell-p, Cob., Coloc., *Dios., Hyper.,* Kali-bi., Kali-c., Kalm., Lyc., Nit-ac., *Plb.,* Puls., *Rhus-t.,* Sep., *Sulph.,* Teucr., Visc.

**Rheumatic:** Berb., *Bry.,* Chel., Colch., Daph., *Dulc.,* Led., *Phyt.,* Merc., *Rhus-t.,* Sang., Stel., Valer. (See **Rheumatism.**)

**Restless, fidgety:** Ars., Carb-v., *Caust.,* Chin., Cimic., Con., Crot-h., Graph., Kali-br., Lil-t., Lyc., *Med., Meny.,* Merc-c., Mygal., Nit-ac., *Phos., Rhus-t.,* Ruta, Scut., *Sep.,* Sulfon., Tarent., *Tarax., Zinc.,* Zinc-val., Ziz.

**Rigidity, stiffness, lameness:** Alum., Ang., *Arg-n.,* Bapt., Bar-m., Calc., *Cic.,* Colch., *Con.,* Dios., *Eup- per.,* Guaj., *Lath.,* Phys., Plat., *Rhus-t., Sarcol-ac.,* Sep., Stry., Xero.

**Sensibility, diminished:** Ox-ac., Phos. (See **NERVOUS SYSTEM.**)

**Sensibility increased:** Lach., Lath. (See **NERVOUS SYSTEM.**)

**Spots on, red:** Calc., Sulph.

**Stretching:** Am-c., *Aml-ns.,* Hell., Helo. (See **FEVER.**)

**Sweat, cold, clammy, at P.M.:** Calc., Merc.

**Sweat extending below knees in A.M.:** Sulph.

**Sweat on thighs, exhausting at P.M.:** Carb-an.

**Swelling:** *Acet-ac., Apis, Ars.,* Aur., *Cact.,* Chel., Colch., *Dig.,* Eup-per., *Ferr.,* Fl-ac., Graph., Kali-c., Lath., *Lyc.,* Merc., Phos., *Rhus-t.,* Samb., Sep., Stront-c., *Staph.,* Sulph., Thyr., Visc. (See **Dropsy, GENERALITIES.**)

**Trembling:** Aesc-g., Arg-met., *Cob., Cocc.,* Cod., Colch., *Con.,* Cur., Dor., *Gels.,* Lol., *Mim-p.,* Nit-ac., Ph-ac., Phos., Tab., Zinc.

**Trickling, as from drops of water:** Acon.

**Ulcers:** *Ars.,* Calc., Carb-v., Cist., Echi., Lyc., Ph-ac., Rhus-t., Sacch., *Sil.,* Trif-p. (See **GENERALITIES.**)

**Weakness, easily fatigued:** Aesc., *Alum., Alumn.,* Am-c., Arg-met., Arg-n., Bar-m., Berb., *Calc-p., Cann-i.,* Cimic., Cob., *Cocc.,* Colch., *Con.,* Cupr., Cur., Dig., Ferr., *Form., Gels.,* Ham., Kali-c., Kalm., Lach., Med., *Nat-m., Nux-v., Olnd.,* Onos., Paeon., *Ph-ac.,* Phel., *Phos., Pic-ac.,* Rhus-t., Ruta, Sarr., *Sarcol-ac.,* Sil., *Stann.,* Sulph., Vib.

**FEET, Affections of ball, and dorsum of toes:** Cann-s.

**Bunions:** Agar., *Benz-ac.,* Hyper., *Kali-i.,* Rhod., *Sil.,* Verat-v. (See **SKIN.**)

**Burning:** Agar., Am-c., *Apis,* Aza., Bran., Borx., Graph., Helo., Kali-c., *Lach.,* Led.., *Med.,* Nat-m., Ph-ac., *Phos.,* Puls., Sec., Sep., Sil., *Sulph.*

**Chilblains:** *Abrot.,* Agar., Petr., Sulph., Tam., Zinc. (See **SKIN.**)

**Coldness:** *Acon.,* Alum., *Ars., Calc.,* Camph., Carb-an., *Carb-v.,* Caust., Chel., Cist., Con., Dig., *Dulc.,* Elaps, Helo., Kali-c., *Lach., Lyc., Meny., Mur-ac.,* Olnd., Petr., Pic-ac., Plat., Puls., Samb., *Sec.,* Sep., *Sil.,* Squil., Sul-ac., Sulph., Trif-p., *Verat.*

**Coldness, clammy:** Bar-c., *Calc.,* Laur., *Sep.,* Stry-p.

**Coldness during day, burning soles at night:** Sulph.

**Coldness of one, warmth of other:** Chel., *Chin.,* Dig., Ip., *Lyc.*

**Enlarged feeling:** Apis.

**Eruptions:** Bism., Elaps, Graph., *Petr.* (See **SKIN.**)

**Fidgety:** *Cina,* Kali-p., *Med.,* Sulph., Tarent., *Zinc., Zinc-val.*

**Itching, worse from scratching, warmth of bed:** Led., Puls., Rhus-t.

**Spasmodic motion of left foot:** Cina.

**Tender feet with shop girls:** Squil.

**HEELS, Blisters:** Squil.

**Burning:** Cycl., Graph. (See **Feet.**)

**Numbness:** *Alum.,* Ign.

**Os calcis, pain:** Aran.

**Purring sensation, extending, to right toes:** Oxyt.

**PAINS, In general:** *Agar., Am-c., Am-m.,* Brom., *Calc-caust., Caul., Caust.,* Colch., *Cycl.,* Ferr., *Graph.,* Kali-i., *Led., Mang-act.,* Nat-ar., Nit-ac., *Ph-ac., Phyt.,* Ran-b., *Rhus-t.,* Sabin., Sep., *Sil.,* Tet., Thuj., Upa., *Valer.,* Zinc.

**Aching, bruised:** Agar., Arn., Laur., Led., *Phyt., Rhus-t.*

**Soreness:** Agar., All-c., Ant-c., Caust., *Cycl.,* Jal., Kali-bi., Med., Ph-ac., Phyt., Valer.

**Soreness, as if stepping on pebbles:** Hep., Lyc.

**Tendo-Achilles, pain:** Arist-m., *Benz-ac.,* Calc-caust., Caust., *Cimic.,* Ign., Med., *Mur-ac.,* Nat-ar., Ruta, Ter., Thuj., Upa., *Valer.*

**Ulcerative:** Am-m., Berb., *Ph-ac.,* Puls., *Ran-b.*

**Ulcers on heels:** All-c., Ars., Arund., Lam.

**Itching of feet:** *Agar.,* Am-m., Ant-s-aur., *Bov.,* Caust., Magn-gr., Nat-s., Sulph., *Tell.*

**Itching, worse on scratching, warmth of bed:** Led., *Puls.,* Rhus-t.

**Joints, gouty, enlarged:** Eucal., Puls-n., Tarent-c., *Zinc.* (See **Joints**.)

**Numbness, formication, go asleep:** Aeth., Am-m., Ars., Calc., *Carb-v.,* Cob., *Cocc.,* Cod., Colch., *Con.,* Fago., Gels., *Hyper.,* Lact., Mag-s., Mez., Nux-v., Onos., Phos., *Phys.,* Pyrog., *Sec.,* Sil., Ulm-c., Upa., Viol-o., *Zinc.*

**PAINS, Aching, bruised:** *Am-m.,* Arn., Aza., Brom., Dros., Euon., Prun., *Verat.*

**Cramps:** Bism., Chin., Cho., *Colch., Cupr.,* Frax., Jatr., Lyc., Nat-c., *Sec.,* Sep., Verb., Zinc.

**Lancinating:** Abrot., *Act-sp.,* Apis, Cedr., Led., Lyc., Nat-c., Sep.

**Rheumatic:** *Act-sp.,* Apis, Berb., *Caul., Caust., Colch.,* Graph., *Led., Lith-c.,* Mang-act., Myric., Phyt., *Puls.,* Ran-b., *Rhus-t.,* Ruta.

**Sensibility, diminished:** Carbn-s.

**SOLES, Blistered:** All-c., Bufo, Calc.

**Burning:** Anac., Apoc-a., Arund., Calc., *Calc-s.,* Canth., *Cham.,* Cupr., Ferr., Graph., Ign., Kreos., *Lach.,* Lachn., Lim., Lyc., Mang-act., *Med.,* Nicc., Petr., Ph-ac., Puls., *Sang.,* Sanic., *Sulph.*

**Callosities:** Anac-oc., *Ant-c.,* Lyc., Ran-b., Sil. (See **SKIN**.)

**Injury, with intolerable pain:** Hyper.

**Itching:** *Agar.,* Anan., Anth., *Calc-s., Hydr.,* Ind., Nat-s., Sil.

**Numbness:** *Cocc.,* Lim., Raph., Sep.

**PAINS, In general:** *Apoc-a.,* Borx., Cann-i., Ferr., *Gua.,* Kali-i., *Led.,* Lim., Mur-ac., Nat-c., Petr., Ph-ac., *Puls.,* Verb.

**Aching:** Lim., Puls.

**Cramps:** Agar., Am-c., Apoc-a., Carb-v., *Colch., Cupr.,* Med., *Nux-v.,* Stront-c., Sulph., Verb., Zinc.

**Cramps, worse at P.M.:** Cupr., *Eug.,* Zing.

**Pains, when walking:** *Aloe,* Caust., Graph., Lyc., Mur-ac., *Petr.,* Ph-ac.

**Ulcerative, unable to walk:** Canth., Ign., Phos.

**Rawness, soreness, tenderness:** Aesc., Alum., *Ant-c.,* Arn., Bar-c., *Calc., Graph.,* Kali-c., *Led.,* Lyc., *Med.,* Nat-c., Nit-ac., *Petr.,* Ph-ac., *Ruta, Sanic.,* Sil.

**Swelling:** Agar., Alum., Arund., Calc., Led., Lyc., Petr. (See **Feet.**)

**Ulcer:** Ars.

**Weakness:** Hipp. (See **Feet.**)

**SWEATING OF FEET:** Alum., Am-c., *Am-m.,* Anan., Apoc-a., Arund., Bar-act., *Bar-c., Calc., Carb-v.,* Cob., *Graph.,* Iod., Lac-ac., *Lyc.,* Mag-m., *Nit-ac.,* Ol-an., *Petr.,* Ph-ac., *Psor.,* Rhus-t., Sal-ac., *Sanic., Sep., Sil., Sulph., Tell.,* Thuj., Zinc.

**Sweating, fetid:** Alum., Am-m., *Bar-c., But-ac.,* Calc., Graph., Kali-c., Nit-ac., Petr., *Psor., Sanic., Sil.,* Zinc.

**Sweating, suppressed:** *Cupr.,* Sep., Sil., *Sulph.,* Zinc.

**Sweating, suppressed, then throat affections:** *Bar-c.,* Graph., Psor., Sanic., Sil.

**Sweating, with soreness of toes:** Bar-c., Iod., Lyc., Nit-ac., *Petr.,* Sanic., *Sil.,* Zinc.

**SWELLING:** *Acet-ac.,* Aesc., Am-c., *Apis, Ars.,* Arund., Bry., *Cact.,* Caust., Chin., Colch., *Dig.,* Ferr., *Graph., Ham.,* Helo., Led., Lyc., Merc., *Merc-c.,* Nat-m., Nat-s., Ph-ac., Plb., *Prun.,* Puls., Sacch., Samb., Sep., Sil., *Stroph-h.,* Verat. (See **Dropsy, GENERALITIES.**)

**TENDERNESS, soreness:** All-c., *Ant-c.,* Arn., Bar-c., Led., Petr., Ph-ac., *Sil.,* Zinc. (See **Pain.**)

**TREMBLING:** *Gels., Phos.,* Sars., Sep., Stram.

**ULCER:** Bar c.

**VARICES:** *Ferr-act.,* Ham. (See **GENERALITIES.**)

**WEAKNESS:** Acon., *Aesc.,* Ant-c., Ars., Bov., Cann-s., *Gels.,* Hipp., Ign., Lyc., Mag-c., Ran-r.

**TOES, Bunion on big toe:** Agar., *Benz-ac.,* Borx., Hyper., Iod., Kali-i., *Rhod.,* Sang., Sars., *Sil.,* Verat-v. (See **SKIN.**)

**Burning:** Alum., Sars.

**Callosities:** Acet-ac., *Ant-c.,* Calc., Cur., *Ferr-pic.,* Graph., Hyper., Lyc., Nit-ac., *Ran-b.,* Ran-s., Semp., Sep., *Sil.,* Sul-ac. (See **SKIN.**)

**Chilblains:** *Nit-ac.,* Sal-ac., (See **SKIN.**)

**Coldness:** Sulph.

**Cracks of skin:** Eug., *Graph., Petr.,* Sabad., Sars.

**Crooked:** Graph.

**Crushed, with intolerable pain:** Hyper.

**Festering:** Graph.

**Itching:** *Agar.,* Kali-c., Maland.

**Joints inflamed:** Am-c., *Benz-ac.,* Borx., Both, Carb-v., *Colch.,* Daph., *Led., Rhod.,* Teucr. (See **Joints.**)

**Nails deformed, thick:** Ant-c., Graph., Sil.

**Nails inflamed:** Sabad.

**Nails, ingrowing:** *Caust., Graph.,* Hep., Mag-p., *M-aust., Nit-ac., Sil.,* Staph., Teucr., Thuj.

**Nails, pain around:** Ant-c., *Fl-ac.,* Hep., Nit-ac., Teucr.

**Numbness:** Con., Nat-m., Phos., Sil., Sulph., *Thal.*

**PAINS, Big toe:** Am-c., Ars., Bar-c., Calc., Elat., Eup-per., Kali-c., Led., Plb., Prim-v., Sep., Sil.

**Cramps:** Cupr., *Cupr-act.,* Dig., *Dios.,* Hyos., Lyc., Rhus-t., Sec., Sep., Sulph.

**Rheumatic:** *Act-sp.,* Apoc-a., *Benz-ac.,* Borx., Both., *Caul.,* Caust., *Colch.,* Daph., *Gnaph.,* Hyper., Kali-c., *Led., Lith-c.,* Nit-ac., Paeon., Ph-ac., *Puls.,* Sabin., *Sil.* (See **Gout.**)

**Rheumatic, in big toe:** Am-be., Arn., *Benz-ac.,* Borx., Both., *Colch.,* Conv., Gnaph., Kali-c., *Led.,* Rhod., Sil.

**Rheumatic, in tips of toes:** Am-m., *Hyper.,* Kali-c., *Sil.,* Syph.

**Tearing:** *Act-sp.,* Am-m., Benz-ac., Brom., *Caul., Colch.,* Pall., Sil., Syph.

**Soreness:** Bar-c., Brom., Nat-ar., Ph-ac. (See **Feet.**)

**Stiffness:** *Caul.,* Graph., Led., Sec. (See **Joints.**)

**Ulcer of big toe:** Sil.

**Ulcer, pemphigus:** *Ars.,* Graph., Petr., Sep.

**Wheals, eroding:** Sulph.

**GAIT: Agility:** Coff.

**Ataxic:** *Arg-n.,* Bell., Helo., Ign., Nux-v., *Sec., Sulfon.* (See **Locomotor Ataxia, NERVOUS SYSTEM.**)

**Sluggish, slow:** Gels., Ph-ac., Phos.

**Spastic, knees knock against each other when walking:** Lath.

**Staggering, unsteady, difficult walking:** Acon., *Agar.,* Agro., Ang., *Arg-n.,* Asar., Aster., *Bell.,* Calc-p., *Carbn-s., Caust., Cocc.,* Colch., *Con.,* Dub., *Gels.,* Helo., Ign., Lac-ac., *Lath.,* Lil-t., Lol., Mang-act., Merc., Morph., Mur-ac., *Mygal.,* Nat-c., Nux-m., *Nux-v.,* Onos., *Oxyt.,* Paeon., Ph-ac., *Phos.,* Rhus-t., *Sec.,* Sep., Stram., Sulfon., Tab., Trion., *Zinc.*

**Staggering, unsteady, when unobserved:** Arg-n.

**Staggering, unsteady, when walking in dark, or with eyes closed:** *Alum., Arg-n.,* Carbn-s., Dub., *Gels.,* Iodof., *Stram.*

**Staggaring, unsteady, with muscular inco-ordination:** Alum., Arag., Arg-n., Aster., *Bar-m.,* Bell., Cocc., *Gels.,* Kali-br., Med., Onos., Oxyt., Ph-ac., *Phys.,* Pic-ac., Plb., Sec., Sil., Trion., *Zinc.*

**Waking backward:** Oxyt.

**Walking backward on metacarpo-phalangeal joint:** Mang-act.
**Walking, child slow to learn:** Bar-c., Calc., Calc-p., Caust., Nat-m., Sil.
**When walking, drags feet:** *Mygal.,* Nux-v., Tab.
**When walking, foot shoots out, or turns:** Acon.
**When walking, heels do not touch gound:** Lath.
**When walking, joints feel painfully tense, as from hamstrings shortened:** Am-m., Caust., Cimx.
**When walking, legs feel heavy as lead:** Med.
**When walking, legs feel as if made of wood, or glass:** Thuj.
**When walking, legs involuntarily thrown forward:** Merc.
**When walking, lifts feet higher than usual, and brings them down hard:** Helo.
**When walking, limps involuntarily:** Bell.
**When walking, must stoop:** Arn., *Lath.,* Mang-act., Phos., Sulph.
**When walking on uneven ground, very difficult:** Lil-t.
**When walking or standing, suddenly falling to ground:** Mag-c.
**When walking, seems to be walking on air:** Dub., Lac-c.
**When walking, stumbles easily, makes missteps:** Agar., Ph-ac.
**When walking, tendency to fall forward, falls when walking backward:** Mang-act.
**When walking, trembles all over:** Lac-ac.

**JOINTS: Burning:** Apis, Ars., *Caust.,* Colch., Mang-act., Merc., *Rhus-t.,* Sulph.
**Bursae:** Benz-ac., Kali-m., *Ruta,* Sil.
**Contraction, painful, of tendons, hamstrings:** Abrot., *Am-m., Caust., Cimx.,* Coloc., Form., *Guaj.,* Kali-i., *Nat-m., Tell.*
**Cracking, on motion:** Acon., Ang., *Benz-ac.,* Calc-f., Camph., *Caust.,* Cocc., Gins., *Graph.,* Kali-bi., Kali-m., Led., Nat-m., *Nat-p., Nit-ac., Petr.,* Thuj., Zinc.
**Dropsy (hydarthrosis):** *Apis,* Bov., Canth., Chin., Chinin-s., Iod.
**Hysterical joints:** *Arg-n.,* Cham., Cot., Hyper., *Ign.,* Zinc.
**Inflammation (ARTHRITIS): Acute:** Abrot., *Acon.,* Arb., Benz-ac., Berb., *Bry.,* Caust., Chin., Cimic., *Colch.,* Gnaph., *Guaj.,* Iod., Kali-bi., Kali-i., Kalm., *Led.,* Lil-t., Lith-c., Mang-act., *Merc.,* Nat-sil., Nit-ac., Phyt., *Puls.,* Rad-br., Rhod., *Rhus-t.,* Sabin., Sal-ac., Solid., *Stel.,* Sul-ter., Viol- t. (See **Rheumatism.**)
**Inflammation, chronic (arthritis deformans):** Am-p., Ant-c., Arb., Arn., *Ars.,* Benz-ac., Calc., Calc-ren., Caul., *Caust., Chin., Cimic.,* Colch., Colchin., Ferr-i., Ferr-pic., *Guaj., Iod., Kali-br., Kali-i.,* Lac-ac., Led., Lyc., Merc-c., Nat-br., Nat-p., Nat-s., *Pipe., Puls.,* Rad-br., Sabin., Sal-ac., Sep., Sulph., *Sul-ter.,* Thyr.

**Inflammation: GOUT:** Abrot., *Acon., Am-be.,* Apis, *Arn.,* Ars., Aur-m., Aur-m-n., Bell., *Benz-ac.,* Berb., *Bry., Caj.,* Calc., Carls., Cham., *Chin., Chinin-s., Colch., Colchin.,* Cupr., Daph., Dulc., Ferr-pic., Form., *Guaj.,* Irid-met., Jab., Kali-bi., Kali-i., Kalm., *Led., Lith-c., Lyc.,* Mang-act., Med., *Merc.,* Nat-lac., Nat-m., Nat-sal., Nux-v., Ox-ac., Pancr., Phyt., *Puls.,* Querc., Rhod., Rhus-t., *Sabin.,* Sil., Spig., Stel., *Sulph.,* Tax., *Ur-ac., Urt-u.*

**Debility after attack:** Bell-p., Cypr.

**Gout of chest:** Colch.

**Gout of eyes:** Nux-v.

**Gout of hands, feet, little swelling, subacute:** Led.

**Gout of heart:** Aur-m., Cact., Conv., Cupr., Kalm.

**Gout of nerves (neuralgia):** *Colch.,* Coloc., Sulph.

**Gout of stomach:** Hydr-ac., Nux-m., Nux-v., Puls.

**Gout of throat:** Colch., Merc.

**Metastasis to heart:** Colch., Kal.

**Metastasis to stomach:** Ant-c., Nux-v.

**Nervous restlessness:** Ign.

**Retrocedent or suppressed:** *Caj.,* Nat-m., Ox-ac., Rhus-t.

**Sub-acute:** Guaj., *Led.,* Puls.

**Uterine disorders:** Sabin.

**INFLAMMATION-SYNOVITIS: Acute:** *Acon., Apis,* Arn., *Bell.,* Berb., *Bry.,* Canth., Fl-ac., *Hep., Iod.,* Led., *Puls., Rhus-t.,* Ruta, *Sabin., Sil.,* Slag, Stict.

**Inflammation, chronic:** *Am-p., Benz-ac., Berb.,* Calc., Calc-f., Calc-p., Caust., Hep., *Iod., Kali-i., Merc.,* Phyt., Puls., *Rhus-t., Ruta,* Sil., Staph., *Stel.,* Sulph., Tub.

**Itching in bends of joints:** Ph-ac.

**Lameness:** Abrot., All-c., *Rhus-t.,* Ruta, Sulph. (See **Stiffness.**)

**NODOSITIES, tophi:** Agn., Am-be., *Am-p.,* Ant-c., Aur., *Benz-ac.,* Berb., Calc., *Calc-ren.,* Caul., Caust., Cimic., *Colch.,* Elat., Eucal., Eup-per., Form., Graph., Guaj., *Hecla,* Iod., Kali-ar., *Kali-i., Kali-sil., Led., Lith-c., Lyc.,* Med., Nat-lac., Nat-uric., Pipe., Rhod., Ruta, *Sabin., Staph.,* Sulph., Urea, Ur-ac.

**PAINS, In general:** Am-c., Am-m., *Arg-met.,* Bar-c., *Bry., Calc-p.,* Cedr., Dios., Dros., Euon., *Iod.,* Kreos., Lappa, Mang-act., Sil., Sulph., Zinc.

**Bruised:** *Arn.,* Bry., Hyper., Kalm., Mez., *Rhus-t.,* Ruta.

**Cutting:** Acon., Bry., *Caul.,* Cimic., Kalm.

**Digging at P.M.:** Kali-i., Mang-ac., *Merc.*

**Drawing, tensive:** *Aloe,* Am-c., Am-m., Apoc-a., Caust., Chin., Cimx., *Colch., Gins.,* Mez., *Puls., Rhus-t., Sulph.*

**Neuralgic:** Arg-met., *Cedr.,* Coloc., Plb., Zinc.

**Rheumatic:** Abrot., *Acon.,* Asc-t., Benz-ac., Berb., *Bry., Caul.,* Caust., Chin., Cimic., *Colch.,* Dig., Dios., Ferr., Form., *Guaj.,* Iod., Kali-bi., *Kalm.,* Lac-ac., Led., *Merc.,* Pin-s., *Puls., Rad-met.,* Rham-cal., Rhod., *Rhus-t., Ruta, Sabin.,* Salol., Staph., Stront-c. (See **Rheumatism**.)

**Soreness, tenderness:** *Acon.,* Am-m., Apis, *Arn.,* Bell., Bell-p., *Bry., Colch.,* Guaj., *Ham.,* Hep., Kalm., Led., Lith-c., Meli., *Phyt.,* Puls., *Rhus-t.,* Sabin., Stict., Verat., *Verb.*

**Stitching, tearing, shifting, erratic:** Apis, Benz-ac., *Bry.,* Caust., Chin., *Cimic., Colch.,* Guaj., Kali-i., *Kalm.,* Led., Lith-c., Magn-gr., *Merc.,* Ph-ac., *Puls., Rhus-t.,* Sulph., Verat-v.

**Stiffness:** Abrot., Ang., Apis, Apoc-a., Arn., Ascl-t., Bar-m., *Bry.,* Caul., *Caust., Colch.,* Coloc., Dios., Form, *Gins., Guaj.,* Iod., *Kali-i.,* Lyc., Magn-gr., Med., *Merc.,* Mez., Nux-v., Ol-j., Petr., *Phyt.,* Pin-s., *Rhus-t.,* Sep., *Stel.,* Stry., *Sulph.,* Thiosin., Trios., Verb.

**Swelling:** Abrot., *Acon., Act-sp.,* Anag., *Apis,* Ars., *Bell.,* Benz-ac., *Bry.,* Caust., Chin., *Colch.,* Dig., *Guaj.,* Iod., *Kali-m.,* Kalm., *Led., Lith-c.,* Mang-act., Med., *Merc., Phyt., Puls.,* Rham-cal., Rhod., *Rhus-t.,* Sabin., *Stel.,* Stict.

**Swelling, dark red:** Bry., Kalm., *Rhus-t.*

**Swelling, pale, white:** *Apis,* Aur., Bry., *Calc.,* Calc-p., Cist., *Colch.,* Con., Dig., Iod., Led., *Merc., Merc-c.,* Ph-ac., Phos., *Puls.,* Rhod., *Sil.,* Sulph., Symph., Tub. (See **Knee**.)

**Swelling, shining:** *Acon., Apis, Bell., Bry.,* Dig., Mang-act., Sabin.

**Ulceration of cartilages:** Merc-c.

**Weakness:** Acon., Bar-m., Bov., *Carb-an., Caust.,* Chin., Euph., Hipp., *Led., Phos.,* Psor., Mez., *Rhus-t.,* Zing.

**Weakness, sprained easily:** Carb-an., Hep., Led.

**ANKLES, Itching:** Puls., Rhus-t., Sel.

**Itching, worse from scratching, warmth of bed:** Led.

**Pain in general:** Abrot., Alum., Am-c., But-ac., Caust., Euon., Lappa, Lath., Nat-m., Sil., Tet., Verb., *Visc.*

**Bruised, dislocated feeling:** Bry., Led., Prun., *Ruta,* Sil., Sulph.

**Rheumatic:** Abrot., *Act-sp., Caul.,* Caust., Colch., Gua., Guaj., *Led.,* Mang-act., Mang-m., Med., *Prop., Puls.,* Rad-br., *Rhod., Ruta,* Sil., Stel., Sulph., Urt-u.

**Sprains:** Carb-an., *Led.,* Nat-ar., *Nat-c., Ruta,* Stront-c.

**Sprains, chronic:** Bov., *Stront-c.*

**Stiffness:** Kali-c., Med., Sep., Sulph., Zinc.

**Swelling:** Apis, *Arg-n.,* Ferr., Ham., *Led.,* Lyc., Med., Mim-h., Plb., Stann., Stront-c. (See **Dropsy**.)

**Ulcer, itching:** Sulph.

**Weakness, "foot turns under":** Calc., *Calc-p., Carb-an., Caust., Cham.,* am., *Led.,* Mang-act., Mang-m., Med., *Nat-ar., Nat-c.,* Nat-m., Phos., *Pin-s., Ruta,* Sil., Sulph.

**ELBOWS, Numbness:** Puls.

**Pains:** Ant-c., *Arg-met.,* Ars., *Caust.,* Cinnb., Colch., *Ferr-m.,* Gua., Kali-c., *Kalm., Lyc.,* Lycpr., *Menis.,* Ol-j., Phos., Sulph., *Visc.,* Zinc-o.

**HIPS, Morbus coxarius, Diseases of:** *Acon., Arg-met.,* Ars., Ars-i., Calc., Calc-hs., Calc-i., *Calc-p., Caust.,* Chin., *Cist., Coloc.,* Ferr., Ferr-p., Fl-ac., Hep., Hippoz., Hyper., Iod., *Kali-c., Kali-i.,* Merc., Merc-i-r., *Ph-ac.,* Phos., Rhus-t., *Sil.,* Staph., Still., *Sulph.,* Tub. (See **Coxalgia**.)

**Luxation:** Coloc.

**Pain (coxalgia):** *Aesc.,* All-s., Arg-met., *Ars.,* Berb., *Bry.,* Calc., *Calc-p.,* Carb-an., Caust., Cham., Chel., Cist., Colch., *Coloc.,* Con., Dros., Elat., Ferr., Form., *Gels.,* Glyc., Gua., *Hyper.,* Kali-c., *Kali-i.,* Led., Lil-t., Lim., Lyc., Mag-m., Mez., Murx., Nat-m., Nat-s., Nux-m., *Puls.,* Rad-br., Sol-n., *Stram.,* Thuj., Tong., Trom.

**Pain, as if broken, as if pelvis was falling apart:** Aesc., *Tril-p.*

**Pain, as if sprained:** *Aesc.,* Am-m., *Calc-p.,* Caust., *Coloc.,* Laur., Nat-m., *Puls.,* Rhus-t., Sarr.

**Pain, in left hip:** Am-m., Coloc., Irid-met., Ovi-p., Sang., Sol-n., *Stram.*

**Pain, in right hip:** Agar., Ant-t., *Chel.,* Graph., Kali-c., Led., *Lil-t.,* Lim., Nux-m., Pall., Stram.

**KNEES, Coldness:** Agn., Apis, Calc., *Carb-v.,* Nat-c. (See **Extremities**)

**Cracking, on motion:** *Benz-ac.,* Caust., *Cocc.,* Croc., Dios., Nat-ar., Nux-v.

**Dislocation of patella, on going upstaris:** Cann-s.

**Dropsy:** Caust., Cedr., Iod.

**Herpes:** Carb-v., Graph., Petr.

**Hygroma patella:** Arn., Calc-p., *Iod.*

**Inflammation (synovitis, bursitis, housemaid's knee): Acute:** *Acon., Apis,* Arn., Bell., *Bry.,* Canth., Cist., Hell., *Hep.,* Iod., Kali-c., *Kali-i.,* Phos., *Puls., Rhus-t.,* Ruta, *Sil., Slag, Stict.,* Sulph. (See **Swelling**.)

**Inflammmation, chronic:** Ant-t., *Benz-ac.,* Berb., *Calc-f.,* Calc-p., Hep., *Iod., Kali-i., Merc.,* Phyt., Rhus-t., Ruta, *Sil.,* Tub.

**Numbness:** Carb-v., Meli.

**Numbness, extends to scrotum, relieved by sitting:** Bar-c.

**PAINS, In general:** Ang., *Apis,* Bell., Benz-ac., *Berb.,* Calc., Cann-i., Dios., *Elaps,* Kali-i., Kreos., Lappa, Mag-m., *Meli.,* Mez., Mur-ac., Phos., Sulph., Xero.

**Aching:** Anac., Con., Led., Meli., Ol-j.

**Boring, relieved by walking:** Indg.

**Bruised:** Ars., *Berb.,* Bry., Sarr.

**Digging, in left knee:** Aur., Caust., Coloc., Rhus-t., Spig., Tarax.

**Drawing:** Calc., Mag-m., Mur-ac., Phos., Sulph.

**Rheumatic:** Arg-met., *Benz-ac.,* Berb., *Bry., Chin.,* Cop., Daph., Elaps, Dios., *Dulc.,* Guaj., Jac-c., *Kali-c., Kali-i., Lac-ac., Led., Mang-act.,* Meli., *Merc.,* Nat-p., *Puls.,* Puls-n., Rad-br., Sabin., Stict., Visc.

**Tearing:** Calc., *Caust.,* Coloc., Gran., Lyc., *Merc.,* Petr., Stict., Tarax., Tong, Verat-v.

**Tensive, crampy:** Anac., Caps., Lath., Paeon., *Puls.,* Sil., *Verb.*

**POPLITEAL SPACE, itching:** Lyc., Sep.

**Popliteal space, pain:** Caust., Lyc., Phys., Rad-met.

**Popliteal space, prurigo:** Ars.

**REFLEXES: Diminished, lost:** *Cur.,* Oxyt., Plb., *Sec.,* Sulfon.

**Reflexes increased:** Anh., Cann-i., Lath., Mang-act. (See **NERVOUS SYSTEM.**)

**Stiffness of knees:** *Berb., Bry.,* Lyc., Mim-h., Petr., Sep., Sulph.

**Swelling:** *Apis,* Arn., Bell., Benz-ac., Berb., *Bry., Calc., Chin.,* Cocc., *Kali-i.,* Lyc., Mag-c., *Rhod.,* Sal-ac., Sil.

**Swelling, white:** Acon., *Apis,* Arn., *Calc.,* Calc-p., *Cist., Kali-i.,* Led., Ph-ac., Phos., *Puls.,* Rhus-t., Sil., Slag, *Stict.,* Sulph., Tub.

**Tenderness:** Apis, Berb., *Bry.,* Chin., *Rhus-t.* (See **Joints.**)

**Ulceration of cartilage:** Merc-d.

**Weakness:** Acon., Anac., Aur., *Cob., Cocc.,* Dios., Hipp., Lac-ac., Nat-m., Nit-ac., Sulph.

**SHOULDERS-SCAPULAE, Deltoid, pain, rheumatism:** Ferr-p., Glyc., Lycpr., Med., Nux-m., Ox-ac., Rhus-t., *Sang.,* Stict., *Syph., Urt-u.,* Viol-o., Zinc-o., Zing.

**PAINS, In general:** Alum., *Am-p.,* Anag., Arn., Aza., Bar-c., *Cann-i., Chel.,* Cocc., Con., *Fago.,* Jug-r., Kreos., Lyc., Menis., *Myric.,* Nat-ar., Nat-c., Nit-ac., *Ran-b.,* Sep., Verat., Visc.

**Pain, between scapulae:** Aesc., Ars., Bry., Camph., *Chen-a.,* Euon., *Gran.,* Guaj., Mag-s.

**Pain burning, in small spots:** Agar., *Phos.,* Ran-b., *Sulph.*

**Pain, drawing:** Ars., Berb., Cham., Coloc., Sulph.

**Pain, in left:** *Acon., Aesc., Agar.,* Ant-t., Aphis, *Aspar.,* Cham., Coloc., Eup-pur., Ferr., Led., Lob-s., Nux-m., *Onos.,* Rhodi., Stram., Sulph.

**Pain, in left, lower angle:** *Aphis.,* Cupr-ar., Ran-b.

**Pain, in right:** Abies-c., Am-m., Aphis, Bry., *Chel., Coloc.,* Ferr-p., Ferr-m., *Gua.,* Ichth., Ipom-p., Jug-c., *Kali-c.,* Kalm., Lycpr., Mag-c., Pall., Phyt., Puls-n., Ran-b., *Sang., Stict.,* Stront-c., *Urt-u.*

**Pain, in right, lower angle:** *Chel.,* Chen-a., Kali-c., *Merc.,* Podo.

**Pains, rheumatic:** Acon., Am-caust., *Berb., Bry.,* Colch., Ferr-m., *Ferr-p.,* Guaj., Ham., *Kali-c.,* Kalm., Lac-ac., *Led.,* Lith-c., *Lith-lac.,* Med., Ol-an., Pall., *Phyt.,* Prim-o., Rad-br., *Ran-b.,* Rhod., *Rhus-t., Sang.,* Stel., *Stict.,* Stront-c., Sulph., Syph., Urt-u., Viol-o.

**Pains, worse singing, using voice:** Stann.

**Stitches, tearing:** Am-m., *Bry.,* Hyper., Kali-c., Lyc., Mag-c., Nit-ac.

**Stiffness:** Cocc., *Dulc.,* Gran., Ind., *Phyt.,* Prim-v., *Sang.,* Senec-j.

**WRISTS, Ganglion, on back:** *Benz-ac.,* Calc-f., Phos., Rhus-t., *Ruta, Sil.,* Thuj.

**Gouty deposits:** Calc., Ruta.

**PAINS, In general:** Abrot., *Act-sp.,* Am-c., Bism., Carb an., *Caul.,* Chel., *Hipp., Kali-c.,* Nat-p., Paeon., *Prop.,* Rhod., *Ruta,* Sep., Sil., Sulph., Urt-u., *Viol-o.*

**Cramps, spasms, painful (writer's cramp):** *Arg-met.,* Arn., Bell., Bell-p., *Caust., Con., Cupr.,* Cycl., Ferr-i., *Gels., Mag-p.,* Nux-v., Pic-ac., Ran-b., *Ruta,* Sec., Sil., *Stann.,* Staph., *Stry.,* Sul-ac., Viol-o., Zinc.

**Rheumatic:** Abrot., *Act-sp.,* Benz-ac., Calc., *Caul., Caust.,* Colch., Hipp., Lac-ac., Lyc., Lycpr., Prop., *Rhod.,* Rhus-t., Rhus-v., *Ruta, Sabin.,* Sep., Stel., Ulm-c., Vario., *Viol-o.,* Wye.

**Sprained, dislocated feeling:** Bry., Cist., *Eup-per., Hipp.,* Ox-ac., *Rhus-t., Ruta,* Ulm-c.

**Paralysis:** *Con., Cur.,* Hipp., Pic-ac., *Plb., Plb-act.,* Ruta, Stann. (See **NERVOUS SYSTEM.**)

**NECK, Burning:** Gua.

**Cracking of cervical vertebrae, on motion:** Aloe, *Cocc., Nat-c.,* Nicc., Ol-an., Thuj.

**Emaciation:** Nat-m. (See **GENERALITIES.**)

**Eruption:** Anac., Clem., Lyc., Nat-m., Petr., *Sep.*

**Fullness, must loosen collar:** *Aml-ns.,* Fel., *Glon., Lach.,* Pyrog., Sep.

**Itching:** Ant-c.

**Muscles, cervical, contraction, rigidity:** *Cic.,* Cimic., Nicot., *Stry.*

**Muscles, cervical, shooting:** Sul-ac.

**Muscles, cervical, twitching:** Agar.

**Muscles, sternocleidomastoid:** *Gels.,* Rhod., Tarax., Trif-p. (See **Torticolis.**)

**NAPE OF NECK, PAINS: In general:** *Acon.,* Aesc., Am-c., *Bell.,* Chinin-ar., *Cimic.,* Coloc., Fel., Ferr-pic., *Gels.,* Graph., Hyper., Jug-c., Lach., Lyc., Myric., *Nat-ch.,* Nat-s., Par., Verat., Vib-o., X-ray, Zinc-val.

**Aching:** Adon., Aesc., Ang., Bapt., Caust., *Con., Gels., Guaj., Par.,* Rad-br., Verat-v., Zinc.

**Dislocated, bruised feeling:** Bell., Caust., Fago., *Lachn.*

**Rheumatic:** Acon., *Bry.,* Calc-p., Caust., *Cimic.,* Colch., *Dulc., Guaj.,* Iod., Kali-i., *Lachn.,* Petr., Puls., Rad-br., Rhod., *Rhus-t.,* Sang., Stel., *Stict.*

**Tearing, shooting, stitching:** *Acon.,* Asar., Bad., Bar-c., Bell., *Berb., Bry.,* Chinin-ar., Colch., Ferr-pic., *Mag-p.,* Nux-v., *Stry.,* Xan.

**Tension:** Con., Sep., Sulph., Tub.

**Tensive numbness:** Plat.

**Stiffness:** Acon., Ant-t., Bell., *Bry.,* Calc., Calc-caust., Calc-p., *Caust.,* Cham., Chel., *Cimic.,* Cocc., Colch., *Dulc.,* Ferr-p., Gels., Guaj., Hyper., Jug-c., Kali-c., Lac-c., *Lachn.,* Lyc., Mag-c., Med., Mentho., *Merc-i-r.,* Nicot., Nit-ac., Nux-v., Pimp., Petr., Phos., Phyt., *Puls.,* Rad-br., Rhod., Rhodi., Rhus-v., Sep., Stel., *Stict.,* Sulph., Trif-p., Vinca, X-ray.

**Swelling:** Calc., Iod., Lyc., Phos., Sil.

**Tenderness:** Aml-ns., *Bry.,* Cimic., Kali-perm., *Lach.,* Tarax.

**Tumor, fatty:** Bar-c.

**Veins, swollen:** Op.

**Weakness, unable to hold head up:** *Abrot.,* Aeth., Colch., Fago., Kali-c., Sil. (See **HEAD.**)

**Wry neck (torticollis):** *Acon.,* Agar., Atrop., *Bell., Bry., Cimic., Colch.,* Guaj., Hyos., Ign., *Lachn.,* Lyc., Mag-p., Mygal., Nux-v., Stry., Thuj.

**RHEUMATISM, TYPE, Articular, acute, RHEUMATIC FEVER:** *Acon.,* Agar., Am-be., Am-caust., Ant-t., *Apis, Arn.,* Ars., *Bell.,* Benz-ac., Berb., *Bry., Cact., Calc.,* Calc-p., Camph., *Casc., Cham.,* Chin., *Chinin-s., Cimic.,* Clem., *Colch., Colchin.,* Coloc., *Dulc., Eup-per., Ferr-p.,* Form., Franc., Gaul., Gels., Gins., *Guaj.,* Ham., Hymos., *Kali-bi.,* Kali-c., Kali-i., Kali-m., Kalm., *Led.,* Lyc., Macrot., *Merc.,* Meth-sal., Nat-lac., Nat-sal., Nux-v., Nyct., Ox-ac., Petr., Phyt., *Prop., Puls.,* Ran-b., *Rham-cal.,* Rhod., *Rhus-t.,* Ruta, *Sal-ac.,* Sang., Spig., *Stel.,* Stict., Still., Stry., *Sulph.,* Syph., Thuj., Til., Verat., *Verat-v., Viol-o.*

**Ascending pains:** Arn., *Led.*

**Descending pains:** Cact., *Kalm.*

**Erratic, wandering pains:** Apoc-a., *Caul.,* Cimic., Colch., Kali-bi., Kalm., Kali-s., *Lac-c.,* Mang-act., Phyt., *Puls.,* Puls-n., Rhod., *Stel.,* Sulph.

**Fibrous tissues (sheaths, tendons):** Arn., Form-ac., Get., Phyt., Rhod., *Rhus-t.*

**Joints, large:** *Acon.,* Arb., Arg-met., Asc-c., *Bry.,* Dros., *Merc.,* Mim-h., Rhus-t., Stict., Verat-v.

**Joints, small:** *Act-sp.,* Benz-ac., Bry., *Caul., Colch.,* Kali-bi., Lac-ac., *Led.,* Lith-c., Lith-lact., *Puls.,* Rhod., Ruta, *Sabin.,* Viol-o.

**Mono-articular:** Acon., Apis, *Bry.,* Caust., Chin., Cop., *Merc.* (See **Joints.**)

**Poly-articular:** Arn., *Bry.,* Guaj., Guaj-c., *Puls.* (See **Erratic pains.**)

**CONCOMITANTS, Alternates with diarrhea, dysentery:** *Abrot., Dulc.,* Gnaph., *Kali-bi.*

**Alternates, with urticaria:** Urt-u.

**Auricular fibrilation following:** Dig.

**Debility:** *Ars.,* Calc-p., *Chin.,* Chinin-s., *Colch.,* Ferr-c., Sulph.

**Fever, adynamic:** Bry., *Rhus-t.*

**Fever, remittent:** Chinin-s.

**Metastasis, to brain:** Bell., Op.

**Metastasis, to heart:** Adon., Aven, Cact., *Kalm.,* Lith-c., Prop., *Spig.*

**Mild cases, in nervous persons:** Viol-o.

**Nervousness, intense pains:** Cham., Coff., Rhus-t.

**Numbness:** Acon., Cham., Led., *Rhus-t.*

**Restlessness:** *Acon.,* Caust., Cimic., Puls., *Rhus-t.*

**Secretions checked:** Abrot.

**Sensitiveness to cold:** Led., *Merc.*

**Sleeplessness:** Bell., Calc., Coff., Ign.

**Skin diseases, acute, after:** Dulc.

**Sweating:** *Calc.,* Hep., Lac-ac., *Merc.,* Rham-cal., Sal-ac., Til.

**Urticarial eruption:** Urt-u.

**AGGRAVATIONS, At night:** *Acon.,* Arn., Cham., *Cimic., Colch.,* Eucal., *Kali-i.,* Kali-m., Kalm., Lac-ac., Led., *Merc.,* Phyt., *Puls.,* Rhod., Rhus-t., Sars., Sil., *Sulph.*

**Before storm:** Puls., *Rhod.,* Rhus-t.

**Colchicum, abuse:** Led.

**Crosswise, side to side:** Lac-c.

**Every other day:** Chin.

**From cold, dry weather:** *Acon.,* Bry., Caust., Nux-m., *Rhod.*

**From damp, wet weather:** Arn., Ars., *Calc-p.,* Cimic., *Colch., Dulc.,* Kali-i., *Merc.,* Nat-s., Nux-m., *Phyt.,* Ran-b., *Rhod., Rhus-t.,* Sars., Verat.

**From melting snow:** Calc-p.

**From motion:** Act-sp., Apis, *Arn., Bry., Calc., Chin.,* Cimic., Clem., Colch., Form., Get., Guaj., Iod., *Kali-m.,* Kalm., Lac-c., Led., *Merc.,* Nux-v., Phyt., Ran-b., Sal-ac., *Stel.*

**From rest:** Euph., Puls., Rhod., *Rhus-t.*

**From sweating:** Hep., *Merc.,* Til.

**From touch:** Act-sp., Acon., Apis, *Arn., Bry., Chin., Colch.,* Iod., Lac-c., Ran-b., Rhus-t., Sal-ac.

**From warmth:** Cham., Kali-m., *Led., Merc., Puls.*

**AMELIORATIONS, From motion, walking:** Cham., Chin., Dulc., Ferr., Lyc., *Puls.,* Rhod., *Rhus-t.,* Verat.

**From pressure:** Bry., Form.

**From rest:** Bry., Get.

**From warmth:** *Ars.,* Bry., Caust., Kali-bi., Nux-m., Rhus-t., *Sil.*

**From water, cold to feet:** *Led.,* Sec.

**In damp weather:** Caust.

**In open air:** Kali-m., Puls.

**ARTICULAR, CHRONIC:** *Am-p.,* Ant-c., Anthraco., Benz-ac., Berb., *Bry.,* Calc., *Calc-caust.,* Carbn-s., Caul., *Caust.,* Cimic., Colch., *Dulc.,* Euon., Ferr., Guaj., Hep., Iod., Kali-bi., Kali-c., *Kali-i.,* Led., *Lith-c.,* Lyc., Med., Merc., Mez., *Ol.j.,* Petr., Phyt., *Puls.,* Rhod., *Rhus-t.,* Ruta, Sil., *Stel.,* Still., Sul-ter., *Sulph.,* Tax. (See **Joints**.)

**ARTHRITIS DEFORMANS:** Arb., *Arn., Ars.,* Benz-ac., Calc., Caps., Caul., *Caust., Cimic., Colch.,* Colchin., *Dulc.,* Ferr-i., Ferr-pic., *Guaj., Iod., Kali-c., Kali-i.,* Lac-ac., Led., Lyc., Mang-act., Methyl., *Merc-c.,* Nat-p., Pip-m., *Puls.,* Rhod., *Sabin.,* Sal-ac., Sep., Sul-ter., *Sulph.,* Thym-gl., Thyr. (See **Joints**.)

**Chronic, secondary to uterine disorder:** Caul., *Cimic., Puls.,* Sabin.

**Gonorrheal:** Acon., *Arg-met.,* Arn., Bry., Caust., Cimic., Clem., Cop., *Daph.,* Guaj., Iod., *Irisin,* Jac-c., Kali-bi., Kali-i., Kalm., *Med.,* Merc., Nat-s., Phyt., *Puls.,* Rhus-t., *Sars.,* Sulph., *Thuj.*

**Intercostal:** Arn., *Cimic.,* Phyt., *Ran-b.,* Rhus-t.

**Muscular (myalgia):** *Acon.,* Ant-t., Apis., Arn., *Bry.,* Calc., *Casc.,* Caust., Chin., Chinin-s., *Cimic.,* Colch., Dulc., *Ferr.,* Gels., Glyc., Gnaph., Ham., Hyper., Jac-c., Lyc., *Macrot.,* Merc., Phos., Phyt., *Ran-b.,* Rhod., Rhus-t., Sang., Sil., Sulph., Syph., Verat-v.

**Paralytic:** Caust., Lath., Phos. (See **Chronic**.)

**Periosteal:** Bell., Cham., Colch., Cycl., Guaj., *Kali-bi.,* Kali-i., Merc., *Mez.,* Phos., Phyt., Sars., Sil.

**Subacute:** Dulc., *Led.,* Merc., *Puls.,* Rhus-t.

**Syphilitic:** (See **Periosteal**.)

■

# NERVOUS SYSTEM

**BRAIN, EPILEPSY, (grand mal):** *Absin.,* Aeth., *Agar.,* Am-br., Aml-ns., Anis., *Arg-n.,* Ars., *Art-v.,* Aster., Atrop., Aur-br., Aven., *Bell.,* Borx., *Bufo, Calc., Calc-ar.,* Calc-p., Camph., Cann-i., *Caust., Cic.,* Cic-m., Cimic., *Cocc.,* Con., *Cupr.,* Cupr-act., *Ferr-cy.,* Ferr-p., Gels., Glon., Hep., *Hydr-ac., Hyos., Ign.,* Indg., Irid-met., *Kali-br.,* Kali-cy., Kali-m., Kali-p., *Lach.,* Mag-c., Mag-p., Meli., Methyl., Nit-ac., *Nux-v., Oena.,* Op., Oest., Passi., Phos., Picro., Plb., Psor., *Salam.,* Santin., Sec., *Sil., Sol-c.,* Spirae., *Stram.,* Stry., *Sulph.,* Sumb., Tarent., Tub., Valer., *Verb.,* Visc., Zinc-cy., Zinc-val., *Ziz.*

**CAUSE, CONCOMITANTS, Aura absent:** Zinc-val.

**Aura absent, several fits, close together:** Art-v.

**Aura begins, as painful spot, between shoulders, or dizziness, flashes of heat, from abdomen to head:** Indg.

**Aura begins, as sensation of mouse running up limb, heat from stomach, visual or aural disturbance:** *Bell.,* Calc., Sulph.

**Aura begins, in brain, as a wavy sensation:** Cimic.

**Aura begins, in knees, ascends to hypogastrium:** Cupr.

**Aura begins, in left arm:** Sil.

**Aura begins, in solar plexus:** Bufo, Calc., Nux-v., Sil.

**Aura begins, in stomach or genitals:** Lyc.

**Aura begins, in upper or lower limbs:** Lyc.

**Aura descends:** Calc.

**Aura felt, in heart region:** Calc-ar.

**During full moon, nocturnal:** Calc.

**During new moon, nocturnal:** Caust., Cupr., Kali-br., Sil.

**During sleep:** Bufo, Cupr., Lach., *Op., Sil.*

**Followed by deep sleep:** Aeth., Hyos., Kali-br., Lach., *Op.*

**Followed by hiccough:** Cic.

**Followed by nausea, vomiting:** Bell.

**Followed by prostration:** Aeth., *Chinin-ar., Cic.,* Hydr-ac., Sec., Sil., *Stry.,* Sulph.

**Followed by rage, automatic impulse:** Op.

**Followed by restlessness:** Cupr.

**Followed by tumor:** Arg-n., Cic.

**From eruptions, suppressed:** Agar., Calc., Cupr., Psor., *Sulph.*

**From fright, emotional causes:** *Arg-n.,* Art-v., Bufo, Calc., Cham., Hyos., *Ign.,* Sil., Stram.

**From hysteria:** Asaf., Cocc., Cupr., Hyos., *Ign.,* Mosch., Oena, *Sol-c.,* Sumb., Tarent., *Zinc-val.*

**From injury:** Con., Cupr., Meli., Nat-s.

**From jealousy:** Lach.

**From menstrual disturbances:** Arg-n., Bufo, Caul., Caust., Cedr., *Cimic.,* Cupr., Kali-br., *Mill.,* Oena., Puls., Sol-c.

**From pregnancy:** Oena.

**From sclerosis, brain tumors:** Plb.

**From sexual disturbances:** Art-v., *Bufo,* Calc., Plat., Stann., Sulph.

**From syphilis, tubercular:** Kali-br.

**From taking cold, nocturnal, worse right side:** Caust.

**From valvular disease:** Calc-ar.

**From vital drains, onanism:** Lach.

**From wet exposure:** Cupr-

**From worms:** Cic., Cina, Indg., Santin., Sil., Stann., Sulph., Teucr.

**In children:** Aeth., Art-v., *Bell.,* Bufo, Calc., Cham., Cupr., Ign., Sil., Sulph.

**Periodical seizures:** Ars., Cupr.

**Preceded, by cold on left side of body:** Sil.

**Preceded, by dilated pupils:** Arg-n.

**Preceded, by gastric flatulency:** *Arg-n.,* Nux-v., Psor., Sulph.

**Preceded, by irritability, rambling:** Bufo.

**Preceded, by malaise:** Cic.

**Preceded, by memory, confused:** Lach.

**Preceded, by palpitation, vertigo:** Lach.

**Preceded, by sudden cry:** Cupr., Hydr-ac.

**Preceded, by tremblings, twitchings:** Absin., Aster.

**Preceded, by vesicular eruption:** Cic.

**Recent cases:** Bell., Caust., Cupr., *Hydr-ac., Ign.,* Op., Plb., Stram.

**Recurrent, several times daily:** Art-v., Cic.

**Status epilepticus:** *Acon.,* Aeth., *Bell.,* Cocc., Oena., Plb., Zinc.

**With consciousness:** Ign.

**With face red, thumbs clenched, jaws locked, foam in mouth, eyes turned downwards, pupils fixed, dilated, pulse small, quick, hard:** Aeth.

**With paralysis following:** *Caust.,* Plb., Sec.

**With swelling of stomach, screaming, unconsciousness, trismus, distorted limbs, frequent during night, recurrent tendency:** Cic.

**With vertigo (epileptic):** Arg-n., Bell., Calc., Caust., Cocc., Cupr., Hydr-ac., Nit-ac., Op., Sil., Stram.

**PARALYSIS, Remedies in general:** Absin., *Acon.,* Agar., Alum., Ang., Arag., Arg-i., *Arg-n.,* Ars-i., Asaf., Aur., *Bar-act., Bar-c., Bar-m., Bell.,* Calc-caust., Calen., *Cann-i.,* Carbn-o., Carbn-s., *Caust.,* Chinin-s., Cic., *Cocc.,* Colch., *Con., Cupr., Dulc., Gels.,* Graph., Grin., *Gua,* Helo., Hydr-ac.,

Hyos., *Hyper.,* Ign., Iris-fl., Kali-br., *Kali-c.,* Kali-i., Kali-p., Lach., Lat-h., Lol., Merc-c., Nat-m., Nux-v., *Olnd., Op., Ox-ac.,* Oxyt., *Phos., Phys.,* Physal., Pic-ac., Plat., Plect., *Plb., Plb-act., Plb-i., Rhus-t.,* Stann., Staph., Sec., Stry-af-cit., Sulph., Tab., *Thal.,* Verat., Xan., Zinc., Zinc-p.

**TYPE, Agitans:** *Agar.,* Ars., *Aur-s.,* Aven., Bufo, *Camph-mbr.,* Cann-i., Cocain., Cocc., *Con., Dub.,* Gels., Helo., *Hyos., Hyosin-hbr.,* Kali-br., Lath., Lol., Mag-p., Mang-act., *Merc.,* Nicot., Phos., Phys., *Plb.,* Scut., Tab., Tarent., Zinc-cy., *Zinc-pic.*

**Ascending spinal:** Alum., Bar-act., *Con.,* Gels., Lath., Led., *Ox-ac., Phos.,* Pic-ac., Sec. (See **Spine**.)

**Bulbar:** Gua., Mang-o., Plb.

**General of insane:** Ant-c., Ars., Aur., Bell., *Cann-i.,* Caust., Hyos., Kali-br., Kali-i., Merc-c., Nat-i., Nux-v., Op., *Phos.,* Phys., Plb., Stram., Sulph., Verat.

**Gradually appearing:** Caust.

**HEMIPLEGIA:** Ambr., *Arn.,* Ars., *Aur.,* Bapt., *Bar-c., Both.,* Carbn-s., *Caust.,* Chen-a., *Cocc.,* Cur., Elaps, Hydr-ac., Irid-met., *Lach., Nux-v., Olnd.,* Phos., Phys., Pic-ac., *Rhus-t., Sec.,* Stann., Stry., Verat-v., Vip., Xan.

**Hemiplegia, left:** Ambr., *Arn.,* Bapt., Bell., Cocc., Cupr-ar., *Lach.,* Lyc., Phys., Verat-v., Xan.

**Hemiplegia, right:** Bell., *Caust,* Chen-a., Cur., Elaps, Irid-met.

**Hysterical:** Acon., Arg-n., Asaf., Cocc., *Ign.,* Phos., *Tarent.*

**Infantile (poliomyelitis, anterior):** *Acon.,* Aeth., Bell., *Calc., Caust.,* Chr-s., *Gels.,* Lath., Nux-v., Phos., *Plb.,* Rhus-t., Sec., Sulph. (See **Spine**.)

**Labio-glosso-pharyngeal:** Anac., Bar-c., *Bell.,* Caust., Cocc., Con., Gels., Mang-o., Nux-v., Olnd., *Plb.*

**Landry's paralysis:** Aconin., Con., Lyss.

**Lead:** *Alumn.,* Caust., Cupr., Kali-i., Nux-v., Op., Plb., Sul-ac.

**LOCALIZED, in ankles, in afternoon:** Cham.

**Localized, in arms, hands:** Cupr., Thyr.

**Localized, in bladder:** Caust., Nux-v.

**Localized, in chest:** Gels.

**Localized, in eye muscles:** Caust., Con., *Gels.,* Phos., Phys., Rhus-t.

**Localized, in face (Bell's palsy):** Acon., *Am-p.,* Bar-c., Bell., Caust., Cur., Gels., Graph., *Kali-chl.,* Nat-m., Physal., Rhus-t., *Zinc-pic.*

**Localized, in feet at night:** Cham.

**Localized, in forearm (wrist drop):** Cur., Ferr-act., Plb., Plb-act., Ruta, Sil.

**Localized, in motor nerves:** Cur., Cystin., *Gels., Ox-ac., Phos., Phys.,* Xan.

**Localized, in neck:** Cocc.

**Localized, in sensory nerves:** *Cocain.,* Cyt-l., Plat.

**Localized, in sphincters:** Ars., *Caust.,* Gels., Naja, Nux-v., Phos., Phys.

**Localized, in throat, vocal cords:** Bell., Both., Canth., *Caust.,* Cocain., Cocc., *Gels.,* Kali-p., Ox-ac., Plb.

**PARAPLEGIA:** Acon., Alum., Anh., *Arg-n.,* Arn., Ars., *Bell.,* Caul., *Caust., Cocc., Con., Cupr.,* Cur., Dulc., Form., *Gels., Hyper.,* Kali-i., *Kali-t.,* Kalm., Lach., *Lath.,* Lat-h., Mang-act., Merc-c., *Nux-v., Ox-ac., Phos.,* Phys., Pic-ac., *Plb-act., Rhus-t.,* Sec., Stry., *Thal.,* Thyr.

**Paraplegia, hysterical:** *Cocc.,* Con., Cupr., *Ign.,* Nux-v., Plb., *Tarent.*

**Paraplegia, spastic:** Gels., Hyper., *Lath.,* Nux-v., Plect., Sec. (See **Sclerosis, Spine**).

**POST-DIPHTHERITIC:** *Arg-n.,* Aur-m., Aven., Botul., *Caust., Cocc.,* Con., *Diph., Gels.,* Kali-i., *Lach.,* Nat-m., Nux-v., Phos., Phyt., Plb., Plb-act., Rhod., Rhus-t., Sec.

**Pseudo-hypertrophic:** Cur., *Phos.,* Thyr.

**Rheumatic:** *Caust.,* Dulc., Lath., Phos., *Rhus-t.,* Sulph.

**Spinal origin:** Alum., Bell., Cann-i., *Con.,* Irid-met., *Lath., Phos.,* Phys., *Pic-ac.,* Plb., Xan.

**PETIT MAL:** *Art-v.,* Bell., Caust., Phos., *Zinc-cy.*

**SLEEP, DROWSINESS:** Aeth., Am-c., Ant-c., *Ant-t., Apis,* Apoc., Arn., Aur., *Aur-m.,* Bapt., Bar-m., Cann-i., *Carbn-o.,* Carbn-s., Caust., *Chin., Clem.,* Coca, Cocc., Corn-f., *Cycl.,* Cyt-l., Dub., Ferr-p., *Gels., Hell.,* Helon., Hydr-ac., Hyper., *Indol.,* Kali-br., Kali-c., Lath., Lina., Lob-p., *Lup., Morph.,* Naja, *Nux-m., Op.,* Ph-ac., Phos., Pyrog., Rhus-t., Rosm., Sarcol-ac., *Scroph-n.,* Sel., Senec., Sulfon., Thea, Zinc.

**Drowsiness, after meals:** Bism., *Chin.,* Graph., Kali-c., *Lyc.,* Nux-m., Nux-v., Paul., *Phos.,* Puls., Scroph-n. (See **Indigestion, STOMACH**.)

**Drowsiness, during day:** *Agar.,* Alum., *Am.c.,* Anac., *Ant-c., Calc.,* Calc-p., Cann-s., Carb-v., *Chin.,* Cinnb., *Colch.,* Euphr., Graph., Indol., Kali-c., Lup., *Lyc.,* Mag-m., Merc., Merc-c., *Nat-c.,* Nat-m., Nux-m., *Op., Phos., Sep.,* Sil., Spong., Staph., *Sulph.,* Tub.

**Drowsiness, during day, wakeful at P.M.:** *Abies-n.,* Cinnb., Colch., Graph., Lach., *Lyc.,* Merc., Ph-ac., Sil., Staph., Thea. (See **Insomnia**.)

**Drowsiness, in A.M. and forenoon:** Alum., Anac., *Am-c.,* Bism., Carb-v., Nat-m., *Nux-v.,* Petr., Zinc.

**Drowsiness, in early evening:** Calc., Mang-act., *Nux-v.,* Phos., Puls., *Sep., Sulph.*

**Drowsiness, in evening, while sitting, reading:** Nux-v.

**Drowsiness, yet cannot sleep:** Ambr., *Apis, Bell.,* Cann-i., Caust., *Cham.,* Coca., Coff., Cupr., Ferr., *Gels.,* Lach., Morph., *Op.,* Sil., Stram.

**INCUBUS (nightmare):** Acon., Am-c., Arn., *Aur-br.,* Bapt., *Cann-i.,* Chlol., *Cina,* Cypr., Daph., *Kali-br.,* Kali-p., Op., *Nux-v.,* Nit-ac., Paeon., Pariet., Phos., Ptel., Scut., Sol-n., Sulph.

**INSOMNIA (sleeplessness), Remedies in general:** *Absin., Acon.,* Agar., Alf., Alum., Ambr., Am-c., *Anac.,* Ant-c., Apis, Apom., Aqui., Arn., Arg-n., *Ars.,* Aur., *Aven.,* Bapt., *Bell.,* But-ac., Cact., *Calc., Camph., Camph-mbr., Cann-i.,* Caul., *Cham.,* Chin., Chinin-s., Chlol., Chrysan., *Cimic., Coca, Cocain., Cocc., Coff.,* Coffin., Coloc., *Cypr.,* Daph., Dip., *Gels., Hyos., Hyosin-hbr., Ign.,* Iod., *Kali-br.,* Kali-p., Lec., Lil-t., *Lup.,* Lyss., Mag-p., Merc., *Nux-v., Op., Passi.,* Phos., Pic-ac., *Puls.,* Sel., *Scut.,* Stann., Staph., Sulfon., *Sulph., Sumb.,* Stram., Tela, Thea, Valer., Xan., Yohim., Zinc-p., Zinc-val.

**CAUSES, OCCURRENCE, Abdominal disturbances:** Ant-t., Cupr.

**Aching in bones:** Daph.

**Aching in legs, yet cannot keep them still:** Med.

**Aching in muscles, too much exhausted, tired out:** Helon.

**Alcoholic, drug, habits:** Ars., Aven., Cann-i., *Cimic., Gels., Hyos., Nux-v.,* Op., Sec., Stram., *Sumb.*

**Anxiety, driving him out of bed, aggravated after midnight:** Ars.

**Aortic disease:** Crat.

**Arterial pulsations:** Acon., *Bell., Cact., Glon.,* Sec., Sel., Sulph., Thea.

**Banqueting, late suppers:** Puls.

**Bed feels too hard, cannot lie on it:** Arn., Bry., *Pyrog.*

**Bed feels too hot, unable to lie on it:** Op.

**Chest oppression:** Physal.

**Chronic nicotinism:** Plan.

**Coffee, abuse:** Cham., *Nux-v.*

**Coldness of body:** *Acon.,* Ambr., Camph., *Carb-v.,* Cist., *Verat.*

**Coldness of knees:** Apis, *Carb-v.*

**Cramps:** Arge., Coloc., Cupr.

**Delirium:** Acon., *Bell.,* Cact., Calc., *Cann-i.,* Gels., *Hyos.,* Kali-br., Phos., *Stram.,* Verat. (See **MIND.**)

**Dentition:** Bell., Borx., *Cham.,* Coff., Cypr. (See **TEETH.**)

**Dry mouth:** Apis, Calc., Caust., Lach., *Nux-m., Par.,* Puls., Tarent.

**Emotional causes (grief, worry, anxiety, over excitement, nervousness):** Absin., *Acon., Alf., Ambr.,* Am-val., Aur., Bry., *Cann-i.,* Cham., Chinin-ar., Chlol., *Cimic.,* Coca, *Coff.,* Coloc., *Gels., Hyos.,* Hyosin-hbr., *Ign., Kali-br.,* Mosch., Nat-m., *Nux-v.,* Op., Passi., Ph-ac., Plat., Senec., *Sep., Stram.,* Sulph., Thea, Valer., Zinc-val.

**Exhaustion, deblity, over-exertion of mind or body:** *Arn., Ars.,* Aven., Cann-i., *Chin.,* Chinin-s., Chlol., *Cimic.,* Coca, *Cocc., Colch.,* Dip., *Gels.,* Hyos., Kali-br., *Nux-v.,* Passi., Pisc., *Phos.*

**Eyes, half open, during:** Bell., *Cham.,* Hyos., Ip., *Op.,* Podo., *Zinc.* (See **EYES.**)

**Every second night:** Chin., Lach.

**Fears suffering from mental and physical exhaustion on waking:** Lach., Syph.

**Formication in calves and feet:** Sulph.

**Grinding of teeth:** *Bell.,* Cic., *Cina,* Hell., Kali-br., *Podo., Santin.,* Spig., Zinc.

**Heat in general:** Acon., Arn., Bar-c., *Bell.,* Borx., Caust., Cham., *Hep.,* Kali-br., Mag-m., Meph., Op., *Sanic.,* Sil., *Sulph.*

**Hunger:** *Abies-n.,* Ap-g., *Cina,* Ign., Lyc., *Psor.,* Sulph.

**Hyperacute senses:** Asar., *Bell.,* Calad., Calc-br., Cham., Cocc., *Coff.,* Ign., Nux-v., *Op.,* Tarent., Valer., Zinc-val.

**In aged:** *Acon.,* Ars., Op., Passi., *Phos.*

**In children:** *Absin., Acon.,* Ars., *Bell.,* Calc-br., *Cham., Cina, Cypr.,* Hyos., Kali-br., *Passi.,* Phos., Puls., Sulph.

**Itching:** Acon., *Agar.,* Alum., Psor., Teucr., Sulph., Valer.

**Itching of anus:** *Aloe,* Alum., Coff., Ign., *Indg.*

**Itching of scrotum:** Urt-u.

**Mental activity, flow of ideas:** Acon., Ap-g., Apis, Bry., Calc., *Chin., Cocc., Coff.,* Gels., Hep., *Hyos.,* Lyc., Meph., *Nux-v.,* Puls., Sep., Verat., Yohim.

**Moaning, whining, during:** Ant-t., Arn., Ars., Aur., *Bapt., Bell.,* Carb-v., *Cham.,* Cic., Cupr-act., *Gels., Hell.,* Hyos., Kali-br., Lach., Lyc., *Mur-ac.,* Nat-m., Nit-ac., *Op., Podo.,* Puls., Rhus-t., Verat.

**Mouth, open:** Merc., Rhus-t., Samb.

**Menopause: women with prolapsus uteri or uterine irritation:** Senec.

**Mouth and throat sore:** Arum-t., Merc.

**Multiple neuritis:** Con.

**Nose stopped up must breathe though mouth:** Am-c., Lyc., Nux-v., Samb.

**Pains:** Ars., Cann-i., *Cham.,* Coloc., Mag-m., Merc., Passi., Puls., Sin-n.

**Palpitation:** Acon., Alum., Am-c., *Cact., Iod.,* Lil-t., Lycps-v., Rhus-t., Sep.

**Picks at bed clothes, during:** Op.

**Weaning of child:** Bell.

**DREAMS, Accidents, falling from height, etc.:** Arn., Bell., Calc., *Dig.,* Lyc., Nit-ac., Sil., Verat.

**Animals, snakes:** Arg-n., Daph., Lac-c., Op., Ran-s.

**Anxious:** Abies-n., *Acon.,* Ambr., Anac., *Apis, Arg-n.,* Arn., *Ars., Bell., Bry.,* Calc., Caust., Cann-i., Canth., *Cham.,* Chin., Euph-l., Ferr-p., Graph., Ign., Kali-c., Lyc., Nat-m., Nit-ac., Nux-v., Oxyt., Puls., *Rhus-t.,* Sec., Sep., *Sil.,* Staph., *Sulph.,* Zinc.

**Business matters he forgets during day:** Sel.

**Confused:** Alum., Chin., Glon., Hell., Hydr-ac., Phos.

**Continues, after being apparently awake:** Calc., Chin., Nat-m.

**Death, or dead persons:** Arn., *Ars.,* Calc., Cann-i., Crot-c., Crot-h., Elaps, *Lach.,* Nit-ac., Ran-s.

**Dreamful:** Alum., Brom., Con., Hyos., Ign., Lyc., Nit-ac., Phos., Sep.

**Drinking:** Ars., Med., Nat-m., Phos.

**Exertion of body, toil, business:** Apis, Ars., Bapt., *Bry.,* Nat-m., Nux-v., Phos., Puls., *Rhus-t.,* Sel., Staph.

**Fantastic, pleasant:** Op.

**Fires, flames, lightening:** Bell., Euphr., Lach., Phos.

**Flying through air:** Apis, *Rhus-g.,* Stict.

**Forgotten matters:** Sel.

**Happy dreams:** Sulph.

**Hemorrhage:** Phos.

**Horrible:** Adon., *Arg-n., Aur.,* Bapt., *Bell., Cact.,* Calc., Cann-i., Castm., *Cham., Chin., Colch.,* Eupi., Graph., *Hyos.,* Kali-br., Kali-c., *Lil-t.,* Lyc., *Merc-c.,* Nux-v., Op., Phos., Psor., Puls., Ran-s., *Rhus-t.,* Sec., Sep., Stram., *Sulph.,* Thea, *Zinc.*

**Images bewildering, figures:** Bell., Hyos.

**Lascivious:** Arg-n., Ars., *Cann-i.,* Canth., *Cob., Dios.,* Ham., *Hyos.,* Ign., Nat-m., Nit-ac., Op., Ph-ac., *Phos.,* Sil., *Staph.,* Thuj., Ust., Verat-v. (See **Emissions, MALE SEXUAL SYSTEM.**)

**Laughs during:** Alum., Caust., Hyos., Lyc.

**Robbers:** Bell., *Nat-m.,* Psor., Verat.

**Vivid:** Agar., *Arg-n.,* Brom., *Cann-i.,* Cench., Cham., Coff., Daph., Dios., Hydr-ac., *Hyos.,* Indol., Iod., Mang-act., Nat-m., Petr., Phos., Puls., Pyrog., *Sulph.,* Tub., Verat-v. (See **Anxious.**)

**POSITION: Must lie in knee-chest positon:** Med.

**Must lie on back:** Am-c., *Ars.,* Cina.

**Must lie on back with thighs drawn upon abdomen, hands above head, disposition to uncover lower limbs:** Plat.

**Must lie on belly:** Acet-ac., Am-c.

**Must lie on hands and knees:** Cina.

**Must lie with hands over head:** Ars., Nux-v., Plat., Puls., Sulph., Verat.

**Must lie with hands under head:** Acon., Ars., Bell., Chin., Coloc., Plat.

**Must lie with legs apart:** Cham., Plat.

**Must lie with legs crossed:** Rhod.

**Must lie with one leg drawn up, other stretched out:** Stann.

**Must move or fidget feet constantly:** Zinc.

**Must stretch violently for hours:** Aml-ns., Plb.

**RESTLESSNESS, awakens frequently (catnaps):** Bar-c., *Calc.,* Dig., Ferr., *Ign.,* Lyc., Nit-ac., Nux-v., *Phos.,* Plat., Sacrol-ac., *Sel.,* Sil., Stram., *Sulph.*

**Restlessness, during:** *Acon., Agar.,* Alum., Ambr., Apis, Apoc., Arg-n., Arn., *Ars., Bapt., Bell.,* Bry., Calc., *Cann-i.,* Castm., Caust., *Cham.,* Chin., *Cimic.,* Cina, Coca, Cocain., *Coff.,* Eup-per., Gels., Glon., Graph., *Hyos., Ign., Jal.,* Kali-br., Lac-d., Lyc., Mentho., Nit-ac., Nux-v., Passi., Psor., Ptel., Puls., Rad-br., *Rhus-t.,* Ruta, Santin., Sarcol-ac., *Scut., Stram.,* Stront-c., Sulfon., *Sulph.,* Tarent., Thea, Zinc.

**Restlessness, kicks off clothes:** Hep., Op., Sanic., *Sulph.*

**Restlessness, rolling head:** Apis, *Bell.,* Hell., *Podo.,* Zinc.

**Sexual causes:** Cann-i., *Canth., Kali-br., Raph.* (See **SEXUAL SYSTEM.**)

**Shocks, electric-like, on falling asleep:** Ant-t., *Cupr.,* Ign., Ip.

**Shrieks, screams, awakens frightened:** Ant-c., Ant-t., *Apis,* Aur., *Bell.,* Borx., *Bry.,* Cham., Chin., *Cic., Cina, Cupr-act.,* Cypr., Dig., *Hell., Hyos.,* Ign., Iodof., Kali-br., Lyc., Nux-m., Phos., Psor., Puls., Spong., Stram., Tub., *Zinc.*

**Singing, during:** Bell., Croc., Ph-ac.

**Singing on awakening:** Sulph.

**Skin dry:** Thea.

**Sleepless, in evening, before midnight:** *Ars.,* Lach., *Lil-t.,* Nat-m., Nux-v., Ph-ac., Phos., *Puls., Rhus-t.,* Sel., Thuj.

**Sleepless, after 2 A.M-to 3 A.M.:** Ap-g., Bapt., Bell-p., Bry., *Calc.,* Chin., *Coff.,* Gels., *Kali-c.,* Kalm., Nat-c., Nat-m., Nit-ac., *Nux-v., Sel.,* Sep.

**Snoring, during:** Chin., Laur., *Op.,* Sil., Stram., Tub., *Zinc.*

**Soporous, deep, heavy sleep:** Am-c., Ant-c., *Apis,* Arn., Chin., *Cupr., Hell.,* Hyos., Kali-br., Lact., Laur., Lon-x., Lup., *Morph.,* Naja, Nux-m., Op., *Ph-ac.,* Pisc., Podo., Rhus-t., Sec., *Stram.,* Sulph.

**Spasmodic symptoms, during (jerkings, twitchings, startings):** *Acon., Aeth., Agar.,* Ambr., Ant-c., *Apis,* Ars., *Bell.,* Borx., Brom., Bry., Calc., Carb-v., Castm., Caust., *Cham.,* Chin., *Cina, Cupr-act.,* Daph., Hell., *Hyos., Ign.,* Kali-c., *Lyc.,* Morph., Nit-ac., Nux-v., Passi., Phos., Samb., Sil., *Stram., Sulph.,* Tarent., Valer., *Zinc.,* Ziz.

**Suddenly wide awake:** Sulph.

**Suffocation, loss of breath, on falling asleep:** *Am-c.,* Ars., *Cur.,* Graph., *Grin.,* Kali-i., *Lach.,* Lac-c., *Merc-p-r.,* Morph., Naja, Op., *Samb., Spong.,* Stront-c., Sulph., Teucr.

**Sweating, during:** Aeth., *Calc., Cham., Chin.,* Op., Ph-ac., Psor., *Sil.,* Verat. (See **Night Sweats, FEVER.**)

**Talking, during:** Bar-c., Bell., Bry., Carb-v., *Cina,* Graph., *Hell.,* Hyos., Kali-c., Lyc., Sep., Sil., Sulph., *Zinc.*

**Tea, abuse:** Camph-mbr., Chin., *Nux-v.*, Puls.

**Tobacco:** Gels.

**Unrefreshing, awakens wretched:** Alum., *Ant-c.*, Ap-g., *Ars.*, Brom., Bry., *Chin.*, Cob., *Con.*, Dig., Ferr., Graph., *Hep.*, *Lach.*, Lil-t., *Lyc.*, Mag-c., Merc-c., Myric., *Nux-v.*, Op., Phos., Ptel., *Puls.*, Rhus-t., Sarcol-ac., Sep., *Sulph.*, Syph., Thuj., Thymol., Tub., Zinc.

**Walking, during (somnambulism):** Art-v., *Bry.*, *Kali-br.*, Paeon., *Sil.* (See **MIND**.)

**Yawning, stretching, limbs:** Acon., *Agar.*, All-c., *Aml-ns.*, Ant-t., Arn., Asar., Calc., Carl., Castm., *Chel.*, *Chin.*, *Cina*, Coca, Crot-h., Cupr-act., Elat., Euphr., *Gels.*, Hep., Hydr-ac., *Ign.*, Kali-c., Lyc., Mang., Morph., *Nat-m.*, *Nux-v.*, Plb., *Rhus-t.*, Sec., *Sil.*, *Sulph.*

**GENERALITIES, ADYNAMIA (general weakness, debility):** Abies-c., *Acet-ac.*, Adren., Aeth., *Ail.*, *Alet.*, Alst., Ambr., Am-c., *Anac.*, *Ant-t.*, *Antip.*, Apis, *Arg-n.*, *Arn.*, *Ars.*, *Ars-i.*, Asaf., Aur., Aur-m., *Aven.*, *Bals-p.*, *Bapt.*, Bar-c., Bell-p., *Bry.*, *Calc.*, Calc-hp., *Calc-p.*, *Camph.*, Cann-s., Canth., *Carb-ac.*, *Carb-v.*, Caul., *Caust.*, *Chin.*, *Chinin-ar.*, *Chinin-fcit.*, *Chinin-s.*, Coca, *Cocc.*, *Colch.*, *Con.*, Crat., Crot-h., *Cupr.*, *Cur.*, *Dig.*, Dip., Diph., Dulc., *Echi.*, *Ferr.*, Ferr-m., Ferr-p., Ferr-pic., *Gels.*, Hell., *Helon.*, Hep., *Hydr.*, Hyos., Ign., *Iod.*, Ip., *Irid-met.*, Iris, Kali-br., *Kali-c.*, Kali-i., *Kali-p.*, Lac-ac., *Lac-c.*, Lach., Lil-t., Lith-c., Lith-chl., Lob-p., *Lyc.*, Mag-m., Mag-p., Meli., Merc., Merc-c., *Merc-cy.*, Merc-i-r., Murx., *Mur-ac.*, *Nat-c.*, *Nat-m.*, *Nat-sal.*, *Nit-ac.*, Nux-v., Op., Orni., Ox-ac., *Ph-ac.*, *Phos.*, Phys., Phyt., *Pic-ac.*, Plb., *Psor.*, Rhus-t., *Ruta*, Sang., *Sarcol-ac.*, Sec., *Sel.*, *Sep.*, *Sil.*, Solid., Spong., *Stann.*, Stroph-h., *Stry.*, *Sul-ac.*, Sulfon., Sulph., *Tab.*, Tanac., Ter., Thea, *Thuj.*, Tub., Uran-n., Valer., *Verat.*, Zinc., *Zinc-ar.*, *Zinc-p.*, *Zinc-pic.*

**Adynamia, collapse:** Acetan., Acon., *Ant-t.*, Arn., *Ars.*, *Camph.*, Carb-ac., *Carb-v.*, Colch., Crat., Crot-h., Cupr-act., *Dig.*, Diph., Hydr-ac., *Laur.*, Lob., Lob-p., Med., Merc-cy., *Morph.*, Mur-ac., Nicot., Op., Phos., *Sec.*, Sul-ac., *Tab.*, *Verat.*, Vip., *Zinc.*

**Adynamia, afebrile:** Ars., Bapt., Carb-v., Chin.

**Adynamia, from acute diseases, mental strain:** Abrot., Alet., *Alst.*, *Anac.*, Aven., *Calc-p.*, Carb-an., *Carb-v.*, *Chin.*, *Chinin-ar.*, Coca, *Cocc.*, Colch., Cupr., Cur., Dig., Fl-ac., Gels., *Helon.*, *Irid-met.*, Kali-fcy., *Kali-p.*, Lath., Lob-p., Macroz., Nat-sal., Nux-v., *Ph-ac.*, *Phos.*, Pic-ac., *Psor.*, Sel., Sil., Staph., Stry-p., Sul-ac., Zinc-ar.

**Adynamia, from anesthetics, surgical shock:** Acet-ac., Hyper.

**Adynamia, from depressing emotions:** Calc-p., Ign., *Ph-ac.*

**Adynamia, from diphtheria, stupor, cold limbs, low temperature, pulse rapid, weak:** Diph.

**Adynamia, from drugging:** Carb-v., Helon., Nux-v.

**Adynamia, from excesses, vital drains:** Agar., *Anac., Calc-p., Carb-v.*, Caust., *Chin.*, Chinin-s., Corn-f., Cur., Gins., Kali-c., Nat-m., *Ph-ac., Phos.*, Sel., Stroph-h.

**Adynamia, from heat of summer:** *Ant-c., Gels.*, Lach., *Nat-c.*, Sel.

**Adynamia, from inebriety, bilious or remittent fevers:** Eup-per.

**Adynamia, from injuries:** *Acet-ac., Arn.*, Calen., Carb-an., *Sul-ac.*

**Adynamia, from jaundice:** Ferr-pic., Pic-ac., Tarax.

**Adynamia, from loss of sleep:** *Cocc.*, Colch., Nux-v.

**Adynamia, from menses, talking even fatigues:** Alum.

**Adynamia, from prolapsus, protracted illness, defective nutrition:** Alet., *Helon.*

**Adynamia, from some deep seated dyscrasia:** Abrot., Eup-per., Hydr., Iod., Nat-m., Nit-ac., *Psor.*, Sul-ac., *Sulph.*, Tub., *Zinc.*

**Adynamia, hysterical:** Nat-m.

**Adynamia, in aged:** Bar-c., Carb-v., *Con.*, Cur., Eup-per., Glyc., Nit-ac., Nux-m., *Phos., Sel.*

**Adynamia, nervous:** Ambr., Anac., Cur., Gels., Kali-br., *Ph-ac., Phos.*, Rhus-t., Sil., Staph., Zinc.

**Adynamia, with erethism:** Ars., Chin., Sil.

**Adynamia, with frequent, faint spells during day:** Murx., Nux-m., Sep., *Sulph.*, Zinc.

**Adynamia, without erethism:** Ph-ac.

**Adynamia, without organic lesion or cause:** Psor.

**Adynamia, worse from ascending:** Calc., Iod., Sarcol-ac.

**Adynamia, worse from descending:** Stann.

**Adynamia, worse from exertion, walking:** *Ars.*, Bry., Calc., Caust., Cycl., Ferr., Lac-d., Merc., Nat-c., Nux-m., Ph-ac., *Pic-ac.*, Sarcol-ac., Sep., Rhus-d., *Stann.*, Thea, Verat.

**Adynamia, worse in A.M.:** *Acal.*, Bar-m., Bry., Calc., Con., Corn-c., Lac c., Lach., Lyc., *Nat-m., Nit-ac.*, Phos., Psor., Sep., Stann., Sulph., Tub.

**Adynamia, worse in women worn out from hard mental and physical work, or from indolence and luxury:** Helon.

**ALCOHOLISM:** Acon., *Agar., Ant-t., Apoc.*, Apom., *Ars., Asar.*, Aur., *Aven.*, Bell., Bism., Calc., Calc-ar., Cann-i., *Caps.*, Chim., *Cimic., Cinch.*, Cocc., Crot-h., *Cupr-ar., Gels.*, Hydr., *Hyos.*, Ichth., Kali-i., Kola, Lach., Led., Lob., Lup., *Nux-v., Op.*, Phos., Psor., *Querc., Ran-b.*, Stram., Stroph-h., *Stry-n., Sul-ac.*, Sulph., Syph., Tub., Zinc. (See **Chronic Gastritis, STOMACH.**)

**Alcoholism, hereditary tendency:** Asar., Psor., Sul-ac., Sulph., Syph., Tub.

**Alcoholism, to overcome habit:** Ange., Bufo, *Cinch.*, Kola, *Querc.*, Sul-ac., Sulph.

**ATHETOSIS:** Lath., Stry.

**BERI-BERI:** *Elat.*, Lath., Rhus-t.

**CHOREA (St.Vitus dance):** Absin., *Agar.*, Agarin., *Arg-n.*, *Ars.*, Art-v., Asaf., Aster., Aven., *Bell.*, Bufo, *Calc.*, Calc-p., *Caust.*, Cham., Chlol., Cic., *Cimic.*, *Cina*, Cocain., *Cocc.*, Con., Croc., *Cupr.*, *Cupr-act.*, Eup-a., Ferr-cy., *Ferr-r.*, *Hipp.*, *Hyos.*, *Ign.*, *Iod.*, Kali-br., Lat-m., *Mag-p.*, *Mygal.*, *Nat-m.*, *Nux-v.*, *Op.*, Phos., Phys., Picro., Psor., Puls., *Santin.*, *Scut.*, Sep., Sol-n., *Spig.*, *Stram.*, *Stry.*, Stry-p., Sulfon., Sulph., *Sumb.*, Tanac., *Tarent.*, Thuj., *Verat-v.*, *Visc.*, *Zinc.*, Zinc-ar, *Zinc-br.*, Zinc-cy., Zinc-val., Ziz.

**CAUSE, OCCURRENCE, Anemia:** Ars., Chin., *Ferr-r.*, Hyos.

**Corybantism:** Bell., Hyos., Stram.

**Eruptions, suppressed:** Zinc.

**Fright:** Calc., Cimic., Cupr., *Ign.*, Laur., Nat-m., Stram., Tarent., Zinc.

**Nervous disturbaces:** *Asaf.*, Bell., *Cimic.*, *Cocc.*, Croc., Gels., Hyos., *Ign.*, Kali-br., Op., Stict., Stram.

**Onanism:** Agar., Calc., Chin.

**Pubertic:** Asaf., Caul., *Cimic.*, Ign., Puls.

**Reflex, from dentition, pregnancy:** Bell.

**Relief, from music, sight of bright colors:** Tarent.

**Relief, from sleep:** *Agar.*, Cupr.

**Rheumatism:** Caust., *Cimic.*, Spig.

**Rhythmical motions:** Agar., Caust., Cham., Cimic., Lyc., *Tarent.*

**Scrofulous, tubercular:** Calc., *Calc-p.*, Caust., *Iod.*, Phos., Psor.

**Worms:** Asaf., Calc., *Cina*, Santin., *Spig.*

**Worse, at approach of thunderstorm:** *Agar.*

**Worse, during sleep:** Tarent., *Ziz.*

**Worse, face:** *Caust.*, Cic., Cupr., Hyos., *Mygal.*, Nat-m., Zinc.

**Worse, from cold, noise, light, emotions:** Ign.

**Worse, in spasms, partial, changing constantly:** Stram.

**Worse, left arm, right leg:** Agar., Cimic.

**Worse, right arm, left leg:** Tarent.

**Worse, right side, tongue affected, staccato speech:** Caust.

**Worse unilaterally:** Calc.

**CONVULSIONS, Remedies in general:** *Absin.*, Acon., *Aeth.*, Agar., Alum-sil., Anis., Antip., Arg-n., Ars., *Art-v.*, Atro., *Bell.*, *Camph.*, Cann-i., Canth., Carb-ac., Castm., *Cham.*, Chlf., *Cic.*, Cic-m., Cimic., *Cina*, *Cocc.*, *Cupr.*, *Cupr-act.*, *Cupr-ar.*, *Cyt-l.*, Dulc., Euon., Gels., *Glon.*, Hell., *Hydr-ac.*, Hyper., *Hyos.*, *Ign.*, Iris-fl., *Kali-br.*, Laur., Lon-x., Lyss., *Mag-p.*, Morph.,

Nat-s., Nux-v., *Oena.,* Op., Ox-ac., Passi., Phos., Phys., Plat., Plb., Plb-chr., *Santin., Sil., Sol-c.,* Sol-ni., *Stram.,* Stry., Sulph., *Upa.,* Upa-a., Verat., Verat-v., Verbe-o., *Zinc.,* Zinc-o., Zinc-s.

**CAUSE AND TYPE, Anger affects mother's milk:** Cham., Nux-v.

**Apoplectic, in inebriates, hemorrhagic or broken down systems:** Crot-h.

**Carpopedal:** Cupr-act., Ign.

**Cataleptic:** Cic., *Mosch.*

**Cerebral sclerosis or tumor:** Plb.

**Children, infants, from reflex causes, dentition:** Absin., Acon., *Aeth.,* Art-v., *Bell.,* Calc., *Camph-mbr.,* Caust., *Cham.,* Chlol., *Cic., Cina,* Cocc., *Cupr.,* Cypr., Glon., Hell., Hydr-ac., *Hyos., Ign., Kali-br.,* Kreos., Laur., *Mag-p.,* Meli., Mosch., Nux-v., *Oena.,* Op., *Santin.,* Scut., Stann., *Stram., Zinc.,* Zinc-s. (See **Worms.**)

**Clonic:** Antip., Apis, Bell., Camph., Carb-ac., Cina, *Cupr.,* Gels., Hyos., Ign., *Nicot.,* Plb., Upa-a.

**Crying, approach of strangers:** Op.

**Exanthemata:** Acon., *Bell.,* Glon., Thea, Verat-v.

**Exanthemata, suppressed:** Apis, Ars., *Cupr.,* Op., Stram., *Zinc.,* Zinc-s.

**Foot sweat, supppressed:** Sil.

**Fright:** Acon., Cupr., Hyos., *Ign.,* Op., Stram.

**Fright, anger or emotional disturbance in nervous, plethoric persons:** Kali-br.

**Grief, or any emotional excitement:** Ign.

**Hypochondriacal:** Mosch., Stann.

**Hysterical:** Absin., Asaf., Asar., Castm., Caul., Cimic., Cocc., *Gels.,* Hydr-ac., *Hyos., Ign.,* Kali-p., *Mosch.,* Nux-m., Plat., Stann., Tarent.

**Injury:** Cic., Hyper.

**Isolated groups of muscles:** Acon., *Cic.,* Cina, Cupr., Ign., Nux-v., *Stram., Stry.*

**Labor:** Acon., Bell., Cic., Cupr., Glon., Hyos., Ign., Kali-br., Oena., Stram., Verat-v. (See **FEMALE SEXUAL SYSTEM.**)

**Meals followed by vomiting, shrieking, spasms:** Hyos.

**Menses suppressed:** Gels., Mill. (See **FEMALE SEXUAL SYSTEM.**)

**Metastasis, from other organs:** Apis, Cupr., Zinc.

**Prodromata:** Acon., Bell., Cham., Ip., Op.

**Reflected light from water, mirror:** Bell., Lyss., *Stram.*

**Sleep, loss of:** Cocc.

**Spinal origin:** Acon., *Cic.,* Cimic., Hydr-ac., *Hyper.,* Ign., Nux-v., Oena., *Phys.*

**Terminal stage:** Op., Plb., Zinc.

**Tonic, Opisthotonos:** Apis, *Cic.,* Cina, Cupr., Cupr-act., *Hydr-ac., Ign.,* Ip., Mag-p., Mosch., Nicot., *Nux-v.,* Phys., Plat., Plb., Sol-c., Sol-n., Stram., *Stry., Upa.,* Verat-v.

**Uremic:** *Carb-ac.,* Cic., *Cupr-ar.,* Glon., Hell., *Hydr-ac.,* Kali-br., Merc-c., Oena., *Op.,* Plb., Pilo., Urt-u. (See **URINARY SYSTEM**.)

**Uterine disease:** Cimic.

**Vaccination:** Sil., Thuj.

**Whooping cough:** Cupr., Kali-br.

**Worms:** Cic., *Cina, Hyos., Indg,* Kali-br., Sabad., *Santin.,* Spig., Tanac.

**CONCOMITANTS: Beginning in face, unilateral, shallow breathing:** Cina.

**Beginning in fingers, toes, radiates all over:** Cupr.

**Bladder, chest, intestines, striated muscles, chiefly involved, drowsiness, rigid limbs, sudden onset, head hot, feet cold:** Bell.

**Calves of legs, clenched thumbs, cyanosis:** Cupr.

**Chorea-like:** Stict.

**Convulsive jerkings, of limbs and head:** Bufo, Cham., *Cic.,* Hyos.

**Cyanosis:** Cupr-act., Hydr-ac.

**Extremities cold:** Bell., Hell., Hydr-ac., *Nicot.,* Oena.

**Eyes half open, upturned, breathing, deep stertorous:** Op.

**Eyes turned downward:** Aeth.

**Fever, skin hot, dry, child frets, screams, gnaws its fists, twitching of single muscles:** Acon.

**Followed by collapse:** Nicot.

**Followed by deep sleep:** Cupr-act., *Op.,* Zinc.

**Followed by paresis:** Acon., *Elaps,* Lon-x., Plb.

**Followed by restlessness:** Cupr.

**No cerebral congestion:** Ign.

**No fever:** Ign., *Mag-p., Zinc.*

**Pale face, rolling eyes, gnashing teeth:** Zinc.

**Preceded, by gastro-intestinal symptoms:** Aeth., Cupr-ar.

**Preceded, by restlessness:** Arg-n., Hyos.

**Shrieks, screams, before, and during:** *Apis,* Cina, Cupr., *Hell.,* Op.

**Terrible pains:** Plb-chr.

**Tremor, spasm of glottis, febrile paroxysm:** Ign.

**Twitchings, cramps, gastro-enteric symptoms:** Nux-v.

**Twitchings of single muscles or groups, especially of upper body:** Stram

**Twitchings over entire body:** Cic., Hyos.

**Twitchings worse upper body, continue after delivery:** Cic.

**Violent vomiting:** Aeth., Upa.

**With consciousness:** Cina, Nux-v., Plat., *Stram., Stry.*

**Without consciousness:** Bell., Calc., Cic., *Cupr.,* Cupr act., Cupr-ar., Glon., Hydr-ac., *Hyos., Mosch.,* Oena., *Op.,* Stram.

**Worse from touch, motion, noise:** Cic., Ign., Lyss., Nux-v., Stram., Stry.

**DEFICIENT REACTION:** Ambr., Am-c., Calc., Camph., Caps., *Carb-v.,* Carbn-s., Caust., Cic., Cupr., Hell., Iod., *Laur.,* Nat-ar., Nat-s., *Op., Psor.,* Rad-br., *Sulph., Tub.,* Valer., X-ray., *Zinc.*

**EXOPHTHALMIC GOITRE (Basedow's disease):** Aml-ns., Antip., Ars., Ars-i., Aur., *Bell.,* Brom., *Cact.,* Calc., Colch., Ephe., *Ferr.,* Ferr-i., Ferr-p., Fuc., *Glon., Iod., Lycps-v.,* Nat-m., *Pilo.,* Pineal., Spartin-s., Spong., *Thyr.*

**MAL-DE-MER: (Sea sickness):** Aml-ns., *Apom.,* Aq-mar., Arn., Cer-ox., Chlol., *Cocc.,* Cuc-p., Glon., Kali-br., Kali-p., Morph., Nicot., *Nux-v., Petr., Staph., Tab.,* Thea, *Ther.* (See **Vomiting, STOMACH.**)

**MORPHINISM:** Apom., *Aven.,* Cann-i., Cimic., Ip., Lob., *Macrot.,* Nat-p., Passi.

**MORVAN'S DISEASE:** Aur., *Aur-m.,* Bar-m., Lach., *Sec.,* Sil., Thuj.

**NERVOUS AFFECTIONS, of cigar makers:** Gels.

**Nervous affections of girls, at puberty:** Caul., *Cimic.*

**Nervous affections of onanists:** *Gels.,* Kali-p.

**Nervous affections from excessive delicacy and sensitiveness of the senses:** Cupr.

**Nervous affections from suppressed discharges, in the psoric:** Asaf., Merc.

**Nervous affections from tobacco in sedentary persons, dyspepsia, right prosopalgia:** Sep.

**Nervous affections from worms:** *Cina,* Psor., Sabad.

**NERVOUSNESS, In general:** Abies-n., Absin., *Acon.,* Alf., Am-val., *Ambr.,* Aml-ns., *Anac.,* Aqui., Arn., Ars., *Asaf., Asar.,* Aven., *Camph-mbr., Cham., Cimic., Coca,* Cocain., *Coff.,* Cupr., Cypr., Eup-ar., *Gels.,* Glyc., Goss., Hedeo., *Hyos., Ign.,* Indol., *Kali-br.,* Kali-c., *Kali-p., Mag-p.,* Nicc., Nux-m., *Nux-v.,* Op., Ov., *Phos.,* Puls., Santin., Senec., Sil., *Stram., Stry.,* Thea, *Ther., Trios., Valer.,* Xan., *Zinc.* (See **Moods, MIND.**)

**Nervousness, hypersensitiveness:** *Acon.,* Ambr., Am-val., Ang., Ant-c., *Apis,* Aqui., *Asaf., Asar.,* Arn., Atro., Aur., *Bell., Borx.,* Bry., Calad., Calc-sil., Camph., Cann-i., Canth., *Cham., Chin.,* Chinin-m., Chrysan., *Cimic., Cocc., Coff., Colch.,* Con., Cupr., Ferr., Glon., *Hep.,* Hyper., *Ign.,* Just., Kali-br., Kali-c., Kali-p., Lac-c., *Lach.,* Lyss., Mag-p., Med., Morph.,

Nit-ac., *Nux-m., Nux-v.,* Op., *Phos.,* Phos-h., Plat., Puls., Sep., *Sil.,* Spig., Stann., *Staph., Stry., Sulph., Tarent.,* Teucr., *Ther., Tub.,* Zinc-

**Nervousness, hypersensitiveness, to cold air, drafts:** Acetan., *Acon.,* Agar., All-s., Am-c., Ambr., Anac., Ant-c., Bac., Bad., *Bar-c.,* Bell., Borx., *Calc., Calc-sil.,* Calen., Camph., *Caps.,* Carb-v., Caust., Cham., *Chin., Cist.,* Con., Cupr., *Graph.,* Ham., *Hep., Kali-c.,* Kali-m., Mag-m., *Merc., Mez.,* Nat-c., *Nat-m.,* Nit ac., Nit-s-d., *Nux-v.,* Phys., *Psor.,* Ran-b., Rhus-t., *Rumx.,* Sel., Sep., *Sil.,* Stry., Sulph., *Tub.*

**Nervousness, hypersensitive, to least pain:** *Acon., Arn.,* Aur., Aur-m., Cact., *Cham., Chin., Coff., Colch., Hep.,* Hyper., *Ign.,* Kali-p., Lat-m., Mag-p., Med., Meli., Mez., *Morph.,* Mosch., Nit-ac., Nux-m., *Nux-v.,* Phos., Ran-s., Valer., Zinc-val.

**Nervousness, tremulousness, faintness:** Abies-c., Ant-t., Aqui., *Arg-n.,* Arn., Ars., Asar., *Caul., Caust., Chin., Cimic.,* Cocc., *Gels., Hyos.,* Lach., Lat-m., *Med., Mosch.,* Murx., *Nux-v.,* Puls., Raph., Sep., Stry., *Sul-ac.,* Sulph., Tarent., Valer., *Zinc.*

**NEURASTHENIA (nervous prostration), Remedies in general:** Agn., Alf., *Anac.,* Anh., *Arg-n.,* Asaf., Asar., *Aven., Calc., Calc-p.,* Cann-i., *Chin.,* Cob., Coca, *Cocc.,* Cupr., Cur., Dam., *Fl-ac., Gels.,* Glyc., Graph., *Helon.,* Hyper., Ign., *Kali-hp., Kali-p.,* Lach., Lath., *Lec.,* Lob-p., Mosch., *Nat-m., Nux-v., Onos., Ox-ac., Phos.,* Phys., *Pic-ac.,* Pip-m., Plb., Puls., Sacch., Sarcol-ac., *Scut., Sil.,* Stann., Staph., *Stry-p.,* Tarent., Tub., Verbe-h., Xan., *Zinc., Zinc-p., Zinc-pic.* (See **Adynamia**.)

**Cerebral symptoms, unable to apply mind:** *Anac.,* Aur., Calc., *Gels., Kali-p.,* Nux-v., *Ph-ac.,* Phos., *Pic-ac.,* Sil., Scut. (See **Brain Fag, MIND**.)

**From long, concentrated grief:** Ign.

**Gastric from›** *Anac.,* Gent-l., Nux-v., Stry-p.

**Hypochondriacal tendency:** *Aur.,* Coca, Con., Kali-br., Nat-m., Sulph.

**In females:** Alet., Aloe, Ambr., Ars., Aur., Bell-p., Calc., Chin., *Cocc., Epiph.,* Ferr., *Helon.,* Hyos., *Ign.,* Iod., Kali-p., *Lach.,* Lyc., *Mag-c.,* Mag-p., Ph-ac., *Pic-ac.,* Puls., *Sep.,* Sil., Sulph., Zinc-val.

**Insomnia:** Ambr., Ars., Aur., *Cimic.,* Coff., Nux-v., Zinc-p. (See **Sleep**.)

**Sexual origin:** Agar., *Agn., Anac.,* Calad., *Chin.,* Coca, Dam., Gels., *Graph.,* Lec., Lyc., Nat-m., Nux-v., Onos., *Ph- ac., Phos., Pic-ac.,* Plat., *Sabal,* Sel., Sep., *Staph.,* Thymol., Zinc-pic. (See **FEMALE SEXUAL SYSTEM.**)

**NEUROSES, Of children:** Passi.

**Neuroses of professional men:** Gels.

**TREMORS, Twitchings, trembling:** *Absin., Agar.,* Agarin., Anac., *Ant-t.,* Apis, *Arg-n.,* Ars., Bell., Camph., Cann-i., *Caust.,* Cham., Chin., Cic., *Cimic., Cocc.,* Cod., Ferr-p., *Gels.,* Hep., *Hyos., Hyosin-hbr., Ign.,* Iod.,

Kali-br., Kali-p., *Lach.*, Lat-m., Lith-chl., Lyc., *Med.*, *Merc.*, Morph., Mosch., Nat-m., *Nux-v.*, Op., Oxyt., *Ph-ac.*, *Phos.*, Phys., Plb., Rhus-t., Sabad., Scut., Sil., *Stram.*, Sulph., Tarent., Tub., Valer., Verin., Verat-v., Visc., *Zinc.*, Zinc-p.

**Alcoholic:** *Ant-t.*, Cocain., Cocc., *Nux-v.*

**Disseminated sclerosis:** Acet-ac., Ars., *Hyosin-hbr.*

**From smoking:** Kali c., Nit-ac., Sep.

**Senile:** Aven., Cann-i., Cocain., *Phos.*

**NERVES, NEURITIS (Inflammation):** *Acon.*, Aesc., *All-c.*, Anan., Arg-n., *Arn.*, *Ars.*, *Bell.*, Bell-p., Ben-d., Berb., *Carbn-s.*, Caust., *Cedr.*, Cimic., Con., Ferr-p., *Gels.*, *Hyper.*, Merc., Nux-v., Pareir., Ph-ac., Phos., *Plb.*, Plb-p., Rhus-t., Sang., *Stann.*, Stront-c., Stry., *Thal.*, Urt-u., Zinc-p.

**TYPE, Alcoholic:** Nux-v., Stry.

**Diphtheritic:** Gels.

**Of anterior crural:** Pareir.

**Of circumflex:** Sang.

**Of lesser sciatic:** Aesc.

**Of lumbo-sacral plexus:** Berb.

**Of upper dorsal roots:** Anan.

**Injuries of nerves:** All-c., Bell-p., *Hyper.*, Ph-ac.

**Multiple:** Bov., Con., Morph., Thal.

**Retro-bulbar, with sudden loss of sight:** Chinin-s.

**Traumatic:** *All-c.*, Arn., Calen., *Hyper.*

**NEURALGIA, Remedies in general:** Acetan., *Acon.*, *Aconin.*, Agar., All-c., Am-pic., Am-val., Aml-ns., Aran., *Arg-n.*, *Arn.*, *Ars.*, Atrop., *Bell.*, *Bry.*, Caj., *Cann-i.*, Caust., *Cham.*, *Chel.*, *Chin.*, *Chinin-ar.*, *Chinin-s.*, *Cedr.*, *Cimic.*, *Coff.*, *Coloc.*, Com., Con., Corn.f., Dios., *Gels.*, Glon., *Gnaph.*, Hyper., *Ign.*, Ip., Kali-ar., *Kali-bi.*, Kali-fcy., Kali-i., *Kalm.*, Lach., Mag-c., *Mag-p.*, Meny., *Mez.*, *Morph.*, Nat-m., Nicc-s., Nux-v., Onos., Ox-ac., Par., *Phos.*, Phyt., Plan., Plat., Prun., *Puls.*, *Ran-b.*, *Rhod.*, Sil., *Spig.*, *Stann.*, Staph., *Sulph.*, Sumb., Thea, Ther., Thuj., Tub., Valer., *Verat.*, *Verb.*, Xan., Zinc-p., *Zinc-val.*

**CAUSE, TYPE, Anemia:** *Ars.*, Chin., *Ferr.*, Kali-fcy., Puls.

**Chronic cases, or later life:** *Arn.*, Kreos., *Phos.*, Sulph., Thuj.

**Climacteric:** Lach.

**Gout, rheumatism:** Cimic., *Colch.*, Coloc., Kalm., Phyt., Ran-b., *Rhod.*, Rhus-t., Sulph.

**Idiopathic cases:** Acon., Ars.

**Influenza, debility:** Ars.

**Malaria:** Aran., *Ars.*, *Cedr.*, Chin., *Chinin-s.*, Meny., Nat-m., *Nicc-s.*, Stann., Sulph.

**Recent origin, occurring in young:** *Acon., Bell.,* Coloc., *Gels.,* Kalm., Spig.

**Syphilis:** *Kali-i.,* Mez., Phyt.

**Traumatic, in amputated limbs:** *All-c.,* Am-m., Arn., *Hyper.,* Kalm., *Ph-ac.,* Symph.

**Zoster, after:** *Mez.,* Morph.

**LOCATION, Brachial plexus, cervico-brachial:** *Acon.,* (prefer tincture of root), All-c., *Bry.,* Cham., Coc-c., Corn-f., Hyper., *Kalm., Merc., Nux-v.,* Par., *Rhus-t.,* Sulph., Ter., *Verat.*

**Cervico-occipital:** Bell., Bry., Chin., Chinin.s., Nux-v., Puls., Zinc-p.

**Ciliary:** *Cimic.,* Gels., Mez., Nat-m., *Spig.* (See **Ciliary Neuralgia, EYE**.)

**Crural, anterior:** Am-m., Coff., *Coloc.,* Gels., *Gnaph., Lim.,* Lycpr., Nat-ar., Oena., Spig., *Staph.,* Sulph., *Xan.*

**Infra-orbital:** *Arg-n.,* Bell., Mag-p., Mez., Nux-v., Phos. (See **Trifacial**.)

**Intercostal:** Acon., Aran., *Arn., Ars.,* Ars-i., *Ascl-t.,* Aster., Bell., Brom., *Bry., Chel., Cimic.,* Gaul., Mag-p., Mentho., *Mez.,* Morph., Nux-v., Par., Phos., Puls., *Ran-b.,* Rhod., Samb., Zinc.

**Lumbo-abdominal:** Aran., Bell., Clem., Coloc., Cupr-ar., Ham., Mag-p., Nux-v.

**Phrenic:** Bell.

**Spermatic cord:** *Clem.,* Coloc., Ham., *Ol-an.,* Ox-ac., Rhod., Spong. (See **MALE SEXUAL SYSTEM.**)

**Spine:** Par. (See **Spine**.)

**Sub-orbital:** Caust., Colch., Con., Kali-c., Phos. (See **Trifacial**.)

**Supra-orbital:** Arg-n., Asaf., *Cedr.,* Chel., *Chinin-s.,* Cimic., *Kali-bi.,* Mag-p., Morph., *Nux-v.,* Ran-b., *Spig.,* Stann., Thein., Tong., Viol-o. (See **Prosopalgia, FACE**.).

**Teeth:** Kreos., Merc., Mez., Plan., Staph., Verb. (See **Odontalgia, TEETH.**)

**Trifacial:** *Acon.,* All-c., Aml-ns., *Aran., Arg-n., Ars.,* Arund., *Bell.,* Cact., Cedr., *Cham., Chel.,* Chin., *Cimic.,* Colch., Coloc., Ferr., *Gels.,* Glon., *Kalm.,* Mag-p., Merc., *Mez.,* Nat-s., *Nux-v.,* Phos., Puls., Rhus-t., Sabal, Sang., *Spig.,* Stann., Thuj., Tong., Verat., *Verb.,* Zinc., *Zinc-val.* (See **Prosopalgia, FACE**)

**Ulnar:** Hyper., Kalm., Lycps-v., Oxyt., Rhus-t.

**SCIATICA:** Acetan., *Acon., Am-m.,* Apoc., Arn., *Ars.,* Ars-met., Ars-s-r., *Bell.,* Bry., Caps., Carbn-o., Carbn-s., *Cham.,* Chin., *Coloc.,* Cot., Dios., Gaul., Gels., *Gins., Gnaph.,* Hymos., Hyper., *Ign., Indg., Iris,* Kali-c., *Kali-i.,* Kali-p., Lac-c., Lyc., Mag-p., Nat-s., Nyct., Nux-v., Pall., Phyt., *Plb.,* Polyg-h., Ran-b., *Rhus-t., Ruta,* Sal-ac., Sep., Staph., Stry., *Sulph.,* Syph., Tell., Ter., Thein., Thuj., Valer., Verat., *Visc.,* Xan., Zinc-val.

**Sciatica, acute cases:** *Acon.,* Bry., Cham., *Coloc.,* Ign.

**Sciatica, chronic cases:** *Ars.,* Calc., Kali-i., Lyc., Phos., *Plb.,* Ran-b., *Rhus-t.,* Sulph., Zinc.

**Sciatica, in summer, croupy cough in winter:** Staph.

**Sciatica, rheumatic:** Acon., Bry., *Cimic.,* Guaj., Hymos., Led., *Rhus-t.*

**Sciatica, syphilitic:** *Kali-i.,* Merc-c., Phyt.

**Sciatica, uterine:** Bell., Ferr., Graph., Merc., *Puls.,* Sep., Sulph.

**Sciatica, vertebral origin:** Lac-c., Nat-m., Phos., Sil., Sulph., Tell.

**TYPE OF PAIN, Bruised:** Apis, Arn., Bell-p., Corn-f., Phyt., Ruta.

**Burning:** Acon., All-c., Anthraci., Apis, *Ars.,* Caps., Sal-ac., Spig.

**Cramp-like, constrictive:** Am-m., *Cact.,* Caul., Cimic., *Coloc.,* Con., Cupr., Gnaph., Iris, *Mag-p.,* Nux-v., *Plat.,* Plb., Stann., Sulph., Thuj., *Verb.*

**Drawing:** *Cham.,* Chin., Coloc., Ph-ac., Phos., *Puls.,* Spig., *Stann.,* Sulph., Verb. (See **Tearing.**)

**Intermittent:** *Ars., Chin.,* Chinin-s., *Coloc.,* Cupr., *Ign.,* Mag-p., Nux-v., *Spig.,* Sulph. (See **Periodical.**)

**Lancinating, electric shock-like:** Acon., *Bell.,* Cact., Caust., Cimic., Coloc., Daph., Gels., Mag-c., *Mag-p., Nux-v.,* Phyt., Plb., *Stry.,* Sul-ac., *Verat., Verb.,* Xan., Zinc-p.

**Localized, in spots:** Ign., Kali-bi., Lil-t., Ox-ac.

**Onset gradual, cessation gradual:** Arg-n., Plat., *Stann.,* Sulph., Verat.

**Onset sudden, cessation sudden:** *Bell.,* Carb-ac., Chr-ac., Coloc., Kali-bi., *Mag-p.,* Ovi-p., Oxyt.

**Periodical:** *Aran., Ars., Cedr.,* Chinin-s., Chr-ac., Kali-bi., *Nicc-s.,* Nux-v., Ox-ac., Parth., Sal-ac., *Spig.,* Sulph., Toxi., *Verb.*

**Plug-like:** Anac.

**Severe, drives him frantic:** *Acon.,* Arg-n., Ars., *Bell., Cham.,* Carb-ac., Chin., Coff., Colch., *Coloc.,* Kreos., *Mag-p.,* Morph., Nux-v., Ox-ac., *Spig.,* Verat.

**Splinter-like:** Ign., Rhus-t.

**Tearing, shifting, darting, shooting:** Aesc., Arg-n., *Ars., Bell.,* Bry., Caust., *Cham.,* Chin., *Coloc.,* Dios., Gels., Gnaph., Ign., Kalm., *Mag-p.,* Mez., Nux-v., Paraf., Phos., Phyt., Puls., Rhus-t., Ruta, Sang., *Spig.,* Ter.

**Tearing, shooting, along tracts, of large nerves:** Gels.

**Tearing, shooting, darting like chain lightening, ending in sharp, vice-like grip:** Cact.

**Tearing, shooting, to chest, trunk:** Corn-f.

**Tearing, shooting, to extremities:** Coloc., Gnaph., Graph., Kalm., Pall.

**Tearing, shooting, to face, shoulder, pelvis:** Arund.

**Tearing, shooting, upwards:** Kalm.

**CONCOMITANTS, Alternates with pain elsewhere, not deeply rooted cases:** Ign.

**Anesthesia:** *Acon.,* Ars., Kalm.

**Anguish, restlessness:** Acon., Ars.

**Arms feel cold, swollen, paralyzed:** Verat.

**Beginning, in pneumogastric nerve disorders:** Arn.

**Cardiac anxiety:** Spig.

**Coldness:** Agar., Ars., *Meny.,* Mez., Nat-m., Nux-v., Plat., Puls., *Rhus-t.,* Sep., Spig., Verat.

**Congestive symptoms:** Acon., Bell., Gels.

**Eructations, gastric symptoms:** Verat., Verb.

**Face pale, restlessness, sweat:** Spig.

**Face red:** Acon., *Bell.,* Cham., Verb.

**Fainting, sudden:** Cham., Hep., Morph.

**Heat of one part, coldness of other:** Pime.

**Hyperesthesia:** *Bell.,* Coff., Ign., Kali-i., Ter.

**Lachrymation:** Chel., Mez., *Puls.,* Rhus-t.

**Mania following:** Cimic.

**Muscular contraction, spasmodic:** Am-m., *Bell.,* Gels., Mag-p., *Nux-v.,* Plat., Plb., Zinc.

**Nervous agitation:** *Acon.,* Am-val., Ars., *Cham., Coff.,* Gels., *Mag-p.,* Spig.

**Numbness:** Acon., Agar., Caust., *Cham., Coloc.,* Glon., *Gnaph.,* Graph., *Kalm.,* Lac c., Led., Lith-c., Merc., Mez., *Plat., Rhus-t.,* Sep., Spig.

**Salivation, stiff neck:** Mez.

**Skin, feels pinched:** Sul-ac.

**Torpor:** Plat.

**Weakness:** *Ars.,* Chin., Colch., Gels., Kalm., *Verat.*

**MODALITIES, AGGRAVATION, Bending back:** Caps.

**Cold:** *Ars.,* Bell., Caps., Chin., Coloc., Kali-bi., *Mag-p.,* Rhus-t., Ruta.

**Exertion, mental:** Kalm.

**Jar, concussion:** *Bell.,* Caps., *Spig., Tell.*

**Left side:** Acon., *Ars.,* Caust., Cedr., Colch., *Coloc.,* Iris, Kali-bi., Mag-c., *Mez.,* Morph., Nux-v., Rhus-t., *Spig.,* Sumb.

**Lying down:** Am-m., Gnaph.

**Lying, on affected side:** Coloc., Kali-i.

**Midnight:** Ars., Bell., Mez., Sulph.

**Morning:** Acon., Chinin-s., Nux-v.

**Morning, 9 A.M-to 4 P.M.:** Verb.

**Motion:** Acon., Ars., Bell., *Bry.,* Chin., Coff., Colch., Coloc., Gnaph., Nux-v., Phyt., Ran-b., *Spig., Verb.*

**Night:** Acon., *Ars.,* Bell., *Cham.,* Cimic., Coff., Gins., Ign., *Kali-i., Mag-p., Merc.,* Mez., Plat., Phyt., Puls., *Rhus-t.,* Ruta, Sal-ac., *Syph.,* Tell.

**Noon (12-1 P.M.):** Nat-m., Sulph.

**Pressure:** Ars., Gels., Plb., Verb., Zinc.

**Rest, first beginning to move:** Lac-c., Rhus-t.

**Rest, sitting:** Am-m., Ars., Mag-c., *Rhus-t., Valer.*

**Right side:** *Bell.,* Chel., Dios., Gnaph., *Kalm., Lyc., Mag-p.,* Morph., Puls., Ran-b., Sul-ac., Tell.

**Standing, resting foot on floor:** Bell., *Valer.*

**Stooping or straightening limb after previous exertion:** Spig.

**Talking, sneezing, change of temperature:** Verb.

**Touch:** Ars., *Bell.,* Bry., *Chin.,* Coloc., *Lach.,* Mag-p., Mez., *Nux-v.,* Plb., *Spig.*

**Touching or closing teeth:** Verb.

**Warmth:** Cham., Mez., Plb., *Puls.,* Xan.

**AMELIORATION, Bending backward:** Dios.

**Bending forward:** Coloc.

**Closing eyes:** Bry.

**Cold:** Ars., Puls.

**Daybreak:** Syph.

**Flexing thigh, on abdomen:** Gnaph.

**Kneeling down, pressing head firmly against floor:** Sang.

**Lying still, rest:** Am-m., Bry., Dios., Kreos., *Mag-p.,* Nux-v.

**Motion, walking:** Am-m., *Ars., Dios., Ign.,* Kali-bi., Kali-i., Mag-c., Ox-ac., *Puls., Rhus-t.,* Sep., Sulph., Valer.

**Pressure:** Ars., Bell., *Bry.,* Coff., *Coloc., Mag-p.,* Meny., *Mez.,* Nux-v., Plb., Spig.

**Rubbing:** Acon.

**Sitting:** Bell., Gnaph.

**Warmth:** *Ars.,* Bell., Coloc., *Mag-p.,* Morph., Nux-v., Phos., Rhus-t.

**SLEEPING SICKNESS:** Ars., Nat-ar. (Atox.)

**SPINAL CORD, Anemia:** Agar., *Plb., Sec.,* Stry-p., Tarent.

**Burning:** Agar., *Alum.,* Alum-sil., Ars., Bell., Gels., *Gua.,* Kali-c., Kali-p., Med., Nux-v., Ph-ac., *Phos.,* Phys., *Pic-ac.,* Stry-p., Sulph., *Zinc.*

**Coldness:** Cimic., Stry.

**Concussion:** *Arn.,* Bell-p., Cic., Con., *Hyper.,* Phys.

**Congestion:** Absin., *Acon.,* Agar., Arn., Bell., *Gels.,* Hyper., *Nux-v.,* Onos., Oxyt., Phos., Phys., Sec., Sil., *Stry.,* Tab., Verat-v.

**DEGENERATION (Softening, sclerosis, etc):** Alum., Alum-sil., Arg-n., Aur., *Aur-m.,* Bar-m., Carbn-s., Naja, Ox-ac., *Phos.,* Phys., *Pic-ac.,* Plb., *Plb-i.,* Zinc. (See **Locomotor Ataxia.**)

**Degeneration, lateral sclerosis:** *Arg-n.,* Cupr., Hyper., Lath., Plb.

**Degeneration, multiple sclerosis:** *Arg-n., Atrop., Aur.,* Bar-c., Bell., Calc., Caust., Chel., *Crot-h.,* Gels., *Lath.,* Lyc., *Nux-v.,* Ox-ac., *Phos., Phys., Plb.,* Sil., *Stry.,* Sulph., Tarent., Thuj.

**Hemorrhage in:** Acon., *Arn., Bell.,* Lach., Nux-v., Sec.

**HYPERESTHESIA:** Abrot., Acon., *Agar.,* Apis, Arg-n., *Ars., Bell.,* Bry., *Chinin-ar.,* Chinin-s., *Cimic., Cocc.,* Crot-h., *Hep., Hyper., Lac-c., Lach.,* Lob., *Ign.,* Med., Menis., Nat-m., *Ox-ac.,* Ph-ac., *Phos., Phys.,* Podo., Ran-b., Rhus-t., Sec., Senec-j., *Sil., Stry-p.,* Sulph., *Tarent.,* Tell., *Ther.,* Visc., *Zinc.*

**Hyperesthesia, between vertebrae:** Chinin-s., Nat-m., Ther.

**Hyperesthesia from using arms in sewing, typewriting, piano playing:** Agar., *Cimic.,* Ran-b.

**Hyperesthesia, mid dorsal:** Stry-p., Tell.

**Hyperesthesia, sacral:** Lob.

**Hyperesthesia, sits sideways to prevent pressure on spine:** Chinin-s., Ther., Zinc.

**Hyperesthesia, spasmodic pain in chest and cardiac region from touch:** Tarent.

**Hyperesthesia, worse from least jar or noise:** Ther.

**INFLAMMATION (meningitis):** Acon., *Bell., Bry.,* Kali-i., Merc., Nat-s., Ox-ac., Verat-v. (See **Myelitis.**)

**Inflammation (myelitis):** *Acon.,* Arg-n., *Arn., Ars., Bell.,* Bell-p., Bry., Chel., *Cic.,* Con., Crot-h., Dulc., Gels., Hyos., Hyper., Kali-i., Lach., *Lath., Merc.,* Naja, Nat-s., *Nux-v., Ox-ac., Phos.,* Phys., Pic-ac., *Plb.,* Rhus-t., *Sec.,* Stram., *Stry.,* Verat., *Zinc-p.*

**Inflammation, chronic (myelitis):** *Ars., Crot-h.,* Lath., *Ox-ac., Plb.,* Stry., Thal.

**Inflammation, spasmodic form:** Arg-n., Ars., Chel., Merc., Verat.

**IRRITATION:** *Agar.,* Ambr., *Arg-n.,* Arn., Bell., *Bell-p.,* Chinin-ar., Chinin-s., *Cimic.,* Cob., *Cocc.,* Cupr., Gels., *Gua., Hyper., Ign.,* Kali-c., Kali-p., Naja, *Nat-m., Nux-v.,* Ox-ac., Phos., *Phys., Pic-ac.,* Plat., Puls., Ran-b., *Sec.,* Sep., *Sil.,* Staph., Stry-p., Sulph., *Tarent., Tell.,* Ther., Tub., *Zinc.,* Zinc-val. (See **Hyperesthesia.**)

**Irritation, from sexual excesses:** Agar., Kali-p., Nat-m.

**LOCOMOTOR ATAXIA:** Agar., *Alum.,* Alumin-m., *Alumn.,* Am-m., Ang., Arag., *Arg-n., Ars.,* Ars-br., *Atrop., Aur-m., Bell.,* Cann-i., Carb-v., Carbn-s., Caust., Chr-s., *Con.,* Cund., Cur., Dub., *Ferr-pic., Fl-ac.,* Gels., Hyos., *Ign.,* Kali-br., *Kali-i.,* Lath., Lyc., *Mag-p.,* Merc-c., Nat-i., Nit-ac., *Nux-v.,* Onos., *Ox-ac.,* Ped., *Phos.,* Phos-h., *Phys., Pic-ac.,* Picrot., *Plb., Plb-p.,* Rhus-t., Ruta, Sabad., *Sec., Sil.,* Stram., *Stry.,* Tarent., Thal., Thiosin., *Zinc-p.,* Zinc-s.

**CONCOMITANTS, Early stage:** Ang., Atrop., *Bell.,* Con., Ign., Nux-v., Sec., Stry., Tarent., Zinc., Zinc-s.

**Enuresis and urinary symptoms:** Bell., Berb., Equis-h., Ferr-p. (See **URINARY SYSTEM.**)

**Fulgurating pains:** *Acetan., Aesc.,* Agar., Alum., *Am-m.,* Ang., Arg-n., *Ars.,* Ars-i., *Atrop.,* Bar-m., *Bell.,* Berb., Dig., *Fl-ac.,* Guaj., Hyos., Ign., *Kalm.,* Lyc., Merc-c., Nit-ac., Nux-m., *Nux-v.,* Ol-sant., *Phos., Phys.,* Pilo., Plb., Plb-i., Sabad., *Sec.,* Sil., *Stront-c.,* Stry., Thal., Thiosin., Zinc., *Zinc-p.,* Zinc-s.

**Gastric symptoms:** *Arg-n.,* Bell., Carb-v., Ign., Lyc., *Nux-v.,* Thiosin.

**Muscular weakness, anesthesia of skin, and muscular sense:** Cann-i.

**Ocular symptoms:** Bell., Con., Ferr-pic., Phos. (See **EYE.**)

**Sexual excitement:** Kali-br., Pic-ac., Phos.

**Syphilitic cases:** *Kali-i.,* Merc-c., Nit-ac., Sec.

**Ulcer of heel:** Sil.

**Vesical and anal symptoms:** Alum., Fl-ac., Ign., Nux-v., Stry., Tarent., Thiosin.

**PAIN IN SPINE:** Abrot., Acon., Adon., *Agar., Arg-n.,* Cact., Cimic., Gels., *Hyper.,* Lact-v., Lob-s., Menis., Nicc-s., *Ox-ac.,* Paraf., Phys., Stry., Sec., Tarent., Ther., *Zinc.* (See **Backache, LOCOMOTOR SYSTEM.**)

**PARESIS:** Cocc., Con., *Irid-met.,* Plect., Plb-i., Sec., *Stry.* (See **Paralysis.**)

**TETANY:** Acon., Cocc., Graph., Lyc., Merc., Plb., Sec., *Sol-n.*

**TETANUS:** *Acon.,* Aconin, Aml-ns., *Ang.,* Arn., Bell., Calen., Camph., Carbn-s., Chlol., *Cic., Cocc.,* Con., Cupr., *Cur., Gels., Hydr-ac., Hyos., Hyper.,* Ign., *Ip.,* Kali-br., Lach., Laur., Led., Lyss., Mag-p., Morph., Mosch., Nicot., *Nux-v.,* Oena., *Op.,* Ox-ac., *Passi., Phys.,* Phyt., Plat., Scor., *Stram., Stry.,* Tab., Ter., Thebin, *Upa.,* Verat., Zinc. (See **Trismus, FACE.**)

**TIC CONVULSIVE:** Arg-n., Hyos., Laur., Lyc., Sep., Tarent., Zinc.

**WEAKNESS OF SPINE:** *Aesc.,* Alum-sil., Arg-n., Bar-c., *Calc-p.,* Cocc., *Con.,* Nat-m., Phos., Pic-ac., Sel., Sil., *Stry.,* Zinc-pic. (See **Back, LOCOMOTOR SYSTEM.**)

■

# FEVER

**CHILLINESS, coldness:** Abies-c., *Acon.*, Aeth., *Agar.*, Alum., *Ant-t.*, Apis, *Aran.*, Arn., *Ars.*, *Ars-i.*, Asar., Astac., Bapt., Berb., Bry., Calc., *Calc-ar.*, *Calc-sil.*, Calen., *Camph.*, Canth., *Caps.*, *Carb-v.*, Castm., Caust., Cedr., Cimx., Cocain., *Colch.*, Corn-f., Crat., Dulc., *Echi.*, Eup-pur., *Ferr.*, *Gels.*, Graph., *Helo.*, *Hep.*, Ip., Jatr., *Kali-c.*, Lac-d., *Laur.*, *Led.*, Lob-p., Lyc., *Mag-p.*, *Meny.*, *Merc.*, Morph., Mosch., *Nat-m.*, *Nux-v.*, Op., Phos., Pimp., Plat., *Puls.*, Pyrus, Rad-br., Sabad., *Sec.*, *Sil.*, Sulph., *Tab.*, *Tela*, Valer., *Verat.*

**Chilliness, after epileptic fit:** Cupr.

**Chilliness, in abdomen, legs:** Meny.

**Chilliness, in arms:** Raph.

**Chilliness, in back and feet:** Bell., Canth.

**Chilliness, in back, between shoulder blades:** *Am-m.*, Castm., *Lachn.*, Pyrog., Tub.

**Chilliness, in back, hips, to legs:** Ham.

**Chilliness, in body and feet, head and face hot:** Arn.

**Chilliness, in body, with face and breath hot:** Cham.

**Chilliness, in bones, extremities, severe, general:** Pyrog.

**Chilliness, in chest, on walking in open air:** Ran-b.

**Chilliness, in forearms:** Carb-v., Med.

**Chilliness, in hands:** Dros.

**Chilliness, in hands and back:** Cact.

**Chilliness, in hands, back, feet and knees:** Benz-ac., *Chinin-ar.*

**Chilliness, in hands, body warm:** Tab.

**Chilliness, in head and limbs:** Calc., Ferr.

**Chilliness, in knees:** *Carb-v.*, Cimx., Phos.

**Chilliness, in lower limbs:** Calc., Cocc.

**Chilliness, in lumbar region:** Agar.

**Chilliness, in single parts:** *Asar.*, Calad., *Calc.*, Kali-bi., Par., Puls.

**Chilliness, in waves, along spine:** *Abies-c.*, *Acon.*, *Aesc.*, *Ars.*, Bol-la., Calen., Conv., Dulc., Echi., Frax., *Gels.*, Helo., *Mag-p.*, Med., Raph., Stry., Tub., *Zinc.*

**Chilliness, with aching in shoulders, joints, small of back, yawning, stretching:** Bol-la.

**Chilliness, with catarrh:** Merc.

**Chilliness, with cough, dry, fatiguing:** Rhus-t.

**Chilliness, with deficient, animal heat:** *Alum.*, Bar-c., Calc., Calc-p., *Calc-sil.*, *Led.*, Lyc., Psor., *Sep.*, *Sil.*, Staph., Thuj., Verat.

**Chilliness, with desire to uncover abdomen:** Tab.

**Chilliness, with evening pains of what ever kind, in warm room:** Puls.

**Chilliness, with face, head, palms hot:** Ferr.

**Chilliness, with face hot:** Dros., Ign.

**Chilliness, with flatulent colic, nausea, vertigo, hot skin, sweat, heat of head:** Cocc.

**Chilliness, with headache:** Conv.

**Chilliness, with headache, extending to parietal region, red eyes:** Cedr.

**Chilliness, with heat and desire to stretch:** Rhus-t.

**Chilliness, with heat, alternately:** Abies-n., Acon., *Apis, Ars.,* Bapt., Bell., Bol-la., Bry., *Cham.,* Dig., Laur., Mag-s., *Merc.,* Merc-c., Phyt., Puls., Sol-n., Solid.

**Chilliness, with ill-humor:** Caps.

**Chilliness, with loquacity:** Podo.

**Chilliness, with nausea:** Echi., *Ip.*

**Chilliness, with nervousness:** *Asar.,* Cimic., Croc., *Gels.,* Goss., Nat-m.

**Chilliness, with no relief from warmth:** Aran., *Cadm-s.,* Caust., Chinin-s., Dros., Laur., Mag-p., *Merc.,* Pulx., Puls., Sil.

**Chilliness, with pain:** Coff., Dulc., *Puls.,* Sil.

**Chilliness, with pain, racking in limbs, anxious restlessness:** Ars.

**Chilliness, with pallor:** Cocain.

**Chilliness, with pruritus:** Mez.

**Chilliness, with rheumatic pain, and soreness:** Bapt., Hom., Rhus-t.

**Chilliness, with septic symptoms:** *Pyrog.,* Tarent-c.

**Chilliness, with suffocative feeling:** Arg-n., Mag-p.

**Chilliness, with thirst:** Acon., *Ars.,* Caps., Carb-v., Conv., Dulc., *Ign., Sec.,* Sep., *Verat.*

**Chilliness, with thirstlessness:** Dros., Gels., Nux-m., *Puls.*

**Chilliness, worse after anger:** Aur., *Bry.,* Cham.

**Chilliness, worse after dinner:** Mag-p.

**Chilliness, worse after drinking:** Caps.

**Chilliness, worse after eating A.M.:** Puls.

**Chilliness, worse from dampness, rain, not relieved by warmth:** Aran.

**Chilliness, worse from least exposure, "air goes right through":** *Acon.,* Agar., Agra., Am-p., Arg-n., *Ars.,* Ars-i., Astac., *Calc., Calc-p.,* Calen., Canch., Caps., Chin., *Hep., Kali-c., Merc.,* Merc-c., Mez., *Nux-v., Psor.,* Sep., *Sil.,* Tub.

**Chilliness, worse from least motion:** Ars., *Nux-v., Spig.*

**Chilliness, worse from touch:** Acon., *Kali-c., Sil.,* Spig.

**Chilliness, worse from warmth, covering:** *Camph.,* Hep., Med., Sanic., *Sec.,* Sulph.

**Chilliness, worse in morning:** Calc.

**Chilliness, worse toward evening and night:** Acon., Alum., Am-c., Ars., Cedr., Dulc., Mag-c., Mag-p., Mentho., *Merc.,* Ol-j., *Phos., Puls.,* Sep.

**FEBRILE HEAT:** Abies-n., Acet-ac., *Acon., Aesc.,* Aeth., *Agar., Agro.,* All-s., Ant-c., Arn., *Bapt., Bell., Bry.,* Calo., Camph., *Canth.,* Carb-v., *Cham.,* Chin., Chinin-ar., *Cimic.,* Dulc., Eucal., *Ferr-p., Gels.,* Glon., Ign., Iod., *Merc.,* Mill., Morph., Nit-ac., Nux-m., *Nux-v.,* Op., Phyt., *Puls.,* Pulx., *Rhus-t., Samb.,* Sep., Sil., *Spira.,* Spirae., Stram., Ter., Thuj., Valer., *Verat-v.*

**Febrile heat, ascends from pelvic organs:** Sep.

**Febrile heat, from anger:** Cham., Cocc., Sep.

**Febrile heat, in evening, falls asleep during, awakens when it ceases:** Calad.

**Febrile heat, in flashes, ebullitions:** Acet-ac., *Aml-ns.,* Antip., *Ars.,* Ars-i., Bol-la., Calc., *Carl.,* Chim., *Dig.,* Erech., Ferr-r., Frax., Hep., Ign., Indg., Iod., Jab., *Kali-c.,* Lach., Lyc., Med., Merc., *Nicc.,* Petr., *Phos.,* Puls., *Sang., Sep., Sul-ac., Sulph.,* Urt-u., Valer., Visc., Yohim.

**Febrile heat, in lower part of back, hip, thighs:** Berb.

**Febrile heat, in palms of hands:** Aphis.

**Febrile heat, in soles of feet:** Canth.

**Febrile heat, in spots:** Agar., Apis.

**Febrile heat, in whole body, face red, hot, yet chilly from least motion or uncovering:** Nux-v.

**Febrile heat, with chill predominant:** Bry.

**Febrile heat, with colic:** Verat.

**Febrile heat, with decline towards A.M., without sweat:** Gels.

**Febrile heat, with delirium, headache:** Agar., Bell.

**Febrile heat, with drowsy stupefaction; agonized tossing about, in search of a cool place, must be uncovered, vomiting, diarrhea, convulsions:** Op.

**Febrile heat, with dryness, during sleep or on falling asleep, deep, dry, cough:** Samb.

**Febrile heat, with dryness, no sweat:** Alum., *Nux-m.*

**Febrile heat, with excitement, nervous agitation:** *Acon.,* Tela.

**Febrile heat, with external coldness:** Ars., Canth.

**Febrile heat, with faintness, sweat:** *Dig.,* Sep., Sul-ac., *Sulph.*

**Febrile heat, with flatulence, bowel movement:** Rad-br.

**Febrile heat, with headache:** Astac.

**Febrile heat, with headache as from thousand hammers:** Nat-m.

**Febrile heat, with hot face, back chilly, feet cold:** Puls.

**Febrile heat, with hot face, cold hands and feet:** Stram.

**Febrile heat, with hot face, cool body, asthenic states:** Arn., Phyt.

**Febrile heat, with hot face, unquenchable thirst, taste of bile, nausea, anxiety, restlessness, dry tongue, after anger:** Cham.

**Febrile heat, with hunger, for days preceding:** Staph.

**Febrile heat, with itching eyes, tearing in limbs, numbness of body, headache:** Cedr.

**Febrile heat, with lassitude, in afternoon, throbs all over:** Lil-t.

**Febrile heat, with night sweats:** *Acet-ac.,* Hep.

**Febrile heat, with palpitation, precordial anguish:** Calc.

**Febrile heat, with prostration:** Ant-t., *Chinin-ar.,* Phyt.

**Febrile heat, with pulsations:** *Bell., Lil-t.,* Puls., Thuj.

**Febrile heat, with pulsations, and distended veins:** *Puls.,* Thuj.

**Febrile heat, with red spot on left cheek:** Acet-ac.

**Febrile heat, with restlessness, cheeks red, apathy:** Iod.

**Febrile heat, with restless sleep:** Calc.

**Febrile heat, with skin dry, hot, face red or red and pale alternately, arterial excitement, anguish, restlessness, tossing about:** Acon.

**Febrile heat, with skin dry, pungent, arterial excitement, distended, superficial vessels:** Bell.

**Febrile heat, with slow, nervous, insidious course, vertigo:** Cocc.

**Febrile heat, smothered feeling, if covered:** Arg-n.

**Febrile heat, with soreness of body:** *Arn.,* Franc., Phyt., *Rhus-t.*

**Febrile heat, with spasms:** Acetan., *Bell.*

**Febrile heat, with stretching of limbs:** Rhus-t.

**Febrile heat, with sudden onset, dry, burning skin, rapid, small, wiry pulse:** Pyrog.

**Febrile heat, with tendency to cover up:** Ign., *Nux-v.,* Samb., Stann.

**Febrile heat, with thirst:** *Acon.,* Ant-c., Bry., Laur., Puls., Ter.

**Febrile heat, with thirstlessness:** *Acet-ac.,* Aeth., Bell., Gels., *Ign.,* Mur-ac., *Nux-m., Puls.,* Samb.

**Febrile heat, worse at night:** Acon., Aesc., Ant-c., Ars., Bell., Calad., *Calc.,* Gels., *Hep.,* Kali-s., Mag-c., *Petr.,* Phos., *Puls.,* Sil., Stann., Urt-u.

**Febrile heat, worse during menses:** Calc., Thuj.

**Febrile heat, worse during sleep:** Acon., Calad., *Samb.*

**Febrile heat, worse covering up:** Ign.

**Febrile heat, worse from motion, then chilly:** Nux-v.

**Febrile heat, worse from uncovering:** *Merc., Nux-v.,* Samb., Stront-c.

**Febrile heat, worse in afternoon:** Aza., Bell., Ferr.

**Febrile heat, worse in morning, in bed:** Kali-c.

**Febrile heat, worse on awaking:** Laur.

**Febrile heat, worse when sitting, walking in open air:** Sep.

**SWEAT, TYPE, Bloody:** *Crot-h.,* Lach., Lyc., Nux-m., Nux-v.

**Cold, clammy:** Abies-c., *Acet-ac., Aeth., Aml-ns.,* Ant-ar., *Ant-t., Ars.,* Benz-ac., Cact., *Calc.,* Calc-p., *Camph.,* Canth., *Carb-v.,* Chin., Corn-f., Crot-h., *Cupr-ar.,* Dig., Dulc., Elaps, Euph-l., Formal., Ign., Ip., Lach., Laur., Lob., Lup., Lyc., Med., *Merc.,* Merc-c., Merc-cy., Nat-c., Pyrog., *Sanic., Sec.,* Sul-ac., *Tab.,* Tela, *Ter., Verat.,* Verat-v.

**Greasy, oily:** Bry., Carb-v., Chin., Lup., Mag-c., *Merc.*

**Hot:** *Aesc.,* Aphis, Carb-v., *Cham., Lach., Op.,* Til., Verat-v.

**LOCALIZED, in general:** Bry., *Calc.,* Chin., *Fl-ac.,* Hep., *Petr.,* Phos., Plec., *Puls.,* Sel., *Sil.,* Sulph.

**Localized, in anterior part of body:** Sel.

**Localized, in axillae:** Calc., Nit-ac., Osm., Petr., Sep., Sil. (See **LOCOMOTOR SYSTEM.**)

**Localized, on chest:** *Calc.,* Cocc., Euphr., *Phos.,* Stann., Stry.

**Localized, on covered parts:** Bell.

**Localized, on extremities, upper right:** Formal.

**Localized, on face, forehead:** *Acet-ac.,* Benz-ac., Calc., Cina, Euph., *Lob.,* Phos., Rheum, Sin-n., Stann., Sulph., Valer., *Verat.*

**Localized, on feet:** Calc., *Graph.,* Lac-ac., Merc., *Petr.,* Phos., Sep., Sil. (See **Feet, LOCOMOTOR SYSTEM.**)

**Localized, on genitals:** Calc., Petr., Ph-ac., Thuj. (See **MALE SEXUAL SYSTEM.**)

**Localized, on hands:** Calc., Cina, Con., Fl-ac., Nit-ac., *Phos.,* Sil. (See **LOCOMOTOR SYSTEM.**)

**Localized, on head, nape of neck:** Bell., *Calc.,* Phos., Puls., Rheum, *Samb., Sanic., Sil.,* Stann., Stry., Verat.

**Localized, on lower body:** Croc., Ran-a., Sanic.

**Localized, on part lain on:** Acon.

**Localized, on parts in contact with each other:** Nicc-s.

**Localized, on posterior part of body:** Sep.

**Localized, on side not reclined upon:** Ben., Thuj.

**Localized, on uncovered parts:** Thuj.

**Localized, on upper body:** Aza., Calc., Cham., Kali-c., Nux-v., Sil.

**Localized, unilaterally:** Jab., Nux-v., Puls.

**ODOR, Fetid, offensive:** Art-v., Bapt., *But-ac.,* Calc., *Carb-an.,* Cimx., Con., Daph., Fl-ac., *Hep.,* Kali-i., *Lyc., Merc., Nit-ac.,* Ol-an., Osm., *Petr.,* Phos., *Psor.,* Puls., *Sep., Sil.,* Sol-t., Stann., *Staph.,* Sulph., *Tax., Thuj.,* Vario. (See **Bromidrosis, SKIN.**)

**Odor musty, mouldy:** Stann.

**Odor sour, acid:** Arn., Bry., *Calc., Cham.,* Fl-ac., Graph., *Hep.,* Kreos., Lac-d., *Mag-c.,* Merc., Nux-v., Pyrog., *Rheum,* Rob., Sanic., Sep., *Sil., Sul-ac., Sulph.,* Thuj.

**Odor sweetish:** *Calad.,* Thuj.

**Odor urinous:** Ery-a., Nit-ac.

**PROFUSE sweat (hyperidrosis):** *Acet-ac., Acon.,* Aesc., *Agarin.,* Am-act., Ant-t., Ars., *Ars-i., Bapt., Bell.,* Bol-la., Bry., *Calc.,* Canth., Cham., *Chin.,* Cocc., Con., Croc., Esin., Ferr., *Ferr-i.,* Fl-ac., Graph., *Hep.,* Hyper., *Iod., Jab., Kali-c.,* Lac-ac., Lob., *Merc.,* Morph., *Nit-ac.,* Nux-v., Op., *Ph-ac., Phos., Pilo.,* Polyp-p., *Psor.,* Puls., Sal-ac., *Samb.,* Sanic., *Sel., Sep., Sil.,* Stann., Sul-ac., Sulph., Thuj., Til., *Verat.,* Zinc.

**Profuse, debilitating (colliquative):** *Acet-ac.,* Camph., Carb-an., *Carb-v.,* Castm., *Chin.,* Chrysan., Eup-per., Ferr., Gels., Kali-n., *Merc.,* Nit-ac., *Op., Ph-ac.,* Phel., Phos., Pyrog., Rhus-g., *Salv., Samb.,* Stann., Sul-ac.

**SCANTY:** Apis, Conv., Lach., *Nux-m.*

**Viscid:** Abies-c., Fl-ac., Hep., *Lyc., Merc.,* Phal., Phos.

**Yellow, staining:** Ars., Carb an., Lach., Lyc., *Merc.*

**OCCURRENCE, After acute diseases:** Psor.

**After eating, drinking:** Carb-v., Cham., Kali-c.

**At end of fever, or only at beginning of sleep:** Ars.

**During climacteric:** Hep., *Jab.,* Til. (See **FEMALE SEXUAL SYSTEM**.)

**During exertion, motion:** Asar., But-ac., *Calc.,* Carb-an., *Chin.,* Eup-pur., *Eupi.,* Graph., *Hep., Iod.,* Kali-c., Lyc., *Merc.,* Merc-c., Nat-c., Nat-m., *Ph-ac., Psor., Sep., Sil.,* Sulph.

**During morning, day time:** Bry., Carb-an., Carb-v., Hep., Lyc., Nat-m., Nux-v., Phos., Sep., Sil., Sulph., Zinc.

**During morning, early:** Stann.

**During sleep (night sweats):** *Acet-ac.,* Agar., *Agarin.,* Aral., *Ars-i.,* Bar-c., Bell., Bol-la., *Calc.,* Carb-an., Carb-v., Cham., *Chin.,* Chrysan., *Con.,* Corn-f., Euphr., Ferr-p., *Hep., Iod.,* Ip., *Jab.,* Kali-c., Kali-i., Lyc., *Merc.,* Myos-s., Nat-tel., Nit-ac., Nux-v., Op., Petr., *Ph-ac., Phos.,* Phyt., Picro., *Pilo., Pop.,* Psor., *Salv.,* Sang., Sanic., Sep., *Sil.,* Stann., Staph., Stront-c., Sulph., *Tarax.,* Thal., *Thuj.,* Til., Zinc.

**During waking hours:** Con., Hep., Merc., Ph-ac., Phos., *Samb.*

**From nervous depression, phthisis, convalescence from acute disease:** Jab.

**From nervous shock, sitting quietly:** Anac., Sep.

**Sweat, affords no relief, or aggravates symptoms:** Ant-t., Bell., Bol-la., Chinin-s., Ferr., Form., *Hep., Merc.,* Ph-ac., Pyrog., Sep., Stram.

**Sweat, affords relief, to symptoms:** *Acon., Ars., Calad.,* Cupr., Eup-per., Franc., *Nat-m., Psor.,* Seneg., *Verat.*

**FEVER TYPE OF, BILIOUS:** *Bapt.,* Bry., *Cham.,* Chin., Coloc., Crot-h., Euon., *Eup-per.,* Gels., Ip., Lept., *Merc., Merc-c.,* Nux-v., Nyct., Podo., Rhus-t., Tarax.

**CATHETER:** *Acon.,* Camph-ac., Petros.

**DENGUE:** *Acon.,* Ars., Bell., Bry., Canth., Chin., *Eup-per., Gels.,* Ip., Nux-v., *Rhus-t.,* Rhus-v.

**DYSENTERIC:** Nux-v.

**ENTERIC, TYPHOiD FEVER:** Agar., Agarin., *Ail., Apis,* Arg-n., *Arn., Ars.,* Arum-t., *Bapt., Bell., Bry.,* Calc., *Carb-v.,* Chin., Cina, Colch., Crot-h., Cupr-ar., Echi., *Eucal., Gels.,* Glon., *Hell.,* Hydr., *Hyos.,* Hyosin-hbr., Iod., Ip., Kali-p., *Lach.,* Laur., *Lyc., Merc.,* Merc-cy., Methyl., Mosch., *Mur-ac., Nit-ac., Nux-m., Op., Ph-ac., Phos., Pyrog., Rhus-t.,* Sel., *Stram.,* Stry., Sul-ac., Sumb., *Ter.,* Vacc-m., Valer., Verat., Xero., Zinc.

**CONCOMITANTS, Biliousness:** *Bry.,* Chel., Hydr., Lept., *Merc.,* Nux-v.

**Carriers: After inoculation with anti-typhoid serum:** Bapt.

**Constipation:** *Bry.,* Hydr., Nux-v., Op.

**Decubitus:** Arn., *Ars.,* Bapt., Carb-v., *Lach.,* Mur-ac., Pyrog., *Sec.*

**Delirium:** Agar., *Agarin.,* Ars., Bapt., *Bell.,* Cann-i., *Hyos., Hyosin-hbr.,* Lach., Methyl., Op., Ph-ac., Phos., Rhus-t., *Stram.,* Ter., Valer.

**Diarrhea:** Arn., *Ars.,* Bapt., Crot-h., *Cupr-ar., Epil.,* Lach., *Merc.,* Ph-ac., Rhus-t.

**Diarrhea, involuntary:** Apis, *Arn.,* Ars., Hyos., Mur-ac., *Ph-ac.*

**Ecchymoses:** *Arn., Ars.,* Carb-v., Mur-ac.

**Epistaxis:** *Acon., Bry.,* Croc., *Ham., Ip.,* Meli., Ph-ac., Rhus-t.

**Fever:** Ars., *Bapt., Bell.,* Gels., Methyl., Rhus-t., Stram.

**Gastric symptoms:** *Bry.,* Canth., Carb-v., *Hydr.,* Merc., Nux-v., Puls.

**Headache:** Acetan., *Bell., Bry.,* Gels., Hyos., Nux-v., Rhus-t.

**Hemorrhage:** Alum., *Alumn.,* Ars., *Bapt.,* Carb-v., Chin., *Crot-h.,* Elaps, *Ham.,* Hydrin-s., Ip., Kreos., Lach., *Mill., Mur-ac., Nit-ac.,* Nux-m., *Ph-ac.,* Sec-*Ter.*

**Insomnia:** Bell., *Coff.,* Gels., *Hyos., Hyosin-hbr.,* Op., Rhus-t.

**Laryngeal affections:** Apis, Merc-c.

**Multiple abscesses:** Ars., Hep., Sil.

**Myocarditis:** Pinealis.

**Nervous symptoms, adynamia:** Agar., *Agarin,* Apis, *Ars.,* Bapt., *Bell.,* Bry., Cocc., Colch., Gels., Hell., *Hyos., Hyosin-hbr., Ign.,* Lach., Lyc., *Mur-ac., Ph-ac., Phos.,* Rhus-t., *Stram.,* Sumb., Valer., Zinc.

**Nervous symptoms, collapse:** *Ars., Camph.,* Carb-v., Chin., Hyosin-hbr., *Laur.,* Mur-ac., Sec., Verat.

**Peritonitis:** Ars., *Bell.,* Carb-v., Coloc., *Merc-c.,* Rhus-t., Ter.

**Pneumonia, bronchial symptoms:** *Ant-t.,* Ars., Bell., *Bry.,* Hyos., *Ip.,* Lach., *Phos.,* Puls., Rhus-t., *Sang.,* Sulph., Ter.

**Putrescent pneumonia:** Ars., Mur-ac.

**Soreness, muscular:** Arn., Bapt., Bry., Gels., *Rhus-t.*

**Stage of convalescence:** Ars-i., Carb-v., *Chin.,* Cocc., Hydr., Kali-p., Nux-v., *Psor.,* Sulph., Tarax.

**Tympanites:** *Asaf., Ars.,* Bapt., *Carb-v.,* Chin., Cocc., Coch., Lyc., Methyl., Mill., Mur-ac., *Nux-m., Ph-ac.,* Rhus-t., *Ter.*

**Ulcer, corneal:** Apis, Ip.

**Urination, profuse:** Gels., Mur-ac., *Ph-ac.*

**Urination, scanty, painful:** Apis, Ars., *Canth.*

**EXANTHEMATA, ERUPTIVE FEVER: RUBELLA, (rothein, German measles):** Acon., Bell., Cop. (See **Rubeola, Measles.**)

**RUBEOLA, MEASLES:** *Acon.,* Ail., Ant-t., *Ars., Ars-i.,* Bell., *Bry.,* Camph., Coff., Dulc., Eup-per., *Euphr.,* Ferr-p., *Gels.,* Ip., *Kali-bi.,* Kali-m., Lach., Merc., Merc-c., Merc-p-r., Op., *Puls.,* Rhus-t., Spong., Squil., *Stict.,* Stram., Sulph., Verat-v., Viol-o.

**CONCOMITANTS: Adenitis:** Kali-bi., Merc-i-r.

**Bronchial and pulmonary symptoms:** *Ant-t.,* Bell., *Bry.,* Chel., Ferr-p., *Ip.,* Kali-bi., *Phos.,* Rumx., *Stict.,* Verat-v., Viol-o.

**Bronchial and pulmonary symptoms persisting:** Calc., Iod., Kali-c., Sil., Sulph.

**Catarrhal symptoms:** All-c., Ars., Dulc., *Euphr.,* Gels., Kali-bi., Merc., *Puls.,* Sabad., *Stict.*

**Cerebral and convulsive symptoms:** Aeth., Apis, *Bell.,* Camph., Coff., *Cupr-act.,* Stram., Verat-v., Viol-o., Zinc.

**Cough, croupy:** Acon., Coff., Dros., Euphr., Gels., *Hep.,* Kali-bi., *Spong.,* Stict.

**Diarrhea:** Ars., Chin., *Ip.,* Merc., *Puls.,* Verat.

**Diphtheritic symptoms:** Lach., Merc-cy.

**Epistaxis:** Acon., Bry., Ip.

**Eye symptoms:** Ars., *Euphr.,* Kali-bi., Puls.

**Gangrene of mouth, vulva:** Ars., Kali-chl., Lach.

**Insomnia, cough:** Calc., Coff.

**Laryngitis:** Dros., Gels., *Kali-bi.,* Viol-o.

**Low fever, toxemia:** *Ail., Ars.,* Bapt., Carb-v., Crot-h., *Lach., Mur-ac., Rhus-t.,* Sulph.

**Malignant types (black or epidemic):** Ail., *Ars.,* Crot-h., Lach.
**Otalgia, rheumatoid symptoms:** Puls.
**Rash, retrocedent, or suppressed:** Ant-t., Apis, *Bry.,* Camph., *Cupr-act., Ip., Lach., Stram.*
**Rash, tardy development:** Ant-t., Apis, *Bry.,* Cupr., Dulc., Gels., Ip., *Stram.,* Sulph., Tub., Verat-v., *Zinc.*
**Sequelae:** Am-c., *Ars.,* Bry., Camph., Coff., *Cupr-act.,* Dros., Kali-c., Merc., Merc-c., Op., *Puls.,* Sang., Stict., *Sulph., Tub.,* Zinc.

**SCARLET FEVER:** *Acon., Ail.,* Am-c., *Apis, Ars.,* Arum-t., *Asim., Bell.,* Bry., Canth., *Carb-ac.,* Chinin-ar., Com., *Crot-h.,* Cupr., Cupr-act., Dub., Echi., Eucal., *Gels.,* Hep., Hyos., Ip., Kali-chl., Kali-s., Lac-c., *Lach.,* Lyc., Merc., Merc-i-r., *Mur-ac.,* Op., Phyt., *Rhus-t.,* Sang., Sil., Sol-n., Spig., *Stram.,* Ter., Zinc.

**CONCOMITANTS, Adenitis, cervical:** Ail., Am-c., Asim., *Bell., Carb-ac.,* Crot-h., Hep., Lach., Merc., *Merc-i-r., Rhus-t.*
**Adenitis, parotid:** Am-c., Phyt., Rhus-t.
**Albuminuria and dropsy:** Acon., Am-c., *Apis,* Apoc., *Ars., Canth.,* Colch., *Dig., Hell.,* Hep., Kali-chl., Lach., Nat-s., *Ter.* (See **Nephritis, URINARY SYSTEM.)**
**Anginosa (sore throat):** Acon., *Ail., Apis,* Ars., *Asim., Bar-c., Bell.,* Brom., Kali-perm., Lac c., *Lach.,* Merc., Mur-ac., *Phyt.,* Rhus-t.
**Anginosa, ulcerativa:** *Am-c.,* Apis, *Ars.,* Arum-t., Bar-c., Crot-h., Hep., *Lach., Merc-cy.,* Merc-i-r., *Mur-ac.,* Nit-ac.
**Cellulitis:** Ail., Am-c., *Apis,* Lach., *Rhus-t.*
**Chronic tendencies aroused:** Calc., Hep., Rhus-t.
**Diarrhea:** Ail., Ars., Asim., Phos., Rhus-t.
**Edema of glottis:** *Apis,* Apisin., Chinin-s., Merc-c.
**Edema of lungs:** *Ant-t.,* Cann-s., Phos., Squil.
**Fever:** Acon., *Apis,* Asim., Bapt., *Bell.,* Gels., Rhus-t.
**Laryngitis:** Brom., Spong.
**Malignant tendency, adynamia:** *Ail.,* Am-c., *Apis,* Ars., Arum-t., Bapt., *Carb-ac.,* Carb-v., *Crot-h.,* Cupr-act., Echi., Hydr-ac., *Lach.,* Merc-cy., *Mur-ac.,* Phos., *Rhus-t.,* Tab., Zinc.
**Miliary type:** *Acon.,* Ail., Am-c., Apis, Ars., Bry., *Coff.,* Kali-ar., Lach., Rhus-t.
**Nervous, convulsive, cerebral symptoms:** Aeth., Ail., Am-c., Apis, Ars., *Bell.,* Camph., Cupr., *Cupr-act., Hyos.,* Rhus-t., *Stram.,* Sulph., Zinc.
**Rash, delayed development:** Apis, Ars., *Bry.,* Lach., Rhus-t., Zinc.
**Rash, hemorrhage in:** Crot-h., *Lach.,* Mur-ac., Phos.
**Rash, livid:** *Ail., Lach.,* Mur-ac., Sol-n.

**Rash, livid, partial, patchy:** Ail.

**Rash, retrocedent, threatened brain paralysis:** *Ail.,* Am-c., Cupr-act., Sulph., Tub., *Zinc.*

**Rash, retrocession of:** Am-c., *Apis,* Ars., Bry., Calc., *Camph.,* Cupr., *Cupr-act., Stram.,* Sulph., Verat., *Zinc.*

**Raw, bloody, itching, painful, surfaces, must pick and bore into them:** Arum-t.

**Rheumatic symptoms:** Bry., *Rhus-t.,* Spig.

**SEQUELAE, Adenitis:** Brom., Hep., Lach., *Merc-i-r.,* Phyt.

**Deafness, sore, bleeding nose:** Mur-ac.

**Desquamation, in large flakes, several times:** Arum-t.

**Ear disorders:** Bell., Carb-ac., Carb-v., Gels., *Hep., Merc.,* Sil., Sulph.

**Nephritis (post-scarlatinal):** Apis, Ars., Arum-t., Canth., Hell. (See **URINARY SYSTEM.**)

**Nose disorders:** Arum-t., Aur-m., Mur-ac., Sulph.

**Stomatitis ulcerative:** Arum-t., Mur-ac.

**Typhoidal symptoms:** Ail., Arum-t., *Hyos.,* Lach., *Rhus-t.,* Stram. (See **malignant.**)

**Vomiting:** Ail., Asim., *Bell.,* Cupr.

**VARICELLA, CHICKENPOX:** *Acon., Ant-t.,* Apis, Bry., *Dulc.,* Kali-m., Led., *Merc.,* Rhus-d., *Rhus-t.,* Urt-u., Vario.

**VARIOLA, SMALLPOX:** Acon., Am-c., Anac., *Ant-t.,* Apis, Ars., *Bapt., Bry., Carb-ac.,* Chinin-s., Cimic., Crot-h., Cupr-act., Gels., *Hep.,* Hydr., *Kali-bi.,* Lach., *Merc.,* Mill., Op., Phos., *Rhus-t., Sarr.,* Sin-n., Sulph., Thuj., *Vario.,* Verat-v.

**TYPE, Confluent:** Ars., Hippoz., *Merc.,* Phos., Sulph., Vario.

**Discrete:** *Ant-t., Bapt.,* Bell., Gels., Sulph.

**Hemorrhage:** Ars., *Crot-h., Ham., Lach., Phos.,* Nat-n., *Sec.,* Sulph.

**Malignant:** Am-c., Ant-t., *Ars.,* Bapt., *Carb-ac., Crot-h., Lach., Mur-ac.,* Ph-ac., Phos., *Rhus-t.,* Sec., Sulph., Vario.

**COMPLICATIONS, Adenitis:** *Merc-i-r.,* Rhus-t.

**Boils:** *Hep.,* Phos., Sulph.

**Collapsic symptoms:** *Ars.,* Carb-v., Lach., *Mur-ac.,* Ph-ac.

**Delirium:** *Bell.,* Stram., Verat-v.

**Dropsical swellings:** *Apis,* Ars., Canth.

**Fever, initial:** *Acon.,* Ant-t., *Bapt., Bell.,* Gels., Vario., *Verat-v.*

**Fever suppurative:** Acon., Bell., Merc., *Rhus-t.*

**Ophthalmia:** Merc., Sulph.

**Pulmonary symptoms:** Acon., *Ant-t.,* Bry., *Phos.,* Sulph., Verat-v.

**Repercussion eruption:** Ars., *Camph.,* Cupr., Sulph., Zinc.

**FEBRICULA (simple continued fever):** *Acon.*, Arn., *Ars.*, *Bapt.*, Bell., Bry., Camph., *Ferr-p.*, Gels., Ip., Kalm., Merc., Nux-v., Puls., *Rhus-t.*

**GASTRIC:** Acon., *Ant-c.*, *Ars.*, *Bapt.*, *Bry.*, Calc., Chin., Hydr., *Ip.*, Lyc., Merc., Nux-v., Ph-ac., *Puls.*, Rhus-t., Santin.

**HECTIC:** Abrot., *Acet-ac.*, Acon., Arg-met., *Ars.*, Ars-i., *Bals-p.*, *Bapt.*, Calc., Calc-i., Calc-s., Carb-v., *Chin.*, *Chinin-ar.*, *Ferr.*, Gels., *Hep.*, Iod., Lyc., Med., *Merc.*, Nit-ac., Ol-j., Ph-ac., Phel., *Phos.*, Pyrog., *Sang.*, Sil., Stann., Sulph.

**INFLAMMATORY:** Acon., Bell., Bry.

**INFLUENZA (grippe):** *Acon.*, Aesc., *All-c.*, Ant-ar., Ant-i., Ant-t., Arn., *Ars.*, *Ars-i.*, Ars-s-r., Asc-t., *Bapt.*, *Bell.*, *Brom.*, *Bry.*, Calc., Camph., Canch., *Carb-ac.*, Card-m., Caust., Chin., *Chinin-s.*, Cupr-ar., Cycl., Dros., *Dulc.*, Ery-a., *Eucal.*, *Eup-per.*, Euph., Euphr., Ferr-p., *Gels.*, Glon., Glyc., Gymno., Influ., Iod., Ip., Kali-bi., Kali-c., Kali-i., Kali-s., Lach., Lob-c., *Lob-p.*, Lyc., Merc-s., *Nat-sal.*, *Nux-v.*, *Phos.*, Phyt., Podo., Psor., Puls., Pyrog., Rhus-r., *Rhus-t.*, Rumx., *Sabad.*, Sal-ac., Sang., *Sangin-n.*, Sarcol-ac., Seneg., Silphu., Spig., Spong., *Stict.*, Sulph., Trios., Verat.

**Influenza, debility of:** Abrot., Adon., *Ars-i.*, *Aven.*, Carb-ac., *Chin.*, *Chinin-ar.*, Chinin-s., Con., Eup-per., Gels., *Iber.*, Lac c., Lath., Phos., Psor., Sal-ac., Sarcol-ac.

**Influenza, pain remaining:** Lycpr.

**INTERMITTENT FEVER (ague, malarial):** Acon., *Alst.*, Am-m., *Am-pic.*, *Aml-ns.*, Ant-c., Ant-t., *Apis*, *Aran.*, Arn., *Ars.*, Ars-br., Aza., Baj., Bapt., Bell., Bol-la., Bry., Cact., *Camph-mbr.*, Canch., *Caps.*, Carb-ac., *Carb-v.*, Cean., *Cedr.*, Cent., *Chin.*, *Chinin-ar.*, *Chinin-m.*, *Chinin-s.*, Chion., Cimx., *Cina*, *Corn-f.*, Crot-h., *Echi.*, Elat., Eucal., *Eup-per.*, *Eup-pur.*, Ferr., Ferr-p., *Gels.*, *Helia.*, Hep., Hydr., *Ign.*, *Ip.*, Kali-n., *Lach.*, Laur., Lyc., Maland., *Meny.*, Methyl., *Nat-m.*, Nat-s., *Nux-v.*, Op., Ost., Pambt., Parth., Petros., *Ph-ac.*, Phel., Podo., Polyp-p., Puls., Rhus-t., Sabad., Spig., Sulph., Tarax., *Tela*, Thuj., Urt-u., Verb., *Verat.*, Verat-v.

**TYPE, Abuse of quinine, cachexia:** Am-m., Aran., Arn., *Ars.*, Ars-i., *Calc-ar.*, Carb-v., Cean., Chelo., *Chinin-ar.*, Eucal., Eup-per., Ferr., *Hydr.*, *Ip.*, *Lach.*, Malar., Maland., *Nat-m.*, *Polym.*, Puls., Sulph., Verat.

**Chronic, inveterate cases:** Abies-n., Am-m., Aran., *Ars.*, Ars-br., Calc-ar., Canch., Carb-v., Corn-c., Corn-f., *Helia.*, Ign., *Nat-m.*, *Puls.*, Pyrog., Querc., Tela. (See **Abuse of Quinine.**)

**Congestive:** Camph., *Op.*, *Verat.*

**Dumb ague:** *Ars.*, Cedr., Chelo., Chinin-s., *Gels.*, *Ip.*, Maland., *Nux-v.*

**Impure cases, in non-malarial regions:** Ip., Nux-v.

**Nervo-hysterical persons:** Aran., Cocc., Ign., Tarent.

**Pernicious cases:** Ars., Camph., Chinin-brh., *Chinin-s.*, Crot-h., *Verat.*

**Recent cases:** Acon., Aran., Ars., Chin., Chinin-s., Ip., Tarent.
**Stages, partial, irregular:** Aran., *Ars.,* Cact., *Carb-v.,* Eup-per., Eup-pur., *Ip.,* Nat-m.
**Stages, regular, well defined:** Chin., *Chinin-s.*

**CHILL, OCCURRENCE, TYPE, Afternoon, 1 P.M-daily:** Ferr-p.
**Afternoon, 2 P.M.:** Calc., Lach.
**Afternoon, 3 P.M.:** Apis, Chinin-s.
**Afternoon, 3 P.M to 4 P.M.:** Lyc., Thuj.
**Afternoon, 4 P.M to 8 P.M.:** Lyc.
**Afternoon, 4 P.M.:** Aesc.
**Afternoon, 5 P.M.:** Chin.
**Afternoon, late, evening, night:** Aran., Bol-la., Cedr., Ip., Petr., Tarent.
**Anticipating:** Chin., *Chinin-s.,* Nux-v.
**Forenoon:** Chin., Formal., Nux-v.
**Hebdomadal:** Chin.
**Midday:** Gels.
**Midnight:** Ars., Nux-v.
**Mingled, with heat:** Ant-t., Apis, *Ars.,* Chin., *Nux-v.,* Tarent., Verat. (See **Chilliness**)
**Morning:** Chinin-s.
**Morning, 1 A.M-to 2 A.M.:** Ars.
**3 A.M.:** Thuj.
**4 A.M.:** Ferr.
**5 A.M.:** Chin.
**6 A.M-to 7 A.M.:** Podo.
**7 A.M-to 9 A.M., at noon following day:** Eup-per.
**9 A.M-to 11 A.M.:** Bapt., Bol-la., Mag-s., *Nat-m.,* Wye.
**11 A.M-and 11 P.M.:** Cact.
**Periodical:** *Aran., Ars.,* Bol-la., Cact., *Cedr.,* Chin., *Chinin-s.,* Cina, *Eucal.,* Ip.
**Periodical, every 7 or 14 days, never at night:** Chin.
**Periodical, every spring:** Carb-v., *Lach.,* Sulph.
**Prolonged:** Aran., Bol-la., Cact., Canch., *Caps., Chinin-s.,* Eup-pur., Ip., Meny., Nat-m., *Nux-v.,* Plb., Podo., Puls., *Pyrog., Sabad., Verat.,* Verat-v.
**Quartan:** Baja, Chin., *Chinin-s.,* Hell.
**Quotidian:** Ars., Bol-la., Chinin-s., Kali-n., Ign., Lob., Nux-v., Plb., Tarent.
**Slight:** *Ars.,* Aza., Carb-v., Cina, Chin., Eup-per., Eup-pur., *Ip.*
**Tertian:** Calc., Chin., *Chinin-s.,* Ip., Lyc.

**LOCATION, Abdomen:** *Apis, Calc.,* Meny.
**Back:** Apis, Bol-la., Conv., Dulc., *Eup-per.,* Eup-pur., *Gels., Lach.,* Mag-s., *Nat-m.,* Pyrog.

**Back, between scapulae:** Am-m., *Caps.,* Pyrog., Sep.
**Back, dorsal region:** Eup-per., Lach.
**Back, lumbar region:** Eup-per., Nat-m.
**Breast:** Chin.
**Feet:** Gels., Lach., Nat-m., Sabad.
**Hand, left:** Carb-v., Nux-m.
**Nose, tip of:** Meny.
**Thigh:** Rhus-t., *Thuj.*

**CONCOMITANTS, Anxiety, exhaustion, hypochrondriacal ideas, mental confusion, vertigo, tension of stomach, no relief from warmth:** Nux-v.
**Anxiety, palpitation, nausea, canine hunger, pressing pain in hypogastrium, congestive headache, distended, painful veins:** Chin., Chinin-s.
**Blue lips, nails:** Eup-per., Eup-pur., Meny., Nat-m., *Nux-v.,* Verat.
**Cardiac region, pain in:** Cact., Tarent.
**Collapsic symptoms; skin icy cold; pallor, cold sweat on forehead:** Verat.
**Cough, dry, teasing:** Rhus-t.
**Diarrhea:** Caps., Elat., Verat.
**Face and hands bloated:** Lyc.
**Face red:** Ferr., Ign., Nux-v.
**Forehead, cold sweat on:** Ip., Verat.
**Gastric symptoms:** *Ant-c.,* Arg-n., Ars., Bol-la., Canch., Eup-per., *Ip.,* Lyc., *Nux-v.,* Puls.
**Hands, feel dead:** Apis, Nux-v.
**Headache:** Bol-la., Chin., Chinin-s., Conv., *Eup-per.,* Eup-pur., Nat-m., Nux-v.
**Headache, vertigo, yawning, stretching, general discomfort:** Ars.
**Heart symptoms, enterrhagia:** Cact.
**Hemorrhoidal symptoms:** Caps.
**Hyperesthesia:** Ign.
**Hyperesthesia of spine:** Chinin-s.
**Loquacity:** Podo.
**Nausea before chill:** Ip.
**No two chills alike:** Puls.
**Pain in bones, limbs, soreness:** Aran., Bol-la., Canch., *Caps.,* Chin., Chinin-s., *Eup-per.,* Eup-pur., Formal., *Gels.,* Nat-m., Nux-v., Phel.
**Pains, in joints:** Chin.
**Pains, in knees, ankles, wrists, hypogastrium:** Podo.
**Restlessness:** Ars., Eup-per., Rhus-t.
**Sighing:** Ign.

**Thirst:** *Apis, Ars., Caps.,* Carb-v., Chin., Cina, Conv., Dulc., *Eup-per., Ign., Nat-m.,* Nux-v., Nyct., Verat., Wye.

**Thirst, after chill:** Ars.

**Thirst, before chill:** Chin., Chinin-s., *Eup-per.,* Gels., Meny., Nyct.

**Thirstlessness:** Chin., Chinin-s., Cimx, *Eup-pur.,* Gels., Nat-m.

**Vehemence, rage, preceding:** Cimx.

**Vomiting, bilious:** *Eup-per.,* Ip., Lyc., Nat-m., Nux-v., Nyct.

**Yawning, somnolency, accelerated breathing:** Nat-m.

**Yawning, stretching:** Ars., Elat., Lyc., Nux-v.

**MODALITIES, Aggravated from acids:** Lach.

**Aggravated, from drink:** Caps.

**Aggravated, from exposure:** Nux-v.

**Aggravated, from exposure, lying down:** Cimx.

**Aggravated, from motion:** Apis.

**Aggravated, from warmth:** Apis, Canch., Chin., Chinin-s., Nux-v.

**Ameliorated from warmth:** Caps., Ign.

**FEVER PAROXYSM, Afternoon, glowing heat, in face, hands, feet:** Aza.

**Anxiety, restlessness, lipothymia, oppression:** Ars.

**Backache:** Eup-per., Nat-m.

**Chill, intermingled:** Ars., Chin., Chinin-s., Nux-v., Tarent.

**Chilliness, after heat of face:** Calc.

**Congestion of head, drowsiness, costiveness, rectal and vesical tenesmus, chilled from uncovering:** Nux-v.

**Delirium:** Ars., Podo., Sabad.

**Desire to be covered:** Nux-v.

**Desire to be uncovered:** Ign., Ip.

**Diarrhea:** Ant-c., Ip., Verat.

**Dyspnea:** Apis, Ars., Conv., Ip.

**Face, hot, feet cold:** Chin., Petr.

**Face pale, insomnia:** Ant-t.

**Gastric symptoms:** Ars., Eup-per., *Ip.,* Nux-v., Puls.

**Hands warm, face cold:** Cina.

**Headache:** Apis, Ars., *Bell.,* Cedr., Chin., Eup-per., *Nat-m.,* Nux-v., Wye.

**Headache, yellowish tongue, nausea, faintness in epigastrium, costiveness:** Polyp-p.

**Heat, burning:** Apis, *Ars.,* Caps., *Eup-per.,* Formal., *Ip.,* Lach., *Nux-v.*

**Hunger:** Chin., Cina.

**Hydroa:** Hep., *Nat-m.,* Rhus-t.

**Lachrymation:** Sabad.

**Loquacity:** Podo.
**Mental confusion:** Formal.
**Nettle rash:** Apis, Ign., Rhus-t.
**Night:** Ars.
**Pain, colicky:** Cina.
**Pain, in head, back, limbs:** Nux-v.
**Pain in the vertebrae, dorsal:** Chinin-s.
**Pain, spasms, paralysis:** Ars.
**Paroysms, frequent, transient:** Carb-v.
**Prolonged heat:** Ars., Bol-la., Ign.
**Prostration, fainting, cold sweat:** Verat.
**Pupils, immobile, pain in abdomen, sopor, tension throughout body:** Op.
**Sighing:** Ign.
**Sleepiness:** Ant-t., Apis, Corn-f., Gels., Op.
**Thirst:** *Ars.,* Chin., Chinin-s., *Eup-per.,* Nat-m., Nux-v., Nyct., Op., Verat.
**Thirstlessness:** Apis, Caps., Chin., Chinin-s., Cimx., *Ign.,* Nat-m., Puls., Sabad., Wye.
**Tongue clean:** Ars., Cina.
**Trembling of limbs, slow pulse:** Chinin-s, Op.
**Unconsciousness:** Nat-m.
**Vomiting:** Ars., Cimic., Cina, Eup-per., *Ip.,* Verat.
**Sweat:** Ant-c., Aran., Aza., *Bol-la.,* Bry., *Chin., Chinin-s.,* Cimx., Cina, Conv., Eup-per., Lyc., Nat-m., Nux-v., Op., *Ph-ac., Verat.,* Wye. (See **Sweat**.)
**Sweat scanty or absent:** *Apis,* Ars., Carb-v., Eup-per., Nux-v.
**Sweat, with coldness:** Plb.
**Sweat, with covering up:** Chin., Hep.
**Sweat, with relief of pains:** Nat-m.
**Sweat, with sleep:** Chin., Con., Podo., Thuj.
**Sweat, with thirst:** Ars., *Chinin s.,* Nux-v.
**APYREXIA, Adynamia, gastro-intestinal pains, sallow face, dropsical swellings, enlarged liver and spleen, restlessness, sleeplessness, spasms, diarrhea, albuminuria:** Ars.
**Adynamia hydremia, chlorosis:** Chin., Puls.
**Adynamia, morning headache, depression, costiveness, amenorrhea, enlarged liver, desire for quiet, sallow face:** Nat-m.
**Gastro-enteric symptoms:** Chin., Hydr., *Ip., Nux-v.,* Puls.
**Jaundice:** Ars., Bol-la., Card-m., Nux-v., Podo.
**Nervous symptoms:** Gels.
**Pains:** Led.

**Relapses from dietetic errors:** Ip.

**Spleen enlarged:** Ars., *Cean.,* Chin., Chinin-s., Ferr., Nat-m.

**Thirst:** Ars., Cimx., Ign.

**Vomiting:** Ip.

**Vomiting, abdominal gripping, pain in back, loins:** Verat.

**LOW FEVERS:** *Ail., Arn., Ars.,* Bapt., Camph., Cocc., Crot-h., Eup-a., *Lach., Mur-ac.,* Nit-s-d., *Ph-ac.,* Phos., Pyrog., *Rhus-t.,* Ter., *Urt-u.* (See **Typhus.**)

**MEDITERRANEAN FEVER:** Bapt., Bry., *Colch.,* Merc., Rhus-t.

**PUERPERAL FEVER,** Acon., Pyrog., Verat. (See **FEMALE SEXUAL SYSTEM.**)

**REFLEX, from local irritation:** *Cham., Cina,* Gels., Ign., Ip., Merc., Nux-v., Sang., Sulph., Verat.

**RELAPSING FEVER:** *Acon.,* Ars., *Bapt., Bry.,* Cimic., *Eucal.,* Eup-per., Rhus-t.

**REMITTENT FEVER:** Acon., Ant-c., *Ars.,* Bell., Bry., Chin., *Chinin-s., Cina,* Crot-h., *Gels.,* Hyos., *Ip.,* Merc., Nit-ac., Nux-v., Nyct., Puls., Rhus-t., Sulph.

**Remittent, bilious, low:** Bry., *Crot-h., Eup-per.,* Gels., Ip., Merc-d., Nyct., Podo.

**Remittent, in children:** Ant-c., Cina, *Gels.,* Lept., Puls., Santin.

**SEPTIC FEVER:** Ail., Anthraci., *Ars.,* Crot-h., Echi., *Pyrog.,* Verat. (See **Pyemia, GENERALITIES.**)

**SYNOCHAL FEVER:** *Acon.,* Bapt., Bell.

**TRAUMATIC FEVER:** Acon., *Arn.,* Ars., Chin., Lach. (See **Injuries, GENERALITIES.**)

**TYPHUS FEVER:** Acet-ac., Agar., *Ail.,* Apis, *Ars.,* Arum-t., *Bapt., Bell.,* Calc., *Camph.,* Chin., Chinin-s., Crot-h., Hell., *Hyos.,* Kreos., *Lach.,* Merc., Merc-i-r., Mur-ac., Nit-ac., *Op., Ph-ac., Phos.,* Pyrog., *Rhus-t.,* Stram., Verat.

**Cellulitis, adenitis (salivary):** Bell., Chinin-s., *Merc-i-r.*

**Nervous symptoms:** Agar., *Bell., Hyos.,* Lach., Op., Ph-ac., Phos., *Stram.*

**Toxemia:** *Ars., Mur-ac.,* Pyrog., Rhus-t. (See **Typhoid.**)

**URETHRAL FEVER:** *Acon.,* Ars., *Chinin-ar., Gels.,* Hep., Lach., Phos., Rhus-t., Sil.

**WORM FEVER:** Bell., *Cina, Merc.,* Santin., Sil., Spig., Stann.

**YELLOW FEVER:** *Acon.,* Ant-t., Apis, *Arg-n., Ars.,* Bell., *Bry., Cadm-s.,* Camph., Canth., Carb-ac., *Carb-v.,* Chin., Chinin-s., Coff., Crot-c., *Crot-h.,* Cupr., Gels., Gua., *Hyos.,* Ip., *Lach.,* Merc., Op., *Phos.,* Plb., Sabin., Sul-ac., Ter., Verat.

■

# SKIN

**ACNE ROSACEA:** Agar., Ars., *Ars-br.,* Ars-i., Bell., *Carb-an.,* Caust., Chrysar., Eug., *Hydrc.,* Kali-br., Kali-i., Kreos., Nux-v., Ov., Petr., Psor., Rad-br., Rhus-r., Rhus-t., Sep., *Sul-i.,* Sulo-ac., Sulph.

**ACNE SIMPLEX:** *Ant-c.,* Ant-s-aur., *Ant-t.,* Ars., *Ars-br.,* Ars-i., Ars-s-r., Asim., *Aster., Bell.,* Bell-p, *Berb-a., Bov., Calc-pic., Calc-s.,* Calc-sil., Carb-ac., *Carb-an., Carb-v.,* Cic., Cimic., Cob., Echi., *Eug.,* Gran., Graph., *Hep., Hydrc., Jug-c., Jug-r.,* Kali-bi., *Kali-br., Kali-i.,* Kali-m., Lappa, *Led., Lyc.,* Nabal., Nat-br., Nat-m., Nit-ac., *Nux-v.,* Olnd., Ph-ac., Psor., Puls., Rad-br., Sel., Sep., Sil., Staph., *Sul-i., Sulph.,* Sumb., Thuj.

**From abuse of KI:** Aur.

**From abuse of mercury:** Kali-i., Mez., Nit-ac.

**From cheese:** Nux-v.

**From cosmetics:** Bov.

**From syphilis:** Aur., *Kali-i.,* Merc., Nit-ac. (See **MALE SEXUAL SYSTEM.**)

**In anemic girls at puberty, with vertex headache, flatulent dyspepsia, better by eating:** Calc-p.

**In drunkards:** Ant-c., Bar-c., *Led., Nux-v.,* Rhus-t.

**In fleshy young people with coarse habits, bluish red, pustules on face, chest, shoulders:** Kali-br.

**In scrofulous:** Bar-c., Brom., *Calc.,* Calc-p., Con., *Iod.,* Merc., Mez., Sil., *Sulph.*

**In tubercular children:** Tub.

**With cachexia:** Ars., Carb-v., Nat-m., Sil.

**With gastric derangements:** *Ant-c., Carb-v.,* Cimic., Lyc., *Nux-v.,* Puls., Rob.

**With glandular swellings:** Brom., Calc-s., Merc.

**With indurated papules:** Agar., Arn., Ars-i., Berb., Bov., Brom., *Carb-an.,* Cob., Con., *Eug.,* Iod., *Kali-br., Kali-i.,* Nat-br., Nit-ac., Rob., *Sulph.,* Thuj.

**With menstrual irregularities:** Aur-m-n., Bell., Bell-p., Berb., *Berb-a.,* Calc., *Cimic.,* Con., Eug., *Graph.,* Kali-br., Kali-c., Kreos., Nat-m., Psor., *Puls., Sang.,* Sars., Thuj., Verat.

**With pregnancy:** Bell., Sabin., Sars., Sep.

**With rheumatism:** Led., Rhus-t.

**With sexual excesses:** *Aur.,* Calc., Kali-br., *Ph-ac.,* Rhus-t., Sep., Thuj.

**With scars unsightly:** Carb-an., Kali-br.

**With symmetrical distribution:** Arn.

**ACTINOMYCOSIS:** Hecla, Hippoz., Kali-i., Nit-ac.

**ALOPECIA:** Alum., Anthraco., *Ars.,* Calc-s., *Fl-ac.,* Manc., *Nat-m., Ph-ac., Phos.,* Pilo., *Pix,* Sel., *Sep.,* Tub., Vinc. (See **Scalp, HEAD**.)

**ANIDROSIS (deficient sweat, dry skin):** Acet-ac., Acon., *Aeth., Alum.,* Apoc., Arg-n., Ars., *Bell., Berb-a.,* Crot-t., *Graph.,* Iod., *Kali-ar., Kali-c.,* Kali-i., Lach., Mag-c., *Maland.,* Nat.c., *Nux-m.,* Op., *Petr.,* Phos., Plb-m., *Psor.,* Sanic., Sars., Sec., *Sulph.,* Thyr.

**ANTHRAX: Carbuncle, Malignant pustule:** Acon., *Anthraci., Apis,* Arn., *Ars.,* Bell., Both., Bry., Bufo, Calc-chln., *Carb-ac.,* Carb-v., *Chin.,* Crot-h., Cupr-ar., *Echi.,* Euph., Hep., Hippoz., *Lach., Lappa, Led.,* Mur-ac., Nit-ac., Phyt., *Pyrog.,* Rhus-t., *Scol.,* Sec., *Sil.,* Sul-ac., Sulph., *Tarent.*

**ATHOPHY of skin:** Ars., Cocc., Graph., Sabad., Sulph.

**BLISTERS, small:** Apis, *Canth.,* Nat-m., *Rhus-t.,* Sec.

**BLOOD BOILS:** *Anthraci.,* Arn., Ars., Crot-h., *Lach.,* Ph-ac., Pyrog., Sec.

**BLUENESS: Lividity:** Agar., *Ail., Ant-t.,* Arn., *Ars.,* Cadm-s., Camph., *Carb-an., Carb-v.,* Chin., Crat., Crot-h., *Cupr., Dig.,* Hell., Ip., Kali-i., *Lach., Laur., Morph.,* Mur-ac., *Sec.,* Sul-ac., *Tarent-c., Verat.,* Vip. (See **FACE.**)

**BROMIDROSIS (offensive sweat):** Art-v., *Bapt.,* Bry., Carb-an., Chin., Con., Graph., *Hep., Lyc., Merc., Nit-ac.,* Osm., *Petr.,* Phos., *Psor.,* Pulx., Sep., *Sil.,* Stann., *Staph.,* Sulph., *Tell.,* Thuj., Vario.

**Bromidrosis, sour odor of body:** *Calc.,* Cham., Colos., Graph., *Hep.,* Kreos., Lac-d., *Mag-c., Rheum, Sul-ac.,* Sulph.

**BURNING:** Acet-ac., *Acon., Agar.,* Anac., *Apis, Ars.,* Bapt., *Bell.,* Bry., *Canth.,* Caps., Caust., Dulc., Euph., *Form.,* Grin., Kali-c., Kreos., Medus., *Nux-v.,* Phos., Rad-br., *Ran-b., Rhus-t.,* Sang., *Sec., Sulph.,* Vesp. (See **Pruritus**.)

**CALLOSITIES (corns):** *Ant-c.,* Elae., *Ferr-pic., Graph.,* Hydr., Lyc., *Nit-ac.,* Petr., *Ran-b.,* Rhus-t., Sal-ac., Sars., Sep., Sil., *Thuj.* (See **Feet, LOCOMOTOR SYSTEM.**)

**CHILBLAINS:** *Abrot., Agar.,* Apis, Ars., Borx., Calc., Calen., *Canth.,* Carb-an., Crot-t., Cycl., Ferr-p., Frag., Ham., *Hep.,* Lach., Led., Merc., *Mur-ac., Nit-ac., Petr.,* Plan., *Puls., Rhus-t.,* Sil., Sul-ac., *Sulph., Tam., Ter.,* Thyr., Verat-v., Zinc.

**CHLOASMA, Liver spots, moth patches:** *Arg-n.,* Aur., Cadm-s., Card-m., *Caul.,* Cob., Cur., Guar., Laur., *Lyc., Nat-hp.,* Paul., Petr., Plb., *Sep.,* Sulph., Thuj. (See **Spots, copper colored**.)

**CICATRICES, Affections:** *Caust., Fl-ac., Graph., Iod.,* Nit-ac., Phyt., Sil., Sul-ac., *Thiosin.*

**COLDNESS:** Abies-c., *Acet-ac.,* Acon., Agar., Ail., Ant-c., Ant-m., *Ant-t., Ars.,* Both., Calc., *Camph., Carb-v.,* Chel., *Chin.,* Chinin-ar., Crat., *Crot-h.,* Dig., Ip., *Jatr-c,* Lach., *Lat-m., Laur.,* Med., Pyrog., Rhus-t., *Sec., Tab., Verat.* (See **Collapse, NERVOUS SYSTEM, Coldness, FEVER**.)

**COMEDO:** *Abrot., Bar-c.,* Bell., Calc-sil., Cic., *Dig., Eug.,* Mez., *Nit-ac.,* Sabin., *Sel.,* Sep., *Sulph., Sumb.*

**DECUBITUS (bed sores):** Arg-n., *Arn.,* Bapt., Carb-ac., Carb-v., Chin., Echi., *Fl-ac.,* Hippoz., *Lach., Mur-ac.,* Nux-m., Paeon., Petr., Pyrog., Sil., *Sul-ac.,* Vip. (See **Ulcer.**)

**DERMAL (trophic lesions):** Thal.

**DERMATALGIA (pain, sensitiveness, soreness):** Agar., Apis, Ars., *Bad.,* Bell., Bell-p., Bov., *Chin.,* Chinin-s., Con., Crot-t., *Dol.,* Euph., Fago., *Hep., Kali-c., Lach.,* Lyc., Nux-m., *Olnd.,* Osm., Paeon., *Petr.,* Phos., *Psor.,* Ran-s., Rhus-d., *Rhus-t.,* Rumx., Semp., Sep., *Sil., Sulph.,* Tarent-c., *Ther., Vinc.,* Xero.

**DRYNESS:** *Acon., Alum., Ars., Bell.,* Calc., *Graph.,* Hydrc., Iod., Lyc., Nat-c., Nit-ac., *Nux-m.,* Pilo., *Plb., Psor.,* Sabad., Sars., Sec.

**ECCHYMOSES:** Aeth., *Arn.,* Ars., Bell-p., Both., Carb-v., Chlor., *Crot-h., Ham.,* Kreos., *Led., Phos.,* Rhus-t., Sec., *Sul-ac.,* Suprar., Ter.

**ECHTHYMA:** Ant-c., *Ant-t., Ars.,* Bell., *Cic.,* Cist., *Crot-t.,* Hydr., Jug-c., *Jug-r.,* Kali-bi., Kreos., *Lach., Merc.,* Nit-ac., Petr., Rhus-t., *Sec., Sil.,* Sulph., Thuj.

**ECZEMA:** *Aethi-m.,* Aln., Alum., *Anac.,* Anthraco., *Ant-c.,* Arb., *Ars.,* Ars-i., *Berb.,* Berb-a., Borx., *Bov., Calc., Canth.,* Caps., *Carb-ac.,* Carb-v., Castor-eq., Caust., Chrysar., *Cic., Clem.,* Com., Con., *Crot-t.,* Dulc., Euph., Fl-ac., Frax., Fuli., *Graph., Hep.,* Hippoz., Hydrc., Jug-c., *Kali-ar.,* Kali-m., Kreos., Lyc., *Mang-act., Merc., Merc-c.,* Merc-d., Merc-p-r., *Mez.,* Mur-ac., Nat-ar., Nat-m., Nux-v., *Olnd., Petr.,* Pilo., *Plb.,* Podo., Polyg-h., Prim-v., *Psor., Rhus-t.,* Rhus-v., Sars., *Sep.,* Skook., *Sul-i., Sulph.,* Thuj., Tub., Ust., *Vinc., Viol-t.,* Xero., X-ray.

**Acute form:** Acon., Anac., Bell., Canth., *Chinin-s., Crot-t.,* Mez., *Rhus-t.,* Sep.

**Eczema, behind ears:** Ars., Arund., Bov., *Chrysar., Graph., Hep.,* Jug-r., Kali-m., Lyc., *Mez., Olnd., Petr.,* Psor., Rhus-t., Sanic., *Scroph-n.,* Sep., Staph., Tub. (See **EARS.**)

**Eczema, of face:** Anac., Ant-c., Bac., Calc., *Carb-ac.,* Cic., Coloc., Corn., *Crot-t.,* Hyper., Kali-ar., Led., Merc-p-r., Psor., Rhus-t., Sep., Staph., *Sul-i., Sulph., Vinc.* (See **FACE.**)

**Eczema, of flexures of joints:** *Aeth.,* Am-c., Caust., *Graph.,* Hep., Kali-ar., Lyc., Mang-act., *Nat-m.,* Psor., *Sep.,* Sulph.

**Eczema, of hands:** Anag., Bar-c., *Berb., Bov.,* Calc., *Graph., Hep.,* Hyper., Jug-c., Kreos., Maland., Petr., *Pix,* Plb., Rhus-v., Sanic., Sel., Sep., Still. (See **Hands, LOCOMOTOR SYSTEM.**)

**Eczema, of neurasthenic persons:** *Anac.,* Ars., Phos., *Stry-ar.,* Stry-p., Viol-t., Zinc-p.

**Eczema of pudendum:** Am-c., Ant-c., Ars., Canth., *Crot-t.,* Hep., Plb., Rhus-t., Sanic., Sep. (See **FEMALE SEXUAL SYSTEM.**)

**Eczema, of rheumatico-gouty persons:** Alum., Arb., Lac-ac., *Rhus-t.,* Ur-ac., Urea.

**Eczema, of scalp:** Astac., Berb-a., *Calc.,* Cic., Clem., Fl-ac., Hep., Kali-m., Lyc., Mez., Nat-m., *Olnd.,* Petr., Psor., Sep., *Sel.,* Staph., Sulph., Tub., *Vinc.,* Viol-o. (See **HEAD**.)

**Eczema, strumous persons:** *Aethi-m., Ars-i.,* Calc., *Calc-i.,* Calc-p., Caust., Cist., Crot-t., *Hep.,* Merc., Merc-c., Rumx., Sep., Sil., Tub.

**Eczema, of whole body:** Crot-t., Rhus-t.

**Eczema, madidans:** Cic., Con., Dulc., Graph., Hep., Kali-m., Merc-c., Merc-p-r., Mez., Sep., Staph., Tub., Viol-t.

**Eczema, with pigmentation in circumscribed areas following:** Berb.

**Eczema, with urinary, gastric, hepatic disorders:** Lyc.

**Eczema, worse after vaccination:** Mez.

**Eczema, worse at menstrual period, menopause:** Mang-act.

**Eczema, worse at seashore, ocean voyage, excess of salt:** Nat-m.

**EDEMA, SWELLING:** Acal., *Acet-ac.,* Acon., *Agar., Anac., Apis, Ars.,* Bell., Bell-p., Both., Bry., *Dig.,* Elat., Euph., Ferr., *Hell.,* Hippoz., Lach., Lyc., Nat-c., Nat-sal., Olnd., Prim-o., *Prun., Rhus-t.,* Samb., *Thyr.*

**EDEMA, ANGIONEUROTIC:** Agar., Antip., Hell.

**ELEPHANTIASIS:** Anac., *Ars.,* Calo., Card-m., *Elae.,* Graph., Ham., *Hydrc.,* Iod., Lyc., *Myris.,* Sil.

**EPHELIS (sunburn):** Bufo, Canth., Kali-c., Rob., Verat.

**EPITHELIOMA:** Abr., Acet-ac., Alumn., *Ars.,* Ars-i., Cic., Con., *Cund.,* Euph., Fuli., Hydr., Kali-ar., Kali-s., Lap-a., Lob., Lyc., Nat-cac., Rad-met., Scroph-n., *Sep.,* Sil., *Strych-g., Thuj.* (See **FACE**.)

**ERUPTIONS, Copper-colored:** Ars., Calc-i., *Carb-an.,* Kreos., Nit-ac.

**Eruptions, dry, scaly:** Alumn., *Anag.,* Ant-c., *Ars.,* Ars-i., *Berb-a.,* Bov., Cadm-s., Canth., Cory., Euph-l., Graph., *Hydrc., Iod., Kali-ar.,* Kali-m., Kali-s., Lith-c., Lyc., *Maland.,* Merc., Nat-m., Nit-ac., *Petr.,* Phos., Phyt., Pip-m., Pix, *Psor., Sars.,* Sel., Sep., *Sulph.,* Tub., Xero.

**Eruptions, humid, moist:** *Aethi-m.,* Ant-c., Ant-t., Bar-c., Bov., Caust., Chrysar., *Clem., Crot-t.,* Dulc., *Graph., Hep.,* Lyc., Manc., Merc., *Mez.,* Nat-m., *Olnd.,* Petr., *Psor., Rhus-t.,* Sep., Staph., Stront-c., Vario., Viol-t.

**Eruptions, pustular:** Aln., *Ant-c., Ant-t.,* Bell., *Berb.,* Bufo, Chel., Cic., *Crot-t.,* Echi., Euph., *Hep.,* Hippoz., Iris, Jug-r., *Kali-bi.,* Kali-i., Kreos., Lach., *Merc.,* Merc-c., Nit-ac., Phyt., *Psor.,* Ran-b., Rhus-v., Sep., *Sil.,* Sul-i., Sulph., Tax., Vario.

**Eruptions, scabby:** Ant-c., Ars., Calc., Chrysar., *Cic.,* Dulc., Graph., *Hep., Lyc.,* Merc., *Mez.,* Mur-ac., Nat-m., Petr., Staph., *Sulph.,* Viol-t., Vinc.

**Eruptions, better in winter:** Kali-bi., Sars.

**Eruptions, worse in spring:** Nat-s., Psor., Sang., *Sars.*

**Eruptions, worse in winter:** Aloe, *Alum.,* Ars., *Petr., Psor.,* Sabad.

**ERYSIPELAS:** *Acon.,* Anac-oc., Anan., *Apis, Arn.,* Ars., Atro., Aur., *Bell.,* Camph., *Canth.,* Carb-ac., Carb-v., *Chin.,* Com., Cop., Crot-h., *Crot-t., Echi., Euph., Graph.,* Hep., Jug-r., *Lach.,* Led., Nat-m., Nat-s., Prim-o., Ran-b., *Rhus-t., Rhus v.,* Samb., Sulph., Tax., Verat-v., *Xero.*

**Afebrile:** *Graph.,* Hep., Lyc.

**Biliary, catarrhal duodenal symptoms:** Hydr.

**Constitutional tendency:** Calen., *Graph.,* Lach., Psor., Sulph.

**Edema, persisting:** *Apis,* Ars., Aur., Graph., Hep., Lyc., Sulph.

**Facial:** Apis, Arn., *Bell.,* Borx., Canth., Carb-an., *Euph., Graph.,* Hep., *Rhus-t.,* Sol-n., sulph.

**Leg, below knee:** Sulph.

**Mammae:** Carb-v., Sulph.

**Neonatorum:** Bell., Camph.

**Phlegmonous:** Acon., Anthraci., Arn., *Ars.,* Bell., Both., Crot-h., Ferr-p., Graph., *Hep.,* Hippoz., *Lach.,* Merc., *Rhus-t.,* Sil., *Tarent-c.,* Verat-v.

**Recurrent and chronic:** Ferr-p., *Graph.,* Nat-m., *Rhus-t., Sulph.*

**Repercussion:** Cupr-act.

**Senile:** *Am-c.,* Carb-an.

**Swelling marked, burning itching, stinging:** Rhus-t.

**Traumatic:** Calen., Psor.

**Traumatic, umbilical, of new born:** Apis.

**Verisular:** Anac-oc., Arn., *Canth., Carb-ac.,* Caust., Crot-t., *Euph.,* Mez., *Rhus-t., Rhus-v.,* Ter., Urt-u., Verb., Verat-v.

**Wandering:** Apis, *Ars.,* Chin., *Graph.,* Hep., Hydr., Puls., Sulph.

**ERYTHEMA, Intertrigo (chafing):** *Aeth.,* Agn., Ars., Bell., Borx., Calc., *Caust., Cham.,* Fago., *Graph.,* Jug-r., Kali-br., *Lyc., Merc.,* Mez., Olnd., Ox-ac., *Petr.,* Psor., Sul-ac., *Sulph.,* Tub.

**Erythema multiforme:** Antip., Bor-ac., Cop., Vespa.

**Erythema nodosum:** Acon., Ant-c., *Apis, Arn.,* Ars., Chin., Chinin-ar., *Chinin-s.,* Ferr., Led., Nat-c., Ptel., *Rhus-t., Rhus-v.*

**Erythema simplex:** Acon., *Antip.,* Apis, *Arn.,* Ars-i., *Bell.,* Bufo, *Canth.,* Chlol., Echi., *Euph-l.,* Gaul., Grin., Kali-c., Lac-ac., *Merc., Mez.,* Narc-ps., Nux-v., Plb-chr., *Rhus-t.,* Rob., Ter., Urt-u., Ust., Verat-v., Xero.

**Fibroma:** Calc-ar., *Con., Iod.,* Kali br., Lyc., Sec., Thuj.

**FISSURES: Rhagades, chaps:** *Alum.,* Anthraci., Ars-s-f., Bad., Bar-c., Calc-f., *Cist., Cund.,* Eug., *Graph., Hep.,* Kali-ar., Led., *Lyc., Maland.,* Mang-act., Merc-i-r., Merc-p-r., *Nat-m.,* Nit-ac., Olnd., *Petr.,* Pix, Ran-b., Rat., Rhus-t., *Sars., Sil.,* Sulph., Xero., X-ray.

**FLABBINESS, Non-tonicity:** *Abrot.,* Aster., Bar-c., Ars., Calc., Chel., *Hep.,* Ip., *Merc.,* Morph., Op., Nat-m., Sanic., Sars., Salv., Thyr., Verat.

**FOREIGN BODIES, To promote expulsion of fish bones, splinters, needles:** Anac., Hep., Sil.

**FORMICATION, Tingling, numbness:** *Acon.,* Ambr., Ap-g., Arund., Calen., *Cocain.,* Cod., Medus., *Mez., Morph.,* Olnd., Ph-ac., Plat., Rumx., Sec., *Sel.,* Sil., Staph., *Sul-ac.,* Valer., Zinc.

**FUNGUS HEMATODES:** *Ars.,* Lach., Lyc., Manc., *Phos., Thuj.*

**FURUNCLE (boil):** Abrot., Aeth., Anan., Anthraci., Ant-c., *Arn.,* Ars., *Bell., Bell-p.,* Calc-hp., *Calc-pic.,* Calc-s., Carb-v., Echi., *Ferr-i.,* Gels., *Hep.,* Hippoz., *Ichth.,* Lach., Lyc., *Med., Merc.,* Ol-myr., Oper., *Ph-ac., Phyt.,* Pic-ac., Rhus-r., Sec., *Sil.,* Sul-ac., Sul-i., *Sulph., Tarent-c.,* Tub., Zinc-o.

**Furuncle, recurrent tendency:** *Arn.,* Ars., Berb., Calc., *Calc-m.,* Calc-p., *Calc-pic.,* Echi., Hep., *Sulph.,* Tub.

**GANGRENE:** Ail., Anthraci., Ant-c., Apis, *Ars.,* Both., Brass., Brom., Calen., Canth., Carb-ac., Carb-an., *Carb-v.,* Chin., Chlor., Chr-o., Crot-t., Cupr-ar., *Echi., Euph.,* Ferr-p., Kali-chl., Kali-p., Kreos., *Lach., Polyg-pe.,* Ran-a., Sal-ac., *Sec., Sul-ac.,* Tarent-c.

**Gangrene, senile:** All-c., Am-c., Ars., Sec., Sul-ac.

**Gangrene, traumatic:** Arn., Lach., Sul-ac.

**HERPES (tetter):** Acon., Aethi-m., Aln., Anac., Anan., Anthraco., Apis, Arn., *Ars.,* Bar-c., Borx., Bry., Bufo, Calc., *Canth., Carb-ac.,* Caust., Chrysar., Cist., Clem., Com., *Crot-t., Dulc.,* Eucal., *Graph., Kali-bi.,* Lith-c., *Merc.,* Mez., Nat-c., *Nat-m., Nit-ac.,* Petr., Ph-ac., Psor., Ran-b., Ran-s., *Rhus-t., Sars., Sep.,* Sil., Sulph., Tell., Vario., Xero.

**Herpes, between fingers:** Nit-ac.

**Herpes, chronic:** Aln.

**Herpes, circinatus, tonsurans:** Ars-s-f., Bar-c., Calc., Calc-act., Chrysar., Equis-a., Hep., Nat-c., Nat-m., *Sep., Tell.,* Tub. (See **Trichophytosis**.)

**Herpes, circinatus, in isolated spots:** Sep.

**Herpes, circinatus, in intersecting rings:** Tell.

**Herpes, dry:** Bov., Fl-ac., Mang-act., Sep., Sil.

**Herpes, of chest, nape of neck:** Nat-m., Petr.

**Herpes, of chin:** Ars., Caust., Graph., Mez., Sil.

**Herpes, of face:** Apis, *Ars.,* Calc-f., Caps., Caust., Clem., Con., Lach., Lim., *Nat-m.,* Ran-b., *Rhus-t.,* Sep., Sulph. (See **FACE**.)

**Herpes, of flexures of knees:** Graph., *Hep., Nat-m., Sep.,* Xero.

**Herpes, of genitals:** Aur-m., Calc., *Caust.,* Crot-t., Dulc., *Hep.,* Jug-r., *Merc., Nit-ac.,* Petr., Ph-ac., *Sars.,* Ter. (See **MALE SEXUAL SYSTEM**.)

**Herpes, of hands:** Cist., Dulc., *Lim.,* Lith-c., Nit-ac.

**Herpes, of knees:** Carb-v., Petr.

**Herpes, of thigh:** Graph., Petr.

**Herpes, neuralgia after:** Kalm., *Mez.,* Ran-b., Still., Vario.

**Herpes, with glandular swelling:** Dulc.

**Herpes, with pimples or pustules surrounding, spread by covalescing:** Hep.

**HERPES ZOSTER, Zona, shingles:** Apis, Arg-n., *Ars.,* Aster., *Canth.,* Carbn-o., *Caust.,* Cedr., *Cist.,* Com., Crot-t., *Dol.,* Dulc., Graph., Grin., Hyper., Iris, Kali-ar., Kali-m., Kalm., Merc., *Mez.,* Morph., Pip-m., *Prun., Ran-b.,* Ran-s., *Rhus-t.,* Sal-ac., Semp., Staph., Stry-ar., Sulph., Thuj., Vario., Zinc-p., Zinc-val.

**Chronic:** Ars., Semp.

**Neuralgia, persisting:** Ars., Dol., *Kalm., Mez.,* Ran-b., Still., Zinc.

**HYDROA:** Kali-i., Kreos., Mag-c., *Nat-m.,* Rhus-v. (See **Herpes**)

**HYPERIDROSIS (Excessive sweating):** *Acet-ac., Aeth., Agarin.,* Am-c., Ant-t., Ars-i., *Bapt.,* Bell., Bol-la., *Calc.,* Cham., *Chin.,* Esin., Ferr., Graph., *Jab.,* Lac-ac., *Merc.,* Nat-c., Nit-ac., Nux-v., Op., *Ph-ac.,* Phos., Pilo., *Samb.,* Sanic., Sel., *Sep., Sil.,* Sul-ac., Sulph., Thuj., Verat. (See **FEVER**.)

**ICHTHYOSIS (fish skin disease):** *Ars., Ars-i.,* Aur., Clem., Graph., *Hydrc.,* Iod., Kali-i., Merc., Nat-c., Oena., Phos., Platan., Plb., Sulph., *Syph.,* Thuj., *Thyr.*

**IMPETIGO:** Aln., *Ant-c.,* Ant-s-aur., *Ant-t.,* Ars., Arum-t., Calc-m., *Cic.,* Clem., *Dulc.,* Euph., Graph., Hep., Iris, Jug-c., *Kali-bi.,* Kali-n., Lyc., *Mez., Rhus-t.,* Rhus-v., Sep., Sil., Sulph., Thuj., *Viol-t.*

**KELOID:** Fl-ac., Graph., Nit-ac., Sabin., Sil.

**LENTIGO (freckles):** Am-c., Bad., Calc., Graph., *Kali-c., Lyc.,* Mur-ac., Nat-c., *Nit-ac.,* Petr., Phos., *Sep., Sulph.,* Tab.

**LEPRA, leprosy:** Anac., *Ars., Bad.,* Calo., Carb-ac., *Chaul.,* Com., Cupr-act., Cur., *Diphterocarpus,* Elae., Graph., Guan., *Gymno.,* Hura, *Hydrc.,* Jatr-g., Lach., Merc., Oena., Phos., *Pip-m.,* Sec., Sep., Sil., *Strych-g.,* Thyr.

**LEUCODERMA:** *Ars-s-f.,* Nat-m., Nit-ac., Sumb., Zinc-p., (See **Pale, FACE**.)

**LICHEN PLANUS:** Agar., Anac., *Ant-c.,* Apis, *Ars., Ars-i.,* Chinin-ar., Iod., *Jug-c., Kali-bi.,* Kali-i., Led., Merc., Sars., Staph., *Sul-i.*

**LICHEN SIMPLEX:** Alum., Am-m., *Anan., Ant-c.,* Apis, *Ars., Bell.,* Bov., Bry., *Calad.,* Castn-v., Dulc., *Jug-c.,* Kali-ar., *Kreos., Led., Lyc.,* Merc., Nabal., Nat-c., *Plan., Phyt., Rumx.,* Sep., Sul-i., *Sulph.,* Til. (See **Acne**.)

**LUPUS ERYTHEMATOSUM:** Apis, Cist., Guar., *Hydrc., Iod., Kali-bi., Phos.,* Sep., *Thyr.*

**LUPUS VULGARIS:** Abr., Apis, *Ars., Ars-i., Aur-ar.,* Aur-i., *Aur-m.,* Calc., Calc-i., Calc-s., *Cist.,* Cund., Ferr-pic., Form-ac., Form., Graph., Guar., *Hep., Hydr., Hydrc.,* Irid-met., *Kali-bi., Kali-i.,* Lyc., Nit-ac., Phyt., Staph., *Sulph.,* Thiosin., Thuj., *Tub.,* Urea, X-ray.

**MILIARIA (prickly heat):** *Acon.,* Am-m., Ars., *Bry.,* Cact., Cent., Hura, *Jab.,* Led., Raph., Syzyg., Urt-u.

**MILIUM:** *Calc-i.,* Staph., Tab. (See **Acne.**)

**MOLLUSCUM:** *Brom.,* Bry., Calc., *Calc-ar.,* Kali-i., Lyc., Merc., Nat-m., *Sil.,* Sulph., Teucr.

**MORBUS SUDATORIUS:** Acon., Ars., Carb-v., Jab., Merc.

**MORPHAEA:** Ars., *Phos.,* Sil. (See **Scleroderma.**)

**NEVUS:** Acet-ac., Calc., *Carb-v.,* Cund., *Fl-ac.,* Lyc., Phos., Rad-br., *Thuj.*

**NAILS, Affections in general:** Alum., *Ant-c.,* Castor-eq., *Graph.,* Hyper., Nit-ac., *Sil.,* Upa., X-ray.

**Affections of pulp, nails recede, leaves raw surface:** Sec.

**Atrophy:** Sil.

**Biting of:** Am-br., Arum-t.

**Blueness:** Dig., Ox-ac., (See **Cyanosis, CIRCULATORY SYSTEM.**)

**Deformed, brittle, thickened (onchogryphosis):** Alum., Anan., *Ant-c., Ars.,* Caust., Dios., Fl-ac., *Graph.,* Merc., Nat-m., Sabad., Sec., Senec., Sep., *Sil.,* Thuj., X-ray.

**Eruptions; Around nails:** Graph., Psor., Stann-m.

**Falling off:** Brass., But-ac., Hell., Hell-f.

**Hangnails:** *Nat-m.,* Sulph., Upa.

**Hypertrophy (Onychauxis):** Graph.

**Inflammation; Around root (paronychia):** Alum., Bufo, Calc-s., *Dios.,* Graph., Hep., *Nat-s.* (See **Felon.**)

**Inflammation of pulp (onychia):** Arn., Calen., *Fl-ac., Graph.,* Phos., Psor., Sars., Sil., Upa.

**Inflammation, under toe nail:** Sabad.

**Ingrowing toe nail:** Caust., M-aust., Nit-ac., *Sil.,* Staph., Teucr., Tet.

**Injury to matrix:** Hyper.

**Irritable feeling under finger nails, relieved by biting them:** Am-br.

**Itching; About roof of:** Upa.

**Pains; burning under:** Sars.

**Pains, gnawing, beneath finger nails:** Alum., Sars., Sep.

**Pains, neuralgic, beneath finger nails:** Berb.

**Pains, neuralgic:** *All-c.,* Alum., Colch.

**Pains, smarting at root:** Sulph.

**Pains, splinter-like, beneath toe nails:** Fl-ac.

**Pains, ulcerative, beneath toe nails:** Ant-c., Graph., Teucr., Graph., Teucr.
**Skin around, dry, cracked:** Graph., Nat-m., Petr.
**Skin around, pigmented:** Naphtin.
**Softening:** Plb., Thuj.
**Spots, white on:** Alum., Nit-ac.
**Trophic changes:** Rad-br.
**Ulceration:** Alum., Graph., Merc., *Phos.,* Psor., Sang., Sars., Sil., Teucr., Tet.
**Yellow color:** Con.

**OILY, Skin:** *Bry., Merc., Nat-m.,* Plb., Psor., Raph., Sanic. (See **Seborrhea.**)

**PELLAGRA:** *Ars.,* Ars-s-r., Bov., Chin., Gels., Ped., Plb-i., Psor., *Sec., Sedi.,* Sulph.
**Pellagra, cachexia:** Ars., Sec.
**Pellagra, fissures, desquamation, skin eruptions:** Graph., *Hep.,* Ign., Phos., Puls., Sep.

**PEMPHIGUS:** Anac., Antip., *Ars.,* Arum-t., Bufo, Calth., *Canth.,* Carbn-o., Caust., Dulc., *Jug-c., Lach., Manc.,* Merc., *Merc-c.,* Merc-p-r., Nat-sal., Ph-ac., Phos., *Ran-a., Ran-b.,* Raph., *Rhus-t.,* Sep., Thuj.

**PETECHIAE:** *Arn.,* Ars., Calc., Cur., Mur-ac., *Phos.,* Sec., *Sul-ac.* (See **Ecchymosis.**)

**PHTHIRIASIS:** Bac., Cocc., Merc., *Nat-m.,* Olnd., Psor., *Sabad., Staph.*

**PITYRIASIS (dermatitis exfoliativa):** *Ars.,* Ars-i., Bac., Berb-a., Calc., Carb-ac., Clem., *Colch., Fl-ac., Graph., Kali-ar.,* Mang-act., Merc-p-r., *Mez.,* Nat-ar., Phos., Pip-m., *Sep.,* Staph., *Sulo-ac.,* Sul-i., *Sulph.,* Tell., Ter., Thyr.

**PRAIRE ITCH:** Led., Rhus-t., Rumx., Sulph.

**PRURIGO:** Acon., Aln., *Ambr.,* Anthraco., *Ars., Ars-i.,* Ars-s-f., Carb-ac., *Chlol.,* Dios., *Dol.,* Kali-bi., *Lyc., Merc., Mez., Nit-ac., Olnd.,* Ov., Ped., *Rhus-t., Rhus-v., Rumx.,* Sil., *Sulph.,* Ter.

**PRURITUS (itching of skin):** Acon., *Agar.,* Alum., *Ambr., Anac.,* Anac-oc., Anag., *Antip.,* Apis, *Ars.,* Calad., Calc., Canth., *Carb-ac.,* Chlol., Chrysar., *Clem., Crot-t., Dol.,* Dulc., Elae., *Fago.,* Fl-ac., Form., Glon., *Graph.,* Gran., Grin., Guan., Hep., *Hydrc.,* Hyper., Ichth., Ign., Kreos., *Lyc.,* Mag-c., Maland., Mang-act., Med., *Merc., Mez., Morph.,* Nicc., Nux-v., Olnd., Op., Petr., *Pix,* Prim-o., Psor., Pulx., *Rad-br.,* Ran-b., *Rhus-t., Rhus-v., Rumx., Sep.,* Staph., Sul-ac., *Sulph.,* Syzyg., Tarent-c., *Urt-u.,* Vesp., Xero.
**Pruritus, of aged:** Bar-act.
**Pruritus, of ankles:** Nat-p., Sel., Sep.
**Pruritus, of bends of elbows, knees:** Sel., Sep.
**Pruritus, of chest, upper limbs:** Arund.

**Pruritus, of ears, nose, arms, urethra:** Sul-i.
**Pruritus, of face, hands, scalp:** Clem.
**Pruritus, of face, shoulders, chest:** Kali-br.
**Pruritus, of feet, ankles:** Led.
**Pruritus, of feet, legs:** Bov.
**Pruritus, of feet, soles of:** Anan., Hydrc.
**Pruritus,, of genitals:** *Ambr.,* Ars-i., Borx., *Calad.,* Carb-ac., Carb-v., Colch., Coll., Crot-t., Dulc., Fuli., Guan., Helon., Kreos., Mez., Nit-ac., Rhus-t., Rhus-v., *Sep.,* Sil., Tarent-c. (See **FEMALE SEXUAL SYSTEM**.)
**Pruritus, of hands, arms:** Pip-m., Sel.
**Pruritus, of joints, abdomen:** Pin-s.
**Pruritus, of knees, elbows, hairy parts:** Dol., Fago.
**Pruritus, of nose:** Morph., Stry.
**Pruritus, of orifices:** Fl-ac.
**Pruritus, of thighs, bends of knees:** Zinc.
**Pruritus, of webs of fingers, bends of joints:** Hep., *Psor.,* Sel., Sep.
**Pruritus, ameliorated from cold:** Berb., Fago., Graph., Mez.
**Pruritus, ameliorated from hot water:** Rhus-v.
**Pruritus, ameliorated from rubbing gently:** Crot-t.
**Pruritus, ameliorated from scratching:** Asaf., Cadm-s., Mang-act., Merc., *Olnd., Rhus-t.*
**Pruritus, ameliorated from warmth:** Ars., Petr., Rumx.
**Pruritus, followed by bleeding, pains, burning:** Alum., *Ars., Crot-t.,* Murx., Pix, Psor., Sep., *Sulph.,* Til.
**Pruritus, followed by, change of site of itching:** Mez., *Staph.*
**Pruritus, without eruption:** Dol.
**Pruritus, worse from contact:** Ran-b.
**Pruritus, worse from exposure, cold air:** Dulc., *Hep.,* Nat-s., *Olnd.,* Petr., Rhus-t., *Rumx.*
**Pruritus, worse from scratching:** *Ars.,* Berb-v., Crot-t., Led., *Mez.,* Sep., Sulph.
**Pruritus, worse from undressing; warmth of bed, at P.M.:** *Alum.,* Ant-c., *Ars.,* Asim., Bell-p., Bov., Carb-v., Card-m., Cist., Dulc., *Jug-c., Kali-ar.,* Kreos., Led., Lyc., *Menis., Merc.,* Merc-i-f., Mez., *Nat-s., Olnd.,* Psor., Puls., Rhus-t., *Rumx.,* Sang., Sep., *Sulph.,* Tub.
**Pruritus, worse from washing, with cold water:** Clem., Tub.

**PSORIASIS:** Ant-t., *Ars., Ars-i.,* Aster., Aur-m-n., Berb-a., *Borx., Carb-ac., Chrysar.,* Cic., Cor-r., Cupr-act., Fl-ac., *Graph.,* Hep., Hydrc., Iris, *Kali-ars., Kali-br.,* Kali-s., *Lyc., Mang-act., Merc.,* Merc-aur., Mur-ac., Naphtin., Nat-ar., Nat-m., Nit-ac., Nit-m-ac., *Petr., Phos.,* Plat., *Sep.,* Stry-ar., Stry-p., Stel., *Sulph.,* Ter., Thuj., *Thyr.,* Tub., Ust.

**Psoriasis of palms:** Calc., Cor-r., *Graph., Hep., Lyc.,* Med., Petr., Phos., Sel.

**Psoriasis, of prepuce, nails:** Graph., *Sep.*

**Psoriasis, of tongue:** Graph., Mur-ac., *Sep.* (See **Tongue, MOUTH.**)

**PURPURA:** Acon., *Arn., Ars.,* Bapt., Bell., Bry., Carb-v., Chinin-s., Chlol., *Crot-h., Ham.,* Jug-r., Kali-i., *Lach.,* Merc., Ph-ac., *Phos.,* Rhus-t., Rhus-v., Sal-ac., Sec., *Sul-ac.,* Sulfon., Ter., Verat-v.

**With colic:** Bov., Coloc., Cupr., Merc-c., Thuj.

**With debility:** Arn., *Ars.,* Carb-v., Lach., Merc., *Sul-ac.*

**PURPURA HEMORRHAGICA:** Aln., *Arn.,* Ars., Both., Bry., *Crot-h.,* Ferr-pic., *Ham.,* Iod., Ip., *Lach.,* Led., Merc., Merc-c., Mill., Naja, Nat-n., *Ph-ac., Phos.,* Rhus-v., Sec., *Sul-ac., Ter.,* Thlas.

**PURPURA RHEUMATICA:** Acon., Ars., *Bry.,* Merc., *Rhus-t.,* Rhus-v.

**RAYNAUD'S DISEASE:** (See **Gangrene**.)

**RHINO-SCLEREMA:** Aur-m-n., *Calc-p.,* Guar., Rhus-r.

**ROSEOLA (rose-rash):** *Acon.,* Bell., Cub.

**RUPIA:** Aethi-m., Ant-t., *Ars.,* Berb-a., Clem., Graph., Hydr., *Kali-i.,* Lach., Merc-i-r., Nit-ac., *Phyt.,* Sec., Syph., Thyr. (See **Syphilis, MALE SEXUAL SYSTEM.**)

**SARCOMA CUTIS:** Calc-p., *Cund.,* Nit-ac., Sil.

**SCABIES (Itch):** Aloe, Anthraco., Caust., *Crot-t., Hep.,* Lyc., Merc., Nux-v., *Psor.,* Rhus-v., Sel., *Sep., Sulph.*

**SCLERODERMA: Scleriasis (hidebound skin):** Alum., *Ant-c.,* Arg-n., Ars., Berb-a., *Bry.,* Caust., *Crot-t.,* Echi., *Elae., Hydr.,* Lyc., Petr., Phos., Ran-b., Rhus-r., Sars., Sil., Still., Sulph., Thiosin., *Thyr.*

**SCROFULODERMA:** Calc-i., *Calc-s.,* Petr., Scroph-n., Ther. (See **Separate Diseases.**)

**SEBACEOUS CYSTS (wen):** *Bar-c.,* Benz-ac., Brom., Calc-sil., *Con.,* Graph., Hep., Kali-br., *Kali-i.,* Nit-ac., Phyt., Thuj. (See **Scalp, HEAD.**)

**SEBORRHEA:** *Am-m., Ars., Bry.,* Bufo, *Calc.,* Chin., Graph., *Iod.,* Kali-br., *Kali-c.,* Kali-s., Lyc., Merc., Mez., *Nat-m., Phos., Plb.,* Psor., *Raph.,* Rhus-t., Sars., *Sel.,* Sep., Staph., Sulph., Thuj., *Vinc.* (See **Scalp, HEAD.**)

**SENSIBILITY OF SKIN: Diminished, or lost (analgesia, anesthesia):** Acet-ac., *Acon.,* Ars., Aur., Bufo, *Cann-i., Carbn-o.,* Carbn-s., Elae., Hyos., *Ign.,* Kali-br., Merc., *Nux-v., Plb.,* Pop-c., Sec., *Zinc.*

**Sensibility of skin increased to atmospheric changes:** Dulc., Hep., Kali-c., Psor., *Sulph.*

**SPOTS, Blue:** Ars., Led., Sul-ac.

**Spots, brown:** Bac., Card-m., Con., Iod., Phos., *Sep.,* Thuj.

**Spots, circumscribed pigmentation following eczematous inflammation:** Berb., Lach., Lyc., Med., Merc., Merc-d., Nit-ac., Sil., Sulph., Ust.

**Spots, copper colored:** *Carb-an.,* Carb-v., *Cor-r.,* Syph.

**Spots, livid:** Agav-a., *Ail., Bapt.,* Both., *Morph.,* Ox-ac., Sec., *Sul-ac.*

**Spots, red:** Agar., Barbit., Bell., Calc., Con., Kali-c., Sulph.

**Spots, white:** Graph., Sulph.

**Spots, yellow:** Nat-p., Phos., Plb., Sep., Sulph.

**Spots, yellow turning green:** Con.

**STROPHULUS (tooth rash):** Apis, *Borx.,* Calc., *Cham.,* Cic., Led., Rhus-t., *Spira.,* Sumb.

**SUDAMINE:** Am-m., Bry., Urt-u.

**SYCOSIS (Barber's Itch):** Anthraco., *Ant-t.,* Ars., Aur., *Calc.,* Calc-s., Chrysar., *Cic.,* Cinnb., Cocc., Cypressus, *Graph., Kali-bi.,* Kali-m., Lith-c., *Lyc.,* Med., *Merc-p-r.,* Nat-s., *Nit-ac.,* Petr., Plan., *Plat.,* Sabin., Sep., Sil., *Staph.,* Stront-c., *Sul-i.,* Sulph., Tell., *Thuj.*

**SYPHILIDAE,** (See **Syphilis, MALE SEXUAL SYSTEM.**)

**TINEA FAVOSA, Favus:** Agar., Ars-i., *Brom.,* Calc., Dulc., Graph., Hep., Jug-r., *Kali-c.,* Lappa, *Lyc.,* Med., *Mez.,* Olnd., Phos., *Sep.,* Sulo-ac., Sulph., Ust., Vinc., *Viol-t.* (See **Scalp, HEAD.**)

**TINEA VERSICOLOR (chromophytosis):** Bac., *Chrysar.,* Mez., *Nat-ar., Sep.,* Sulph., Tell.

**TRICHOPHYTOSIS, Ringworm:** Ant-c., Ant-t., *Ars., Bac.,* Calc., Calc-i., *Chrysar., Graph.,* Hep., Jug-c., Jug-r., Kali-s., Lyc., Mez., Psor., Rhus-t., Semp., *Sep.,* Sulph., *Tell.,* Tub., Viol-t. (See **Scalp, HEAD.**)

**Trichophytosis, in intersecting rings over great portion of body, fever, great constitutional disturbances:** Tell.

**Trichophytosis, in isolated spots on upper part of body:** Sep.

**ULCERS:** Anac-oc., *Anan., Anthraci.,* Arn., *Ars.,* Aster., Bals-p., Bell., *Calc., Calc-p., Calc-s., Calc-sil.,* Calen., *Carb-ac., Carb-an., Carb-v.,* Carbn-s., Caust., Cist., *Clem.,* Com., Con., Crot-h., Cupr-ar., *Echi., Fl-ac.,* Gali., *Gaul., Ger.,* Graph., Ham., *Hep.,* Hippoz., *Hydr.,* Iod., Jug-r., Kali-ar., *Kali-bi.,* Kali-i., *Lach., Merc.,* Merc-c., *Mez.,* Nat-s., *Nit-ac., Paeon.,* Petr., Ph-ac., Phos., *Phyt.,* Psor., Rad-br., Ran-a., Scroph-n., Sep., *Sil.,* Sul-ac., Sulph., *Syph.,* Tarent-c., Thuj.

**Bleeding, easily, when touched:** Ars., *Carb-v.,* Dulc., Hep., Kreos., *Lach.,* Merc., Mez., *Nit-ac., Petr., Phos.*

**Burning:** Alumn., *Anthraci., Ars., Carb-v.,* Hep., Kreos., Mez., Thuj.

**Cancerous, malignant:** Anthraci., *Ars., Aster.,* Carb-an., Chim., Clem., Cund., Fuli., *Gali.,* Hydr., Kreos., Lach., Tarent-c., Thuj.

**Deep:** Asaf., Com., *Kali-bi.,* Kali-i., Mur-ac., *Nit-ac.,* Tarent-c.

**Eroding, of face:** Con.

**Fistulous:** *Calc-f.,* Calen., Kali-i., Nit-ac., Phyt., *Sil.,* Thuj.

**Indolent, torpid:** *Anag.,* Aster., Bar-c., Calc-f., *Calc-i., Calc-p.,* Carb-v., Chel., Con , Cupr., Eucal., Euph., Fl-ac., Fuli., *Ger.,* Graph., Hydr., Kali-bi., *Kali-i.,* Lach., Lyc., *Merc.,* Nit-ac., Paeon., Phyt., *Psor.,* Pyrog., *Sil., Sulph.,* Syph., Syzyg.

**Inflamed:** *Ars., Bell.,* Calen., Carb-an., Phyt. (See **Sensitive.**)

**Phagedenic:** *Ars.,* Carb-v., *Crot-h.,* Kali-ar., Merc., Merc-c., Merc-d., *Nit-ac.* (See **Gangrenous.**)

**Scrofulous:** *Calcareas,* Chin., Hep., Iodides, Mercuries, Nit-ac., *Sil.,* Sulph.

**Sensitive:** Ang., *Arn., Ars., Asaf., Calen.,* Dulc., Graph., *Hep., Lach., Mez., Nit-ac.,* Paeon., Sil., Tarent-c.

**Smooth, pale, shallow, on scalp, penis:** Merc.

**Superficial, flat:** Ars., Cor-r., Lach., Nit-ac., Thuj.

**Superficial, serpiginous:** Chel., *Merc.,* Merc-c., Ph-ac.

**Syphilitic:** Ars., *Asaf.,* Carb-v., *Cinnb.,* Cist., Cor-r., *Fl-ac.,* Graph., Hep., *Iod., Kali-bi., Kali-i.,* Lach., Lyc., Merc., *Merc-c., Merc-i-r., Nit-ac.,* Phyt., Sars., Still.

**Traumatic:** Arn., Con.

**Varicose:** Calc-f., Calen., *Card-m., Carb-v.,* Clem-vit., Cund., Eucal., *Fl-ac., Ham.,* Lach., Phyt., Psor., Pyrog., *Sec.*

**Verrucous, on cheek:** Ars.

**Ulcers, from pemphigus blisters on toes, with ulcerated borders, moist, red, flat surface:** Petr.

**Ulcers, from scarlet fever:** Cham.

**Ulcers, with base, blue or black:** *Ars.,* Calc-f., Carb-an., Lach., Mur-ac., Tarent-c.

**With base, dry, lardaceous:** Phyt.

**With base, indurated:** *Alumn, Calc-f.,* Com., Con.

**With base, lardaceous, surrounded with dark halo, dirty, unhealthy look, apt to coalescence:** Merc.

**With base, like raw flesh:** Ars., Merc., *Nit-ac.*

**With discharge, fetid, purulent, sloughing:** *Anan., Anthraci.,* Ars., Asaf., Bapt., Calc-f., *Calen., Carb-ac., Carb-v.,* Con., Crot-t., *Echi.,* Eucal., Fl-ac., Gels., *Ger., Hep.,* Lach., *Merc.,* Merc-c., *Mez.,* Mur-ac., *Nit-ac.,* Paeon., Ph-ac., Psor., Pyrog., Puls., Sil., Sulph., *Thuj.*

**With discharge, glutinous:** *Graph.,* Kali-bi.

**With discharge, ichorous:** Aster., *Carb-ac.,* Carb-v., Cor-r., *Mez.*

**With discharge, ichorous, foul:** Anthraci., *Ars.,* Asaf., Mez.

**With discharge, thin, acrid, foul:** Ars., Asaf., Kali-i., Nit-ac.

**With edges, deep regular, "punched out":** Kali-bi., Phos.

**With edges, eczematous, copper colored:** Kali-bi.

**With edges, gangrenous:** Anthraci., *Ars., Carb-v.,* Kreos., Lach., Nit-ac., Sec., *Sul-ac.,* Tarent-c.

**With edges, indurated:** Calc-f., *Carb-an.,* Com., Nit-ac., Paeon., Ph-ac.

**With edges, irregular, undefined:** *Merc.,* Nit-ac.

**With edges, raised:** Ars., Calen., Nit-ac., Ph-ac., *Sil.* (See **Granulations.**)

**With fungus growths:** Mur-ac.

**With glazed, shining appearance:** Lac-c.

**With granulations, exuberant:** Ap g., *Ars.,* Carb-an., *Caust.,* Fl-ac., *Nit-ac.,* Petr., Ph-ac., *Sil.,* Thuj.

**With itching:** Mez., Ph-ac., Sil.

**Without pain or redness, uneven, jagged base, dirty pus:** Ph-ac.

**With pain, in small spot, lightening-like, worse from warmth:** Fl-ac.

**With pain, splinter-like:** Ham., Hep., *Nit-ac.*

**With pimples surrounding it:** Grin., *Hep.,* Lach., Merc-

**With small ulcers, surrounding it:** Phos., Sil.

**With stupor, low delirium, prostration:** Bapt.

**With vesicles, surrounding it, red shining areolae:** Fl-ac., Hep., *Mez.*

**UNHEALTHY SKIN: Every scratch festers, or heals with difficulty:** *Borx.,* Bufo, Calc., Calc-s., Calen., Carbn-s., Cham., *Graph., Hep.,* Hydr., Lyc., *Merc., Petr.,* Pip-m., Psor., *Pyrog., Sil., Sulph.*

**URTICARIA (hives, nettle rash):** Acon., Anac., Anthraco., *Ant-c., Antip.,* Ap-g., *Apis, Ars., Astac.,* Berb., *Bomb-pr., Bov.,* Calc., *Camph.,* Chinin-s., *Chlol., Cimic,* Cina, Con., *Cop.,* Crot-t., Cund., *Dulc.,* Fago., *Frag.,* Hep., Hom., *Ichth.,* Ign., Ip., Kali-c., Kali-chl., Medus., Nat-m., *Nat-p.,* Nit-ac., Nux-v., Petr., *Puls., Rhus-t.,* Rhus-v., Rob., Sanic., Sep., Stann., Stroph-n., Stry-p., *Sulph.,* Ter., Tet., *Trios., Urt-u.,* Ust., Vesp.

**Chronic:** *Anac., Ant-c.,* Antip., *Ars., Astac., Bov.,* Calc., *Chlol.,* Cund., *Cop., Dulc.,* Hep., Ichth., *Lyc.,* Nat-m., *Rhus-t.,* Sep., Stroph-h., *Sulph., Urt-u.*

**Nodosa:** Bov., Urt-u.

**Tuberosa:** *Anac.,* Bol-lu.

**CAUSE, CONCOMITANTS, From emotion:** Anac., Bov., Ign., Kali-br.

**From exertion, excessive:** Con., Nat-m.

**From exposure:** Chlol., *Dulc.,* Rhus-t.

**From gastric derangement:** *Ant-c.,* Ars., Carb-v., Cop., Dulc., Nux-v., *Puls.,* Rob., Trios.

**From menstrual conditions:** Bell., *Cimic., Dulc.,* Kali-c., Mag-c., Puls., Ust.

**From shellfish, roe:** Camph.

**From suppressed malaria:** Elat.

**From sweat:** Apis.

**With catarrh:** All-c., Dulc.
**With chill, of intermittents:** Ign., Nat-m.
**With constipation, fever:** Cop.
**With croup, alternating:** Ars.
**With diarrhea:** Apis, Bov., *Puls.*
**With edema:** *Apis,* Vesp.
**With erosion, on toes:** Sulph.
**With itching, burning after scratching, no fever:** Dulc.
**With liver disturbance:** Astac.
**With petechial disturbance or erysipelatous eruption:** Frag.
**With rheumatic lameness, palpitation, diarrhea:** *Bov.,* Dulc.
**With rheumatism, alternating:** Urt-u.
**With sequelae,from suppressed hives:** Apis, Urt-u.
**With sudden coming and going:** Antip.
**With sudden, violent onset, syncope:** Camph.

**MODALITIES, AGGRAVATIONS, At climacteric:** Morph., Ust.
**At menstrual period:** *Cimic., Dulc.,* Kali-c., Mag-c.
**At night:** Ant-c., Ars.
**From bathing, walking in A.M.:** Bov.
**From cold:** Ars., Dulc., Rhus-t., Rumx., Sep.
**From exertion, exercise:** Apis, Calc., Hep., Nat-m., Psor., Sanic., Urt-u.
**From fruit, pork, buckwheat:** Puls.
**From open air:** Nit-ac., Sep.
**From spirituous drinks:** Chlol.
**From warmth:** Apis, Dulc., Kali-c., Lyc., Sulph.
**In children:** Cop.
**Periodically, every year:** Urt-u.

**AMELIORATIONS, From cold water:** Apis, Dulc.
**From hot drinks:** Chlol.
**From open air:** Calc.
**From warmth:** Ars., Chlol, Sep.

**VACCINIA:** *Acon.,* Ant-t., Apis, *Bell.,* Merc., Phos., *Sil.,* Sulph., *Thuj.,* Vac.

**VERUCCA (warts):** Acet-ac., Am-c., Anac-oc., Anag., *Ant-c.,* Ant-t., Ars br., Aur-m-n., Bar-c., *Calc.,* Castm., Castor-eq., *Caust.,* Chr-o., Cinnb., *Dulc., Ferr-pic.,* Kali-m., Kali-perm., Lyc., *Mag-s., Nat-c.,* Nat-m., Nat-s., *Nit-ac.,* Ran-b., Semp., Sep., *Sil.,* Staph., Sul-ac., Sulph., *Thuj.,* X-ray.
**Bleed easily:** Cinnb.
**Bleed easily, jagged, large:** Caust., *Nit-ac.*
**Condylomata, fig warts:** Calc., *Cinnb.,* Euphr., Kali-i., Lyc., Med., Merc., Merc-c., Nat-s., *Nit-ac.,* Ph-ac., *Sabin.,* Sep., Sil., *Staph., Thuj.*
**Cracked, ragged, with furfuraceous areola:** Lyc.

**Flat, smooth, sore:** Ruta.
**Horny, broad:** Rhus-t.
**Large, seedy:** Thuj.
**Large, smooth, fleshy, on back of hands:** Dulc.
**Lupoid:** Ferr-pic.
**Moist, itching, flat, broad:** Thuj.
**Moist, oozing:** Nit-ac.
**Painful, hard, stiff, shining:** Sil.
**Painful, sticking:** *Nit-ac.,* Staph., Thuj.
**Pedunculated:** Caust., Lyc., *Nit-ac.,* Sabin., Staph., *Thuj.*
**Situated, on body, general:** Nat-s., Sep.
**Situated, on breast:** Castor-eq.
**Situated, on face, hands:** Calc., Caust., Carb-an., Dulc., Kali-c.
**Situated, on forehead:** Cast-m.
**Situated, on genito-anal surface:** Nit-ac., Thuj.
**Situated, on hands:** Anac., *Bufo,* Ferr-ma., Kali-m., Lach., Nat-c., *Nat-m.,* Rhus-t., Ruta.
**Situated, on neck, arms, hands, soft, smooth:** Ant-c.
**Situated, on nose, finger tips, eye brows:** Caust.
**Situated, on prepuce:** Cinnb., Ph-ac., Sabin.
**Small, all over body:** Caust.
**Smooth:** Calc., Ruta.
**Sycotic, syphilitic:** Nit-ac.

**WHITLOW: felon, panaritium:** All-c., Alum., Am-c., *Anthraci.,* Apis, Bell., *Bry.,* Bufo, Calc-f., Calc-s., Calen., Crot-h., *Dios., Fl-ac., Hep.,* Hyper., Led., Merc., Myris., Nat-s., Ol-myr., Phos., *Sil.,* Tarent-c.
**Malignant tendency:** Anthraci., *Ars.,* Carb-ac., *Lach.*
**Predisposition to:** Dios., Hep.
**Recurrence:** Sil.
**Traumatic:** Led.

■

# GENERALITIES

**ABSCESS, Acute:** Acon., *Anan.*, Anthraci., Apis, *Arn.*, Ars., *Bell.*, Calc-hp., *Calc-s.*, Calen., *Carb-ac.*, Chin., Chinin-s., Crot-h., Fl-ac., *Hep.*, Hippoz., *Lach.*, Lap-a., Lyc., *Merc.*, *Myris.*, *Nit-ac.*, Ph-ac., Phos., *Rhus-t.*, *Sil.*, Sil-mar., Syph., *Sulph.*, *Tarent-c.*, Vesp.

**About bones:** Asaf., *Aur.*, Calc-f., Calc-hp., Calc-p., Fl-ac., Mang., *Phos.*, Puls., *Sil.*, Symph.

**About joints:** Calc-hp., Sil.

**Chronic:** Arn., Calc., *Calc-f.*, Calc-i., Calc-p., Carb-v., Cham., Chin., Fl-ac., Graph., Hep., *Iod.*, Iodof., Kali-i., *Merc.*, Merc-i-r., Ol-j., Phos., *Sil.*, Sulph.

**Muscles, deep:** Calc.

**Psoas abscess:** Sil., Symph.

**To abort:** Apis, Bell., Bry., *Hep.*, *Merc.*

**To hasten suppuration:** Guaj., *Hep.*, Lach., *Merc.*, Oper., Phos., Phyt., *Sil.*

**ACROMEGALY:** Pitu-gl., Thyr.

**ADDISON'S DISEASE:** *Adren.*, Ant-c., Apom., *Arg-n.*, *Ars.*, Ars-i., Bac., Bell., Calc., Calc-ar., Hydr-ac., *Iod.*, Kreos., Nat-m., Nit-ac., Phos., Sec., *Sil.*, Spig., Sulph., *Suprar.*, Thuj., *Tub.*, Vanad.

**ANEMIA, Chlorosis:** Acet-ac., *Alet.*, Alum., *Arg-n.*, *Arg-o.*, Arn., *Ars.*, Aur-ar., Bism., *Calc.*, Calc-ar., Calc-lac., Calc.p., Calo., Carb-v., *Chin.*, *Chinin-ar.*, Chinin-fcit., *Chinin-s.*, Cic., Con., Crat., Crot-h., *Cupr.*, Cupr-ar., *Cycl.*, *Ferr.*, Ferr-act., *Ferr-ar.*, Ferr-c., Ferr-p., *Ferr-i.*, Ferr-m., Ferr-ox., *Ferr-r.*, Goss., *Graph.*, *Helon.*, Hydr., Iod., *Irid-met.*, Kali-bi., *Kali-c.*, Kali-p., Lec., *Lyc.*, *Mang-act.*, Merc., Nat-c., *Nat-m.*, *Nit-ac.*, Nux-v., Petr., *Phos.*, Phyt., Pic-ac., Plat., *Plb-act.*, *Puls.*, Rub-t., Sacch., *Sec.*, *Sep.*, Sil., *Stry-et-ferr-cit.*, *Sulph.*, Thyr., Vanad., Zinc-ar., Zinc-m.

**From cardiac disease:** Ars., Crat., Stroph-h..

**From grief:** Nat-m., *Ph-ac.*

**From malaria:** Alst., *Ars.*, *Nat-m.*, Ost., Rob.

**From menstrual derangements:** Arg-o., Ars., *Calc.*, Calc-p., Crat., *Cycl.*, *Ferr.*, *Graph.*, *Kali-c.*, Mang-act., *Nat-m.*, *Puls.*, Sep.

**From nutritional disturbance:** Alet., Alum., *Calc-p.*, Ferr., Helon., Nux-v.

**From suboxidation:** Pic-ac.

**From syphilis:** Calo.

**From vital drains, exhausting disease:** Acet-ac., Alst., *Calc-p.*, *Chin.*, Chinin-s., *Ferr.*, Helon., Kali-c., *Nat-m.*, *Ph-ac.*, Phos.

**Hemorrhagic chlorosis:** *Arg-o., Ars.,* Calc., Crot-h., Ign., Nat-br.

**Pernicious anemia:** *Ars., Phos.,* Pic-ac., Thyr.

**Type, erythistic; worse in winter:** Ferr.

**ASPHYXIA:** Am-c., *Ant-t., Hydr-ac.,* Sul-h., Upa.

**Asphyxia neonatorum:** *Ant-t.,* Laur.

**BLOOD, Disorganization:** Ail., Am-c., *Anthraci.,* Arn., *Ars.,* Ars-h., *Bapt.,* Carb-ac., *Crot-h., Echi.,* Kreos., *Lach., Mur-ac.,* Phos., Psor., *Pyrog., Rhus-t.,* Tarent-c. (See **Pyemia.**)

**BONES, Club foot:** Nux-v., Phos., Stry.

**Cold feeling:** Zinc.

**Condyles, epiphyses, swollen:** Conch., Rhus-t.

**Condyles, sutures, affected:** Calc., Calc-p.

**Cranial bones, thin, soft:** Calc., *Calc-p.*

**Crooked:** Am-c., Calc., Calc-p., Iod., Sil.

**Development, tardy:** *Calc.,* Calc-f., *Calc-p.,* Sil.

**Enlargement (acromegaly):** Pitu-gl., Thyr.

**Exostoses:** Arg-met., Aur., Calc., *Calc-f.,* Fl-ac., *Hecla, Kali-bi., Kali-i.,* Lap-a., Maland., Merc., Merc-c., *Merc-p.,* Mez., *Phos., Plb-act.,* Ruta, *Sil.,* Still., Sulph., Zinc.

**Fractures, shock:** Acon., Arn.

**Fractures, slow union:** *Calc.p.,* Calen., Iod., Mang-act., *Mez.,* Ph-ac., *Ruta, Sil., Symph.,* Thyr.

**Inflammation (osteitis):** Asaf., *Aur.,* Aur-i., Conch., Hecla, Hep., Iod., *Kali-i., Merc.,* Mez., *Nit-ac.,* Ph-ac., Phos., Staph., Still., Stront-c.

**Inflammation, chronic (osteitis deformans):** Aur., Calc-p., Hecla, Nit-ac.

**Inflammation (osteomyelitis):** Acon., Chinin-s., Gunp., Phos.

**NECROSIS:** Ang., *Arg-met.,* Ars., *Asaf.,* Aur-i., *Aur.,* Calc., *Calc-f.,* Calc-hp., Calc-p., Calc-sil., Chin., Con., *Fl-ac.,* Graph., Hecla, *Hep.,* Iod., Kali-bi., Kali-i., Lach., Med., *Merc.,* Mez., *Nat-sil-f., Nit-ac.,* Ph-ac., *Phos.,* Plat-m., *Sil.,* Staph., Sul-ac., Sulph., Symph., Syph., Thea, Ther., *Tub.,* Vitr-an.

**Facial:** Hep., Mez., Sil.

**Femur:** Stront-c.

**Long bones:** Ang., Asaf., *Fl-ac.,* Mez., Stront-c.

**Mastoid, palatine, cranial, nasal:** Aur.

**Mastoid, temporal:** Calc-f., Caps.

**Nasal:** Aur., Kali-bi.

**Skull:** Fl-ac.

**Sternum:** Con.

**Tarsus:** Plat-m.

**Tibiae:** Asaf., Carb-ac., Hep., Lach., Nit-ac., Phos.

**Vertebrae:** Calc., Nat-m., Ph-ac., Sil., Stict., Syph.

**Vertebrae, inferior maxilla:** Phos.

**NODES:** Asaf., *Aur-m., Cinnb.,* Fl-ac., *Kali-bi., Kali-i.,* Merc., Mez., Nux-v., Phyt., *Sil., Still.* (See **Syphilis, MALE SEXUAL SYSTEM.**)

**PAIN:** Agar., Ang., Asaf., *Aur.,* Aur-m., Bry., Castor-eq., Caust., Chin., Crot-c., Crot-h., *Eup-per.,* Euph., *Fl-ac.,* Guaj., Hep., Iod., Ip., *Kali-bi., Kali-i.,* Lyc., Lyss., Mang-act., Merc., Merc-c., *Mez.,* Ph-ac., Phos., *Phyt., Rhod.,* Rhus-t., *Ruta,* Sil., *Staph.,* Sulph., *Symph.,* Syph., Ther., Vitr-an.

**Burning:** Aur., Euph., Fl-ac., Kali-i., Ph-ac., Sulph.

**Constricting, band-like:** *Apis,* Carb-ac., Hep., Nit-ac., Sulph.

**Drawing, pressing, sensitiveness:** Nit-ac.

**Gnawing, digging:** *Aur.,* Carb-ac., Kali-i., Mang-act., Merc., Symph.

**Growing:** Guaj., Mang-act., Ph-ac.

**In coccyx:** Castor-eq.

**In face, feet:** Aur.

**In long bones:** Cinnb., Eup-per., Staph., Stront-c., Syph.

**In shin bones:** Arag., Asaf., Castor-eq., Carb-ac., Dulc., *Mez.,* Staph., Still., Syph.

**In skull:** Eup-per., Kali-bi.

**In vertebrae:** Agar.

**Influenzal:** Eup-per.

**Localized in spots, worse, from weather changes:** Rhod.

**Nocturnal:** *Asaf., Aur.,* Fl-ac., Hep., Iod., *Kali-i.,* Lach., Mang-act., *Merc., Mez.,* Ph-ac., Phyt., Rhod., Still., Syph.

**Pricking:** Arn., *Symph.*

**Sore, bruised, aching:** Chin., Conch., Eup-per., Lyss., Phyt., Ruta.

**Sore, bruised, as if scraped:** *Ip.,* Par., *Ph-ac.,* Rhus-t.

**Sore, bruised, worse, from cold, wandering:** Kali-bi.

**Tearing:** Caust., Colch., Fl-ac., Ph-ac.

**Throbbing, jerking, darting, drawing, hypersensitiveness:** Asaf.

**Worse, from damp weather:** Merc., Mez., Nit-ac., Phyt., Rhus-t., Still., Syph.

**PERIOSTITIS, And periosteal affections:** Apis, Aran., *Asaf., Aur., Aur-m.,* Calc., Chin., Clem., Colch., Con., Ferr-i., Graph., *Guaj.,* Hecla, Iod., *Kali-bi., Kali-i.,* Mang-act., *Merc., Mez., Nit-ac.,* Ph-ac., Phos., *Phyt.,* Plat-m., Rhod., Rhus-t., *Ruta,* Sars., *Sil.,* Still., Symph.

**SOFTENING, Mollities ossium:** Calc., *Calc-i.,* Calc-p., Guaj., Iod., Merc., *Phos.*

**SPINAL bifida:** Bry., *Calc.p.,* Psor., Tub.

**Spinal caries (Pott's disease):** Arg-met., Aur., Calc., Calc-i., *Calc-p.,* Con., *Iod.,* Kali-i., Merc-i-r., *Ph-ac., Phos.,* Pyrog., *Sil.,* Still., Sulph., *Syph.,* Tub., Vit-an.

**Spinal curvature:** Calc., *Calc-p.,* Ferr-i., Phos., *Sil.,* Sulph., Ther.

**Wounds:** Ruta, Symph.

**BUBONIC PLAGUE:** Anthraci., Ant-t., *Ars.,* Bapt., Bell., Carb-v., Chin., *Crot-h.,* Ign., Iod., *Lach.,* Naja, Oper., *Phos., Pyrog.,* Rhus-t., *Tarent-c.,* Yers.

**CANCER, Remedies in general:** Acet-ac., Anan., *Ant-m.,* Apis, *Ars.,* Ars-br., Ars-i., *Aster.,* Aur-ar., Aur-m-n., Bapt., Bism., Brom., Calc., Calc-i., Calc-ox., Calen., Carb-ac., *Carb-an.,* Carbn-s., Carc., Cholin., Cic., Cinnm., *Cist., Con., Cund.,* Cupr-act., Eos., Euph., Form., Form-ac., Fuli., *Gali.,* Guaj., Graph., Ham., *Hydr., Iod.,* Kali-ar., *Kali-cy.,* Kali-i., *Kreos.,* Lach., Lap-a., Lyc., Maland., Med., Phos., Phyt., Rad-br., Rumx-act., Sang., *Semp.,* Scirr., Sed-r., Sep., Sil., *Strych-g.,* Sulph., Symph., Tax., *Thuj.*

**Cancer, of antrum:** Aur., Symph.

**Cancer, of bone:** Aur-i., Phos., Symph.

**Cancer, of bowel, lower:** Ruta.

**Cancer, of breast:** Ars-i., Bar-i; Brom., Bufo, *Carb-an.,* Carc., *Con.,* Cund., Form-ac., Graph., *Hydr.,* Phyt., *Plb-i.,* Nat-cac., Scir. (See **FEMALE SEXUAL SYSTEM**.)

**Cancer, caecum:** Orni.

**Cancer, of glandular structures:** Strych-g.

**Cancer, of omentum:** Lob-e.

**Cancer, of stomach:** Acet-ac., *Ars.,* Bism., Cadm-s., *Cund.,* Form-ac., *Hydr.,* Kreos., Orni., Phos., Sec. (See **STOMACH**.)

**Cancer, of uterus:** *Aur-m.n.,* Carb-an., Carc., Fuli., Hydr., Iod., Lap-a., Nat-cac., Nit-ac., Sec. (See **FEMALE SEXUAL SYSTEM.**)

**Cancer, to relieve pains:** *Apis,* Anthraci., *Ars.,* Aster., Bry., Calc., *Calc-act.,* Calc-ox., Carc., Cedr., Cinnm., Con., Cund., Echi., *Euph.,* Euph-he., *Hydr.,* Mag-p., Morph., Op., Ovi-p., Ph-ac., Sil.

**CARTILAGES (perichondritis), Inflammation:** Arg-met., Bell., Cham., Cimic., Olnd., Plb., *Ruta.*

**Cartilages, pains:** Arg-met., Ruta.

**Cartilages, ulceration:** Merc.

**CELLULAR TISSUE, Indurated:** *Anthraci.,* Carb-an., Graph., *Kali-i.,* Kreos., Merc., Plb-i., *Rhus-t.,* Sil.

**CELLULITIS:** Apis, Arn., *Ars.,* Bapt., Crot-h., *Lach.,* Mang-act., *Merc-i-r., Rhus-t.,* Sil., Vesp.

**COMPLAINTS, ABUSE of alcoholic beverages:** *Agar.,* Ant-c., Apom., *Ars.,* Asar., Aur., Calc-ar., Carb-v., Carbn-s., Card-m., Coca, Cocc., Colch.,

Eup-per., Hydr., Ip., Lach., Led., *Lob.*, Lyc., *Nux-v.*, Querc., *Ran-b.*, Stry., Sul-ac., Sulph., *Verat.* (See **Alcoholism, NERVOUS SYSTEM.**)

**Absue of aconite:** Sulph.

**Absue of arsenic:** Carb-v., Ferr., Hep., *Ip.*, Samb., Verat.

**Absue of belladonna:** Hyos., Op.

**Absue of bromide of potassium:** Camph., Helon., Nux-v., Zinc.

**Absue of camphor:** Canth., Coff., Op.

**Absue of cantharis:** Apis; Camph.

**Absue of chamomilla:** Chin., Coff., Ign., Nux-v., Puls., Valer.

**Absue of chloral:** Cann-i.

**Absue of chlorate of potash:** Hydr.

**Absue of cod liver oil:** Hep.

**Absue of coffee:** Cham., Guar., *Ign.*, *Nux-v.*

**Absue of colchicum:** Led.

**Absue of condiments:** Nux-v.

**Absue of digitalis:** Chin., Nit-ac.

**Absue of drugs in general:** Aloe, Hydr., *Nux-v.*, Teucr.

**Absue of ergot:** Chin., Lach., Nux-v., Sec., Sol-n.

**Absue of iodides:** Ars., Bell., *Hep.*, Hydr., Phos.

**Absue of iron:** Chin., *Hep.*, *Puls.*

**Absue of lead (plumbism):** *Alum.*, Bell., Carbn-s., Caust., *Coloc.*, Iod., Kali-br., *Kali-i.*, Merc., Nux-v., *Op.*, Petr., Plat., Sul-ac.

**Absue of magnesia:** Nux-v., Rheum.

**Absue of mercury:** Ang., Ant-t., Arg-met., Asaf., *Aur.*, Carb-v., Caust., Chin., Clem., Dulc., Fl-ac., Guaj., *Hep.*, *Iod.*, *Kali-i.*, Lach., Mez., *Nit-ac.*, Op., Plat-m., Phyt., Podo., Puls., Rhus-g., Sars., Sulph.

**Absue of narcotics:** Acet-ac., Apom., Aven., Camph., Cann-i., *Cham.*, Cimic., Ip., Macro., Mur-ac.

**Absue of nitrate of silver:** Nat-m.

**Absue of phosphorus:** Lach., Nux-v.

**Absue of quinine:** *Ars.*, Bell., Coloc., Carb-v., Eucal., Ferr., *Ip.*, Lach., Meny., *Nat-m.*, Parth., *Puls.*, Sel.

**Absue of salt (halophagia):** Ars., Carb-v., Nat-m., *Nit-s-d.*, *Phos.*

**Absue of stramonium:** Acet-ac., Nux-v., Tab.

**Absue of stychinine:** Cur., *Eucal.*, Kali-br., Phys.

**Absue of sugar:** Merc., Nat-p.

**Absue of sulphur:** Puls., Sel.

**Absue of tar, locally:** Bov.

**Absue of tea:** Abies-n., *Chin.*, *Dios.*, Ferr., Puls., *Sel.*, Thuj.

**Absue of tobacco:** *Abies-n., Ars.,* Calad., Calc-p., Camph., Chin., Chinin-ar., Coca, *Gels., Ign., Ip.,* Kalm., Lyc., Mur-ac., *Nux-v., Phos., Plan.,* Plb., *Sep., Spig.,* Staph., Tab., Verat.

**Absue of tobacco, in boys:** Arg-n., Ars., Verat.

**Absue of turpentine:** Nux-m.

**Absue of vegetable medicines:** Camph., *Nux-v.*

**Absue of veratrum:** Camph., Coff.

**Absue of anesthetic vapors, antidote:** *Acet-ac.,* Am-caust., Aml-ns., Hep., Phos.

**BITES of insects, snakes, dogs:** Acet-ac., Am-c., Am-caust., Anthraci., *Apis,* Arn., *Ars.,* Bell., Calad., Camph., *Cedr.,* Crot.h., *Echi.,* Euph-po., Gaul., *Grin.,* Gua., Gymne., Hydr-ac., *Hyper.,* Kali-perm., *Lach., Led.,* Mosch., Pyrog., Selag., Sisy., Spirae., Strych-g.

**CHARCOAL fumes, illuminating gas, ill effects:** Acet-ac., Am-c., Arn., Bell., Bov., Coff., Op.

**CHECKED disharges, ill effects:** Abrot., Asaf., Aur-m., *Bar-c.,* Bry., *Graph.,* Lach., *Lob.,* Med., Merc., *Psor.,* Sanic., *Sil.,* Stram., Sulph., Zinc.

**Checked foot sweat, ill effects:** *Bar-c.,* Cupr., Form., Graph., Psor., Sanic., *Sil.,* Zinc.

**Checked gonorrhea, ill effects:** Graph., Psor., *Med., Thuj.,* X-ray.

**Checked, sweats, ill effects:** *Acon.,* Bell-p., Dulc., Rhus-t.

**CHRONIC DISEASES, to begin treatment:** Calc., Calc-p., *Nux-v.,* Puls., *Sulph.*

**CICATRICES, affections:** Calc-f., *Fl-ac.,* Hyper., Phyt., Sil., *Thiosin.*

**Cicatrices, freshen up, reopen:** *Caust.,* Fl-ac., *Graph.,* M-ambo., Sil.

**Cicatrices, itch:** Fl-ac.

**Cicatrices, pain during change of weather:** Nit-ac.

**Cicatrices, turn green:** Led.

**Cicatrices, turn red or blue:** Sul-ac.

**COMPLAINTS, Appear, atypically:** Mosch.

**Complaints, appear, diagonally, upper left, lower right side:** *Agar.,* Ant-t., Stram.

**Complaints, appear diagonally, upper right, lower left side:** Ambr., Brom., Med., Phos., Sul-ac.

**Complaints, appear, from above downwards:** Cact., *Kalm.*

**Complaints, appear, from below, upwards:** Led.

**Complaints, appear, gradually:** Calc-sil., Chin., Rad-br., Tell.

**Complaints, appear, gradually, cease gradually:** Arg-n., *Plat., Stann.,* Stront-c., Syph.

**Complaints, appear, gradually, cease suddenly:** Ign., *Puls.,* Sul-ac.

**Complaints, appear, in small spots:** Coff., *Ign., Kali-bi.,* Lil-t., *Ox-ac.*

**Complaints, appear, suddenly, cease gradually:** Puls., Sul-ac.

**Complaints, appear, suddenly, cease suddenly:** *Bell.,* Cact., Carb-ac., Eup-per., Eup-pur., Ictod., Ign., Kali-bi., Lyc., *Mag-p.,* Nit-ac., Oxyt., Petr., *Stry.,* Tub.

**Complaints, appear, suddenly, tension acutely increases, leaves with a snap on first motion:** Puls., Rhus-t.

**Complaints, fatal issue; to induce "euthanasia":** Aml-ns., Ant-t., *Ars.,* Carb-v., Lach., Tarent.

**Complaints, from chilling:** *Acon.,* Coff., Dulc., Nux-v., Sil.

**Complaints, from exposure of feet:** *Calc.,* Cupr., Nux-m., Sil.

**Complaints, from exposure, to cold dry wind:** *Acon.,* Bry., Caust., Hep., *Rhod.*

**Complaints, from living in cool, damp places:** Ant-t., *Aran.,* Ars., Ars-i., Calc., Calc-sil., *Dulc., Nat-s.,* Nux-m., *Rhus-t.,* Ter.

**Complaints, from overlifting:** *Arn., Carb-an.,* Carb-v., Kali-c., Lyc., *Nat-c.,* Nat-m., Phos., *Rhus-t.,* Sep., Sulph.

**Complaints, from working, in clay, cold water:** Calc., Mag-p.

**Complaints, improve, then relapse continually:** Sulph.

**Complaints, improve, then remain stationary:** Caust., Psor., *Sulph.*

**Complaints, in extremes of life:** Ant-c., *Bar-c.,* Lyc., Mill., Op., *Verat.*

**Complaints, in fleshy persons:** All-s., Am-c., Am-m., *Ant-c.,* Aur., Bar-c., Blatta-o., *Calc.,* Calc-ar., *Caps.,* Carb-v., Ferr., *Graph.,* Kali-bi., Kali-br., *Kali-c.,* Lob., Op., Phyt., Puls., Thuj. (See **Obesity**.)

**Complaints, in old people:** Agar., Aloe, *Alum.,* Alumn., *Ambr.,* Ant-c., Ars., Aur., *Bar-c., Bar-m.,* Caps., *Carb-an.,* Carb-v., Cit-v., Colch., *Con.,* Crot-h., Fl-ac., Hydr., Iod., Kali-c., Lyc., Mill., Nit-ac., Nux-m., *Op.,* Phos., Sec., Sul-ac., *Verat.*

**Complaints, wander, or shift about, erratic, changeable:** Apis, Bell., Benz-ac., Berb., *Dios., Ign., Kali-bi., Kali-s., Lac-c.,* Lil-t., Mag-p., Magn-gr., *Mang-act.,* Phyt., *Puls.,* Sanic., Syph., *Tub.*

**Complaints, with painlessness:** Op., *Stram.*

**ERUPTIONS, exanthemata, suppressed, or repercussed, ill effects:** *Apis,* Ars., Asaf., *Bry., Camph.,* Caust., *Cic., Cupr., Hell.,* Mag-s., Op., Psor., Puls., Stram., *Sulph., Tub.,* X-ray, *Zinc.*

**Foreign bodies, in larynx, trachea:** Ant-t., Ip., Sil.

**Growth, too rapid, ill effects:** *Calc., Calc-p.,* Ferr-ac., Irid-met., Kreos., *Ph-ac., Phos.*

**Mental labor, sufferings from:** *Arg-n., Gels.,* Graph., Lyc., Nat-c., *Nux-v.,* Ph-ac., Sil.

**Mining, ill effects:** Card-m., Nat-ar.

**Mountain climbing, aviation, ill effects:** Ars., Coca.

**Night watching, mental strain, ill effects:** Bell-p., Caps., Caust., *Cocc., Colch.,* Cupr., Dip., *Gels., Ign., Lac-d.,* Nit-ac., *Nux-v., Ph-ac., Zinc-act.* (See **Neurasthenia, NERVOUS SYSTEM**.)

**Nutritional disturbances, development tardy:** Bac., *Bar-c., Calc., Calc-p.,* Caust., Kreos., Lac-d., Med., Nat-m., Pin-s., *Sil.,* Thyr.

**Poison oak, and rhus poisoning:** Am-c., *Anac.,* Apis, Arn., Astac., Cimic., *Crot-t.,* Cypr., Echi., Erech., Euph-l., Graph., *Grin.,* Hedeo., Hydro-v., *Led.,* Mez., Plan., Prim-o., Rhus-d., *Rhus-t., Sang.,* Sep., Tanac., Urt-u., Vanil., Verb., *Xero.*

**PTOMAINE poisoning (decayed food):** Absin., Acet-ac., All-c., *Ars.,* Camph., Carb-an., Carb v., Crot-h., *Cupr-ar.,* Gunp., Kreos., Pyrog., Urt-u., *Verat.*

**Ptomaine poisoning (mushrooms):** Agar., Atrop., *Bell.,* Camph., Pyrog.

**Sewer gas, or noxious effluvia, ill effects:** Anthraci., *Bapt.,* Phyt., Pyrog.

**SUN exposure, ill effects: SUNSTROKE (coup-de-soleil):** Acon., *Ant-c., Bell.,* Bry., Cact., Camph., *Gels., Glon.,* Hydr-ac., Lach., *Nat-c.,* Op., Stram., Usn., *Verat-v.* (See **Collapse, NERVOUS SYSTEM; MODALITIES.**)

**VACCINATION, ill effects:** Acon., *Ant-t.,* Apis, Bell., Crot-h., Echi., *Maland.,* Merc., *Mez.,* Sars., Sep., *Sil.,* Sulph., Thuj.

**VITAL drains, ill effects:** Calc-p., *Chin.,* Ham., *Kali-c., Kali-p.,* Nat-m., *Ph-ac.,* Phos., Psor., Sep., Staph.

**DEGENERATION, Fatty:** *Ars.,* Aur., *Cupr.,* Kali-c., *Phos.,* Vanad.

**DROPSY:** Acetan., *Acet-ac.,* Acon., *Adon.,* Am-be., Ampe-tr., *Apis, Apoc.,* Arg-p., *Ars.,* Ars-i., Asc-c., Benz-ac., *Blatta-a.,* Brass., Bry., Cact., Calc., Calc-ar., *Cain.,* Card-m., *Chin.,* Coch., Coffin., *Colch., Conv.,* Cop., *Crat., Dig.,* Dulc., Elat., Eup-pur., Euph., Ferr., *Fl-ac.,* Gali., *Hell.,* Hep., Iod., Iris, Iris-g., Jatr-u., *Juni-c.,* Kali-act., Kali-ar., Kali-c., *Kali-i., Kali- n.,* Lac-d., *Lach.,* Lact., *Liat.,* Lyc., Merc-d., Nast., Nit-s-d., Onis., *Oxyd., Phase.,* Phos., *Pilo.,* Prun., Psor., Querc., Rhus-t., Samb., *Samb-c.,* Sol-n., Solid., *Squil., Stroph-h.,* Stry-ar., *Ter.,* Teucr-s., Thlas., Toxi., Ur-ac., Urin., Vince.

**From abuse of quinine:** Apoc.

**From alcoholism:** Ars., Fl-ac., Sulph.

**From eruption suppressed, sweat, rheumatism:** Dulc.

**From heart disease:** *Adon.,* Apis, Apoc., Arn., *Ars.,* Ars-i., Asc-t., Aur., *Cact., Coffin.,* Coll., *Conv., Crat., Dig., Digin.,* Iod., Kalm., Liat., Merc-d., *Stroph-h.* (See **Heart, CIRCULATORY SYSTEM**.)

**From kidney disease:** Ampe-tr., Ant-t., *Apis,* Apoc., Ars., Asc-c., Aspar., Chim., *Dig.,* Digin., Eup-pur., Helon., Lac-d., Liat., *Merc-c.,* Merc-d., Plb., Ter., Ur-ac. (See **URINARY SYSTEM**.)

**From liver disease:** *Apoc.,* Ars., Asc-c., Aur., Card-m., Cean., Chel., Chim., Lac-d., Liat., *Lyc.,* Mur-ac., Polym. (See **Liver, ABDOMEN**.)

**From menstrual disorder at puberty, or menopause:** Puls.

**From spleen disease:** Cean., Liat., Querc., Squil. (See **Spleen, ABDOMEN**.)

**From remittent fever:** Hell.

**From scarlet fever:** Acon., *Apis,* Apoc., *Ars.,* Asc-c., Colch., Dig., Dulc., *Hell., Hep.,* Juni-c., Lach., Pilo., Squil., *Ter.*

**From suppressed exanthemata:** Apis, Hell., Zinc.

**From suppressed intermittents:** Carb-v., Chin., Ferr., Hell., Lac-d.

**Dropsy, in newborn:** Apis, Carb-v., Coffin., Dig., Lach.

**Dropsy, with diarrhea:** Acet-ac.

**Dropsy, with serum oozing:** Ars., Lyc., Rhus-t.

**Dropsy, with soreness in uterine region:** Conv.

**Dropsy, with suppressed urine, fever, debility:** Hell.

**Dropsy, with thirst:** *Acet-ac.,* Acon., *Apoc.,* Ars.

**Dropsy, without thirst:** Apis; Hell.

**LOCATION, Abdomen: ASCITES:** *Acet-ac., Adon., Apis, Apoc., Ars.,* Aur., Aur-m-n., *Blatta-a.,* Cain., Canth., *Chin.,* Cop., *Dig., Digin.,* Fl-ac., *Hell.,* Iod., Kali-c., Lact., Led., *Lyc.,* Nat-chor., Oxyd., *Prun.,* Samb., *Senec.,* Sep., Ter., Uran-n.

**Chest (hydrothorax):** *Apis,* Apoc., *Ars.,* Ars-i., Colch., *Dig.,* Hell., Kali-c., Lach., Lact., *Merc-sul.,* Squil., Sulph. (See **Chest, RESPIRATORY SYSTEM**.)

**Extremity, left:** Cact.

**General, ANASARCA:** Acetan., Acet- ac., Acon., Aeth., *Apis,* Apoc., Arn., *Ars.,* Cain., *Chin., Conv.,* Cop., Crat., *Dig.,* Dulc., Ferr., *Hell.,* Kali-c., *Liat.,* Lyc., *Merc-c.,* Oxyd., Pic-ac., Prun., Ter., Uran-n. (See **Dropsy**.)

**EFFUSION, Threatening:** *Apis, Bry.,* Chin., Cic., *Hell.,* Iodof., Op., Tub., *Zinc.*

**GLANDERS:** Acon., Ars., Chinin-s., *Crot-h.,* Hep., Hippoz., *Kali-bi.,* Lach., *Merc.,* Phos., Sep., Sil., Thuj.

**GLANDS, Abscess:** Bell., Calc., Calc-i., Cist., Hep., Lap-a., *Merc.,* Nit-ac., Rhus-t., *Sil.*

**Affections, traumatic:** Aster., Con.

**Atrophy:** Iod.

**Induration:** Alumn., Ars., Ars-br., *Aster.,* Aur-m., Bad., *Bar-c., Bar-i.,* Bar-m., Bell., Berb-a., *Brom.,* Calc., Calc-chln., *Calc-f., Carb-an.,* Chin., *Cist.,* Clem., *Con.,* Dulc., Graph., *Hecla, Iod.,* Kali-i., *Lap a.,* Merc-i-f., Merc-i-r., Oper., Phyt., *Rhus-t., Spong.,* Thyr., Trif-r.

**Inflammation (ADENITIS): Acute:** Acon., Ail., Alumn., Anan., *Apis,* Ars-i., Bar-c., Bar-i., *Bell., Cist.,* Clem., *Dulc.,* Graph., *Hep.,* Iod., *Iodof., Kali-i., Merc., Merc-i-r.,* Oper., *Phyt.,* Rhus-t., Sil., *Sil-mar.*

**Inflammation, chronic, GLANDULAR SWELLINGS:** Acon-l., *Ail., Aln.,* Apis, Ars., Ars-br., *Ars-i.,* Arum-t., Astac., Aur-m., *Bad., Bar-c., Bar-i.,* Bar-m., *Brom., Calc., Calc-f., Calc-i.,* Calc-p., Calen., *Carb-an., Cist., Clem., Con.,* Cory., Crot-h., Dulc., Ferr-i., Fil., Graph., Hep., *Iod., Kali-i.,* Lach., *Lap-a.,* Lyc., Med., Merc., Merc-cy., Merc-i-f., *Merc-i-r.,* Nit-ac., *Phyt.,* Psor., Rhus-t., *Rumx.,* Sal-mar., Scir., *Scroph-n., Sil.,* Sil-mar., *Spong., Sulph.,* Tax., Thiosin., Thuj., Tub.

**LOCATION, OF GLANDULAR AFFECTION, Axillary:** Acon-l., *Aster., Bar-c.,* Bell., Calc., Carb-an., *Con.,* Elaps, Graph., Hep., Jugl-r., *Lac-ac.,* Nat-s., Nit-ac., Phyt., Raph., Rhus-t., Sil., Sulph.

**Bronchial:** Bell., Calc., Calc-f., *Iod.,* Merc-c., Tub.

**Cervical:** Acon-l., *Am-c.,* Astac., Bac., *Bar-c.,* Bar-i., *Bell., Brom.,* Calc., Calc-chl., Calc-f., Calc-i., *Carb an.,* Caust., *Cist.,* Dulc., Graph., Hecla, *Hep.,* Iod., Kali-i., Kali-m., *Lap-a.,* Mag-p., Merc., *Merc-i-f., Merc-i-r.,* Nit-ac., *Rhus-t.,* Rhus-r., Rhus-v., Sal-mar., Sil., Spong., *Still.,* Sulph.

**Inguinal:** Apis, Ars., Aur., Bac., *Bar-c.,* Bar-m., Bell., *Calc.,* Carb-an., Clem., Dulc., Graph., Kali-i., *Merc., Merc-i-f., Nit-ac.,* Oci., Pall., Pin-s., Rhus-t., Sil., Sulph., Xero.

**Mesenteric:** *Ars.,* Ars-i., Bac., Bar-c., Bar-m., *Calc.,* Calc-f., *Calc-i.,* Con., Graph., *Iod.,* Iodof., Lap-a., *Merc-c.,* Mez., Tub. (See **Tabes mesenterica.**)

**Parotid, Inflammation (Parotitis, Mumps):** *Acon.,* Ail., Am-c., Anthraci., Ant-t., Aur-m., *Bar-c.,* Bar-m., *Bell., Brom.,* Calc., Carb-an., Cham., Cist., Dulc., Euphr., *Ferr-p.,* Hep., *Kali-bi.,* Kali-m., Lach., Mag-p., *Merc., Merc-c.,* Merc-cy., Merc-i-f., Merc-i-r., *Phyt.,* Pilo., *Puls., Rhus-t., Sil.,* Sul-i., Sulph., Trif-p., Trif-r.

**Parotitis, gangrenous:** Anthraci.

**Parotitis, metastasis to brain:** Apis, Bell.

**Parotitis, metastasis to mammae, ovaries:** Con., Jab., Puls.

**Parotitis, metastasis to testis:** Aur., *Clem., Ham., Puls.,* Rhus-t.

**Parotitis, persistent:** Bar-act., Bar-c., *Con., Iod.,* Sil.

**Sebaceous glands:** Lyc., Psor., Raph., Sil., Sulph. (See **SKIN.**)

**Submaxillary:** Aln., *Arum-t.,* Asim., *Bar-c.,* Brom., Calc., Calen., Cham., Cist., Clem., Iod., *Kali-bi.,* Kali-m., Lyc., Mag-p., Merc., Merc-cy., *Merc-i-r.,* Nat-m., Petr., Pin-s., Phyt., *Rhus-t.,* Sil., Staph., Sulph., Trif-p., Trif-r.

**Thyroid (Goitre, bronchocele):** Adren., Am-c., Am-m., Apis, Aur-s., Bad., Bar-i., *Bell., Brom., Calc.,* Calc-f., Calc-i., Caust., Chr-s., Cist., *Crot-c.,*

Ferr., *Fl-ac., Fuc.,* Glon., Hep., *Hydr.,* Hydr-ac., Iod., *Iris,* Kali-c., *Kali-i., Lap-a.,* Mag-p., Merc-i-f., *Nat-m.,* Phos., Phyt., Pineal., Puls., Sil., *Spong.,* Sulph., *Thyr., Thyroiod.*

**Thyroid, (EXOPHTHALMIC GOITRE, Basedow's disease):** Aml-ns., Ars., Ars-i., Aur., Bad., Bar-c., *Bell.,* Brom., *Cact., Calc.,* Cann-i., Chr-s., Colch., Con., Echi., Ephe., *Ferr.,* Ferr-i., Ferr-p., *Fl-ac.,* Fuc., *Glon., Iod.,* Jab., *Lycps-v.,* Nat-m., *Pilo.,* Spartin-s., Spong., Stram., *Thyr.*

**Paroxysm:** Cact., Dig., Glon., Samb.

**GRANULATIONS, Exuberant:** Calen., Nit-ac., Sabin., *Sil.,* Thuj. **(See Ulcers.)**

**GREASE, in horse:** Thuj.

**HEMOPHILIA, Small wounds, bleed profusely, or protractedly:** *Adren.,* Ail., Ars., Bov., Calc-lac., Chin., *Crot-h.,* Ferr., *Ham.,* Kreos., *Lach.,* Merc., Mill., *Nat-sil., Phos., Sec.,* Ter.

**HEMORRHAGES:** Acal., *Acet-ac., Acon., Adren.,* Alum., Alumn., Anthraci., *Arn.,* Ars-h., Bell., Both., *Bov., Cact.,* Canth., Carb-v., *Chin.,* Chinin-s., *Cinnm.,* Croc., *Crot-h.,* Dig., Elaps, Erech., Ergot., *Erig.,* Ferr., *Ferr-p.,* Fic-r., Gal-ac., Gelatin., *Ger., Ham., Hydrin-s., Ip.,* Kali-c., Kreos., Lach., Meli., Merc-cy., *Mill.,* Mur-ac., Nat-sil., *Nit-ac.,* Op., *Phos.,* Puls., *Sabin.,* Sanguiso., *Sec., Sul-ac.,* Sulph., *Ter.,* Thlas., Til., *Tril-p.,* Ust., Verat., Xan.

**Hemorrhage, chronic effects:** Stront-c.

**Hemorrhage, from traumatism:** Aran., *Arn.,* Bov., Euph-pi., Ham., *Mill.,* Tril-p.

**Hemorrhage, hysterical (hemosialemesis):** Bad., Croc., Hyos., Ign., Kali-i., Merc., Stict., Sulph.

**Hemorrhage, with face intensely red, preceding:** Meli.

**Hemorrhage, with fainting, tinnitus, loss of sight, general coldness, even convulsions:** *Chin.,* Ferr., Phos.

**Hemorrhage, with no mental anxiety:** Ham.

**Hemorrhage, with putrescence; tingling in limbs; debility:** Sec.

**Hemorrhage, without fever or pain:** Mill.

**Blood, bright red:** *Acon.,* Bell., Erech., *Erig.,* Ferr., *Ferr-p., Ip.,* Led., *Mill.,* Nit-ac., Ph-ac., Phos., Sabin., *Tril-p.,* Ust.

**Blood, clotted, partly fluid:** Erig., Ferr., Plat., Puls., Rat., *Sabin.,* Ust.

**Blood, dark, clotted:** Alum., Anthraci., Chin., *Croc.,* Crot-h., *Elaps,* Merc., Merc-cy., Mur-ac., Plat., *Sul-ac.,* Ter., *Thlas.,* Tril-p.

**Blood, decomposes rapidly:** Acet-ac., Am-c., Anthraci., *Crot-h.,* Lach., Ter.

**Non-coagulable; intermittent:** Phos.

**Non-coagulable, thin, dark:** *Crot-h.,* Elaps, *Lach., Sec.,* Sul-ac.

**Thin, pale, fluid:** Ferr., Til.

**Venous, dark, clotted:** Ham., Mang-i.

**Vicarious:** Acet-ac., Ham.

**HODGKINS DISEASE (pseudo-leukemia):** Acon., Acon-l., *Ars., Ars-i., Bar-i.,* Calc-f., Ferr-pic., *Iod.,* Kali-m., Nat-m., Phos., Scroph-n.

**HOOKWORM DISEASE:** Carbn-tm., Chen-a., Thymol.

**INFLAMMATIONS:** Abrot., *Acon., Agrosti-a.,* Apis, Arn., Ars., *Bell., Bry.,* Canth., Chel., Chin., *Ferr-p.,* Hep., *Iod.,* Kali-bi., Kali-c., Kali-i., Kali-m., Kali-s., *Nat-n., Spira.,* Sulph., *Verat-v.,* Vib-o.

**Inflammation, passive:** *Dig., Gels.,* Puls., Sulph.

**Inflammation surgical:** Acon., *Anthraci.,* Arn., Ars., Ars-i., *Bell.,* Bell-p., Calen., Calc-s., Echi., Gunp., *Hep.,* Hyper., Iod., Merc-c., Merc-i-r., Myris., *Pyrog.,* Rhus-t., *Sil.* (See **Pyemia.**)

**Inflammation, to favor absorption:** Ant-t., Apis, *Kali-i.,* Kali-m., Lyc., Phos., Sulph.

**INJURIES (traumatism):** Acet-ac., Acon., Ang., *Arn., Bell-p.,* Bufo, *Calen., Cic.,* Crot-t., Euphr., Glon., *Ham., Hyper., Led.,* Mag-c., Mill., Nat-s., Phys., *Rhus-t.,* Ruta, Stront-c., Sul-ac., Verb.

**Bruises, contusions:** Acet-ac., *Arn.,* Bell-p., *Con.,* Echi., Euphr., *Ham., Hyper.,* Led., *Rhus-t., Ruta,* Sul-ac., *Symph.,* Verb.

**Bruises, of bone:** Arn., Calc-p., *Ruta, Symph.*

**Bruises, of breast:** Bell-p., *Con.*

**Bruises, of eye:** Acon., *Arn.,* Ham., *Led., Symph.*

**Bruises, of parts, rich in sentient nerves:** Bell-p., *Hyper.*

**Bruises, with persistence of ecchymosis:** Arn., Led., *Sul-ac.*

**Burns, scalds:** Acet-ac., Acon., Arn., *Ars.,* Calc-s., Calen., Camph., *Canth.,* Carb-ac., *Caust.,* Gaul., Grin., Ham., *Hep.,* Jab., *Kali-bi.,* Kreos., Petr., Rhus-t., Ter., *Urt-u.*

**Burns, fail to heal, or ill effects:** Carb-ac., Caust.

**Chronic effects of injuries:** *Arn.,* Carb v., Cic., *Con.,* Glon., Ham., Hyper., Led., *Nat-s., Stront-c.*

**Mental symptoms, from injuries:** Cic., *Glon.,* Hyper., Mag-c., *Nat-s.*

**Post-operative disorders:** Acet-ac., Apis, *Arn., Bell-p.,* Berb., *Calen.,* Calc-f., Camph., Croc., Ferr-p., *Hyper.,* Kali-s., Mill., Naja, Nit-ac., Raph., Rhus-t., *Staph., Stront-c.,* Verat.

**Prostration, from injuries:** *Acet-ac.,* Camph., Hyper., *Sul-ac.,* Verat.

**Sprains, strains:** Acet-ac., *Acon.,* Agn., *Arn.,* Bell., *Bell-p., Calc.,* Calc-f., Calen., *Carb-an.,* Form., *Hyper.,* Mill., Nux-v., Rhod., *Rhus-t., Ruta,* Stront-c., *Symph.*

**Sprains, tendency to:** Nat-c., Nat-m., Psor., *Sil.*

**Tetanus prevented:** Hyper., Phys.

**Wounds, bleed profusely:** Arn., *Crot-h.,* Ham., Kreos., *Lach.,* Mill., *Ph-ac.*

**Wounds, bleed profusely, after a fall:** *Arn.,* Ham., Mill.

**Wounds, bluish, discolored:** *Lach.,* Lyss.

**Wounds, bullet, from:** Arn., Calen.

**Wounds, contused:** *Arn.,* Ham., Sul-ac., Symph.

**Wounds, dissecting, post-mortem:** *Anthraci., Apis, Ars.,* Crot-h., *Echi., Lach., Pyrog.* (See **Pyemia.**)

**Wounds, incised:** Arn., Calen., Ham., Hyper., Led., *Staph.*

**Wounds, involving muscles, tendons, joints:** Calen.

**Wounds, lacerated:** Arn., *Calen.,* Carb-ac., Ham., Led., *Hyper.,* Staph., Sul-ac., Symph.

**Wounds, punctured:** Apis, Hyper., *Led.,* Phase.

**Wounds, with burning, cutting, shooting:** Nat-c.

**Wounds, with gangrenous tendency:** Calen., Sal-ac., Sul-ac. (See **Dissecting.**)

**LEUCOCYTHEMIA, Leukemia:** Aran., *Ars., Ars-i.,* Bar-i., Benzo., Bry., Calc., Cean., Chinin-s., Con., *Ferr-pic.,* Ip., Merc., *Nat-m.,* Nat-s., Nux-v., Phos., *Pic-ac.,* Thuj. (See **Anemia.**)

**Leucocythemia, splenic:** *Cean.,* Nat-s., Querc., Succ.

**LYMPHANGITIS:** Anthraci., *Apis,* Ars-i., *Bell.,* Both., Bufo, Crot-h., Echi., Hippoz., *Lach.,* Lat-k., *Merc.,* Merc-i-r., Mygal., Pyrog., *Rhus-t.*

**MARASMUS (emaciation, atrophy, wasting):** *Abrot., Acet-ac.,* Ant-i., Arg-met., *Arg-n., Ars.,* Ars-i., *Bar-c., Calc., Calc-p., Calc-sil.,* Carb-an., Carb-v., Caust., Cetr., Chin., Clem., Ferr., *Ferr-p.,* Fl-ac., Glyc., Helon., *Hep., Hydr., Iod.,* Kali-i., Kali-p., Kreos., Led., *Lyc.,* Mang-act., Merc., *Merc-c.,* Nat-c., *Nat-m., Ol-j.,* Op., *Ph-ac.,* Phos., Phyt., *Plb., Plb-act.,* Plb-i., Plb-n., Psor., Ric., Rhus-t., *Samb., Sanic., Sars.,* Sec., Sel., *Sil.,* Stann., Staph., *Sulph., Syph.,* Ter., *Thuj., Tub.,* Uran-n., Vanad., *Verat.,* Zinc.

**Affected parts, atrophy:** Ars., *Caust.,* Graph., Led., Sel.

**Atrophy of children:** *Abrot.,* Arg-n., *Ars.,* Ars-s-f., Bac., Bar-c., *Calc-p., Calc-sil., Iod., Nat-m., Ol-j.,* Phos., Podo., Psor., Sanic., Sars., *Sulph.,* Thyr., *Tub.*

**Atrophy of face, hands, legs, feet, single parts:** Sel.

**Atrophy of legs:** *Abrot., Am-m., Arg-n.,* Iod., Pin-s., Sanic., Tub.

**Atrophy of mesenteric glands (tabes mesenterica):** Ars., Bapt., Bar-c., *Calc.,* Calc-ar., Calc-chl., Calc-hp., Calc-i., *Calc-p.,* Con., Hep., *Iod.,* Merc-c., Plb-act., Sacch., Sil.

**Atrophy of neck, flabby, loose skin:** Abrot., Calc-p., Iod., *Nat-m., Sanic.,* Sars.

**Atrophy, from above downwards:** Lyc., Nat-m.

**Atrophy, from below upwards:** Abrot.

**Atrophy, neck so weak, unable to hold head up:** *Abrot.,* Aeth., Calc-p.

**Atrophy, progressive, muscular:** Ars., Carbn-s., Hyper., Kali-hp., *Phos.,* Phys., *Plb.,* Sec.

**Atrophy, rapid:** Iod., Plb., Samb., *Thuj., Tub.*

**Atrophy, rapid, with cold sweat, debility:** *Ars., Tub., Verat.*

**Atrophy, with bulimia:** *Abrot.,* Acet-ac., Ars-i., Bar-c., Calc., Con., *Iod., Nat-m.,* Sanic., Tub., Thyr.

**Atrophy, with shrivelled up look:** Abrot., *Arg-n.,* Fl-ac., Kreos., Op., Sanic., Sars., Sil., *Sulph.*

**MUSCLES, Inflammation (myositis):** *Arn.,* Bell., *Bry.,* Hep., Kali-i., Merc., *Mez., Rhus-t.*

**Muscles, pain (myalgia):** *Acon.,* Ant-t., *Arn.,* Ars., Bell., Bell-p., *Bry.,* Carbn-s., Caust., *Cimic.,* Colch., *Dulc., Gels.,* Led., *Marco.,* Merc., Morph., Nux-v., *Ran-b., Rham-cal., Rhus-t., Ruta,* Sal-ac., Stram., *Stry.,* Valer., *Verat.,* Verat-v. (See **Rheumatism, LOCOMOTOR SYSTEM.**)

**Muscles, pain cramp-like:** Ant-t., Cho., *Cimic.,* Colch., Coloc., *Cupr., Mag-p.,* Nux-v., Op., Plb-act., Sec., *Sulph.,* Syph., Verat.

**Muscles, pain, hysterical:** Ign., Nux-v., Plb., Puls.

**Muscles, soreness, stiffness:** Ang., *Arn.,* Bad., *Bapt.,* Bell., *Bell-p., Bry.,* Caust., Cic., *Cimic.,* Cupr-act., *Gels.,* Guaj., Ham., *Helon.,* Jac-c., *Magn-gr.,* Merc., Myric., *Phyt.,* Pyrog., *Rhus-t., Ruta,* Sang.

**Muscles, twitchings:** Acon., *Agar.,* Ang., Apis, Ars., Asaf., Atrop., *Bell.,* Bry., Caust., *Cham., Cic., Cimic.,* Cina, *Cocc.,* Cod., *Coloc.,* Croc., *Cupr.,* Ferr-r., Gels., Hell., *Hyos., Ign.,* Kali-br., Kali-c., Lup., Mez., *Morph., Mygal., Nux-v.,* Op., Phos., Phys., Plb-act., Puls., *Santin.,* Sec., Spig., *Stram., Stry.,* Tarent., Verat-v., *Zinc.,* Ziz.

**Muscles, weakness, debility:** Acet-ac., *Alet.,* Alum., *Alumn.,* Am-caust., Anh., *Ant-t.,* Arg-n., Ars., Bry., Calc, Carb-v., Caust., Colch., Coll., *Con., Gels., Hell.,* Helon., Hep., Hydr., Ign., Kali-c., Kali-hp., *Kali-p.,* Kalm., Lob., Mag-p., Merc., *Mur-ac.,* Nux-v., Onos., Pall., Phys., Physal-al., *Pic-ac.,* Plb-act., Rhus-t., Sabad., *Sarcol-ac.,* Sil., *Stry.,* Tab., *Verat., Verat-v., Zinc.* (See **Adynamia, NERVOUS SYSTEM.**)

**MUTINISM of childhood:** Agra.

**MYXEDEMA:** Ars., Prim-o., *Thyr.*

**OBESITY (adiposis, corpulence):** *Am-br.,* Am-c., Ant-c., Ars., *Calc., Calc ar., Calo.,* Caps., Coloc., *Fuc.,* Graph., Kali-br., Kali-c., Lac-d., Mang-act., *Phos., Phyt.,* Sabal, *Thyr., Thyroiod.,* Tus-fr.

**Obesity, in children:** *Ant-c.,* Bar-c., *Calc., Caps., Ferr.,* Kali-bi., Sacch.

**POLYCYTHEMIA:** Phos.

**PROPHYLACTICS, Catheter fever:** Camph-ac.

**Cholera:** Ars., Cupr-act., Verat.

**Diphtheria:** Apis (30); Diph.(30).

**Erysipelas:** Graph. (30).

**Hay fever:** Ars., Psor.

**Hydrophobia:** Bell., Canth., Hyos., Stram.

**Intermittent fever:** Ars., Chinin-s.

**Measles:** Acon., Ars., Puls.

**Mumps:** Trif-r.

**Pus infection:** Arn.

**Quinsy:** Bar-c. (30).

**Scarlet fever:** Bell. (30), Eucal.

**Sunstroke:** Ilx-p.

**Variola:** Ant-t., Hydr., Kali-cy., *Maland.,* Thuj., *Vac.,* Vario.

**Whooping cough:** Dros., Vac.

**PYEMIA, SEPTICEMIA:** *Acon., Anthraci.,* Apisin., *Arn., Ars.,* Ars-i., Atrop., *Bapt.,* Bell., Both., *Bry.,* Calen., *Carb-ac., Chinin-ar., Chinin-s.,* Crot-h., *Echi.,* Gunp., Hippoz., Hyos., Irid-met., *Lach.,* Lat-h., Merc., Merc-cy., Methyl., Mur-ac., Nat-s-c., *Pyrog., Rhus-t., Sec.,* Sil., Streptoc., Tarent-c., Verat.

**RACHITIS (rickets):** *Ars.,* Ars-i., *Calc.,* Calc-act., Calc-hph., *Calc-p.,* Calc-sil., Ferr-p., Fl-ac., Hecla, Hep., *Iod.,* Kali-i., Mag-m., Med., Merc., Nit-ac., *Ph-ac., Phos.,* Pin-s., Sanic., *Sil.,* Sulph., Suprar., Ther., Thuj., *Thyr., Tub.* (See **Scrofulosis.**)

**SCROFULOSIS:** *Aethi-m.,* Aln., Alum., Ars., *Ars-i., Aurums,* Bac., Bad., *Barytas,* Brom., *Calcareas,* Caps., Carb-an., *Caust.,* Cinnb., Cist., Clem., Con., Diph., *Dulc., Ferrums,* Fl-ac., *Graph.,* Hell., *Hep.,* Hydr., *Iodides,* Iodof., Kali-bi., Kali-i., Kreos., Lap-a., Lyc., Mag-m., *Mercuries,* Mez., Nit-ac., Ol-j., Petr., Ph-ac., Phos., *Pin-s.,* Plb-i., Psor., Ruta, Samb., Sed-ac., *Sil.,* Sil-mar., Still., *Sulph.,* Ther., *Tub.,* Viol-t.

**SCURVY (scorbutus):** Acet-ac., *Agav-a.,* Aln., *Ars.,* Bov., Carb-v., Chin., Chinin-s., *Ferr-p.,* Gali., Ham., Kali-ch., Kali-p., Kreos., Lach., *Merc., Mur-ac.,* Nat-m., Nit-ac., Nit-m-ac., Ph-ac., *Phos.,* Rhus-t., Staph., Sul-ac., Sulph., Urin.

**SENILE DECAY:** *Agn., Arg-n.,* Ars., *Bar-c.,* Cann-i., *Con.,* Fl-ac., Iod., *Lyc., Ov.,* Phos., Thiosin.

**SENSATION, of burning:** *Acon., Agar.,* Agro., *All-c.,* Anthraci., *Apis, Ars.,* Bell., *Calad., Canth., Caps.,* Carb-an., *Caust.,* Cham., *Dory.,* Eos., Kreos., Ol-an., Ph-ac., *Phos.,* Pip-m., Pop-c., Rhus-t., *Sang.,* Sec., *Sulph.,* Tarent.

**Sensation, of constriction:** Alum-sil., *Anac.,* Asar., *Cact.,* Caps., *Carb-ac.,* Coloc., Iod., Lach., Mag-p., Naja, Nat-m., *Nit-ac.,* Plb., Sec., *Sulph.*

**Sensation, of numbness:** *Acon., Agar.,* Alum-sil., *Ambr.,* Ars., Bov., *Calc-p., Cedr., Cham.,* Cic., *Cocain.,* Cod., *Con.,* Helo., Ign., Irid-met., Kali-br., Nux-v., *Olnd.,* Onos., Ox-ac., *Phos., Plat.,* Plb., Raph., *Rhus-t.,* Sec., Stann., Thal.

**Sensation, of numbess, attending pains:** *Acon.,* Cann-i., *Cham.,* Cimic., *Kalm., Plat., Rhus-t.,* Stann., Staph.

**Sensation, of stitching:** Acon., *Asc-t., Bry., Kali-c.,* Mag-p., Nat-s., Nit-ac., *Ran-b.,* Rumx., Squil.

**TUMORS:** Anan., Aur-m-n., *Bar-c.,* Bar-i., Bar-m., Bell-p., *Calc.,* Calc-ar., *Calc-f., Cist.,* Coloc., *Con.,* Eucal., *Ferr-i.,* Ferr-pic., Form-ac., Gali., *Graph., Hecla,* Hydr., *Kali-br.,* Kali-i., Kreos., Lach., *Lap-a., Lob-e.,* Lyc., Maland., Manc., Med., Merc-i-r., Merl., Nat-cac., Nat-sil., *Phos.,* Phyt., *Plb-i.,* Psor., *Semp., Sil.,* Thiosin., *Thuj., Thyr., Ur-ac.,* Urea. (See **Cancer.**)

**Cystic:** Apis, *Bar-c.,* Calc., Calc-p., Calc-s., *Iod., Kali-br.,* Platan., Sil., Staph. (See Scalp, **HEAD, SKIN.**)

**Bone like, protuberances:** *Calc-f., Hecla,* Lap-a., Maland., Ruta, Sil.

**Enchondroma:** Calc-f., Lap-a., Sil.

**Epithelial:** Acet-ac., Ferr-pic. (See **SKIN.**)

**Epulis:** Calc., Plb-act., *Thuj.*

**Erectile:** Lyc., *Phos.*

**Fibroid:** *Calc-i.,* Calc-s., Chr-s., Graph., Hydrin-m., *Kali-i.,* Lap-a., Sec., *Sil.,* Thiosin., Thyr. (See **Uterus.**)

**Fibroid, hemorrhage:** *Hydrin-m.,* Lap-a., Sabin., Thlas., *Tril-p.,* Ust.

**Fungoid:** Clem., Manc., Phos., *Thuj.*

**Ganglion:** Benz-ac., Kali-m., *Ruta, Sil.*

**Lipoma:** *Bar-c.,* Calc., Calc-ar., Lap-a., Phyt., *Thuj.,* Ur-ac.

**Nevus on right temple, flat; in children:** Fl-ac.

**Neuroma:** All-c., Calen.

**Nodulated, of tongue:** Gali.

**Papillomata:** Ant-c., Nit-ac., Staph., *Thuj.*

**Polypi:** All-c., *Calc., Form.,* Kali-bi., Kali-s., Lem-m., Nit-ac., *Phos.,* Psor., Sang., *Sangin-n.,* Sil., Teucr., *Thuj.* (See **NOSE; EAR, UTERUS.**)

**Ranula:** Ambr., Thuj.

**Sarcocele:** Merc-i-r. (See **MALE SEXUAL SYSTEM.**)

**Tumors of urinary passages:** Anil.

**Vascular in urethra:** Cann-s., *Eucal.*

**Wen:** Bar-c., Benz-ac., Calc., Con., Daph., Graph., Hep., Kali-c., Mez.

■

# MODALITIES

**AGGRAVATION: Acids:** *Ant-c.,* Ant-t., Ferr., Lach., Merc-c., Nux-v., Phos., *Sep.* (See **STOMACH.**)

**Afternoon:** Aesc., Alum., Am-m., Ars., *Bell.,* Cench., Coc-c., Cocc., Fago., Kali-bi., Kali-c., Kali-cy., Kali-n., Lil-t., Lob., *Rhus-t.,* Sep., Sil., Still., *Thuj.,* Verb., Xero., X-ray.

**Afternoon, late:** *Apis,* Aran., Carb-v., Colch., *Coloc., Hell., Lyc.,* Mag-p., Med., Meli., Ol-an., *Puls.,* Sabad., Zinc. (See **Evening.**)

**Air cold, dry:** Abrot., *Acon.,* Aesc., Agar., Alum., *Ars., Asar.,* Aur-m., Bac., *Bar-c.,* Bell., *Bry.,* Calc., *Camph.,* Caps., Carb-an., *Caust., Cham., Chin., Cist.,* Cupr., Cur., Euph-l., *Hep.,* Ign., *Kali-c.,* Mag-p., *Mez.,* Nat-c., *Nux-v.,* Plb., *Psor., Rhod., Rumx.,* Sel., Sep., *Sil., Spong.,* Tub., Urt-u., Viol-o., Visc.

**Air, open:** *Acon.,* Agar., Benz-ac., Bry., Cadm-s., *Caps.,* Carbn-s., *Cham.,* Cic., Cocc., Coff., Cor-r., Crot-h., *Cycl.,* Epiph., Euphr., Ign., Kalm., Kreos., Lina, Mosch., *Nux-v.,* Ran-b., *Seneg.,* Lycpr., Thea, X-ray. (See **Air, cold.**)

**Anger:** *Bry., Cham.,* Coloc., Ign., *Nux-v., Staph.* (See **Emotions, MIND.**)

**Arms moved backward:** Sanic.

**Ascending stairs:** Am-c., *Ars.,* But-ac., Cact., *Calc.,* Cann-s., Coca, Glon., *Kali-c.,* Meny., Spong.

**Autumn; warm days, cold, damp nights:** Merc.

**Bathing:** *Ant-c.,* Bell-p., Calc., Caust., Form., Mag-p., Nux-m., Phys., *Rhus-t.,* Sep., *Sulph.* (See **Water.**)

**Bed, turning in:** *Con.,* Nux-v., Puls.

**Beer:** Bry., *Kali-bi.,* Nux-m.

**Bending double:** Dios.

**Bending forward:** *Bell.,* Kalm., Nux-v.

**Biting hard:** Am-c., *Verb.*

**Breakfast, after:** Cham., *Nux-v.,* Phos., *Thuj.,* Zinc. (See **Eating.**)

**Breakfast, before:** Croc.

**Bright objects:** *Bell., Canth.,* Cocc-s., *Lyss., Stram.*

**Brushing teeth:** Coc-c., Staph.

**Celibacy:** Con.

**Coffee:** Aster., Cann-i., *Canth.,* Carb-v., Caust., *Cham.,* Ign., Kali-c., *Nux-v.,* Psor., Thuj.

**Coitus, after:** Agar., *Calad.,* Calc-s., *Chin., Kali-c.,* Nux-v., *Ph-ac.,* Phos., *Sel.,* Sep.

**Cold:** *Acon.,* Agar., *Alum.,* Alumn., Am-c., Ant-c., *Ars.,* Bad., *Bar-c.,* Bell., *Bry.,* Calc., *Camph.,* Caps., *Caust., Cham.,* Coll., Cocc., Coff., Con., Crot-c., *Dulc.,* Form., *Hep.,* Ign., *Kali-c.,* Kali-p., Kreos., Lach., Lob., *Mag-p.,* Merc., *Mez.,* Mosch., Nit-ac., Nux-m., *Nux-v.,* Ran-b., *Rhod., Rhus-t., Rumx.,* Ruta, Sabad., Sel., *Sep., Sil.,* Spig., Stram., Stront-c., Sul-ac., Tab., Verat., Xero.

**Concussion:** Cic. (See **Jar.**)

**Consolation:** Cact., Graph., *Hell.,* Ign., Lil-t., *Nat-m.,* Sabal, *Sep.,* Sil.

**Contact, of clothing, about neck:** Glon., *Lach.,* Sep. (See **Touch.**)

**Conversation:** Ambr., Cocc., *Ph-ac., Stann.* (See **Talking.**)

**Cough:** Ars., Bry., *Cina,* Hyos., *Phos.,* Sep., *Tell.* (See **RESPIRATORY SYSTEM.**)

**Damp living houses:** Ant-t., *Aran.,* Ars., *Dulc., Nat-s.,* Ter.

**Dampness:** Amph., *Aran., Ars-i.,* Aster., Bar-c., *Calc.,* Calen., Carb-v., Chim., Chin., Chinin-s., *Colch.,* Crot-h., Cur., *Dulc.,* Elat., Euphr., Form., Gels., Kali-i., Lath., Lem-m., Magn-gr., Meli., Mur-ac., *Nat-s.,* Nux-m., *Petr., Phyt.,* Rad-br., Rhod., *Rhus-t.,* Ruta, Sep., Sil., Still., Sulph., Tub.

**Dampness, cold:** Am-c., Ant-t., Aran., Arn., Asc-t., Aster., Borx., *Calc., Calc-p., Dulc.,* Gels., *Guaj.,* Mang-act., *Merc.,* Nux-m., Nux-v., Physal-al., Phyt., *Rhus-t.,* Sil., Thuj., Urt-u., Verat.

**Dampness, warm:** Bapt., Brom., Carb-v., Carbn-s., *Gels.,* Ham., Phos., Sep.

**Dark:** *Ars.,* Calc., Carb-an., Phos., *Stram.* (See **Emotions, MIND.**)

**Daylight to sunset:** Med.

**Defecation, after:** *Aesc.* (See **Stool, ABDOMEN.**)

**Dentition:** Aeth., *Bell.,* Borx., Calc., Calc-p., *Cham., Kreos.,* Phyt., *Podo., Rheum,* Zinc. (See **TEETH.**)

**Dinner, after:** Ars., *Nux-v.* (See **STOMACH.**)

**Direction, diagonally:** *Agar.,* Both.

**Direction, diagonally, upper left, lower right:** Agar., Ant-t., Stram.

**Direction, diagonally, upper right, lower left:** Ambr., Brom., Med., Phos., Sul-ac.

**Direction, downward:** *Borx.,* Cact., Kalm., Lyc., *Sanic.*

**Direction, outwards:** Kali-c., *Sulph.*

**Direction, upwards:** Ben., Eup-per., *Led.*

**Drinking, during:** Bell.

**Eating:** Abies-n., Aesc., Aeth., Agar., *Aloe,* Ant-c., *Arg-n., Ars., Bry., Calc., Carb-v.,* Caust., *Chin.,* Chion., Cina, Cocc., *Coloc.,* Con., *Crot-t.,* Dig., *Graph.,* Hyos., Ign., *Ip.,* Kali-bi., *Kali-c.,* Kali-p., Kreos., Lach., *Lyc.,* Mag-m., Nat-m., Nit-ac., *Nux-v.,* Ol-an., Petr., Phos., *Puls.,* Rheum, Rumx., Samb., *Sep.,* Sil., *Staph.,* Stry., Sulph., Thea, Zinc. (See **Indigestion, STOMACH.**)

**Emotional excitement:** Acon., *Ambr., Arg-n.,* Aur., Chin., Cob., *Coff., Colch.,* Coll., Coloc., Con., Cupr-act., *Gels., Hyos., Ign.,* Kali-p., Lyss., Nit-s-d., *Nux-v.,* Petr., Ph-ac., *Phos.,* Sil., *Staph.* (See **MIND.**)

**Erratic, shifting, constantly changing, symptoms:** Apis, Berb., *Ign., Kali-bi., Kali-s., Lac-c.,* Lil-t., *Mang-act.,* Paraf., Phyt., *Puls.,* Sanic., *Tub.*

**Evening:** *Acon.,* Alf., *All-c.,* Am-br., Am-m., *Ambr.,* Apis, Ant-t., Arn., *Bell.,* Bry., Caj., Carb-v., Caust., Cham., Colch., Crot-h., *Cycl.,* Dios., Euon., Euphr., Ferr-p., *Hell., Hyos., Lyc., Kali-s., Merc.,* Merc-c., Mez., Nit-ac., *Phos.,* Plat., Plb., *Puls.,* Ran-b., *Rumx.,* Ruta, *Sep.,* Sil., Stann., Sul-ac., *Syph.,* Tab., Vib., X-rāy., Zinc.

**Eyes, closing:** Bry., Sep., Ther.

**Eyes, motion of:** *Bry.,* Nux-v., Spig.

**Eyes, opening of:** Tab.

**Fasting:** Croc., Iod.

**Fats:** Carb-v., *Cycl.,* Kali-m., *Puls.,* Thuj.

**Feet, exposure:** Con., Cupr., *Sil.*

**Feet hanging down:** Puls.

**Fish:** Nat-s., Urt-u.

**Fog:** Bapt., Gels., Hyper. (See **Dampness.**)

**Fright:** *Acon.,* Gels., *Ign.,* Op., Verat.

**Fruit:** *Ars.,* Bry., *Chin., Coloc.,* Ip., Samb., *Verat.*

**Gaslight:** Glon., Nat-c.

**Grief:** Aur., Gels., *Ign., Ph-ac.,* Staph., Verat. (See **Emotions,MIND.**)

**Hair cut:** Acon., *Bell.,* Glon.

**Head, uncovering:** Bell., Sil. (See **Air, cold.**)

**High altitudes:** Coca.

**Hot drinks:** Chion., Lach., Stann.

**Inspiration:** *Acon., Bry.,* Phos., Ran-b., Spig. (See **RESPIRATORY SYSTEM.**)

**Intermittently:** Anac., *Chin.,* Stry. (See **Periodical.**)

**Jar:** Arn., *Bell.,* Berb., *Bry., Cic.,* Crot-h., Glon., Ign., Nux-v., *Spig.,* Ther.

**Laughing:** Arg-met., *Dros.,* Mang-act., *Phos.,* Stann., Tell.

**Laundry work:** Sep.

**Left side:** Agar., Arg-met., Arg-n., Asaf., Aster., *Bell-p., Cean.,* Chim., Cimic., Colch., Cupr., Erig., *Lach.,* Lepi., *Lil-t., Ox-ac.,* Pulx., Rumx., Sapo., Sep., Ther., Thuj., Ust.

**Left side, then right side:** Lac-c., *Lach.*

**Light:** *Acon., Bell.,* Calc., Coca, *Con., Colch.,* Graph., Ign., *Lyss., Nux-v., Phos.,* Spig., *Stram.*

**Liquors:** *Agar.,* Ant-c., *Cann-i., Carb-v.,* Cimic., *Lach.,* Led., *Nux-v.,* Ran-b., Stram., *Sul-ac., Zinc.* (See **Alcoholism, NERVOUS SYSTEM.**)

**Localized spots:** Coff., *Ign., Kali-bi.,* Lil-t., Ox-ac.
**Looking downwards:** Acon., *Kalm.,* Olnd., *Spig.,* Sulph.
**Looking, intently, at objects:** Cina, Croc.
**Looking upwards:** Benzo., Calc., *Puls.,* Sulph.
**Lower half of body:** Bac-t.
**Lying down:** Ambr., Ant-t., Arn., *Ars.,* Arum-t., Aur., *Bell.,* Cann-s., Caust., Cench., *Con.,* Croc., *Dios.,* Dros., Dulc., *Glon., Hyos.,* Iber., Ip., Kreos., *Lach.,* Lyc., Meny., Nat-m., Nat-s., Plat., *Phos., Puls., Rhus-t., Rumx.,* Ruta, Samb., Sil., Tarax., *Trif-p.,* X-ray.
**Lying, on back:** Acet-ac., *Nux-v.,* Puls., Rhus-t.
**Lying, on left side:** Arg-n., *Cact.,* Calad., Coc-c., Iber., *Kali-c.,* Lyc., Magn-gr., *Phos.,* Plat., *Ptel.,* Puls., *Spig.,* Visc.
**Lying, on painful, or affected side:** Acon., Ars., *Bar-c.,* Calad., *Hep., Iod., Kali-c., Nux-m., Phos.,* Ruta, Sil., Tell., Vib.
**Lying, on painless side:** *Bry.,* Cham., Coloc., Ptel., *Puls.*
**Lying, on right side:** Cann-i., *Mag-m., Merc., Rhus-t.,* Scroph-n., Stann.
**Lying, with head low:** Ars.
**Masturbation:** Calc., *Chin.,* Con., *Nux-v., Ph-ac.,* Sep., *Staph.*
**Medicines, patent, aromatic, bitter, vegetable, pills:** Nux-v.
**Menses, after:** Alum., *Borx., Graph.,* Kreos., Lil-t., Nat-m., Nux-v., *Sep., Zinc.*
**Menses, at beginning, and close:** Lach.
**Menses, before:** Am-c., *Bov., Calc.,* Cocc., Con., Cupr., *Gels., Lach.,* Lyc., Mag-m., *Puls.,* Sars., *Sep.,* Verat., *Zinc.*
**Menses, during:** Am-c., Arg-n., *Bell.,* Bov., Cham., *Cimic.,* Con., Graph., Ham., Hyos., *Kali-c.,* Mag-c., *Nux-v., Puls., Sep.,* Sil., Sulph., Verat., *Vib.* (See **Menstruation, FEMALE SEXUAL SYSTEM.**)
**Mental exertion:** Agar., Aloe, Aml-ns., *Anac., Arg-n.,* Aur., Calc., Calc-p., Cimic., *Cocc.,* Cupr., *Gels.,* Ign., Kali-p., *Nat-c.,* Nat-m., *Nux-v.,* Ph-ac., *Phos., Pic-ac.,* Sabad., Sep., *Sil.,* Thymol. (See **MIND.**)
**Midnight, after:** Apis, *Ars.,* Bell., Carb-an., *Dros.,* Ferr., *Kali-c.,* Kali-n., Nit-ac., *Nux-v.,* Phos., *Podo.,* Rhus-t., Sil., Thuj.
**Midnight, at:** Aran., *Ars.,* Mez.
**Midnight, before:** Arg-n., Brom., Carb-v., Cham., *Coff.,* Led., Lyc., *Merc.,* Mur-ac., Nit-ac., Phos., *Puls.,* Ran-s., *Rhus-t., Rumx., Spong.,* Stann.
**Milk:** *Aeth.,* Ant-t., Calc., *Carb-v.,* Chin., Hom., Mag-c., Nit-ac., Sep., *Sulph.*
**Misdeeds of others:** Colch., *Staph.*
**Moon, full:** *Alum.,* Calc., Graph., Sabad., *Sil.*
**Moonlight:** Ant-c., Thuj.
**Moon, new:** Alum., Caust., Clem., *Sil.*
**Morning:** *Acal.,* Alum., Ambr., *Am-m.,* Arg-n., Aur., *Bry., Calc.,* Cann-i.,

Croc., Crot-h., Fl-ac., Glon., Ign., *Kali-bi.,* Kali-n., Lac-c., *Lach.,* Lil-t., Lith-c., Magn-gr., Med., Mygal., *Nat-m.,* Nicc., *Nit-ac.,* Nuph., *Nux-v.,* Onos., Ph-ac., *Phos.,* Podo., *Puls.,* Rhus-t., Rumx., Sep., Sil., Stel., Stry., *Sulph., Verb.*

**Morning, early (2 A.M-to 5 A.M.):** Aeth., Aesc., *Aloe,* Am-c., Bac., Bell., Chel., Cina, Coc-c., Cur., *Kali-bi., Kali-c.,* Kali-cy., Kali-p., Nat-s., *Nux-v.,* Ox-ac., *Podo.,* Ptel., Rhod., *Rumx., Sulph.,* Thuj., Tub.

**Morning, (10 A.M-to 11 A.M.):** Gels., *Nat-m., Sep.,* Sulph.

**Mortification from an offense:** *Coloc.,* Lyc., Staph.

**Motion:** Aesc., Agar., Aloe, Am-c., Aml-ns., Anh., Apis, *Bell., Berb.,* Bism., *But-ac.,* Cact., Cadm-s., *Calad.,* Calc-ar., Camph., Cean., *Cimic.,* Chin., *Cocc., Colch.,* Cupr., Dig., Equis-h., Ferr-p., *Gels.,* Get., Guaj., Helon., *Iber.,* Ip., Jug-c., Kali-m., *Kalm.,* Lac-c., *Led.,* Lina., Lob., Lycpr., Mag-p., Med., Meli., *Merc.,* Mez., *Nat-m.,* Nat-s., Nit-ac., Nux-m., *Nux-v.,* Onos., Pall., Petr., *Phyt.,* Phos., Pic-ac., Plat., Plb., Pulx., Puls-n., *Ran-b.,* Rheum, Ruta, *Sabin.,* Sang., *Sec.,* Seneg., Sil., *Spig.,* Squil., Still., Stry., Sulph., Tab., *Tarent.,* Thea, Thymol., Verat., Visc.

**Motion, downward:** *Borx.,* Gels., Sanic.

**Motion, on beginning:** Puls., *Rhus-t.,* Stront-c.

**Mountain climbing:** *Ars.,* Coca. (See **Ascending.**)

**Music:** *Acon.,* Ambr., Dig., *Graph., Nat-c.,* Nux-v., Pall., Ph-ac., *Sabin.,* Sep., *Thuj.*

**Narcotics:** Bell., *Cham., Coff.,* Lach., *Nux-v.,* Thuj.

**Night:** *Acon.,* Ant-t., Arg-n., Arn., *Ars.,* Aster., Bac., Bell., Bry., But-ac., Caj., Camph., Caust., Cench., *Cham., Chin.,* Chion., Cina, Clem., *Coff., Colch.,* Com., *Con.,* Crot-c., Cupr., *Cycl.,* Dios., Dol., *Dulc., Ferr.,* Ferr., p., Gamb., *Graph.,* Guaj., *Hep., Hyos., Iod.,* Iris, *Kali-i.,* Lach., Lil-t., Mag-m., Mag-p., *Merc.,* Merc-c., Mez., Nat-m., *Nit-ac.,* Nux-m., *Phos.,* Phyt., Plat., Plb., Psor., *Puls., Rhus-t.,* Rumx., Sep., *Sil.,* Sulph., *Syph.,* Tell., Thea, Thuj., Verat., Vib., X-ray, *Zinc.* (See **Evening.**)

**Noise:** Acon., Asar., *Bell., Borx., Calad.,* Cham., *Chin.,* Cocc., *Coff., Colch.,* Ferr., Glon., *Ign.,* Lyc., Lycpr., Mag-m., Med., Nux-m., *Nux-v.,* Onos., Phos., *Spig.,* Tarent., *Ther.*

**One half of body:** *Cham.,* Ign., Mez., *Puls.,* Sil., Spig., Thuj., Valer.

**Overeating:** Ant-c., *Nux-v.,* Puls. (See **Eating.**)

**Overheating:** Acon., *Ant-c.,* Bell., Brom., *Bry.,* Calc., Carb-v., Glon., Lyc., Nux-m., *Nux-v.*

**Pastry, rich food:** Carb-v., Kali-m., *Puls.*

**Peaches:** All-c., Glon.

**People, presence of:** Ambr.

**Periodically:** Alum., *Aran., Ars.,* Ars-met., *Cact.,* Carls., *Cedr.,* Chr-ac.,

*Chin.,* Cupr., *Eup-per.,* Ign., Ip., Kali-bi., *Nat-m.,* Nicc., Prim-o., Nit-ac., Ran-s., Sep., Sil., Tarent., *Tela,* Thuj., Urt-u.

**Periodically, every alternate day:** *Alum.,* Chin., Fl-ac., Nit-ac., Oxyt.

**Periodically, every two weeks:** Nicc.

**Periodically, every 2-3 weeks:** Ars-met.

**Periodically, every 2-4 weeks:** Carls., Ox-ac., Sulph.

**Periodically, every 3 weeks:** Ars., *Mag-c.*

**Periodically, every year:** *Ars.,* Carb-v., Crot-h., *Lach.,* Nicc., Sulph., *Thuj.,* Urt-u.

**Periodically, 4 P.M-to 8 P.M.:** Lyc., Sabad.

**Periodically, new and full moon:** Alum.

**Plants, growing near water:** Nat-s.

**Potatoes:** Alum.

**Pressure:** Acon., Agar., *Apis,* Arg-met., Bar-c., Borx., Calc., Cench., Cina., Equis-h., Guaj., *Hep.,* Iod., Kali-c., *Lach.,* Led., Lyc., *Merc-c.,* Nat-s., *Nux-v.,* Onos., Ovi-p., Phyt., Ran-b., Sil., *Ther.* (See **Touch**.)

**Rest:** Acon., *Arn., Ars.,* Asaf., Aur., Calc-f., Caps., Com., Con., *Cycl.,* Dulc., Euph., *Ferr.,* Indg., Iris, Kali-c., Kreos., Lith-lac., Lyc., Mag-c., Meny., *Merc.,* Olnd., *Puls., Rhod., Rhus-t.,* Sabad., *Samb.,* Seneg., *Sep.,* Stront-c., Sulph., Tarent., Tarax., Valer.

**Riding:** Arg-met., Berb., Caust., *Cocc.,* Lyss., Nux-m., *Petr., Sanic.,* Ther.

**Right side:** *Agar.,* Am-c., Anac., Apis, Ars., *Bell.,* Both., *Bry., Caust., Chel.,* Cinnb., Con., Crot-h., Cur., Dol., Equis-h., Ferr-p., Iod., *Kali-c.,* Lith-c., *Lyc.,* Lycpr., *Mag-p., Merc.,* Phyt., Podo., Rhus-t., *Sang.,* Tarent., Viol-o.

**Rising:** *Acon.,* Am-m., Ars., Bell., *Bry.,* Caps., Carb-v., *Cocc.,* Con., Dig., Ferr., Lach., Lyc., *Nux-v.,* Phos., *Phyt.,* Puls., Rad-br., *Rhus-t.,* Sulph.

**Room, heated:** Acon., *All-c.,* Alum., Ant-c., *Apis,* Aran-sc., Bapt., Brom., Bufo, Crat., *Croc.,* Euphr., *Glon.,* Hyper., *Iod.,* Kali-i., *Kali-s.,* Lil-t., *Merc., Puls.,* Sabin., Vib. (See **Warmth**.)

**Scratching:** Anac., Ars., Caps., *Dol., Merc.,* Mez., *Puls.,* Rhus-t., *Staph., Sulph.*

**Sea bathing:** Ars., Lim., Mag-m.

**Seashore:** *Aq-m.,* Ars., Brom., *Nat-m., Nat-s.,* Syph.

**Sedentary habits:** Acon., Aloe, Am-c., Anac., Arg-n., Bry., Con., *Nux-v.,* Sep.

**Shaving, after:** Caps., *Carb-an.,* Ox-ac., Plb.

**Sitting:** Alum., *Bry.,* Caps., Con., *Cycl.,* Dig., Dios., Dulc., Equis-h., Euph., Ferr., Hydrc., Lyc., Indg., Kali-c., Nat-c., Nux-v., Phyt., *Plat.,* Puls., *Rhus-t., Sep.,* Sulph., Tarax., Valer.

**Sitting, on cold steps:** Chim., *Nux-v.*

**Sleep, after:** Ambr., *Apis,* Bufo, Cadm-s., Calc., Coc-c., *Cocc.,* Crat., Epiph., Hom., *Lach.,* Merc-c., Morph., *Op.,* Parth., Pic-ac., Rhus-t., Sel., *Spong.,* Stram., Sulph., Syph., Tub., Valer., Ziz.

**Smoking:** *Abies-n.,* Borx., Cann-i., Chinin-ar., *Cic.,* Cocc., *Gels., Ign.,* Kalm., *Lac-ac.,* Lob., *Nux-v.,* Puls., Sec., Spig., Spong., *Staph.,* Stel.

**Sneezing:** *Ars.,* Bry., Kali-c., Phos., *Sulph., Verb.* (See **Jar**.)

**Snow, melting:** Calc-p.

**Snow storm:** Con., Form., Merc., Sep., Urt-u.

**Solitude:** *Bism.,* Kali-c., Lil-t., Lyc., Pall., Stram. (See **Fears, MIND**.)

**Soup:** Alum., Kali-c. (See **Fats**.)

**Spices:** *Nux-v.,* Phos.

**Spring:** All-c., Ars-br., Aur., Calc-p., Crot-h., Dulc., Gels., Kali-bi., *Lach., Nat-m.,* Nat-s., Nit-s-d., Rhus-t., *Sars.*

**Standing:** Aesc., Aloe, *Berb.,* Calc., Con., *Cycl.,* Lil-t., Plat., *Sulph.,* Valer.

**Stimulants:** Ant-c., Cadm-s., Chion., Fl-ac., *Glon.,* Ign., Lach., Led., Naja, *Nux-v.,* Op., *Zinc.*

**Storm, before:** *Bell-p.,* Meli., *Nat-s.,* Psor., *Rhod.,* Rhus-t.

**Stooping:** *Aesc.,* Am-c., Bry., Calc., Glon., Lyss., Merc., Ran-b., Spig., *Sulph.,* Valer.

**Straining, overlifting:** Arn., Carb-an., *Rhus-t.,* Ruta.

**Stretching:** Med., Rhus-t.

**Sun:** *Ant-c., Bell.,* Bry., Cact., Fago., *Gels., Glon.,* Lach., Lyss., *Nat-c.,* Nat-m., Puls., Sel. (See **Weather, hot**.)

**Sun, pain:** *Glon.,* Nat-m., *Sang.,* Spig., Tab.

**Swallowing:** Apis; *Bell.,* Brom., Bry., *Hep.,* Hyos., *Lach., Merc.,* Merc-i-f., Merc-i-r., Nit-ac., Stram., Sulph. (See **Dysphagia, THROAT**.)

**Sweating:** Ant-t., Chinin-s., *Hep., Merc.,* Merc-c., Nit-ac., Op., Ph-ac., *Sep.,* Stram., Verat.

**Sweets:** *Ant-c., Arg-n.,* Ign., *Lyc.,* Med., Sang., *Zinc.*

**Talking:** Ambr., Am-c., Anac., *Arg-met.,* Arum-t., Calc., Cann-s., Chinin-s., *Cocc.,* Mag-m., *Mang-act.,* Nat-c., *Nat-m.,* Ph-ac., Rhus-t., *Sel., Stann.,* Sulph., Verb.

**Tea:** *Abies-n., Chin.,* Dios., Lob., Nux-v., Puls., *Sel.,* Thuj.

**Temperature, extremes of:** Ant-c., Ip., Lach.

**Thinking of symptoms:** Bar-c., *Calc-p.,* Caust., *Gels., Helon., Med.,* Nux-v., *Ox-ac.,* Oxyt., Pip-m., Sabad., Staph.

**Thunderstorm, before, during:** Agar., Gels., Med., Meli., *Nat-c.,* Petr., *Phos.,* Phyt., Psor., *Rhod.,* Sep., Sil.

**Tobacco chewing:** *Ars.,* Ign., Lyc., Sel., *Verat.*

**Tobacco smoke:** Acon., Cic., Cocc., *Ign.,* Staph. (See **Smoking**.)

**Touch:** Acon., Ang., *Apis,* Arg-met., *Arn.,* Asaf., *Bell.,* Borx., *Bry.,* Calc., Camph., Caps., Carb-an., *Cham., Chin.,* Cic., Cocc., *Colch.,* Coloc., Com., *Cupr.,* Cupr-act., Equis-h., Euph-l., Euphr., Ferr-p., Guaj., Helon., *Hep.,* Hyos., Ign., *Kali-c., Lach., Lil-t.,* Lob., Lyc., Mag-p., Mez., Murx., *Nit-ac., Nux-v.,* Olnd., *Ox-ac.,* Phos., *Plb.,* Puls., *Ran-b., Rhod.,* Rhus-t., Sabin., Sang., Sep., *Sil., Spig.,* Staph., *Stry.,* Sulph., *Tarent.,* Tell., *Ther.,* Urt-u., Zinc.

**Touch of hat:** Glon.

**Travelling:** Coca, Plat.

**Twilight, to daylight:** Aur., *Merc.,* Phyt., *Syph.*

**Uncovering:** Ars., Bell., Benz-ac., Caps., Dros., Hell., *Hep.,* Kali-bi., *Mag-p., Nux-v.,* Rheum, *Rhus-t., Rumx., Samb.,* Sil., Stront-c.

**Vaccination, after:** Sil., Thuj.

**Veal:** Ip., *Kali-n.*

**Vital drains:** Calc., *Calc-p., Carb-v., Chin.,* Con., *Kali-c., Kali-p.,* Nux-v., *Ph-ac., Phos.,* Puls., *Sel.,* Sep., *Staph.*

**Voice, using:** Arg-met., Arg-n., Arum-t., Carb-v., *Dros.,* Mang-act., Nux-v., *Phos.,* Sel., *Stann.,* Wye.

**Vomiting:** Aeth., Ant-t., *Ars.,* Cupr., *Ip., Nux-v.,* Puls., Sil.

**Waking:** Ambr., Lach., Nit-ac., Nux-v. (See **Sleep.**)

**Warmth, heat:** Acon., Aeth., Agar., *All-c.,* Alum., Ambr., Anac., *Ant-c.,* Ant-t., *Apis,* Arg-n.,Asaf., Bell., *Bry.,* Calc., Camph., *Cham.,* Chin., Clem., *Com.,* Conv., *Dros.,* Euphr., Ferr., Fl-ac., Gels., Glon., *Graph.,* Guaj., Helia., Hyos., Iber., *Iod.,* Jug-c., Just., Kali-i., *Kali-m.,* Lach., *Led.,* Lyc., Med., *Merc., Nat-c.,* Nat-m., Nit-ac., Nux-m., Op., *Puls., Sabin., Sec.,* Stell., Sul-ac., Sulph., Tab. (See **Weather, hot.**)

**Warmth of bed:** Alum., Apis, Bell-p., Calc., *Cham.,* Clem., *Dros., Led.,* Lyc., Mag-c., *Merc.,* Mez., *Puls.,* Sabin., *Sec., Sulph.,* Thuj., Visc.

**Washing, water:** *Am-c., Ant-c.,* Ars-i., Bar-c., Bell., *Calc.,* Canth., Cham., Clem., *Crot-c.,* Ferr., Kreos., Lil-t., Mag-p., *Merc.,* Mez., *Nat-s.,* Nit-ac., Rhus-t., Sep., Sil., Spig., *Sulph.,* Urt-u.

**Water, drinks cold:** Ant-c., Apoc., Arg-n., *Ars.,* Calc., *Canth.,* Clem., Cocc., *Crot-t.,* Cycl., Dros., Ferr., Lob., Lyc., Nux-m., *Rhus-t.,* Sabad., Spong., Sulph.

**Water, drinks warm:** Ambr., Bry., *Lach.,* Phos., *Puls.,* Sep., Stann.

**Water, seeing or hearing:** Lyss..

**Water, working:** *Calc.,* Mag-p.

**Weather changes:** *Am-c.,* Bry., Calc., Calc-f., *Calc-p.,* Chel., Chin., *Dulc.,* Mang-act., Mag-c., *Merc.,* Nat-c., Nit-ac., *Nux-m., Phos., Psor., Ran-b., Rhod., Rhus-t.,* Ruta, Stict., Stront-c., Sulph., Tarent. (See **Dampness.**)

**Weather changes, in spring:** All-c., Ant-t., Gels., Kali-s., Nat-s.

**Weather, dry, cold:** Agar., Alum., Apoc., *Asar., Aur., Caust.,* Dulc., Ip., *Kali-c.,* Kreos., Nit-s-d., *Nux-v., Petr.,* Rhus-t., Visc. (See **Air, cold**.)

**Weather, hot:** *Acon.,* Aeth., Aloe, *Ant-c., Bell.,* Borx., *Bry.,* Croc., Crot-h., Crot-t., *Gels., Glon.,* Kali-bi., Lach., *Nat-c., Nat-m.,* Nit-ac., Phos., Pic-ac., *Podo.,* Puls., Sabin., Sel., Syph. (See **Sun**.)

**Weather, stormy:** Nux-m., Psor., Ran-b., *Rhod.,* Rhus-t.

**Weather, windy, dry:** *Acon.,* Arum-t., Cham., Cupr., *Hep.,* Lyc., Mag-c., *Nux-v.,* Phos., Puls., *Rhod.*

**Weather windy, moist:** All-c., Dulc., *Euphr.,* Ip., *Nux-m.,* Rhod.

**Weeping:** Cham., *Nat-m.,* Puls., *Sep.,* Stann.

**Wet application:** *Am-c., Ant-c.,* Calc., *Clem.,* Crot-h., *Merc.,* Rhus-t., *Sulph.* (See **Washing**.)

**Wet exposure:** All-c., Am-c., Ant-c., Apis, Aran., Ars., *Calc.,* Caust., *Dulc., Elaps,* Meli., *Merc.,* Narc-ps., Nat-s., Nux-m., *Phyt.,* Pic-ac., Ran-b., Rhod., *Rhus-t.,* Ruta, Sep. (See **Dampness**.)

**Wet feet:** All-c., Calc., Puls., *Rhus-t., Sil.*

**Wine:** *Alum.,* Ant-c., Arn., *Ars.,* Benz-ac., *Carb-v.,* Con., Fl-ac., Led., Lyc., *Nux-v.,* Op., Ran-b., Sel., Sil., *Zinc.*

**Yawning:** Cina; *Ign.,* Kreos., *Nux-v.,* Rhus-t., *Sars.*

**Yearly:** Lach., Rhus-r.

**AMELIORATIONS, Acids:** Ptel., Sang.

**Air, cool, open:** *Acon.,* Aesc., Aeth., *All-c.,* Aloe, *Alum.,* Am-m., Ambr., *Aml-ns.,* Ant-c., Ant-t., *Apis, Arg-n.,* Asaf., Bar-c., Bry., Bufo, Cact., Cann-i., *Chin.,* Clem., Coca, Com., Conv., Crat., Croc., Dig., Dios., Dros., Dulc., Euon., Euphr., Gels., *Glon.,* Graph., Iod., *Kali-i., Kali-s.,* Lil-t., *Lyc., Mag-c.,* Mag-m., Merc-i-r., Mez., Mosch., Naja, *Nat-m.,* Nat-s., Ol-an., Phos., *Pic-ac.,* Plat., *Puls.,* Rad-br., Rhus-t., *Sabad.,* Sabin., Sec., *Sep.,* Stel., Stry., Sulph., *Tab., Tarent.,* Vib. (See **Warmth, Aggravation**.)

**Air, cool, must have windows open:** *Aml-ns., Arg-n.,* Bapt., Calc., *Lach.,* Med., *Puls., Sulph.* (See **Asthma, RESPIRATORY SYSTEM**.)

**Air, warm:** Aur., Calc., Caust., Led., Mag-c., Merc., Petr., Rhus-t. (See **Warmth**.)

**Bathing:** Acon., Apis, Ars., *Asar., Caust.,* Euphr., *Puls.,* Spig.

**Bathing, cold:** Apis, Asar., Bufo, Meph., Nat-m., Sep.

**Bathing, vinegar:** Vesp.

**Bathing, warm:** Ant-c., Bufo, Rad-br., *Stront-c.,* Thea.

**Bending, double:** Aloe, Chin., *Coloc., Mag-p.* (See **Pressure**.)

**Bending, forward:** Gels., *Kali-c.*

**Boring into, nose, ears:** Nat-c., Spig.

**Breakfast, after:** Nat-s., Staph. (See **Eating.**)

**Carrying:** Ant-t., *Cham.*

**Chewing:** Bry., Cupr-act.
**Coffee:** Euphr., Fl-ac.
**Cold:** All-c., Bell-p., Borx., *Bry.,* Fag., Iod., *Led.,* Lyc., Onos., Op., *Phos., Sec.*
**Cold applications, washing:** Alum., *Apis,* Arg-n., Asar., Bell., Ferr-p., Kali-m., Merc., Phos., *Puls.,* Sabin. (See **Bathing**.)
**Cold water:** Agar-em., Aloe, Ambr; *Bry.,* Camph., Cann-i., *Caust.,* Cupr., Fago., *Led., Phos.,* Pic-ac., *Puls., Sep.*
**Colors, objects, bright:** *Stram.,* Tarent.
**Combing hair:** Form.
**Company:** Aeth., *Bism.,* Kali-c., Lil-t., Lyc., *Stram.*
**Consolation:** Puls.
**Conversation:** Eup-per.
**Coughing:** Apis, Stann. (See **RESPIRATORY SYSTEM.**)
**Covering light:** Sec.
**Dark:** Coca, Con., *Euphr.,* Graph., Phos., *Sang.*
**Day, during:** Kali-c., Syph. (See **Aggravations**.)
**Days, alternating:** Alum.
**Descending:** Spong.
**Discharges, appearances of:** *Lach.,* Mosch., Stann., *Zinc.*
**Drawing limbs up:** Sep., Sulph., Thuj.
**Drinks, cold:** Ambr., *Cupr.*
**Drinks, warm:** Alum., Ars., Chel., *Lyc.,* Nux-v., Sabad., *Spong.* (See **Warm**.)
**Eating:** Acet-ac., *Alum.,* Ambr., *Anac.,* Brom., Cadm-met., Caps., *Chel.,* Cimic., Cist., Con., Ferr., Ferr-act., Graph., *Hep.,* Hom., *Ign., Iod., Kali-p.,* Lach., *Lith-c., Nat-c.,* Nat-m., Onos., *Petr.,* Phos., Pip-n., *Psor.,* Rhod., Sep., *Spong.,* Zinc.
**Eructations:** Ant-t., *Arg-n.,* Bry., *Carb-v.,* Dios., *Graph.,* Ign., *Kali-c.,* Lyc., Mosch., Nux-v., Ol-an., Sang.
**Evenings:** Borx., Lob., Nicc., Nux-v., Stel.
**Excitement, pleasurable:** Kali-p., Pall.
**Exercise:** Alumn., Brom., Plb., *Rhus-t.,* Sep. (See **Walking**.)
**Expectoration:** Ant-t., Hep., *Stann.,* Zinc. (See **RESPIRATORY SYSTEM.**)
**Expulsion of flatus, per ano:** Aloe, Arn., Calc-p., Corn., Grat., Hep., Iris, Kali-n., Mez.
**Fanned, being:** *Arg-n., Carb v.,* Chin., Lach., Med.
**Fasting:** Cham., Con., *Nat-m.*
**Feet in ice water:** *Led.,* Sec.
**Food cold:** Ambr., Bry., Lyc., Phos., Sil.
**Food warm:** Kreos., Lyc. (See **Aggravations**.)

**Forenoon, in:** Lil-t.
**Head bent backward:** Hyper., Seneg.
**Head bent forward, while lying:** Coloc.
**Head, wrapped up warm:** Hep., Psor., Rhod., Sil.
**Head elevated:** Ars., Gels.
**Heat:** *Ars.,* Caps., Gymno., Xero. (See **Warmth.**)
**Ice, holding in mouth:** Coff.
**Inland, mountains:** Syph.
**Inspiration:** Colch., Ign., *Spig.* (See **RESPIRATORY SYSTEM.**)
**Lemonade:** Cycl.
**Light:** Stram.
**Limb hanging down:** Con.
**Lying down:** Acon., Anh., Arn., *Bell.,* Bell-p., Brom., *Bry.,* Calad., Calc., Coff., *Colch.,* Equis-h., Ferr., *Mang-act., Nat-m.,* Nux-v., Onos., *Pic-ac.,* Pulx., *Puls.,* Rad-br., *Stann.,* Stry., Symph.
**Lying, on back with shoulders raised:** Acon., Ars.
**Lying, on left side:** Ign., Mur-ac., Nat-m., Stann. (See **Aggravations.**)
**Lying, on painful side:** Ambr., Am-c., Arn., Borx., *Bry.,* Calc., *Coloc.,* Cupr-act., Ptel., *Puls.,* Sul-ac. (See **Pressure.**)
**Lying, on right side:** Ant-t., Nat-m., *Phos.,* Sulph., Tab. (See **Aggravations.**)
**Lying on right side, with head high:** Ars., Cact., *Spig.,* Spong.
**Lying, on stomach:** *Acet-ac.,* Am-c., Ant-t., *Coloc.,* Med., *Podo., Tab.*
**Lying, with head high:** Petr., Puls., Spig.
**Lying with head low:** Arn., Spong.
**Magnetized:** Phos.
**Menses, between:** Bell., Bov., Elaps, Ham., Magn-gr.
**Menses, during:** Am-c., Cycl., *Lach., Zinc.* (See **FEMALE SEXUAL SYSTEM.**)
**Mental occupation:** Ferr., Kali-br., *Helon.,* Nat-c.
**Midnight, after:** Lyc. (See **Night.**)
**Midnight, until noon:** Puls.
**Mind being diverted:** Calc-p., Helon., Ox-ac., Pip-m., Tarent.
**Mornings:** Apis, Jug-c., Still., Xero.
**Motion:** Abrot., Aesc., *Alum.,* Arn., Ars., Asaf., *Aur.,* Bell., Bell-p., **Brom.,** *Caps.,* Chin., Coca, Coc-c., Com., Con., *Cycl., Dios., Dulc.,* Euph., *Ferr.,* Fl-ac., Gels., *Helon.,* Hom., Ign., Indg., Iris, Kali-c., Kali-i., **Kali-p.,** Kreos., Lith-c., Lith-lac., Lob., Lyc., *Mag-c.,* Mag-m., Magn-gr., Meny., Nat-c., Op., Parth., Pip-m., Plat., *Puls.,* Pyrog., Rad-met., Rhod., *Rhus-t.,* Ruta, Sabad., *Samb., Sep.,* Stel., Sulph., Syph., *Valer.,* Verat., Xer., Zinc.
**Motion, slow:** Agar., Ambr., *Ferr.,* Ferr-act., Plat., Stann., Zinc.

**Mouth, covered:** Rumx.
**Music:** Tarent.
**Night:** Cupr-act.
**Oil applications:** Euph-l.
**Position, change of:** Apis, Caust., *Ign.,* Nat-s., Ph-ac., *Rhus-t.,* Valer., Zinc.
**Position, hands and feet:** Eup-per.
**Position, semi-erect:** Ant-t., Apis, Bell. (See **Rest**.)
**Pressure:** *Arg-n.,* Asaf., Borx., *Bry., Caps.,* Chel., *Chin., Coloc.,* Con., Cupr act., *Dios.,* Dros., Euon., Form., Guaj., *Ign.,* Indg., *Lil-t.,* Mag-m., *Mag-p.,* Meny., Nat-c., Nat-m., Nat-s., Nux-v., Pic-ac., *Plb., Puls.,* Rad-met., *Sep.,* Sil., *Stann.,* Verat.
**Putting feet on chair:** Con.
**Rest:** Aesc., Ant-c., Bell., *Bry.,* Cadm-s., Cann-i., *Colch.,* Crat., Get., Gymno., Kali-p., Merc., Merc-c., *Nux-v.,* Phyt., Pulx., Squil., Staph., Stry-p., Vib.
**Riding in carriage:** Nit-ac.
**Rising:** Ambr., Am-c., *Ars.,* Calc., Lith-c., Parth., Samb., Sep.
**Rocking:** Cina, Kali-c.
**Room close, in:** Euph-l. (See **Warmth**.)
**Rubbing:** Anac., Calc., *Canth.,* Carb-ac., Dios., Form., Indg., *Mag-p.,* Nat-c., Ol-an., Phos., Plb., *Podo.,* Rhus-t., Sec., *Tarent.*
**Scratching:** Asaf., *Calc.,* Com., Cycl., *Jug-c.,* Mur-ac., Nat-c., Phos., Sulph.
**Sea, at:** Brom.
**Seashore, at:** Med.
**Shaving, after:** Brom.
**Sipping water:** Kali-n.
**Sitting erect:** Ant-t., Apis, Bell.
**Sitting up in bed:** *Kali-c.,* Samb.
**Sleep:** Calad., Colch., Merc., Mygal., *Nux-v.,* Phos., *Sang.,* Sep.
**Smoking:** Aran., Tarent-c.
**Standing erect:** Ars., Bell., *Dios.,* Kali-p.
**Stimulants:** Gels., Glon.
**Stooping:** Colch.
**Storm, after:** Rhod.
**Stretching limbs:** Aml-ns., Plb., Rhus-t., Sec., Teucr.
**Summer, during:** Alum., Aur., Calc-p., Ferr., Sil. (See **Warmth**.)
**Sweat:** Acon., Ars., Calad., *Cham.,* Cupr., Franc., Rhus-t., *Verat.* (See **FEVER**.)
**Taking hold of anything:** Anac.
**Thinking of symptoms:** *Camph.,* Hell.
**Touch:** Asaf., Calc., Cycl., Mur-ac., Tarax., Thuj.
**Uncovering:** Apis, Camph., Lyc., Onos., *Sec., Tab.* (See **Aggravations**.)

**Urination:** *Gels.,* Ign., *Ph-ac.,* Sil.

**Vomiting:** Helia.

**Warmth, heat:** *Ars.,* Aur., Bad., Bell., Bry., Calc-f., Camph., Caust., Cimic., *Coloc., Coll.,* Coff., Cor-r., Cupr act., Cycl., *Dulc.,* Form., *Hep.,* Ign., Kali-bi., Kali-p., Kreos., Lach., Lob., Lyc., Lycpr., *Mag-p.,* Nux-m., *Nux-v.,* Ph-ac., Phyt., Psor., Rhod., Rhus-t., *Rumx.,* Sabad., Sep., Sil., Staph., Stram., Sul-ac., Thea, Verat.

**Warmth, heat of, applications:** Ars., Bry., Calc-f., *Lach., Mag-p.,* Nux-m., Rad-br., Rhus-t., Sep.

**Warmth, of head:** Bell., Graph., *Hep., Psor.,* Sanic., *Sil.*

**Water, cold:** Aloe, *Bry.,* Caust., *Jatr-c., Phos.,* Pic-ac., Sep.

**Water, hot:** Spig.

**Weather, damp, wet:** Alum., Asar., *Caust., Hep.,* Med., Mur-ac., Nux-v.

**Weather, damp, warm:** Cham., Kali-c., Sil.

**Weather, dry:** Am-c., Calc., Kali-c., Magn-gr., Petr., Still. (See **Aggravations.**)

**Weather, dry, warm:** Alum., *Calc-p.,* Nat-s., Nux-m., Rhus-t., *Sulph.* (See **Summer.**)

**Wine:** Coca.

**Winter, during:** Ilx-a.

■

# INDEX TO THE REPERTORY

# INDEX TO THE REPERTORY

[Number within square brackets shows the page number of repertory]

**ABORTION** [773]: Premature expulsion of a fetus.

**ABSCESS** [895]: A circumscribed cavity containing pus, buries in the tissues.

**ABSCESS, RETROPHARYNGEAL** [685]: Abscess behind the pharynx, a suppurative inflammation of lymph nodes in the posterior and lateral walls of the pharynx.

**ACIDITY** [696]: Sourness, containing acid.

**ACNE** [879]: Inflammation of the sebaceous glands from retained secretion.

**ACNE ROSACEA** [879]: Chronic hyperemic disease of the skin especially of the face.

**ACROMEGALY** [895]: Enlargement of many parts of the skeletal system especially of the face and extremities, associated with the hypersecretion of the pituitary growth hormone.

**ACTINOMYCOSIS** [880]: An infectious disease of cattle and man due to the ray-fungus (Actinomyces).

**ADDISON'S DISEASE** [895]: A disorder characterised by hypotension, weight loss, anorexia, weakness and bronze like hyperpigmentation of the skin caused by deficiency of adrenocortical hormone.

**ADENITIS** [904]: Inflammation of a gland or lymph node.

**ADENOIDS** [684]: Hypertrophied adenoid tissue, as in the pharynx. (Adenoid: resembling a gland.)

**ADYNAMIA** [849]: A deficiency or loss of vital power.

**AFTER-PAINS** [776]: Postpartum pains.

**AGALACTEA** [778]: Absence or failure in secretion of milk.

**AGGRAVATIONS** [911]: Worsening of patient's condition.

**AGORAPHOBIA** [607]: A dread of open, public spaces or crossing open spaces.

**AGUE** [873]: Malarial or intermittent fever.

**ALAE NASI** [654]: The cartilaginous wing of the nose.

**ALBUMINURIA** [745]: The prescence of albumin and globulin in urine.

**ALCOHOLISM** [850]: Symptoms of the excessive use of alcohol.

**ALOPECIA** [880]: Loss of hair, baldness

**AMBLYOPIA** [646]: Dimness of vision.

**AMELIORATIONS** [919]: Improvement, of the condition of the patient.

**AMENORRHEA** [764]: Absence or abnormal stoppage of menses

**ANASARCA** [903]: General dropsy.

**ANEMIA** [895]: Deficiency of blood or red corpuscles and hemoglobin.

**ANEMIA, PERNICIOUS** [895]: A megaloblastic anemia usually in older adults due to impaired interstitial absorption of Vit B12 caused by lack of intrinsic factor. Characterized by pallor, acidity, glossitis, weakness, gastric mucosal atropy, etc.

**ANEURISM** [809]: A sac formed by the dilatation in the wall of an artery.

**ANGER, ILL EFFECTS** [606]

**ANGINA PECTORIS** [812]: Pain and oppression around the heart.

**ANIDROSIS** [880]: Absence or deficiency of sweat.

**ANKLES, WEAK** [835]

**ANTHRAX** [880]: A carbuncle; the disease is produced by Bacillus anthracis.

**ANTHROPOPHOBIA** [607]: Fear of society or of people.

**ANTRUM AFFECTIONS** [661]: (Antrum: a cavity, especially in the bone.)

**ANURIA** [743]: An absence or deficiency of urine.

**ANUS, AFFECTIONS** [714]: (Anus: the rectal exit.)

**AORTITIS** [809]: Inflammation of the aorta.

**APHASIA** [616]: Loss of power of speech from a cortical lesion.

**APHONIA** [802]: Loss of voice, due to a peripheral lesion.

**APHTHAE** [673]: Thrush: small white ulcers in the mouth.

**APOPLEXY** [809]: A sudden neuralgic impairment due to a cerebrovascular disorder, either an arterial occlusion or an ultra cranial hemorrhage.

**APPENDICITIS** [733]: Inflammation of appendix vermiformis.

**APPETITE DISORDERS** [692]: (Appetite: a desire for food; lust.)

**ARTERIOSCLEROSIS** [809]: Thickening and loss of elasticity of arterial walls. (Sclerosis: induration and overgrowth of the connective tissue of an organ.)

**ARTERITIS** [809]: Inflammation of an artery.

**ARTHRITIS** [832]: Inflammation of a joint.

**ARTHRITIS DEFORMANS** [840]: Chronic inflammation of a joint, with deformity.

**ASCARIDES** [733]: A family of nematode worms, to which belongs the round worm (Ascaris lumbricoides) and the thread worm (Oxyuris vermicularis)

**ASCITES** [903]: Dropsy of the abdomen.

**ASPHYXIA** [896]: The condition caused by non oxygenation of the blood resulting in hypoxia and hypercapnia.

**ASTHENOPIA** [647]: Weak or painful vision.

**ASTHMA** [786]: Paroxysmal dyspnea with oppression.

**ASTIGMATISM** [647]: A condition in which the rays of light from a point do not converage at a point on the retina due to the unequal curvature of the refractive surfaces of the eye.

**ATHEROMA** [809]: A soft encysted tumor; fatty degeneration of the arterial walls.

ATHETOSIS [851]: A disease in which there is an inability to maintain one position, withering movements especially of fingers and toes. Post hemiplegic chorea.

AURICLE, AFFECTIONS [649]: (Auricle: the external ear; one of the upper cavities of heart.)

AVERSIONS [692]: Noxious, tendency to avoid.

AXILLA, AFFECTIONS [817]: (Axilla: the armpit.)

AZOTURIA [747]: An increase of urea in the urine.

BACKACHE [817]

BAKER'S ITCH [885]: Lichen: eczema caused by handling yeast.

BALANITIS [752]: Inflammation of the glans penis.

BALANOPOSTITIS [752]: The same as balanitis.

BARBER'S ITCH (Sycosis) [890]: A chronic inflammation of hair follicles.

BASEDOW'S DISEASE [905]: Exophthalmic goitre.

BED SORES [881] Decubitus ulcer.

BELL'S PALSY [667]: Unilateral facial paralysis due to a lesion in the facial nerve resulting in characteristic distortions of the face.

BERI BERI [851]: An east Indian disease, characterized by polyneuritis, cardiac pathology and edema. A deficiency disease due to lack of vitamins in the diet.

BILIARY COLIC [728]: Paroxysms of pain from the passage of gall stones through the gall duct.

BILIOUS FEVER [869]: Fever with vomiting of bile.

BILIOUSNESS [695]: The condition marked by constipation, adrenal discomfort, headache and anorexia, due to excess of bile.

BLACK EYE [638]: Extravasation of blood around the eye, after an injury.

BLADDER, AFFECTIONS [734]: Diseases of the bladder.

BLADDER, INFLAMMATION [735]

BLADDER, IRRITABLE [735]: A state marked by a constant desire to micturate with an increased frequency.

BLADDER, PARALYSIS [736]

BLEPHARITIS [639]: Inflammation of the eye lids.

BLEPHAROSPASM [640]: Spasm of the orbicularis oculi muscle producing more or less complete closure of the eyes.

BLINDNESS [646]: Loss of ability to see. (Amaurosis: partial or total blindness.)

BLOOD, DISORGANIZATION [896].

BONE, AFFECTIONS [896].

BORBORYGMI [713]: (Borborygmus: the rumbling noise caused by the propulsion of gas through the intestines.)

BOWEL OBSTRUCTION [730]

**BRACHIALGIA** [822]: Pain in the arm.

**BRADYCARDIA** (Slow pulse) [815]: Abnormal infrequency of the pulse.

**BRAIN FAG** [605]: Brain-tire; cerebral asthenia.

**BRAIN, CONCUSSION** [617]

**BRAIN, CONGESTION** [617]

**BRAIN, INFLAMMATION** [617]

**BRAIN, SOFTENING** [617]

**BREATH, OFFENSIVE** (Halitosis) [671]: Foul breath.

**BRIGHT'S DISEASE** [737]: A generic term for acute and chronic disease of the kidneys, usually associated with dropsy and albuminuria.

**BROMHIDROSIS** [880]: Fetid perspiration, especially in the armpits due to bacterial decomposition.

**BRONCHIECTASIS** [788]: Chronic dilatation of the bronchi with fetid breath, paroxysmal cough and muco purulent expectoration.

**BRONCHITIS** [788]: Inflammation of the bronchial tubes.

**BRONCHITIS, ACUTE** [788]: Bronchitis with a short, more or less severe course.

**BRONCHITIS, CHRONIC** [788]: Long continued with a tendency to recurrence.

**BRONCHITIS, CROUPOUS** [788]: Bronchitis characterised by violent cough with paroxysms of dyspnea.

**BRONCHORRHEA** [788]: A profuse discharge of mucus from the air passages.

**BRUISES** [906]: A flesh injury; contusion.

**BUBO** [749]: An inflammation and swelling of the lymphatic glands of the groin, axilla due to infections like gonorrhea, syphilis, plague, tuberculosis, chancroid.

**BUBONIC PLAGUE** [898]: A contagious, epidemic disease with fever, delirium and buboes.

**BULBAR PARALYSIS** [843]: A progressive atrophy and paralysis of the muscles of the tongue, lips, palate, pharynx and larynx.

**BUNIONS** [830]: A swelling of a bursa of the foot.

**BURNS, SCALDS** [906]: A lesion of tissue from dry heat or flame.

**BURSITIS** [835]: Inflammation of a bursa.

**CALCULI, BILIARY** [728]: A gall stone.

**CALCULI, RENAL** [736]: A stone in the kidney.

**CANCER** [898]: Carcinoma; a malignant tumor with an uncontrollable production of epithelioid cells.

**CANCER PAINS** [898]

**CANCRUM ORIS** [673]: Gangrenous ulceration of the mouth.

**CANKER SORES** [672]: A cancerous or gangrenous sore.

**CARBUNCLES** [880]: Necrotising infection of the skin and subcutaneous tissue, composed of a cluster of boils with incipient draining sinuses.
**CARDIAC DROPSY** [903]: An effusion of fluid into the tissues or cavities of the body due to a cardiac disease. (Cardiac: Pertaining to the heart.)
**CARDIAC NEUROSES** [811]: (Neurosis: A nervous affection without lesion.)
**CARDIALGIA** [695]: Pain in the heart.
**CARIES** [680, 896]: Decay or death of bone substance in which it becomes softened, discolored and porous.
**CARPHOLAGIA** [605]: Delirious (picking at the bed clothes.)
**CARTILAGE:** A non-vascular elastic tissue softer than bone.
**CARTILAGES, AFFECTIONS** [898]
**CATALEPSY** [605]: A neurosis associated with muscular rigidity and loss of will, without alteration in circulation, etc.
**CATARACT** [635]: Opacity of the crystalline lens.
**CATARRH, BLADDER** [735]
**CATARRH, BRONCHI** [788]
**CATARRH, LARYNX** [800]
**CATARRH, NOSE** [657]
**CATARRH, STOMACH** [700]
**CATARRH, THROAT** [687]
**CATARRH, UTERUS** [781]
**CATARRH:** Inflammation of a mucous membrane.
**CATHETERISM** [869]: The use of catheter.
**CELLULITIS** [898]: Inflammation of cellular tissue.
**CEREBROSPINAL MENINGITIS** [617]: Inflammation of meninges of the brain and cord.
**CHANCRE** [755]: The painless primary lesion of syphilis at the site of entry of infection.
**CHANCROID** [749]: A sexually transmitted disease with a painful primary ulcer at the site of inoculation, generally on the external genitalia with local lymphadenopathy or the "soft" chancre.
**CHANGE OF LIFE** [763]: Menopause.
**CHAPPED, HANDS** [823]: (Chap: Rough or cracked skin generally from cold or frequent wetting.)
**CHECKED DISCHARGES** [900]
**CHECKED ERUPTIONS** [901]
**CHEEKS, AFFECTIONS** [665]: (Cheek: The fleshy protuberance on the side of the face.)
**CHEYNE-STOKES RESPIRATION** [806]: Rythemic waxing and waning in the depth of respiration, with regularly recurring periods of apnea.

**CHICKEN POX** [872]: Varicella; infectious eruptive disease due to Varicella zoster virus.

**CHILBLAINS** [880]: Localised erythema and edema caused by exposure to cold especially in hands, feet and ears.

**CHILLINESS** [863]

**CHLOASMA** [880]: Pigmentation of the skin; liver spots.

**CHLOROSIS** [895]: Iron deficiency anemia, most common in young women, marked by greenish color of the skin and menstrual disturbances.

**CHOLERA** [717]: A disease characterised by emesis, rice water diarrhea, cramps and prostration.

**CHOLERA INFANTUM** [717]: The summer complaint of children.

**CHOLERA MORBUS** [717]: Acute gastroenteritis.

**CHORDEE** [750]: Painful, down curved erection of penis in gonorrhoea.

**CHOREA** (St. Vitus Dance) [851]: Involuntary muscular twitchings.

**CHOROID, AFFECTIONS** [635]

**CHOROID:** The second or vascular tunic of the eye.

**CICATRICES** [900]: Plural of cicatrix.

**CICATRIX:** The scar of a wound.

**CILIARY MUSCLE, SPASM** [635]: Spasm of the muscle of accomodation in the eye.

**CILIARY NEURALGIA** [635]: (Neuralgia: Pain in a nerve.)

**CIRRHOSIS OF LIVER** [731]: Diffuse interfacing hands of fibrous tissue dividing the hepatic parenchyma into micro and macronodular areas.

**CLAIRVOYANCE** [605]: An extra sensory perception in which knowledge of objective events is acquired without the use of senses. Telepathy.

**CLERGYMAN'S SORE THROAT** [687]: A granular form of pharyngitis.

**CLIMACTERIC DISORDERS** [763]

**CLIMACTERIC FLUSHINGS** [763]: Rush of blood to the head and face with a sensation of heat during menopause.

**CLIMACTERIC:** A critical period in life; menopause.

**COCCYGODYNIA** [820]: Pain in the coccyx and the neighbouring region.

**COLIC** [709]: Acute spasmodic pain in the abdomen.

**COLIC, BABIES** [709]

**COLIC, BILIARY** [728]: Pain due to the passage of a gall stone through the gall duct.

**COLIC, LEAD** [710]: Intestinal colic due to lead poisoning.

**COLIC, RENAL** [738]: Pain due to a calculus in the ureter.

**COLITIS** [728]: Inflammation of the colon.

**COLLAPSE** [849]: Marked depression of the vital activities of the body.

**COLOR BLINDNESS** [646]: Abnormalism or deficiency of color perceptions.

**COMA** [606]: Stupor.

**COMA VIGIL** [605]: Delirious lethargy with open eyes.

**COMEDO** [881]: Blackhead; a worm-like mass in an obstructed sebaceous duct. A non-inflammatory lesion of acne.

**COMPLAINTS, GENERAL** [898]

**CONDYLOMATA** [893]: (Condyloma: a wart like growth near the anus.)

**CONJUNCTIVITIS** [636]: Inflammation of the conjunctiva.

**CONSTIPATION** [717]: A sluggish action of the bowels.

**CONSUMPTION** [804]: Phthisis; wasting, atrophy.

**CONTUSIONS** [906]: A bruise from a blow by a blunt object.

**CONVULSIONS** [851]: A violent involuntary contraction of voluntary muscles, a spasm, fit or seizure.

**CONVULSIONS, PUERPERAL** [775]: Involuntary spasms in women, just before, during or after child birth.

**CONVULSIONS, SUPPRESSED ERUPTION** [852]: Spasms due to suppression of skin symptoms.

**CONVULSIONS, TEETHING** [852]: Spasm during dentition.

**CONVULSIONS, UREMIC** [853]: Due to uremia. A convulsion due to renal disease.

**CORNEA, AFFECTIONS** [636]: (Cornea: The transparent anterior part of the eye ball.)

**CORNS** (Callosities) [880]: A local thickening and induration of the epidermis, as on the toes caused by friction and pressure.

**CORYZA** [658]: Catarrhal inflammation of the nose.

**COUGH** [791]: A sudden, forced expiratory noise; tussis.

**COUGH, DRY** [795]

**COUGH, HOARSE** [795]

**COUGH, LARYNGEAL** [795]

**COUGH, LOOSE** [795]

**COUGH, NERVOUS** [796]

**COUGH, PHTHISICAL** [795]

**COWPERITIS** [750]: Inflammation of Cowper's gland. (Cowper's gland: two compound, tubular glands situated between the two layers of the triangular ligament, anterior to the prostate gland.)

**COXALGIA** [835]: Pain in the hip joint. Hip joint disease.

**CRACKED LIPS** [671]

**CRAMPS IN CALVES** [827]: (Cramp: A spasmodic muscular contraction with pain.)

**CRETINISM** [605]: A chronic condition due to congenital lack of thyroid secretion. Marked by arrested mental and physical development, dystrophy of bones and soft parts and lowered basal metabolism.

**CROUP** [800]: Inflammation of the larynx and trachea with dyspnea and membranous deposit.

**CROUP, MEMBRANOUS** [800]: Diphtheria.

**CRUSTA LACTEA** [629]: Seborrhea of the scalp in infants.

**CYANOSIS** [810]: Blue discoloration of skin from non-oxidation of blood.

**CYSTITIS, ACUTE** [735]: (Cystitis: Inflammation of the bladder.)

**CYSTITIS, CHRONIC** [735]

**CYSTS** [771, 889, 910]: A membraneous sac containing fluid or a semi-solid material.

**DANDRUFF** [629]: Scruf on the head, coming off as small scales.

**DAY BLINDNESS** [646]: Subnormal vision in daylight.

**DEAFNESS** [649]: The condition of being deaf.

**DEBILITY** [849]: (Asthenia: loss of strength; adynamia.)

**DECUBITUS** (Bed sores) [881]: Act of lying down.

**DELIRIUM** [605]: Mental aberration due to disease.

**DELIRIUM TREMENS** [605]: Delirium due to cessation or reduction in alcohol consumption. In alcoholics with 10 yrs. or more of heavy drinking.

**DELUSIONS** [608]: False judgement of objective things with a firm belief in it.

**DEMENTIA** [606]: Profound mental incapacity.

**DENGUE** [869]: An acute self limiting disease. Symptoms of fever, prostration, headache, myalgia, rash, lymphadenopathy and leucopenia appear.

**DENTITION** [680]: The cutting of teeth, and the period of the same.

**DERMATALGIA** [881]: Neuralgia of the skin.

**DIABETES MELLITUS** [748]: An excessive flow of sugar containing urine.

**DIABETES, INSIPIDUS** [741]: Polyuria.

**DIABETES**: A disease characterized by an excessive flow of urine.

**DIAPHRAGMITIS** [720]: Inflammation of the diaphragm.

**DIARRHEA, ACUTE** [720]: (Diarrhea: morbidly frequent evacuation of the bowels.)

**DIARRHEA, CHRONIC** [720]

**DIARRHEA, TEETHING** [722]: Diarrhea during dentition.

**DIPHTHERIA** [684]: An infectious, depressing disease with a membranous exudation on the mucous membranes, commonly on the fauces, and often ending fatally.

**DIPLOPIA** [647]: Double vision.

**DISSECTING WOUNDS** [907]

**DREAMS** [846]: Thoughts and images experienced in sleep; any imaginary vision.

**DROPSY** [902]: An effusion of fluid into the intercellular space or cavities of the body.

**DROWSINESS** [844]: (Drowsy: Heavy with sleepiness.)

**DRUGS, ABUSE** [697]

**DUODENITIS** [727]: Inflammation of the duodenum.

**DYSENTERY** [727]: Inflammation and ulceration of the intestinal mucous membrane with bloody evacuations.

**DYSMENORRHEA** [766]: Painful menstruation.

**DYSPEPSIA** [696]: Impaired digestion.

**DYSPHAGIA** [685]: An inability to swallow.

**DYSPNEA** [806]: Difficult or labored breathing.

**DYSPNEA, CARDIAC** [810]: Labored breathing due to heart disease.

**DYSURIA** [741]: Difficult or painful micturition.

**EARACHE** (Otalgia) [652]

**ECCHYMOSES** [881]: An extravasation of blood into areolar tissue.

**ECLAMPSIA** (Convulsion) [775]: A convulsive or epileptiform seizure occurring in women during pregnancy, labor or puerperium.

**ECLAMPSIA, PUERPERAL** [776]

**ECTHYMA** [881]: An ulcerative pyoderma usually caused by group A beta hemolytic streptococci at the site of minor trauma. Heals with scar formation.

**ECTROPION** [639]: Eversion of the eyelid, or endometrium.

**ECZEMA** [881]: Inflammation of the skin with exudation of lymph. Tetter. Salt rheum.

**EDEMA** [882, 902]: Accumulation of serum in the cellular tissue.

**EDEMA, LARYNX** [800]

**EDEMA, LUNGS** [803]

**EDEMA, PEDES** [830]: Edema of lower extremities.

**ELEPHANTIASIS** [882]: A chronic edematous disease of the skin with hypertrophy of the cellular tissue.

**EMISSIONS** [754]: An ejaculation.

**EMPHYSEMA** [803]: Distention of the tissues with air or other gases.

**EMPYEMA** [805]: Pus in the pleural cavity.

**ENCEPHALITIS LETHARGICA** [860]: An epidemic form. A peculiar epidemic disease characterized by increasing languor, apathy, drowsiness, passing onto lethargy.

**ENCEPHALITIS:** Inflammation of the brain.

**ENDOCARDITIS** [811]: Inflammation of the endocardium.

**ENDOCARDIUM:** The transparent lining membrane of the heart.

**ENDOCERVICITIS** [779]: Inflammation of the mucosa of cervix uteri.

**ENDOMETRITIS** [781]: Inflammation of the endometrium.

**ENDOMETRIUM:** Lining membrane of the uterus.

**ENTERALGIA** [710]: Pain in the bowels.

**ENTERITIS, ACUTE** [720]: Inflammation of the intestine.
**ENTERITIS, CHRONIC** [720]
**ENTROPION** [639]: Inversion of the margins of the eyelids.
**ENURESIS** [734]: Incontinence of urine.
**EPHELIS** (Sunburn) [882]: A freckle.
**EPIDIDYMIS:** A small body attached to the posterior border of the testis.
**EPIDIDYMITIS** [757]: Inflammation of the epididymis.
**EPILEPSY** (Grand mal) [841]: A nervous disease with loss of consciousness, and tonic and clonic convulsions.
**EPIPHORA** [641]: An overflow of tears.
**EPISTAXIS** (Nose bleed) [655]: Hemorrhage from the nose.
**EPITHELIOMA** [882]: A cancerous growth of the skin.
**EROTOMANIA** [610]: Insanely uncontrollable sexual passion.
**ERUCTATIONS** [698]: Belching.
**ERYSIPELAS** [883]: An acute specific inflammation of the skin and subcutaneous tissues, accompanied by fever and constitutional disturbances.
**ERYTHEMA** [883]: Non-contagious superficial hyperemia of the cutaneous surface; redness and swelling of the skin.
**ERYTHEMA NODOSUM** [883]: This form is usually ushred in with chills, fever, rheumatic pains, gastric disturbances.
**ESOPHAGUS, AFFECTIONS** [684]: Affections of the canal from the pharynx to the stomach.
**EUSTACHIAN DEAFNESS** [650]: Hearing loss due to a defect in the eustachian canal.
**EUSTACHIAN TUBE:** The canal from the tympanum to the pharynx.
**EYELIDS, AFFECTIONS** [639]
**FACE, ERUPTIONS** [665]
**FAINTING** [816]: Swooning; syncope.
**FALSE LABOR PAINS** [776]
**FATTY DEGENERATION** [902]: The conversion of an organ into oil.
**FEARS** [606]
**FEBRICULA** [873]: A mild fever of short duration. Indefinite origin or pathology.
**FELON** (Whitlow) [894]: Infection of a finger usually terminating in an abscess; paronychia.
**FEVER** [863]: Rise in body temperature, with associated symptoms.
**FIBROID TUMORS** [783]: (Fibroma: A tumor of fibrous tissue.)
**FISSURES** [883]: A groove or cleft
**FISSURES, ANUS** [715]: A linear ulcer at the margin of the anus.

**FISTULA IN ANO** [715]: An opening near the anus that may or may not communicate with the bowel.
**FISTULA LACHRYMALIS** [641]: An abnormal passage communicating with the lachrymal sac or duct.
**FISTULA, DENTALIS** [681]
**FISTULA:** An abnormal tube, like a passage in the body between two internal organs or from an internal organ to the surface of the body.
**FLATULENCE** [713]: The presence of gas in the digestive canal.
**FLOATING KIDNEY** [737]: A movable or misplaced kidney.
**FRACTURE** [896]: The breaking of a bone.
**FRECKLES** (Lentigo) [885]: A benign, small, tan to brown macule occurring on the skin exposed to the sun usually in children, fading in adult life.
**FRIGHT, ILL EFFECTS** [606]
**FUNGUS HEMATODES** [884]: A bleeding and ulcerated vascular tumor.
**FURUNCLE** (Boil) [884]: A boil; a circumscribed abscess.
**GAIT, DISORDERS** [831]
**GAIT:** A mode of walking or running
**GALACTORRHEA** [778]: An excessive flow of milk.
**GALL COLIC** [728]
**GALL STONES** [728]: Calcareous concretions in the gall bladder and its ducts.
**GANGLION** [837]: An encysted tumor on a tendon or on an aponeurosis.
**GANGRENE** [884]: The mortification or death of soft tissue.
**GAS FUMES, ILL EFFECTS** [902]
**GASTRALGIA** [696]: Pain in the stomach.
**GASTRIC FEVER** [873]: Fever with gastric derangement.
**GASTRIC ULCER** [705]: An ulcer on the gastric or duodenal mucosa.
**GASTRITIS, ACUTE** [700]: (Gastritis: Inflammation of the stomach.)
**GASTRITIS, CHRONIC** [700]
**GASTROENTERITIS** [700]: Inflammation of the stomach and bowel.
**GLANDERS** [903]: Disease of horses, often transmitted to man.
**GLANDS, AFFECTIONS** [903]: (Gland: A secreting organ; a lymphatic node.)
**GLANDS, SWOLLEN** [904]
**GLAUCOMA** [640]: A disease of the eye, characterized by increased intraocular tension.
**GLEET** [750]: Chronic stage of gonorrhea with mucopurulent discharge.
**GLOSSITIS** [677]: Inflammation of the tongue.
**GOITRE** [905]: An enlargement of the thyroid gland.
**GOITRE, EXOPTHALMIC** [854, 905]: Goitre with abnormal protrusion of eyeballs and cardiac palpitation; Basedow's disease.

**GONORRHEA** (Specific urethritis) [750, 759]: A contagious inflammation with a purulent discharge from the genitals. A sexually transmitted disease.

**GOUT** [833]: A disease associated with joint inflammation, swelling especially of the big toe with high uric acid in the blood.

**GRAVEL** [747]: A sand-like deposit in the urine.

**GRIEF, ILL EFFECTS OF** [606]

**GROWING PAINS** [821]: Neuralgic pains in the limbs during youth, growing years.

**GUM AFFECTIONS** [679]

**GUM BOIL** [679]: An abscess of the jaw; parulis.

**HAIR, DISORDERS** [630]

**HALITOSIS** [671]: Foul breath.

**HALOPHAGIA** [899]: Abuse of salt.

**HAMSTRING, CONTRACTIONS** [832]: Contractions of the tendons which form the sides of the ham (the back part of thigh), behind the knee.

**HAY FEVER** [657]: Seasonal disease of nasal mucous membrane, with coryza. Allergic.

**HEADACHE, ANEMIC** [619]: Due to anemia.

**HEADACHE, CHRONIC** [619]: Long standing with a tendency to recur.

**HEADACHE, CONGESTIVE** [619]: Headache ascribed to hyperemia or congestion.

**HEADACHE, NERVOUS** [620]

**HEADACHE, SICK** [620]: A headache accompanied by a stomach disorder.

**HEADACHES** [618]: Pain in the head.

**HEART AFFECTIONS** [809]

**HEART DILATATION** [810]

**HEART FAILURE** [810]

**HEART, FATTY DEGENERATION** [810]: Fatty degeneration of the muscular fibres of the heart; increase in the quantity of subpericardial fat.

**HEART, HYPERTROPHY** [811]: Abnormal enlargement of the heart.

**HEARTBURN** (Pyrosis) [699]: A burning sensation the epigastrium and lower part of chest due to hyperchlorhydria.

**HECTIC FEVER** [873]: The protracted fever of phthisis.

**HEMATEMESIS** [696]: The vomiting of blood.

**HEMATURIA** [745]: Blood in urine.

**HEMICRANIA** [620]: Migraine; neuralgia of half the head.

**HEMIOPIA** [647]: Blindness of one-half of the visual field.

**HEMIPLEGIA** [843]: Paralysis of one side of the body.

**HEMOGLOBINURIA** [747] : The presence of hemoglobin in urine.

**HEMOPHILIA** [905]: Abnormal tendency to hemorrhage. Hereditory disease.

**HEMOPTYSIS** [803]: The spitting of blood.

**HEMORRHAGES** [905]: A flow of blood.

**HEMORRHOIDS** [728]: Piles. A varicose dilatation of a vein resulting from a persistant increase in venous pressure in the anus.

**HEPATITIS** [731]: Inflammation of the liver.

**HERNIA** [730]: The protrusion of a viscus from its normal position through an abnormal opening.

**HERPES** [884]: A skin disease with patches of distinct vesicles along the course of a nerve. An acute, non-contagious, inflammatory disease, characterized by clusters of vesicles on a hyperemic base with burning and severe pain.

**HERPES LABIALIS** [671]: Herpes on the lips.

**HERPES ZOSTER** (Shingles) [885]: An acute typical inflammatory disease of the skin, appearing in the course of certain cutaneous nerves, accompanied by severe neuralgic pains, and by the presence of groups of firm, tense vesicles rising from an edematous base.

**HICCOUGH** [696]: A spasmodic inspiration suddenly arrested by an involuntary closure of the glottis.

**HIP JOINT DISEASE** [835]: A tubercular lesion of the hip joint.

**HIVES** (Urticaria) [892]: A vesicular cutaneous eruption.

**HOARSENESS** [802]: Roughness and hoarseness in the voice.

**HODGKIN'S DISEASE** (Pseudoleukemia) [906]: A form of malignant lymphoma characterised by painless, progressive enlargement of the lymph nodes, spleen and general lymphoid tissue.

**HOME SICKNESS** (Nostalgia) [606]: Longing for home.

**HOOKWORM DISEASE** [906]: Ankylostomiasis (an ailment marked by progressive anemia and digestive disturbances.)

**HOUSEMAID'S KNEE** [835]: An inflammation of the patellar bursa.

**HYDARTHROSIS** [832]: White swelling; a serous effusion in a joint.

**HYDROA** [885]: Certain vesicular or bulbous eruptions with erythematous lesions.

**HYDROCELE** [753]: A collection of serum in the tunica vaginalis or in connection with the testicle or cord.

**HYDROCEPHALUS** [628]: A collection of water in the head. Dropsy of the brain.

**HYDROPHOBIA** [607]: Fear of water; a symptom of rabies.

**HYDROTHORAX** [805]: Dropsy of the chest.

**HYGROMA PATELLA** [835]

**HYGROMA:** A serous cyst.

**HYPERCHLORHYDRIA** [696]: An excess of gastric hydrochloric acid. Acidity.

**HYPERIDROSIS** [868]: Excessive sweating.

**HYPERMETROPIA** [647]: Far sightedness; an abnormal refraction of the eye due to a short anterio-posterior diameter, the focus of parallel rays of light being behind the retina.

**HYPERTROPHY OF HEART** [811]: Abnormal enlargement of the heart.

**HYPOCHONDRIASIS** [607]: Extreme depression with morbid anxiety regarding the health.

**HYSTERALGIA** [782]: Pain in the womb.

**HYSTERIA** [607]: A functional neurosis with abnormal sensations, emotions or paroxysms.

**ICHTHYOSIS** [885]: Fish skin disease, a chronic cutaneous hypertrophy and induration, with scale formation

**IMPACTED BOWELS** [730]: Overloaded and obstructed intestines.

**IMPETIGO** [885]: An acute pustular disease of the skin, characterised by the formation of discrete, round or oval pustules, situated on a slightly inflamed base.

**IMPOTENCE** [751]: Lack of sexual power.

**INCUBUS** (Nightmare) [845]: Oppression with horror during sleep.

**INDIGESTION** [696]: Dyspepsia.

**INFANTILE PARALYSIS** [843]: Acute anterior poliomylitis.

**INFLAMMATION** [906]: A morbid condition with hyperemia, pain, heat, swelling and disordered function.

**INFLUENZA** (Grippe) [873]: A contagious epidemic catarrhal fever with great prostration and varying symptoms and sequele.

**INFRAMAMMARY PAINS** [762]: (Inframammary: below the mammae.)

**INGROWN TOE NAIL** [886]

**INJURIES** [906]: Damage or harm to the body.

**INSANITY** (See Dementia, Mania, Melancholia) [609]: Mental derangement; madness

**INSECT BITES** [900]

**INSOMNIA** [845]: Inability to sleep.

**INTERMITTENT FEVER** [873]: A fever with periods of apyrexia.

**INTERTRIGO** (Chafing) [883]: Erythema from friction.

**INTUSSUSCEPTION** [730]: Slipping of one part of intestine into another.

**IRITIS** [640]: Inflammation of the iris.

**ISCHURIA** (Retention of urine) [742]: Retention or suppression of urine.

**JAUNDICE** [730]: A syndrome characterised by hyperbilirubinemia and deposition of bile pigment in the skin mucous membrane and sclera, resulting in a yellowish appearance of the patient.

**JAUNDICE, INFANTILE** [730]

**JAWS, AFFECTION** [666]

**KELOID** [885]: A sharply elevated, irregularly shaped, progressively enlarging scar due to the formation of excess collagen during connective tissue repair.

**KERATITIS** [636]: Inflammation of the cornea.

**KIDNEYS, CALCULI** [736]

**KIDNEYS, CONGESTION** [737]

**KIDNEYS, FLOATING** [737]: Loosened and displaced kidney.

**KIDNEYS, INFLAMMATION** [737]

**LABOR** [775]: Parturition; bringing forth of the young.

**LABYRINTHINE AFFECTIONS** [651]: (Labyrinth: the cavities of the internal ear, comprising of the vestibule, cochlea, and semicircular canals.)

**LACHRYMAL FISTULA** [641]: (Lachrimal: pertaining to tears.)

**LACHRYMAL SAC, INFLAMMATION** [641]: (Lachrimal sac: the dilated upper portion of the lacrimal duct storing tears.)

**LACHRYMATION** [641]: An excessive secretion of tears.

**LACTATION** [778]: The formation or secretion of milk; at the time of suckling.

**LAGOPHTHALMOS** [641]: An inability to close the eyes.

**LANDRY'S PARALYSIS** [843]: Acute ascending paralysis.

**LARYNGISMUS STRIDULUS** [801]: Spasmodic contracture of the glottis.

**LARYNGITIS, ACUTE** [800]: (Laryngitis: Inflammation of the larynx.)

**LARYNGITIS, CHRONIC** [800]

**LARYNGITIS, TUBERCULAR** [801]

**LEAD COLIC** [710]: Colic from lead poisoning.

**LENTIGO** (Freckles) [885]: Circumscribed spots on the skin, like freckles, but histologically distinct from it due to the presence of an increased number of normal appearing melanocytes along the dermo epidermal junction. Do not darken on exposure to sunlight.

**LEPROSY** [885]: An endemic, chronic, malignant disease with cutaneous and other lesions, due to Bacillus leprae.

**LEUCOCYTHEMIA** [907]: An abnormal increase in the number of white blood corpuscles, with glandular enlargement.

**LEUCODERMA** [885]: A condition of defective pigmentation of the skin, especially congenital absence of pigment in patches.

**LEUCORRHEA** [759]: A whitish, viscid discharge from the vagina and uterine cavity.

**LICHEN** [885]: A papular skin disease in which the lesions are typically small, firm papules which are usually set very close together.

**LIENTERIA** [725]: (Lientery: diarrhea with undigested food.)

**LIPOMA** [910]: A fatty tumor.

**LIPS, AFFECTIONS** [671]

**LITHEMIA LITHIASIS** [747]: (Lithemia: an excess of uric acid in the blood. Lithiasis: the formation of calculi in the body.)

**LIVER SPOTS** (Chloasma) [880].
**LIVER, FATTY** [731]: Marked with fatty degeneration and infiltration.
**LIVER, ACUTE YELLOW ATROPHY** [731]
**LIVER, CANCER** [731]
**LIVER, CIRRHOSIS** [731]
**LIVER, CONGESTION** [731]
**LIVER, HYPERTROPHY** [731]: Abnormal enlargement of the liver.
**LIVER, INFLAMMATION** [731]
**LOCHIA, DISORDERS** [777]: (Lochia: a vaginal discharge after labor.)
**LOCOMOTOR ATAXIA** [861]: Disease of the posterior columns of spinal cord.
**LOW FEVERS** [878]
**LUMBAGO** [826]: Pain in the lower part of the back.
**LUNG, PARALYSIS** [804]
**LUNGS, CONGESTION** [803]
**LUNGS, INFLAMMATION CROUPOUS** [804]
**LUNGS, INFLAMMATION, CATARRHAL** [804]
**LUNGS, EDEMA** [803]
**LUPUS** [886]: Localised destruction or degenration of the skin caused by various cutaneous diseases.
**LYING-IN PERIOD** [776]: Being in child-birth.
**LYMPHANGITIS** [907]: Inflammation of the lymphatics.
**MALARIA** [873]: An infectious disease caused by a protosoan parasite which is transmitted by mosquitoes, characterised with periodic fever and chills.
**MALNUTRITION** [902]: Poor nutrition.
**MAMMARY GLANDS, AFFECTIONS** [762]: Affections of the milk secreting glands.
**MANIA** [609]: Delirium or madness.
**MANIA-A-POTU** [605]: Delirium tremens; delirium due to alcoholic poisoning.
**MARASMUS** [907]: Wasting or emaciation.
**MASTITIS** [762]: Inflammation of the breast.
**MASTODYNIA** [762]: Pain in the breast.
**MASTOID, AFFECTIONS** [651]: (Mastoid: shaped like a breast, as the mastoid process pertaining to the mastical process.)
**MASTURBATION, ILL EFFECTS** [751]: (Masturbation: causing venereal orgasm by the hand.)
**MEASLES** (Rubeola) [870]: An exhanthematous contagious disease in children.
**MEGRIM** (Migraine) [620]: A paroxysmal headache, usually unilateral, attended with gastric and visual disturbances.

**MELANCHOLIA** [610]: Depression of spirits; gloominess.
**MENIERE'S DISEASE** [632]: Hearing loss, tinnitus and vertigo resulting from non suppurative disease of the labyrinth.
**MENINGITIS** [617]: Inflammation of the meninges.
**MENINGITIS, CEREBRO SPINAL** [617]: That affecting the membranes of the brain and cord.
**MENINGITIS, SPINAL** [861]: That affecting the membranes of the spinal cord.
**MENINGITIS, TUBERCULAR** [617]: A severe bacterial meningitis caused by Mycobacterium tuberculosis, usually spreading from a primary lesion in the lungs.
**MENOPAUSE** [763]: Cessations of the menstrual or reproductive life.
**MENORRHAGIA** [766]: Profuse menstrual flow.
**MENSTRUATION, DELAYED** [764]
**MENSTRUATION, PAINFUL** [765]
**MENSTRUATION, PROFUSE** [766]
**MENSTRUATION, SUPPRESSED** [765]
**MENSTRUATION** [764]: Monthly discharge of bloody fluid from the womb between puberty and the menopause.
**METRITIS** [781]: Inflammation of the uterus.
**METRITIS, CHRONIC** [782]
**METRORRHAGIA** [780]: Uterine hemorrhage between menstrual periods.
**MILIARIA** (Prickly heat) [886]: Sudamina; a disorder of the sweat glands with obstruction of their ducts.
**MILK FEVER** [777]: Fever attending the establishment of lactation after delivery.
**MILK LEG** (Phlegmasia alba dolens) [778]: An acute edema, especially of the leg, from venous obstruction.
**MISCARRIAGE, HABIT** [774]: Tendency to expulsion of the fetus between the fourth and the sixth months of pregnancy; abortion.
**MISCARRIAGE, THREATENDED** [774]
**MODALITIES** [911]
**MOLLITIES OSSIUM** [897]: Osteomalacia. (Mollities: softness.)
**MOODS** [611]
**MORNING SICKNESS** [775]: Morning nausea and vomiting of pregnancy.
**MORPHINISM** [854]: The morbid state produced by the excessive use of morphine.
**MORVAN'S DISEASE** [854]: A form of syringomyelia. (Syringomyelus: an abnormal dilatation of the central canal of the spinal cord.
**MOUNTAIN SICKNESS** [902]: A condition marked by dyspnea, nausea, rapid pulse and headache, due to rarified air at high altitude.

**MUMPS** [904]: An acute infectious disease marked by swelling of the parotid glands.

**MUSCAE VOLITANTES** [648]: Floating spots in the visual field.

**MUSHROOM POISONING** [902]

**MUTINISM** [908]: (Mute: dumb; without the power of speech.)

**MYALGIA** [908]: Pain in the muscles.

**MYELITIS** [861]: Inflammation of the spinal cord.

**MYOCARDITIS** [811]: Inflammation of the cardiac muscular tissue.

**MYOPIA** [647]: Near sightedness

**MYOSITIS** [908]: Inflammation of the muscle tissue.

**MYXEDEMA** [908]: Due to decrease or absence of thyroid hormone; characterized by a sallow, puffy appearance, low metabolic rate, increased sensitivity to cold, dryness of skin, absence of sweating, brittle nails and hair, lethargy and apathy.

**NAILS, AFFECTIONS** [886]

**NAUSEA** [700]: Desire to vomit.

**NECROSIS** [896]: The death of a circumscribed piece of tissue.

**NEPHRALGIA** [738]: Pain in the kidney.

**NEPHRITIS, ACUTE** [737]: Acute inflammation of kidneys.

**NEPHRITIS, CHRONIC** [738]: Chronic inflammation of the kidneys.

**NEPHROLITHIASIS** [736]: Formation of renal stone.

**NEURALGIA** [856]: Pain in a nerve.

**NEURALGIA, BRACHIAL** [857]: Pain in the arm.

**NEURALGIA, CILIARY** [635, 857]

**NEURALGIA, FACIAL** [667]

**NEURALGIA, GASTRIC** [702]

**NEURALGIA, INTERCOSTAL** [857]

**NEURALGIA, SCIATIC** [857]: (Sciatica: neuralgia of the sciatic nerve.)

**NEURALGIA, SPERMATIC CORD** [754, 857]

**NEURALGIA, SUPRAORBITAL** [643, 857]: Nerve pain above the bony cavity of the eyeball.

**NEURALGIA, UTERINE** [782]

**NEURASTHENIA** [855]: Exhaustion of nerve-force.

**NEURITIS** [856]: Inflammation of a nerve.

**NEVUS** [886]: A birth mark.

**NIGHT SWEATS** [868]: Excessive sweating at night.

**NIGHT TERRORS** [614]: Excessive nightmares, especially in children.

**NIPPLES, AFFECTIONS** [762]

**NIPPLES, ULCERATED** [762]

**NODES** [897]: A small mass of tissue in the form of a swelling, knot or protuberance, either normal or pathological.

**NODOSITIES, TOPHI** [833]: (Tophi: calcareous deposits in gout, generally around joints, in cartilage bone, tissue and extenal ear.)

**NOSE EXTERNAL, AFFECTIONS** [654]

**NOSTALGIA** [606]: Home sickness.

**NYCTALOPIA** [646]: Night blindness.

**NYMPOMANIA** [771]: Excessive sexual desire in women.

**OBESITY** [908]: Fatness; corpulence.

**ODONTALGIA** (Toothache) [681]

**ONYCHIA** [886]: Chronic inflammation of matrix of a nail.

**OPHTHALMIA** [642]: Severe inflammation of the eye or the conjunctiva or deeper structures of the eye.

**OPTIC NEURITIS** [642]: Inflammation of the optic nerve.

**OPTICAL ILLUSIONS** [647]

**ORCHITIS** [757]: Inflammation of the testicle.

**OSTEITIS** [896]: Inflammation of bone.

**OSTEOMYELITIS** [896]: Inflammation of the bone caused by a pyogenic organism. It may remain localised or may spread to the entire bone.

**OTITIS MEDIA, ACUTE** [652]: Acute inflammation of the middle ear.

**OTITIS MEDIA, CHRONIC** [652]: Chronic inflammation of the middle ear.

**OTORRHEA** [652]: A discharge from the external auditory meatus.

**OVARALGIA** [772]: Pain in an ovary.

**OVARIAN CYST** [771]

**OVARITIS** [771]: Inflammation of an ovary.

**OXALURIA** [747]: The presence of calcium oxalate in urine.

**OXYURIS** [733]: A genus of nematode worms.

**OZENA** [660]: Atrophic rhinitis marked by a thick muco purulent discharge, mucosal crusting and fetor.

**PALATE, AFFECTIONS** [673]: Affection of the roof of the mouth and floor of the nose.

**PALPITATION** [812]: Violent pulsation of the heart.

**PANARITIUM** (Felon's whitlow) [894]: An extremely painful abscess on the palmer aspect of the fingertip, as a result of infection in the closed space of the terminal phalanx.

**PANCREAS, AFFECTIONS** [732]: Affection of the racemose gland in the abdomen.

**PANNUS** [645]: Superficial vascularization of the cornea with infilteration of granulation tissue.

**PARALYIS, LEAD** [843]: Paralysis due to lead poisoning, peripheral neuritis, marked by wrist drop.

**PARALYSIS** [843]: Loss or impairment of motor function in a part due to a lesion in the neural or muscular mechanism. Also impairment of sensory function.

**PARALYSIS AGITANS** [843]: Paralysis with constant tremor of the muscles, mask like facies, slowing of voluntary movements, festinating gait, peculiar posture and weakness of muscles. Usually occuring late in life. Parkinsonism of unknown etiology.

**PARALYSIS INFANTILE** (Poliomyelitis) [843]: Acute anterior poliomyletis, a disease marked by sudden paralysis of one or more limbs or of individual muscle groups, followed by rapid wasting of the affected parts.

**PARALYSIS, ACUTE ASCENDING** [843]: A form of paralysis marked by loss of motor power in the legs, gradually extending upward.

**PARALYSIS, FACIAL** (Bell's Palsy) [667, 843]: Unilateral facial paralysis due to lesion of the facial nerve.

**PARALYSIS, GENERAL OF INSANE** [843]

**PARALYSIS, HEMIPLEGIA** [843]: Paralysis of one side of the body.

**PARALYSIS, HYSTERICAL** [843]: Paralysis associated with hysteria, apparent loss of power for movement in a part, in the absence of an organic lesion.

**PARALYSIS, LANDRY** [843]: Acute ascending paralysis, acute idiopathic polyneuritis.

**PARALYSIS, PARAPLEGIA** [844]: Paralysis of the legs.

**PARALYSIS, PNEUMOGASTRIC** [804]: (Pneumogastric: pertaining to the lungs and the stomach.)

**PARALYSIS, POST-DIPHTHERITIC** [844]: A form of paralysis sometimes following diphtheria; it is primarily a multiple neuritis, due to the toxin of diphtheria.

**PARALYSIS, SPINAL** [843]

**PARALYSIS, TYPISTS, PIANISTS** [843]: Paralysis in typists and pianists.

**PARAPLEGIA** [844]: Paralysis of the legs.

**PARAPLEGIA, SPASTIC** [844]: Lateral sclerosis.

**PAROTITIS** (Mumps) [904]: Inflammation of the parotid.

**PELLAGRA** [887]: A clinical deficiency syndrome, due to deficiency of niacin, characterized by digestive disturbances, skin lesions, and nervous symptoms. Now said to be a deficiency disease.

**PELVIC, AFFECTIONS** [773]

**PELVIC, CELLULITIS** [773]

**PEMPHIGUS** [887]: A chronic skin disease characterized by a successive formation of irregularly scattered, variously sized vescicles and bullae.

**PENIS, AFFECTIONS** [751]: Affections of the male organ of copulation.

**PERICARDITIS** [811]: Inflammation of the pericardium.

**PERIOSTITIS** [897]: Inflammation of the periostium.

**PERITONITIS** [732]: Inflammation of the peritonium (serous membrane lining the abdomen.)

**PERITYPHILITIS** [732]: Inflammation of the peritonium surrounding the caecum.

**PERTUSSIS** (Whooping cough) [796]: A contagious convulsive cough.

**PETICHIAE** [887]: A small pin point ecchymosis under the skin.

**PETIT MAL** [844]: Absence of seizures, usually has the onset at childhood or adolecence.

**PHARYNGITIS, ACUTE** [687]: Acute inflammation of the pharynx.

**PHARYNGITIS, CHRONIC** [687]: The result of repeated, acute attacks of pharyngitis, with hypertrophy of the mucous membrane.

**PHARYNGITIS, FOLLICULAR** [687]: (Follicle: a small secretory cavity or sac). Sore throat with enlargement of the pharyngeal glands.

**PHARYNGITIS, SICCA** [687]: The chronic form with a dry state of mucous membrane.

**PHIMOSIS, PARAPHIMOSIS** [752]: Stenosis of the preputial orifice.

**PHLEBITIS** [816]: Inflammation of a vein.

**PHLEGMASIA ALBA DOLENS** [778]: An acute edema, especially of the leg, from venous obstruction; milk leg.

**PHOBIAS** [606]: Fears.

**PHOSPHATURIA** [748]: The presence of phosphates in urine.

**PHOTOPHOBIA** [645]: A hyperesthetic sensitiveness to light.

**PHTHISIS** [804]: Pulmonary tuberculosis.

**PHTHISIS, LARYNGEAL** [801]: Laryngeal tuberculosis.

**PICA** (Craving) [693]: A depraved appetite for unnatural food.

**PITYRIASIS** [887]: A scaly skin disease with hypopigmented patches, usually involving the face especially the cheeks and the area around the mouth.

**PLACENTA, RETAINED** [776]: (Placenta: a feto-maternal organ joining the mother and offspring, providing the fetus nourishment and removing the wastes.)

**PLAGUE** [898]: A contagious, malignant, epidemic disease transmitted by the bite of a rat flea.

**PLEURISY** [805]: Inflammation of the pleura.

**PLEURODYNIA** [790]: Pain in the intercostal muscles.

**PLICA POLONICA** [629]: Verminous matting of hair.

**PNEUMONIA CROUPOUS** [804]: Lobar pneumonia, generally due to a specific microorganism.

**PNEUMONIA, CATARRHAL** [804]: Broncho-pneumonia.

**PNEUMONIA:** Inflammation of the lungs.

**POISON OAK, ANTIDOTES** [902]

**POLIOMYELITIS, ANTERIOR** [843]: Acute inflammation of the anterior horns of the gray matter in the spinal cord.

**POLIOMYELITIS**: Inflammation of the gray matter in the cord.

**POLYCHROME SPECTRA** [647]: (Polychromatic: many colored.)

**POLYPI** [910]: A pedunculated tumor found in the nose, ear, rectum, etc.

**POLYPI, NASAL** [657]

**POLYPI, UTERINE** [783]

**POLYURIA** [741]: Excessive secretion of urine, characteristic of diabetes.

**PORTAL CONGESTION** [816]: Congestion of the portal vein, the vein carrying blood to the liver.

**POST- PARTUM HEMORRHAGE** [776]: Hemorrhage after labor.

**POST-NASAL AFFECTIONS** [660]

**POST-OPERATIVE DISORDERS** [906]

**PREGNANCY, DISORDERS** [773]

**PRIAPISM** [751]: Painful erection of the penis.

**PROCITITIS** [715]: Inflammation of the rectum.

**PROLAPSUS ANI** [716]: (Prolapsus: falling down of a part.)

**PROLAPSUS UTERI** [780]

**PROPHYLACTICS** [909]: Pertaining to the prevention of a disease.

**PROSOPALGIA** (Face ache) [667]: Tic douloureux; spasmodic facial neuralgia.

**PROSTATE AFFECTIONS** [752]: Affections of the glandular body situated around the neck of the bladder in a male.

**PROSTATE, HYPERTROPHY** [752]: Hypertrophy of the prostate gland.

**PROSTATITIS** [752]: Inflammation of the prostate gland.

**PRURIGO** [887]: A chronic papular skin disease with intense itching.

**PRURITUS VULVAE** [784]: Intense itching of vulva.

**PRURITUS** [887]: Intense itching.

**PRURITUS ANI** [715]: Intense itching of anus.

**PSORIASIS** [888]: A chronic inflammatory skin disease with scale formation.

**PTERYGIUM** [645]: A chronic thickening of the conjunctiva, usually triangular and situated at the inner canthus.

**PTOMAINE POISONING** [902]: (Ptomaina: a crystallizable, nitrogenous basic substance, produced by bacteria in dead animals or vegetable matter.)

**PTOSIS** [639]: Drooping of the upper eyelid due to paralysis.

**PTYALISM** (Salivation) [673]: An excessive secretion of saliva.

**PUERPERIUM DISORDERS** (Lying-in period) [777]: The period from delivery to the completion of involution.

**PULMONARY EDEMA** [803]: Edema of the lungs.

**PULSE DISTURBANCES** [814]: Disturbances of the expansile impulse of the arteries.

**PUPILS, CONTRACTED** (Myosis) [645]: Abnormally small pupils.
**PUPILS, DILATED** (Mydriasis) [645]: Dilatation of the pupil.
**PURPURA** [889]: Small hemorrhages about 1 cm in diameter on the skin, mucous membrane or serosal surface. It maybe caused by various factors like blood disorders, vascular abnormalities, trauma, etc.
**PURPURA HEMORRHAGICA** [889]: A grave form of purpura with mucous hemorrhages, thrombocytopenic.
**PURPURA RHEUMATICA** [889]: A form of purpura with fever and rheumatic pains.
**PYELITIS** [739]: Inflammation of the pelvis of the kidney.
**PYEMIA** [909]: A condition in which pyogenic bacteria circulate in the blood, and form abscesses wherever they lodge.
**PYLORUS, AFFECTIONS** [704]: Affections at the opening of the stomach into the duodenum.
**PYORRHEA ALVEOLARIS** [679]: Progressive necrosis of the dental alveoli, periodontitis.
**PYROSIS** [699]: Gastric burning pain with eructations; heartburn.
**PYURIA** [748]: Presence of pus in urine.
**QUINSY** [690]: Peritonsillar abscess.
**RACHITIS** [909]: Rickets. Inflammatory disease of the vertebral column.
**RANULA** [676]: A cystic tumor beneath the tongue.
**RAYNAUD'S DISEASE** [889]: Intermittent, bilateral attacks of ischemia in fingers and toes, sometimes ears and nose, marked by severe pallor, paresthesia and pain. Brought on by cold or emotional stimuli. Relieved by heat.
**RECTAL POCKETS** [715]
**RECTUM, AFFECTIONS** [714]: Affections of the lower part of the large intestines.
**REFLEXES, DISTURBANCES** [836]: (Reflex: an involuntary action from nerve stimulus.)
**RELAPSING FEVER** [878]: A fever recurring during convalescence.
**REMITTENT FEVER** [878]: Fever alternately abating and returning.
**RENAL COLIC** [738]: Pain due to a calculus in the ureter.
**RETINA, AFFECTIONS** [645]
**RETINITIS** [645]: Inflammation of the retina.
**RETROPHARYNGEAL ABSCESS** [685]: Abscess behind the pharynx.
**RHEUMATIC GOUT** [833]
**RHEUMATISM, ACUTE** [838]: (Rheumatism: disorder with inflammation, degeneration or metabolic derangement of the connective tissue structure of the body, especially the joints and related structures like, bursa, tendons, muscles and fibrous tissues.

**RHEUMATISM, CHRONIC** [840]

**RHEUMATISM, GONORRHEAL** [840]: Arthritis associated with gonorrheal urethritis, frequently producing ankylosis of the joints.

**RHEUMATISM, MUSCULAR** [840]: Muscular pain with or without fever and other rheumatic symptoms.

**RHEUMATISM, PERIOSTEAL** [840]

**RHINITIS, ACUTE** [659]: Inflammation of the nasal mucous membrane; coryza.

**RHINITIS, CHRONIC** [659]

**RHINITIS, SICCA** [659]: Atrophic rhinitis in which the secretion is entirely absent.

**RIGG'S DISEASE** [683]: Pyorrhea alveolaris; progressive necrosis of the dental alveoli, marginal periodontitis.

**RIGID OS** [776]: Rigid mouth of the uterus.

**RING WORM** [890]: Ring shaped configuration of lesions, popular name for tinea.

**ROSE COLD** [657]: Hay fever.

**ROSEOLA** [889]: Rose coloured rash on the skin.

**RUBELLA** (Rolheln) [870]: Infectious fever of childhood, resembling mild measles; German measles.

**RUBEOLA** (Measles) [870]: An exanthematous, contagious disease of children.

**RUPIA** [889]: A syphilitic eruption with dark, encrusted, foul ulcers.

**SALPINGITIS** [779]: Inflammation of a fallopian tube.

**SATYRIASIS** [749]: Excessive, insatiable sexual desire in males.

**SCABIES** [889]: The itch, a contagious parasitic skin disease caused by the itch mite.

**SCALP, AFFECTIONS** [629]: Affections of the integument covering the cranium

**SCARLET FEVER** [871]: An epidemic, exanthematous, contagious disease with fever and a erythematous rash.

**SCIATICA** [857]: Neuralgia of the sciatic nerve.

**SCLERODERMA** [889]: A chronic hardening and thickening of the skin. (Sclerosis: induration and, or hardening of the connective tissue of an organ.)

**SCLEROSIS, MULTIPLE** [861]: Demylination of the white matter. Occasionally extends to the grey matter. Characterised by weakness, incoordination, paraesthesias, speech disturbance and visual complaints.

**SCLEROTIC, AFFECTIONS** [646]: Hard; indurated, Pertaining to the sclera.

**SCROFULOSIS** (Scrofula) [909]: A constitutional condition with glandular tumors and a tuberculous tendency.

**SCROTUM, AFFECTIONS** [753]: Affections of the pouch containing the testes.

**SCURVY** (Scrobutus) [909]: A form of purpura due to deficiency of ascorbic acid.

**SEA SICKNESS** (Mal-de-mer) [854]: Nausea produced by motion in a vessel on sea/ocean.

**SEBACEOUS CYST** [889]: A retention cyst of a sebaceous gland.

**SEBACEOUS**: Pertaining to sebum.

**SEBORRHEA** [889]: Excess secretion of sebum, seborrhic dermatitis.

**SEMINAL VESICULITIS** [753]: Inflammation of the seminal vesicles.

**SENILE DECAY** [909]: Old age.

**SENSATIONS** [909]: A mental condition or a perception arising as the result of the stimulation of an afferent nerve.

**SEPTICEMIA** [909]: An infection characterized by the presence of bacteria in the blood.

**SEPTICEMIA, PUERPERAL** [777]: Infection following childbirth.

**SEPTUM, ULCERATION** [655]

**SINUS AFFECTIONS** [661]: (Sinus: a hollow, cavity, recess or pocket.)

**SLEEPING SICKNESS** [860]: A peculiar epidemic disease caused by the bite of Tsetse fly, characterized by increasing somolence.

**SLEEPLESSNESS** [845]

**SMALL POX** (Variola) [872]: A specific infection with fever and papules followed by vesicles, pustules and pits. Now completely erradicated.

**SMELL, DISORDERS** [661]: (Smell: the perception of odor; the olfactory sense.)

**SNAKE POISON, ANTIDOTES** [900]

**SNEEZING** [661]: An explosive expulsion of air through the nasal passages and mouth.

**SOMNAMBULISM** [616, 849]: Sleep walking.

**SPERMATIC CORD AFFECTIONS** [754]: (Spermatic cord: the suspensory cord of the testes conveying blood, lymph vessels, nerves, and the vas deferens.)

**SPERMATORRHEA** [754]: Involuntary, frequent and excessive discharge of semen.

**SPINAL BIFIDA** [897]: A cleft of the spine, a congenital anomaly.

**SPINAL CORD, CONCUSSION** [860]

**SPINAL CORD, DEGENERATION** [860]: (Degeneration: deterioration in the structure of a tissue.)

**SPINAL CORD, HYPERESTHESIA** [861]

**SPINAL CORD, INFLAMMATION** [861]

**SPINAL CORD, IRRITATION** [861]: A neurasthenic condition with spinal tenderness.

**SPLEEN, AFFECTIONS** [732]: (Spleen: a large ductless gland in the upper part of the abdominal cavity on the left side, lateral to the stomach.

**SPRAINS** [906]: A joint injury in which some fibres of a supporting ligament are ruptured but the continuity of the ligament remains the same.

**STAGE FRIGHT** [607]: Nervous/scared of being on stage.

**STERILITY** [759]: Inability to produce offsprings.

**STOMACH, DILATATION** [696]

**STOMATITIS** [673]: Inflammation of the mouth.

**STRABISMUS** (Squint) [646]: Deviation of the visual axis which cannot be overcome.

**STRANGURY** [743]: Slow and painful discharge of urine due to spasm of the urethra and bladder.

**STROPHULUS** (Tooth rash) [890]: A red papular eruption in infants, papular urticaria.

**STYE** [639]: Hordeolum; furuncle on the eyelid.

**SUB-INVOLUTION** [779]: Imperfect involution, failure of a part to return to its original shape and size after enlargement due to a functional activity, like the subinvolution of the uterus after pregnancy.

**SUDAMINE** [890]: A whitish vesicle caused by retention of sweat in the sudorific ducts or in the layers of epidermis.

**SUPPRESSED ERUPTIONS** [901]

**SUPPRESSED MENSES** [765]

**SUPPRESSED MILK** [778]

**SUPPURATION** [895]: The formation of pus.

**SURGICAL SHOCK** [849]

**SWEAT, DISORDERS** [867]

**SYCOSIS** (Barber's itch) [890]: A chronic inflammation of the hair follicles, especially of the beard.

**SYNCOPE** (Fainting) [816]: Swooning or fainting; a temporary suspension of respiration and circulation.

**SYNOCHAL FEVER** [878]: (Synocha: a continuous fever.)

**SYNOVITIS** [833]: Inflammation of the synovial membrane.

**SYPHILIDAE** [756]: A syphilitic skin disease.

**SYPHILIS** [755]: A chronic, infectious, veneral disease, which may also be hereditory, inducing cutaneous and other lesions, caused by a spirochete, Treponema pallidum.

**SYPHILIS, CONGENITAL** [756]: (Congenital: existing since birth.)

**TABES DORSALIS** (Locomotor ataxia) [861]: Degeneration of the posterior columns of the spinal cord.

**TABES MESENTERICA** [907]: Infantile tuberculosis of the mesenteric glands.

**TACHYCARDIA** (Rapid pulse) [815]: Abnormally rapid cardiac action.

**TAENIA** (Tapeworm) [733]: A flat band or strip of soft tissue.

**TASTE DISORDERS** [678]: Disorders in the sense by which savors are perceived.

**TEETH, AFFECTIONS** [680]

**TENESMUS** [726]: Straining, ineffectual and painful straining at stool or in micturition.

**TENESMUS VESICAE** [736]: Tenesmus of the bladder.

**TESTALGIA** [758]: Pain of the testes.

**TESTES, AFFECTIONS** [757]

**TETANUS** [862]: A disease with spasmodic and continuous contraction of the muscles. A fatally infectious disease caused by Clostridium tetani.

**THIRST** [705]

**TICS** [670]: An involuntary, convulsive, repetitive movement of the face or shoulder, resembling a purposeful movement.

**TINEA** [890]: A skin disease from fungi.

**TINEA VERSICOLOR** [890]: A contagious vegetable parasitic disease of the skin, appearing as an erythematous, scaly patch, occurring anywhere on the body and is due to the microsporon furfur.

**TINNITUS** (Noises in ears) [653]

**TOBACCO ABUSE** [900]

**TONGUE, AFFECTIONS** [675]

**TONSILS, DEPOSITS** [689]: (Tonsil: a glandular, lymphatic organ on each side of the fauces.)

**TONSILS, HYPERTROPHY** [690]

**TONSILS, INFLAMMATION** (Tonsillitis) [690]

**TONSILS, INFLAMMATION, PHLEGMONOUS** (Quinsy) [690]

**TORTICOLLIS** [838]: Contraction of cervical muscles leading to twisting of the neck in an unnatural position of the head.

**TRACHEA, AFFECTIONS** [808]

**TRACHOMA** (Granular lids) [639]: A chronic infectious disease of the conjunctiva and cornea, producing photophobia, pain and lachrymation caused by Chalamydia trachomatis.

**TRAUMATISM** [906]: The physical of psychic state resulting from an injury or wound.

**TRICHINAE** [733]: A genus of Nematode worms.

**TRICHOPHYTOSIS** (Ringworm) [890]: A contagious disease of the skin and hair due to the invasion of Trichophyton, a fungal disease.

**TRISMUS** (Lockjaw) [666]: A spasm of the muscles of mastication.

**TUBERCULOSIS** [804]: An infectious disease due to a Mycobacterium tuberculosis, characterized by the formation of tubercles.

**TUMORS** [910]: A swelling; an abnormal enlargement; A new growth not the result of inflammation.

**TYMPANITES** [713]: Gaseous distention of the abdomen.

**TYPHOID FEVER** [869]: A continuous, acute, infectious fever with intestinal lesions, eruptions, etc.; enteric fever, caused by Salmonella typhi.

**TYPHUS** [878]: Infection by Tickettsial, characterised by severe headache, chills, fever, stupor and papulo-vesicular eruptions.

**ULCER** [890]: A local defect or excavation on the surface of an organ or tissue, produced by the sloughing of inflammatory necrotic tissue.

**UMBILICUS, AFFECTIONS** [733]: Affections to the navel; the round, depressed cicatric in the median line of the abdomen, marking the site of attachment of the umbilical cord in the fetus.

**UREMIA** [738]: Azotemia. Excess of urea, creatinine and other nitrogenous end products in blood.

**URETHRA, AFFECTIONS** [739]: Affections to the excretory canal of the bladder.

**URETHRAL CARUNCLE** [740]

**URETHRAL FEVER** (Catheterism) [878]

**URETHRITIS, SPECIFIC** [750]: Inflammation of the urethra.

**URTICARIA** (Hives) [892]: Nettle rash; a vascular reaction, usually transient, involving the upper dermis with localised edema due to dilatations and increased permeability of capillaries. Marked by the development of wheals.

**UTERUS, AFFECTIONS** [779]: (Uterus: the womb, the female organ of gestation.)

**UTERUS, CANCER** [783]

**UTERUS, DISPLACEMENTS** [780]

**UTERUS, INFLAMMATION** [781]

**UVULA, AFFECTIONS** [691]: Affections of the conic, membranous appendix from the free edge of palate.

**UVULA, ELONGATED** [691]

**VACCINATION, ILL EFFECTS** [902]: (Vaccination: inoculation with vaccine to protect against small pox, protective inoculation with any vaccine.)

**VACCINIA** [893]: Cow pox, a vesicular disease of cows.

**VAGINISMUS** [784]: Painful vaginal spasms.

**VAGINITIS** [784]: Inflammation of the vagina.

**VALVULAR DISEASES** [816]

**VARICELLA** (Chickenpox) [872]: Infectious, eruptive disease of childhood.

**VARICOCELE** [753]: A dilation of the scrotal veins.

■

# THERAPEUTIC INDEX

# THERAPEUTIC INDEX

Any attempt to select the proper homoeopathic remedy for any case except by the study of the totality of symptoms will prove futile. In order to prescribe homoeopathically, the essentials for doing so must be observed, i. *e, to let the characteristic symptoms of the individual patient, largely independent of the pathological nature of the case, be paramount in selecting the remedy.*

Such characteristics are found especially

1. In the location or part affected;
2. In the sensations;
3. In the modalities.

The study of the repertory alone will give the indicated remedy. But throughout this work are numerous suggestions for remedies based on clinical observations or deductions from partial provings, all of which may prove very valuable additions to our materia medica if further verified at the bedside. As many of them have no place as yet in our published repertories, I have thought it advisable to give them a place with others in this therapeutic index, in order to bring them to the attention and further study of the physician. At best, a clinical index is but suggestive.

**Abortion, threatened**: Caul., Vib.
**Abscess**: Anan., Bell., *Hep.,* Merc., Sil.
**Acidity**: Calc., Nux-v., *Rob.,* Sul-ac.
**Acne**: Ant-c., *Berb-a.,* Hydrc., Cimic., Led., Kali-br.
— **rosacea**: Carb-an., Kreos., Ov., Rad-met., Sulph.
**Acromegaly**: Chrysar., Thyr.
**Actinomycosis**: Hecla, Hippoz., Nit-ac.
**Addison's disease**: Adren., Ars., Calc-ar., Phos.
**Adenitis**: Bell., Cist., Iod., Merc.
**Adenoids**: Agra., Calc-i.
**Adiposity**: Fuc., Phyt.
**Adynamia**: Chin., Ph-ac.
**After-pains**: Caul., Mag. p.
**Agalactia**: Lact., Agn., Urt-u.
**Ague**: Nat-m., Chin., Cedr.
**Albuminuria**: Ars., Kalm., Merc-c.
**Alcoholism**: Aven., Caps., Nux-v., Querc.
**Alopecia**: Fl-ac., Pix.

**Amenorrhea**: Graph., Nat-m., Puls.
**Anasarca**: Elat., Liat., Oxyd.
**Anemia**: Calc-p., Chin., Ferr-cit., Nat-m.
— **pernicious**: Ars., Trinit.
**Aneurism**: Bar-c., Lyc.
**Angina pectoris**: Bry., Cact., Glon., Haem., Lam-m., Ox-ac., Spig.
**Angioma**: Abrot.
**Ankylostomiasis**: Card-m.
**Anorexia**: *Chin., Hydr.,* Nux-v.
**Anthrax**: *Echi.*
**Aortitis**: *Aur-ar.*
**Antrum**: Amyg., Euph., Hep., Kali-bi., Nit-ac.
**Aphasia**: Both., Kali-br., Stram.
**Aphonia**: Alumn., Arg-m., Aur., Caust., Nit-ac., Ox-ac., Spong.
**Aphthae**: Aeth., *Borx.,* Hydrin-m., Kali-m., *Merc.,* Nit-ac.
**Apoplexy**: Arn., Bell., Op., Phos.
**Appendicitis**: Bell., Echi., Lach., Iris-t.
**Arterial tension lowered**: Gels.
**Arterial tension raised**: Verat-v., Visc.
**Arteriosclerosis**: Am-i., Aur., Bar-c., Card-m., Glon. 2x., Plb-i., Polyg-a., Sumb.
**Arthritis**: Arb., Bry., Elat., Sulph.
**Ascarides**: Abrot., Cina, Sabad., Spig.
**Ascites**: Acet-ac., Apoc., Apis, Ars., *Dig.,* Hell.
**Asthenopia**: Croc., Nat-m., Ruta, Seneg.
**Asthma**: *Adren.,* Ars., Eucal., Ip., Nat-s.
— **cardiac**: Ars-i., Conv., Iber.
**Astigmatism (myopic)**: Lil-t.
**Atrophy**: Ars., Iod., Ol-j.
**Auricular fibrillation**: Dig., Quin.
**Auto-intoxication**: Indol., Skat., Sulph.
**Azoturia**: Caust., Senn.
**Backache**: Aesc., Ant-t., Cimic., Kali-c., Nux-v., Ox-ac., Puls., Rhus-t., Vario.
**Balanitis**: Merc.
**Barber's itch**: Sul-i., Thuj.
**Bed-sores**: Arn., Fl-ac., Sul-ac.
**Bell's paralysis**: Am-p., *Caust.,* Zinc-pic.
**Beri Beri**: Ars., Elat., Rhus-t.,
**Bilharziasis**: Ant-t.

**Biliousness**: Bry., Chel., Euon., Merc., Nux-v., Nyct., Podo., Sulph., Yuc.
**Bladder (irritable)**: Apis, Cop., *Eup-pur.,* Ferr., Nux-v., Sars.
**— hemorrhage**: Amgd-p., Ham., *Nit-ac.*
**Blepharitis**: Graph., Merc., Puls.
**Blepharospasm**: Agar., Phys.
**Blood pressure: high**: Aur., Bar-m., Glon., Visc.
**Boils**: *Bell.,* Bell-p., Calc-pic., Ferr-i., *Hep.,* Ichth., Ol-myr., Sil.
**Bone affections**: Aur., Calc-p., Fl-ac., Mez., Ruta, Sil., Symph.
**Borborygmi**: Haem.
**Bradycardia (slow pulse)**: Abies-n., Apoc., *Dig.,* Kalm.
**Brain, softening**: Bar-c., Phos., Salam.
**Brain-fag**: Anac., Anh., Phos., Sil., Zinc.
**Bright's disease**: Apis, Ars., Kali-cit., Merc-c., Nat-m., Ph-ac., Ter.
**Bromidrosis**: Calc., But-ac., Sil.
**Bronchitis**: Acon., Ant-t., *Bry., Ferr-p.,* Phos., Pilo., Sang.
**— (chronic)**: Ammc., Ars., Ant-i., Seneg., Sulph.
**Broncho-pneumonia**: Ant-t., Kali-bi., Phos., Squil., Tub.
**Bronchorrhea**: Ammc., Bac., *Bals-p.,* Eucal.,Stann.
**Bulbar paralysis**: Botul., Gua., Plb.
**Bubo**: Carb-an., Merc., Nit-ac., Phyt.
**Burns**: Canth., Pic-ac., Urt-u.
**Bursae**: Benz-ac., Ruta, Sil.
**Calculi (biliary)**: Berb., Chel., Chin.
**— (renal)**: Berb., Pareir., Sars.
**Cancer, (bladder)**: Tarax.
**— (epithelial)**: Acet-ac.
**— (gastric)** : Ger.
**— (rectal)**: Hydr., Kali-cy., Ruta
**— (tongue)**: Fuli.
**Cancer**: Ant-m., *Ars.,* Gali., Hydr., Semp.,
**— mammae**: Aster., Carc., Con., Plb-i.
**— pains**: Euph.
**Cancrum oris**: Ars., Bapt., Kreos., Sec.
**Capillary stasis**: Caps., Echi.
**Carbuncles**: *Anthraci., Ars.,* Lach., Led., Sil., Tarent-c.
**Cardiac dropsy**: Adon., Dig.
**Cardiac dyspnea**: Acon-f., Queb.
**Cardialgia**: Ferr-t.
**Cardio-vascular spasm**: Act-sp.

— **(membranous)**: Borx., Calc-act.
**Dyspepsia**: *Anac.,* Carb-v., Graph., Hom., Hydr., Lyc., *Nux v.,* Petr., Puls.
**Dyspepsia, (acid)**: Rob.
— **(atonic)**: Hydr.
— **(fermentative)**: Sal-ac.
— **(nervous)**: Anac., Ign.
**Dysphagia**: Bell., Caj., Cur., Epil., Lach., Merc.
**Dyspnea**: Apis, Ars., Ip., Queb., Spong.
**Dysuria**: Apis, Bell., Camph., *Canth.,* Fab., Sars., Tritic.
**Earache**: Bell., Cham., Verb-ol.
**Ear, (discharges)**: Kali-m.
— **(very offensive)**: Elaps.
**Ecchymosis**: Aeth., *Arn.,* Rhus-t., Sul-ac.
**Eczema**: Aln., *Anac.,* Arb., *Ars.,* Bov., Clem., Dulc., Graph., Nat-ar., Olnd., Petr., *Psor., Rhus-t.,* Sulph.
**Edema**: Apis, Ars., Dig.
— **(of lungs)**: Ant-t.
— **(pedum)**: Prun.
**Esophagus**: Bapt., Caj., Cund.
**Elephantiasis**: Ars., Elae, Hydrc., Lyc.
**Emphysema**: Am-c., Ant-ar., Lob.
**Empyemia**: Arn.
**Enteritis (acute)**: Chin., Crot-t., Podo.
— **(chronic)**: Arg-n., Ars., Sulph.
**Enuresis**: Bell., Benz-ac., Caust., Equis-h., Lup., Physal., Rhus-a., Sulph., Uran-n.
**Epididymitis.**: Puls., Sabal.
**Epilepsy**: Absin., Art-v., Calc-ar., Cupr., Ferr-cy., Hydr-ac., *Oena.*, Sil., Sol-c.
**Epistaxis**: Ambro., *Arn.,* Bry., Ferr-p., Ham., Ip., Nat-n., *Nit-ac.,* Phos.
**Epithelioma**: Abr., Ars., Chr-ac., Thuj.
**Erotomania**: Orig., Phos., Pic-ac., Plat., Stram.
**Erysipelas**: Anan., *Apis,* Bell., Canth., Graph., *Rhus-t.,* Verat-v.
**Erythema**: Antip., Bell., Mez.
— **nodosum**: Apis, Rhus-t.
**Eustachian deafness**: Kali-s., Hydr., Ros.
**Exophthalmic goitre**: Lycps-v., Pilo.
**Exostosis**: Calc-f., Hecla.
**Exudative pleurisy**: Abrot.
**Eyes, (inflamed)**: Acon., Euphr., Ruta.
— **(detachment of retina)**: Naphtin.
**Fever**: *Acon.,* Agrosti-a., Bapt., Ferr-p., Gels., Spira., Verat-v.

**Fibroids**: Calc-i.
**Fibroma**: Ergot., Lap-a., Tril-p.
**Fissures**: Graph., Led., Petr.
**Fistula**: Fl-ac., Nit-ac., Sil.
**Flatulence**: Arg. n., *Asaf.,* Caj., Carb-ac., Carb-v., Chin., Lyc., Mosch., *Nux-m.*
**Framboesia**: Jatr-c., Merc-n.
**Freckles**: Bad., Sep.
**Galactorrhea**: Calc., Salv.
**Gall-stones**: Berb., Calc., Cal-ren. (8-10x trit.), Chin., Chion.,
**Ganglion**: Benz-ac., Ruta.
**Gangrene**: Euph., Carb-v., Lach., *Sec.*
**Gastralgia**: Bism., Carb-v., Cocc., Cupr-ar., Nux-v., Petr., Phos.
— **(recurring)**: Graph.
**Gastric ulcer**: Arg-n., Ars., *Atrop.,* Ger., Kali-bi., Uran-n.
**Gastritis**: Ars., Hydr., Nux-v., Ox-ac., Phos.
**Gastro-enteritis**: Arg-n., Ars.
**Glanders**: Hippoz., Merc.
**Glands, swollen**: Aln., Bell., Kali-i., Merc-i., Phyt.
**Gleet**: Abies-c., Puls., Santal., Sep., Thuj.
**Glossitis**: Apis., Lach., Mur-ac.
**Globus hystericus**: Asaf., Ign.
**Gonorrhea**: Cann-s., Gels., Merc., Ol-sant., Petros., Tus-p.
**Gout**: Am-be., Colch., Form., Frax., Led., Lith-c., Lyc., Urt-u.
— **(retrocedent)**: Caj.
**Gravel**: Berb., Hydrang., Lyc., Solid.
**Growing pains**: Calc-p., Guaj., Ph-ac.
**Gumboil:** Bell., Hecla, Merc., Phos.
**Hallucinations**: Antip., Bell., Stram.
**Halophagia**: Ars., Nit-s-d., Phos.
**Hay-fever**: Ambro., Aral., Arund., Cupr-act., Lina., Naphtin., Phle., Rosa., *Sabad.*
**Headaches**: **(anemic)**: Chin., Ferr-p.
— **(bursting)**: Glon., *Usn.*
— **(congestive)**: Acon., Bell., Gels., Glon., Lach., Meli.
— **(nervous)**: Cann-i., Cimic., Coff., Guar., Ign., Nicc., Zinc.
— **(sick)**: Chion., Iris, Nux-v., Sang.
**Heart affections**: Acon., Adon., *Cact.,* Conv., *Crat., Dig.,* Lyc., *Naja,* Phase., Spig., Spong.

**Heartburn**: Carb-v., Ger.

**Heart failure**: Agarin. (l/10 gr.), hypodermically, Spartin-s. (1/4 gr.), Stry-s. (1/60-1/30 gr.);

**Hectic fever**: Ars., Bapt., Chinin-ar.

**Hemicrania**: Coff., Ol-an., Onos., Sep., Stann.

**Hemiplegia**: Both., Cocc., Olnd.

**Hemopia (vertical)**: Titan.

**Hematemesis**: Ham., Ip., Mill., Phos.

**Hematuria**: Canth., Ham., Nit-ac., Ter.

**Hemoglobinuria**: *Phos., Pic-ac.*

**Hemophilia**: Nat-sil., Phos.

**Hemoptysis**: Acal., All-s., Erig., Ger., Ferr-p., Hydrin-m., Ip., Mill., Sec.

**Hemorrhages**: Adren., Chin., Crot-h., Ham., Hydrin-s., Ip., Mill., Sabin., Tril-p.

— **(chronic sequelae)**: Stront-c.

**Hemorrhoids**: Aesc., *Aloe,* Coll., Fl-ac., *Ham., Mur-ac.,* Neg., *Nux-v.,* Scroph n.

**Hepatitis**: Bry., Lach., Merc., Nat-s.

**Herpes**: **(circinatus)**: Sep., Tell.

**Herpes labialis**: Caps., Nat-m., Rhus-t.

— **(preputialis)** : Hep., Nit-ac.

— **(pudendi)**: Calad., Nat-m., Nit-ac.

— **zoster**: Carbn-o., Menth., Ran-b., Rhus-t.

**Hiccough**: Gins., Nux-v., Rat., Sul-ac.

**Hoarseness**: Acon., Bry., Carb-v., Dros., Caust., Phos.

**Hodgkin's disease**: Ars-i., Iod., Phos.

**Homesickness**: Caps., Ign.

**Hookworm**: Chen-a., Thymol.

**Housemaid's knee**: Slag, Stict.

**Hydrocephalus**: Hell., Iodof., Zinc.

**Hydrocele**: Graph., Puls., Rhod.

**Hydrophobia**: Anag., Canth., Xanth.

**Hydrothorax**: Adon., Fl-ac., Kali-c., Lact., Merc-sul., Ran-b.

**Hyperchlorhydria**: Anac., Arg-n., *Atro.,* Chinin-ar., Iris, Orex., Rob.

**Hysteria**: Aqui., Asaf., Castm., Ictod., Ign., Mosch., Plat., Sumb., Valer.

**Hysterical joint**: Cot.

**Ichthyosis**: Ars-i., Syph.

**Impetigo**: Ant-t., Ars., Mez.

**Impotence**: Agn., Calad., Con., Lyc., Onos., *Ph-ac.,* Sel., *Yohim.*

**Megrim (migraine)**: Coff., Menis., Sep., Stann.
**Meniere's disease**: Carbn-s., Chen-a., Nat- sal., Pilo-m., Sal-ac., Sil.
**Meningitis (tubercular)**: Bac., Cupr-cy., Iodof.
**Menorrhagia**: Calc., Chin., Croc., Plat., Sabin., Sed-ac., Sanguiso., Tell.
**Menstruation, (cessation)**: Graph., Lach., Puls., Sang.
— **(delayed)**: Calc-p., Caul., Nat-m., Puls.
— **(painful)**: Bell., Mag-p., Vib.
— **(profuse)**: Bell., Cham., Ip., Sabin., Tril-p.
**Metritis, chronic**: Aur-m-n., Mel-c-s., Merc.
**Milk-leg**: Ars., Bufo, Ham., Puls., Rhus-t.
**Miscarriage**: **(repeated)**: Bac., Syph.
— **(threatened)**: Sabin., Vib.
**Morning sickness**: Alet., Amgd-p., Apom., Cocc., Cuc-p., Ip., Nux-v.,
**Morphine habit**: Aven.
**Morvan's disease**: Aur-m., Thuj.
**Mountain sickness**: Coca.
**Mumps**: Bell., Merc., Pilo., Rhus-t.
**Muscae volitantes**: Caust., Chin., Cypr.
**Mushroom poisoning**: Absin.
**Myalgia**: Acon., Bry., Macro., Rhus-t.
**Myelitis**: Ars., Dulc., Ox-ac., Plb., Sec.
**Myocardial degeneration after influenza**: Gels., Nux-v.
**Myocarditis**: Ars-i., Aur-m., Dig.
**Myositis**: Arn., Mez., Rhus-t.
**Myxedema**: Thyr.
**Nephritis**: Apis, Berb., Canth., Eucal., Kali-chl., Merc-c., Methyl., Phos., Ter., Tub-k.
**Nephrolithiasis**: Pareir., Senec.
**Neuralgia**: *Acon.,* Am-val., *Ars.,* Bell., Coloc., Kalm., Phos., *Spig.,* Zinc-val.
— **(lumbo-abdominal)**: Aran.
— **(periodic)**: Ars., Cedr., Nicc-s.
— **(spermatic cord)**: Clem., Ol-an., Ox-ac.
**Neurasthenia**: Anac., Phys., Stry-p., *Zinc-pic.*
— **(gastric)**: Anac., Gent-l.
**Neuritis**: Ars., Plb., Hyper., Stann., Thal.
**Nevus**: Fl-ac., Thuj.
**Night-sweats**: Acet-ac., Agar., Nat-tel., Picro., Pilo., Pop., Salv.
**Nipples, ulcerated**: Castor-eq., Eup-a., Rat.
**Nodosities of joints**: Am-p.

**Tympanitis**: Asaf., Erig., Lyc., Ter.
**Typhoid**: Ars., Bapt., Bry., Mur-ac., Ph-ac.
— **(diarrhea)**: Epil.
**Ulcers**: Ars., Calen., Com., Kali-i., Lach., Nit-ac., Paeon., Sil.
**Uremia**: Am-c., Cupr-ar., *Morph.*
**Urethral caruncle**: Cann-s., *Eucal.*
**Urethritis**: Acon., Apis, *Canth.*
— **(in children)**: Dor.
**Uric acid diathesis**: Oci., Hed.
**Urticaria**: Ant-c., Antip., Apis, Astac., Bomb-pr., Cop., Frag., Nat-m.
**Uterine displacement**: Abies-c., Eup., Ferr-i., Frax., Helio., Puls., Sep.
— **(induration)**: Aur-m., Kalm.
— **(tumors)**: *Aur-m-n.*
**Vaginismus**: Bell., Cact., Plb.
**Varicose veins**: Calc-f., Ham., Puls.
**Variola**: Ant-t., Sarr.
— **(hemorrhage)**: Ars., Crot-h., Phos.
**Vascular tension**: Acon., Bell., Verat-v.
— **(with arterial lesion)**: Adren., Bar-m., Plb., Tab.
— **(rapid reducers)**: Aml-ns., Glon., Nat-n., Trinit.
**Vertigo**: Cocc., Con., Gels., *Gran.,* Phos.,
**Venous stasis**: *Aesc.*
**Warts**: Ant-c., Caust., Nit-ac., Sal-ac., *Thuj.*
**Wens**: Bac., Benz-ac., Thuj.
**Whooping cough**: Castn-v., Cupr., *Dros.,* Mag-p., Pert.
**Worms**: Calc., Cina, Naphtin., Santin., Spig., Teucr.
**Wrist rheumatism**: Act-sp., Viol-t.
**Writers' cramp**: Arg-met., Sul-ac.
**Weil's disease**: Chel., Phos.
**Yellow fever**: Ars., Cadm-s., Crot-h.

■

# SOME INDIAN DRUGS

# ABROMA AUGUSTA

(Olat Kambal) **Abrom-a.**

Olat Kambal, Devil's Cotton, Olat Tambol.

N.O.: Sterculiaceae. (N.O.: Natural Order)

**Clinical:** Albuminuria; sleeplessness; amenorrhea; carbuncle; diabetes mellitus and insipidus; debility; dysmenorrhea; weakness of brain.

Great uneasiness; feeling of extreme prostration. Inability to do any work; disinclination to work. Great loss of flesh; rapid emaciation; parasitic weakness. Burning sensation all over the body with thirst for large quantities of water.

**Mind:** Irritable; excitable angry mood; ill humor; forgetfulness; absent minded; depression; morose; anxious; moody, cannot bear contradiction.

**Head:** Empty feeling; rolling of the head and vertigo; heaviness and discomfort; marked giddiness. Pain at the back of the head.

**Eyes:** Weakness of vision; puffiness of the lids; heaviness; eyes easily tire; inclination to close the eyes; pain over both the eyes lachrymation; conjunctiva, pale.

**Ears:** Shortness of hearing; buzzing in the ears (tinnitus) and otorrhea.

**Nose:** Sneezing several times; watery nasal discharge; dryness of the nose with a desire to rub.

**Face:** Pale, yellow, wrinkled, old looking; itching eruptions on the face with a burning sensation; furuncles on the face.

**Mouth:** Almost constant dryness of the mouth; drinks large quantities of cold water at a time, which does not relieve the dryness; dry and clean tongue; indistinct speech; lips dry and pale or bluish. Insatiable thirst.

**Throat:** Dry; burning sensation; painful; difficulty in swallowing solids but drinking relieves the throat symptoms temporarily. Painful deglutition.

**Stomach:** Unnatural appetite, insatiable hunger, hungry shortly after eating a good meal. Desire for sweets. Hungry with a faint feeling; desire for all kinds of food; sensation of emptiness in the stomach, food does not seem to stay long in the stomach. No dyspeptic symptoms.

**Abdomen:** Flatulence with distention of the abdomen. Pain in the abdomen during peristalsis; free passage of flatus.

**Stool:** Constipation; brownish, black, knotty, hard; lumpy stool with much straining. Dryness of the rectum.

**Urinary:** Profuse and frequent micturition day and night (polyuria) dryness of the mouth and great thirst; desire to drink after micturition which relieves thirst; micturition leads to exhaustion; fishy odor in urine; a slight sediment; diabetes mellitus; nocturnal enuresis; urethritis, burning in the urethra; white ulcers at the mouth of prepuce caused by excessive passage of sugar in the urine; inability to retain urine; urgent desire to pass urine; high specific gravity.

**Male:** Absence of sexual desire, impotence, becomes exhausted after coition; swelling and hanging of the testies (orchitis).

**Female:** Irregular catamenia; menstrual blood is dark, clotted, profuse or scanty and pale; amenorrhea or dysmenorrhea; leucorrhea profuse, white, thin, watery; chlorosis; colicky pain in the lower abdomen, 2-3 days before menses; hysteria associated with menstrual disorders.

**Respiratory:** Cough with purulent expectoration and pain in the chest; lumpy sputum, white or yellowish in color, worse in cold air, in the evening and at night; patient holds his chest while coughing. Bronchitis and broncho-pneumonia with profuse expectoration.

**Heart:** Weakness of the heart; palpitations, worse on movement; faint feeling.

**Sleep:** Drowsiness, but cannot sleep; insomnia, prostration and aversion to do any labour; unrefreshed sleep, sleeps better in the early part of the morning.

**Fever:** Dry heat over the whole body; great thirst.

**Skin:** Dry skin, scratching; burning; small boils in summers, carbuncles, an outcome of diabetes.

**Relationship:** Compare: *Bry.*

**Dose:** Mother tuncture, 2x, 3x.

---

## ABROMA AUGUSTA RADIX

(Olat Kambal Root) **Abrom-a-r.**

Olat Kambal Mul, Devil's Cotton. N.O.: Sterculiaceae.

**Clinical:** Female disorders.

The efficacy of *Abrom-a-r.* is marked in all female diseases especially those connected with the uterus. Also useful in some cases of chlorosis. Mental and other symptoms tally with those of *Abrom-a.*

**Female:** Irregular menstrual disorder; dysmenorrhea; colicky pains in the lower abdomen, before and during menses; menstrual flow may be copious or scanty; the discharge is black and mixed with clots. Leucorrhea.

**Relationship:** Compare: *Puls., Vib-c.*

**Dose:** Mother tincture, 2x, 3x.

---

# ACALYPHA INDICA

(Muktajhuri or Muktabarshi) **Acal.**

Aritta Manjarie, Khokali, N.O.: Euphorbiaceae.
Indian Acalypha, Kuppaimeni,
Haritaki Manjiri, Vahchni Kanto,
Indra Maris.

**Clinical:** Cough; diarrhea; flatulence; hemoptysis; phthisis.

It has a marked influence on the alimentary canal and respiratory organs. It is employed in the beginning of phthisis with hemoptysis and arterial hemorrhage, but no febrile disturbance. Burning sensation in the pharynx, esophagus, stomach and intestines. Dryness of the mouth and throat. Weak in the morning. Gains strength during the day. It is of great importance in progressive emaciation and all pathological hemorrhages having a morning aggravation.

**Head:** Head and eyes seem dull and heavy. Feels sleepy but cannot sleep due to oppressive frontal headache.

**Nose:** Sneezing; catarrh; thin watery discharge from the nose and eyes.

**Mouth:** Dryness of the tongue. Toothache with swelling of gums.

**Throat:** Tickling sensation bringing on cough and a sticky sputa. Dryness.

**Stomach:** Nausea with a diminished appetite. Great desire for acid fruits and drinks. Fullness of the stomach followed by eructations.

**Abdomen:** Fullness with griping; flatulence; burning; rumbling and distention.

**Rectum:** Hemorrhage, morning aggravation.

**Stool:** Spluttering diarrhea with forcible expulsion of flatus, bearing down pain and tenesmus. Stools, watery, mucoid, frothy, warm. Thirsty after stools.

**Respiratory:** Violent, dry cough followed by bloody expectoration; pure blood comes in the morning and dark lumps of clotted blood in the evening, cough becomes violent at night; constant and severe pain in the chest. Pulse is soft and compressible. Dullness of the chest on percussion.

**Sleep:** Fitful due to cough; unrefreshing.

**Skin:** Jaundice; circumscribed furuncle-like swelling; itching, etc.

**Modalities:** Worse, in the morning.

**Relationship:** Compare: *Ham., Ip., Fic-r., Mill., Phos.*

Antidoted by: *Calc.*

**Dose:** Mother tincture, 3x, 6x, are generally used.

## ACHYRANTHES ASPERA

(Apamarga) **Achy-a.**

Apang, Latjira, Aghada, Kutri, Na-yuivt, Apa-kharevazhun. N.O.: Amaranthaceae.

**Clinical:** Astringent; diarrhea; diuretic; dysentery; menorrhagia; bad effects of dog and snake bites; burns.

**Stomach:** Sour belching, heartburn. Nausea and vomiting of water and mucus; thready pulse. Extreme thirst.

**Stool:** Acute diarrhea and cholera; watery stool; yellowish and mixed with flakes of mucus, profuse in quantity; associated with a burning sensation all over the body, scanty urine, and extreme thirst, followed by extreme exhaustion, weakness and giddiness.

**Skin:** Boils, carbuncles; foul smelling, poisonous ulcers, etc. Can be used internally and externally; red spot on the skin, burning pain all over the body.

**Dose:** Mother tincture, 3x, 3, 6.

---

## AEGLE FOLIA

(Bel Fruit) **Aegle-f.**

Sriphala, Bilwa, Bengal-quince, Bilinu-phal, Vilwa-pazhan, Bilwa-pandu. N.O. : Rutaceae.

**Clinical:** Bleeding piles; diarrhea; dysentery; fever with dropsy; impotence.

It is a useful remedy in dropsy, bleeding piles, diarrhea and dysentery. Acts as a mild stimulant to the intestinal mucous membrane. A full, regular and strong pulse is the characteristic symptom of this drug. An excellent remedy for dropsy and beri-beri with decreased urine. Pain in all the limbs is aggravated after 4 p.m.

**Mind:** Commits mistakes in spelling.

**Head:** Headache appears between 4-8 p.m. Heat in the vertex appears in the evening which is better by eating. Headache is due to congestion.

**Eyes:** Upper lids of eyes swollen.

**Face:** Flushes of heat from face, eyes and ears, disappears after eating.

**Abdomen:** Waterbrash; abdomen distended especially lower abdomen (*Lyc.*); flatus expelled with a loud noise especially in the afternoon. Useful in indigestion, colic, piles and constipation. It is considered as a anti-bilious and febrifuge remedy. Amoebic and bacillary dysentery.

**Urinary:** Urine decreased considerably due to cardiac disease or dropsy;

patient feels a slight pain in the back and lumbar region, which is worse in the afternoon.

**Male:** Sexual impotency.

**Respiratory:** Catarrh; bronchitis; pneumonia; cough.

**Fever:** With catarrhal symptoms like influenza and dropsy, especially in children. Continuous fever with edema of hands, legs and face, present along with diarrhea; chronic fever associated with splenic or hepatic disorders.

**Skin:** Itching; ringworm.

**Relationship:** Compare: *Nux-v., Dig., Lyc. Aegle marmalos* (indicated in diarrhea and dysentery of a chronic nature).

**Dose:** Mother tincture, 3x, 6, 30, 200.

---

# ANDERSONIA Or AMOORA ROHITAKA

(Rohitaka) **Anders.**

Royna, Rohera, Rohido, Harinhara, Pitaraja. N.O.: Mediaceae.

**Clinical:** Chronic fever; general debility; enlarged glands; liver and spleen disorders; leucorrhea.

A splendid remedy for hepatic and splenic disorders, especially if associated with chronic malarial fevers. Hepato-splenomegaly with tenderness. Constipation is a characteristic symptom. Particularly useful in patients with a bilious temperament.

**Mind:** Memory becomes dull and disordered; makes mistakes in spelling, very lazy especially on getting up in the morning; can't fix the mind on any subject; easily angered.

**Head:** Heat in the vertex; giddiness; pain in the temples associated with heat which is relieved by cold air and cold application.

**Face:** Flushes of heat in the face; burning sensation in the face including eyes.

**Mouth:** Insipid taste in the mouth; bad and bitter taste in the morning.

**Stomach:** Sensation of heat with spasmodic colic due to indigestion.

**Abdomen:** Burning sensation in the stomach; enlargement of the liver and spleen; nausea and vomiting.

**Fever:** Feverish with headache; aching pains during fever; burning in hands and feet.

**Modalities:** Relief when body coverings are removed.

**Relationship:** Compare: *Cephd-i., Kalm., Aza., Nyct.*

**Dose:** 3x, 6x, 30, etc.

# ANDROGRAPHIS PANICULATA

(Kalmegh)

**Androg-p.**

Mahatekta, Kiryat, Kirata,
The Great Bhunimba,
Kalpanath, Kiryato, Olenkirayet,
Nalavemu, Nilavambu, Nilavoepu,
The Great King of Bitters, etc.

N.O.: Acantheceae.

**Clinical:** First stage of cold and cough; convalescence after prolonged fever; general debility; infantile liver; jaundice.

A highly efficacious remedy in all types of liver disorders. General burning sensation especially in the palms is a keynote symptom. Washes hands and feet with cold water in order to relieve the burning sensation. In slow fevers of children with a deranged or enlarged liver. Infantile jaundice. Efficacious in Kala azar of infants.

**Mind:** Despondency; no desire to do any work or to talk; restless; easily angered.

**Head:** Giddiness; heaviness and throbbing pain in the occiput.

**Eyes:** Redness of the eyes, yellowish tinge in the eyes.

**Nose:** Watery discharge from the nose with occasional sneezing.

**Mouth:** Bitter taste in the mouth with dryness and burning in the throat. Tongue coated white.

**Abdomen:** Burning in the chest; heaviness of the abdomen without any appetite; hepatomegaly, infantile jaundice. Indicated in torpidity of the liver, neuralgia, dyspepsia and in general debility.

**Stool:** Alternate diarrhea and constipation; frequent urging for stool without evacuation; black, hard stool; yellowish loose stool. Flatulence and diarrhea in children. An anti-helmintic indicated in the fully developed stage of dysentery.

**Urinary:** High colored urine; thick and yellow in color.

**Fever:** Fever with chilliness and heat all over the body; there is headache with thirst; burning all over the body relieved by cold air, water; fever comes at 11 a.m., and then again at 7-8 p.m.; intermittent or remittent fever; disinclined to move during fever.

**Modalities:** Better, cold water, sweat, cold. Worse, during fever.

**Dose:** Mother tincture, 3x, 6x, 30.

# ATISTA INDICA Or GLYCOSMIS PENTAPHYLLA

(Ash-sheora) **Atis.**

Bannimbu, Vanamenibuka, Keimira. N.O.: Rutaceae.

**Clinical:** Biliary colic; diarrhea; flatulence; tinnitus; scurvy; scorbutic teeth.

An excellent remedy in breaking and stopping fevers which appear on alternate days or on every third day with or without malarial infection, especially during autumn. In diseases of children with signs and symptoms of worms. Convulsions due to worms. Biliary colic and gastric colic.

**Mind:** Weak memory; indifferent mood; vigorless.

**Head:** Vertigo in the morning; gnawing pain in one temple at a time.

**Eyes:** Photophobia; on opening the eyes, light trembles before him for a few seconds, obliging him to shut his eyes; trembling of light before eyes, after sleep. Burning in the eyes.

**Ears:** Unusually increased hearing, humming sound in the ears.

**Nose:** Epistaxis; dry coryza.

**Face:** Pale, with a yellowish countenance. Spasm of facial muscles.

**Mouth:** Bleeding from gums; dull pain at the root of the teeth. Halitosis; bitter taste after the paroxysm of fever is over. Dryness of the mouth with unbearable thirst during the hot stage. Constant spitting in the morning with occasional belching of salty water. Sour waterbrash.

**Throat:** Inflammation of the tonsils persist few weeks after fever. Tonsillitis.

**Stomach:** Canine hunger; aversion to liquid foods and strong desire for lime juice; throbbing at the pit of the stomach, heaviness in the stomach after a meal; flatulence temporarily relieved by eructations; indigestion due to worms; frequent eructations after a meal; heartburn 3-4 hours after food. Sour vomiting and eructations immediately after eating. Worm symptoms.

**Abdomen:** Colicky pain around the navel makes the patient senseless; tenesmus and drawing pain in the renal region. Flatulence; burning in region of liver and spleen; aggravation in the evening. Distention and indigestion.

**Stool:** Constipation and watery diarrhea during the entire episode of fever; pale earthly stool; bloody, mucoid stool with or without force. Dysentery with mucus and blood, amoebic or bacillary; cholera.

**Male:** No sexual desire; erection at night without any cause; peculiar electric-like throbbing in the urethra for a few seconds, coming like lightening.

**Back:** Pain in the neck and under the scapula; pain in the limbs, sacral region. Stiffness while stooping.

**Extremities:** Weakness and heaviness of the limbs; legs 'go to sleep'; cramping while getting them straight. Legs seem to give away at every step.

**Sleep:** Transient; unrefreshing.

**Fever:** Chill without thirst, heat with intense thirst, fever comes between 5-10 a.m. and subsides around 3-4 a.m., fever appears every alternate day. Periodicity is not marked.

**Relationship:** Antidote: *Nux-v., Camph., Bell., lime juice.*

**Dose:** Mother tincture, 2x, 3x, 6, etc.

---

## ATISTA RADIX

(Root of Ash-sheora) **Atis-r.**

Bannimbu, Vanamenibuka. N.O.: Rutaceae.

**Clinical:** Dysentery; worm complaints.

**Stool:** It is more powerful than *Atista indica* when used in dysentery, both amoebic and bacillary; patient passes only blood along with pain around the naval; dysentery appearing in autumn; also used for worm complaints; flatulence and biliary colic.

**Dose:** Mother tincture, 3x, 12, 30.

---

## AZADIRACHTA INDICA Or MELIA AZADIRACHTA

(Nim) **Aza.**

Nimba, Margosa Tree, Vembaka, Bal-nimb, Vembu, Vepa, The Neem. N.O.: Meliaceae.

**Clinical:** Ozena; pemphigus; scabies; leprosy; helminthiasis; gonorrhea; glossitis.

It is a well known tonic. antiseptic, astringent and an antiperiodic remedy of great use in ophthalmia, asthma, cough, catarrh, constipation, uterine debility and helminthiasis. It is a grand remedy in chronic fever. Locally, it helps in the removal of slough and promotes healthy granulation and healing.

**Mind:** Depressed; forgetful, makes mistakes in writing and spelling; forgets the names of very familiar people, or what has been done the previous day. Loss of memory; weak; dull; full of anxiety. Inactive; no desire to go out.

**Head:** Giddiness, especially at 10 a.m., worse when rising from a sitting posture; throbbing headache; especially right sided; worse in the open air, aggravated by stooping; scalp is painful and sensitive to touch, even hair is painful.

**Eyes:** Eyes are red, congested, burn; dull and heavy; pressive pain in the right eyeball.

**Ears:** Buzzing in the ears; a cracking sound is heard in the ears as if being tickled by a feather; worse on opening the mouth.

**Nose:** Watery discharge from the nose.

**Face:** Hot flushes.

**Mouth:** Putrid taste in the mouth; no thirst but mouth is clammy and bitter; tongue is painful with a burning sensation, as if scalded; papillae seem enlarged and prominent, saliva tastes salty; dysphagia, especially when swollowing water and meat; very thirsty, especially at long intervals or sometimes thirstless.

**Throat:** Left sided sore throat.

**Stomach:** Good, keen appetite. Thirst for large quantities of cold water. Heartburn and waterbrash.

**Abdomen:** Great uneasiness in abdomen with flatulence, passes offensive flatus; twisting pain in the epigastrium; clutching pain in the umbilical region, must bend forward which relieves; distention.

**Stool:** Insufficient stool; small, hard and knotty when constipated but natural stools are copious, soft and semi-solid; burning in the bowels.

**Urinary:** Scanty, high colored, scalding; white, clear and copious; strong odor.

**Male:** Great excitement of sexual organs.

**Respiratory:** Very troublesome cough after bathing at 1 p.m.; sputa is white, thick and in small lumps, expelled with much difficulty. Deep, sighing respiration. Hoarseness.

**Chest:** Aching in the lower part of the right side of chest, below the nipple; stitches especially on the right side, crampy pains in the lower part.

**Extremities:** Numbness of the limbs especially right hand; sensation as if paralysed; burning of the soles and hands; rheumatic pain in the lower extremities. Strength of hands diminished.

**Sleep:** Sleeplessness and tossing in bed; dreamy, interrupted sleep; dreams of quarrels, beating, etc. in the latter part of the night.

**Fever:** Fever with chill or without chill from 4.30 p.m. and abates from 7.30 p.m.; glowing heat with burning in various parts of the body, even in open air; copious sweat, especially on the forehead, neck, upper part of the body; no sweat on the lower parts of the body, commences on the forehead.

**Modalities:** Worse, open air; in the afternoon.

**Relationship:** Compare: *Ars., Chin., Ip., Nat-m., Puls., Rhus-t., Sulph., Cedr.*

**Dose:** 6, 30, 200.

## BLUMEA ODORATA

(Kuksima) **Blum-o.**

Kukundar, Kukurmota. N.O.: Compositae.

**Clinical:** Cough; fever; hemorrhage; hoarseness.

It has got reputation in bleeding piles; diarrhea or dysentery associated with blood; excellent results in miscarriage when hemorrhage is profuse; in bloody leucorrhea and menorrhagia it exerts a powerful influence to arrest bleeding.

**Throat:** Controls cough; hoarseness due to cough; trumpet-like sound or barking sound associated with cough.

**Fever:** In tertian fever.

**Dose:** Mother tincture, 2x, 3x.

---

## BOERHAAVIA DIFFUSA

(Punarnava) **Boerh-d.**

Sothaghni, Sant, Ghetuli, Itsit, Mukukrattai. N.O.: Nyctagineae.

**Clinical:** Asthma; beri-beri; dropsy; jaundice; gonorrhea; heart problems; hypertension; bites of venomous animals, etc.; ascitis; cirrhosis.

Has marked diuretic properties. Dropsy associated with healthy kidneys and early liver and peritonial conditions. Ascitis due to cirrhosis of liver. Kala azar. Swelling in eyelids, hands and feet.

**Head:** Severe; bursting; right sided headache better by cold application; giddiness.

**Throat:** Coryza with dry cough and thick white expectoration.

**Stomach:** Nausea; vomiting mixed with bile.

**Abdomen:** Slight pain in the hepatic region was felt on touch, movement or pressure and better by hard pressure; cirrhosis of liver.

**Urinary:** Scanty, high colored urine; strangury.

**Heart:** Frequent palpitations and intermittent, throbbing pain in the cardiac region. Hypertension with ringing in the ears and heat in the vertex.

**Back and Extremities:** Rheumatic-like pains all over

**Dose:** Mother tincture.

---

## BRAHMI

**Brahmi**

**Clinical:** Impaired memory; whooping cough.

It is mostly used as a tonic for absent mindedness and for a short, weak memory. It is also used for whooping cough.

**Dose:** Mother tincture.

---

## CAESALPINIA BONDUCELLA

(Nata) **Caesal-b.**

Kuberakshi, Nata-karanja, Sugar-ghota, Fever Nut, Physic nut, Bonduc Nut, Devil's Testicle, Kazhar-shikkay.

N.O.: Leguminosae.

**Clinical:** Fever, headache, etc.

Of great value in chronic intermittent fever and hepatosplenomegaly.

**Mind:** Mental depression; lack of enthusiasm. No desire to take a bath.

**Head:** Severe headache; better by wrapping, by pressure.

**Eyes:** Severe pain, as if they were burnt, before and during the invasion of fever, relieved by cold applications.

**Nose:** Hot breath. Frequent and hurried respiration during fever.

**Mouth:** Mildly coated, white tongue; bloodless, pale, white, moist tongue; thirst for cold water during the heat stage of fever.

**Stomach:** Desire for boiled rice, meat or other hard substances; aversion to liquid food.

**Abdomen:** Gurgling in the lower abdomen. Tenderness in the hepatic region; Lower lobe is enlarged. Uneasiness in the hepatic region before the onset of fever. Splenomegaly with hardness and tenderness.

**Stool:** Hard, saffron colored or liquid, slimy and yellow colored stool.

**Back:** Drawing pain in the back after a cold bath.

**Fever:** Irregular, comes on at anytime. Accompanied by chills and shivering on one day and on the other with hardly any chills. Character of fever is very changeable. Fever appears between 8 and 10 a.m. or between 2 and 4 p.m. No thirst in afternoon fever but marked thirst during the heat in morning fever.

Sweat stage lasts for a short time. Sweat breaks out over the face, chest, neck and shoulder. Fever does not last for more than 6 hours. After fever there is extreme prostration; patient lies down quietly in bed with eyes closed; cannot even talk. Useful in intermittent fever and remittent fever of malarial origin.

**Skin:** Dry, dirty, small eruptions like mosquito bites.

**Dose:** Mother tincture, 2x, 3x.

---

# CALOTROPIS GIGANTEA

(Akanda) **Calo.**

Arka, Mandara, Gigantic Swallow-woop, Ekke, Jellude, Badabadam, Madar, Mudar, Akadu. N.O.: Asclepiadeae.

**Clinical:** Asthma; ascites; cough; catarrh; chronic rheumatism; diarrhea; dysentery; elephantiasis; pneumonic tuberculosis; poisonous snake bite; leprosy; intestinal worms; skin diseases; syphilis; splenomegaly; otalgia; piles.

An excellent remedy for skin and eye affections. Sensation of warmth in the scrobiculous cordis is the characteristic symptom of this remedy. In severe and advanced cases of syphilis with thickening of the ends of nails. Decreases obesity while the muscle mass becomes harder and firmer.

**Head:** Dizziness; dull occipital headache from 11 a.m.; head hot till midnight, throbbing painful, confusion; faint and giddiness with an inclination to vomit.

**Face:** Face hot, cheeks burn like fire; lips and throat dry.

**Mouth:** Foul breath; pain on moving the jaw, soreness and swelling on the right side of palate.

**Stomach:** Constant eructations; nausea.

**Urinary:** Frequent micturition; urine dark red with a strong smell.

**Respiratory:** Oppression of chest, short respiration.

**Heart:** Pulse quickened.

**Extremities:** Cramping pain in the centre of the right palm when grasping anything, lasts for many days. Pain in the wrist joint, aggravated on movement. Slight pain on moving the inside of right thigh, just below the groin followed by swelling and tenderness, thigh is sore making turning irksome; cannot bend leg while walking. Intermittent cramping pain, moves the foot continously in bed for relief. Pain in foot so severe when at rest, that it brings tears to the eyes; worse from drinking coffee. Places the foot very gently on the ground, can stand without pain but pain returns on taking the weight off the foot. Foot red and swollen, not tender.

**Sleep:** Restless and feverish; tossing from side to side.

**Fever:** Frequent chills passing up the spine; head hot, body cold; cheeks burn like fire, chills return towards bedtime even when close to fire; fits of perspiration alternate with chills.

**Skin:** In all ulcers especially gangrenous ulcers, ulcers of leprosy; elephantiasis of the leg and scrotum; of use in scorpion and bites of other poisonous insects.

**Dose:** Mother tincture, 2x, 3x, 6.

---

## CALOTROPIS LACTUM

(Glue of Calotropis) **Calo-l.**

Akanda, Madar, Gigantic, Swallow-woop, Arka. N.O.: Asclepiadeae.

It is prepared from milk, juice or glue of *Calotropis gigantea* and usually the cases which are not benefitted by the employment of *Calotropis gigantea* yield to the therapeutic properties of *Calotropis lactum.* Purging; vomiting; toothache; splenomegaly; diseases of the eye and skin are successfully treated by this drug.

**Dose:** 3x, 6x.

---

## CARICA PAPAYA

(Penpay) **Asim.**

Popaiya, Papend, Aranda, Kharguza, Poppayi, Boppaiya, Papaya, Kappalam, Pappayam, Paputn, Melonenbum. N.O.: Passifloreae.

**Clinical:** Abortion; dyspepsia; hepatomegaly; splenomegaly; uterine disorders; jaundice.

An efficacious remedy helping digestion in very weak patients.

**Abdomen:** Enlarged liver and spleen with fever, dyspepsia, indigestion and weakness. Pain in the hepatic region; complications of liver; jaundice, conjunctiva yellow, tongue coated white, intolerance of milk, even a small quantity causes indigestion and pain in the hepatic region.

**Stool:** Lienteric in small quantity passed several times a day.

**Female:** It aids menstrual discharge; helps uterine contraction and induces abortion when locally applied to the mouth of the uterus.

**Dose:** Mother tincture, 1x, 3x (trituration).

---

# CEPHALANDRA INDICA

(Telakucha) **Cephd-i.**

Bimba, Kanduri ki-bill, Korai, Kabare-hindi. N.O.: Cucurbitaceae.

**Clinical:** Diabetes mellitus and insipidus; skin affections; jaundice; dropsy; dysentery; sunstroke; boils; abscesses; carbuncles.

The grand medicine for diabetes mellitus and insipidus; glycosuria. Intolerable burning sensation all over the body, especially adapted to people, oversensitive to noise and external impressions.

**Mind:** Morose, fretful; disinclined to do any work, gloomy; memory partially gone; oversensitiveness (mentally and physically).

**Head:** Giddiness worse after micturition; weakness.

**Eyes:** Burning in the eyes.

**Face:** Red and burning.

**Mouth:** Dryness of mouth with great thirst for large quantity of water at a time, worse after micturition.

**Throat:** Dryness of the throat.

**Stomach:** Loss of a appetite.

**Abdomen:** Flatulence, distended.

**Stool:** Greenish mucoid; tinged with blood and, pain before and during stool.

**Urinary:** Profuse micturition; weakness and exhaustion after micturition; sugar in the urine; diabetes mellitus. Polyuria.

**Modalities:** Worse after micturition, better cold application.

**Dose:** Mother tincture, 1x, 3x.

---

# CLERODENDRON INFORTUNATUM

(Bhat) **Clerod-i.**

Bhanta, Ghantakarna, Bhandira, Karo. N.O.: Leguminosae.

**Clinical:** Gastric problems; worms.

A remedy for gastric derangements and chronic fever.

**Abdomen:** Hepatomegaly; splenomegaly; no appetite, indigestion. Worm symptoms; colic due to worms in children. Waterbrash.

**Stool:** Diarrhea with nausea. Stools are liquid, deep yellow in color and frothy. Loose evacuation with worm infestation. Occasionally constipation.

**Fever:** Fever with enlargement of the liver and spleen, fever comes in the afternoon; burning sensation in the eyes and face.

**Relationship:** Compare: *Ip., Puls.*

**Dose:** Mother tincture, 3x, 6, 30.

## COLEUS AROMATICUS

(Pashanbhedi) **Coleus-a.**

Himsagara, Patharkuchi, Pather-chu.

**Clinical:** Gonorrhea; urinary problems.

Action on the genito-urinary organs, however requires extensive trial.

**Urinary:** Strangury, suppression or retention of urine; gonorrhea with burning sensation during and after micturition; cystitis, vesical catarrh.

**Dose:** Mother tincture, 2x.

---

## CYNODON DACTYLON

(Durba) **Cyn-d.**

Hurialee-grass, Granthi, Doorva, Garika, Arugu, Talla. N.O.: Gramineae.

**Clinical:** Hemorrhage; dysentery; dropsy; leucorrhea; scabies.

An excellent hemorrhagic remedy in hematemesis, epistaxis, hemoptysis, bleeding from cuts or wounds or bleeding piles. In the latter two, it can be used internally and locally. Dropsy and general anasarca.

**Eyes:** Catarrhal ophthalmia, internally and externally.

**Stomach and Abdomen:** Chronic diarrhea; bilious vomiting

**Urinary:** Retention and suppression of urine with dropsy and general anasarca. Vesical calculus; dysuria; irritation of urinary organs. Secondary syphilis and gleet.

**Dose:** Mother tincture, 3x.

---

## DESMODIUM GANGETICUM

(Shalpani) **Desm-g.**

Sarivan, Shalaparni, Gitanaram. N.O.: Leguminosae.

**Clinical:** Fever; headache; meningitis; typhoid; wry neck.

A neuralgic remedy; pain all over the body, cannot sit straight due to spinal pain, Neuralgic pain in the stomach and knee joint. Burning sensation in hands and feet.

**Head:** Cerebrospinal meningitis, headache associated with a sensation as if all sides of the head are bound with a tape or rope.

**Sleep:** Sleeplessness, comatose sleep.

**Fever:** Intermittent and remittent fever in children with sleepiness, drowsiness and pain all over the body, especially over the spine. Typhoid; cerebrospinal meningitis. Fever comes on at 7 a.m. with mild chills, lasting for two to three hours, with a burning sensation over the face, eyes, hands and feet. Remission of fever with perspiration over the forehead and back part of hands and feet. Fever returns regularly everyday.

**Relationship:** Compare: *Aza., Kalmegh, Sulph., Gels.*

**Dose:** Mother tincture, 3x, 6x, 30.

---

## EMBELIA RIBES

(Biranga) **Emb-r.**

Beberang, Vidanga, Baburung, Karkannic, Vayuvilamgan. N.O.: Myrsineae.

**Clinical:** Children's remedy; worm killer; diarrhea; dyspepsia and flatulence due to worms.

`Kriminga' literally means 'killer of worms'. It is an efficent vermifuge.

**Mind:** Morose; irritable, fretful; ill humored; restless.

**Nose:** Itching sensation, picks at the nose.

**Mouth:** Dry tongue; grinding of teeth.

**Stomach:** Flatulence, diarrhea, dyspepsia, severe nausea; great hunger, soon after a meal. Worms.

**Rectum:** Itching in the rectum; lienteria with expulsion of worms.

**Urinary:** Pungent, bloody or red colored.

**Sleep:** Shrieks out during sleep, disturbed sleep.

**Fever:** Fever comes in the morning, ranging between 101-103° F.

**Relationship:** Compare: *Cina, Sant., Nux-v.*

**Dose:** Mother tincture, 3x, 6, 30.

---

## FICUS INDICA Or BENGALENSIS

(Bot) **Opun-f.**

Bor, Banyan Tree, Vata, Bar, Mari. N.O.: Urticaceae.

**Clinical:** Hemorrhages.

It possesses greater anti-hemorrhagic properties than *Ficus religiosa.* Hemorrhage from the throat or mouth due to any cause, when the color of blood is pure red, hemorrhage before any evacuation; bloody leucorrhea, etc. Successfully arrests hemorrhage from piles, and in chronic bloody dysentery; hemorrhage during menses.

**Stool:** Acute or chronic dysentery; profuse bright red blood; associated with tenesmus, urging and colic.

**Urinary:** Gonorrhea and diabetes; associated with a burning sensation during micturition; haematuria.

**Male:** Nervous debility due to seminal loss.

**Relationship:** Compare: *Merc-c., Fic-r., Tril-p., Thlas., Ham., Sab.*

**Dose:** Mother tincture, 3x, 6.

---

# FICUS RELIGIOSA

(Ashwatta) **Fic-r.**

Pippala, Pipal, Sacred Fig, Arshemaran, Areyal, Jeri.

N.O.: Urticaceae.

**Clinical:** Hemorrhage arrester; bleeding piles; epistaxis; dysentery; hemoptysis; hematemesis; hematuria; menorrhagia; metrorrhagia; typhoid.

A great anti-hemorrhagic remedy; bright red blood is passed from all the orifices. Has been used successfully in phthisical hemoptysis, where other remedies have failed. Patient is very weak and restless.

**Mind:** Unwilling to move, sad, melancholic; very sensitive to noise.

**Head:** Nausea; vertigo; burning in the vertex; vertigo with a slight headache.

**Nose:** Epistaxis.

**Mouth:** White tongue with profuse saliva.

**Stomach:** Vomiting of bright red blood; great repungance to all kinds of foods; sick feeling in the stomach.

**Stool:** Bloody dysentery; dysentery with menorrhagia.

**Urinary:** Frequent micturition; hematuria.

**Female:** Menorrhagia, bright red; bearing down pain in the lower abdomen.

**Respiratory:** Difficulty in breathing; cough; hemoptysis.

**Relationship:** Compare: *Ham., Thlas., Tril-p.*

**Dose:** Mother tincture, 3x, 6, 30.

---

## GENTIANA CHIRATA Or SWERTIA CHIRATA

(Chirata) **Gent-ch.**

Nela-verun, Kirata-tikla. N.O.: Gentianaceae.

**Clinical:** Anti-pyretic or febrifuge (fever killer); dyspepsia; hyperacidity; functional inactivity of the liver; flatulence; anorexia; worms; chronic fever.

A noted 'fever killer', in both acute and chronic malarial fevers. The keynote symptom accompanying the fever is burning in the eyes for as long as the fever lasts. Kala azar, with hepatomegaly and splenomegaly. Wards off debility after fever.

**Mind:** Dullness of mind, desire to lie down all the time, lazyness.

**Head:** Coldness of the head; dull pain in the temples, gradually extends to the whole head.

**Eyes:** Burning sensation.

**Ears:** Hissing sound in the ears.

**Nose:** Flushes of heat from the nostrils.

**Mouth:** Bad taste in the mouth, in the morning with halitosis. Yellowish coating in the centre of the tongue; difficulty in speech; tongue feels heavy.

**Throat:** Pain, better by hot drinks, worse morning and evening; dry hacking cough.

**Abdomen:** Flatulence; pain with an enlarged liver and spleen, especially, right sided renal pain; desire for bitter substances and meat.

**Urinary:** Red colored urine; burning during micturition.

**Male:** Weakness of the organ, impotence; slight discharge of semen.

**Extremities:** Aching pain in the extremities; weakness in legs; difficulty in walking.

**Fever:** Cold stage lasts long with nausea and bilious vomiting; no thirst but desire for hot water. The heat stage lasts for about three hours with slight thirst. Sweat after heat stage with little perspiration, only on the axilla, chest and thighs. Fever may appear at any time with burning in the eyes from its onset and lasts as long as it persists.

**Dose:** Mother tincture, 3x, 6.

---

## GYMNEMA SYLVESTRE

(Meshasringi or Gurmar) **Gymne.**

Mesha-sringa (Ram's Horn), N.O.: Asclepiadceae.

Chotta-dudhilata, Shiru-kuranja, Kavali.

**Clinical:** 'Sugar killer': diabetes mellitus; poisonous snake bites.

Is almost specific for diabetes mellitus. Diminishes sugar in the urine, patient puts on flesh and weight, appetite improves; assumes a healthy look. Improves his mental, physical and sexual faculties. Is able to work hard, is not exhausted after a little exertion as before. Prolongs a diabetic patients life. All symptoms accompanied with a burning sensation all over the body. Relaxation of all muscles.

**Mind:** Despondent; hopeful of recovery even on the death bed.

**Stomach:** Drinks large amounts, often.

**Urinary:** Profuse micturition loaded with sugar; extreme weakness after passing large quantities of urine. Color of urine is white with high specific gravity. Polyuria; day and night. Coitus increases the flow of urine and sugar. Sexual power almost lost.

**Skin:** Sensation of burning all over; diabetic carbuncles and boils burn.

**Modalities:** Worse coitus.

**Dose:** Mother tincture, 3x, 6.

---

# HOLARRHENA ANTIDYSENTERICA Or WRIGHTIA TINCTO

(Kurchi) **Kurch.**

Kutaji, Kaluoga, Indrayava, Indrajaveru, Pandrakura, Kurchi-conessi, Tellicherry Bark. N.O.: Apocynaceae.

**Clinical:** Acute and chronic dysentery.

Indicated in acute or chronic dysentery with profuse mucus and blood; associated with pinching, griping colic around the naval, prostration, emaciation, loss of appetite and a bitter taste in the mouth. Tenesmus; eructations and proctalgia with a constant urging to stools.

**Dose**: Mother tincture, 3x, 6x.

---

# HYDROCOTYLE ASIATICA

(Thankuni) **Hydrc.**

Indian Pennywort, Kurivana, Valla-rai, Tholkuri. N.O.: Umbelliferae.

**Clinical:** Dysentery; jaundice; gonorrhea; dropsy; leprosy; secondary syphilis; elephantiasis; gangrene after amputation; acne rosacea; gout; leucorrhea; lupus; ringworm.

The skin and female generative organs are the chief centers of attack. Also in intestinal inflammation and cellular proliferation; there is hypertrophy and induration of connective tissue; scleroderma. Affections of the trigeminal nerve. A great tonic to keep up strength and memory.

**Mind:** Gloomy; misanthropy; desire for solitude; indifference; loquacity; weakness of memory (Sushruta found it useful in increasing the memory).

**Head:** Vertigo with torpor; neuralgic pain in the external frontal nerve; occiput acutely sensitive to touch. Constriction in the occiput and integuments; swelling in the posterior part of the skull. Painful drawing in almost all cranial nerves.

**Eyes:** Dim vision; hyperemia of the palpebral conjunctiva; neuralgia orbitalis.

**Ears:** Otitis media; ringing in the left ear with stoppage and a blowing sound. Throbbing in the right ear.

**Nose:** Swollen; tickling, worse in left nostril; coryza, dry; stoppage of nose; epistaxis.

**Face:** Trigeminal neuralgia, especially on the left side. Intoxicated expression.

**Mouth:** Syphilitic affections, stomatitis, apthae, thrush on the left upper and under side of tongue. Impairment of speech; dysphagia; ptyalism. Taste insipid or bitter in the morning.

**Throat:** Tonsils inflamed, hyperemic; prickling in the larynx. Esophagus dry, rough with prickling and burning.

**Stomach:** Loathes food; anorexia followed by a good appetite; aversion to tobacco smoke. Acrid frequent eructations, globus hystericus. Heat in the stomach region.

**Abdomen:** Borborygmi, flatus with violent contractions in the intestines; pain especially in the transverse colon. Sensation as if all the organs were in motion. Pain in the upper part of liver; cirrhosis; obstructive jaundice.

**Rectum:** Sensation of weight; burning and itching in the anus.

**Stool:** Ineffectual desire; dry; hard.

**Urinary:** Irritation of the neck of the bladder and urethra. Frequent desire to micturate; urine profuse; becomes brown on cooling; turbid with sediment.

**Male:** Drawing pain in the spermatic cords; impotency; indifference to intercourse. Left scrotum relaxed; prostrate feels heavy.

**Female:** Leucorrhea; heaviness in uterus; vulva, vagina and cervix are red, severe labor-like pain in the uterus and appendages. Prickling and itching at the vulval orifice.

**Respiratory:** Dryness of larynx; weak voice; talking causes fatigue; difficulty in expectorating the bronchial mucus; shortness of breath. Oppression of chest; irritation of the air passages.

**Heart:** Constriction of the heart; cardiac spasm; irregular beating; pulse quiet and regular.

**Extremities:** Revival of old rheumatic pains. Contraction of forearms and legs; irresistible desire to stretch. Pain in all the joints, worse left side. Sensation as if hot water running through the marrow of bones, myalgia with weariness and crampy numbness in all muscles. Rheumatoid arthritis; gout, inability to stand.

**Sleep:** Yawning and stretching; sleepy during the day; heavy dreamless sleep or dreams all the while he is asleep.

**Fever:** Shivering in the afternoon; hands and feet cold, ameliorated by rubbing and becomes cold on ceasation of rubbing. Profuse sweat.

**Skin:** Multiplicity of skin affections. Circular spots with raised scaly edges. Erythema with severe itching and copious sweat. Miliary eruptions on the neck, back and chest. Itching at the tip of the nose. Thickening of the epidermoid layer with exfoliation of scales; elephantiasis, scleroderma, eczema, pemphigus, lupus. Acne rosacea; pustules on the chest. Syphilitic affections.

**Modalities:** Worse left side.

**Dose:** Mother tincture, 3x, 6x.

---

## HYGROPHILIA SPHINOSA

(Kule Khara) **Hydroph-s.**

Kokilaksha, Talmakhana, Gokshura, Tolimkhana, Nirguviveru, Gokhulajanum. N.O.: Acanthaceae.

**Clinical:** Anasarca and dropsy; gonorrhea; insomnia; impotency; rheumatism; leucorrhea; skin problems; renal calculus; hepatic obstruction.

Useful in skin affections which are worse by warmth and ameliorated by cold applications in gonorrhea; urinary affections; rheumatism and insomnia.

**Urinary:** Renal calculus, dropsy.

**Sleep:** Insomnia. An infaliable remedy for sleep.

**Fever:** Malaria associated with urticaria. With the rise in temperature, there is intense itching and urticaria like eruptions which are relieved by cold applications; fever appears in the morning without chill or thirst.

**Skin:** Urticaria, appears in summers, worse from heat and warmth; small red pimples and eruptions all over resembling measles; prickly heat. Ulcers due to impurity of blood.

**Modalities:** Worse heat, summers. Better cold application.

**Relationship:** Compare: *Rhus-t., Apis.*

**Dose:** Mother tincture, 3x, 6x, 30.

# JANOSIA Or JOANESIA ASOCA Or SARACA INDICA

(The Asoka Tree) **Joan.**

Asoka, Kankeli, Asok, Ashopalava. N.O.: Leguminosae.

**Clinical:** Uterine disorders; menorrhagia.

An ancient medicine of great repute for menstrual and uterine disorders. A sovereign remedy for amenorrhea and scanty menses with intolerable pain and burning sensation during micturition. A uterine tonic, giving strength to the uterus which has been weakened by chronic ailments.

**Mind:** Good natured; affectionate; lachrymose; timid; excitable and fatigued, does not like to do any work; absent minded; slow to understand; hysterical; impatient; satisfied with small things; disturbed sleep, insomnia; dreams of travelling or of fear; not very imaginative, exaggerated suffering.

**Head:** Stupefying or congestive headache; headache better by free menstrual flow; periodical headache better by bathing; heaviness of head; vertigo.

**Eyes:** Conjunctiva hyperemic, with burning and itching; lachrymation; photophobia; styes on the upper eyelids; short sighted; tired feeling in the eyes on least exertion.

**Ears:** Otalgia; hardness of hearing after a severe cold.

**Nose:** Catarrh, profuse watering from the nose, sneezing; soreness of the nostrils; obstruction of the nose; anosmia; epistaxis.

**Face:** Pale face; alternately hot and red; pimples on the face.

**Mouth:** Dryness with excessive thirst, drinks large quantities of water at a time; thickly white or brown coated tongue; bleeding gums; toothache.

**Throat:** Redness of the throat with a sore feeling; takes cold easily; cough, troublesome.

**Stomach:** Excessive nausea, sometimes with bilious vomiting, pain in the epigastrium; colicky pain; no desire for food; eats little. Eructations. Desire for sweet, sour acid things; disinclined to drink milk. Drinks large quantities of water. Want of appetite, dislikes food.

**Abdomen:** Hard, distended with passage of foul smelling flatus worse in the evening. Soreness in the lower abdomen. Flatulent colic.

**Stool:** Obstinate constipation; passes stool on every third or fourth day; pain before stool; soreness in the anus; blind or bleeding piles with itching and smarting; large, hard stools covered with mucus.

**Urinary:** Frequent, bloody, scanty and involuntary micturition at night; tenderness in bladder and pain in the lion. Nocturnal enuresis; profuse emission of watery urine.

**Male:** Orchitis; drawing pain in the spermatic cord; itching in the scrotum; seminal discharge with or without dreams.

**Female:** Headache due to suppression of menses; delayed or irregular menses; menstrual discharge is scanty, pale, watery; foul smelling, blackish; amenorrhea at puberty with headache; palpitations, hysteria with loss of appetite. Better by commencement of free flow; menorrhagia; profuse, long lasting menses making the female weak and anemic; menorrhagia due to uterine fibroids. Dysmenorrhea with constipation and a burning sensation over the face and eyes. Cessation of menses when colicky, abdominal pains supervene. Has a stimulating effect on the endometrium and ovarian tissue. Useful in sterility and menopause. Leucorrhea from delayed menses or in place of menses; infantile leucorrhea, small girls become emaciated despite regular nourishment; menstrual colic; headache due to scanty flow of menses with severe pain in the lower parts of the abdomen and back.

**Respiratory:** Hurried respiration; difficulty in breathing when walking and worse in the afternoon, evening; hacking cough.

**Heart:** Pain over the precordium; palpitations of the heart, worse on movement, walking or bending forward; tight feeling across the chest; pulse full; hard, quick.

**Back:** Pain in the back and sacrum, radiating towards the abdomen and thighs.

**Extremities:** Weak feeling in the limbs; pain in the small joints; shifting pain; numbness of the limbs.

**Sleep:** Disturbed; sleeplessness. Dreams of fear, travelling.

**Fever:** Chill without thirst; dry heat with restlessness; red cheeks; flushed face; running nose.

**Dose:** Mother tincture, 2x, 3x.

---

## JUSTICIA ADHATODA

(Vasaka) **Just.**

Baidyamata, Arusha, Adhatodai, Malabar-nut.

N.O.: Acanthaceae.

**Clinical:** Cough; coryza; bronchitis; pneumonia; phthisis; hemoptysis; jaundice; vomiting; constipation.

Excellent in all sorts of coughs and cold. It is proclaimed that no death can take place from cough of any kind, if Vasaka can display its healing properties.

**Mind:** Low spirited; oversensitive to external impressions; anxious; no desire to talk; irritable; despondent.

**Head:** Burning sensation over the forehead; heaviness and fullness of head; hot sensation; pulsations in both the temples.

**Eyes:** Lachrymation with coryza; burning in the eyes; dimness of vision.

**Ears:** Sound intolerable.

**Nose:** Profuse coryza with sneezing and headache. Pain and swelling in the nose; anosmia; loss of taste; obstruction of the nose with snuffles; dryness of the nose.

**Face:** Red; burning, hot; gnawing pains.

**Mouth:** Shooting pains in teeth radiating to the cheeks. Dryness of the mouth and tongue; marked thirst. White coating on the tongue.

**Throat:** Dry; pain during empty swallowing; tenacious mucus which cannot be raised by coughing.

**Stomach:** Loss of appetite; putrid taste in the mouth. Nausea; vomiting during cough; vomiting of mucus; weakness after vomiting.

**Abdomen:** Gnawing pain in the hepatic region; jaundice. Abundant flatus; gurgling; distention.

**Stool:** Obstinate constipation. Loose, mixed with mucus.

**Respiratory:** Highly efficacious in cold, coryza, cough, bronchitis, pneumonia, phthisis and hemoptysis. Audible rattling of mucus in the chest; difficult expectoration; loosened only by repeated hawking; expectoration of tough, yellow mucus. Dry, spasmodic cough; sense of constriction; dyspnea associated with cough; threatened suffocation. Whooping cough; child looses breath, turns pale, becomes still and blue, rigidity of the body. Vomiting with cough; no food or drink is retained in the stomach.

First stage of phthisis, hemoptysis. Hoarseness, larynx painful to touch. Tightness across the chest; asthmatic attacks, cannot endure a close, warm room; cough with wheezing.

**Fever:** Chills every evening with night sweats, also useful in consumption and other lung affections, attended with cough and hectic fever.

**Dose:** 3x, 6x, 30.

---

## JUSTICIA RUBRUM

(Rakta Vasaka) **Just-r.**

**Clinical:** Hemoptysis; hematemesis.

*Justicia rubrum* is highly efficacious where *Justicia adhatoda* fails; used where there is more hemoptysis and hematemesis.

**Relationship:** Compare: *Mill., Ip., Acal., Fic-r.*

**Dose:** Mother tincture, 3x, 6.

---

## LEUCAS ASPERA

(Drona) **Leucas-a.**

Dronapushpi, Dandakalasa, N.O.: Labiatae.
Guldera, Kulannaphul, Kumki.

**Clinical:** Intermittent fever; asthma; cough; dysentery; jaundice; hepatomegaly; splenomegaly; bite of venemous animals; skin problems.

Useful in cases of snake bites; mother tincture is applied both externally and internally; 10-15 drops per dose, at 15-20 minutes interval, till the patient feels better. In case of scorpion bites also, its action is noticed the burning pains disappears within a short period.

Also useful in intermittent fevers, asthma, nasal catarrh, scabies and complaints due to bilious disorders like jaundice. Bloody dysentery; splenic affections, induration and enlargement.

**Dose:** Mother tincture, 2x, 3x.

---

## LUFFA AMARA

(Titpolla) **Luf-am.**

Dhamarjab. N.O.: Cucurbitaceae.

**Clinical:** Splenomegaly; fever; hepatic congestion.

Of use in loose stools and vomiting with a marked burning sensation all over the body. Sometimes chills are felt. The pulse is weak and feeble, face is pale and the extremities are cold with clammy perspiration.

**Mind:** Anxious and dejected.

**Mouth:** Dry with excessive thirst, bitter taste in the mouth.

**Stomach:** Vomiting, sometimes every half hour, of bile and water. Simultaneous vomiting and purging.

**Abdomen:** Pain the hepatic and splenic regions; relieved by pressure.

**Stool:** Loose; rice water like; every 20-30 minutes; sometimes mixed with mucous. No pain is associated with stools; profuse, painless evacuations.

**Dose:** Mother tincture, 3x, 6x.

---

## LUFFA BINDAL

(Ghosalata) **Lub-b.**

Debdali, Koshataki. N.O.: Cucurbitaceae.

**Clinical:** Chronic malarial fever; gall stone colic; dropsy; acute and chronic nasal catarrh; enlarged liver and spleen (some authors also recommend its use externally over piles).

Those who are very susceptible to cold or to changes in the weather, or those who are attacked by catarrh off and on, are specially benefited by this drug.

**Nose:** Acute and chronic nasal catarrh; tendency to take on cold.

**Abdomen:** Splenomegaly; can replace *Ceanothus americanus* admirably. Gall stone colic, problems due to liver disorders.

**Rectum:** Controls piles satisfactorily (can be used externally over piles).

**Fever:** Chronic malarial fever associated with dropsy, hepatomegaly and splenomegaly.

**Dose:** Mother tincture, 3x, 6.

---

## MENISPERMUM COCCULUS

(Rakta Kanthalia) **Menis.**

**Clinical:** Menorrhagia. A great remedy for uterine hemorrhages.

**Mind:** Despondent.

**Head:** Giddiness of the head.

**Ears:** Ringing in the ears.

**Stool:** Lienteric with thirst and want of hunger.

**Female:** Menorrhagia; patient becomes extremely weak due to excessive bleeding; blood continuously oozes out of the uterus, hemorrhage worse from or during movement; color of blood is bright red and is mixed with clots; copious, bleeding; pain in the lower abdomen; excessive hemorrhage after delivery.

**Modalities:** Worse movement.

**Relationship:** Compare: *Sab., Tril-p., Ham., Ip.*

**Dose:** Mother tincture, 3x, 6x.

---

## NYCTANTHES ARBORTRISTIS

(Shephalika) **Nyct.**

Siuli, Harsinghar, N.O.: Jasminaceae.

Paghala Malli.

**Clinical:** Remittent fever; rheumatism; sciatica; constipation; headache. Bilious and obstinate, remittent fever, sciatica, rheumatism and constipation in children.

**Mind:** Anxious; restless.

**Head:** Dull headache; giddiness.

**Mouth:** Thickly coated with a white or yellowish fur.

**Stomach:** Burning sensation in the stomach, better by cold applications; profuse bilious vomiting with nausea; bitter vomiting.

**Abdomen:** Tenderness in the liver region, sensitive to touch, stitches in the liver region.

**Stool:** Constipated, profuse, bilious stools accompanied by nausea.

**Urinary:** High colored urine.

**Fever:** Useful in all fevers with a predominance of bilious symptoms. Insatiable thirst exists before and during chill and heat; nausea may or may not be present; drinking causes bilious vomiting. Sweat not marked.

**Relationship:** Compare: *Eup-per.*

**Dose:** Mother tincture.

---

# OCIMUM CARYOPHYLLATUM

(Dulal Tulasi) **Oci-car.**

**Clinical:** Spermatorrhea; gonorrhea; hematuria; bloody dysentery; nephritis; pyuria.

Frequent micturition; extreme burning during micturition, passage of pus with urine; hematuria. Has decided action upon the kidney, bladder and urethra. Inflammation and congestion of kidneys. In gonorrhea, in the first stage when there is excessive burning during micturition which is mixed with pus. Spermatorrhea; bloody dysentery. Fever may accompany all complaints.

**Dose:** Mother tincture, 3x, 6x.

---

# OCIMUM GRATISSIMUM

(Ram Tulsi) **Oci-g.**

**Clinical:** Gonorrhea; pyuria; dysuria; nasal catarrh; cough; fever.

The therapeutic properties that are attributed to *Oci-sa.* are present in this variety of Tulsi also. Nasal catarrh, cough and fever in children. Also used in gonorrhea with difficulty in micturition, burning while micturating and pyuria.

**Dose:** Mother tincture, 3x, 30.

---

# OCIMUM SANCTUM

(Tulsi) **Oci-sa.**

Vishnupriya, Tulasi, N.O.: Labiaceae.
Divya, Bharati, Krishna-mul,
Kala Tulasi, Shiva Tulasi, Holy Basil.

**Clinical:** Asthma; catarrh; cold; opthalmia neonatorum; typhoid; worm affections; tonsillitis; pleurisy.

In remittent fever associated with cold, cough or diarrhea, pneumonia, bronchitis and asthma. Remittent fever in children during dentition, diarrhea or worm complaints. Gastric and intestinal catarrh with fever and diarrhea.

**Mind:** Patient is very forgetful; forgets to perform his usual duties, makes mistakes; peevish during worm complaints. Starts from sleep, does not let the doctor examine them; does not like to lie in bed. Lack of concentration; drowsiness; prostration; falls asleep while answering (*Bapt.*).

**Head:** Head heavy, throbbing pain, as if a nail was driven into it, relieved by pressure, application of cold water and by fanning the head; worse while walking, better by wrapping up the head; heat on the vertex, better by pouring cold water over the head and fanning.

**Eyes:** Pain, hyperemia; lachrymation due to nasal catarrh; ophthalmia especially in infants, mist before the eyes when fixing them on something.

**Ears:** Noise in the ears; loud sound appears to be very painful. Watery discharge from the ear; offensive otorrhea; shortness of hearing; hot flushes in the ear. Otalgia due to nasal catarrh.

**Nose:** Nasal catarrh associated with frequent sneezing; white or yellow discharge from the nose; nostrils ulcerated; epistaxis. Influenza.

**Face:** Pale with a reddish hue or red.

**Mouth:** Lips are bright red; watery, profuse salivation; putrid and bitter taste in the mouth; aphthae in the mouth; the entire tongue is bright red or the sides are red but middle portion is thickly coated; lips dry and black, as if burnt. Toothache, severe, worse at night, on touch and from cold. Halitosis.

**Throat:** Pain and hyperemia of throat with dysphagia. Pain while coughing, hoarseness. Ulceration of the throat; glairy mucus; tonsillitis, voice altered.

**Stomach:** Eructations, hiccough, want of appetite.

**Abdomen:** Flatulent, distended, gurgling sound on pressure; heaviness. No relief despite frequent passages of stool. Griping pain in the hepatic and splenic regions. Pain in the right iliac fossa.

**Stool:** Copious, very offensive, watery, mucoid or bloody, yellow or greenish; involuntary during high fever; diarrhea in the rainy season or autumn.

**Urinary:** Enuresis in children, burning while micturating, frequent desire to micturate.

**Female:** Lochia, terribly offensive, of an unnatural color, lasts long; mixed with pus, blood and mucus, resembles washing of a fish. Menses are irregular. Leucorrhea and uterine complications avoided if used after delivery.

**Respiratory:** Of benefit in diarrhea and fever associated with cold, cough, bronchitis; eases difficult respiration. In cases of asthma where the patient sits bent forward and supports the head with the hands while the elbows rest on the knee; cannot lie quiet in bed. Wheezing and rattling. Pain in the chest while coughing or sneezing; pain in the middle of the sternum; pleuritic pains.

**Fever:** Excellent remedy in influenza and fevers associated with cough and diarrhea; acute pains all over the body; bone pains; soreness of the muscles and severe headache. Typhoid fever with chilliness; burning sensation all over the body; delirium; drowsiness and a comatose condition, with keynote symptoms of tongue and lips. Intermittent fever, comes on in the afternoon with extreme chilliness, hands and feet become cold, numb and tingle, do not become warm easily. Sensation of extreme heat and flashes of heat during the hot stage, burning in palms and soles relieved by a cool breeze and cold washing. Along with heat, sweat breaks out.

**Modalities:** Relieved by cold water application.

**Relationship:** *Cham., Cina, Bapt., Lob., Blatta-o., Eup-per.*

**Dose:** Mother tincture, 3x.

---

## OLDENLANDIA HERBACEA

(Khatpapra) **Olden-h.**

Kshetra-parpata, Daman-papar, Veno-nela Vemy, Poriengo, Kazuri, Two Flowered Indian Madder. N.O.: Rubiaceae.

**Clinical:** Low form of fevers; gastric problems; nervous depressions; jaundice.

Rise of temperature early in the morning with chill, thirst, headache and a burning sensation all over the body. Intensity of fever gradually lessens. Fever either remittent or intermittent coming on with bilious symptoms. Fever appears with greater intensity one day and on the next day it is of a milder character. Bilious vomiting; bilious loose stool, jaundice and gastric irritability. Increases the flow of urine and is a valuable remedy in nervous depression.

**Dose:** Mother tincture, 3x, 6x, 30.

---

## PSORALEA CORYLIFOLIA

(Babchi) **Psoral-c.**

Vakuchi, Lata Kasturi, Bavachi, Bawachi, Karpo-karishi, Kani Bogi. N.O.: Leguminoceae.

**Clinical:** Leucoderma; streptococci.

Has a powerful action against the skin streptococci. Locally beneficial in the treatment of leucoderma of a non-syphilitic origin. It dilates the arterioles of the subcapillary plexus; plasma content in the area is increased and it becomes hyperemic; the melanoblasts are stimulated leading to pigment formation; it diffuses into the decolorised leucodermic patches.

**Dose:** Mother tincture.

---

## RAUWOLFIA SERPENTINA

(Chandra) **Rauw.**

Sarpagandha, Chandrika, Chandra, Chotachand, Dhanmarna, Dhanbarua, Covannmilpori, Patalagandhi.

N.O.: Apocynaceae.

**Clinical:** Hypertension; mania.

Irritative condition of the central nervous system; insanity with violent maniacal symptoms. Fever during puerperium. In high blood pressure without marked atheromatous changes in the vessels. It also acts as a sedative.

**Dose:** Mother tincture.

---

## SOLANUM XANTHOCARPUM

(Kantikari) **Sol-x.**

Nidigdhika, Katele, Bhuringni, Warumlea, Kandankattiri, Pinna-mulaka.

N.O.: Solanaceae.

**Clinical:** Hoarseness; aphonia; bronchitis; pneumonia; broncho-pneumonia; asthma; fever; suppression of urine; renal calculi.

An excellent remedy for hoarseness with cough. Respiratory diseases with aphonia. Catarrhal fever. A sure preventive against small pox.

**Urinary:** Stricture, retention or suppression of urine. Renal calculus.

**Respiratory:** Hoarseness due to any cause with cough; bronchitis, pneumonia and broncho-pneumonia associated with aphonia. A sovereign remedy in asthma.

**Fever:** Fever with thirst; aversion to food; burning sensation and pain all over the body.

**Relationship:** Compare: *Caust., Phos., Sel., Berb., Canth., Sars., Lyc.*

**Dose:** Mother tincture, 2x, 3x.

---

# SYZYGIUM JAMBOLANUM

(Kala Jam) **Syzyg.**

Nilaphala, Jaman, Jambudo, Nacraedu, Navil, Nagum, Naval, Sittalchini, Black Plum. N.O.: Myrtaceae.

**Clinical:** Diabetes mellitus and insipidus; prickly heat; diarrhea; dysentery; scorbutic gums.

The most powerful remedy in diabetes mellitus; causes a marked diminution and disappearance of sugar in the urine; polydipsia; polyuria; profound prostration and emaciation. In cases of sore throat and spongy gums, a decoction of its bark is used as a gargle. Especially suited to patients who suffer from chronic dyspepsia.

**Mouth:** Scorbutic gums.

**Stool:** In all sorts of bloody dysentery; chronic diarrhea and dysentery.

**Urinary:** Polyuria; glycosuria; increased frequency and quantity day and night; high specific gravity.

**Skin:** Prickly heat on the upper body and arms; skin covered with small red papules which itch intensely. Chronic ulcers; diabetic ulcers.

**Relationship:** Compare: *Abrom-a.; Gymne.; Ceph-i.*

**Dose:** Mother tincture, 2x, 3x.

---

# TERMINALIA ARJUNA

(Arjuna) **Term-a.**

Vellaimarudamarum, Shardul, Sajadan. N.O.: Combretaceae.

**Clinical:** Angina pectoris; fractures; ecchymosis; gonorrhea; spermatorrhea; vertigo.

Diseases of the heart, both organic and functional; angina pectoris; suffocation; vertigo. In fractures, pain all over the body owing to a fall and all sorts of ecchymosis, the action of this drug in such cases is supreme. It is also efficacious in spermatorrhea and in gonorrhea.

**Mind:** Nervous.

**Head:** Giddiness.

**Ears:** Ringing in the ear.

**Mouth:** Bitter taste in the mouth; dryness.

**Urinary:** Scanty urine.

**Heart:** Palpitations, angina pectoris, weakness and sudden jerking pains in the heart.

**Dose:** Mother tincture, 3x.

---

## TERMINALIA CHEBULA

(Haritaki) **Term-c.**

Abhaya, Pathya, Har, Harara, Harrar, Hirda, Harda, Kadakai, Kadut-key (tree), Kadut-kaypinji (fruit), Karaka, Kurka (tree).

N.O.: Combrataceae.

**Clinical:** Bleeding piles; diarrhea; chronic dysentery; constipation; biliary colic; headache; vertigo; dropsy; skin diseases; glossitis.

Remedy for piles, constipation, chronic dysentery, dropsy, chronic diarrhea and some skin diseases.

**Mind:** Indifferent, easily indisposed with constant yawning, single minded.

**Head:** Vertigo, remains the whole day and night aggravated by hot, sun rays; aggravations from motion, hard pressure, ameliorated by cold bathing, in the evening, from dry cold air, sleep, eating. Slight headache in the occiput and right cranium.

**Mouth:** Profuse salivation with intense thirst for cold water; sensation of dryness in the upper jaw; gums swollen and hard; foul breath; fetid eructation. Acrid, empty eructation in the morning. Flabby, dry, brown coating on the tip of the tongue; sore and raw tongue.

**Stomach:** Sensation of fullness in the stomach.

**Abdomen:** Distention; rumbling and gurgling. Pain in the epigastrium and right lower abdomen. Slight pain in the region of liver (the large lobe); ameliorated temporarily by external pressure.

**Stool:** Frequent ineffectual desire for stool but passes only a small quantity with great force or nothing comes out at all; sweat during stool; pressive pain; itching and sensation of fullness in the rectum. In diarrhea; small quantity of feces mixed with mucus, flatulence associated with burning in the stomach. In constipation, small hard stool.

**Urinary:** Scanty urine, frequency of micturation increases at night.

**Respiratory:** Deep breathing.

**Heart:** Intense, pressive pain on the right side of chest; pressure, pain in the cardiac region; some heart beats are feeble or have a low sound, some are normal and some have a loud sound. Pulse for some moments is rapid and hard, and for some moments it is weak.

**Back:** Intense pain in the right lumbar region and lower spinal column aggravated on sitting, better by lying down in bed or by sleeping; pain in the back of the neck.

**Extremities:** Muscular pain in the right deltoid muscle; itching better by scratching.

**Modalities:** Worse by hot, sun rays; motion, hard pressure and exertion. Ameliorated by cold bathing, evening cold dry air, during sleep, by eating; closing the eyes and during complete mental and physical rest.

**Dose:** Mother tincture, 3x, 6x, 30.

---

## TINOSPORA CORDIFOLIA

(Gulancha) **Tinas.**

Ninjara, Guluchee, Guruchi, Gilo, Gularich, Gulwali, Gharol, Gula-veli, Shindil, Kodi, Tippa-tige, Guluchi, Amritvel, Heart-leaved. N.O.: Menispermaceae.

**Clinical:** Seminal debility; fevers; intermittent fevers; jaundice; splenic affections; leprosy; leucorrhea; rheumatism; skin diseases; secondary syphilis; genito-urinary problems; gonorrhea; dysuria; pyuria; etc.

A tonic, patient is extremely weak owing to repeated attacks of fever and exhausting seminal emissions. An excellent remedy for intermittent fever, jaundice, torpidity of the liver, bilious vomiting and leprosy.

**Urinary:** Frequent passage of small quantities of urine with burning during micturition, dysuria, urine mixed with pus. Gonorrhea and secondary syphilis.

**Heart:** Excessive palpitations due to severe weakness or excessive seminal emissions.

**Fever:** Acute or chronic malarial fever; temperature rises in the afternoon with chills and shivering, bilious vomiting with thirst and headache. Chronic, slow fever with history of gonorrhea and weakness due to seminal loss. Bad effects of quinine which causes continuation of fever with burning in hands, feet and face, jaundice, loss of appetite and headache.

**Dose:** Mother tincture, 2x, 3x, 6x.

---

## TRICHOSANTHES DIOICA

(Patal) **Trich.**

Patola, Parver, Palwal, Kombu-pudalai, Kammu-potla, Wild Snakegourd. N.O.: Cucurbitaceae.

**Clinical:** Chronic and acute malarial fever, kala-azar; nausea and vomiting; cholera; dysentery; hepatomegaly; jaundice; splenomegaly.

Burning sensation all over the body with thirst and a desire for cold things. In all kinds of fever with predominance of bilious symptoms. Extreme weakness, restlessness and sleepiness.

**Mind:** Despondent, yawning and stretching of limbs. No desire to cover the body, desire to have a bath.

**Head:** Vertigo while lying in bed, terrible headache during fever.

**Eyes:** Dilated pupils. Yellow discoloration during fever with hepato-splenomegaly.

**Mouth:** Thirst; with dryness of throat; slimy salivation; constant waterbrash; bitter, insipid taste in the mouth.

**Stomach:** Nausea from the smell of medicine; waterbrash; vomiting of stringy mucus streaked with blood. Hematemesis. Pulse almost imperceptible with vomiting and purging. Eructations; extreme hunger; desires cold things.

**Abdomen:** Empty feeling; distention; uneasiness; hot feeling in the abdomen at 11 a.m.; pain and gurgling. Hepatomegaly, tender; worse sneezing, coughing and movement. Splenomegaly. Jaundice.

**Stool:** Copious, painless, greenish-yellow, liquid, mixed with bile and mucus; bloody stool, becomes exhausted due to frequent passage of stool. After stool, urging and straining continue for a long time; rectal prolapse; burning in the anus; smarting pain after stools is the characteristic symptom for its application; passage of involuntary, bloody, stools. In cholera with copious stools and vomiting; associated with restlessness, thirst, burning sweat extreme prostration; coldness of extremities and pulselessness.

**Urinary:** Scanty; red urine, retention of urine along with purging and vomiting.

**Extremities:** Swelling of the lower extremities.

**Fever:** Comes around 11 a.m. - 12 noon with chills; during fever, burning sensation all over the body; rise in temperature is associated with headache, and burning thirst. Acute fever is associated with vomiting, nausea and a constant waterbrash. Chronic fever with hepato-splenomegaly and jaundice; chronic malarial fevers and Kala-azar. Fever of short duration one day and of greater intensity the next day. Rise or fall in temperature is directly proportional to headache. Used in all kinds of fever with predominance of bilious symptoms. Headache, waterbrash and nausea are the keynote symptoms for its administration.

**Relationship:** Compare: *Ip., Podo.*

**Dose:** Mother tincture, 3x, 6x, 30.

# VERNONIA ANTHELMINTICA

(Somaraja) **Vern-a.**

Somraj, Bakchi; N.O.: Compositae.
Kali-jiri, Kadvo-jiri,
Kattu-shiragam, Adavi-jilakara.

**Clinical:** Anti-helmintic; threadworms; worm problems.

It has a remarkable anti-helmintic property and it is distinctly effective in threadworm infection. It is also useful in problems arising as a consequence to worm problems; nocturnal enuresis, grinding of teeth at night, etc.

**Dose:** Mother tincture, 3x.

■

# SOME IMPORTANT NOSODES & SARCODES

# AVIAIRE

(Tuberculinum Avis) **Tub-a.**

**Source:** Prepared from of chicken tuberculosis

**Clinical:** Bronchitis; influenza; measles; phthisis; meningitis; broncho-pneumonia; infantile asthma; acute rhinitis; acute sinusitis; acute blepharitis; conjunctivitis; acute otitis; mastoiditis; cervical adenopathy.

*Aviaire* is indicated in acute pulmonary affections. Marked asthenia, anorexia and emaciation. Cervical micro-adenopathy. Problems arising after measles.

**Head:** *Frontal headache* with a hot forehead. Meningitis, especially following measles, convustions.

**Eyes:** *Conjunctiva congested;* lachrymation.

**Ears:** Acute otitis media; otorrhea; acute mastoiditis.

**Nose:** Anosmia; muco-purulent catarrh with continuous sneezing; sinusitis, *pain at the root of the nose.*

**Throat:** Laryngitis; *hoarseness.*

**Respiratory:** Acts most prominently on the apices. In broncho-pulmonary diseases of children and acute affections of adults; bronchitis following measles; infantile broncho-pneumonia. Dry, painful cough, thoracic wall painful; polypnea, with fan-like motion of alae nasi. Tuberculosis ; asthma in children.

**Heart:** Tachycardia with a rapid, bounding pulse. Cynosis especially of extremities.

**Fever:** General uneasines with chills and general muscular pains. Temprature ranges between 39° C and 40° C

**Relationship:** Compare : *Ferr-p., Puls., Ars-i., Sulph-i., Bac., Tub.*

**Dose:** In acute cases: 4C or 5C every 2 hours.

In chronic cases: 7 C.

(C - centecimal potency)

---

# BACILLUS 7 (PATERSON)

**Bacls-7**

**Source:** Gram negative bacilli whose characters are similar to *Aerobacter aerogenes*. It is isolated from water, soil and very rarely from the fecal matter of men and animals.

**Clinical:** Hypothyroidism; lumbago; flat foot; rheumatism.

It is named so, as it was the 7th non-lactose, fermenting type of bacillus to be observed in the laboratory, and as it did not conform to any of the previously known groups, it was given the number 7.

*Mental and physical fatigue* is the red line symptom of this drug. Tubercular constitution, premature aging; walks slowly like an old man, is swollen, slow and pale. Worn out subjects, fatigued at the idea of an effort. Muscular and *sexual weakness.*

**Eyes:** Thrombosis of the central vein in retina. Eyes feel heavy; dropsy, edematous eyelids.

**Ears:** Deafness of catarrhal origin.

**Throat:** Hypothyroidism, tonsillitis.

**Abdomen:** All symptoms are related to general lack of nerve and muscle tone. Sensation of fullness after meals; flatulent distention, ptosis of intestines. Pain in the liver region; constipation; hemorrhoids.

**Urinary:** Feeble flow or oliguria.

**Respiratory:** Bronchitis; asthma; tough mucus, difficult to raise.

**Heart:** Arterial hypotension; myocardial weakness with a slow pulse. Profuse sweat.

**Back:** Backache, cannot stand for long without feeling faint; stiffness of the neck; 'cracks like a nut'. Relaxed fibrous tissue with a tendency to form '*rheumatic nodules*'. *Fibrosity of the neck and shoulders.* Pain better, rest and *heat;* worse, humid and *cold weather.*

**Extremities:** Arthritis and stiffness of knees, heels shoulders, elbows and wrist; edema of the articulations of the legs; gout. Swollen fingers; *throbbing in the capillary vessels of the fingers.*

**Sleep:** Takes long to fall asleep, around 2 hours. Light sleepers, wakes up around 2-3 a.m.

**Skin:** Fissures on palms and finger tips, paronychia.

**Modalities:** Worse, cold, humidity, beginning movement. Better, heat and rest.

**Relationship:** Compare: *Kali-s., Calc-f., Calc., Rhus-t., Caust.*

**Dose:** 6C, 30C, 200C, 1M, 10M, 50M, and CM.

---

## BACILLUS 10 (PATERSON)

**Bacls-10**

**Source:** Does not exist in its bacteriological nomenclature. Is prepared by the Nelson pharmacy.

**Clinical:** Anorexia; cholecystitis; asthma; lipoma; warts; dermatitis.

Suited to anxious, irritable and depressed people, especially blondes.

**Mouth:** Halitosis; *spongy gums.*

**Stomach:** Anorexia; aversion to breakfast; desires chocolate, sugar and fried fish; cannot digest eggs and fat. Nausea; vomiting.

**Abdomen:** Occasional cholecystitis; intestinal paresis . Anal pruritus.

**Female:** Pruritus vulva; *leucorrhea smells like fish; greenish and corrosive.*

**Respiratory:** Asthma; difficult expectoration; cough worse in the morning.

**Extremities:** Pain in the iliac fossa, thighs, coccyx and left knee.

**Skin:** Lipoma, warts on hands, numerous, flat or pointed. Dermatitis in the folds.

**Dose:** 6C, 12C, 30C, 200C, 1M, 10M, 50M and CM.

---

# BACILLUS DYSENTERIAE (BACH)

(Dysenteriae Compound—Bach) **Dys.**

**Source:** Prepared from *Bacillus dysenteriae,* which is eliminated in the fecal matter of infected people.

**Clinical:** Chorea; gastric and duodenal ulcer; bronchitis; pharyngitis; cystitis; dysmenorrhea; osteoarthritis; osteoporosis; herpes; eczema; urticaria.

The keynote of this nosode is anticipatory *nervous tension.* Tubercular constitutions similar to *Phosphorus,* with a *restless mind.*

**Mind:** Nervous tension, mental uneasiness in anticipation of some event. Claustrophobia, uneasy and shy among strangers. This mental uneasiness manifests itself as physical restlessness. Cannot keep still, fidgets; *choreic twitching of facial muscles, limbs.* Hypersensitive to criticism. Nervous stammering; restless; depressed; embarrased.

**Head:** Headache, frontal, over the eyes or in the vertex; brought on by excitement; periodic headache occurring every to 7 to 14 days. Integument sensitive and tender on combing. Abundant dandruff.

**Eyes:** Conjunctivitis; blepharitis; styes. Vision yellow, sees floating bodies.

**Ears:** Otorrhea.

**Nose:** *Pain at the root* of nose; acute catarrh of acute nasal mucous membranes; *rhinorrhea*, hay fever.

**Face:** Trembling of facial muscles.

**Mouth:** Dry, fissured lips. Bad taste; tongue as if scorched and burning.

**Throat:** Hypertrophy of the thyroid gland with tachycardia. Repeated and frequent attacks of tonsillitis; pharyngitis.

**Stomach:** Has a selective action on the pylorus causing spasm and retention of digested contents; dilatation of stomach. Awakened around 12 midnight and 1 a.m. due to acute pain in the stomach; relieved by profuse mucoid vomiting. *Dys.* has been successfully used in *congenital pyloric stenosis* when the reason is spasm of the pylorus. Gastralgia and gastric ulcer. Desires fats, sweetened food, salty food and milk.

**Abdomen:** Distention with flatulence and uneasiness after meals. Duodenal ulcer with history of nervous tension.

**Rectum:** Sensation of throbbing; sensation of a plug in the rectum, sensation of diarrhea.

**Stool:** Diarrhea, frequent stools for 5-6 days.

**Urinary:** Urgent desire to micturate while travelling by train, aeroplane, etc., due to anticipatory tension, cystitis.

**Female:** *Irregular menses,* dysmenorrhea.

**Respiratory:** Sensation of constriction in the lower ribs; dry pleurisy, pleurodynia; chronic bronchitis with repeated attacks; spasmodic cough with expectoration, tinged with blood.

**Heart:** Functional disturbance of the heart with precordial uneasiness before important events.

**Extremities:** *Osteoarthritis* especially of the knees. Periostitis of the heel. Osteoporosis.

**Skin:** Herpes especially on the upper half of the body. Vesicles or eczema between fingers. Psoriasis; urticaria. Dry dermatitis of the hands with painful fissures.

**Modalities:** Worse, in a crowd, during a journey; at night, between 1-2 a.m. Better, while eating.

**Relationship:** Compare: *Ars., Arg-n., Kalm.*

**Dose:** 12C, 30C, 200C, 1M, 10M, 50M and CM.

---

## BACILLUS GAERTNER (BACH)

(Gaertner (Bach) or Salmonella Enteriditis) **Gaert.**

**Source:** *Salmonella enteriditis* is a serotype of *Salmonella,* frequently found in animals, which cause food intoxication in men.

**Clinical:** Precancerous state; coeliac disease; furunculosis; rheumatism; gastroenteritis; pancreatic diseases; malnutrition.

The keynote is *malnutrition*, thus it is applicable in the treatment of several diseases of childhood. Also valuable in extremes of life associated with malignancy. Marked emaciation can be considered as an indication for the use of this nosode. Great deficiency of connective tissue. People, especially children are hypersensitive.

**Mind:** Symptoms mostly observed in children, *hypersensitive* to all mental and physical impressions; over active brain with an under nourished body. *Intelligent*, nervous with *restlessness of hands and feet* especially when crossing the road or when alone, chews his nails.

**Eyes:** Styes.

**Nose:** Catarrh; polyp.

**Mouth:** Perilabial herpes; dry eruptions with desquamation of lips. Tongue fissured, teeth black; profuse salivation.

**Stomach:** *Cannot digest fatty food.* Desires cheese, eggs, milk, puddings, sugar and sweets. Vomits after eating sweets. Hyperchlorhydria.

**Abdomen:** Chief seat of action; often manifests itself around the age of 6 months when the infant is put on top feed. *Coeliac disease;* ketosis; chronic gastroenteritis; tabes mesentrica.

**Stool:** Fetid diarrhea, every 15 days; stools mixed with mucus and blood. Threadworms.

**Urinary:** Urethritis; blood and mucus in urine.

**Female:** Profuse, fetid leucorrhea; pruritus vulva.

**Back:** Severe backache with pain in hips.

**Extremities:** Fibrous rheumatism of the shoulder; worse at night. Rheumatism of hands and feet.

**Sleep:** *Sleeps for a long time;* wants light and company while sleeping; cannot sleep alone. Fear at night with profuse sweat.

**Skin:** Chapped hands in winters, furuncles on arms and legs; round, urticarious patches.

**Modalities:** Worse, when nervous, at night and in winters. Better, when someone is near.

**Relationship:** Compare: *Phos., Sil., Merc., Tub., Syph.*

**Dose:** 12C, 30C, 10M, 50M and CM.

---

# BACILLUS MORGAN (BACH)

**Morg.**

**Source:** A gram negative bacilli isolated from faecal matter of children suffering from summer diarrhea caused by these bacilli.

**Clinical:** Migraine; Meniere's disease; cholelithiasis; chronic cholecystitis; aphthae; fissures; varices; hemorrhoids; hypertension; cerebral thrombosis; broncho-pneumonia; bronchitis; emphysema; warts; acne rosacea; chilblains; arthritis; renal stone; dysparunia, sinusitis; rhinitis; etc.

The keynote for the *Morgan* group is *'congestion'*. If this is used in the study of the various parts affected, it will give a good symptom picture of the pathogenesis of this drug. It is prescribed when there is a history of repeated congestions in any part.

**Mind:** *Anxious* and apprehensive about health. Irritable; avoids company but gets anxious if left alone, *agoraphobia*; *fear of a crowd.* Depressed with suicidal tendency.

**Head:** Congestive headache with a flushed face; worse heat, thunderstorm, excitement and travelling. Vertigo from high blood pressure or intense nervous excitement. Migraine at the beginning of menses and due to hepatic problems.

**Eyes:** Chalazion; conjunctivitis; styes. Phlyctenular keratitis.

**Ears:** Tinnitus; deficent hearing; catarrh and otorrhea. Furuncle of the meatus. Alopecia.

**Nose:** Anosmia, sinusitis of frontal and maxillary sinuses. Epistaxis.

**Mouth:** Lips red, *fissures at the corners of lips.* Halitosis, pyrosis; dirty tongue. Bitter taste in the morning with accumulation of mucus, resulting in gagging as soon as one rises from the bed. Stomatitis; aphthae. Warts on the tongue.

**Throat:** Dry, burning and congested; tonsillitis, quinsy; cervical lymphadenopathy. Hoarseness in the morning, difficult expectoration. Laryngitis, pharyngitis and tracheitis.

**Stomach:** Congestion of gastric mucosa; heartburn. Desires fats, sweets, eggs and butter. Pain in the epigastrium. Acidity and pain relieved by eating.

**Abdomen:** Borborygmi. Congestion of the liver; bilious vomitings, especially at menopause. Tenderness in the hepatic region; cholecystitis, cholelithiasis.

**Rectum:** *Anal fissures.* Anal pruritus. Hemorrhoids.

**Stool:** Constipated with fissures. Diarrhea in the morning and after meals.

**Urinary:** Dysuria; frequent micturition. Glycosuria; strong smelling and corrosive urine. Renal stone and cystitis.

**Male:** Vesicular, desquamous, oozing, red, eczematous *eruptions on the scrotum,* perineum and groin.

**Female:** Congestive dysmenorrhea; menorrhagia and metrorrhagia. Intense vagino–vulvar pruritus; *corrosive leucorrhea,* fetid, yellow, brownish-green. Furuncle on the vulva. Congestive flushing of menopause; congestive headache before menses. Dysparunia. Bartholinitis.

**Heart:** Hypertension, venous congestion resulting in varices; venous stasis especially of legs and feet.

**Back:** Rigidity of the back and shoulders.

**Extremities:** Chronic congestion around joints, usually affecting the knee and phalangeal joints. *Rheumatism of hands with painful swelling;* nodosities of fingers. Painful swelling of knees, osteoarthritis; fibrous arthritis. Soles painful. Pain worse at night, by heat and on beginning movement. Offensive foot sweat. Chilblains of feet and toes due to erythro-cynosis. Varices with a bluish discoloration of the legs.

**Skin:** The most prominent sphere of action is seen here when there is congestion of the skin with itchy eruptions, worse from heat. *Acne rosacea.* Skin sensitive to touch of linen and sun. Eczema on the buttocks of children, especially during dentition. Furuncles.

**Modalities:** Worse, heat, at night and by washing. Better, while eating and prolonged movement.

**Relationship:** Compare: *Sulph., Psor., Puls., Graph., Sep., Calc., Rhus-t., Nat-s., Med., Sil., Petr., Lyc. Bacillus Morgan pure* (*Paterson*) (*Morg-p.*) – Indicated in marked skin eruptions, liver disturbances, bilious headache and cholelithiasis. *Bacillus Morgan – Gaertner* (*Paterson*)*-Morg-g.* –Also indicated in liver and skin affections. However it is more useful in acute inflammatory attacks as in cholecystitis. Can also be considered in cases of renal colic due to renal stone.

**Dose:** 30C, 200C, 1M, 10M, 50M and CM.

---

# BACILLUS MORGAN GAERTNER (PATERSON)

(Morgan-gaertner—Paterson) **Morg-g.**

**Clinical:** Claustrophobia; cholecystitis; anal fissures; angina pectoris; myocarditis; sinusitis; otitis; chalazion; styes; renal stone; pyelitis; alopecia; warts; psoriasis; eczema; polyarthritis.

Suited to subjects with a pale face and fine brown hair. Indicated in liver and skin diseases where there is an evidence of acute inflammatory attacks. A good remedy for renal colic. Predominently a right sided remedy.

**Mind:** *Impatient, tense and irritable;* reacts strongly; gets excited in company; apprehensive; chews nails. Claustrophobia.

**Eyes:** Blepharitis of a chronic origin; styes; chalazions. Corneal ulcer, vitrous opacity.

**Ears:** Buzzing in the ears. Furuncles in the auditory conduit.

**Nose:** Maxillary sinusitis, rhinitis, profuse flow. Ulceration of the nose, epistaxis. Nasal herpes.

**Face:** Facial neuralgia especially left sided. Sudden edema of the face. Herpes of the left side.

**Mouth:** Pyorrhea, gingivitis. Tongue burns, as if pricked by needles; bitter taste; thick saliva. Fissures at the corner of lips.

**Throat:** Tonsillitis. Edematous uvula. Burning sensation at the base of throat.

**Stomach:** *Desires sweets;* noisy eructations with an offensive smell. Fullness of the epigastrium without eating. Vomiting after meals; dyspepsia.

**Abdomen:** Flatus, especially in the left and right hypochondrial region. *Cholecystitis.*

**Rectum:** Anal fissure; and pruritus. Painful, bleeding hemorrhoids. Ano-rectal prolapse.

**Stool:** Constipation due to intestinal lethargy; dry, hard stool with mucus; spontaneous expulsion of mucus through the rectum even when the patient is not constipated.

**Urinary:** Cystitis with frequent micturition. Burning urine; pain in the region of kidney. Renal colic especially associated with lithiasis; pyelonephritis. Enuresis.

**Female:** *Irritation at the approach of menses;* dysmenorrhea. Vulvar pruritus. Warts on the breast.

**Respiratory:** Pleurodynia; tickling cough in the morning and evening. Asthma.

**Heart:** Angina pectoris; constriction in the chest; pain radiates to the left arm. Sensation of coldness in the chest. Nocturnal palpitations wake the patient up; bitter eructations, passing flatus and by movement.

**Back:** Cervical spondylosis.

**Extremities:** Progressive polyarthritis. Thumb swollen. Excessive heat of feet at night.

**Sleep:** *Fear of the night;* cries out in sleep.

**Skin:** Alopecia areata; integument sensitive. Psoriasis, eczema and urticaria. Big, flat or lacerated warts on the hands. Herpetic eruptions on left side of face and on the soles.

**Modalities:** Worse, in company, after meals, before menses, by heat of bed and at night. Better, motion, passing flatus and eructations.

**Relationship:** Compare: *Lyc., Puls., Sil., Kali-bi., Nat-m., Nux-v., Sulph., Sep., Graph., Calc.*

**Dose:** 6C, 12C, 30C, 200C, 1M, 10M, 50M and CM.

---

# BACILLUS PROTEUS (BACH)

**Prot.**

All the symptoms are associated with the central and peripheral nervous system, the keynote being *"suddenness"*. For instance; *"brain storm"*, violent upset of the nervous system. The patient displays a violent temper especially when opposed. Patient becomes violent, throws everything that comes in hand; kicks and strikes. The child throws a tantrum by lying on the floor, screams and kicks. Emotional hysteria. Convulsions, and epileptiform seizures. Meningitis in children during fever is observed.

Further indication for the use of this nosode is in disturbance of the peripheral nervous system as evidenced by spasm of the peripheral circulation. For example – intermittent claudication of lower limbs; anginal attacks due to spasm of coronary capillaries; etc. There are two well known diseases associated with capillary spasm where nosode *Prot.* has been found useful:

1. Raynaud's disease (spasm of the capillaries supplying the extremities) and ;
2. Meniere's disease (spasm of capillaries supplying the brain resulting in vertigo).

Symptoms are also manifested in the digestive tract but are secondary to the action of the central nervous system. Prolonged nervous strain or tension is an important cause of duodenal ulcers.

Muscular cramps are characteristic of this nosode. Also seen is, angioneurotic edema and a tendency for herpetic eruptions at the muco-cutaneous margins. Marked sensitivity to ultra violet rays.

**Relationship:** Compare: *Ign.* (in emotional hysteria); *Nat-m.* (duodenal ulcer); *Apis* (in angioneurotic edema); *Cupr.* (muscular cramps).

**Dose:** High potencies.

---

# BACILLUS SYCOCCUS (PATERSON)

(Sycotic Co. or Sycotic Compound or Sycoccus—Paterson) **Syc.**

**Source:** A non-lactose fermenting coccus found in the intestinal tract. It is a gram-negative diplococcus. Morphologically similar to *gonococcus*.

**Clinical:** Glossitis; worms; hepatitis; asthma; sinusitis; conjunctivitis; otorrhea; nephritis; cystitis; polyarthritis; rheumatism; herpes zoster; acne rosacea; paronychia.

The characteristic symptom is irritability in special reference to the mucus and synovial membranes. Tubercular constitution; a pale anemic subject having a swollen face, yellowish discoloration and premature graying of hair.

**Mind:** Nervous irritability; chews nails; angry; fear of the dark, of being alone. Tense, tearful, timid, hypersensitive.

**Head:** *Premature graying of hair,* profuse sweat on the head at night. Irritation of meninges, sub-acute or chronic. Headache every fortnight, frontal and congestive, due to sinusitis or tubercular meningitis; better rest and heat; worse noise.

**Eyes:** *Blinking of lids,* painful; photophobia, hemiopia. Chalazion; conjunctivitis; vitreous opacity.

**Ears:** Excess of cerumen. Otorrhea; diminished hearing. Fissures behind the ear; eczema of the auditory conduit.

**Nose:** *Sinusitis;* frontal and maxillary sinuses involved. Coryza, anosmia, epistaxis. *Dryness of the nose* with crusts; *fissures* of the nostrils.

**Face:** Hirsutism in women, left sided, facial neuralgia; pale anemic, edematous; yellowish discoloration.

**Mouth:** *Lips and tongue dry and fissured.* Tongue sticks to the palate; ulcers and warts on the tongue; diminution of taste; sialorrhea.

**Throat:** Tonsillitis and adenoids; dysphagia; easily choked.

**Stomach:** Chronic irritation of the alimentary tract. Hyperchlorhydria; heartburn, vomiting at night which ameliorates. Capricious appetite. Desires butter, fat, cheese, milk and sweets. Aversion to eggs; nausea at the smell of food, after eating eggs.

**Abdomen:** Distended with pain in the iliac fossa. Gastroenteritis; hepatitis.

**Stool:** Urgent desire for stool on waking up; loose, offensive stool, excoriating; constipation is unusual, diarrhea is common. Ano-rectal prolapse.

**Urinary:** Marked action on the urinary tract causes irritation of the mucous membranes from the kidneys to the urethral tract; pyelitis, cystitis and urethritis. Irritating urine with a strong smell; frequent proteinuria.

**Male:** Balanitis, sexual weakness.

**Female:** Delayed menstrual cycle irritation of the female sexual system; endocervicitis; metritis, ovaritis. Pain in the left ovary; left salpingo-ovaritis; cystic ovary; leucorrhea, profuse, yellowish, fetid, corrosive pruritis.

**Respiratory:** Asthma and bronchitis aggravated during frost and humid weather; better at seaside. Dyspnea in the morning; easy expectoration; fits of spasmodic, weakening cough. *Fibrosis of the thoracic walls;* intercostal pain; pleurodynia.

**Back:** Stiffness, rheumatic fibrositis of the neck, shoulder and back. Pain in the hips and lumbosacral region; worse, prolonged sitting in one position, at night and on first movement, amelioration by heat and continuous motion.

**Extremities:** Nocturnal pain in arms, wrist, hands and fingers. General rheumatic fibrositis. *Painful swollen heel.* Slight edema of extremities, especially feet. Profuse sweat on hands, feet and head.

**Sleep:** Restless, fear of the night; cannot stay alone. Takes a long time to fall asleep; dreams of dead people.

**Skin:** Sallow complexion. Warts on muco-cutaneous surfaces; *flat warts on hands and feet.* Vesicular eruptions in the body and face; worse by heat, at night and by detergents; herpes zoster; chickenpox. Erythmatous dermatitis, fissured; fissures on finger tips and heels. Alopecia, brittle nails and acne rosacea. Chilblains, intertrigo of breasts; chronic and acute eczema. *Fibrositic induration of skin;* scleroderma.

**Modalities:** Worse, cold, humidity, sitting in one position; first movement and at night. Better, at the sea side, by heat and prolonged movement.

**Relationship:** Compare: *Puls., Thuj., Lyc., Sep., Nat-m., Tub., Bac., Kali-bi., Sulph., Sil., Calc., Med.*

**Dose:** 6C, 12C, 30C, 200C, 1M, 10M, 50M and CM.

---

# BOTULINUM

**Botul.**

**Source:** *Clostridium botulinum* elaborated on putrified pork.

**Clinical:** Dysphagia; diplopia; mask facies; uremia.

It is an extremely toxic substance, a type of pyrogenum. It is characterised by paralysis, poliomyelitis, mask-like face due to facial paralysis, ptosis, diplopia, respiratory paralysis, paralysis of vocal cords and legs. Complaints are accompanied by retention of urine and stool; dysphagia and marked thirst.

**Relationship:** Compare: *Benzinum nitricum.*

**Dose:** 30C to 1M.

---

# BRUCELLA MELITENSIS

**Brucel.**

**Source:** Melitine is the filterate of a 21 days old culture of the fever microbe.

**Clinical:** Chronic fevers; myalgia,; neurasthenia; subacute polyartaritis; orchitis, epididmitis.

Indicated in *chronic febrile states* with *profuse sweat* on the least exertion, and at night. *Muscular* and *articular pains* especially in the lower limbs . Marked anorexia and emaciation . Tendancy to constipation with dry, hard stools.

**Mind:** Irritable, nervous, emotional instability with insomnia, vertigo and headache.

**Modalities:** Worse, prolonged exercise , in a hot room, breeze from the sea, humidity and during a storm. Better, heat and in the sun.

**Relationship:** Compare : *Nat-m., Gels., Ferr-p.*

**Dose:** 30 C potency and above.

---

# COLIBACILLINUM

**Coli.**

**Source:** From the culture of three stocks of *Escherichia coli.*

**Clinical:** Chronic renal and intestinal diseases; typhoid; Addison's disease; colibacillary myelitis; colibacillary meningitis; colibacillary encephalitis; schizophrenia; cholecystitis; chronic appendicitis; worms; colibacillary pyelonephritis; cystitis; inflammation of male and female genital organs; rheumatism.

A state of permanent asthenia with mental and physical weakness. General fatigue and depression which is proportional to digestive and urinary problems.

All complaints date back to a digestive or urinary problem.

**Mind:** *Amnesia;* forgets recent incidents; cannot find the right word; forgets names. Constant mental confusion due to loss of memory. *Subsitutes one word for another.* Empty feeling in the head; *timidity; indecision.* Depressed, confused, delirious and obsessional neurosis . *Schizophrenia.*

**Head:** *Frontal* and *supraorbital* headache; worse, humidity, cold, contradictory and strong emotions.

**Eyes:** *Unilateral swelling of upper eyelids.*

**Mouth:** White coated tongue; united glossy patches without pappillae on the median strip.

**Stomach:** Capricious appetite or anorexia.

**Abdomen:** Heaviness of the abdomen. Distended with flatus; expulsion of putrid gas. Sensation of coldness and chills immideatly after meals. Hepatomegaly; liver sensitive; cholecystitis. Spasms; slow intestinal movement; spasmodic colitis. Chronic appendicitis; rumbling in the right caeco-colic region.

**Stool:** Constipation. Profuse, prostrating diarrhea in infants and small children with hypothermia, bradycardia and dehydration.

**Urinary:** Inflammation of the entire urinary tract i.e. pyelonephritis, urethritis, cystitis, etc. *Frequent micturition; passes small quantities* at a time; sensation as if he *must go again to micturate immideatly after passing urine.* Dysuria; burning at the end of flow. Pain in region of kidney and along the urethra; painful on palpation . Offensive urine; occasionally, hematuria, sensation of heat and burning after micturition.

**Male:** Erection and ejaculation painful; burning in the urethra after coition. Relapsing epididmitis; prostration.

**Female:** Lower abdomen feels heavy; bilateral ovarian pain; salpingitis, metritis, vaginitis. Yellow , mildly irritating leucorrhea . Burning in the vulva and vagina during coition. Subacute puerperal fever.

**Heart:** Hypotension; tendancy to collapse; paleness and anxiety.

**Extremities:** Joints of hands and legs swollen; polyarthritis; chronic degenerative rheumatism.

**Sleep:** Hypersomnia, heavy somnolence.

**Modalities:** Worse cold, humidity, on the seaside, after rest, milk. Better, by heat .

**Relationship:** Compare: *Psor., Med., Anac., Lyc., Sep., Thuj., Thymol., Cyn-d.*

**Dose:** 6C to 30C.

---

## D.T.T.A.B.

(Diphthero-tetano-typho-paratyphoidi) **Diph-t-tpt.**

**Source:** Obtained from anti-diphitheric, anti-tetnic and anti-typho-paratyphoid mixed vaccine.

**Clinical:** Allergy; epilepsy; tetnus; paralysis; hematuria ; nephritis; herpes zoster.

Indicated in various types of paresis viz, monoplegia, hemiplegia, etc. in over worked people. Also in epileptiform and tetaniform convulsions. Chorea. Symptoms are accompanied by fever, headache, bodyache and lumbago.

**Mind:** Amnesia and confusion.

**Eyes:** Optic neuritis; paralysis of optic nerve with glaucoma and exophthalmos.

**Abdomen:** Colic; pain in the right iliac fossa. Hepatic congestion; jaundice; nausea and diarrhea.

**Urinary:** Chronic albuminuria. Acute nephritis, tenderness, fever, oliguria, proteinuria and hematuria.

**Heart:** *Sudden hypotension.*

**Skin:** Urticaria ; facial herpes; erythema nodosum; purpura. Allergic eruptions.

**Relationship:** Compare: *Pic-ac., Phos., Zinc.*

**Dose:** 6C.

---

## ELECTRICITAS

(Electricity, Effects of Atmospheric and Static Electricity) **Elec.**

**Source:** Attenuations are made from sugar of milk saturated with the current.

**Clinical:** Chorea; hysteria; paralysis; rheumatism; otorrhea; asthma; convulsions; syncope; enuresis; hematuria.

Presents a general picture of *nerve and muscle relaxation;* fainting, stiffness, paralysis, tremors, chorea, spasms, convulsions, epilepsy, etc. General depression and weariness with giddiness or drowsiness; syncope with a tendency to fall down; decrease in body weight. Tingling sensation in the electrified parts. *Dreads the approach of a thunderstorm.*

**Mind:** Intense nervous anxiety, screams with nervous fear; restless, uneasy. Timid, fearful, sighing and lachrymose; paroxysms of crying. Violent agitation. Dreads the approach of a thunderstorm; mentally tortured before and during a thunderstorm. Involuntary, hysterical, laughter; ill humor; rage. Slow and difficult comprehension, insensible, loss of memory. Looses consciousness and sensibility; stupefaction; looks around with haggard eyes. *Elec.* should not be used when suffering from a cold, especially if the chest is involved; fatal results have been observed.

**Head:** Giddiness, especially on stooping; dullness. Scurf on the scalp; promotes hair growth. Pain in the head; bruised pain in the occiput; tearing pain from the nape of the neck to the occiput. Violent pulsations or sensation of heat throughout the head. Tingling and prickling under the scalp.

**Eyes:** Inflammation of the eyes and profuse lachrymation, especially of the right eye. Edges of eyelids and external angle swollen. Clouded vision, dim sighted. Blindness. Objects appear yellow and a dark room appears illuminated. Gnawing sensation in the left eye; or violent, drawing pain, extending to the forehead.

**Ears:** Otorrhea with small pustules in the auditory duct. Augmented secretion of wax, whizzing in the ears; sensation as if obstructed by a plug. Swelling in the inner ear; pulsations in the ear with hyperemia and heat. Vesicles full of an acrid serum, behind the ears.

**Nose:** Anosmia; milky discharge from the nose. Tingling in the nose with sneezing.

**Face:** Expression of alarm or terror. Face red and swollen. Scabby eruptions on the face; lips are cracked; upper lip is swollen. Shocks throughout the body, proceeding from the malar bone.

**Mouth:** Tearing pain in upper teeth with headache. Pain from a subcutaneous ulceration in an old socket of molar teeth. Teeth grow rapidly in children. Increased secretion of saliva; foam in the mouth. Prominent papillae on the tongue; red and sensitive tongue, especially on the tip. Vesicles on the palate and tongue. Inability to articulate, results in loss of speech.

**Throat:** Irritation; pharyngitis; laryngitis.

**Stomach:** Increased appetite; heartburn. Nausea, retching and vomiting; with profuse salivation; hematemesis. Sensation of fullness even after eating a small amount.

**Abdomen:** Spasmodic tension and contraction at the approach of a storm. Borborygmi with distention.

**Stool:** Diarrhea, hot yellowish-black, fetid, with drawing up of testicles during stool and tenesmus. Constriction of the anus after stool, burning in the anus. Hemorrhoids.

**Urinary:** Frequent micturition; enuresis; bloody urine with mucus or a white sediment. Sensation as if the bladder would burst.

**Female:** Catamenia. Profuse menses with pressure in the rectum. Leucorrhea, first serous then thick with coagula, the size of a hazel nut.

**Respiration:** Short, irritable cough with tickling in the throat. Hemoptysis. Asthma with rapid respiration and tendency to syncope. Oppression of the chest.

**Heart:** Palpitations especially at the approach of a storm with a tendency to syncope. Lancinating pain spreads from the heart to the chest.

**Back:** Boils on the back and nape of neck. Difficulty in moving the neck; darting pain in the enlarged cervical glands. Tingling along the vertebral column.

**Extremities:** *Severe pain in the arms and legs.* Paralysis; sensation of numbness in the finger tips and feet, as if gone off to sleep. Trembling of hands and feet with a feeling of weariness. Hands red and swollen. Burning in feet upto the knees; tingling, knees down; and soles

**Sleep:** Yawning and shuddering all over the body; great drowsiness. Sleeplessness for two months. Confused dreams.

**Fever:** Shuddering all over, in the morning with yawning. At first shivering, then dry, transient heat with inflammation of the throat. Augmentation of internal heat; *internal heat of parts which have sustained an electric shock;* circulation of blood accelerated. Profuse perspiration, especially at night.

**Skin:** *Blackish discoloration;* ecchymosis. Itching or tingling all over the body. Miliary or measle-like eruptions.

**Relationship:** Compare: *X-ray, Psor., Tub., Phos.*

Antidoted by: *Morph-act.*

Antidotes: *Merc.*

---

# ENTEROCOCCINUM

**Enteroc.**

**Source:** It is prepared from a mixture of three stocks which are cultured for 24 hours at 37°C.

**Clinical:** Colitis; proctitis; dysentery; allergies.

The digestive system is the primary seat of action for this drug. The tongue is *white, like milk.* Anorexia, nausea, eructations and flatulence is marked. Colitis and enterocolitis, which keeps relapsing due to an allergic condition. Hemorrhagic recto-colitis. Rectal tenesmus.

Stools resemble cow dung. *Morning diarrhea* with a great urgency, between 4-9 a.m. Dentitional, emotional and menstrual diarrhea with profuse mucus. Diarrhea accompanied by hypotension, slow pulse, fatigue, and irritability.

**Relationship:** Compare: *Sulph., Podo., Crot-t., Dios., Cyn-d., Prot.*

**Dose:** 4C to 9C.

---

# EPIHYSTERINUM

**Epih.**

**Source:** Obtained from a case of hemorrhage suffering from fibroids with possibly, malignant elements. Of great value in controlling hemorrhages especially uterine, with or without fibroids. Menses are profuse and frequent.

**Clinical:** Fibroma; menorrhagia; metrorrhagia.

**Relationship:** Compare: *Carc., Frax., Hydr., Thlas.*

**Dose:** 30C upwards.

---

# FLAVUS

**Flav.**

**Source:** *Flavus* is a bacteria called *Neisseria pharingis.*

**Clinical:** Coryza; sinusitis; conjunctivitis; loose teeth; dysmenorrhea; endometritis ; arthritis; sciatica; ecchymosis .

Of marked value in eye, nose and throat affections. Left sided remedy.

**Mind:** Bad morals; exaggerates problems. Sensitive to emotions and contradictions; depressed.

**Eyes:** *Right sided, periorbital headache* (*Sang.*). Asthenopia, marked in the evening . Eyes swollen in the morning; eyelids heavy; conjuctivitis.

**Ears:** Repeated attacks of otitis media. Right sided otalgia .

**Nose:** Dry with crusts. Epistaxis in the morning; ozena (*Kali-bi.*). Sinusitis; frontal and maxillary sinuses tender; congestion of the nose at night; one nostril stops and the other opens. Sneezing; better in the morning after sneezing.

**Face:** Flushes of heat at night.

**Mouth:** *Loose teeth.*

**Throat:** Dysphagia; globus hystericus; sensation of a feather in the throat (*Kali-bi.*) ; heaviness of the larynx after prolonged talking . Pain in the throat after getting feet wet. Inflammation of the throat; sensation as if the palate is touching the tongue; dryness, worse at night. Frequent loss of voice.

**Stomach:** Poor digestion ; frequent nausea after meals; aggravated by wine (*Zinc., Nux-v.*).

**Female:** Irregular menses; dymenorrhea; menorrhagia ; early with profuse, pale blood. *Bleeding during ovulation.* Delayed menses with pre-menstrual syndrome. Endometrosis.

**Respiratory:** Takes cold easily. Cough wakes him up between 1-1.30 a.m. Dyspnea, worse towards 2 a.m. ; wakes up suffocated. Dry cough, worse in the morning.

**Back:** *Arthrosis* of the vertebral column; cracking. Cervico-brachial neuralgia.

**Extremities:** Left sided sciatica; pain in the left arm. Mild tremors, localized to the fingers.

**Skin:** Frequent ecchymosis; sweaty palms.

**Modalities:** Worse, cold, heat, in the morning on waking up. Better, after a hot bath, in the spring and autumn.

**Relationship:** Compare: *Kali-bi., Zinc., Luff-a.*
**Dose:** 6C. Can be taken as drops, upto 30 C also.

---

# INFLUENZINUM

**Influ.**

**Source:** 3 parts of Asiatic virus and 1 part of the European virus is mixed and cultured on a chicken embryo. Only prepared by the Pasteur Institute.

**Clinical:** Influenza; measles; encephalitis; meningitis; entero-colitis; varicose ulcers; rhino-pharyngitis; bronchial asthma; nasal polyp; sinusitis; otitis; conjunctivitis; blepharitis; rheumatism.

Has a stimulating action in extreme weakness, prostration and fatigue. Asthenia and anorexia. General stiffness and ill feeling, with chills and headache. Hypothyroidism.

**Mind:** Neurotic and depressed.

**Head:** Meningitis and encephalitis with vomiting. Headache due to influenza.

**Eyes:** Heavy; sensitive to movement; stiffness on movement. Conjunctivitis of influenza.

**Ears:** Otitis media with influenza.

**Nose:** Oculo-nasal catarrh; *influenza*; *sinusitis*; nasal polyp; chronic atrophic rhinitis. *Nasal voice.*

**Throat:** Stridulous laryngitis in children; chronic laryngitis; pharyngitis.

**Abdomen:** Colic, weakness of anal sphincter with weakening diarrhea.

**Respiratory:** *Bronchial asthma*; broncho-pneumonia; bronchitis; dry, hard cough.

**Heart:** Tendency to hypotension. *Weakness of myocardia.* Leucopenia with mononucleosis.

**Extremities:** *Venous and arterial congestion of lower limbs.* Rheumatism during humid and cold weather.

**Relationship:** Compare: *Mim-p., Luff-a.*
**Dose:** 6C.

---

# LAC FELINUM

(Cat's Milk)

**Lac-f.**

**Source:** A dilution of cat's milk.

**Clinical:** Ciliary neuralgia; dysmenorrhea; styes; keratitis; leucoma.

Head and eye symptoms are most marked. The *right half of the body,* from head to foot feels extremely weak, heavy and distressed, as a result, it is difficult to walk. Constant nervous trembling, especially of hands.

**Mind:** Severe depression. Fear of falling down, without vertigo. Extremely conscientious, every little fault seems like a crime. Illusions that the corners of furniture or any pointed object will run into her eyes. Very cross at everyone.

**Head:** Dull pain and heaviness in the forehead and region of eyebrows. Pulsations in the head . Intense pain early in the morning, in the vertex and left side of head, involving the left half of nose and jaws; extends to the left ear. Pain never crosses the median line. Patient must close her eyes tightly due to the intensity or she holds her head firmly with her hands and rushes from one room to another, screaming; the severity of pain along the jaw causes the mouth to fill up with saliva.

**Eyes:** Sharp lancinating pain through the center of left eyeball leaving it sore internally, resulting in profuse lachrymation. Eyes feel sunken. Similar pain in the center of right eyeball extending externally to the temple and frontal region over the eyes, with intense *photophobia,* redness of the conjunctiva and *lachrymation*, worse reading or writing. Pain appears to be in the interior of the eyeball; *choroiditis.* Muscular *aesthenopia* of the eye. Severe photophobia to natural and artificial light; eyes ache in gaslight. Styes; keratitis. Corneal ulceration. Eyes get bad every September.

**Nose:** Smell of clams (which she is fond of) is unbearable, making them unedible also.

**Mouth:** Hyperemia of the buccal cavity; aphthae on the tongue and palate, stomatitis. Parts of mouth seem to stick together. Loss of taste.

**Throat:** Stringy, tough mucus in the pharynx, cannot hawk it up, must swallow. Yellowish expectoration, if and when expectorated. Posterior pharyngeal wall slightly inflamed.

**Stomach:** Anorexia; desire to eat paper. Soreness and sensitiveness in the epigastrium.

**Abdomen:** Distention after eating, must loosen clothing. Colic.

**Stool:** Normal stool at 2 a.m. On ceasing to strain, stool slips back, as if the rectum is unable to expel its contents.

**Urinary:** Frequent desire, urine very pale.

**Female:** Dysmenorrhea. Leucorrhea ceases on third, and reappears on the fourth day; yellowish discharge. Intense pruritus vulva. Dragging sensation down the pelvis, as if the uterus would come out.

**Respiratory:** Oppressed breathing, difficulty in taking a deep breath.

**Sleep:** Heavy, profound sleep, cannot be awakened easily. Dreams of earthquakes.

**Relationship:** Compare: *Lac-c., Lac-d., Staph., Puls., Hep., Spig.*

**Dose:** 30C to 1M.

---

# LAC VACCINUM

(Cow's Milk) **Lac-v.**

**Source:** Prepared from pure cow's milk.

**Clinical:** Albuminuria; diabetes; rheumatism; aphthae.

The keynote symptom of this drug is that *pain is felt simultaneously on both sides of the body.* Sudden, mental and physical prostration to such an extent that she cannot even collect her thoughts or pick up a pencil to write her symptoms; even answering questions relating to her health, seems like an enormous effort. Intolerance to milk with headache, biliousness, flatulence and constipation. Aggravates uric acid diathesis, thus increasing the rheumatic tendency. Also indicated in diabetes with increased thirst and polyuria. In some highly sensitive women, the effect on the sexual organs is pronounced. Burnett remarks that children who drink too much milk after their teeth are fully grown, develop a tendency to take on colds easily.

**Mind:** *Severe mental prostration;* confusion, cannot express herself. General nervousness with depression of spirits; anticipates bad news.

**Head:** Vertigo with a tendency to fall back when eyes are closed. A creeping sensation from above the left eye to the vertex, then from 2 inches behind the left ear to the vertex; pressure on vertex with a sensation of heat. All these symptoms pass away except for pain on top of the head.

**Eyes:** Dull pain especially over the right eye. Blurring or dimness of vision, off and on for a few moments; blindness coming on three or four times in succession, lasting only a second at a time, leaving a pain in both the temples, on top of the head and left ear.

**Ears:** Feel stopped up.

**Mouth:** Dirty, yellow coated tongue; sour taste; aphthae on the tongue; glossitis; halitosis; stomatitis. Acrid saliva staining the handkerchief yellow.

**Throat:** Sensation of a plug in the throat.

**Stomach:** Thirst for cold water in large quantities. Eructations, nausea without vomiting. Contracting, pressing pain in the stomach, better external pressure.

**Abdomen:** Constant flatulence, an hour after drinking milk for lunch, passed with great difficulty. Pain from the sternum extends across the abdomen, about an inch below the umbilicus.

**Stool:** Obstinate constipation; hard, dry, like impacted balls; passed only after great straining. Passage of flatus which relieves.

**Urinary:** Diabetes. Urine not increased in the morning; in the afternoon, micturates every fifteen minutes. Albuminuria with a specific gravity of 1030.

**Female:** White, watery leucorrhea; pain in the sacrum. Drinking a glass of water suppresses menses till the next menstrual period.

**Chest:** Pain followed by burning in a spot on each side of the sternum, around the middle of the chest with a sense of suffocation.

**Back:** Lumbago, pain in sacrum.

**Extremities:** Fingers of both hands, especially when stretched out, tremble and quiver from extreme weakness. Sharp pain under the left scapula, extending upwards to the left shoulder and then down the left arm. Cold, clammy stickiness in both hands and feet. Lancinating and aching pain in both hip joints; spreads along the thighs up to the knees. Osteoarthritis of the knees; knees feel weak and powerless. Rheumatic pain in knees and tarsal joints when walking.

**Sleep:** Drowsy, sleeps well at night; must force herself to keep awake. Even after seven hours of sleep, can fall asleep any minute during the day. General restlessness and bad dreams, dreams of trying to lay out a corpse.

**Fever:** Hands become hot and dry during fever, with aching in legs from the thighs to the knees. Fever at night with profuse sweat all over. Fever is preceded by chills, commencing in the shoulder.

**Relationship:** Compare: *Lac-c., Lac-f., Lac-v-g.*

**Dose:** 6C, 30C, 200C.

---

## LAC VACCINUM COAGULATUM

(Curd) **Lac-v-c.**

**Source:** Prepared from curd.

**Clinical:** Nausea of pregnancy.

Nausea during pregnancy with a desire for food; better by drinking milk.

**Relationship:** Compare: *Chel.*

**Dose:** 6C, 30C, 200C.

---

## MAGNETIS POLI AMBO

(The Magnet) **M-ambo.**

**Source:** The potencies are prepared by triturating sugar of milk which has been saturated when exposed to the emanations of a magnet.

**Clinical:** Syncope; hemorrhage; orchitis; paraphimosis; prolapsus ani; rheumatism; ulcers.

Bruised pain in the joints where the cartilages of two bones touch each other, in the morning or on the side lain on. Joints are painful when touched; dull, numb pain; paralytic pain in all joints. *Intolerable burning* from head to feet. Sensation as if every part was cut up. *Shuddering movement throughout the body. Spasmodic jerking and rising of the body* from a recumbant position during shock or fright followed by loss of consciousness and then sensation of great heat. Fits of fainting with palpitations and suffocation; insensibility or deadly sopor.

**Mind:** Talks aloud, to himself while working, without being aware of it; says and does something different; tries to do something but ends up doing something contrary; omits letters, words, syllables. Inclined to be angry, vehement. Absent minded.

**Head:** Vertigo, especially in the evening on lying down, staggers while walking. Headache follows least chagrin or from over strained memory. Pain as is bruised; digging, stupefying headache, as if a nail was driven into the head. Sensation on top of the head, as if the head and body were pressed down.

**Eyes:** Dilated pupils when cheerful; contraction during spasmodic attacks or syncope. Fiery sparks before the eyes, like shooting stars at twilight. Itching in the eyes, especially lids and inner canthi; sensation as if lids were dry.

**Ears:** Hardness of hearing. Humming in the ears with headache on the same side. Itching and burning in the auditory meatus.

**Nose:** Illusions of smell; a smoky or mouldy smell like manure.

**Face:** Sweat without heat, early in the morning. Violent, burning, lancinating pain in the facial muscles.

**Mouth:** Toothache after taking anything cold or from cold air; teeth loose. Shocks in the jaw and teeth with burning. Inflammation of submaxillary glands; profuse salivation *especially in the evening with swollen lips. Halitosis* which he himself does not perceive.

**Stomach:** Hungry in the evening; has an appetite but no taste. Metallic taste. Aversion to tobacco although he relishes it. *Eructations;* tasting of ingesta which is spoiled or smells like saw dust. Acrid risings on stooping. Sensation of pressure on the stomach with cramps towards the upper part. Distention in the diaphragmatic region. Speedy satiety.

**Abdomen:** Borborygmi; noisy, rumbling; flatulent colic. Qualmish, painful sensation in the intestine with emission of hot, putrid flatus; especially during mental exertion. Burning pain in the abdomen; itching around the umbilicus.

**Stool:** Constipation, as if the rectum was constricted and contracted, with headache lasting for several day. Hemorrhoids, with severe pain after stools and burning in the anus when sitting; itchy; blind with soft stool. Prolapsus recti on straining for stool.

**Urinary:** Cystitis with burning in the neck of the bladder, a few minutes after micturating.

**Male:** Want of sexual desire; aversion to coition; penis relaxed, despite sexual excitement. Erection without amorous thoughts, early in the morning. *Nocturnal emission. Burning sensation* in the region of spermatic vesicles, which excites sexual desire. *Prepuce retreats entirely behind the glans.* Epididymitis.

**Female:** Metrorrhagia in old women. Menses which had ceased a few days before, return a day after imposing a magnetic surface.

**Respiratory:** Convulsive cough at night; short attacks which do not wake him, with hemoptysis; shocks in the chest, anxious breathing and oppression of the chest. Mucus in the trachea is easily hawked up in the morning and evening. Asthma after midnight due to mucus in the chest, better coughing.

**Back:** Pain in the lumbosacral joint, in the morning when lying on a side and when stooping for a long time. Shocks or jerks in the lumbo-sacral region, almost arresting breathing. Twitching in muscles of the back, sensation as if something alive in them.

**Extremities:** Drawing pain in joints and muscles of arms; tearing, jerking pain after some exposure to cold. Cramps in the calves and toes on waking up in the morning. Heels burn; corns.

**Sleep:** Disturbed; talks, snores and, keeps tossing about. Wakes up at 3 a.m. Sleeps on the back early in the morning, with one hand under the occiput and the other on the abdomen, knees are slightly apart, half opened mouth with muttering and snoring; amorous dreams of emissions, without any actual emission. Lascivious dreams, even during a siesta with prostratic discharge. Vivid dreams; dreams of boasting, bragging and feasting. Body jerks several times before going to sleep.

**Fever:** Shuddering all over the body with profuse sweat. Fever after midnight has no shuddering but a sensation of heat all over. Heat without thirst at night, with a desire to be uncovered.

**Skin:** Old wounds bleed afresh. Boils on various parts of the body. Continuous itching and pricking here and there followed by burning.

**Relationship:** Compare: *M-arct., M-aust., Zinc., Anac., Podo., Caust., Ign., Bell., Lyc., Nux-v.*

Antidoted by: *Ign., Zinc., Elec.*

Action lasts for 10 to 14 days.

---

# MAGNETIS POLUS ARCTICUS

(North Pole of the Magnet) **M-arct.**

**Source:** Sugar of milk charged with the north pole of a magnet is used for triturations.

**Clinical:** Amenorrhea; inguinal hernia; somnambulism; toothache; cervical spondylosis; exophthalmos; asthma.

Great lassitude and a painful, bruised sensation all over the body especially in the morning and open air. Over excitement with trembling, uneasy restlessness of limbs and great nervous weakness. Tremulousness throughout the body, especially in the feet; accompanied with a numb sensation. Tremors of the part, touched by a magnet, with a sensation of coldness; warmth. Tensive, bruised sensation in the adjoining parts. Dryness and tightness of the body with want of strength. Drawing sensation in the periosteum of all bones, as at the commencement of fever.

**Mind:** *Indolent.* When sitting, feels he has lost all power of motion; feels stuck to the chair. Sad in the evening, weeps despite his will; with chilliness. Anxious, despondent, inconsolable. Irritated; doesn't like to be interrupted in his work, which he does not accomplish. Alternately cheerful and sad; great strength and weakness. *Makes mistakes while writing; talks aloud to himself* while attending to business. Calm, composed mood, devoid of care. Weak memory; sensation of intoxication.

**Head:** Vertigo with staggering; as if she would fall in any direction. *Sensation as if the head was being pressed down* by a load. Violent headache, as if the brain was going to brust out. *Rush of blood* to the head with suffusion of heat in the cheeks. Tension of the scalp, as if firmly adherent to the skull.

**Eyes:** Exophthalmos; *starring look. Intense itching* in the inner canthi and margin of lids, *dryness* of the eyelids with a *prickling* sensation and profuse lachrymation early in the morning. Sunlight intolerable. Sensation of coldness in the weak eye; as if the eye was a piece of ice. Sensation of a cobweb in front of the eyes. Formication between the eyes.

**Ears:** *Whizzing* in ears with internal heat, as if from boiling water. Deafness, as if caused by a band over the ears.

**Nose:** *Abberation of smell;* imagines the room smells of fresh white wash and dust, or of rotten eggs. *Severe epistaxis* for three successive days, worse in the afternoon, preceded by an ache in the forehead. *Tip of the nose red* and hot, followed by hot circumscribed spots on the cheeks.

**Face:** Intensely painful tightness of the face; trismus. Suffusion of heat in cheeks with rush of blood to the head.

**Mouth:** Symptoms of mouth are most prominent. Caries; toothache, especially in carious teeth, as if the tooth would be torn out; pain extends upwards, towards the eye; gums inflamed with burning in the cheeks; pain worse after a meal, in a smoky room; better walking in open air. Toothache with jerks through the periosteum of the jaw. Accumulation of a lot of saliva in the mouth at night; pillow becomes wet because of it. Itching in the forepart of the tongue, obliging one to rub and scratch.

**Stomach:** Voracious appetite at supper, eats well, but develops a flat taste in the mouth immediately after, with a sensation of heat in the ear lobules. Tobacco disagrees. Long continuous, rancid heartburn. Frequent eructations of mere air with painful jerks. Sensation of weight in the stomach. Sudden griping and throbbing in the pit of the stomach.

**Abdomen:** *Incarcerated flatus* with gurgling and a withering sensation. Marked pressure in the abdomen from within outward due to flatus, which wakes the patient up at night. Sensation as if the abdomen would burst; *flatulent colic.* Continuous aching and pinching in the entire hypogastric region. *Inguinal hernia;* threatens to protrude especially when coughing.

**Stool:** Obstinate constipation; large, hard, difficult to evacuate, often preceded by drawing, dysenteric pain in the hypogastrium. Blood with stools twice a day.

**Urinary:** Dark urine; copious emission.

**Male:** *Nocturnal, involuntary emissions.* Excessive desire.

**Female:** Feeble or suppressed menses.

**Respiratory:** Suffocative, spasmodic cough around midnight, hindering sleep. Dry, asthmatic cough, worse walking in open air. Unceasing irritation which induces cough, this irritation can only be removed by suppressing the cough by will power.

**Heart:** Sudden oppression and sharp stitches on the left side of chest. Anxiety and qualmishness.

**Back:** Crackling in the cervical vertebra, especially the atlas, during motion. Backache, feels as if broken.

**Extremities:** Sensation of cramps along the arm with prickling as if it had gone off to sleep. Soreness of the right shoulder. Pain and stiffness in the finger joints, especially of the right side. Fracture-like pain in the hip joints and lower limbs. Sensation of great lassitude in legs, as if they would break when walking. Tearing pain with pressure on the outer side of the knee, extending down to the ankle. Burning, pulsative stitches in the calves; rigid tension in hamstrings, feel too short. Corns.

**Sleep:** Spasmodic yawning with pain in the articulation of left jaw; feels dislocated. Constantly drowsy during the day. Lascivious dreams; vivid dreams. Sleeps well at night, generally on his back. Sings while sleeping, which usually wakes him up. Half awake at 2 a.m., filled with great ideas, in a state of perfect inner consciousness. However when fully awake, cannot remember those ideas or thoughts clearly. Restless sleep, tosses about as the bed feels too warm.

**Fever:** Sensation of coldness, chills. Sensation of heat all over the body with cool *hands and feet; cool perspiration* on palms and soles.

**Skin:** Formication; tingling with a crawling itch, as of a fly or flea, followed by soreness.

**Modalities:** All symptoms are better by uncovering.

**Relationship:** Compare: *Ip., Con., Cupr., Ferr-m., Cham.*

Antidoted by: *M-aust., Ign., Zinc.*

# MAGNETIS POLUS AUSTRALIS

(South Pole of the Magnet) **M-aust.**

**Source:** Sugar of milk is charged by the south pole of a magnet and then triturated for further potencies.

**Clinical:** Frostbite; hernia; ingrowing toe nails; menorrhagia; varicosis; enuresis; balanitis; orchitis.

Laziness and heaviness of the body, with a feeling on anxiety; as if threatened with paralysis, as if he would fall. Bruised pain all over, as if he had been lying on stones. Stiffness and cracking in joints during motion. Legs feel bruised while walking in open air, becomes faint or is suddenly attacked by an inclination to sleep. Body feels light.

**Mind:** Morose, despondent, has an aversion to conversation and cheerful faces. Dislikes society. Passion and rage. Instability of ideas.

**Head:** Vertigo; as if intoxicated, staggers. Rush of blood to the head, without heat in the morning, in bed. Formication in the brain. Pressure and headache in the occiput. Jerks in the head.

**Eyes:** Dryness and smarting of eyelids, noticeable when moving them in the morning and evening. Lachrymation; amblyopia; diplopia. Swelling of the Meibomian glands of the lower lid, as if a stye would form, but it merely passes away.

**Ears:** Roaring; sensation of air; whizzing in the ears in the morning. Tearing pain in the cartilage of the outer and inner ear. Inflammation of the outer ear with rhagades.

**Mouth:** Inflammation of the submaxillary glands; profuse salivation. Swollen tongue impedes speech. Jerks in the upper jaw.

**Throat:** Burning in the pharynx; sensation of strangulation.

**Stomach:** Indifferent to eating or drinking; relishes food but has no desire for it; indifference to milk, bordering on an aversion. Food appears incipid. Nausea when stooping forward; inclination to vomit. Pain in the pit of the stomach.

**Abdomen:** Noisy borborygmi, flatulent colic, worse at night and early in the morning; portions of flatus spring up from here and there, which is painful. Pinching in the abdomen, brought on by a draft of air. Distended abdomen with emission of a large quantity of air. Sensation as if the hernia would protrude.

**Stool:** Soft, loose stools preceded by griping. Frequent and sudden desire, but expelled with difficulty. Constriction and contraction of the rectum, preventing even flatus from passing. Itching hemorrhoids.

**Urinary:** *Enuresis* due to relaxation of sphincter vesicae. Urethritis.

**Male:** Impotence, sudden cessation of all enjoyment at climaxis. Pain in the penis, as if some fibres were torn. Balanitis, orchitis; painful retraction of testies at night with drawing of spermatic cord. Emissions in a hemiplegia patient; paralysis worse after emission.

**Female:** Menorrhagia, prolonged flow only during motion, ceases at rest. Discharge of blood accompanied with pain in the abdomen.

**Respiratory:** Cough and coryza with expectoration of a greenish mucus and dyspnea. Nocturnal paroxysm of fetid cough. Oppression of chest. Sighing respiration with involuntary deglutition.

**Heart:** *Violent palpitations.*

**Back:** Gnawing and smarting; pain as if sprained. Sensation of heat, commensing in the cervical vertebrae and extending down the back.

**Extremities:** Sensation as if small snakes crawling down the left arm. Painful jerks in the arms from above downwards. Tingling, like little shocks along the arm. Cracking in the knee joints during motion; arthritis; tearing pain in the patella while walking. Jerks in the hamstring with contraction of the leg.

Throbbing in the leg muscles after walking. Easy dislocation of a foot joint on making a false step. Varices; legs pain when left hanging down. *Ingrown toe nails. Shoe bite* on top and on the sides of the toes when walking.

**Sleep:** *Dreams of fire,* quarrels and fights. Sleepless and awake before midnight; desire to sleep at day break. Restless, frequently turns sides.

**Fever:** Ache in long bones before an attack of fever or ague. Thirst at the commencement of chills. Chills in a room, especially after an evening nap, without thirst. Internal coldness, is actually quite warm, but must lie down and cover himself; followed by profuse sweat and shuddering over the perspiring parts.

**Skin:** Corrosive itching in the evening, in bed.

**Modalities:** Worse, walking in open air, sitting, and hanging limbs down.

**Relationship:** Compare: *M-ambo., Elec., Caps., Graph., Sil., Nit-ac., Thuj.*

Antidoted by: *M-arct., Ign., Zinc.*

---

## MALARIA OFFICINALIS

**Malar.**

**Source:** Is prepared from decayed vegetable matter, taken from a marsh, during the dry season, when the malarial parasite is most active. This vegetable matter is then placed in a glass jar filled with water and allowed to decompose for 12 weeks.

**Clinical:** Anemia; neuritis; sciatica; bronchitis; beginning of tuberculosis; entero-colitis; liver affections; splenic affections; cholecystitis; ague.

Great exhaustion even after a short walk; as though had suffered from a long illness with anorexia; strong desire to lie down. Typhoidal, semi-paralytic state. Rheumatism; rheumatic paralysis and emaciation.

**Mind:** Feels stupid and sleepy, very forgetful.

**Head:** Sensation as if he would become dizzy; dizziness on rising from a recling position. Dull headache with drowsiness; sensation as if the head would burst; frequent attacks beginning in the forehead.

**Eyes:** Aching above the inner canthi of right eye. Eyes feel heavy and sleepy. Asthenopia with blurring of vision.

**Ears:** Drawing pain in right external ear.

**Nose:** Congestive feeling at the root of the nose, as in severe colds. Epistaxis in the morning; occasionally stopped up.

**Face:** Right cheek and malar bone itchy; better by gently nibling or scratching. Face warm as if flushed, this sensation spreads all over the body.

**Mouth:** Pain in left upper teeth. Saliva more than usual; must swallow frequently. Sensation as if a few specs of pepper were on the tip of the tongue. Tongue coated white; bitter taste.

**Stomach:** Continuous nausea; retching, vomiting of bile. Easy, bland belching. Odor or cooking is pleasing but does not have a desire to eat; on sitting down eats a good dinner with relish. Thirsty, craves cold drinks, especially lemonade.

**Abdomen:** Rumbling and burning in the abdomen; sense of heat. Sensation as if loose stools will come (but they do not come); sensation as if the spleen would ache. Cannot breathe on account of pain in the liver; better hard pressure, worse lying down. Aching under right scapula. Uneasiness in lower abdomen. Tired feeling in the abdomen and chest.

**Stool:** Diarrhea in the morning; bloody; yellow; foul smelling. Long standing hemorrhoids; bleeding but, no pain.

**Urinary:** Highly colored urine like strong tea, strong ammoniacal smell; frequent, scanty micturition. Ineffectual desire.

**Respiratory:** Shallow breathing; frequent sighing. Malaria antidotes phthisis and a tubercular constitution is protected against malaria.

**Back:** Neck and back feels tired; stiffness and lameness; cervical spondylosis. Lumbago; pain radiates up the back, worse lying down, walking; better lying on the abdomen.

**Extremities:** Aching, tired feeling in the arms, hands and legs. Legs weary from a short walk. Legs restless, feels like stretching and moving them.

**Sleep:** Must lie down. Sense of dizziness on falling asleep, thus preventing sleep. Sleepy all the time; can go to sleep while standing. Sleep does not relieve drowsiness, wakes up unrefreshed. Constant yawning and a desire to stretch.

**Fever:** Chills all over, ascending from the legs. Face feels warm, as if flushed or feverish, spreads all over the body. Intermittent quotidian and tertiary fever. Ague, every alternate day; weak and drowsy between attacks. High fever at night and in the morning. Chills begin at noon; icy cold from hips down. Profuse perspiration.

**Modalities:** Worse least effort, in a closed room and lying down. Better, by rest, fresh air and hard pressure.

**Relationship:** Compare: *Ars., Eup-per., Nat-m., Chin., Chinin-s., Ip., Puls., Acet-ac.*

**Dose:** 30C, 200C, 400C.

---

## MENINGOCOCCINUM

**Meningoc.**

**Source:** Prepared from *Neisseria meningotides.*

**Clinical:** Cerebro-spinal meningitis; rhino-pharyngitis; septicemia.

It presents a picture of acute meningitis. Is a valuable remedy for it, and often gives unexpected results. Can also be used as a prophylaxis in cerebrospinal meningitis.

**Relationship:** Compare: *Hell., Op., Nux-m.*

**Dose:** Use high dilutions, 30C. For prophylaxis, a single, drop dose is directly dropped on the tongue; the duration of immunity provided is 3 months.

---

## MONILIA ALBICANS

(Candida Albicans) **Moni.**

**Source:** It is a mushroom which appears in a culture, like oval or round yeast. The homoeopathic preparation is made from the alcoholic mother tincture (1/10) of the culture supplied by the Pasteur Institute.

**Clinical:** Aphthae; gingivitis; enterocolitis; allergic asthma; vulvo-vaginitis; polyarthritis.

Has an affinity for the skin and mucous membrane, especially of the digestive tract and female genitals.

**Mouth:** Tongue dry, thick, cracked and red; posterior part white. Oral candidiasis; aphthous stomatitis; halitosis. Gingivitis, bleeding gums. Lips dry, cracked and crusty.

**Abdomen:** Painful, spasmodic enterocolitis; tendency to constipation, especially after antibiotics.

**Female:** Vulvitis; vaginitis with vesicles and pustules. Vulva fissured; pruritus vulva with oozing which may end in keratinisation. Candidiasis. Kraurosis of the vulva.

**Skin:** *Eczema with linear fissures in the folds of skin and mucous membranes;* interdigital eczema with a linear, red, fine, painful crack. Interdigital eruptions; vesicles itching and onyxis. Peri-ungual inflammation; keratine of nails affected, develops furrows. Dermatosis after antibiotics.

**Relationship:** Compare: *Thuj., Med.*

**Dose:** 15 C.

---

## MORBILLINUM

**Morb.**

**Source:** Is prepared from the exudate of the mouth and pharynx of patients suffering from measles and not yet treated.

**Clinical:** Measles; phlyctenular conjunctivitis; acute coryza; acute otitis; erythematous lupus; spontaneous abortion.

Nasal voice with nasal and ocular catarrh. Hyperthermia upto 30° – 39°C.

**Head:** Meningitis; convulsions especially in a grumbling child.

**Eyes:** Optic neuritis; photophobia; lachrymation.

**Nose:** Snoring; flapping of alae nasi; polypnea. Catarrh.

**Mouth:** *Koplic's spots.*

**Throat:** *Red; irritated; hypertrophy of the superficial glands in the neck. Stridulous laryngitis.*

**Abdomen:** Pain especially in the appendicular region. Adeno-splenomegaly.

**Respiratory:** *Diffused bronchial rales*; purulent pleurisy. Radiograph shows hilar opacities. *Feline cough.*

**Skin:** Rosy, round and oval maculae; disappear on pressure. Ecchymosis; miliary, confluent, red eruptions.

**Dose:** 6C.

---

## OSTEO-ARTHRITIC NOSODE

(Osteo-arthriticum) **Osteo-a.**

**Source:** There are two preparations; one comes from the knee of a patient suffering from osteoarthritis, and the other from the hip of a similar case.

**Clinical:** Arthritis; styes; furuncles; tendinitis; cramps.

Weakness with a state of indifference and irritability, aggravated in the evening; and, redness with swelling of the joints, especially right side, are the keynote symptoms of this drug. Right sided remedy.

**Mind:** Extreme weakness with indifference towards others. Has taste for nothing; irritable; especially towards the evening.

**Eyes:** Styes on the upper eyelid of left eye.

**Male:** Increased sexual desire.

**Extremities:** Redness, pain and swelling of the right shoulder, forearm and wrist. Muscular pain in the right hip. Pain in tendo-Achellis. Pain aggravated by first movement and ameliorated by continuous motion.

**Skin:** Tendency to furuncles.

**Modalities:** Worse, first movement and at night. Better prolonged movement.

**Relationship:** Compare: *Rhus-t., Anthraci., Rheumatic arthritis nosode.*

**Dose:** 6C to 200C.

---

## PARATYPHOIDINUM - B

**Parat-b.**

**Source:** A mixture of various strains of *Paratyphoidinum bacilli* is cultured on a maceration of chopped meat for 24 hours.

**Clinical:** Encephalitis; meningitis; cholecystitis; enterocolitis; bradycardia; phlebitis; bronchitis; pyelocystitis; polyarthritis, typhoid and para typhoid.

Chronic *emaciation with a history of Salmonella infection;* typhoid or paratyphoid. Malnutrition with a tendency towards general marasmus. Pre-cancerous state. Intense fatigue and general sweat.

**Mind:** *Depressed*; pessimistic, sees the negative side of everything, future appears dark; afraid of catastrophy, cannot tolerate noise.

**Head:** Continuous headache; generalised; with or without vertigo and epistaxis. Headache accompanied with anorexia and nausea. Meningitis; encephalo-myelitis, post infectious encephalitis in children (measles, diphtheria, whooping cough, etc.); epileptic attacks.

**Eyes:** Conjunctivitis.

**Ears:** Acute, sub-acute or chronic otitis.

**Nose:** Epistaxis.

**Mouth:** Stomatitis, parotiditis. Saburrale tongue with aphthae.

**Throat:** Pharyngitis.

**Abdomen:** State of malnutrition and emaciation. Colic and sensation of burning in the intestines, enterocolitis; hemorrhagic recto-colitis. Acute, subacute or chronic cholecystitis; pancreatitis. Hepato-spleno-megaly.

**Stool:** Morning diarrhea; acute or subacute *with fever and vomitings;* gastroenteritis in summers. Stubborn constipation also seen.

**Urinary:** Pyelocystitis; relapsing cystitis; pain in the bladder region.

**Respiratory:** Bronchitis; cough without any expectoration, diffused bronchial rales. Pulmonary congestion and broncho-pneumonia appear and disappear rapidly. Pulmonary abscess.

**Heart:** Dull heart sounds; arrythmias. Bradycardia; sometimes irregular.

**Back:** Osteoarthritis of the back with deformity. Myelitis especially post infection in children.

**Extremities:** Erratic osteoarthritis of joints, purulent arthritis of knees. Slow, insiduous phlebitis of the lower limbs, especially of the left leg.

**Sleep:** Insomnia.

**Fever:** *Prolonged pyrexia,* with or without any cause, with dehydration and pallor. Typhoid and paratyphoid fever. Toxicosis in babies.

**Skin:** Peri-buccal herpes.

**Relationship:** Compare: *Coli., Eberth., Achy., Paro-i.*

**Dose:** 4C to 9C. In a case with a history of paratyphoid, 30C may be prescribed.

---

# PAROTIDINUM

**Parot.**

**Source:** It is a nosode of mumps.

**Clinical:** Meningitis; mumps; orchitis.

Indicated in mumps, can be repeated every four hours; can also be given in complication of mumps-like orchitis and cerebral inflammation. It is used as a prophylactic against mumps.

**Relationship:** Compare: *Merc.*

**Dose:** 6C–30C as prophylactic; 30C-200C in mumps.

---

# PNEUMOCOCCINUM

**Pneu.**

**Source:** A gram-positive diplococcus. Found in the saliva of 50% healthy people. Also in the nasal mucosa, pharyngeal mucosa and conjunctiva.

**Clinical:** Migraine; sinusitis; bronchitis; emphysema; constipation; trachitis.

A depressive state with pain, especially in the cervico-dorsal region. Respiratory problems, especially of the bronchi.

**Mind:** Depressed and anxious; no thirst of life. Loss of memory. *Fear of falling ill and death. Desire to remain at home, horror of going out;* feels as if he is going to break down, that he can walk no more.

**Head:** *Right sided migraine;* worse walking. Headache continuous for 3-4 days, frequent; in the nape of the neck; worse noise, coughing, bending the head. Pain as if caught in a vice, *aggravated by rest at night, ameliorated by movement. Vertigo. Sensation of liquid in the head, when bending down.*

**Ears:** Inflammatory otalgia.

**Nose:** Pain in the left frontal sinus.

**Mouth:** Aphthae.

**Stomach:** Poor digestion, frequent nausea after meals, better eating. Cramps in the stomach with sensation of burning. Gastralgia when hungry.

**Abdomen:** Bloating and pain in the left hypochondrium; better by passing wind; insufficient liver.

**Stool:** Constipation, especially during a journey. Gas alternating with constipation and fetid stools.

**Urinary:** Enuresis while coughing .

**Female:** Premenstrual aggravation; menstrual migraine; *short menstrual cycle,* 22-24 days; oligomenorrhea. **Burning** *sensation during coition; sensation of heaviness in the uterus.*

**Respiratory:** *Sensation of a feather in the throat.* Bronchitis; trachitis; *incessant cough without expectoration, especially at night with nausea.* Cough especially while entering a hot room, *or metro;* scrapes the throat; bends own while coughing; no cough after 9 a.m.

**Heart:** Frequent palpitations, anytime during the day, patient must stop while walking or going upstairs. Emotional palpitations. E.C.G. reveals right focal block. *Precordial, puncturing pain;* angina pectoris.

**Back:** Spondylosis; cannot stand erect on account of pain.

**Extremities:** Legs restless before menses; heavy in the morning on waking up. Cramps and pain in legs. Pain in arms.

**Modalities:** Worse, entering a hot room, by inactivity, by rest, at night, prolonged sitting position, immobility, humidity; before menses. Better, open air, in the fields, by a short nap, after meals, by a hot foot bath.

**Relationship:** Compare: *Med., Thuj., Nat-s., Hip-ac., Zinc.*

**Dose:** 6C to 30C.

---

## STAPHYLOCOCCINUM

**Staphycoc.**

**Source:** It is prepared from a culture of *Staphylococcus pyrogens aureus* without the addition of an antiseptic.

**Clinical:** Furuncle; osteomyelitis; anthrax; herpes zoster; pericarditis; endocarditis; meningitis; myelitis.

It is indicated in conditions of acute septicemia; oscillating fever with marked chills. The general condition is weakened. Pre-diabetic conditions.

**Head:** Meningitis; myelitis. Abscess of the brain.

**Eyes:** Styes.

**Nose:** Abscess of the nasal fossa; sinusitis.

**Urinary:** Pyuria; Pyelo-nephritis.

**Male:** Acute prostatic abscess; prostatitis.

**Respiratory:** Purulent, pleural exudation; multiple abscess in the lungs.

**Heart:** *Endocarditis* followed by valvular insufficiency. *Pericarditis* with pericardial rubbing. Hypotension; arrythmias.

**Back:** Spondylitis; myelitis.

**Extremities:** Osteitis; osteomyelitis.

**Skin:** Folliculitis; sycosis of the moustach. Adenitis in the armpits; anthrax; purpura; paronychia; herpes zoster.

**Relationship:** Compare: *Rhus-v., Sil., Hep., Merc-s.*

**Dose:** 6C, 9C.

---

# STREPTOCOCCINUM

**Streptoc.**

**Source:** Is obtained from the culture prepared from a mixture of many stocks of streptococcinum without the addition of an antiseptic.

**Clinical:** Erysipelas; migraine; Sydenam's chorea; appendicitis; phlebitis; glossitis; pyorrhea; pericarditis; lymphadenitis; sinusitis; otitis mastoiditis; nephritis; arthritis; rheumatism; eczema.

The patient is intolerant to noise light and the current of air caused by the movement of a person. Asthma is very marked, it may be muscular cardiac or nervous. *Audio-visual hallucinations.*

**Mind:** Vertigo while rising and lying down. Severe migraine with vomiting of bile; sensation as if the head is going to burst. Epileptiform attacks. Hair fall.

**Eyes:** Glaucoma; asthenopia with a need for spectacles.

**Ears:** Otalgia especially when lying on the left side. Acute and chronic otitis and mastoiditis.

**Nose:** Acute and chronic rhinitis, mucopurulent discharge with crusts. Sinusitis with fever and headache.

**Mouth:** White coated tongue with a red tip, without papillae in the front and back part. Painful gums; alveolo-dental pyorrhea; glossitis.

**Throat:** Adenopathies of the neck. Quinsy; acute and chronic laryngitis. Persistant redness and pain in the throat, palate and uvula.

**Stomach:** Esophagitis; pain in the esophagus after meals radiating to the back. Nausea and vertigo with bilious vomiting.

**Abdomen:** Deep , dull pain in the epigastric region. Cannot even bear the weight of the hand on the abdomen while lying down. Chronic appendicitis.

**Urinary:** Acute glomerulo-nephritis; interstitial nephritis.

**Heart:** Angina pectoris with anaemia and hypercholestrolemia. Heart feels weak. Partial right sided block. Myocardial asthenia.Arrhythmic pericarditis.

**Back:** Backache sensation of vibrations in the vertebral column and limbs.

**Extremities:** Muscular asthenia. Arthritis of small jcints. Choreiform movements . Paraesthesia of limbs. Chronic edema of lower limbs.

**Sleep:** Agitated sleep with dreams of scuffles and violence.

**Skin:** Repeated eczema; desquamating and dry. Streptococcal nodular erythema.

**Modalities:** Worse, consolation, humid weather. Better, beginning movement especially in open air.

**Relationship:** Compare: *Ail., Bell., Ars., Rhus-t., Pyrog., Enteroc.*

**Dose:** 6C to 9C. For psychotic conditions 30C.

---

# TOXOPLASMA GONDII

**Toxo-g.**

**Source:** The human toxoplasma has an essentially alimentary origin due to the ingestion of infected pork or meat. *Toxoplasma gondii* is diluted and dynamised according to the homoeopathic pharmacopiea.

**Clinical:** Lymphadenitis; tuberculosis; infectious mononucleosis; encephalo-myelitis; chorea; epilepsy; multiple sclerosis; hepatitis; Wilson's disease; Crohn's disease; myocarditis; myositis; arthritis purpura.

*Toxoplasma gondii* has polychrest indications but lacks a well proved pathogenesis. It has a slow and deep action on the tissues with genetic repercussion. Tuberculosis and pre-cancerous states with isolated and persistent, non-suppurating *adenopathies* of the periphery with *asthenia.* Burnt out condition. General toxoplasmosis in immuno suppressed cases. Children have mental and physical retardation with a tendency to repeated attacks of rhino-pharyngitis. Infectious mononucleosis in children with sub-febrile states; discrete adenopathy and eosinophilia. Neonatal septicemia with hepatitis, hepato-splenomegaly and purpura. Hodgkin's disease; *acute lymphocytosis.*

**Mind:** Depression; mental retardation in children. Mongolism.

**Head:** Meningo-encephalitis; post-infectious epileptiform convulsions in babies, *convulsions in children*; hydrocephalus; chorea, multiple sclerosis.

**Eyes:** Iridocyclitis, chorio-retinitis and uveitis. Optic neuritis.

**Abdomen:** Hepatitis with hepatomegaly, Wilson's disease. Diffuse abdominal pain, not localised. Acute or sub-acute mesenteric lymphadenitis; Crohn's disease. Follicular inflammation of the ileum.

**Female:** Repeated abortions, especially during the first three months. Normal pregnancy with congenital toxoplasmosis. Menorrhagia; metrorrhagia.

**Heart:** Precordial pain, *palpitations, dyspnea* on any effort, *orthopnea* and cough. Nocturnal polypneic attacks. Tachycardia with occasional arrhythmia; galloping sound with systolic murmer. *Hyptension.* E.C.G. shows changes in the ST segment and T wave; left ventricular hypertrophy, problems in conduction; fibrillation or auricular flutter due to bundle branch block, extra systoles; subacute myocarditis. Hereditory cardiomegaly. Congenital cardiopathies.

**Back:** Myelitis in children and adults. Hemiplegia, paraplegia. Arthritis and myositis.

**Skin:** Maculo-papular or vesiculous exanthema; polymorphus erythema. Purpura.

**Relationship:** Compare: *Carc.*

**Dose:** 6C, 9C, 30C, 100C, 200C.

---

# V.A.B.

(Vaccin att, nu, bili or B.C.G.,) **V-A-B.**

**Source:** It is prepared from the vaccine B.C.G.

**Clinical:** Hyperthyroidism; colitis; tonsillitis; adenoids; pleurisy; whooping cough; tuberculosis; nasal polyp; blepharitis; conjunctivitis; anal fissures.

A polycrest remedy with *persistent asthenia. Marked fatigue* and a heavy head. *Great chilliness,* cannot get warm enough. A tuberculous constitution of lean subjects, always fatigued and suffering from chronic constipation; hypersensitive and restless; constitution similar to *Phosphorus.* Sarcoidosis or Schaumann's disease.

**Mind:** Easily angered or depressed. *Every noise irritates. Intellectual excitability.* Brain feels benumbed; difficulty in finding words, to under take intellectual work, which makes him weak. Anxiety, vertigo, sensation of imminent death.

**Head:** *Headache towards the end of afternoon and in the evening* students headache, in over worked intellectuals.

**Eyes:** Conjunctivitis; blepharitis, eczema of the lids; swollen eyelids. Interstitial keratitis.

**Ears:** Acute otalgia.

**Nose:** Sneezing. Chronic rhinitis; nasal polyp; repeated attacks.

**Face:** Pain in left temporomaxillary joint, worse mastication. Pale face.

**Mouth:** Bitter taste, saburral tongue with a yellowish white coating. Distaste for cigarette.

**Throat:** Hyperthyroidism, chronic tonsillitis, pain while swallowing, especially in the right side. Adenopathy of the neck; maybe suppurative. Scraping and pain in the posterior part of throat.

**Stomach:** *Anorexia with nausea or unceasing hunger;* nausea on waking up, while standing, better eating, slow digestion.

**Abdomen:** Prickling pain in the liver region, better on lying down Atony of the gall bladder. Intestinal sluggishness resulting in constipation. Gastro-colitis.

**Respiratory:** Pleuritis; sero-fibrinous pleurisy; pleurodynia. Terminal stage of whooping cough. Terminal stage of whooping cough; repeated attacks bronchitis; cough rough, dry and fatiguing. Infantile asthma. Loeffler's syndrome, pneumonia with eosinophilia.

**Heart:** Chronic hypotension with emaciation and hyposthenia.

**Blood:** Marked leucocytosis; increased E.S.R. Arneth formula is *deviated to the left* (Arneth formula is a method of determining the percentage of neutrophils having the same number (1-5) of nuclear lobes. An increase in the percentage with fewer lobes is termed as a *shift to the left*).

**Back:** Cervical pain, worse turning towards the right, better slow, continuous movement. Schaurmann's disease or painful, dorsal kyphosis in children. Calve's diseases, osteochondritis of the vertebra in children between 5-10 years.

**Extremities:** Polyarthritis. Cramps in fingers and left leg.

**Sleep:** Restless with erotic dreams, prolonged insomnia in the second part of the night.

**Skin:** Skin and lips dry. Ichthyosis. *Cracks and fissures at labial commissures.*

**Modalities:** Worse, noise, towards the end of the day and by exercise. Better by stretching and eating.

**Relationship:** Compare: *Dros., Calc-p., Nat-m., Aq-mar., Hed.*

**Dose:** 6C to 30C.

■

# SOME IMPORTANT MOTHER TINCTURES

## ABROMA AUGUSTA

### Clinical

- Diabetes mellitus.
- Dysmenorrhea

### Urinary System

- Profuse urination day and night.
- Fishy odor of the urine.
- Diabetes mellitus.
- White ulcers in the mouth of prepuce.

### Female

- Affects instant cure and relief in dysmenorrhea.
- Chlorosis, hysterical spasms, irregular menses and leucorrhea.
- Colicky pain in lower abdomen 2-3 days before menses.

### Dose

- In diabetes mellitus administer *Abroma augusta* Q drops, 3 times a day and Syzygium jambolanum Q (Jamun) 5 drops twice daily.
- In dysmenorrhea and all complication associated with it, give *Abroma augusta* Q 10 drops every hour or oftener according to the severity of the pain.

## ABROMA RADIX

### Clinical

- Female disorders.

### Symptoms

- A great uterine tonic.
- Very efficacious in dysmenorrhea.

## ABROTANUM

### Clinical

- Marasmus.
- Peritonitis.

### Symptoms

- Marvelous action in consumption (wasting) with peritonitis, emaciation and marasmus from feet upward with constant distention and acidity in abdomen, face shriveled, dry cold and pale with characteristics that the patient losses flesh rapidly while living well with a ravenous hunger.

### Dose

- Give 1x, 2 drops 4 times a day or according to the severity of the case.

## ABSINTHIUM

### Clinical

- Seizures.
- Sleeplessnes.

### Symptoms

- A very good medicine in epileptiform seizures.
- Nervous excitement and sleeplessness.
- Cerebral irritation, hysteria, infantile spasms, chorea, tremors.
- Vertigo, with tendency to fall backward.

### Dose

- Give *Absinthium* Q, 2 to 4 drops or 1x, 1 drop during paroxysm every 10 to 15 minutes otherwise 4 times a day.

## ACALYPHA INDICA

### Clinical

- Bronchietasis.
- Cough.
- Hemoptysis.
- Incipient phthisis.

### Symptoms

- Hemorrhage from lungs.
- Employed in the beginning of phthisis.
- Expectoration of pure bright red blood comes on in morning and dark clotted blood in the evening, while violent teasing cough at night.
- It is indicated in incipient phthisis with hard, racking cough, bloody expectoration, arterial hemorrhage but without febrile disturbances.

### Dose

- Used as Q; in the beginning 5 drops, 4 times a day in an ounce of water and afterwards 1x, 2 drops, 4 times a day.

## ACONITUM NAPELLUS

### Clinical

- Rheumatic fever.
- Collapse condition.

### Symptoms

- Coldness of body, face cyanotic and like a corpse, great agony, restlessness, fear of death, weakness of heart with regular beat but imperceptible pulse."
- In fever, cold stage more marked.

- Evening chilliness. Cold waves pass through him.
- Thirst and restlessness always present.
- Sweat drenching on parts lain on; relieving all symptoms.

**Dose**

- Give 1 drop of *Aconite* Q with cool water every 15 minutes.
- In rheumatic fever when the temperature rises higher than 105 °F, give *Aconite* Q drop in cool water every 15 minutes.

## ADONIS VERNALIS

**Clinical**

- Heart disorders.

**Symptoms**

- It acts predominantly on the heart when it is affected after rheumatism, influenza or nephritis, where the muscles of the heart are in the stage of fatty degeneration.
- It regulates the pulse, increases the contracting power of the heart, with increased urinary secretion.
- Cardiac dropsy, hydrothorax; ascites and anasarca.
- Compensatory hypertrophy of heart in cardiac stenosis and mitral regurgitation.

**Dose**

- 5 to 10 drops of the tincture 4 times a day.

## AEGELE FOLIA AND AEGELE MARMELOS

**Clinical**

- Dropsy.

**Symptoms**

- Dropsy of any part of the body; upper part of the eyelid swollen; dropsical swelling due to heart diseases.
- Excellent medicine in beri-beri; ascites.

**Dose**

- 5 drops of mother tincture of *Aegele folia* should be used two times a day.

## AESCULUS HIPPOCASTANUM

**Clinical**

- Hemorrhoids.
- Backache.

**Rectum**

- Engorged hemorrhoidal veins, with characteristic backache, and absence of actual constipation.

- Dry, aching. Feels full of small sticks; hemorrhoids, with sharp, shooting pains up the back; blind and bleeding.
- Burning in anus with chills up and down the back.

**Back**

- Back and legs give out. Backache affecting sacrum and hips.

**Dose**

- 5 to 10 drops, three times a day in an ounce of cool water.

## AGARICUS MUSCARIUS

**Clinical**

- Chorea.
- Paralysis.

**Symptoms**

- It corresponds to various forms of cerebral excitement rather than congestion.
- Involuntary movements while awake; ceases during sleep.
- Burning, itching and redness of various parts as if frostbitten.

**Dose**

- Give 5 drops in an ounce of cool water thrice daily.

## ALETRIS FARINOSA

**Clinical**

- Leucorrhea.
- Disturbed menstrual flow.
- Prolapsus.
- Sterility.

**Female**

- A great uterine tonic.
- It is successfully used in the weakness of the uterus caused by frequent child bearing and over work.
- Premature and profuse menses, with labor-like pains. Leucorrhea associated with debility and anemia.
- Uterine displacement and prolapsus uterus with pain in right inguinal region.
- Tendency of habitual abortion.
- Sterility and chlorosis.
- Gastric derangement connected with uterine disorders.
- Obstinate vomiting of pregnancy.

**Dose**

- 5 drops in cool water thrice daily.

## ALFALFA

**Clinical**

- Marasmus.
- Deficient development.

**Symptoms**

- Favorably influences nutrition; "toning up" of appetite and digestion.
- A tissue builder. Greatly increases weight. It is highly efficacious in anemia, chlorosis, marasmus, deficient development, phthisis and all conditions characterized by tissue waste.
- Increases quality and quantity of milk in nursing mother.

**Dose**

- 5-10 drops of mother tincture, 3-4 times a day in cool water.

## ALOE SOCOTRINA

**Clinical**

- Dysentery.
- Hemorrhoids.

**Stool**

- Dysenteric stools with mucus and blood with prolapsus ani, loss of control over sphincter ani.
- Stool passes without effort almost unnoticed. Jelly-like stools, with soreness in rectum after stools.

**Rectum**

- Hemorrhoids better cold water application. Burning in anus and rectum.

**Dose**

- 2 drops with cool water 4 times a day.

## AMALAKI

**Clinical**

- Spermatorrhea.
- Cough.
- Grey hair.

**Dose**

- Mother tincture of *Amlaki* is prepared by mixing 1 part of amla with 1 part of alcohol. Give 3 drops thrice daily.

## AMYGDALUS PERSICA

**Clinical**

- Vomiting.
- Morning sickness of pregnancy.

**Gastro-intestinal**

- Valuable remedy in vomiting of various kinds.
- Very efficacious in gastric irritation of children. Gastric and intestinal irritation when the tongue is elongated and pointed, tip and edges red.

**Dose**

- Give 2 drops of tincture every 2 hours or thrice daily.

## ANACARDIUM ORIENTALE

**Clinical**

- Elephantiasis.

## APOCYNUM CANNABINUM

**Clinical**

- Dropsy.
- Ascites.
- Digestive complaints.
- Bright's disease.

**Symptoms**

- Dropsy with or without organic disease.
- Scanty urine and sweat, feels if he could only sweat he would get well.

**Dose**

- Ten drops of tinctrure three times daily.

## ARALIA RACEMOSA

**Clinical**

- Asthma.
- Hay fever suppressed menses.
- Leucorrhea.

**Respiratory**

- Dry cough coming on after first sleep, about middle of night.
- Asthma worse after first sleep, with tickling in throat.
- Constriction of chest.
- Hay fever. Rawness and burning behind sternum.
- The least current of air causes sneezing with copious, watery, excoriating nasal discharge of salty acrid taste.

**Female**

- Leucorrhea foul smelling, acrid, with pressing down pain.

**Dose**

- Give *Aralia* Q, 5 drops 4 times a day.

## ARANEA DIADEMA

**Clinical**

- Malarial poisoning.

**Fever**

- It is a very useful remedy in intermittent fever with swollen spleen.
- Periodicity and coldness with great susceptibility to dampness.
- Coldness to the very bone.
- Inability to live near fresh water, lakes, rivers etc. or in damp, marshy chilly places.
- Coldness not relieved by anything.
- Wakes up at night with hands feeling twice their natural size.
- Sensation of a stone in the abdomen at the same hour daily.
- Important note: All symptoms of *Aranea* are characterised by periodicity, coldness and susceptibility to dampness.

**Dose**

- Give *Aranea* Q, 3-5 drops, thrice daily.

## ARJUNA - TERMINALIA ARJUNA

**Clinical**

- Heart diseases.
- Fracture pain.

**Heart**

- "Feeling as if heart would stop beating at any moment; palpitation violent; patient faints.
- Patient obliged to lie on the left side.
- Feeling as if too much blood has accumulated in the heart and expects relief if vomiting of blood takes place.
- Piercing in the heart with violent palpitation before coughing.
- Pulse very irregular, sometimes very quick and sometimes very feeble and slow."
- Ecchymosis.

**Dose**

- Q dilution, 5 drops thrice daily.

## ASARUM EUROPAEUM

**Clinical**

- Nervous affection.
- Vomiting.

**Symptoms**

- A remedy for nervous affection, loss of energy and excessive erethism. Always feels cold.
- Oversensitiveness of nerves.
- Desire for alcoholic drink.
- It is of great service in pregnancy of early month in vomiting of whatever kind in nervous women.

**Dose**

- Give 3x, 2 drops 4 times a day.

## ASCLEPIAS SYRIACA

**Clinical**

- Urinary disorder.
- Rheumatic inflammation.

**Symptoms**

- It especially acts on urinary system.
- A good remedy for dropsy, hepatic, renal or cardiac and post-scarlatinal disease.

**Dose**

- 5 drops of mother tincture, thrice daily.

## ASOCA JOANESIA

**Clinical**

- Uterine and menstrual disorders.

**Female**

- Violent pain in pelvic region due to sudden suppression of menstrual flow with extension of this pain in the whole abdominal region and violent pain in head and lumbar region.
- Most inveterate cases of chronic leucorrhea with sterility.
- Very fetid, long lasting, black lochia.
- Thirst, weakness; vertigo, diarrhea, etc. due to uterine disorders.
- Anemia; chlorosis in lean and thin hysterical women.

**Dose**

*Asoka* Q, 5 drops, thrice daily.

## ASPARAGUS OFFICINALIS

**Clinical**

- Heart affections.

**Symptoms**

- Violent palpitation of the heart; pain about left shoulder.
- Oppression in breathing due to hydrothorax.

**Dose**

- One drop of 1x dilution thrice daily.

## ASPIDOSPERMA

**Clinical**

- Asthma.

**Respiratory**

- Pulmonary stenosis.
- Thrombosis of pulmonary artery.
- "Want of breath" during exertion.

**Dose**

- First trituration (1x) or tincture every hour for a few days.

## ASWAGANDHA

**Clinical**

- Weak memory.
- Spermatorrhea.
- Impotency.
- Menstrual disorders.

**Symptoms**

- A great mental tonic. Acts like magic in slowly advancing mental inertia, imbecility, with loss of comprehension and expression.
- For a student who cannot fix his attention on any subject nor can memorise his lesson, nor express what he has read.
- For impotency and all kind of seminal deficiencies.

**Dose**

- Use 5 drops of mother tincture, thrice daily.

## ATISTA INDICA OR GLYCOSMIS PENTAPHYLLA

**Clinical**

- Biliary colic, diarrhea, flatulence.

**Stomach**

- Strong desire for lime juice.

- Worms.
- Heartburn 3-4 hours after food.

**Abdomen**

- Colicky pain round the naval.

**Stool**

- Constipation or watery diarrhea during the whole period of fever.

**Dose**

- 2-5 drops of mother tincture in an ounce of cool water thrice daily.

## ATISTA RADIX

**Clinical**

- Dysentery.
- Worm - complaints.

**Stool**

- Dysentery both amoebic and bacillary.
- Dysentery appearing in autumn.

**Dose**

- It should be used in mother tincture form, 2 drops per dose 4 times a day.

## AVENA SATIVA

**Clinical**

- Alcoholism.
- Bad effect of morphine habit.
- Debility.
- Neuroasthenia.
- Palpitation.
- Sexual excess.
- Sleeplessness.
- Cold.
- Spermatorrhea.
- Prostate enlargement.

**Symptoms**

- Best remedy for debility after exhausting diseases.
- Post-diphtheritic paralysis.
- Rheumatism of heart.
- Sleeplessness, especially of alcoholics, bad effects of morphine habits.
- Nervous exhaustion.
- Excessive indulgence in sexual intercourse with mental depression and physical prostration with amenorrhea.

- Enlargement of the prostate.

**Dose**

- Tincture ten to twenty drops, preferably in hot water thrice daily.

## AZADIRACHTA INDICA

**Clinical**

- Malaria.
- Skin diseases.

**Fever**

- In chronic malarial fever.
- The liver and spleen are enlarged and indurated.

**Chill**

- Rise of temperature with slight chill in the afternoon.

**Sweat**

- It is very beneficial in fever with burning, thirstlessness.

**Skin**

- Itching without eruptions; scabies, leprosy.

**Dose**

- Give one drop of this drug in 1x or 3x dilutions, 4 times a day.

## BACOPA MONNIERI OR BRAHMI

**Clinical**

- Impaired memory.
- Whooping cough.

**Symptoms**

- It has significant influence on learning abilities.
- Anxiety, impaired memory, tension due to mental over work.

**Dose**

- 10-15 drops in water twice daily.

## BAPTISIA TINCTORIA

**Clinical**

- Malarial fever.
- Typhoid fever.

**Symptoms**

- Septic conditions of the blood, malarial poisoning.
- Headache; furious delirium; sensation as if the limbs were, apart from him and an attempt to gather the scattered limb.

- Putrid fever in typhoid state.
- Watery, very offensive black stools; foul smell in breath.
- Sore and bruised feeling of the parts rested upon in whatever position he lies.

**Dose**

- Give *Baptisia tinctoria* Q, 3 drops every 2 hours.

## BELLADONNA

**Clinical**

- Opium poisoning.

**Symptoms**

- In opium poisoning when the patient in unconscious and drifting towards death.
- In stiff-neck when the pain comes and goes like electric shocks with intermittency.

**Dose**

- *Belladonna* 1x, 3 drops every 3 hourly.

## BELLIS PERENNIS

**Clinical**

- Injury.
- Sprain.
- Nocturnal emissions.

**Symptoms**

- Acts upon the muscular fibres of the blood vessels.
- First remedy in injuries to the deeper tissues, after surgical works.
- Results of injuries to nerves with intense soreness and intolerance of cold bathing.
- Excellent remedy for sprains and bruises.
- Traumatism of the pelvic organs.
- Ill effects from masturbation.
- Nocturnal emission, spermatorrhea, discharge of prostatic fluid in the urine.

**Dose**

- Mother tincture, 5 drops, twice daily.

## BERBERIS AQUIFOLIUM

**Clinical**

- Skin affections.

**Symptoms**

- Stimulate all glands and improve nutrition.

### Face

- Acne, blotches and pimples.
- Clears the complexion.

### Skin

- Pimples, dry, rough, scaly.
- Eruptions on scalp extending to the neck and face.
- Psoriasis.
- Acne.
- Dry eczema.
- Pruritus.

### Dose

- 5 to 10 drops in an ounce of cool water 4 times a day.

## BERBERIS VULGARIS

### Clinical

- Hepatic disorders.
- Renal disorders.

### Gall Stone Colic

- Short, sudden, stabbing, puncturing type of pain in the liver region.
- Gall stone colic is often associated with jaundice.

### Urinary

- Renal colic.
- Dysuria.

### Dose

- *Berberis vulgaris* Q, 5 drops every hour or more oftener according to the severity of the case.

## BETONICA AQUATICA

### Clinical

- Pain in various parts.

### Dose

- Give 5 drops of mother tincture thrice daily.

## BLATTA ORIENTALIS

### Clinical

- Asthma.

### Respiratory

- Asthma, especially when associated with bronchitis.

- Much pus-like mucus.
- Asthma worsened during night; and lying down; better by expectoration.

**Dose**

- *Blatta* Q, 10 drops frequently (2-4 times) during an attack. After the spasm for the remaining cough use the higher potency. Stop with improvement to prevent return of aggravation.

## BOERHAAVIA DIFFUSA

**Clinical**

- Asthma.
- Beri-beri.
- Dropsy.
- Jaundice.
- Heart troubles.

**Symptoms**

- Attack of beri-beri and dropsy in every rainy season.
- Dropsy in feet, up to thigh.
- Retention of urine.
- Cirrhosis of liver.
- Swelling of eyelids; hands; abdomen; legs and feet.

**Dose**

- *Boerhaavia* Q, 5 drops in cool water thrice daily for some time.

## BRYOPHYLLUM CALYCINUM

**Clinical**

- Cholera.

**Stool**

- In the first stage of cholera, serious diarrhea and dysentery with mucus or bloody stools.

**Dose**

- Give *Bryophyllum* Q, 5 drops in an ounce of cool water after each stool in cholera, diarrhea and dysentery and it will instantly cure the cases.

## BUFO RANA

**Clinical**

- Epilepsy.
- Masturbation.
- Paralytic affections.
- Whitlow.

### Epileptic Symptoms

- Convulsive seizures occur during sleep at night.
- Epilepsy at the time of menses.
- Epilepsy due to masturbation.

### Male

- Involuntary emissions; impotency.
- Buboes.
- Disposition to handle organs. Seek a solitary place for masturbation.

### Female

- Epilepsy at the time of menses.

### Skin

- In whitlow, after blow, the pain ascends upward from the site of blow.

### Dose

- *Bufo* Q, 5 drops thrice or 4 times daily.

## CACTUS GRANDIFOLIUS

### Clinical

- Heart disorders.

### Heart

- It has a direct action on heart, sensation as if the heart is caged with wire bands, each wire being twisted tighter.
- Endocardities with mitral insufficiency.
- Heart weakness of arteriosclerosis.
- Violent palpitation; worse lying on left side.
- Angina pectoris. Pain in apex, shooting down left arm.
- Constriction; very acute pains and stitches in heart. Endocardial murmurs; precordial dullness, enlarged ventricles.
- Low blood pressure.

### Dose

- *Cactus* Q, 5 drops thrice daily.

## CAFFEINUM

### Clinical

- Heart complaints.

### Preparation

- Mix 1 part of Caffein with a part of sugar of milk and get it well triturated and the 1x trituration is prepared.

### Symptoms

- Threatening heart failure due to frequent motion.

### Dose

- Give 1 grain over 10 to 15 minutes intervals.

## CALADIUM SEGUINUM

### Clinical

- Asthma.
- Male complaints.
- Skin complaints.
- Tobacco chewing habit.

### Respiratory

- In asthma, patient afraid to go to sleep.

### Male

- Pruritus, erection when half-asleep, cease when fully awake.
- Impotency; relaxation of penis during excitement.
- Spermatorrhea and nocturnal emission.

### Skin

- Sweet sweat attracts flies.
- Tobacco craving; it diminishes and modifies tobacco craving.

### Dose

- 2-5 drops of the tincture in an ounce of boiled water after meals and at bed time.

## CALOTROPIS GIGANTEA

### Clinical

- Syphilis.
- Leprosy.
- Fever.

### Symptoms

- Useful in purifying blood and efficacious in curing syphilis in all its stages, leprosy in feet, around nails, fingers etc.
- Putrid gangrenous ulcers and leprosy.
- Chilliness prominent in intermittent fever, chilliness and shivering start from feet and ascend upward through spinal cord.

### Dose

- *Calotropis* 1x, 3 drops thrice or four times a day.

## CALOTROPIS LACTUM

### Symptoms

- It is more efficacious and acts more promptly than *Calotropis gigantea* in all its characteristics.

**Dose**

- 1x, 2x, 1gr. or 1 drop, thrice daily.

## CAMPHORA OFFICINALIS

**Clinical**

- Cholera.
- Collapsed condition.

**Symptoms**

- Cholera infantum, cholera asiatica.
- Priapism.
- Spasmodic stricture of urethra.

**Dose**

- Mother tincture Q, 5 drops repeated frequently.
- In convulsion of children, if symptoms correspond smelling of spirits of Camphora is also very effective.

## CANNABIS INDICA

**Clinical**

- Headache.

**Symptoms**

- Dr. Cowperthwaite suggests to give *Cannabis indica* Q, 3 drops thrice daily in violent pains of hemicrania of any side.

## CARDUUS MARIANUS

**Clinical**

- Hepatic disorders.
- Varicose veins.
- Hemorrhagic piles.

**Abdomen**

- Left lobe very sensitive.
- Constipation; stools hard, difficult, knotty; alternates with diarrhea.
- Swelling of gall bladder.
- Hyperemia of liver, with jaundice, cirrhosis with dropsy.

**Rectum**

- Hemorrhagic piles.
- Rectal cancer.

**Skin**

- Varicose veins, also varicose ulcers.

**Dose**

- *Carduus* Q, 5 drops thrice daily.

## CASCARA AMARGA

**Clinical**

- Syphilis.

**Symptoms**

- Specific action on syphilis in all its stages and development. It cures the disease by purifying the blood.

**Dose**

- *Cascara amarga* Q, 5 drops twice daily.

## CASCARA SAGRADA

**Clinical**

- Gastric disorders.
- Rheumatism.

**Symptoms**

- Chronic indigestion, cirrhosis and jaundice.
- Constipation.
- Gastric headache.
- Rheumatism of muscles and joints, with obstinate constipation.

**Dose**

- 5 drops mother tincture thrice daily.

## CASTANEA VESCA

**Clinical**

- Whooping cough.

**Symptoms**

- Whooping cough, especially in the early stage.
- Desire for warm drink.
- Very thirsty with loss of appetite.

**Dose**

- Q, 5 drops thrice daily.

## CASTOREUM

**Clinical**

- Hysteria.

**Symptoms**

- A great remedy for hysteria.
- Prostration marked.
- Day blindness.

### Dose

- Give Q, 5 drops, thrice daily.

## CATARIA NEPETA

### Clinical

- Colic.

### Symptoms

- Children's remedy for colic, and also for nervous headache and hysteria.

### Dose

- Give 5 to 10 drops of Q, thrice daily.

## CAULOPHYLLUM THALICTROIDES

### Clinical

- False labor pains.
- Habitual abortion
- Dysmenorrhea
- Prolapse uteri.

### Female

- False labor pains. "Labor pains weak and deficient, fetus does not pass downward.
- Spasmodic rigidity of os, delaying labor.
- Needle-like pains in cervix.
- In prolapse uteri when the uterus is retroverted or prolapsed due to defective nutrition.
- In climacteric period there is great tension, unrest, indisposition to work and worry about trifles.

### Abortion

- Habitual abotion from uterine debility.
- Threatening abortion, spasmodic bearing down pains.
- Passive hemorrhage after abortion.

### Rheumatism

- Rheumatism of phalangeal and metacarpal joints in females.

### Dose

- Q 5 drops, 10-15 minute intervals in urgency to thrice daily in chronic complaints.

## CEANOTHUS AMERICANUS

### Clinical

- Spleenic affections.
- Hair fall.

### Symptoms

- Enormous enlargement of the spleen.
- Splenitis pain in left hypochondrium.
- Leucemia.

### Dose

- *Ceanothus* Q 2 to 5 drops three times a day. It can be applied locally on scalp as hair tonic.

## CEDRON

### Clinical

- Fever especially malaria.
- Clock like periodicity of the paroxysm.
- Malarial affections, especially neuralgia.
- Chilliness towards evening, then frontal headache extending into parietal region.

### Dose

- *Cedron* Q, 5 drops or 1x, one drop thrice daily.

## CHAPARRO AMARGOSO

### Clinical

- Diarrhea.

### Stool

- In chronic diarrhea when all indicated remedies fail.

### Dose

- Give Q, 2 to 4 drops, 3 to 4 times a day.

## CHELIDONIUM MAJUS

### Clinical

- Liver disorders.

### Symptoms

- A prominent liver remedy.
- Liver enlarged.
- Jaundiced skin, and constant pain under the inferior angle of right scapulae.
- General lethargy and indisposition to make any effort is also marked.
- Bilious complication during gestation.

### Dose

- Give Q, 5 drops, thrice daily.

## CHELONE GLABRA

### Clinical

- Liver affection.
- Worms.

### Symptoms

- Pain or soreness of the left lobe of the liver.
- Malaise.
- Dyspepsia with hepatic torpor.
- Jaundice.
- Round and thread worms.

### Dose

- Tincture, one to five drops.

## CHIMAPHILA UMBELLATA

### Clinical

- Urinary complaints.
- Prostate enlargement.
- Tumor breast.

### Urinary

- Chronic cystitis.
- Acute prostatitis, retention and feeling of a ball in perineum.
- Unable to urinate without standing with feet wide apart and body inclined forward.

### Male

- Loss of prostatic fluid, prostatic enlargement and rotation.

### Female

- Mammae, with tumor not ulcerated, with undue secretion.
- Rapid atrophy of breast.

### Dose

- 5 drops of mother tincture thrice daily.

## CHIONANTHUS LATIFOLIA

### Clinical

- Headache.
- Hepatic derangement.
- Gall stones.

### Head

- Dull frontal headache, chiefly over eyes. Eyeballs very painful, with pressure over root of nose.

**Abdomen and Liver**

- Feels as if a string were tied in a slip-knot, around intestines which is suddenly drawn tight and then gradually loosened.
- Jaundice and constipation.
- Bilious colic. Gall stones.

**Dose**

- *Chionanthus latifolia* Q, 10 drops in an ounce of cool water every hour during paroxysm of pain.
- To stop recurrence of stones and pain give *Chionanthus latifolia* Q, 5 drops thrice daily.

## CHIRATA OR GENTIANA CHIRATA

**Clinical**

- Malaria.
- Scabies.

**Dose**

- Give 5 drops of Q or 1x, 2 drops thrice daily.

## CHOLESTRINUM

**Clinical**

- Gall stones.
- Liver cancer.

**Liver**

- Obstinate hepatic engorgements.
- Burning pain in side; on walking holds his hand on side, hurts him so.
- Jaundice, gallstones.

**Dose**

- *Cholestrinum* 1x, 5 drops or 5 grains every half an hour or oftener during paroxysm of pain and give it's 2x trituration 1 grain liquid or 1 drop thrice daily for radical cure.

## CHRYSOPHANICUM ACIDUM

**Clinical**

- Dandruff.

**Symptoms**

- Dandruff and peeling of the skin of palms.

**Dose**

- Give 3 drops thrice daily.

## CINA

**Clinical**

- Gastric complaints.
- Worms infestation.

**Symptoms**

- All ailments dependent on worms such as fever, derangement of stomach and bowels, epilepsy, tetanic spasms and convulsion, unconsciousness; constant picking at nose, itching at the anus, grinding of teeth in sleep, etc.

**Dose**

- Cina Q or 1x, one drop, thrice daily.

## CINNAMONUM

**Clinical**

- Hemorrhage.
- Cancer.
- Hiccough.

**Symptoms**

- Cancer where pain and fetor are present. Best when skin is intact.
- Hemorrhage from bowels, hemoptysis, nose bleed. Post-partum hemorrhage.
- Uterine hemorrhage caused by overlifting, during puerperal state.

**Dose**

- For cancer, strong decoction, one-half pint in a day.
- Three drops on sugar for hiccough.

## CLEMATIS ERECTA

**Clinical**

- Urethral pain.
- Swollen testes.

**Male**

- Burning at orifice.
- Testicles indurated with bruised feeling, swelling of scrotum.
- Testicles heavy with pain along spermatic cord.

**Dose**

- In urethral pain *Clematis erecta* Q, 3 drops every three hours acts like magic.

## CLERODENDRON INFORTUNATUM

**Clinical**

- Worm infestation.

**Symptoms**

- It is useful in worms of children with foamy, watery, diarrhoeic stools and water brash.

**Dose**

- Tincture 5 drops or 1x, 2 drops thrice daily.

## COCA

**Clinical**

- Mountaineer's complaints.
- Aphonia.

**Symptoms**

- Useful in a variety of complaints incidental to mountain climbing, such as palpitation, dyspnea, anxiety and insomnia.
- Loss of voice.
- Weak vocal cords.

**Dose**

- Give Q, 5 drops three or four times a day.
- In loss of voice give 5-6 drops, every half hour, two hours before expected demand on voice.

## COFFEA MOCHA

**Clinical**

- Cholera.

**Symptoms**

- It is a specific remedy for cholera.

**Dose**

- Give 10 drops in an ounce of water every 10 minutes, and 3 doses are more than sufficient.

## CUNDURANGO

**Clinical**

- Gastric disorders.
- Cancer of stomach.

**Gastro-intestinal**

- Stimulates the digestive functions and improves the general health.
- Stricture of esophagus, with burning pains behind sternum, where food seems to stick.

- Vomiting of food, and induration in left hypochondrium with constant burning pain.

**Dose**

- *Cundurango,* Q 5 drops, thrice daily.

## CONVALLARIA MAJALIS

**Clinical**

- Heart disorders.

**Heart**

- Valvular diseases especially mitral.
- Pericardial adhesion rather than tissue degeneration of use when the ventricles are over-distended and dilatations begins, and when there is an absence of compensatory hypertrophy, and when venous stasis is marked.
- Endocarditis, with extreme orthopnea.
- Palpitation from the least exertion. Tobacco heart, especially when due to cigarettes.
- Angina pectoris.
- Extremely rapid and irregular pulse.

**Dose**

- *Convallaria* Q, 5 drops in an ounce of cool water thrice daily.

## CORNUS ALTERNIFOLIA

**Clinical**

- Skin disorder.

**Skin**

- Serious discharge from chilblains or broken skin; eczema.

**Dose**

- *Cornus alternifolia* Q, 5 drops, thrice daily.

## CRATAEGUS OXYACANTHA

**Clinical**

- Heart complaints.

**Heart**

- Cardiac dropsy.
- Fatty degeneration.
- Aortic disease.
- Extreme dyspnea without much increase of pulse.
- Pain in region of heart and under left clavicle.
- Heart dilated; first sound weak.
- Valvular murmurs, angina pectoris.

- *Crataegus oxyacantha* is said to have solvent power upon crustaceous and calcareous deposits in arteries.

**Dose**

- *Crataegus* 10-15 drops in an ounce of warm water every 10-15 minute in emergency cases.
- Otherwise 5-10 drops thrice daily. Must be used for some time in order to obtain good results.

## CYNODON DACTYLON

**Clinical**

- Hemorrhage.
- Dysentery.
- Dropsy.

**Hemorrhage**

- Hemorrhage from any orifice of the body.
- Urinary and Genito-urinary System
- Retention of urine.
- Vesical calculus.
- Secondary syphilis.

**Abdomen**

- Chronic diarrhea; anasarca; bilious vomiting.

**Dose**

- *Cynodon dactylon* Q, 5 drops or 1x in 2 drops three hourly, then thrice daily.

## DAMIANA

**Clinical**

- Impotency.
- Prostatic discharge.
- Spermatorrhea.
- Sexual debility.

**Sexual Neurasthenia; Impotency**

- Sexual debility from nervous prostration.
- Spermatorrhea in weak, exhausted subjects

**Dose**

- *Damiana* Q, 10 drops in an ounce of cool water, 3 or 4 times a day.

## DIOSCOREA VILLOSA

**Clinical**

- Gastric disorders.
- Gall bladder colic.

**Symptoms**

- It affords prompt relief in colic, painful affections of abdominal and pelvic viscera.
- Aggravation by lying down and doubling up, better by standing erect or bending backward.
- Pain suddenly shifts to different parts. Pain from gall-bladder to chest, back and arms.

**Dose**

- *Dioscorea* Q, 5 drops thrice daily.
- In acute pain 5 drops Q, every 10 to 15 minutes.

## ECHINACEA ANGUSTIFOLIA

**Clinical**

- Blood dyscrasia.

**Symptoms**

- Symptoms of blood poisoning, septic conditions.
- Boils, erysipelas and foul ulcers. Gangrene. Pustules.
- Tendency of malignancy. Last stage of cancer, to ease pain.
- Venom infection. Irritation from insect bites and poisonous plants.
- Lymphatic inflammation; crushing injuries.
- Snake bite and stings generally

**Dose**

- Tincture, one to ten drops, every three hour.

## EMBELIA RIBES

**Clinical**

- Worm infestation.

**Symptoms**

- In all abnormalities dependent worms, especially in children.
- Itching in rectum, undigested stool with worms.

**Dose**

- Give Q, 10 drops every 3 hourly with fasting for 24 hours. Then 5 drops Q, thrice daily.

## EPIGEA REPENS

**Clinical**

- Urinary complaints.

**Urinary**

- Chronic cystitis, with dysuria; muco-pus and uric acid deposits, gravel, renal calculi, fine sand in urine of a brown color.
- Pyelitis.

**Dose**

- Tincture 5 drops, after every three hours.

## EQUISETUM HYEMALE

**Clinical**

- Dysuria.

**Urinary**

- Frequent urging with severe pain at the close of urination.
- Urine flows only drop by drop.
- Incontinence in children with dreams or night mares when passing urine.
- Incontinency in old women.
- Retention and dysuria during pregnancy and after delivery.

**Dose**

- Mother tincture, 5-7 drops in hot water.

## ERIODICTYON CALIFORNICUM

**Clinical**

- Asthma.

**Respiratory**

- Asthmatic and bronchial affections.
- Chronic bronchitis, bronchial tuberculosis, with profuse, easily raised bronchial secretion, giving relief.

**Dose**

- Give Q, 5 - 10 drops, thrice daily.

## ERYNGIUM AQUATICUM

**Clinical**

- Urinary disorders.

**Urinary**

- Tenesmus of bladder and urethra.
- Spasmodic stricture.
- Renal colic. Congestion of kidneys.

**Dose**

- Give Q, 5 drops, thrice daily.

## ESCULENTINE

**Clinical**

- Obesity.
- Rheumatism.

**Symptoms**

- Esculentine is of great service in reducing fat. It reduced bulk and converts flabby, fatty tissues into healthy muscular tissues.
- It strengthens the heart and improves the general health.
- It also controls the intolerable rheumatic pain of obese subject.

**Dose**

- Give one tablespoonful of Q in an ounce of hot water twice daily before meals.

## EUPATORIUM AYAPANA

**Clinical**

- Snake bite.
- Hemorrhage.

**Symptoms**

- Efficacious remedy in snake bite.
- Useful in bleeding from lungs with cough in consumption and bleeding from bowels in dysentery due to ulcers therein.

**Dose**

- Q, 5 drops every 10 to 15 minutes in snake bites.
- In pulmonary hemorrhage, 2x, 1 drop 4 times a day.
- Give 1x, 1 drop thrice daily in dysentery.

## EUPATORIUM PERFOLIATUM

**Clinical**

- Fever.

**Fever**

- Intermittent fever, chill; intense aching in all bones before chill, soreness in bones, bruised feeling everywhere.
- Insatiable thirst before and during chill and fever, periodicity third or seventh day.

**Dose**

- *Eupatorium* Q, 5 drops or 1x, 2 drops every 15 minutes during paroxysm of fever and 4 times during prodromal stage.

## EUPHORBIA PILULIFERA

**Clinical**

- Asthma.

**Respiratory**

- Humid asthma, cardiac dyspnea, hay fever and bronchitis.
- It has cured desperate cases of asthma.

**Dose**

- Tincture 10 drops, 10 minutes apart during paroxysm and thrice daily when paroxysm is over.

## EUPHORBIUM OFFICINARUM

**Clinical**

- Skin complaints (topical use).

**Skin**

- It has been used topically for cancer, epithelioma, gangrene, pustular and eczematous eruptions.

**Dose**

- Give Euphorbium officinarum 1x, 1 drop every half hour in severe diarrhea and eczematous eruptions.

## EUPHRASIA

**Clinical**

- Eye affections.

**Eyes**

- Catarrhal conjunctivitis, discharge of acrid matter.
- Acrid lachrymation; bland coryza.
- Traumatic conjunctivitis, blepharitis; corneal ulcers. Rheumatic iritis.
- Dr. Clarke says; As an eye lotion Euphrasia has great value, I have seen corneal opacities removed by it."

**Dose**

- Give *Euphrasia* 1x, one drop every two hours or four times a day according to the severity of the case.
- Mix one part of *Euphrasia* Q with nine parts of rose water, 3 drops three times a day should be instilled into the eyes with the aid of dropper.

## FICUS INDICA

**Clinical**

- Hemorrhage.
- Dysentery.
- Spermatorrhea.

**Symptoms**

- Has anti-hemorrhagic property.

**Dose**

Give Q, 5 drops or 1x, 2 drops 4 times a day with an ounce of cool water.

## FICUS RELIGIOSA

**Clinical**

- Hemorrhagic tendency.

- Epistaxis.
- Hemoptysis.
- Hematemesis.
- Hematuria.

**Symptoms**

- Hemorrhage of bright red blood from any orifice of body

**Dose**

- Give Q, 5 drops or 1x, 2 drops every 10 to 15 minutes or four times a day according to the nature of the case.

## FRAXINUS AMERICANA

**Clinical**

- Female complaints.

**Female**

- Fibrous growth, subinvolution and prolapse, with bearing down sensations.
- Dysmenorrhea.

**Dose**

- Ten to fifteen drops of tincture, three times a day.

## FUCUS VESICULOSUS

**Clinical**

- Obesity.
- Non-toxic goitre. Flatulency.
- A remedy for obesity and non-toxic goitre. It increases the rapidity of digestion.
- Thyroid enlargement in obese people.

**Dose**

- Give 5 drops of tincture twice daily for a long time for reduction of fat.

## GALIUM APARINE

**Clinical**

- Cancer.

**Symptoms**

- Has power to suspend or modify cancerous action.
- Favors healthy granulation on ulcerated surfaces.

**Dose**

- Give Q, 30 to 60 drops mixed with water or milk, four times a day.

## GELSEMIUM SEMPERVIRENS

**Clinical**

- Deafness.

- Rheumatism.
- Paralysis.
- Convulsions.
- False labor pains.

**Symptoms**

- Deafness resulting from abuse of quinine.
- Useful in paralysis affecting single groups of muscles, more especially about the mouth, eyes, throat, larynx, chest, extremities and sphincters.
- In post-diphtheritic paralysis.
- An excellent remedy in false labor pains.

**Dose**

- Give Q, 5 drops or 1x, 2 drops every 15 minutes in emergency cases and thrice daily in other cases.

## GERANIUM MACULATUM

**Clinical**

- Hemorrhage.
- Gastric ulcer.

**Hemorrhage**

- Hemorrhages, pulmonary and from different organs, vomiting of blood.
- Ulceration of stomach.

**Stomach**

- Tendency to ulceration and passive hemorrhages.

**Female**

- Menses too profuse.
- Post-partum hemorrhage.

**Dose**

- 10 to 15 drops, 3 or 4 times a day.

**External Use**

- Tincture should be applied on chronic ulcers either pure or mixed with olive oil or coconut oil, one in ten.
- The tincture should be applied over the nasal polyp once a day, the tumor will shrink speedily.

## GLONOINUM

**Clinical**

- Effect of heat.

- Angina.
- Sunstroke.
- Congestion.
- Apoplexy.

**Symptoms**

- In insanity caused by long continued exposure to heat of the sun.
- In angina with fluttering of the heart and violent beating as if it would burst.
- In threatened apoplexy.
- For affects of sun stroke, a rapid and efficient remedy.
- For the congestive form of puerperal convulsions with rush of blood to the head.
- Cerebral congestion or alternate congestion of head and heart.
- Intense congestion of brain from delayed or suppressed menses.

**Dose**

- Put 10 drops of *Glonoinum* 2x, 3x, or 4x in 4 ounces of water and give a teaspoonful every hour or 4 times a day according to the nature of the case.

## GRINDELIA ROBUSTA

**Clinical**

- Asthma.

**Respiratory**

- For wheezing and oppression in bronchitis patients.
- Sibilant rales.
- Asthma, with profuse tenacious expectoration.
- Cannot breathe when lying down.
- Cheyne - stokes respiration.

**Dose**

- *Grindelia* Q, 5-10 drops every 15 minutes during paroxysm and thrice daily in normal state.

## GUAIACUM

**Clinical**

- Rheumatic sore throat.
- Rheumatism.

**Throat**

- Rheumatic sore throat with weak throat muscles.
- Specially valuable in follicular tonsillitis, rheumatic pharyngitis and tonsillitis when there is violent burning in the throat.

- Extremely offensive expectoration of phthisis.

**Extremities**

- Chronic rheumatism of the upper extremities.
- Lumbago especially after abuse of mercury or dependent on syphilis.

**Dose**

- *Guaiacum* Q, 5 drops or 1x, 2 drops, thrice daily.

## GYMNEMA SYLVESTRE

**Clinical**

- Diabetes mellitus.

**Diabetes**

- After passage of urine, patient feels very weak.
- Burning all over the body; diabetic carbuncles.

**Dose**

- Give Q, 5 drops thrice daily.

## HAMAMELIS VIRGINICA

**Clinical**

- Hemorrhage.
- Varicose vein.
- Hemorrhoids.

**Symptoms**

- An important venous remedy.
- Venous congestion, hemorrhages, varicose veins, and hemorrhoids, with bruised soreness of affected parts.
- Piles, bleeding profusely with burning, soreness, fullness.

**Dose**

- Give tincture 5 to 10 drops, 15 minutes or oftener, or 3 times a day.

## HELONIAS

**Clinical**

- Uterine derangement.

**Female**

- A great uterine tonic.
- Prolapsus uteri and ulceration of cervix.
- Prolapse from atony.
- Constant dark fetid bloody discharge, after parturition.
- Of great service in excessive uterine hemorrhage.

- Threatened abortion, especially in habitual abortion.
- Uterine derangement with tired backache in females.

**Dose**

- 5 drops of Q, twice daily for a longer time.

## HEMIDESMUS INDICA

**Clinical**

- Blood poisoning.

**Symptoms**

- A very efficacious remedy in curing all diseases dependent on blood poisoning as it renders the blood free from septic conditions.
- It has cured eruptions due to abuse of mercury.

**Dose**

- Give Q, 5 drops or 1x, 2 drops thrice daily.

## HOANG-NAN

**Clinical**

- Skin complaints.

**Skin**

- Pustules and boils.
- Eczema, prurigo, old ulcers, leprosy, cancer of glandular structures and bites of serpents.
- Removes fetor and hemorrhages in cancer, revives the healing process.

**Dose**

- Give 5 drops of Q, thrice daily.

## HOLARRHENA ANTIDYSENTERICA

**Clinical**

- Dysentery.

**Stool**

- Effective remedy in all kinds of acute and chronic dysentery.

**Dose**

- Q, 5 drops every 2 hourly.
- In chronic case 1x, 2 drops, 4 times a day.

## HYDRANGEA ARBORESCENS

**Clinical**

- Urinary affections.

**Urinary**

- For gravel and profuse deposit of white amorphous salts in urine.
- Calculus, renal colic, bloody urine.
- Acts on ureter.
- Urine hard to start.

**Dose**

- Give Q, 4-5 drops thrice daily.

## HYDRASTIS CANADENSIS

**Clinical**

- Cancer.
- Tumor.
- Leucorrhea.
- Constipation.
- Stomatitis.
- Gall stone colic.
- Skin complaints.

**Cancer**

- In cancer and pre-cancerous states, before ulceration when pain is the principal symptom.

**Tumor**

- Scirrhous tumors developing in glandular tissue.
- Goitre of puberty and pregnancy.
- Tumor of breast.

**Abdomen**

- Liver torpid, tender.
- Jaundice.
- Gall stones.
- Loss of appetite in cancerous and phthisical patients.
- Stomatitis in nursing women, especially after abuse of mercury or chlorate of potash.

**Rectum**

- Constipation dependent on inertia or congestion of the lower abdomen due to sedentary life style or purgative medicines.

**Female**

- Erosion and excoriation of cervix.
- Leucorrhea.

**Skin**

- Ulcers; cancerous formations.
- Unhealthy skin.

**Dose**

- *Hydrastis* Q, 5 drops thrice daily in cancer of soft palate.
- *Hydrastis* 1x, 2 drops every 3 hourly in cancer of last part of intestine.
- When *Arsenic* fails in cancer with intense burning, *Hydrastis can.* Q, 5 drop, 4 times a day.
- In other cases Q, 5 drops 3 to 4 times a day.

## HYDROCOTYLE ASIATICA

**Clinical**

- Leprosy.
- Elephantiasis.
- Granular cancer of uterus.

**Skin**

- Thickness of epidermoid layer of skin and exfoliations in scales.
- Psoriasis.
- Dry eruptions.
- Erythema on face, neck, back, chest, arms, thighs with much itching with copious sweat.
- Miliary eruptions. Intolerable itching specially of soles.

**Female**

- Pruritus of vagina.
- Granular ulceration of womb.
- Profuse leucorrhea.

**Dose**

- Give tincture, 5 drops or 1x, 2 drops, thrice daily.

## HYMOSA

**Clinical**

m.

**Symptoms**

- It quickly brings down rheumatic fever, diminishes pain and cures the inflammation of the joints.
- Prevents rheumatic heart fever. Acute and chronic arthritis and muscular rheumatism.
- In gout it nerutralises the acidity of thre blood, removes deposits from joints.
- It marvelously cures sciatica.

**Dose**

- *Hymosa* Q, 1 dram in an ounce of hot water, followed by plenty of hot water or soda water, every 3 hourly in acute stage and 4 times a day in chronic cases.

## HYPERICUM PERFORATUM

**Clinical**

- Nerve injury.

**Symptoms**

- For injuries to nerves, especially of fingers, toes and nails.
- Crushed fingers, especially tips.
- Excessive painfulness.
- To remove pain following surgical operations, especially amputations, lock jaw.
- Numbness and crawling in the limbs, hands and feet.

**Dose**

- Give Q, 5 drops at an interval of 10 minutes, 3 to 4 times a day.
- In chronic lock-jaw, after amputation, 200 or higher potencies should be tried if Q is not sufficient.

## IBERIS AMARA

**Clinical**

- Cardiac diseases.

**Heart**

- Conscious of heart's action.
- Palpitation.
- Stitching pain in cardiac region.
- Worse, least motion and in warm room.
- Dropsy with enlarged heart.
- Cardiac dyspnea.
- Dilatation of heart.

**Dose**

- Give Q, 5 drops thrice daily.

## JABORANDI

**Clinical**

- Perspiration.
- Hair fall.
- Mumps.

**Symptoms**

- It is a very effective remedy for profuse debilitating sweats of phthisis.
- Abnormal sweats especially at night.
- A valuable remedy in limiting the duration of mumps.
- A good hair restorer and blackens white hair.

**Dose**

- Use 1x or 2x, 2 drops 4 times a day.
- In hair complaints, apply externally on scalp mixed with oil.

## JACARANDA CAROBA

**Clinical**

- Gout, rheumatism.
- Male complaints.

**Symptoms**

- Has a good reputation in venereal diseases and rheumatism.

**Extremities**

- Rheumatic pain in right knee.
- Morning soreness and stiffness of muscles.
- Gonorrheal and syphilitic arthritis.

**Dose**

- Tincture, 5 drops, thrice daily.

## JUGLANS REGIA

**Clinical**

- Skin eruptions.

**Symptoms**

- Comedones and acne of the face.
- Crusta lactea.
- Axillary glands suppurate.

**Dose**

- Give Q, 5 drops, thrice daily.

## JUSTICIA ADHATODA

**Clinical**

- Respiratory complaints.

**Respiratory**

- Used in teasing cough, in coryza, pneumonia, bronchitis, phthisis and for clearing the lungs.
- Very beneficial in the first stage of phthisis and all kinds of pulmonary diseases with discharge of blood in the phlegm.
- Whooping cough of children with gagging after coughing and a cyanotic face.

**Dose**

- Give 3 drops of Q or 1 drop of 1x, 4 times a day.

## JUSTICIA RUBRUM

**Clinical**

- Hemoptysis.

**Symptoms**

- A successful remedy in profuse hemoptysis, and hemorrhage from lungs during paroxysm of cough in pthisical patients where *Justicia adhatoda* is used but has failed.

**Dose**

- Give Q, 3 drops or 1x, 2 drops, 4 times a day.

## KALMEGH

**Clinical**

- Kala azar.
- Malaria.
- Jaundice.

**Symptoms**

- It is an effective medicine in kala azar, malaria and in intermittent fever with double paroxysm. Chronic malaria and kala-azar.
- Its specific action is on the liver, especially in children.
- Jaundice of infants.
- Infantile liver, enlargement of liver and spleen with pain in them.

**Dose**

- Give 2 to 5 drops of mother tincture or one drop of 1x, 4 times a day.

## LATHYRUS SATIVUS

**Clinical**

- Beri-beri.
- Paralysis of lower extremities.
- Dropsy.

**Extremities**

- Excessive rigidity of legs; spastic gait.
- Knees knock against each other when walking.
- Gluteal muscles and lower limbs emaciated.

**Dose**

- Give Q, 5 drops or 1x, 2 drops, thrice daily.

## LAUROCERASUS

**Clinical**

- Cardio-respiratory disorder.

**Symptoms**
- Cyanosis and dyspnea; worse sitting up. Patient puts hands on heart.
- Cough with valvular diseases.
- Threatening paralysis of lungs. Gasping for breath; clutches at heart.
- Mitral regurgitation.
- Cyanosis neonatorum.

**Dose**
- Give Q, 2 to 5 drops thrice daily or 1x, 1 drop twice or thrice daily.

## LOBELIA INFLATA

**Clinical**
- Vomiting.
- Dyspnea.

**Symptoms**
- Vomiting of pregnancy with violent nausea, morning sickness.
- Dyspnea from constriction of chest, worse by exertion.
- Sensation of pressure or weight in chest; better by rapid walking.
- Asthma attacks with weakness preceded by pricking all over.

**Dose**
- Give Q, 5 drops or 1x, 2 drops, thrice daily.

## MAKARADHWAJA

**Clinical**
- Cough.
- Prostration after long lasting disease.

**Symptoms**
- It is a great cardiac, mental, nervous and seminal tonic with violent palpitation of heart, indigestion and vertigo.
- Stimulates the system in convalescents after long lasting diseases.
- Also valuable in spasmodic cough and asthma with aggravation at night.

**Dose**
- Give 1x, 2 drops every 10-15 minutes in emergency cases, otherwise thrice daily.

## MENISPERMUM CANADENSE

**Clinical**
- Menorrhagia.

**Female**
- Copious, bright red bleeding during menses; patient becomes extremely weak due to excessive bleeding; blood oozes out of the uterus; worse from

or during movement.

- Excessive hemorrhage after delivery.

**Dose**

- Give 1x every hour, 2 drops. Then thrice daily.

## MENTHA PIPERITA

**Clinical**

- Respiratory complaints.

**Respiratory**

- Voice husky.
- Dry cough, worse from air into larynx, tobacco smoke, fog, talking; with irritation in suprasternal fossa.
- Trachea painful to touch.

**Dose**

- Give Q, 5 drops thrice daily.

## MILLEFOLIUM

**Clinical**

- Hemorrhage.

**Hemorrhage**

- It is an invaluable remedy for various types of hemorrhage; blood bright red.
- Hemoptysis in incipient pthisis.
- Cough with bloody expectoration, in suppressed menses or hemorrhoids.
- Hemorrhages from uterus; bright red fluid.

**Dose**

- Give 5 drops of mother tincture, thrice daily.

## MITCHELLA REPENS

**Clinical**

- Irritation of urinary bladder.

**Urinary**

- Urging to urinate.
- Dysuria.
- Catarrh of bladder.

**Dose**

- Give Q, 5 drops, thrice daily.

## MOMORDICA BALSAMINA

### Clinical

- Colic.

### Symptoms

- Griping colic, pain in back and hypogastrium with painful and excessive menses.
- Accumulation of flatus in splenic flexure of colon.

### Dose

- Give Q, 5 drops half hourly in emergency and thrice daily in other complaints.

## MULLIEN OIL

### Clinical

- Enuresis.

### Urine

- Constant dribbling of urine or frequent urging to urinate.

### Dose

- 2 drops of Q, 4 times a day.

## MUTHA

### Clinical

- Digestive disorders.

### Gastro-intestinal

- A great tonic for the digestive system.
- Very efficacious in indigestion, dyspepsia, acidity, diarrhea and flatulence.

### Dose

- 5 drops of tincture, 4 times a day or 2 drops of 1x, 4 times a day.

## MYOSOTIS

### Clinical

- Bronchitis.

### Respiratory

- Chronic bronchitis.
- Cough with profuse muco-purulent expectoration.
- Bronchorrhea.

### Dose

- Give Q, 5 drops or 1x, 2 drops thrice daily.

## MYRICA CERIFERA

**Clinical**

- Jaundice.

**Dose**

- Give Q, 5 drops thrice daily.

## NUPHAR LUTEUM

**Clinical**

- Male sexual complaints.

**Male**

- Nervous weakness, with marked symptoms in sexual sphere.
- Complete absence of sexual desire; parts relaxed; penis retracted.
- Impotency, with involuntary emissions during stool, when urinating.
- Spermatorrhea.

**Dose**

- Mother tincture, 5 drops or 1x, 2 drops, 4 times a day.

## NUX JUGLANS

**Clinical**

- Respiratory complaints.
- Acne.

**Symptoms**

- In consumption with cough, aphonia; heaviness in chest, distention and hardness of abdomen, diarrhea, indigestion, glandular swelling with pus in axilla and its vicinity.
- Acne in young girls at puberty.

**Dose**

- *Nux juglans* Q or 1x, 2 drops 4 times a day.

## NUX VOMICA

**Clinical**

- Tetanus.

**Symptoms**

- At the very commencement of tetanus

**Dose**

- *Nux vomica* Q or 1x in 2 drop doses, promptly arrests the progress of the case.

## NYCTANTHES ARBOR TRISTIS

**Clinical**

- Bilious fever.
- Hepatic disorder.

**Symptoms**

- Bilious fever with vomiting and purging of bile or constipation; insatiable thirst before chill.
- Thick white or yellow coating on the tongue.

**Dose**

Give Q, 5 drops or 1x, 1 drop, 4 times a day.

## OCIMUM CARYOPHYLLATUM

**Clinical**

- Urinary complaints.

**Urinary**

- Frequent micturition; extreme burning during urination, passage of pus with urine; hematuria.
- Has decided action upon the kidney, bladder and urethra.
- In first stage of gonorrhea.

**Dose**

- Give Q, 5 drops thrice daily.

## OCIMUM SANCTUM

**Clinical**

- Malaria.
- Tuberculosis.

**Fever**

- Intermittent fever.
- Constantly yawning and stretching during chill.
- Thirst increased, with the rise of temperature, flashes.

**Tuberculosis**

- First stage of consumption, distressing dry cough, expectoration of phlegm streaked with blood.

**Dose**

- Tincture 5 drops or 1x, 2 drops 4 times a day.

## OENANTHE CROCATA

**Clinical**

- Epilepsy.

**Epilepsy**

- Epileptiform convulsions; worse during menstruation and pregnancy.
- Puerperal eclampsia; uremic convulsions.

**Dose**

- Q, 2 drops or 1x, 1 drop in an ounce of cool water, thrice daily.

## OLEUM SANTALI

**Clinical**

- Urinary complaints.

**Urinary**

- Frequent, burning, smarting, swelling and redness of meatus.
- Stream slow and small.
- Sensation of ball pressing against the urethra.

**Dose**

- Give 5 drops of Q three times a day.

## ORIGANUM MAJORANA

**Clinical**

- Excessively aroused sexual impulse.

**Dose**

- Tincture, 5 drops or 1x, 2 drops thrice daily.

## ORNITHOGALUM UMBELLATUM

**Clinical**

- Chronic gastric indurations.

**Gastro-intestinal**

- Useful in chronic gastric and other abdominal indurations, possibly cancer of intestinal tract and especially of stomach and caecum.
- Gastric ulceration with hemorrhage.
- Frequent belching of offensive flatus.

**Dose**

- Give single dose of mother tincture and await action.

## OVA TOSTA

**Clinical**

- Leucorrhea.
- Cancer of os uteri.

**Female**

- Leucorrhea profuse and offensive with sensation as if the back were broken into two and tied with a string.

- Controls hemorrhage from the uterus.
- Has cured cases of cancer of os uteri.

**Dose**

- 1 grain of 3x, 4 times a day.

## PAREIRA BRAVA

**Clinical**

- Renal colic.
- Urinary affections.

**Urinary**

- Very beneficial in renal colic.
- Difficult micturition with strong urging for urination.
- Red sand or brick – dust in the urine.

**Dose**

- Give Q, 30 drops in hot water every half an hour in emergency and thrice daily in chronic complaints.

## PASSIFLORA COMPOUND

**Clinical**

- Impaired nerve function.
- Convulsions.
- Asthma.

**Symptoms**

- Good nerve sedative.
- Important in insomnia, convulsions, epilepsy, tetanus, chorea, paralysis agitans, locomotor ataxia, in spasmodic and non-spasmodic asthma.
- Important remedy in convulsions of childhood and epilepsy.
- All nervous disorders due to derangement of the genito-urinary systems are amenable to it.

**Dose**

- 15 drops to 1 dram of Q every 15 minutes or thrice daily.

## PASSIFLORA INCARNATA

**Clinical**

- Cough.
- Insomnia.
- Tetanus.
- Asthma.
- Morphine addiction.

**Symptoms**

- Delirium tremens.
- Convulsions in children; has a quieting effect on the nervous system.
- Insomnia, produces normal sleep, no disturbance of cerebral function.
- Restless and wakeful, resulting from exhaustion, mental worry and overwork.

**Dose**

- 30 to 60 drops in an ounce of hot water every 15 minutes to 3 times a day according to the nature of the disease.

## PHYTOLACCA

**Clinical**

- Obesity.
- Breast tumor.

**Female**

- Mastitis; mammae hard and very sensitive.
- Tumor of the breast with enlarged axillary glands.
- Cancer of breast.
- Mammary abscess.
- While child nurses, pain goes from nipple to all over body.
- Galactorrhea.
- Obesity. It is a fat reducer.
- Rheumatism and gout associated with obesity.
- Sterility of obese people.

**Dose**

- 2 drops in an ounce of hot water, 4 times a day.

## PINUS SILVESTRIS

**Clinical**

- Emaciated child.

**Symptoms**

- Useful in treatment of weak ankles and tardiness in walking, in scrofulous and rachitic children.
- Emaciation of lower extremities.
- The chest seems very thin.

**Dose**

- Give Q, thrice daily.

## PLANTAGO MAJOR

**Clinical**

- Earache.
- Toothache.

**Symptoms**

- Pain plays between teeth and ears.
- Neuralgic earache.
- Toothache better while eating.
- Profuse flow of saliva.
- Toothache, with reflex neuralgia of eyelids.

**Dose**

- Give Q, 10 drops thrice daily.
- Of local use in hollow teeth, otorrhea, pruritus and poison oak.

## PULSATILLA

**Clinical**

- Amenorrhea.

**Female**

- Suppressed menses from wet feet, nervous debility, chlorosis or any other cause.

**Dose**

- Give Q, 5 drops thrice daily.

## RAUWOLFIA SERPENTINA

**Clinical**

- High blood pressure
- Nerous symptoms.

**Symptoms**

- High blood pressure without marked atheromatous changes in the vessels.
- Irritative condition of central nervous system; insanity; violent maniacal symptoms.

**Dose**

- Give 5 to 10 drops of tincture twice daily in the beginning, then give 1x, 2 drops, twice daily.

## RICINUS COMMUNIS

**Clinical**

- Suppression of milk.

**Symptoms**

- Efficacious in suppression of milk with amenorrhea. It increases the quantity of milk in nursing women with commencement of menstrual flow.

**Dose**

- *Ricinus* Q, 5 drops every four hour for increasing flow of milk.
- External application and massage of Q in breast stimulates the secreting power of mammary glands.

## RUTA GRAVEOLENS

**Clinical**

- Gangrenous tumor.
- Cancer of bone.

**Dose**

- Give 1x, 2 drops thrice daily. Locally the tincture for ganglia and as a lotion for the eye.

## SABAL SERRULATA

**Clinical**

- Prostate enlargement.
- Undeveloped breast.

**Dose**

- Give Q, 10 to 20 drops, 3 or 4 times a day.

## SALIX NIGRA

**Clinical**

- Male and female sexual complaints.

**Female**

- Nervous disturbances before and during menses.
- Ovarian congestion and neuralgia.
- Nymphomania.

**Male**

- In acute gonorrhea, with much erotic troubles.
- After masturbation; spermatorrhea.
- Painful movements of the testicles.

**Dose**

- Give Q, 10 drops thrice daily.

## SANGUINARIA

**Clinical**

- Headache.

**Symptoms**

- Sun headache, worse right side. Periodical sick headache; pain begins in occiput, spreads upward, and settles over eyes, especially right.
- Headache returns at climacteric.
- Pain at the back of head, "like flash of lightening."

**Dose**

- Give Q, 5 – 10 drops thrice daily.

## SANTONINUM

**Clinical**

- Worm infestation.

**Symptoms**

- Of unquestioned value in the treatment of worm diseases, as gastrointestinal irritation, itching of nose, restless sleep, twitching of muscles.
- Ascaris lumbricoides and thread worm.

**Dose**

- *Santoninum* 1x, 2 grains, 4 doses in a day.
- Note: Do not give to a child with fever or constipation.

## SCROPHULARIA NODOSA

**Clinical**

- Enlarged glands.

**Symptoms**

- A powerful medicine whenever enlarged glands are present.
- Hodgkin's disease has a specific affinity for the breast; very useful in the dissipation of breast tumor. Nodosities in the breast.

**Dose**

- Tincture 5 drops or 1x, 2 drops thrice daily.
- It is also used locally over cancerous gland.

## SECALE CORNUTUM

**Clinical**

- Amenorrhea.

**Female**

- Amenorrhea due to any cause with intense burning and great longing for cold things in weak, delicate subjects.

**Dose**

- Give Q, 10 drops thrice daily.
- Note: First ascertain the pregnancy before using this drug as it causes abortion.

## SEDUM ACRE

**Clinical**

- Hemorrhoidal pain.
- Fissures.

**Rectum**

- Hemorrhoidal pains, like those of anal fissures; constricting pains, worse few hours after stool.

**Dose**

- Give Q, 5 drops or 1x, 2 drops thrice daily.

## SEMPERVIVUM TECTORUM

**Clinical**

- Herpes zoster.
- Cancerous tumor.
- Scirrhous induration of tongue.

**Mouth**

- Malignant ulcers of mouth, cancer of tongue.

**Dose**

Give Q, 5 drops or 1x, 2 drops thrice daily.

It is applied locally for bites of insects, stings of bees, poisoned wounds and warts.

## SENEGA

**Clinical**

- Respiratory complaints.

**Respiratory**

- Hoarseness. Loss of voice, hacking cough. Thorax feels too narrow.
- Cough often ends in a sneeze.
- Bronchial catarrh with much mucus; sensation of oppression and weight on chest.
- Difficult raising of tough, profuse mucus, in the aged.
- Complaints aggravated during walking and ameliorated by bending head backward.

**Dose**

- Give Q, 5 drops, 4 times a day.

## SENECIO AUREUS

**Clinical**

- Menstrual complaints.
- Male complaints.

**Female**

- Menses retarded, suppressed.
- Functional amenorrhea of young girls with backache.
- Anemic dysmenorrhea.

**Male**

- Lascivious dreams, with involuntary emissions.
- Prostate enlarged.

**Dose**

- Give Q, 5 drops, 4 times a day.

## SPIRITUS GLANDIUM QUERCUS

**Clinical**

- Alcohol addiction.

**Symptoms**

- It antidotes effects of alcohol.
- It is used for removing craving for alcohol.

**Dose**

- Ten drops to a teaspoonful of Q, three to four times a day.

## SPONGIA TOSTA

**Clinical**

- Skin disease.

**Skin**

- According to Dr. Persey, any kind of skin disease is cured by *Spongia.*

**Dose**

- Q, 2 drops, thrice daily.

## STERCULIA ACUMINATA

**Clinical**

- Weakness.
- Alcoholic craving.

**Symptoms**

- Neurasthenia.
- Regulates the circulation, is a tonic and regulates cardiac rhythm.
- Weak heart.
- Promotes appetite and digestion, and lessens the craving for liquor.

**Dose**

- 3 to 5 drops of Q, even one dram doses, three times a day.

## STROPHANTHUS HISPIDUS

**Clinical**

- Heart complaints.
- Alcohol craving.

**Heart**

- Mitral regurgitation, where edema and dropsy have supervened.
- Arterio-sclerosis; rigid arteries of aged.
- Irritable heart of tobacco smokers.
- Anemia with palpitations and breathlessness.
- Heart's action weak, rapid, irregular due to muscular debility.

**Alcohol**

- Diminishes the craving for spiritus liquor slowly but surely.

**Dose**

- Give Q, 10 drops, thrice daily.

## STRYCHNINUM PHOSPHORICUM

**Clinical**

- Paralysis.

**Symptoms**

- Burning, aching and weakness of spine; pain extends to front of chest.

**Dose**

- 2x or 3x trituration thrice daily.

## SYMPHORICARPUS RACEMOSA

**Clinical**

- Morning sickness.
- Vomiting.

**Dose**

- Give Q, 5 drops or 1x, 2 drops, thrice daily.

## SYMPHYTUM OFFICINALE

**Clinical**

- Injury.
- Cancer.

**Symptoms**

- Great use in wounds penetrating the perineum and bones, and in non-union of fractures; irritable stump after amputation.
- Psoas abscess.
- It is efficacious in treating cancer due to injury.

**Dose**

- Give Q, 10 drops, 4 times a day.

## SYZYGIUM JAMBOLANUM

**Clinical**

- Diabetes mellitus.

**Symptoms**

- Most useful remedy in diabetes mellitus. It causes marked degree of diminution and disappearance of sugar in urine.
- Great thirst, weakness, emaciation.
- Very large amount of urine, specific gravity high.
- Prickly heat in upper part of the body; small red pimples itch violently.
- Diabetic ulceration.

**Dose**

- Give Q, 5 drops, 4 times a day.

## THLASPI BURSA PASTORIS

**Clinical**

- Female complaints.
- Urinary complaints.

**Symptoms**

- It is an anti-hemorrhagic and anti-uric acid remedy.

**Female**

- Metrorrhagia. Hemorrhage with violent uterine colic. Every alternate period very profuse. Scarcely recovers from one period before another begins.

**Urinary**

- Frequent desire; urine heavy, phosphatic.
- Chronic cystitis.
- Hematuria.
- Brick-dust sediments.
- Albuminuria during gestation.

**Dose**

- Give Q, 5 drops every hour or thrice daily according to severity of disease.

## TONGO ODORATA

**Clinical**

- Neuralgia.

**Symptoms**

- Tearing pain in supra-orbital nerve, with heat and throbbing pain in head and epiphora.
- Trembling in right upper lid.

**Dose**

- Tincture 5 drops, 3 or 4 times a day.

## TRIBULUS TERRESTRIS

**Clinical**

- Genito-urinary complaints of male.

**Male**

- Dysuria.
- Debilitated state of the sexual organs.
- Seminal weakness.
- Prostatitis, calculous affections and sexual neurasthenia.
- Auto-traumatism of masturbation, correcting the emissions & spermatorrhea.
- Partial impotence caused by over-indulgence.

**Dose**

- Ten to twenty drops of tincture three times daily.

## TRIFOLIUM PRETENSE

**Clinical**

- Ptyalism.

**Symptoms**

- Feeling of fullness with congestion of salivary glands, followed by increased copious flow of saliva.
- Feeling as if mumps were coming on.

**Dose**

- Tincture 5 drops, thrice daily.

## TRIFOLIUM REPENS

**Clinical**

- Mumps.
- Glands affection.

**Symptoms**

- Prophylactic against mumps.

**Dose**

- Tincture 5 drops, thrice daily.

## TRILLIUM PENDULUM

**Clinical**

- Female complaints.

**Female**

- Uterine hemorrhages, with sensation as though hips and back were falling to pieces; better tight bandages.
- Gushing of bright blood on least movement.
- Hemorrhage from fibroids.
- Prolapse.
- Dribbling of urine after labor.

**Dose**

- Give Q or 1x, 2 drops thrice daily.

## URTICA URENS

**Clinical**

- Rheumatism.
- Urticaria.
- Ill effects of shell fish.

**Skin**

- Itching blotches.
- Consequence of suppressed nettle-rash.
- Rheumatism alternates with nettle rash.
- Burns confined to skin. Burns and scalds.
- Urticaria nodosa.
- Erythema, with burning and stinging.
- Chicken pox.
- It antidotes ill effects of eating shellfish.

**Dose**

- 2-5 drops of Q, thrice daily.

## USNEA BARBATA

**Clinical**

- Congestive headache.
- Sunstroke.

**Head**

- Bursting feeling, as if temples would burst, or the eyes would burst out of the sockets. Throbbing carotids.

**Dose**

- Give Q, 5 drops every half hourly in an acute headache.

## UVA URSI

**Clinical**

- Urinary complaints.

**Urinary**

- Cystitis, with bloody urine.
- Uterine hemorrhage.
- Chronic vesical irritation.
- Burning after the discharge of slimy urine.
- Pyelitis.
- Calculous inflammation.

**Dose**

- Tincture, 5 to 30 drops thrice daily.

## VALERIANA OFFICINALIS

**Clinical**

- Hysteria. Hysterical flatulency.

**Symptoms**

- Hysteria, oversensitiveness, nervous affections, hysterical spasms and affections generally.
- Changeable disposition.

**Dose**

- Give Q, 5 drops thrice daily for a long time.

## VERBENA

**Clinical**

- Nervous affections.

**Symptoms**

- Nervous depression, weakness, irritation and spasms.
- Epilepsy, insomnia, mental exhaustion.
- In epilepsy, it brightens up the patient's mental power.

**Dose**

- Single dose of 5 drops tincture.

## VERNONIA ANTHELMINTICA

**Clinical**

- Worm infestation.

**Symptoms**

- Remarkable anti-helmintic property. Distinctly effective in thread worm infections.

- In troubles arising as consequence with worm troubles.

**Dose**

- Q, 5 drops thrice daily.

## VESICARIA COMMUNIS

**Clinical**

- Urinary complaints.

**Symptoms**

- Cystitis; irritable bladder.
- Prevents uric acid diathesis.
- It controls the suppurative stage of urethra due to T.B. or gonorrhea.

**Dose**

- Give Q, 10 drops every hour in emergency cases and 5 drops every 3 hours in ordinary cases.

## VIBURNUM OPULUS

**Clinical**

- Dysmenorrhea.
- Leucorrhea.
- Abortion.

**Female**

- Spasmodic and membranous dysmenorrhea.
- Leucorrhea, excoriating.
- Frequent and very early miscarriage causing seeming sterility.

**Dose**

- Give Q, 10 drops every half an hour, otherwise 5 drops thrice daily.

## VISCUM ALBUM

**Clinical**

- Rheumatism.

**Symptoms**

- Rheumatic and gouty complaints.

**Dose**

Give Q, 5 drops thrice daily.

## ZINCUM VALERIANICUM

**Clinical**

- Neuralgia.

**Symptoms**

- Neuralgia, hysteria and other painful affections, notably in ovarian affections.
- Facial neuralgia.
- Ovalgia.

**Dose**

- Give 1x and 2x trituration. Must be continued for sometime in treatment of neuralgia.

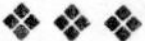

# RELATIONSHIP OF REMEDIES

# RELATIONSHIP OF REMEDIES

Dr. R. Gibson Miller, Glasgow, Scotland

### Authorities

1. Hering's Guiding Symptoms and Condensed Materia Medica.
2. J.T. Kent's Lectures on Materia Medica.
3. Guernsey's Key-notes to Materia Medica.
4. Boenninghausen's Manual.

| Remedy | Comple-mentary remedies | Remedies that follows well | Inimicals | Antidotes | Duration |
|---|---|---|---|---|---|
| Acet-ac. | Chin. | | After Borx., Caust., Nux-v., Ran-b., Sars. | Acon., Nat-m., Nux-v., Sep., Tab. | 14-20 d. |
| Acon. | Arn., Coff., Sulph. | Abrot., Arn., Ars., Bell., Bry., Cact., Calc., Canth., Cocc., Coff., Hep., Ip., Kali-br., Merc., Puls., Rhus-t., Sep., Spig., Spong., Sulph., Sil. | | Acet-ac., Bell., Berb., Coff., Nux-v., Par., Sulph., Vinum, Wine. | 1 hour to several weeks. |
| Aesc. | | | | Nux-v. | 30 d. |
| Aeth. | Calc. | | | Vegetable acids | 20-30 d. |
| Agar. | | Bell., Calc., Cupr., Merc., Op., Puls., Rhus-t., Sil., Tub. | | Calc., Puls., Rhus-t., Vinum. | 40 d. |
| Agn. | | Ars., Bry., Calad., Ign., Lyc., Puls., Sel., Sulph. | | Camph., Nat-m., Nux-v. | 8-14 d. |
| All-c. | Phos., Puls., Sars., Thuj. | Calc., Sil. | All-s., Aloe, Squil. | Arn., Cham., Nux-v., Thuj., Verat. | 1 d. |
| All-s. | Ars. | | All-c., Aloe, Squil. | Lyc. | |
| Aloe | Sulph. | Kali-bi., Sep., Sulph., Sul-ac. | All-s. | Camph., Lyc., Nux-v., Sulph. | 30-40 d. |
| Alum. | Bry., Ferr. | Arg-met., Bry. | | Bry., Camph., Cham., Ip. | 40-60 d. |

| Remedy | Comple-mentary remedies | Remedies that follows well | Inimicals | Antidotes | Duration |
|---|---|---|---|---|---|
| Alumn. | | | | Cham., Nux-v., Ip., Sulph. | Long acting. |
| Ambr. | | Lyc., Puls., Sep., Sulph. | | Camph., Coff., Nux-v., Puls., Staph. | 40 d. |
| Am-c. | | Bell., Bry., Calc., Lyc., Phos., Puls., Rhus-t., Sep., Sulph., Verat. | Lach. | Arn., Camph., Hep. | 40 d. |
| Am-m. | | Ant-c., Coff., Merc., Nux-v., Phos., Puls., Rhus-t., Sanic. | | Coff., Hep., Nux-v. | 20-30 d. |
| Anac. | | Lyc., Puls., Plat. | | Clem., Crot-t., Coff., Jug., Ran-b., Rhus-t. | 30-40 d. |
| Ang. | | Bell., Ign., Lyc., Sep. | | Coff. | 20-30 d. |
| Ant-c. | Squil. | Calc., Lach., Merc., Puls., Sep., Sulph. | | Calc., Hep., Merc. | 40 d. |
| Ant-t. | Ip. | Bar-c., Camph., Carb-v., Cina, Ip., Puls., Sep., Sulph., Ter. | | Asaf., Chin., Cocc., Ip., Laur., Op., Puls., Rhus-t., Sep. | 20-30 d. |
| Apis | Nat-m. | Arn., Ars., Graph., Iod., Lyc., Puls., Nat-m., Stram., Sulph. | Phos., Rhus-t. | Canth., Carb-ac., Ip., Lac-ac., Lach., Led., Nat-m., Plan. | |
| Arg-met. | | Calc., Puls., Sep. | | Merc., Puls. | 30 d. |
| Arg-n. | | Bry., Calc., Kali-c., Lyc., Lyss., Merc., Puls., Sep., Sil., Spig., Spong., Verat. | | Ars., Calc., Iod., Lyc., Merc., Nat-m., Phos., Puls., Rhus-t., Sep., Sil., Sulph. | 30 d. |
| Arn. | Acon., Hyper., Ip., Rhus-t., Verat. | Acon., Ars., Bar-m., Bell., Berb., Bry., Cact., Calc., Calen., Cham., Chin., Con., Cur., Hep., Iod., Ip., Nux-v., Phos., Led., Puls., Psor., Rhus-t., Ruta, Sul-ac., Sulph., Verat. | | Acon., Ars., Camph., Chin., Ign., Ip. | 6-10 d. |

| Remedy | Complementary remedies | Remedies that follows well | Inimicals | Antidotes | Duration |
|---|---|---|---|---|---|
| Ars. | All-s., Carb-v., Nat-s., Phos., Pyrog., Thuj. | Apis, Aran., Arn., Bar-c., Bell., Cact., Calc-p., Cham., Chel., Chin., Cic., Ferr., Fl-Chin., Hep., Iod., Ip., Kali-bi., Lach., Lyc., Merc., Nat-s., Nux-v., Phos., Ran-s., Sulph., Thuj, Verat. | | Camph., Carb-ac., Chin., Chinin-s., Euph., Ferr., Graph., Hep., Iod., Ip., Kali-bi., Merc., Nux-m., Nux-v., Op., Samb., Sulph., Tab., Verat. | 60-90 d. |
| Arum-t. | | Euphr. | Calad. | Acet-ac., Bell., Lac-ac., Puls. | 1-2 d. |
| Asaf. | | Chin., Merc., Puls. | | Caust., Camph., Chin., Merc., Puls., Valer. | 20-40 d. |
| Asar. | | Bism., Caust., Puls., Sil., Sul-ac. | | Acet-ac., Camph., | 8-14 d. |
| Asc-t. | | | | | 40-60 d. |
| Aster. | | | Coff., Nux-v. | Plb., Zinc. | |
| Aur-m-n. | | | Coff. | | |
| Aur. | | Acon., Bell., Calc., Chin., Lyc., Merc., Nit-ac., Puls., Rhus-t., Sep., Sulph., Syph. | | Bell., Chin., Cocc., Coff., Cupr., Merc., Puls., Sol-ni. Spig., | 50-60 d. |
| Bad. | Iod., Merc., Sulph. | Lach. | | | |
| Bapt. | | Crot., Ham., Nit-ac., Pyrog., Ter. | | | 6-8 d. |
| Bar-c. | Dulc. | Ant-t., Calc., Con., Chin., Lyc., Merc., Nit-ac., Phos., Psor., Puls., Rhus-t., Sep., Sil., Sulph., Tub. | After Calc. | Ant-t., Bell., Camph., Dulc., Merc., Zinc. | 40 d. |
| Bell. | Calc. | Acon., Ars., Cact., Calc., Carb-v., Cham., Chin., Con., Cur., | Acet-ac., Dulc. | Acon., Camph., Coff., Hep., Hyos., Merc., | 1-7 d. |

| Remedy | Comple-mentary remedies | Remedies that follows well | Inimicals | Antidotes | Duration |
|---|---|---|---|---|---|
| | | Dulc., Hep., Hyos., Lach., Merc., Merc-i-r., Mosch., Mur-ac., Nux-v., Puls., Rhus-t., Seneg., Sep., Sil., Stram., Sulph., Valer., Verat. | | Op., Puls., Sabad., Vinum. | |
| Berb. | | | | Bell., Camph. | 20-30 d. |
| Bism. | | Bell., Calc., Puls., Sep. | | Calc., Caps., Coff., Nux-v. | 20-50 d. |
| Borx. | | Ars., Bry., Calc., Lyc., Nux-v., Phos., Sil. | Acet-ac., Wine. | Cham., Coff. | 30 d. |
| Bov. | | Alum., Calc., Rhus-t., Sep., Verat. | Coff. | Camph. | 7-14 d. |
| Brom. | | Arg-n., Kali-c. | | Am-c., Camph., Mag-c., Op. | 20-30 d. |
| Bry. | Alum., Rhus-t. | Alum., Ars., Abrot., Ant-t., Bell., Berb., Cact., Carb-v., Dros., Dulc.,Hyos., Kali-c., Mur-ac., Nux-v., Phos., Puls., Rhus-t., Sabad., Sep., Sil., Squil., Sulph. | | Acon., Alum., Camph., Cham., Chel., Clem., Coff., Ign., Mur-ac., Nux-v., Puls., Rhus-t., Seneg. | 7-21 d. |
| Cact. | | Dig., Eup-per., Lach., Nux-v., Sulph. | | Acon., Camph., Chin. | 7-10 d. |
| Cadm. | | Bell., Carb-v., Lob. | | | |
| Calad. | Nit-ac. | Acon., Canth., Caust., Puls., Sep., Sel. | Arum-t. | Camph., Caps., Carb-v., Ign., Hyos., Merc. | 30-40 d. |
| Calc-ar. | | Con., Glon., Op., Puls. | | Carb-v., Glon., Puls. | |
| Calc. | Bell., Rhus-t. | Aran., Agar., Bell., Borx., Bism., Dros., Dulc., Graph., Ip., Kali-bi., Lyc., Nat-c., Nit-ac., Nux-v., Phos., Plat., Podo., Puls., Rhus-t.,Sars., Sep., Sil., Ther., Tub. | Bar-c., Nit-ac. & Sulph. do not follow. After Kali-bi. & Nit-ac. | Bry., Camph., Chin., Iod., Ip., Nit., ac., Nit- s-d., Nux-v., Sep., Sulph. | 60 d. |

| Remedy | Complementary remedies | Remedies that follows well | Inimicals | Antidotes | Duration |
|---|---|---|---|---|---|
| Calc-f. | | Calc-p., Nat-m., Ph-ac., Sil. | | | |
| Calc-p. | Hep., Ruta, Sulph., Zinc. | Iod., Psor., Rhus-t., Sanic., Sulph. | Coff. | | 60 d. |
| Calen. | Hep. | Arn., Ars., Bry., Nit-ac., Phos., Rhus-t. | Camph. | Arn. | |
| Camph. | Canth. | Ant-t., Ars., Bell., Cocc., Nux-v., Rhus-t., Verat. | After Kali-n. | Canth., Dulc., Nit-s-d., Op. Phos. | 1 d. |
| Cann-s. | | Bell., Hyos., Lyc., Nux-v., Op., Puls., Rhus-t., Verat. | | Camph., Merc. | 1-10 d. |
| Canth. | Camph. | Bell., Kali-bi., Kali-i., Merc., Phos., Puls., Sep., Sulph. | Coff. | Acon., Apis, Camph., Kali-n., Laur., Puls., Rheum. | 30-40 d. |
| Caps. | | Bell., Cina, Lyc., Puls., Sil. | | Calad., Camph., Chin., Cina, Sul-ac. | 7 d. |
| Carb-an. | Calc-p. | Ars., Bell., Bry., (Carb-v.), Nit-ac., Phos., Puls., Sep., Sil., Sulph., Verat. | Carb-v.? | Ars., Camph., Nux-v., Vinum. | 60 d. |
| Carb-v. | Dros., Kali-c., Phos. | Acon., Ars., Chin., Dros., Kali-c., Lyc., Merc., Nux-v., Ph-ac., Puls., Sep., Sulph., Verat. | Carb-an.? Kreos. does not follow. | Ars., Camph., Coff., Lach., Nit-s-d. | 60 d. |
| Caul. | | | Coff. | | |
| Caust. | Carb-v. Coloc., Petros. | Ant-t., Arum-t., Coloc., Calc., Guaj., Kali-i., Lyc., Nux-v., Puls., Rhus-t., Ruta, Sep., Sil., Stann., Sulph. | Acet-ac., Coff., Ph-ac., Phos. | Asaf., Coff., Coloc., Dulc., Guaj., Nit-s-d., Nux-v. | 50 d. |

| Remedy | Comple-mentary remedies | Remedies that follows well | Inimicals | Antidotes | Duration |
|---|---|---|---|---|---|
| Cham. | Bell., Mag-c. | Acon., Arn., Bell., Bry., Cact., Calc., Cocc., Form., Merc., Nux-v., Puls., Rhus-t., Sep., Sil., Sulph. | Zinc. | Acon., Alum., Borx., Camph., Chin., Cocc., Coff., Coloc., Con., Ign., Nux-v., Puls., Valer. | 20-30 d. |
| Chel. | | Acon., Ars., Bry., Cor-r., Ip., Led., Lyc., Nux-v., Sep., Spig., Sulph. | | Acon., Acids, Cham., Coff., Wine. | 7-14 d. |
| Chin. | Ferr. | Acet-ac., Arn., Ars., Asaf., Bell., Calc., Calc-p., Carb-v., Ferr., Lach., Merc., Ph-ac., Phos., Puls., Sulph., Verat. | After Dig. and Sel. | Apis, Aran., Arn., Ars., Asaf., Bell., Bry., Calc., Caps., Carb-an., Carb-v., Caust., Cedr., Cina, Eup-per., Ferr., Ip., Lach., Led., Lyc., Meny., Merc., Nat-c., Nat-m., Nux-v., Puls., Rhus-t., Sep., Sulph., Verat. | 14-21 d. |
| Cic. | | Bell., Hep., Op., Puls., Rhus-t., Sep. | | Arn., Coff., Op., Tab. | 35-40 d. |
| Cimic. | | | | Acon., Bapt. | 8-12 d. |
| Cina | | Calc., Chin., Ign., Nux-v., Plat., Puls., Rhus-t., Sil., Stann. | | Arn., Camph., Caps., Chin., Pip-n. | 14-20 d. |
| Cist. | | Bell., Carb-v., Mag-c., Phos. | Coff. | Rhus-t., Sep. | |
| Clem. | | Calc., Rhus-t., Sep., Sil., Sulph. | | Anac., Bry., Camph., Cham., Crot-t., Ran-b., Rhus-t. | 14-20 d. |

| Remedy | Comple-mentary remedies | Remedies that follows well | Inimicals | Antidotes | Duration |
|---|---|---|---|---|---|
| Cob. | | | | | 30 d. |
| Cocc. | | Ars., Bell., Hep., Ign., Lyc., Nux-v., Puls., Rhus-t., Sulph. | Coff. | Camph., Cham., Cupr., Ign., Nux-v. | 30 d. |
| Coff. | Acon. | Acon., Aur., Bell., Fl-ac., Lyc., Nux-v., Op., Sulph. | Canth., Caust. Cocc., Ign. | Acet-ac., Acon., Cham., Chin., Grat., Ign., Merc., Nux v., Puls., Sulph. | 1-10 d. |
| Colch. | | Carb-v., Merc., Nux-v., Puls., Rhus-t., Sep. | | Bell., Camph., Cocc., Led., Nux-v., Puls., Spig. | 14-20 d. |
| Coll. | | Aesc., Aloe, Con. | | Nux-v. | 30 d. |
| Coloc. | | Bell., Bry., Caust., Cham., Merc., Nux-v., Puls., Spig., Staph. | | Camph., Caust., Cham., Coff., Op., Staph. | 1-7 d. |
| Con. | Bar-m. | Arn., Ars., Bell., Calc., Calc-ar., Cic., Dros., Lyc., Nux-v., Phos., Psor., Puls., Rhus-t., Stram., Sulph. | | Coff., Dulc., Nit-ac., Nit-s-d. | 30-50 d. |
| Cor-r. | | Sulph. | | Calc., Merc. | |
| Croc. | | Chin., Nux-v., Puls., Sulph. | | Acon., Bell., Op. | 8 d. |
| Crot-h. | | | | Lach. | 30 d. |
| Crot-t. | | Rhus-t. | | Anac., Ant-t., Clem., Ran-b. Rhus-t. | 30 d. |
| Cupr. | Calc. | Apis, Ars., Bell., Calc., Caust., Cic., Hyos., Kali-n., Puls., Stram., Verat., Zinc. | | Bell., Camph., Cic., Chin., Cocc., Con., Dulc., Hep., Ip., Merc., Nux-v., Puls., Verat. | 40-50 d. |
| Cycl. | | Phos., Puls., Rhus-t., Sep., Sulph. | | Camph., Coff., Puls. | 14-20 d. |

| Remedy | Comple-mentary remedies | Remedies that follows well | Inimicals | Antidotes | Duration |
|---|---|---|---|---|---|
| Dig. | | Acet-ac., Bell., Bry., Cham., Chin., Lyc., Nux-v., Op., Phos., Sep., Sulph., Verat. Puls. | Chin., Nit-s-d. | Apis, Camph., Calc., (Colch.), Nit-ac., Nux-v., Op. | 40-50 d. |
| Dios. | | | | | 1-7 d. |
| Dros. | Nux-v. | Calc., Cina, Con., Puls., Sulph., Verat. | | Camph. | 20-30 d. |
| Dulc. | Bar-c., Calc., Kali-s., Sulph. | Bell., Calc., Lyc., Rhus-t., Sep. | Acet-ac., Bell., Lach. | Camph., Cupr., Ip., Kali-c., Merc. | 30 d. |
| Eup-per. | | Nat-m., Sep., Tub. | | | 1-7 d. |
| Euph. | | Ferr., Lach., Puls., Sep., Sulph. | | Acet-ac., Camph. | 50 d. |
| Euphr. | | Acon., Alum., Calc., Con., Lyc., Merc., Nux-v., Phos., Puls., Rhus-t., Sil., Sulph. | | Camph., Caust., Puls. | 7 d. |
| Ferr. | Alum., Chin., Ham. | Acon., Arn., Bell., Chin., Con., Lyc., Merc., Phos., Puls., Verat. | Acet-ac. | Arn., Ars., Bell., Beer, Chin., Hep., Ip., Puls., Sulph., Thea, Verat. | 50 d. |
| Fl-ac. | Coca, Sil. | Graph., Nit-ac. | | Sil. | 30 d. |
| Gamb. | | | | Camph., Coff., Coloc., Kali-c., Op. | 1-7 d. |
| Gels. | | Bapt., Cact., Ip. | | Atro., Chin., Coff., Dig., Nat-m. | 30 d. |
| Glon. | | | | Acon., Camph., Coff., Nux-v. | 1 d. |
| Graph. | Aran., Ars., Caust., Ferr., Hep., Lyc. | Euphr., Nat-s., Sil. | | Acon., Ars., Nux-v. | 40-50 d. |
| Guaj. | | Calc., Merc. | | Nux-v. | 40 d. |
| Ham. | Ferr. | Arn. | | | |

| Remedy | Complementary remedies | Remedies that follows well | Inimicals | Antidotes | Duration |
|---|---|---|---|---|---|
| Hell. | | Bell., Bry., Chin., Lyc., Nux-v., Phos., Puls., Sulph., Zinc. | | Camph., Chin. | 20-30 d. |
| Hep. | Calen. | Abrot., Acon., Arn., Arum-t., Bell., Bry., Calen., Hell., Iod., Lach., Merc., Nit-ac., Nux-v., Puls., Rhus-t., Sep., Sil., Spong., Sulph., Zinc. | Spong. does not follow (C. C. Smith). | Acet-ac., Ars., Bell., Cham., Sil. | 40-50 d. |
| Hyos. | | Bell., Puls., Stram., Verat. | | Acet-ac., Bell., Chin., Cit-ac., Stram. | 6-14 d. |
| Hyper. | | | | Ars., Cham., Sulph. | 1-7 d. |
| Ign. | Nat-m. | Ars., Bell., Calc., Chin., Cocc., Lyc., Nux-v., Ph-ac., Puls., Rhus-t., Sep., Sil., Sulph. | Coff., Nux-v., Tab. | Acet-ac., Arn., Camph., Cham., Cocc., Coff., Nux-v., Puls. | 9 d. |
| Iod. | Bad., Lyc. | Acon., Arg-n., Calc., Calc-p., Kali-bi., Lyc., Merc., Nux-v., Phos., Puls., Rhus-t., Sep., Sil., Sulph. | | Acon., Ant-t., Apis., Ars., Bell., Camph., Chin., Chinin-s., Coff., Ferr., Graph., Grat., Hep., Op., Phos., Spong., Sulph., Thuj. | 30-40 d. |
| Ip. | Ant-t., Arn., Cupr. | Ant-c., Ant-t., Apis, Aran., Arn., Ars., Bell., Bry., Cact., Cadm., Calc., Cham., Chin., Cupr., Ign., Nux-v., Phos., Podo., Puls., Rheum, Sep., Sulph., Tab., Verat. | | Arn., Ars., Chin., Nux-v., Tab. | 7-10 d. |
| Kali-bi. | Ars. | Ant-t., Berb., Puls. | Does not follow Calc. | Ars., Lach., Puls. | 30 d. |
| Kali-br. | | Cact. | | Camph., Helon., Nux-v., Zinc. | |

| Remedy | Comple-mentary remedies | Remedies that follows well | Inimicals | Antidotes | Duration |
|---|---|---|---|---|---|
| Kali-c. | Carb-v., Nux-v. | Ars., Carb-v., Fl-ac., Lyc., Nit-ac., Phos., Puls., Sep., Sulph. | | Camph., Coff., Dulc., Helon., Nit-s-d. | 40-50 d. |
| Kali-i. | | | | Am-m., Ars., Chin., Merc., Rhus-t., Sulph., Valer. | 20-30 d. |
| Kali-n. | | Bell., Calc., Puls., Rhus-t., Sep., Sulph. | Camph. does not follow. | Nit-s-d. | 30-40 d. |
| Kali-s. | | Acet-ac., Ars., Calc., Hep., Kali-c., Puls., Rhus-t., Sep., Sil., Sulph. | | | |
| Kalm. | Benz-ac. | Calc., Lith-c., Lyc., Nat-m., Puls., Spig. | | Acon., Bell., Spig. | 7-14 d. |
| Kreos. | | Ars., Bell., Calc., Kali-c., Lyc., Nit-ac., Nux-v., Rhus-t., Sep., Sulph. | After Carb-v. | Acon., Nux-v. | 15-20 d. |
| Lac-ac. | | Psor. | Coff. | Bry. | |
| Lach. | Hep., Lyc., Nit-ac. | Acon., Alum., Ars., Bell., Brom., Cact., Calc., Carb-v., Caust., Chin., Cic., Con., Euphr., Hep., Hyos.,Kali-bi., Lac-c., Lyc., Merc., Merc-i-f., Nat-m., Nit-ac., Nux-v., Olnd., Phos., Puls., Rhus-t., Sil., Sulph., Tarent. | Acet-ac., Am-c., Carb-ac., Dulc., Nit-ac., Psor., Sep. | Alum., Ars., Bell., Calc., Cham., Carb-v., Cocc., Coff., Hell., Hep., Led., Merc., Nit-ac., Nux-v., Op., Ph-ac. | 30-40 d. |
| Laur. | | Bell., Carb-v., Phos., Puls., Verat. | | Camph., Coff., Ip., Nux-m.,Op. | 4-8 d. |
| Led. | | Acon., Bell., Bry., Chel., Nux-v., Puls., Rhus-t., Sul-ac., Sulph | Chin. | Camph. | 30 d. |
| Lil-t. | | | | Helon., Nux-v., Plat., Puls. | 14-20 d. |

| Remedy | Comple-mentary remedies | Remedies that follows well | Inimicals | Antidotes | Duration |
|---|---|---|---|---|---|
| Lyc. | Iod., Lach., Puls. | Anac., Bell., Bry., Calc., Carb-v., Colch., Dros., Dulc., Graph., Hyos., Kali-c., Lach., Led., Nux-v., Phos., Puls., Sep., Sil, Ther., Stram., Verat. | After Sulph. except in cycle of Sulph., Calc., Lyc., Sulph. etc., Coff. | Acon., Camph., Caust., Cham., Coff., Graph., Puls. | 40-50 d. |
| Mag-c. | Cham. | Caust., Phos., Puls., Sep., Sulph. | | Ars., Cham., Merc., Nux-v., Puls., Rheum. | 40-50 d. |
| Mag-m. | | Bell., Lyc., Nat-m., Nux-v., Puls., Sep. | | Ars., Camph., Cham., Nux-v. | 40-50 d. |
| Manc. | | | | | 30-40 d. |
| Mang. | | Puls., Rhus-t., Sulph. | | Camph., Coff. | 40 d. |
| Med. | | Sulph., Thuj. | | Ip. | |
| Meny. | | Caps., Lyc., Puls., Rhus-t. | | Camph. | 14-20 d. |
| Meph. | | | | | 1 d. |
| Merc. | Bad. | Ars., Asaf., Bell., Calc.,Calc-p., Carb-v., Chin., Dulc., Guaj., Hep., Iod., Lach., Lyc., Mur-ac., Nit-ac., Phos., Puls., Rhus-t., Sep., Sulph., Thuj. | Acet-ac., Sil. disagrees before or after poten-tised Mer-cury but an-tidotes the crude substance. | Aran., Ars., Asaf., Aur., Bell., Bry., Calad., Calc., Carb-v., Chin., Clem., Con., Cor-r., Cupr., Daph., Dulc., Ferr., Guaj., Hep., Iod., Kali-bi., Kali-chl., Kali-i., Lach., Mez., Nit-ac., Nux-m. Op., Phyt., Podo., Rat., Ruta, Sars., Sep., Spig., Staph., Still., Stram., Sulph., Thuj., Valer. | 30-60 d. |
| Mez. | | Calc., Caust., Ign., Lyc., Merc., Nux-v., Phos., Puls. | | Acids., Acon., Bry., Calc., Kali-i., Merc., Nux-v. | 30-60 d. |

| Remedy | Comple-mentary remedies | Remedies that follows well | Inimicals | Antidotes | Duration |
|---|---|---|---|---|---|
| Mill. | | | Coff. | Arum-m. | 1-3 d. |
| Mosch. | | | | Camph., Coff. | 1 d. |
| Mur-ac. | | Calc., Kali-c., Nux-v., Puls., Sep., Sil., Sulph. | | Bry., Camph. | 35 d. |
| Nat-c. | | Calc., Nit-ac., Nux-v., Puls., Sel., Sep., Sulph. | | Camph., Nit-s-d. | 30 d. |
| Nat-m. | Apis, Ign., Sep. | Apis, Bry., Calc., Hep., Kali-c., Puls., Rhus-t., Sep., Sulph., Thuj. | | Ars., Camph., Phos., Nit-s-d., Nux-v., Sep. | 40-50. |
| Nat-s. | Ars., Thuj. | Bell., Thuj. | | | 30-40 d. |
| Nit-ac. | Ars., Calad. | Arn., Arum-t., Bell., Calc., Carb-v., Kali-c., Kreos., Merc., Phos., Puls., Sec., Sep., Sil., Sulph., Thuj. | Lach., after Calc. (Hahnemann) | Acon., Calc., Con., Hep., Merc., Mez., Sulph. | 40-60 d. |
| Nux-m. | | Ant-t., Lyc., Nux-v., Puls., Rhus-t., Stram. | | Camph., Gels., Laur., Nux-v., Op., Valer., Zinc. | 60 d. |
| Nux-v. | Kali-c., Sep., Sulph. | Act-sp., Aesc., Aran., Ars., Bell., Bry., Cact., Calc., Carb-v., Cob., Cocc., Colch., Hyos., Lyc., Ph-ac., Phos., Puls., Rhus-t., Sep., Sulph. | Acet-ac., Ign., Zinc. | Acon., Ars., Bell., Camph., Cham., Cocc., Coff., Euphr., Ign., Op., Puls., Thuj. | 1-7 d. or 15-21 d. |
| Olnd. | | Con., Lyc., Nat-m., Puls., Rhus-t., Sep., Spig. | | Camph., Sulph. | 20-30 d. |
| Op. | | Acon., Ant-t., Bell., Bry., Hyos., Nux-m., Nux-v., Samb. | | Acet-ac., Bell., Cham., Cic., Coff., Cupr., Gels., Ip., Merc., Mur-ac., Nux-v., Puls., Verat., Wine, Zinc. | 7 d. |

| Remedy | Comple-mentary remedies | Remedies that follows well | Inimicals | Antidotes | Duration |
|---|---|---|---|---|---|
| Sars. | All-c., Merc., Sep. | All-c., Bell., Hep., Merc., Phos., Rhus-t., Sep., Sulph. | Acet-ac. | Bell., Merc., Sep. | 35 d. |
| Sec. | | Acon., Ars., Bell., Chin., Merc., Puls. | | Camph., Op. | 20-30 d. |
| Sel. | | Calc., Merc., Nux-v., Sep. | Chin., Wine. | Ign., Puls. | 40 d. |
| Seneg. | | Arum-t., Calc., Lyc., Phos., Sulph. | | Arn., Bell., Bry., Camph. | 30 d. |
| Sep. | Nat-m., Nux-v., Sabad. | Bell., Calc., Carb-v., Con., Dros., Dulc., Euphr., Graph., Lyc., Nat-c., Nux-v., Petr., Puls., Rhus-t., Sars., Sil., Sulph., Tarent. | Bry., Lach. | Acon., Ant-c., Ant-t., Nit-s-d., Sulph. Vegetable acids. | 40-50 d. |
| Sil. | Calc., Fl-ac., Puls., Sanic., Thuj. | Aran., Ars., Asaf., Bell., Calc., Clem., Fl-ac., Graph., Hep., Lach., Lyc., Nux-v., Phos., Puls., Rhus-t., Sep., Sulph., Thuj.,Tub. | Merc. | Camph., Fl-ac., Hep. | 40-60 d. |
| Spig. | | Acon., Arn., Ars., Bell., Calc., Cimic., Dig., Iris, Kali-c., Kalm., Nux-v., Puls., Rhus-t., Sep., Sulph., Zinc. | | Aur., Camph., Cocc., Puls. | 20-30 d. |
| Spong. | | Brom., Bry., Carb-v., Con., Fl-ac., Hep., Kali-br., Nux-v., Phos., Puls. | | Camph. | 20-30 d. |
| Squil. | | Ars., Bar-c., Ign., Nux-v., Rhus-t., Sil. | All-s. | Camph. | 14-20 d. |
| Stann. | Puls. | Calc., Kali-c., Lyss., Nux-v., Phos., Puls., Rhus-t., Sulph. | | Puls. | 35 d. |
| Staph. | Caust., Coloc. | Calc., Caust., Coloc., Fl-ac., Kali-c., Ign., Lyc., Nux-v., Puls., Rhus-t., Sel., Sulph. | Ran-b. | Ambr., Camph. | 20-30 d. |

| Remedy | Comple-mentary remedies | Remedies that follows well | Inimicals | Antidotes | Duration |
|---|---|---|---|---|---|
| Stram. | | Acon., Bell., Bry., Cupr., Hyos., Nux-v. | Coff. | Acet-ac., Bell., Hyos., Nux-v., Op., Puls., Tab. | |
| Stront-c. | | Bell., Caust., Kali-c., Puls., Rhus-t., Sep., Sulph. | | Camph. | 40 d. |
| Sulph. | Acon., Aloe, Ars., Bad., Nux-v., Psor. | Acon., Aesc., Alum., Apis, Ars., Bar-c., Bell., Berb., Borx., Bry., Calc., Carb-v., Euphr., Graph., Guaj., Kali-c., Merc., Nit-ac., Nux-v., Phos., Podo., Puls., Rhus-t., Samb., Sars., Sep. | Sulph., follows Lyc., but Lyc. does not follow Sulph. (Kent). Ran-b. | Acon., Ars., Camph., Caust., Cham., Chin., Con., Merc., Nux-v., Puls., Rhus-t., Sep., Sil., Thuj. | 40-60 d. |
| Sul-ac. | Puls. | Arn., Calc., Con., Lyc., Plat., Sep., Sulph. | | Puls. | 30-40 d. |
| Tab. | | Carb-v., Lyss. | | Acet-ac., Ars., Clem., Cocc., Ign., Ip., Lyc., Nux-v., Phos., Puls., Sep., Staph., Verat. | |
| Tarax. | | Ars., Asaf., Bell., Chin., Lyc., Rhus-t., Staph., Sulph. | | Camph. | 14-21 d. |
| Tell. | | | | Nux-v. | 30-40 d. |
| Teucr. | | Chin., Puls., Sil. | | Camph. | 14-21 d. |
| Ther. | | | | Acon., Graph., Mosch. | 30 d. |
| Thuj. | Ars., Med., Nat-s., Sabin., Sil. | Asaf., Calc., Ign., Kali-c., Lyc., Merc., Nit-ac., Puls., Sabin., Sil., Sulph. | | Camph., Cham., Cocc., Merc., Puls., Staph., Sulph. | 60 d. |
| Tub. | Bell., Calc., Hydr., Psor., Sulph. | Bar-c., Calc., Calc-p., Sil. | | | |

| Remedy | Comple-mentary remedies | Remedies that follows well | Inimicals | Antidotes | Duration |
|---|---|---|---|---|---|
| Valer. | | Phos., Puls. | | Bell., Camph., Coff., Merc., Puls. | 8-10 d. |
| Verat. | Arn. | Acon., Arg-n., Arn., Ars., Bell., Carb-v., Cham., Chin., Cupr., Dros., Dulc., Ip., Puls., Rhus-t., Samb., Sep., Sulph. | | Acon., Ars., Camph., Chin., Coff. | 20-30 d. |
| Verb. | | Bell., Chin., Lyc., Puls., Rhus-t., Sep., Stram., Sulph. | | Camph. | 8-10 d. |
| Vesp. | | | Arg-n. | Acet-ac., Apis. | |
| Viol-o. | | Bell., Cina, Cor-r., Nux-v., Puls. | | Camph. | 2-4 d. |
| Viol-t. | | Puls., Rhus-t., Sep. Staph. | | Camph., Merc., Puls., Rhus-t. | 8-14 d. |
| Zinc. | | Hep., Ign., Puls., Sep., Sulph. | Cham., Nux-v. | Camph., Hep., Ign., Wine. | 30-40 d. |

# THE SIDES OF THE BODY AND DRUG AFFINITIES

(From Boenninghausen's Lesser Writings)

The action of most drugs is more or less manifested on either side of the body as seen during drug proving and during their use in disease. The question thus arising is, for which side of the body does the drug have a particular affinity. This distinction, as well as the degree of action is best indicated by different fonts.

It seems impossible that in an arrangement like this, incorrect statements should have occurred; on the other hand, finding a remedy is facilitated by the alphabetical order which has been uniformly observed.

In the second part of this work, 'The Drug Affinities', the remedies which belong to the lowest degree, have been omitted for the purpose of avoiding unnecessary crowding of mere names which would simply embarrass the reader; the other three degrees have been distinguished by the same varieties of print, as in the first part. This second part contains the result of examination to which I have been subjected, for a number of years, my former labors in reference to the same subject have convinced me that an excessive number of remedies rendered their proper application in disease so much more difficult.

In conclusion, I need scarcely remark that body parts of this little work, should only be looked upon and used as means of facilitating the selection of the proper remedy, and that the homoeopathic law— 'Similia Similibus' should always remain the supreme guide in the treatment of disease whenever the characteristic symptoms of the drug are indicated with sufficient clarity to enable us to decide that the spirit of the remedy which we select, is in harmony with the character of the disease.

The four different kinds of type used here are in accordance to the Synthesis:

1. Common type, like: Agar., Alum., Ang., Ant-t., Aur., etc., indicate the lowest degree of action.
2. Italics, such as: *Acon., Ammc.,* etc. indicate the second degree, which has been pretty thoroughly verified and confirmed by experience.
3. Bold type, such as; **Ambr., Ammc., Anac.,** etc. indicates the next higher degree of action.
4. Bold capitals such as: **BROM., SEP.,** etc., highest and most distinguished degree.

# THE SIDES OF THE BODY

## INTERNAL, HEAD

### Left Side

*Acon.*, Agar., Alum., **Ambr.**, *Ammc.*, **Am-m.**, *Anac.*, Ang., **Ant-c.**, Ant-t., **Apis, Arg., Arn.**, *Ars.*, **Asaf.**, **Asar.**, Aur., Bar-c., Bell., Bism., Borx., **Bov., BROM.**, *Bry.*, Calad., **Calc.**, Camph., Cann-s., Canth., **Caps.**, *Carb-an.*, Carb-v., *Caust.*, **Cham.**, Chel., *Chin.*, **Cic.**, Cina, *Clem.*, Cocc., Coff., *Colch.*, **Coloc.**, Con., **Croc.**, *Cupr.*, **Cycl., Dig.**, Dros., *Dulc.*, **Euph.**, Euphr., Ferr., Fl-ac., **Graph., Guaj.**, Hell., Hep., Hyos., Ign., **Iod.**, *Ip.*, **Kali.**, *Kali-n.*, *Kreos.*, **Lach.**, *Laur.*, Led., Lyc., M-arct., **M-aust.**, *Mag.*, *Mang.*, *Meny.*, **Merc., Mez.**, Mill., Mosch., *Mur-ac.*, Nat., Nat-m., **Nit-ac., Nux-m.**, *Nux-v.*, **Olnd.**, Op., **Par.**, *Petr.*, *Phos.*, *Ph-ac.*, **Plat.**, Plb., **Psor.**, *Puls.*, Ran-b., Ran-s., Rheum, **Rhod.**, *Rhus-t.*, Ruta, Sabad., *Sabin.*, **Samb.**, *Sars.*, Squil., Sec., **Sel.**, Seneg., **SEP.**, Sil., **Spig.**, *Spong.*, *Stann.*, *Staph.*, Stram., Stront., **Sulph.**, *Sul-ac.*, *Tarax.*, Teucr., Thuj., Valer., *Verat.*, Verb., Viol-o., Viol-t., Vit., **Zinc.**

### Right Side

Acon., *Agar.*, **Alum.**, Ambr., Ammc., *Am-m.*, Anac., Ang., Ant-c., Ant-t., *Apis*, Arg., *Arn.*, Ars., *Asaf.*, Asar., Aur., Bar-c., **BELL., Bism.**, **Borx.**, Bov., Brom., **Bry.**, *Calad.*, **CALC.**, Camph., *Cann-s.*, **Canth.**, *Caps.*, Carb-an., **CARB-V., Caust.**, *Cham.*, **Chel.**, Chin., Cic., **Cina**, Clem., Cocc., Coff., *Colch.*, Coloc., Con., Croc., Cupr., Cycl., Dig., *Dros.*, **Dulc.**, Euph., Euphr., Ferr., **Fl-ac.**, *Graph.*, Guaj., *Hell.*, **Hep.**, *Hyos.*, IGN., Iod., Kali., Kali-n., Kreos., *Lach.*, Laur., Led., **Lyc.**, M-arct., M-aust., *Mag.*, Mang., Meny., Merc., Mez., *Mill.*, **Mosch.**, Mur-ac., Nat., Nat-m., Nit-ac., *Nux-m.*, **Nux-v.**, *Olnd.*, Op., Par., Petr., *Phos.*, *Ph-ac.*, *Plat.*, **Plb.**, Psor., *Puls.*, **Ran-b.**, *Ran-s.*, *Rheum*, *Rhod.*, **Rhus-t., SABAD.**, **Sabin.**, Samb., Sars., *Squil.*, Sec., Sel., Seneg., *Sep.*, **SIL.**, *Spig.*, Spong., Stann., **Staph.**, *Stram.*, *Stront.*, *Sulph.*, **Sul-ac.**, Tarax., **Teucr., Thuj., Valer.**, Verat., **Verb.**, Viol-o., Viol-t., *Vit.*, *Zinc.*

## EXTERNAL HEAD

### Left Side

*Acon.*, Agar., Alum., *Ammc.*, Anac., *Ang.*, *Ant-c.*, *Ant-t.*, Arg., **Ars.**, **Asar.**, Aur., *Bar-c.*, Bell., **Borx.**, Calc., Caps., **Carb-an.**, *Carb-v.*, *Caust.*, *Cham.*, **Chel.**, **Chin.**, **CLEM.**, *Cocc.*, *Coloc.*, **Dig., Dulc.**,

### Right Side

**Agar.**, *Alum.*, *Ambr.*, Ammc., *Am-m.*, **Anac.**, Ang., *Aur.*, *Bell.*, Borx., *Brom.*, **Bry.**, **CALC.**, **CANTH.**, Caps., Carb-an., Carb-v., Caust., **Chel.**, Chin., Clem., Coloc., **CON.**, Dig., **Dros.**, Graph., *Guaj.*,

*Euph.*, **Graph.**, *Hep.*, Iod., Kali., Kali-n., Laur., *Lyc.*, *Mag.*, Mag-m., Mang., Meny., **Merc.**, Mill., *Mur-ac.*, Nat., **Nat-m.**, Nit-ac., *Olnd.*, *Petr.*, **Phos.**, *Ph-ac.*, *Plat.*, *Rhod.*, Rhus-t., **RUTA**, *Seneg.*, Sep., *Sil.*, *Spig.*, Staph., Stront., **Sulph.**, *Tarax.*, **THUJ.**, *Verb.*, Viol-t., Zinc.

Hep., *Iod.*, **Kali.**, *Kali-n.*, *Kreos.*, Laur., *Led.*, *Lyc.*, Mag-m., *Mang.*, **Meny.**, Merc., **MEZ.**, Mur-ac., *Nat.*, Nat-m., **Nit-ac.**, Petr., Phos., Ph-ac., Plat., Psor., **Puls.**, Ran-b., *Ran-s.*, Rhod., **Rhus-t.**, *Sabad.*, **Sars.**, **Sep.**, **Sil.**, Spig., *Spong.*, Stann., **Staph.**, Stront., Thuj., *Verat.*, Viol-t., *Vit.*, *Zinc.*

## EYES

### Left Side

**Acon.**, *Agar.*, Alum., Ambr., Ammc., Am-m., Anac., *Ant-c.*, Ant-t., Apis, *Arn.*, **Ars.**, **Asaf.**, **Asar.**, *Aur.*, Bar-c., *Bell.*, *Borx.*, Bov., Brom., **Bry.**, Calad., *Calc.*, Camph., Canth., Caps., *Carb-an.*, Carb-v., **Caust.**, **Chel.**, **Chin.**, Cina, *Clem.*, Colch., *Con.*, *Croc.*, *Dros.*, Euph., *Euphr.*, Ferr., *Fl-ac.*, *Hell.*, **HEP.**, Ign., Iod., Kali., Kali-n., **Laur.**, *Lyc.*, *M-arct.*, **M-aust.**, *Mag.*, *Meny.*, *Merc.*, **Mez.**, **Mill.**, Mur-ac., *Nat-m.*, *Nit-ac.*, **Nux-v.**, *Olnd.*, *Op.*, Par., Petr., *Phos.*, *Ph-ac.*, Plat., **Plb.**, *Psor.*, **Puls.**, Ran-b., Ran-s., Rheum, Rhod., *Rhus-t.*, *Ruta*, Sabad., *Sabin.*, Sars., **Squil.**, *Sel.*, Seneg., **Sep.**, *Sil.*, **Spig.**, **SPONG.**, **Stann.**, Staph., Stram., *Stront.*, **SULPH.**, Sul-ac., **Tarax.**, Teucr., **Thuj.**, Valer., Verat., *Viol-o.*, *Viol-t.*, *Zinc.*

### Right Side

*Acon.*, Agar., *Alum.*, Ambr., **Ammc.**, Am-m., Anac., Ang., Ant-c., *Ant-t.*, Apis., *Arn.*, *Ars.*, *Asaf.*, Asar., Aur., *Bar-c.*, **BELL.**, *Bism.*, Borx., *Bov.*, Brom., Bry., Calad., **CALC.**, **Camph.**, **CANN-S.**, **Canth.**, Caps., Carb-an., **Carb-v.**, *Caust.*, *Cham.*, Chel., Chin., **Cic.**, Cina, **Clem.**, Coff., *Colch.*, **COLOC.**, **Con.**, **Croc.**, *Cycl.*, **Dig.**, Dros., *Euph.*, **Euphr.**, *Ferr.*, **Fl-ac.**, *Graph.*, *Guaj.*, *Hep.*, *Hyos.*, *Ign.*, Iod., **Kali.**, **Kali-n.**, *Kreos.*, Laur., *Led.*, **LYC.**, *M-arct.*, M-aust., *Mag-m.*, **Mang.**, **Merc.**, Mill., *Mur-ac.*, **Nat.**, **NAT-M.**, **NIT-AC.**, *Nux-m.*, Nux-v., Olnd., **Par.**, **PETR.**, **Phos.**, Ph-ac., **PLAT.**, **Plb.**, *Psor.*, *Puls.*, *Ran-b.*, **Ran-s.**, Rheum., **Rhod.**, **RHUS-T.**, Ruta, Sabad., Sars., Squil., Sel., **SENEG.**, *Sep.*, **SIL.**, *Spig.*, Spong., Stann., **Staph.**, Stram., *Sulph.*, Sul-ac., Tarax., *Teucr.*, Thuj., *Valer.*, **Verat.**, Viol-t., *Vit.*, *Zinc.*

## EARS

### Left Side

*Acon.*, Agar., Alum., *Ambr.*, **Ammc.**, Am-m., **ANAC.**, Ang., Ant-c., **Apis**, Arg., **Arn.**, *Ars.*, **ASAF.**,

### Right Side

**Acon.**, *Agar.*, **Alum.**, Ambr., Ammc., **Am-m.**, Anac., **Ang.**, **Ant-c.**, Apis, Arg., Arn., Ars., Asaf., *Asar.*,

Asar., **Aur.,** Bar-c., Bell., *Bism.,* **BORX., Brom., Bry.,** Calad., *Calc.,* **Camph.,** Cann-s., Canth., *Caps.,* Carb-an., *Carb-v., Caust.,* Chel., Chin., Cic., Clem., Colch., Con., Croc., Cupr., Cycl., Dig., Dros., **Dulc.,** Euph., Euphr., Ferr., Fl-ac., **GRAPH., GUAJ.,** Hep., **IGN.,** Iod., Kali., Kali-n., *Kreos.,* Lach., **Laur.,** Lyc., Mang., Meny., **Merc., Mez., Mill.,** *Mur-ac.,* Nat., Nat-m., *Nit-ac.,* Nux-m., **OLND.,** *Par.,* Petr., *Phos.,* Ph-ac., Plat., Plb., **Psor.,** *Puls,* Ran-b., Ran-s., Rheum., *Rhod., Rhus-t.,* Sabad., Sabin., Sars., Squil., Sel., Seneg., *Sep.,* Sil., *Spig.,* Spong., *Stann.,* **Staph.,** *Sulph.,* Tarax., Teucr., Thuj., Valer., Verat., **Verb., VIOL-O.,** Viol-t., Vit., Zinc.

*Bar-c.,* **BELL.,** Borx., **Bov.,** Brom., Bry., *Calad.,* **Calc.,** *Cann-s.,* **Canth., Carb-an.,** Carb-v., *Caust., Cham.,* **Chel.,** Chin., *Cic.,* Clem., *Cocc., Colch.,* Coloc., *Con.,* Croc., *Cupr., Cycl.,* Dig., Dros., Dulc., Euph., Euphr., Ferr., **FL-AC.,** Graph., *Hell.,* **Hep.,** *Hyos.,* **IOD.,** *Ip.,* **Kali., Kali-n.,** Kreos., *Lach.,* Laur., *Led.,* Lyc., *M-arct.,* Mag., Mang., Meny., Merc., Mez., Mill., Mur-ac., Nat., Nat-m., Nit-ac., *Nux-m.,* **NUX-V.,** Par., *Petr.,* **Phos.,** *Ph-ac.,* **PLAT., Plb.,** Psor., **Puls,** *Ran-b.,* **Ran-s.,** Rheum., Rhod., **Rhus-t.,** Ruta, Sabad., Sabin., *Samb.,* **Sars.,** Squil., Sel., *Seneg., Sep.,* **SIL., SPONG.,** Stann., Staph., **Sulph., Sul-ac.,** Tarax., Teucr., **Thuj.,** Valer., *Verat.,* Verb., Zinc.

## NOSE

### Left Side

*Agar.,* **Ammc.,** *Am-m.,* Anac., Ant-c., *Apis,* **Ars.,** Asar., **Aur., Bell., Borx., Bov.,** Brom., *Bry.,* Calc., Canth., Caps., Carb-an., **CARB-V., Caust.,** Chel., Chin., Cina, Cocc., **Coff., Coloc.,** Dros., *Dulc.,* Fl-ac., Graph., *Hell.,* Hep., Kali., Laur., Lyc., M-arct., *Mag., Mag-m.,* **Merc., NAT-M.,** Nit-ac., **Nux-m.,** *Nux-v., Olnd.,* Petr., *Phos.,* **Plat.,** Psor., Puls., **RHOD.,** *Rhus-t.,* Sabin., *Sars.,* **SEP., Sil.,** *Spong.,* Stann., **Staph.,** Sulph., Tarax., Teucr., *Thuj.,* Viol-t., Zinc.

### Right Side

**Acon.,** *Alum.,* Ambr., **Ammc.,** Am-m., Anac., Ant-c., *Asaf., Aur.,* **Brom., Bry.,** *Calad.,* **Calc.,** *Canth.,* Carb-an., Carb-v., Caust., **Chel.,** Cic., Cocc., Colch., CON., Croc., Dros., **Fl-ac., Graph.,** Hep., *Iod.,* **Kali.,** *Kali-n.,* Laur., **Lyc.,** *M-arct., Mang.,* Merc., *Nat.,* Nat-m., **Nit-ac.,** *Nux-v.,* Petr., **Phos., Ph-ac.,** Plat., **Psor., Puls., Ran-b.,** *Ran-s.,* **Rhus-t.,** Sabin., Sars., Sep., *Sil.,* Stann., **Sulph.,** Sul-ac., Tarax., *Teucr.,* Thuj., *Verat., Viol-o.,* Viol-t., *Vit.,* Zinc.

## FACE

### Left Side

Acon., Alum., *Ammc.,* Anac., *Ant-c.,* Ant-t., *Apis,* Arg., *Arn.,* Ars.,

### Right Side

Acon., *Agar., Alum.,* Ammc., **Am-m.,** *Anac.,* Ant-c., Ant-t., Apis,

**Asaf.,** *Asar.,* Aur., *Bar-c., Bell., Borx., Bov.,* **Brom.,** Bry., *Calc.,* **Cann-s.,** Canth., **Caps., Carb-an.,** *Caust.,* Cham., Chel., Chin., **Cic.,** *Cina,* **Clem.,** Cocc., *Coff.,* Colch., **Coloc., Con.,** *Cupr.,* **Dig.,** Dros., *Dulc., Euph., Euphr.,* Fl-ac., Graph., Guaj., *Hell.,* Hep., **Hyos.,** *Ign.,* Iod., Kali., Kali-n., Kreos., *Lach.,* Laur., *Led.,* Lyc., **M-ARCT.,** Mag., Mag-m., Mang., Meny., *Merc., Mez., Mill.,* Mosch., **Mur-ac.,** Nat., *Nat-m.,* Nit-ac., Nux-m., Nux-v., **Olnd., Par.,** Petr., Phos., *Ph-ac., Plat.,* Plb., Psor., *Puls.,* Ran-b., **Rhod.,** *Rhus-t., Ruta, Sabad., Sabin., Samb., Seneg.,* **Sep.,** Sil., Spig., **Spong.,** Stann., Staph., Stram., Stront., **Sulph.,** Sul-ac., Tarax., Teucr., *Thuj.,* Valer., *Verat., Verb., Viol-o.,* **Viol-t.,** Zinc.

*Arg.,* Arn., **Ars.,** Asaf., Asar., **Aur.,** *Bar-c.,* **BELL.,** *Bism.,* Borx., Brom., **Bry., CALC.,** Cann-s., **CANTH.,** Caps., Carb-an., Carb-v., *Caust.,* Cham., *Chel.,* **Chin.,** Cina, **Cocc.,** *Colch.,* Coloc., *Con.,* Cupr., *Cycl.,* Dig., *Dros., Dulc.,* Euph., **Fl-ac.,** *Graph., Guaj.,* **Hep.,** Hyos., Iod., *Kali., Kali-n.,* **Kreos.,** *Lach.,* Laur., Led., **LYC.,** M-arct., *Mag.,* Mag-m., *Mang., Meny.,* **Merc.,** *Mez.,* Mill., *Mosch.,* **Nat.,** Nat-m., **Nit-ac.,** *Nux-m.,* **NUX-V.,** Olnd., Par., Petr., **Phos.,** Ph-ac., Plat., **Plb., Psor., Puls.,** Ran-b., Ran-s., *Rheum,* **Rhus-t.,** Sabad., Sabin., *Sars., Sep.,* **Sil., Spig.,** Spong., Stann., **Staph.,** Stram., Stront., *Sulph.,* Sul-ac., *Tarax., Teucr., Thuj., Valer.,* Verat., *Verb.,* **Vit.,** Zinc.

## TEETH

### Left Side

*Acon.,* **Agar.,** *Alum.,* Ambr., *Ammc., Am-m.,* Anac., **Apis, Arn.,** *Asaf., Asar., Aur.,* **Bar-c.,** Bell., **Borx.,** *Brom., Bry., Calc.,* Cann-s., Canth., **Carb-an., Carb-v., CAUST., CHEM.,** *Chel.,* **Chin., CLEM.,** *Colch.,* **Con.,** *Croc., Cycl.,* **EUPH.,** Fl-ac., Graph., **Guaj.,** *Hyos.,* Iod., Kali., *Kali-n.,* Kreos., **Laur.,** *Led.,* Lyc., **M-arct., Merc., MEZ.,** *Mill.,* Nat-m., **Nux-m.,** *Nux-v., Olnd.,* **Phos.,** *Puls.,* Ran-s., *Rheum,* **Rhod., Rhus-t.,** Sabad., *Sabin., Samb.,* **Sel.,** *Seneg.,* **SEP., Sil., Spig.,** Spong., *Staph.,* Stront., **SULPH.,** Teucr., **THUJ.,** *Verat.,* Verb., **Zinc.**

### Right Side

Agar., Alum., *Ambr., Ammc.,* Anac., **Ang.,** Apis, *Aur.,* Bar-c., **BELL.,** *Bov.,* Brom., **Bry., Calc.,** *Camph., Cann-s.,* Canth., Carb-an., Carb-v., *Caust., Chin., Coff.,* Colch., *Coloc.,* Con., **FL-AC.,** *Graph.,* **Hell., Iod.,** Kali., **Kreos.,** Lach., Laur., Lyc., **Mag.,** *Mang., Merc.,* Mez., *Nat., Nat-m., Nit-ac.,* **Nux-v.,** Olnd., **Petr.,** *Ph-ac.,* **Psor.,** *Puls.,* Ran-b., Ran-s., Rhod., *Rhus-t., Ruta,* **Sabad., Sars.,** *Sep., Sil.,* Spig., Spong., **STAPH.,** Stront., Sulph., **Tarax.,** *Teucr.,* Thuj., *Valer.,* **Verb.,** *Vit.,* Zinc.

## MOUTH AND FAUCES

### Left Side

*Acon.*, Alum., *Ang.*, Ant-c., *Ant-t.*, *Apis*, *Aur.*, Bar-c., **BELL.**, Bov., Calc., *Carb-an.*, Carb-v., **Caust.**, *Colch.*, *Croc.*, *Cupr.*, Dros., *Euph.*, Fl-ac., **Graph.**, **Hep.**, Iod., **Kali.**, Kreos., **Lyc.**, *M-aust.*, *Meny.*, *Mez.*, Mill., Nat-m., *Nit-ac.*, *Nux-m.*, **Nux-v.**, Olnd., *Phos.*, Ph-ac., Plat., Psor., **Puls.**, Rhod, **Rhus-t.**, Sabad., *Sabin.*, **Seneg.**, **SEP.**, *Sil.*, Spig., **Sulph.**, *Tarax.*, *Teucr.*, *Thuj.*, *Verat.*, Zinc.

### Right Side

*Alum.*, **Ammc.**, Ant-c., *Ars.*, Aur., Bov., *Brom.*, *Calc.*, **Carb-v.**, *Caust.*, *Chin.*, *Coloc.*, **Dros.**, **Fl-ac.**, Graph., Iod., **Kreos.**, Lach., *M-arct.*, **MERC.**, Mill., *Nat-m.*, *Nit-ac.*, *Nux-v.*, *Petr.*, Plat., *Plb.*, *Psor.*, *Ran-b.*, Rhus-t., *Sabad.*, *Sep.*, Sil., *Spig.*, *Stann.*, *Sulph.*, Teucr., *Thuj.*, Zinc.

## HYPOCHONDRIA

### Left Side

Acon., *Agar.*, Alum., Ammc., **Am-m.**, *Anac.*, **Ant-c.**, **Apis**, *Arg.*, **Arn.**, **Ars.**, **ASAF.**, **Asar.**, *Aur.*, Bell., **Borx.**, Brom., *Bry.*, Calad., *Calc.*, **Cann-s.**, Carb-an., **Carb-v.**, **Caust.**, **Cham.**, *Chel.*, **Chin.**, *Cocc.*, *Coff.*, *Con.*, **Cupr.**, *Dig.*, Dulc., **Euph.**, **Ferr.**, **FL-AC.**, *Graph.*, *Hep.*, **IGN.**, Iod., *Ip.*, *Kali.*, *Kali-n.*, *Kreos.*, Laur., Lyc., Mang., Merc., **Mez.**, **Mill.**, Mosch., **Mur-ac.**, *Nat.*, *Nat-m.*, **NIT-AC.**, *Nux-v.*, *Olnd.*, *Par.*, Petr., Phos., Ph-ac., *Plat.*, *Plb.*, *Puls.*, **Psor.**, **Ran-b.**, *Ran-s.*, **Rheum**, *Rhod.*, Rhus-t., *Ruta*, Sabad., *Sars.*, *Squil.*, *Sec.*, *Seneg.*, **Sep.**, *Sil.*, *Spig.*, *Stann.*, *Staph.*, **SULPH.**, *Sul-ac.*, Teucr., Valer., **Verb.**, *Viol-t.*, **Vit.**, **Zinc.**

### Right Side

**ACON.**, *Agar.*, **Alum.**, **Ambr.**, **AMMC.**, Am-m., **Anac.**, *Ang.*, *Ant-c.*, Apis, *Arn.*, *Ars.*, *Asaf.*, **BAR-C.**, **BELL.**, Borx., **BRY.**, Calad., **Calc.**, **Canth.**, **Carb-an.**, *Carb-v.*, Caust., Chel., *Chin.*, **Clem.**, **COCC.**, **Colch.**, **Con.**, **Dig.**, Dulc., *Ferr.*, Fl-ac., *Graph.*, *Hep.*, *Hyos.*, *Ign.*, *Iod.*, **KALI.**, Kreos., **Lach.**, **Laur.**, *Led.*, **LYC.**, *M-arct.*, *M-aust.*, **MAG-M.**, Mang., Merc., Mill., **Mosch.**, *Nat.*, **Nat-m.**, Nit-ac., *Nux-m.*, **NUX-V.**, Par., Petr., Phos., Ph-ac., Plat., *Plb.*, Psor., *Puls.*, *Ran-b.*, *Ran-s.*, Rhod., *Rhus-t.*, *Ruta*, **Sabad.**, *Sabin.*, **Sec.**, **Sel.**, *Sep.*, **Sil.**, Spig., **Stann.**, Staph., *Sulph.*, *Sul-ac.*, *Teucr.*, Valer., **Verat.**, Verb., *Vit.*, Zinc.

## ABDOMEN

### Left Side

*Acon.*, Agar., *Alum.*, Ambr., **Ammc., Am-m.,** Anac., Ang., Ant-c., **Ant-t, Apis, Arg.,** Arn., Ars., **ASAF.,** *Asar., Aur.,* Bar-c., *Bell.,* **Bov.,** *Brom.,* **Bry., Calc.,** Camph., *Cann-s.,* Canth., *Caps.,* Carb-v., Caust., **Cham.,** Chel., Chin., Cina, Cocc., Colch., Coloc., *Con.,* Croc., Cupr., *Dig.,* **DULC.,** *Euph.,* **FL-AC., GRAPH., Guaj., HEP.,** *Ign., Iod.,* **Kali.,** *Kreos.,* Laur., *Led.,* Lyc., *M-arct.,* M-aust., Mag-m., *Mang., Meny.,* Merc., *Mez.,* **Mill.,** *Mur-ac., Nat.,* **Nat-m.,** Nit-ac., Nux-m., *Nux-v., Olnd., Op.,* **Par.,** Petr., *Ph-ac.,* Plat., **PLB.,** *Psor.,* **Puls., Ran-b., RHEUM,** Rhod., Rhus-t., *Ruta, Sabad.,* Sabin., *Samb.,* **Sars.,** Squil, *Sel.,* Sep., Sil., **Spig.,** *Spong.,* Stann., *Staph.,* **SULPH.,** *Sul-ac.,* **TARAX.,** Teucr., Thuj., **Valer.,** *Verb.,* Viol-t., Vit., Zinc.

### Right Side

Agar., **Ambr.,** Am-m., Anac., *Ang., Ant-c.,* Apis, Arg., *Arn.,* **ARS.,** Asaf., Aur., **Bar-c.,** Bell., *Bism., Bry., Calad.,* Calc., Camph., Cann-s., **Canth., Carb-an., Carb-v., Caust.,** Chel., Chin., *Cic., Clem.,* Cocc., *Colch.,* **Coloc.,** Con., *Croc.,* Cupr., *Cycl.,* Dig., *Dros.,* Dulc., Fl-ac., Graph., Guaj., **Ign.,** Iod., *Ip.,* Kali., **Kali-n.,** Kreos., **Lach.,** Laur., **Lyc.,** M-aust., **Mag-m.,** Meny., *Merc.,* Mez., Mill., *Mosch.,* Nit-ac., Nux-m., *Nux-v.,* Olnd., Petr., *Phos.,* Ph-ac., *Plat.,* Plb., Psor., *Puls.,* Ran-b., *Ran-s.,* Rhod., **Rhus-t.,** Sabad., *Sabin.,* Samb., Squil., **Seneg., Sep.,** Sil., Spig., Spong., **Stann.,** *Stront.,* Sulph., Tarax., *Teucr.,* **Thuj.,** Verb., *Viol-t., Vit.,* Zinc.

## ABDOMINAL RINGS

### Left Side

*Agar., Alum, Ambr.,* **Ammc.,** Am-m., Ant-c., **Apis., Arg.,** Arn., *Asar.,* Aur., Bell., Calc., Camph., Cann-s., Canth., Carb-an., *Chel.,* Cocc., *Dig.,* **Dulc., EUPH.,** Fl-ac., Graph., **Ign.,** Kali., Laur., Lyc., **M-arct.,** *M-aust.,* **MAG.,** *Mag-m., Merc.,* **Nit-ac.,** Nux-m., *Nux-v., Par., Phos.,* Rhod., Rhus-t., *Sabad.,* Sabin., Sars., *Sep.,* Sil., *Spig.,* Spong., *Stann., Staph.,* **Sulph.,** *Sul-ac., Tarax., Verat.,* Viol-t., Vit., *Zinc.*

### Right Side

Alum., Amm-c., **Am-m.,** *Apis., Ars.,* **Aur.,** *Bell., Borx.,* **CALC.,** Camph., Cann-s., Canth., Carb-an., **Carb-v.,** *Cic., Clem., Cocc.,* **Coloc.,** *Con.,* Dig., *Dros.,* Dulc., Fl-ac., Graph., *Hell., Iod., Ip.,* **KALI., LACH., Laur., LYC.,** *Mang., Merc., Mez.,* **NUX-V.,** *Op.,* **Petr.,** *Ph-ac., Psor.,* **PULS.,** *Ran-b.,* **RHOD., RHUS-T.,** *Ruta, Sabin.,* Sars., **Seneg.,** *Sep.,* **Sil.,** Spig., Spong., Stann., **Staph., Stront.,** Sulph., **SUL-AC.,** *Teucr.,* **THUJ.,** *Valer.,* **Verat.,** Vit., Zinc.

## SEXUAL ORGANS

### Left Side

*Agar.*, Alum., Ambr., *Am-m.*, **Ang.**, *Ant-c.*, **Apis,** *Arg.*, *Aur.*, *Bar-c.*, **Brom.**, *Bry.*, *Calc.*, Cann-s., **Chin.**, Clem., *Colch.*, *Con.*, *Euph.*, **Fl-ac.**, Graph., **Kali.**, Lyc., M-arct., **Mag.**, Meny., *Merc.*, Mez., **Nat.**, **Nit-ac.**, Petr., **Ph-ac.**, *Plb.*, *Puls.*, **Rhod.**, *Rhus-t.*, *Sabad.*, Sel., *Sep.*, Sil., Spig., Staph., Tarax., Teucr., **THUJ.**, Zinc.

### Right Side

**Acon.**, Alum., *Apis,* **Arn.**, **Aur.**, *Bism.*, **CALC.**, *Cann-s.*, *Canth.*, **CAUST.**, **Clem.**, *Coff.*, **Coloc.**, **Con.**, *Croc.*, Graph., **HEP.**, **Iod.**, **Lach.**, **Lyc.**, M-arct., **Meny.**, **Merc.**, Mez., *Mur-ac.*, Nit-ac., **NUX-V.**, Petr., **Puls.**, *Rhod.*, **Sabin.**, *Sec.*, *Sel.*, Sil., **Spig.**, **SPONG.**, **Staph.**, **Sulph.**, **SUL-AC.**, Tarax., Teucr., *Valer.*, **VERAT.**, **Zinc.**

## NECK AND NAPE OF THE NECK

### Left Side

*Alum.*, *Ammc.*, Anac., Ang., Ant-c., *Ant-t.*, Apis, *Arg.*, Asaf., Aur., **Bell.**, **Bism.**, Bry., *Calc.*, *Camph.*, Canth., *Caps.*, Carb-v., **CAUST.**, *Chel.*, **Chin.**, *Cina,* Cocc., **Colch.**, Coloc., **Con.**, *Cupr.*, *Dulc.*, **FL-AC.**, Guaj., **Hep.**, **Iod.**, **Kali.**, *Kali-n.*, **Lach.**, **Laur.**, *Led.*, *Lyc.*, *M-aust.*, *Meny.*, **MERC.**, **Mez.**, *Nat.*, *Nat-m.*, **NIT-AC.**, **Nux-v.**, Olnd., *Petr.*, Ph-ac., *Plat.*, *Plb.*, *Puls.*, Rhod., Sabin., **Sars.**, **Seneg.**, **Sil.**, *Spig.*, **Spong.**, Staph., *Sulph.*, **Sul-ac.**, *Teucr.*, Thuj., Vit., Zinc.

### Right Side

*Acon.*, Alum., *Am-m.*, *Anac.*, *Ang.*, **APIS.**, *Ant-c.*, Arg., *Arn.*, Ars., **ASAF.**, **Asar.**, Aur., *Bar-c.*, Bell., *Borx.*, *Bov.*, *Brom.*, *Bry.*, **CALC.**, *Canth.*, *Carb-an.*, *Carb-v.*, Caust., *Cic.*, Cocc., Colch., *Coloc.*, *Croc.*, *Cycl.*, Fl-ac., **Guaj.**, *Hyos.*, *Ign.*, Kali., Lach., Laur., **Lyc.**, Merc., Mez., *Mosch.*, *Nux-v.*, **Olnd.**, *Par.*, Ph-ac., *Psor.*, Rhod., *Rhus-t.*, **Sabin.**, *Squil.*, **Sel.**, *Sep.*, *Sil.*, Spig., *Spong.*, *Staph.*, **Stram.**, **SULPH.**, *Sul-ac.*, **Tarax.**, Teucr., **Thuj.**, *Verat.*, *Viol-t.*, Vit., Zinc.

## CHEST

### Left Side

**Acon.**, *Agar.*, Alum., Ambr., *Ammc.*, **AM-M.**, *Anac.*, Ang., *Ant-c.*, **Ant-t.**, **Apis,** Arg., **Arn.**, *Asaf.*, Asar., *Aur.*, *Bar-c.*, *Bell.*, *Bism.*, Borx., *Bov.*, Brom., *Bry.*, *Calad.*, **CALC.**, *Camph.*, **Cann-s.**, *Canth.*, **Caps.**,

### Right Side

*Acon.*, Agar., *Alum.*, Ambr., **Ammc.**, Am-m., Anac., Ang., Ant-c., Ant-t., *Arg.*, **ARN.**, *Ars.*, **Asaf.**, Asar., **Aur.**, Bar-c., **BELL.**, Bism., **Borx.**, Bov., **Brom.**, **BRY.**, Calad., *Calc.*, Camph., *Cann-s.*, **Canth.**, Caps.,

*Carb-an.,* **Carb-v., Caust., Cham.,** *Chel.,* **Chin.,** Cic., **Cina,** Clem., **Cocc.,** Colch., Coloc., *Con., Croc., Cupr., Cycl.,* Dig., *Dros.,* **Dulc., EUPH., FL-AC., Graph., Guaj.,** *Hep.,* Hyos., **Ign., KALI., Kali-n., Kreos.,** Lach., **LAUR.,** Led., **LYC.,** M-ambo., **M-arct., M-aust.,** *Mag.,* Mang., **Meny., Merc.,** Mez., Mill., *Mosch.,* Mur-ac., *Nat.,* **Nat-m., NIT-AC.,** Nux-m., **NUX-V., Olnd.,** Par., Petr., **Phos., Ph-ac.,** *Plat.,* **Plb.,** Psor., Puls., **Ran-b.,** Ran-s., *Rheum,* **Rhod., RHUS-T.,** Ruta, Sabad., Sabin., Sars., *Squil.,* **SENEG., Sep.,** *Sil.,* **Spig., Spong., STANN.,** *Staph.,* Stront., **SULPH., Sul-ac.,** Tarax., Teucr., **Thuj., Valer.,** *Verat.,* **Verb., Viol-t.,** Vit., ., **Zinc.**

**CARB-AN.,** *Carb-v.,* Caust., *Cham.,* Chel., Chin., Cic., Cina, Clem., *Cocc.,* **Colch., COLOC.,** Con., Croc., Cupr., Cycl., **Dig.,** Dros., *Dulc.,* Euph., Fl-ac., *Graph.,* **Hep., Hyos.,** Ign., **IOD.,** *Ip.,* Kali., Kali-n., Kreos., **LACH.,** Laur., **Led., M-ambo.,** *M-arct.,* M-aust., **Mag-m.,** Mang., Meny., *Merc.,* Mez., Mill., **Mur-ac.,** Nat., *Nat-m., Nit-ac., Nux-m., Nux-v.,* Olnd., **Op.,** *Par.,* Petr., **Phos.,** *Ph-ac.,* Plat., Plb., *Psor.,* **PULS.,** *Ran-b., Ran-s.,* Rheum, *Rhus-t.,* Ruta., *Sabad.,* Sabin., Sars., **Squil.,** Seneg., *Sep.,* **SIL.,** *Spig.,* Spong., Stann., Staph., Stront., *Sulph.,* Sul-ac., **Tarax.,** *Teucr.,* Thuj., Valer., **Verat.,** *Viol-t., Vit.,* Zinc.

## BACK

### Left Side

**Acon., Agar., Alum.,** Ambr., *Ammc.,* Am-m., **Anac.,** Ang., Ant-c., Ant-t., **Apis,** Arg., *Ars., Asaf.,* Aur., **Bar-c.,** Bell., **Bism., Bry.,** Calc., Cann-s., Canth., Carb-an., *Carb-v.,* **Caust.,** Chel., **Chin.,** Cina, *Cocc.,* Colch., *Coloc.,* Con., *Croc., Cupr., Dig.,* **DROS.,** *Dulc.,* Euph., *Ferr., Fl-ac.,* **Graph.,** Guaj., *Hell.,* **Hep., Ign.,** Iod., **Kali.,** *Kali-n., Kreos.,* Laur., *Led., Lyc., M-ambo., M-aust.,* **Mang.,** Meny., Merc., Mez., *Mill., Mosch.,* Mur-ac., *Nat-m.,* Nit-ac., Nux-v., Olnd., **Par.,** *Petr.,* Phos., *Ph-ac.,* Plat., Plb., *Psor.,* **Puls.,** Ran-s., *Rhod., Rhus-t.,* **Ruta,** Sabad., **Sabin.,** Sars., **Squil., Seneg.,** Sep., **SIL.,** *Spig.,* **Spong., Stann.,** *Staph., Stront.,* **Sulph., Sul-ac.,** Tarax., **Teucr.,** *Thuj.,* **Valer., Verat.,** Verb., Viol-t., Vit., Zinc.

### Right Side

Acon., Agar., Alum., Ambr., Ammc., *Am-m.,* Anac., Ang., *Ant-c., Ant-t.,* Apis, *Arg.,* **Arn., Ars.,** Asaf., *Asar., Aur.,* Bar-c., Bell., *Borx., Brom., Bry.,* **CALC.,** Cann-s., **Canth., Carb-an.,** Carb-v., Caust., Chel., *Chin.,* **CIC.,** Cina., Cocc., *Colch.,* **Coloc., Con.,** Cupr., Dig., Dros., Dulc., **Euph.,** FL-AC., **Guaj.,** Hep., *Iod., Kali.,* **Laur., Lyc., M-arct.,** M-aust., Meny., Merc., Mez., Mill., Mur-ac., **Nat-m.,** Nit-ac., **Nux-v., Olnd.,** Petr., **Phos.,** Plat., **PLB., Ran-b.,** Ran-s., Rhod., **Rhus-t.,** Ruta, *Sabad.,* **Samb.,** Sars., *Sep., Sil.,* Spig., Spong., Stann., Staph., *Sulph.,* Sul-ac., **Tarax.,** Teucr., Thuj., Verb., Viol-t., Vit., **ZINC.**

## UPPER EXTREMITIES

### Left Side

Acon., Agar., **Alum.**, Ambr., Ammc., Am-m., **ANAC.**, Ang., Ant-c., *Ant-t.*, **Apis**, Arg., **ARN.**, *Ars.*, **ASAF.**, Asar., Aur., **Bar-c.**, *Bell.*, Bism., Borx., Bov., *Brom.*, *Bry.*, *Calad.*, *Calc.*, *Camph.*, Cann-s., Canth., **Caps.**, Carb-an., *Carb-v.*, Caust., **Cham.**, Chel., *Chin.*, *Cic.*, *Cina.*, Clem., *Coca*, *Coff.*, Colch., Coloc., *Con.*, *Croc.*, Cupr., **Cycl.**, Dig., Dros., Dulc., Euph., **Euphr.**, Ferr., **Fl-ac.**, Graph., Guaj., Hell., Hep., *Hyos.*, *Ign.*, *Iod.*, **IP.**, **KALI.**, *Kali-n.*, **Kreos.**, *Lach.*, *Led.*, **Lyc.**, M-ambo., **M-arct.**, **M-AUST.**, Mang., **Mag-m.**, *Meny.*, *Merc.*, Mez., Mill., *Mosch.*, *Mur-ac.*, Nat., *Nat-m.*, *Nit-ac.*, *Nux-m.*, *Nux-v.*, **Olnd.**, *Op.*, Par., **Petr.**, Phos., **Ph-ac.**, Plat., Plb., *Psor.*, *Puls.*, Ran-b., Ran-s., Rheum, Rhod., **RHUS-T.**, Ruta, Sabad., **SABIN.**, Samb., Sars., **SQUIL.**, Sec., *Sel.*, **Seneg.**, *Sep.*, *Sil.*, Spig., Spong., **STANN.**, *Staph.*, *Stram.*, *Stront.*, **SULPH.**, Sul-ac., **Tarax.**, **Teucr.**, *Thuj.*, **Valer.**, *Verat.*, **Verb.**, Viol-o., **Viol-t.**, Vit., *Zinc.*

### Right Sise

*Acon.*, Agar., Alum., **Ambr.**, Ammc., *Am-m.*, Anac., **Ang.**, *Ant-c.*, Ant-t., *Apis*, Arg., Arn., **Ars.**, Asaf., Asar., **Aur.**, Bar-c., **BELL.**, **BISM.**, **Borx.**, **Bov.**, Brom., **BRY.**, Calad., **CALC.**, Camph., **Cann-s.**, **Canth.**, Caps., Carb-an., **Carb-v.**, **CAUST.**, *Cham.*, *Chel.*, Chin., Cic., Cina, Clem., **Cocc.**, Coff., **Colch.**, **COLOC.**, *Con.*, Croc., **Cupr.**, Cycl., *Dig.*, *Dros.*, *Dulc.*, Euph., Euphr., *Ferr.*, Fl-ac., **GRAPH.**, Guaj., Hell., Hep., Hyos., **Ign.**, Iod., *Ip.*, Kali., Kali-n., Kreos., **Lach.**, Laur., Led., *Lyc.*, *M-ambo.*, M-arct., M-aust., *Mag.*, Mag-m., **Mang.**, Meny., Merc., Mez., Mill., Mosch., Mur-ac., **Nat.**, Nat-m., Nit-ac., Nux-m., Nux-v., Olnd., Op., Par., *Petr.*, **PHOS.**, *Ph-ac.*, Plat., **Plb.**, **Psor.**, **PULS.**, Ran-b., Ran-s., *Rheum*, **RHOD.**, *Rhus-t.*, Ruta., Sabad., Sabin., Samb., *Sars.*, Squil., Sec., Sel., Seneg., **SEP.**, **SIL.**, Spig., Spong., Stann., *Staph.*, Stram., Stront., *Sulph.*, **Sul-ac.**, Tarax., Teucr., *Thuj.*, Valer., Verat., Verb., *Viol-o.*, Viol-t., *Vit.*, *Zinc.*

## LOWER EXTREMITIES

### Left Side

Acon., **Agar.**, Alum., **AMBR.**, *Ammc.*, *Am-m.*, *Anac.*, Ang., Ant-c., **Ant-t.**, **Apis**, **Arg.**, Arn., *Ars.*, **ASAF.**, *Asar.*, Aur., *Bar-c.*, *Bell.*, Bism., *Borx.*, *Bov.*, Brom., *Bry.*, **Calad.**, **CALC.**, Camph., Cann-s., Canth., Caps., Carb-an., *Carb-v.*, **Caust.**, Cham., *Chel.*, Chin., **Cic.**, **CINA**,

### Right Sise

Acon., Agar., *Alum.*, Ambr., Amm-c., Am-m., Anac., *Ang.*, Ant-c., Ant-t., *Apis*, *Arg.*, **Arn.**, **ARS.**, Asaf., Asar., **Aur.**, Bar-c., **BELL.**, Bism., Borx., Bov., **Brom.**, **BRY.**, Calad., *Calc.*, *Camph.*, Cann-s., **Canth.**, Caps., *Carb-an.*, *Carb-v.*, *Caust.*, Cham., Chel., *Chin.*, Cic., Cina,

# DRUG AFFINITIES

Acon: **Arn., Ars., BELL., BRY., Canth., CHAM., COFF.,** *Croc., Dulc., Graph.,* **Lyc., MERC., Mill., Nux-v., Op., Phos., Ph-ac., Puls., RHUS-T.,** *Ruta,* **SEP., Sulph., Valer.,** *Verat.*

Agar: **Bell., CALC., Cocc.,** *Coff.,* **LYC., Nit-ac., NUX-V., Petr., Phos., Puls., Sep., SIL., Sulph.**

Alum: **BRY., Calc., Cham.,** *Ign.,* **Ip.,** *Lach.,* **Lyc., Nat-m.,** *Phos., Plb.,* **Puls.,** *Verat.*

Ambr: **Bell., Calc., Lyc., Nux-v., Puls.,** *Staph.,* **Sulph.**

Ammc: **Brom., Calc.,** *Fl-ac.,* **Hep., Phos., Sec.**

Am-m.: **Ars.,** *Nux-v.,* **Puls., Rhus-t.**

Anac: *Calc.,* **Coff., Con., Nat-m.**

Ang: *Bry., Calc., Lyc.,* **Rhus-t,** *Verb.*

Ant-c.: **Ars.,** *Bism., Brom.,* **HEP.,** *Ip.,* **MERC.,** *Puls.,* **Sep., SULPH.**

Ant-t.: **BELL., Chin., Cocc.,** *Con.,* **Ip., Op., Puls., Sep.**

Apis: **ARS., Bell., Canth., Chin.,** *Ferr., Graph., Hep., Iod., Kali., Lach.,* **Lyc.,** *Merc., Mill.,* **PULS., Sep., Sulph.**

Arg.: *Merc.*

Arn.: **Acon., Arn.,** *Bry., Cann-s., Caps.,* **Chin., CIC., Ferr., Ign., IP.,** *Merc., Mill.,* **Puls.,** *Rhus-t., Sabin., Samb.,* **Squil., Seneg., Verat., ZINC.**

Ars.: *Acon., Am-m.,* **Ant-t., Arn., APIS, Bar-c.,** *Brom.,* **Bry.,** *Calc.,* **Carb-v., CHAM., CHIN.,** *Coff.,* **Dig.,** *Colch., Dulc., Euph.,* **FERR., Graph., HEP., Ign., IOD., IP.,** *Kali.,* **Lach., LYC.,** *Mag.,* **MERC.,** *Mosch., Mur-ac.,* **Nat-m., NUX-V., Petr., Phos.,** *Ph-ac., Plb., Ran-s.,* **Samb., Squil., Sec., Sep., Sil.,** *Stann.,* **Staph., SULPH.,** *Sul-ac.,* **Verat.**

Asaf.: *Aur.,* **Caust., CHIN.,** *Meny.,* **MERC., Nit-ac., Ph-ac.,** *Plat.,* **Puls., Sep.**

Asar.: *Cup., Nux-v., Phos.*

Aur.: *Asaf., Calc., Coff.,* **Merc., Nux-v., Puls., Phos.**

Bar-c.: **Ars.,** *Calc., Nux-v., Sep., Zinc.*

Bell: **ACON., Agar., Ambr., Ant-t., Apis, Bry., CALC., Cann-s., Canth., Caust., Cham., Chin.,** *Cic., Cina,* **Coff., Colch., Coloc., Croc., Cupr.,** *Dig.,* **Graph.,** *Hell.,* **HEP.,** *Hyos.,* **Iod., LACH., Merc., MOSCH., Nit-ac., NUX-V., Op., Ph-ac.,** *Plat.,* **Plb., PULS., Rheum, Rhus-t., Sars., Seneg., SEP.,** *Sil.,* **Stram.,** *Sulph.,* **Valer.**

Bism: *Ant-c.,* **CALC.,** *Cocc., Ign., Spig., Staph.*

Borx: **Bry., Calc., Cham.,** *Coff.,* **Sil.,** *Sulph.*

Bov.: *Nit-ac.,* **Sel.,** *Sil.*

Brom: **AMMC., Ant-c.,** *Ars., Camph., Coff.,* **Hep., Iod.,** *Mag., Nat-m., Op., Phos.,* **Spong.**

Bry.: **ACON., ALUM.,** *Ang.,* **Ars.,** *Bell., Borx.,* **Calc., Carb-v.,** *Caust.,* **Chin., Clem.,** *Coloc.,* **Dulc.,** *Guaj.,* **Iod.,** *Ip.,* **Kali., Led., Lyc., Mez., MILL.,** *Phos.,* **PULS., Ran-b., RHOD., RHUS-T.,** *Squil.,* **Seneg., Sep., Verat.**

Calad.: *Canth.,* **CAPS.,** *Ign., Nux-v.*

Calc.: **AGAR.,** *Alum.,* **Ambr., Ammc.,** *Anac., Ang., Ars., Aur., Bar-c.,* **BELL., BISM., Borx., Bry., Cann-s.,** Caust., *Chel.,* **Chin., Cocc.,** *Cupr.,* **Fl-ac.,** *Graph., Ign., Iod., IP., Kali., Kali-n.,* **LYC., Mag-m.,** *Meny., Merc.,* **NAT., NIT-AC., NUX-V., Petr., Phos., Ph-ac., PULS., Rhus-t.,** *Sabin.,* **SARS., Sel., Sep., SIL., SULPH.,** *Verat., Vit.*

Camph.: **Brom., Canth., OP.,** *Verat.*

Cann-s.: *Arn.,* **Bell., Calc.,** *Canth., Coloc.,* **Euph.,** Meny., *Nat-m.,* **Nit-ac., Puls., Thuj.**

Canth.: **ACON., Apis, Bell.,** *Calad.,* **Camph.,** *Cann-s., Laur.,* **LYC., PULS.**

Caps.: *Arn.,* **CALAD.,** *Cham., Chin.,* **CINA,** *Ign., Nux-v., Puls.*

Carb-an.: *Carb-v., Rhod.,* **THUJ.**

Carb-v.: **Ars., Bry.,** *Carb-an.,* **CHIN.,** *Dulc.,* **Ferr., Ign.,** *Ip., Kali.,* **Lach., MERC., Nat-m.,** *Nit-ac.,* **Nux-v.,** *Op.,* **Petr., Puls.,** *Rhod., Sep.,* **Sulph.,** *Verat.*

Caust.: **Asaf., Bell., Bry.,** *Calc., Cocc.,* **Clem.,** *Coloc.,* **Cupr., Graph.,** *Hep.,* **Ign.,** *Kreos.,* **LACH.,** *Lyc.,* **NAT., Nux-v., Phos., Plat., Puls., Rhod., Rhus-t., SEP., Sil., SULPH.**

Cham.: **ACON.,** *Alum.,* **Ars., Bell., Borx.,** *Caps.,* **Chin., Cina, COCC., Coff.,** *Coloc.,* **HEP., IGN.,** *Ip., Lyc., Mag.,* **NUX-V.,** *Petr.,* **PULS.,** Rheum, *Rhus-t., Stram.,* **Sulph., Valer.**

Chel.: *Calc., Lyc., Puols., Sulph.*

Chin.: *Ammc.,* **Ant-t., Apis, ARN., ARS., ASAF., BELL., Bry., Calc.,** *Caps.,* **CARB-V., Cham., Cina, Cupr.,** *Cycl., Dig.,* **FERR.,** *Fl-ac.,* **Hell., Iod., IP., LACH., MERC.,** *Mill.,* **Nat-m.,** *Nux-v., Phos.,* **Ph-ac.,** *Plb.,* **PULS.,** *Samb.,* **Sep.,** *Stann.,* **Sulph.,** *Sul-ac.,* **VERAT.**

Cic.: **ARN.,** *Bell., Dulc., Lyc., Merc., Op., Rhus-t., Stram., Verat.*

Cina.: *Bell.,* **CAPS., Chin.,** *Dros., Hyos., Merc., Phos., Verat.*

Clem.: **Bry., Graph., Merc., RHOD., Rhus-t.**

Cocc.: *Agar.,* **Ant-t.,** *Bism.,* **Calc.,** *Caust.,* **CHAM., Cupr., IGN., IP.,** *Kali., Mosch., Nux-m.,* **Nux-v.,** *Olnd.*

Coff.: **Acon.,** *Agar., Anac., Ars., Aur.,* **Bell.,** *Borx., Brom., Caps.,* **Cham., COLOC.,** *Con.,* **Ign.,** *Mag., Merc., Mosch.,* **Nux-v., Op., Puls.,** *Sulph., Teucr.,* **Valer., Verat.**

Colch.: *Ars.,* **Bell., Fl-ac.,** *Merc.,* **Nux-v.,** *Op.,* **Puls.**

Coloc.: **Bell.,** *Bry., Cann-s.,* **Caust.,** *Cham.,* **COFF.,** *Mag.,* **Rheum, Sec., STAPH.**

Con.: *Anac., Ant-t., Coll., Cupr., Cycl., Dig., Dulc.,* **LACH., Lyc., Nit-ac.,** *Nux-v.,* **Puls.,** *Vit.*

Croc.: *Acon., Bell., Op., Plat.*

Cupr.: **Bell.,** *Calc.,* **Caust., Chin., Cocc.,** *Con., Dulc.,* **HEP., Hyos., Ign., Ip., Lyc., Merc., Nux-v., Op.,** *Ph-ac.,* **PULS.,** *Sep., Sil., Sulph.,* **VERAT.**

Cycl.: *Con.,* **Puls.**

Dig.: **Ars.,** *Bell., Chin., Con., Merc.,* **Nux-v., Op.,** *Phos., Ph-ac.,* **Plat., Puls.,** *Spig., Sul-ac.*

Dros.: *Cina, Hep.,* **Ip.,** *Nux-v., Sep.,* **Spong., Verat.**

Dulc.: *Acon., Ars.,* **Bry.,** *Cic., Con.,* **Cupr.,** *Led.,* **Merc.,** *Nux-v., Ph-ac., Puls.,* **Rhus-t., Sep.,** *Sulph.*

Euph.: *Ars., Lyc.,* **Merc.,** *Mez.,* **Puls.,** *Rhus-t., Sep.,* **Zinc.**

Euphr.: **Cann-s., Hep., Nux-v.,** *Spig.*

Ferr.: *Apis,* **Arn., ARS.,** *Carb-v., Chin.,* **HEP., Ip., Puls., Sulph.,** *Sul-ac.,* **Verat.**

Fl-ac.: *Ammc.,* **Calc.,** *Chin.,* **Colch., GRAPH., NIT-AC., Sil.**

Graph.: *Acon., Apis,* **Ars., Bell.,** *Calc.,* **Caust., FL-AC.,** *Guaj., Kali.,* **Lyc.,** *Mag.,* **NAT.,** *Nit-ac.,* **Nux-v., Phos., PULS., Sep.,** *Sil., Sulph.,* **Thuj.,** *Vit.*

Guaj.: *Bry., Graph., Merc.*

Hell.: *Bell.,* **Chin.,** *Phos.*

Hep.: **Ammc., ANT-C.,** *Apis,* **ARS., BELL., Brom.,** *Caust.,* **CHAM., CUPR.,** *Dros.,* **Euphr., FERR.,** *Ign.,* **IOD., LACH.,** *Lyc.,* **MERC., Nit-ac., Rhus-t., Sep., SIL., SPONG.,** *Sulph.,* **Thuj., ZINC.**

Hyos.: **BELL., Cina, Cupr.,** *Op.,* **Ph-ac., Plb., STRAM., Valer., Verat.**

Ign.: *Alum.,* **Arn., Ars., Bism.,** *Calad., Calc., Caps.,* **Carb-v., Caust., CHAM.,** *Cocc.,* **Coff., Cupr.,** *Hep., Ip., Lyc.,* **M-ambo., M-arct., M-aust., Nux-v.,** *Ph-ac.,* **Plat., Puls.,** *Ruta,* **Sel.,** *Stram., Teucr., Valer.,* **ZINC.**

Iod.: *Apis,* **ARS., Bell., Brom., Bry.,** *Calc.,* **Chin., HEP.,** *Kali., Lyc.,* **Merc., Par., Phos.,** *Sil.,* **Spong.,** *Sulph.*

Ip.: **Alum.,** *Ant-c.,* **ANT-T., ARN., ARS.,** *Bry.,* **CALC.,** *Carb-v., Cham.,* **Chin.,** *Cocc.,* **Cupr., Dros., Ferr., Ign., Kali-n., Laur., NUX-V.,** *Op., Phos.,* **Puls.,** *Sul-ac.,* **Verat.**

Kali.: *Apis,* **Ars., Bry., Calc.,** *Carb-v., Cocc., Laur.,* **Lyc., Mag., Nat., Nat-m., NIT-AC.,** *Nux-v.,* **Phos., PULS.,** *Sil.*

Kali-n.: *Calc.,* **Ip.**

Kreos.: *Caust.,* **Nat-m., NUX-V., Sep., Sulph.**

Lach.: *Alum., Apis,* **Ars., BELL.,** *Carb-v.,* **CAUST.,** *Chin.,* **CON., HEP., LYC., MERC., Nux-v., Ph-ac., PLAT., PULS., Stann.,** *Zinc.*

Laur.: **Canth., Ip.,** *Kali., Merc., Spig.*

Led.: **Bry.,** *Dulc., Lyc., Puls.*

Lyc. *Acon.,* **Agar.,** *Alum., Ambr., Ang.,* **Apis, ARS.,** *Bry.,* **CALC., CANTH.,** *Caust.,* **CHAM.,** *Chel., Chin., Cic.,* **Con., Cupr.,** *Euph.,* **Graph.,** *Hep., Ign., Iod.,* **Kali., LACH.,** *Led., Mag-m.,* **Mang.,** *Merc.,* **Mur-ac., NAT.,** Nit-ac., **NUX-V., Petr.,** *Phos., Ph-ac.,* **PULS., Rhus-t., Sep.,** *Sil., Vit.*

M-ambo.: **Ign.,** *Zinc.*

M-arct.: *Bell.,* **Ign., M-aust., Puls., Zinc.**

M-aust: **Ign., M-arct., Nux-v., Zinc.**

Mag.: **Ars.,** *Brom.,* **Cham.,** *Coff.,* **Coloc.,** *Graph.,* **Kali.,** *Mag-m.,* **Nux-v., Puls., Rheum.**

Mag-m.: **Calc.,** *Lyc., Mag., Nux-v.,* **SEP.,** *Sulph.*

Mang.: *Bry.,* **Lyc.,** *Puls*

Meny.: *Asar., Calc., Cann-s., Plat., Sep.*

Merc.: *Acon.,* **ANT-C.,** *Apis, Arg., Arn., Ars.,* **ASAF., Aur., BELL.,** *Bry.,* **Calc., CARB-V., CHIN.,** *Cic., Cina, Clem., Coff., Colch.,* **Cupr.,** *Dig.,* **Dulc., EUPH.,** *Guaj.,* **HEP., Iod., LACH.,** *Laur., Lyc.,* **Mez., NIT-AC.,** *Nux-v.,* **OP.,** *Ph-ac., Plat.,* **Puls.,** *Rheum, Rhod., Rhus-t.,* **Sars.,** *Sel., Sep.,* **Sil., Spig., STAPH., SULPH., Thuj.,** *Valer., Verat., Vit.,* **Zinc.**

Mez.: **Bry.,** *Euph.,* **Merc.,** *Mur-ac.,* **Nit-ac., Rhus-t.,** *Sil., Verb.*

Mill.: **Acon.,** *Apis, Arn.,* **BRY.,** *Chin.,* **NUX-V., PULS., Squil.**

Mosch.: **BELL.,** *Cocc., Coff., Nux-v., Op., Phos.*

Mur-ac.: **Ars., BRY., Lyc.**

Nat.: **CALC.,** *Caust.,* **Graph.,** *Kali.,* **LYC., Nat-m., PULS., Sep.,** *Sil.,* **Spig.,** *Sulph.*

Nat-m.: *Alum., Anac.,* **Ars.,** *Brom., Cann-s.,* **Carb-v., Chin., Kali., Kreos., Nat.,** *Nux-v., Petr.,* **PULS., Ruta,** *Spig., Vit.*

Nit-ac.: *Agar.,* **Asaf., Bell.,** *Bov.,* **CALC., Cann-s.,** *Carb-v.,* **Con.,** Fl-ac., *Graph.,* **HEP., KALI.,** *Lyc.,* **MERC.,** *Mez.,* **PETR., Puls., Rhus-t., SEP.,** *Sulph., Thuj.*

Nux-m.: *Cocc., Ign., Nux-v., Sep.*

Nux-v.: **Acon., AGAR., Ambr.,** *Am-m.,* **ARS.,** *Asar., Aur., Bar-ac.,* **BELL.,** *Calad.,* **CALC.,** *Caps., Carb-v.,* **Caust., CHAM.,** *Chin.,* **Cocc., Coff., Colch.,** *Con.,* **Cupr., Dig.,** *Dros., Dulc.,* **Euphr., Graph.,** *Guaj., Ign.,* **IP.,** *Kali.,* **KREOS., Lach., LYC.,** *M-aust., Mag., Merc.,* **MILL.,** *Mosch., Mur-ac., Nat-m.,* **OP.,** *Par.,* **PETR., PHOS.,** *Plb.,* **Puls., Rheum, RHUS-T., Sel.,** *Sep., Sil.,* **Stram., Sulph., Valer.**

Olnd.: *Cocc.,* **Vit.**

Op.: **Acon., Ant-t., BELL.,** *Brom.,* **CAMPH.,** *Carb-v., Cic.,* **Coff.,** *Colch.,* **Croc., Cupr., Dig.,** *Hyos., Ip.,* **MERC.,** *Mosch.,* **Nux-v.,** *Phos., Ph-ac.,* **PLB.,** *Stram.*

Par.: **Iod.,** *Nux-v., Phos.*

Petr.: *Agar.,* **Ars., Calc.,** *Carb-v., Cham.,* **Lyc.,** *Nat-m.,* **Nit-ac., NUX-V.,** *Phos., Puls.,* **Sil.,** *Sulph.,* **Thuj.**

Phos.: *Acon., Agar., Alum.,* **Ammc., Ars.,** *Aur., Brom.,* **Calc., Caust.,** *Chin., Cina, Dig.,* **Graph.,** *Hell.,* **Iod.,** *Ip.,* **Kali.,** *Lyc., Mosch.,* **NUX-V.,** *Op., Par., Petr.,* **PULS.,** *Sec.,* **Sep.,** *Sil., Stront., Verat., Verb.*

Ph-ac.: *Acon.,* **Ars., Asaf., Bell., Calc., Chin.,** *Cupr.,* **Dig.,** *Dulc.,* **Hyos.,** *Ign.,* **Lach.,** *Lyc., Merc., Op.,* **Rheum,** *Rhus-t.,* **Staph.,** *Verat.,* **Zinc.**

Plat.: *Asaf., Bell.,* **Caust.,** *Croc.,* **Dig., Ign., LACH.,** *Meny., Merc.,* **PLB., PULS.,** *Sabad., Sabin., Stront., Vit.*

Plb.: **Alum., Ars., Bell.,** *Chin., Hyos.,* **Nat-m.,** *Nux-v.,* **OP., PLAT., Stram.,** *Sulph.,* **Sul-ac.**

Puls.: *Acon.,* **Agar., Alum., Ambr.,** *Am-m., Ant-c.,* **Ant-t., Apis, Arn., Asaf., Aur., BELL., BRY., Calc.,** *Cann-s.,* **CANTH.,** *Caps.,* **Carb-v., Caust., CHAM.,** *Chel.,* **Chin., Coff., Colch., Con., CUPR., Cycl., Dig.,** *Dulc.,* **Euph., Ferr., GRAPH.,** *Ign., Ip.,* **KALI., LACH.,** *Led.,* **LYC.,** *M-arct., Mag., Mang., Merc.,* **MILL., NAT., NAT-M., NIT-AC., Nux-v.,** *Petr.,* **Phos., PLAT., Ran-b.,** *Rheum,* **Rhus-t., Sabad., SEP., Sil.,** *Spig.,* **STANN.,** *Sulph.,* **SEC.,** *Valer., Verb., Vit.*

Ran-b.: **Bry., Puls.,** *Sulph., Staph., Verb.*

Ran-s.: *Ars., Puls., Verat.*

Rheum.: **Bell., Cham., Coloc.,** *Mag.,* **Merc., NUX-V., Ph-ac., Puls.**

Rhod.: **BRY.,** *Calc., Carb-an., Carb-v.,* **Caust., CLEM.,** *Merc., Nux-v.,* **RHUS-T.,** *Sep.*

Rhus-t.: **ACON.**, *Am-m.*, **Ang.**, *Arn.*, **ARS.**, **Bell.**, **BRY.**, **Calc.**, **Caust.**, *Cham.*, *Cic.*, **Clem.**, **Coff.**, *Dulc.*, *Euph.*, **Hep.**, **Lyc.**, *Merc.*, **Mez.**, *Nit-ac.*, **NUX-V.**, *Phos.*, *Ph-ac.*, **Puls.**, **RHOD.**, *Samb.*, **SEP.**, *Sil.*, **Sulph.**, *Verat.*

Ruta: *Ign.*, **Nat-m.**

Sabad.: *Plat.*, **Puls.**

Sabin.: *Arn.*, *Calc.*, *Plat.*

Samb.: *Arn.*, **Ars.**, *Chin.*, *Rhus-t.*

Sars.: *Bell.*, **CALC.**, *Merc.*, **Sulph.**

Sec.: *Ammc.*, **Ars.**, **Bell.**, **Coloc.**, *Phos.*, *Verat.*

Sel.: **ALUM.**, **Bry.**, **Bov.**, **Calc.**, **Ign.**, *Merc.*, **Nux-v.**, **Puls.**, **Sep.**, *Sulph.*, *Thuj.*

Seneg.: **Arn.**, **Bell.**, **Bry.**, *Stann.*

Sep.: **ACON.**, *Agar.*, *Ant-c.*, **Ant-t.**, *Apis*, **Ars.**, *Asaf.*, *Bar-c.*, **BELL.**, *Bry.*, **Calc.**, *Carb-v.*, **CAUST.**, **CHIN.**, *Clem.*, *Cupr.*, *Dros.*, **Dulc.**, *Euph.*, **Graph.**, **Hep.**, **Kreos.**, **Lyc.**, **MAG-M.**, *Meny.*, *Merc.*, **Nat.**, **NIT-AC.**, *Nux-v.*, **Phos.**, **PULS.**, *Rhod.*, **RHUS-T.**, *Sel.*, **SIL.**, **SULPH.**, *Verat.*, *Vit.*

Sil.: **Agar.**, *Ars.*, *Bell.*, **Borx.**, **CALC.**, **Caust.**, *Cupr.*, **Fl-ac.**, *Graph.*, **HEP.**, *Iod.*, *Kali.*, *Lyc.*, **Merc.**, *Mez.*, *Nat.*, *Nux-v.*, **Petr.**, *Phos.*, *Puls.*, *Rhus-t.*, **SEP.**, **Staph.**, *Sulph.*

Spig.: *Bism.*, *Dig.*, *Euph.*, *Laur.*, **Merc.**, **Nat.**, ***Nat-m.***, ***Puls.***, ***Verat.***

Spong.: **Brom.**, **Dros.**, **HEP.**, *Iod.*

Squil.: **Arn.**, **Ars.**, *Bry.*, **Mill.**

Stann.: *Ars.*, *Chin.*, **Lach.**, **PULS.**, *Seneg.*, *Sulph.*, *Valer.*

Staph.: **Ars.**, *Bism.*, **COLOC.**, **Merc.**, **Ph-ac.**, *Ran-b.*, **Sil.**, *Sulph.*, *Thuj.*

Stram.: **Bell.**, ***Cham.***, *Cic.*, *Hell.*, **HYOS.**, *Ign.*, **Nux-v.**, *Op.*, **Plb.**, **Verat.**

Stront.: *Phos.*, *Plat.*, *Sulph.*

Sulph.: *Acon.*, *Ambr.*, *Ant-c.*, **Apis.**, **ARS.**, *Bell.*, *Borx.*, **CALC.**, **Carb-v.**, **CAUST.**, **Cham.**, *Chel.*, **Chin.**, *Coff.*, *Dulc.*, **Ferr.**, *Graph.*, *Hep.*, *Iod.*, *Kreos.*, **MERC.**, *Nit-ac.*, **Nux-v.**, *Petr.*, **PULS.**, *Ran-b.*, *Rhus-t.*, *Sars.*, *Sel.*, **SEP.**, *Sil.*, *Stann.*, *Staph.*, *Stront.*, **Thuj.**, **Valer.**, **Vit.**

Sul-ac.: *Ars.*, *Chin.*, *Dig.*, *Ferr.*, *Ip.*, **Plb.**, **PULS.**

Tarent.: *Con.*, *Kali.*, *Puls.*, *Valer.*

Teucr.: *Coff.*, *Ign.*

Thuj.: **Cann-s.**, **CARB-AN.**, **Hep.**, **Graph.**, **Merc.**, **Nit-ac.**, **Petr.**, *Puls.*, *Sel.*, *Staph.*, **Sulph.**

Valer.: *Acon.*, **Bell.**, **Cham.**, **Coff.**, **Hyos.**, *Ign.*, *Merc.*, **Nux-v.**, *Puls.*, *Stann.*, **Sulph.**

Verat.: **Acon.,** *Alum.,* **Arn., Ars.,** *Bry., Calc., Camph., Carb-v.,* **CHIN.,** *Cic.,* **Cina, Coff., CUPR., Dros., Ferr., Hyos., Ip.,** *Merc., Phos., Ph-ac., Sec., Sep., Spig., Stram.*

Verb.: *Ang., Mez., Phos., Puls., Ran-b.*

Viol-o.: *Nux-v., Phos.*

Viol-t.: *Bar-c., Nit-ac., Rhus-t.*

Vit.: *Calc., Con., Graph., Lyc., Merc., Nux-v.,* **Olnd.,** *Puls., Rhod., Sep., Sulph.*

Zinc.: **ARN., BAR-C.,** *Carb-v.,* **Euph., HEP., IGN.,** *Lach.,* **M-ambo., M-arct., M-aust., MERC., Ph-ac.**

■ ■ ■

# LIST OF REMEDY ABBREVIATIONS

# LIST OF REMEDY ABBREVIATIONS

| | |
|---|---|
| | 10 (Paterson)→bacls-10. |
| | 7 (Paterson)→bacls-7. |
| abel. | abelmoschus |
| abies-a. | abies alba |
| abies-c. | abies canadensis |
| abies-n. | abies nigra |
| abrom-a-r. | abroma augusta radix |
| abrom-a. | abroma augusta |
| abrot. | abrotanum |
| abr. | abrus precatorius |
| absintls. | absintalsem |
| absin. | absinthium |
| acac-f. | acacia farnesiana |
| acal. | acalypha indica |
| | acanthia lectularia→cimx. |
| | acanthus mollis→bran. |
| | acarus of the fly; red→trom. |
| acenoc. | acenocoumarol |
| acer-c. | acer campestre |
| acetan. | acetanilidum |
| acetars. | acetarsolum |
| acetaz. | acetazolamide |
| acetontl. | acetonitrilum |
| aceton. | acetonum |
| acetoph. | acetophenonum |
| acetylar. | acetylarsan |
| acetylch-m. | acetylcholinum muriaticum |
| acetyls-ac. | acetylsalicylicum acidum |
| acet-ac. | aceticum acidum |
| | achillea millefolium→mill. |
| achil-m. | achillea moschata |
| achil-n. | achillea nana |
| achil-p. | achillea ptarmica |
| achras | achras sapota |
| achy-a. | achyranthes aspera |
| achy. | achyranthes calea |
| acicl. | aciclovir |
| | acidum ascorbicum→ascor-ac. |
| | acidum benzoicum→benz-ac. |
| | acidum boricum→bor-ac. |
| | acidum butyricum→but-ac. |

| | |
|---|---|
| | acidum hydroiodicum→iod-h. |
| | acidum pantothenicum→pant-ac. |
| | acidum picronitricum→pic-ac. |
| acioa-d. | acioa dewevrei |
| aclad. | acladium castellanii |
| | acokanthera schimperi→car. |
| aconin. | aconitinum |
| acon-ac. | aconiticum acidum |
| acon-a. | aconitum anthora |
| acon-co. | aconitum columbianum |
| acon-c. | aconitum cammarum |
| acon-f. | aconitum ferox |
| acon-l. | aconitum lycoctonum |
| acon-s. | aconitlim septentrionale |
| acon. | aconitum napellus |
| | acorus calamus→calam. |
| acrol. | acroleinum |
| | actaea racemosa→cimic. |
| | actea racemosa→cimic. |
| | actea spicata→act-sp. |
| actinid-ctx. | actinidiae cortex |
| actin-a. | actinomyces albus |
| actin-c. | actinomyces citreus |
| actin-g. | actinomyces griseus |
| actin-l. | actinomyces luteus |
| act-sp. | actaea spicata |
| adam. | adamas |
| adans-d. | adansonia digitata |
| adax. | adaxukah |
| adel. | Adelheid aqua |
| adenin. | adeninum |
| adenyl-ac. | adenylicum acidum |
| | adeps suillus→adeps-s. |
| adeps-s. | adeps suis |
| | adhatoda→just. |
| | adhatoda vasika→just. |
| adiant. | adiantum capillus veneris |
| adlu. | adlumia fungosa |
| | adn→des-ac. |
| adonin. | adonidinum |

| | |
|---|---|
| adon-ae. | adonis aestivalis |
| adon. | adonis vernalis |
| adox. | adoxa moschatellina |
| adp. | adenosinum diphosphoricum acidum |
| | adp→adp. |
| | adrenal cortex→adr-ctx. |
| adren-bt. | adrenalinum bitartaricum |
| adren. | adrenalinum |
| adr-ctx. | adrenalis-cortex |
| | adrenocorticotropinum→cortico. |
| aegle-f. | aegle folia |
| aegle-m. | aegle marmelos |
| aegop-p. | aegopodium podagraria |
| aesc-c. | aesculus cornea |
| aesc-g. | aesculus glabra |
| aesc. | aesculus hippocastanum |
| | aethanolum→alco. |
| aether | aether |
| | aether aethylicus→aether |
| | aether sulphuricus→aether |
| aethi-a. | aethiops antimonialis |
| aethi-m. | aethiops mineralis |
| | aethylicum→aethyl. |
| aethyl-act. | aethylium aceticum |
| aethyl-br. | aethylium bromidum |
| aethyl-m. | aethylium muriaticum |
| aethyl-n. | aethylium nitricum |
| aethyl-s-d. | aethylium sulfuricum dichloratum |
| aethyl-s. | aethylium sulfuricum |
| aethyl. | aethylium |
| | aethylium nitrosum→nit-s-d. |
| aeth. | aethusa cynapium |
| | aethylum aceticum→aethyl-act. |
| | aethylum nitricum→aethyl-n. |
| | aethylum oxidum→aether |
| agap. | agapanthus |
| agarin. | agaricinum |
| agar-ac. | agaricicum acidum |
| | agaricus bulbosus→agar-ph. |
| agar-cit. | agaricus citrinus |
| agar-cpn. | agaricus campanulatus |
| agar-cps. | agaricus campestris |
| agar-em. | agaricus emeticus |
| | agaricus laricis→bol-la. |
| agar-pa. | agaricus pantherinus |
| agar-ph. | agaricus phalloides |

| | |
|---|---|
| agar-pr. | agaricus procerus |
| agar-r. | agaricus rubescens |
| agar-se. | agaricus semiglobatus |
| agar-st. | agaricus stercorarius |
| agar-v. | agaricus vernus |
| agar. | agaricus muscarius |
| agav-a. | agave americana |
| | agave rigida→agav-t. |
| agav-t. | agave tequilana |
| ager-c. | ageratum conyzoides |
| agn. | agnus castus |
| agra. | agraphis nutans |
| agre. | agremone ochroleuca |
| agri. | agrimonia eupatoria |
| | agropyrum repens→tritic. |
| agrosti-a. | agrostis alba |
| agrosti-vg. | agrostis vulgaris |
| agro. | agrostema githago |
| | agrostemna githago→agro. |
| ag-ag. | agar agar |
| aids. | aids nosode |
| | ailanthus altissima→ail. |
| ail. | ailanthus glandulosa |
| aira-fl. | aira flexuosa |
| aju-c. | ajuga chamaepitys |
| aju-r. | ajuga reptans |
| alam. | alamanitra |
| alan-d. | alaninum D |
| alan-l. | alaninum L |
| | alarconia helenoides→wye. |
| album. | albuminum |
| albz-f. | albizzia fastigiata |
| alchem-a. | alchemillia alpina |
| alchem-vg. | alchemilla vulgaris |
| alchor-c. | alchornea cordifolia |
| alco-s. | alcoholus sulphuris |
| alco. | alcoholus |
| aldos. | aldosteron |
| ald. | aldehydum |
| alet. | aletris farinosa |
| | aleurisma canis→aleur-l. |
| | aleurisma castellanii→aclad. |
| aleur-l. | aleurisma lugdunense |
| alf. | alfalfa |
| alh. | alhanodium |
| | alhenna→henna |
| alis-p. | alisma plantago |
| | alkana tinctoria→anch-t. |
| | alkekengi→physal-al. |
| allant. | allantoinum |

| | |
|---|---|
| alliar-o. | alliaria officinalis |
| allox. | alloxanum |
| all-a. | allium ascalonicum |
| all-c. | allium cepa |
| all-f. | allium fallax |
| all-p. | allium porrum |
| all-s. | allium sativum |
| all-u. | allium ursinum |
| all-v. | allium victorialis |
| aln-g. | alnus glutinosa |
| aln. | alnus rubra |
| | alnus serrulata→aln. |
| | aloe ferox→aloe |
| | aloe perryi→aloe |
| aloe | aloe socotrina |
| alop-p. | alopecurus pratensis |
| | alpina officinarum→galan. |
| | alpinia officinarum→galan. |
| | alsidium helminthocorton →helm. |
| | alsine media→stel. |
| alst-b. | alstonia boonei |
| alst-s. | alstonia scholaris |
| alst. | alstonia constricta |
| alth-r. | althaea rosea |
| alth. | althaea officinalis |
| | alumen chronicum→kali-s-chr. |
| | alumen crudum→alumn. |
| alumin-act. | aluminium aceticum |
| alumin-br. | aluminium bromatum |
| | aluminium chloridum→ alumin-m. |
| alumin-gl. | aluminium gluconicum |
| alumin-l. | aluminium lacticum |
| alumin-m. | aluminium muriaticum |
| alumin-o. | aluminium oxydatum |
| alumin-p. | aluminium phosphoricum |
| alumin-s. | aluminium sulfuricum |
| alumin. | aluminium metallicum |
| alumn. | alumen |
| alum-p. | alumina phosphorica |
| alum-sil. | alumina silicata |
| alum. | alumina |
| | aluminium silico-sulpho-calcite→slag |
| | aluminum chloridum→ alumin-m. |
| | amanita bulbosa→agar-ph. |
| aman-c. | amanita citrina |
| | amanita muscaria→agar. |
| | amanita phalloides→agar-ph. |
| aman-r. | amanita rubescens |
| | amanita verna→agar-v. |
| | amara→ign. |
| | amaranthus→amar-h. |
| amary-e. | amaryllis equestris |
| amar-h. | amaranthus hypochondriacus |
| amar-s. | amaranthus spinosus |
| amar-t. | amaranthus tristis |
| ambro-r. | ambrosia chamissonis |
| ambro. | ambrosia artemisiaefolia |
| ambr. | ambra grisea |
| amfep-m. | amfepramonum muriaticum |
| | aminoaceticum acidum→ glyco. |
| | aminobenzene→anil. |
| amgd-p. | amygdalus persica |
| amibe-ac. | aminobenzoicum acidum |
| | aminobenzolum→anil. |
| amicap-ac. | aminocaproicum acidum |
| amidop. | amidopyrinum |
| amisuc-ac. | aminosuccinicum acidum |
| ami-ncap-ac. | amino-n-caproicum acidum |
| | ammoniacum→ammc. |
| | ammonium auricum→aur-fu. |
| | ammonium chloratum→am-m. |
| | ammonium chloridum→am-m. |
| | ammonium hydratum→am-caust. |
| | amoora rohikata→anders. |
| | amoracia→coch. |
| | amp→amp. |
| | amygdala amara→amyg. |
| | amygdala communis dulcis →amyg-d. |
| | amygdalae→tonsi. |
| | amygdalae amarae aqua→ amyg. |
| | amygdalus communis amara →amyg. |
| aml-act. | amylium aceticum |
| aml-ns. | amylenum nitrosum |
| ammc. | ammoniacum gummi |
| ammi-m. | ammi majus |
| ammi-v. | ammi visnaga |
| amm-fml. | ammonium formaldehydum |
| amn-l. | amnii liquor |
| amoeb-h. | amoeba hystolytica |
| amor-r. | amorphophallus riviere |
| ampe-qu. | ampelopsis quinquefolia |

| | |
|---|---|
| ampe-tr. | ampelopsis trifoliata |
| ampe-w. | ampelopsis weitchii |
| amphet-s. | amphetaminum sulfuricum |
| amph. | amphisbaena vermicularis |
| amp. | adenosinum monophosphoricum acidum |
| amyg-d. | amygdalus dulcis |
| amyg. | amygdalus communis |
| amylam. | amylaminum hydrochloricum |
| amyloc-m. | amylocainum muriaticum |
| amyls. | amylase |
| amylu-t. | amylum tritici |
| am-act. | ammonium aceticum |
| am-ar. | ammonium arsenicicum |
| am-be. | ammonium benzoicum |
| am-bi. | ammonium bichromicum |
| am-br. | ammonium bromatum |
| am-caust. | ammonium causticum |
| am-c. | ammonium carbonicum |
| am-f. | ammonium fluoratum |
| am-hox. | ammonium hydroxynum |
| am-i. | ammonium iodatum |
| am-mlb. | ammonium molybdicum |
| am-m. | ammonium muriaticum |
| am-n. | ammonium nitricum |
| am-ox. | ammonium oxalicum |
| am-pic. | ammonium picricum |
| am-p. | ammonium phosphoricum |
| am-sel. | ammonium selenicosum |
| am-s. | ammonium sulfuricum |
| am-t. | ammonium tartaricum |
| am-val. | ammonium valerianicum |
| | amylium nitricum→aml-ns. |
| | amylium nitrosum→aml-ns. |
| am-van. | ammonium vanadinicum |
| anacy-p. | anacyclus pyrethrum |
| anac-oc. | anacardium occidentale |
| anac. | anacardium orientale |
| anagy. | anagyris foetida |
| anag. | anagallis arvensis |
| | anagyroides→cyt-l. |
| | anamirta cocculus→cocc. |
| anans-d. | ananassa domosus |
| anans-s. | ananassa sativa |
| anan. | anantherum muricatum |
| anchi-s. | anchieta salutaris |
| | anchusa italica→anch-o. |
| anch-o. | anchusa officinalis |
| anch-t. | anchusa tinctora |
| | ancistrodon contortrix→cench. |
| | ancistrodon mokeson→cench. |
| ancis-p. | ancistrodon piscivorus |
| | andalusite→alum-sil. |
| anders. | andersonia |
| | andira araroba→chrysar. |
| | andira inermis→geo. |
| androc. | androctonus amoreuxii hebraeus |
| | androctonus amurreuxi hebraeus→androc. |
| | androctonus australis→buth-a. |
| androg-p. | andrographis paniculata |
| | andromeda arborea→oxyd. |
| | andropogon muraticus→anan. |
| | andropogon muricatus→anan. |
| | andropogon nardus→cymbop-n. |
| androp-sn. | andropogon schoenantus |
| | andropogon squarrosus→ anan. |
| androst. | androsteron |
| andr. | androsace lactea |
| | anemone hepatica→hepat. |
| | anemone ludoviciana→puls-n. |
| | anemone montana→puls-m. |
| | anemone nuttaliana→puls-n. |
| | anemone pratensis→puls. |
| | anemone pulsatilla→puls-vg. |
| | anemone pulsatilla→puls. |
| anemps. | anemopsis californica |
| anetho-g. | anetholum graveolens |
| aneur. | aneurinum |
| ane-n. | anemone nemorosa |
| ane-r. | anemone ranunculoides |
| | anethum foeniculum→foen-an. |
| | anethum vulgare→foen-an. |
| ange-ar. | angelica archangelica |
| ange-b. | angelicae brasiliensis |
| ange-s. | angelicae sinensis |
| ange. | angelica atropurpurea |
| | angelicae sinensis radix→ange-s. |
| ango. | angophora lanceolata |
| | anguillae serum→ser-ang. |
| | angustura falsa→bruc. |
| | angustura spuira→bruc. |
| | angustura spuria falsa→bruc. |
| ang. | angustura vera |
| anh. | anhalonium lewinii |
| anil-s. | anilinum sulphuricum |
| anil. | anilinum |
| | anisum pimpinella→pimp-a. |
| anis. | anisum stellatum |

| Abbreviation | Remedy |
|---|---|
| | ankistrodon contortrix→cench. |
| | ankistrodon contortrix mokeson →cench. |
| anona | anona muricata |
| | anona triloba→asim. |
| | antennaria dioica→gnaph. |
| | anthemis pyrethrum→pyre-p. |
| antho. | anthoxanthum odoratum |
| anthraci. | anthracinum |
| anthraco. | anthracokali |
| anthraq. | anthraquinone |
| | anthrakokali→anthraco. |
| anthyl. | anthyllis vulneraria |
| anth. | anthemis nobilis |
| | anthrokokali→anthraco. |
| | antiaris toxicaria→upa-a. |
| | antifebrinum→acetan. |
| | antimonium arsenicicum→ ant-ar. |
| | antimonium chloridum→ant-m. |
| | antimonium sulphuratum aureum→ant-s-aur. |
| | antimonium sulphuratum nigrum→ant-c. |
| antip-sal. | antipyrinum salicylicum |
| antip. | antipyrinum |
| antirr. | antirrhinum majus |
| ant-ac. | antimonium acidum |
| ant-ar. | antimonium arsenicosum |
| ant-c. | antimonium crudum |
| ant-f. | antimonium fluoratum |
| ant-i. | antimonium iodatum |
| ant-met. | antimonium metallicum |
| ant-m. | antimonium muriaticum |
| ant-n. | antimonium nitricum |
| ant-o. | antimonium oxydatum |
| ant-s-aur. | antimonium sulphuratum auratum |
| ant-s-r. | antimonium sulfuratum rubrum |
| ant-t. | antimonium tartaricum |
| aphis | aphis chenopodii glauci |
| aphlo-t. | aphloia theaeformis |
| apiol. | apiolum |
| apis | apis mellifica |
| apisin. | apisinum |
| | apium petroselinum→petros. |
| | apium virus→apisin. |
| apoc-a. | apocynum androsaemifolium |
| apoc. | apocynum cannabinum |
| apom-m. | apomorphinum muriaticum |
| apom. | apomorphinum hydrochloricum |
| ap-d. | apium dulce |
| ap-g. | apium graveolens |
| aqui. | aquilegia vulgaris |
| aq-calc. | aqua calcarea |
| aq-chl. | aqua chlorata |
| | aqua glandium quercus→ querc. |
| aq-mar. | aqua marina |
| aq-pet. | aqua petra |
| aq-pur. | aqua pura |
| | aqua regia→nit-m-ac. |
| | aqua sanicula→sanic. |
| aq-sil. | aqua silicata |
| | aqueous calendula→calen. |
| arab. | arabinosum |
| arag. | aragallus lamberti |
| aral-c. | aralia californica |
| | aralia ginseng→gins. |
| aral-h. | aralia hispida |
| | aralia quinquefolia→gins. |
| aral. | aralia racemosa |
| | aranea avicularia→mygal. |
| aranin. | araninum |
| aran-ix. | aranea ixobola |
| aran-sc. | aranea scinencia |
| aran. | aranea diadema |
| | araneae tela→tela |
| | aranearum tela→tela |
| | araroba→chrysar. |
| | arbor tristis→nyct. |
| arbin. | arbutinum |
| arb-m. | arbutus menziesii |
| arb-u. | arbutus unedo |
| arb. | arbutus andrachne |
| | arbutus uva ursi→uva |
| | arctium lappa→lappa |
| | arctium majus→lappa |
| | arctostaphylos manzanita→ manz. |
| | arctostaphylos uva ursi→ uva |
| ard-l. | ardesius lapis |
| areco-bh. | arecolinum bromhydricum |
| arec. | areca catechu |
| aren-r. | arenaria rubra |
| aren-s. | arenaria serpyllifolia |
| aren. | arenaria glabra |
| arge. | argemone mexicana |

| | |
|---|---|
| argin. | argininum |
| argon | argon |
| arg-act. | argentum aceticum |
| arg-ars. | argentum arsenicicum |
| | argentum chloratum→arg-mur. |
| arg-br. | argentum bromaturn |
| arg-col. | argentum colloidale |
| arg-cy. | argentum cyanatum |
| arg-f. | argentum fluoratum |
| arg-i. | argentum iodatum |
| arg-met. | argentum metallicum |
| arg-mur. | argentum muriaticum |
| arg-n. | argentum nitricum |
| arg-o. | argentum oxydatum |
| arg-pr. | argentum proteinatum |
| arg-p. | argentum phosphoricum |
| arg-s. | argenturn sulfuricurn |
| | argilla→alum. |
| arg-vi. | argentum vitellinicum |
| arion | arion empiricorum |
| | arisaema atrorubens→arum-t. |
| aristl. | aristol |
| arist-cl. | aristolochia clematitis |
| arist-cl. | aristolochia colombiana |
| arist-co. | aristolochia colombiana |
| | aristolochia cymbifera→arist-m. |
| | aristolochia infesta→arfst-cl. |
| arist-m. | aristolochia milhomens |
| arist-r. | aristolochia rotunda |
| | aristolochia serpentaria→ serp. |
| | armoracia lapathifolia→coch. |
| | armoracia rusticana→coch. |
| armo-r. | armoracia rusticana |
| | armoracia sativa→coch. |
| arn. | arnica montana |
| | arrhenal→nat-meth-ar. |
| arrh-e. | arrhenaterum elatius |
| ars-ac. | arsenicum acidum |
| ars-br. | arsenicum bromaturn |
| | arsenicum citrinum→ars-s-f. |
| ars-h. | arsenicum hydrogenisatum |
| ars-i. | arsenicum iodatum |
| ars-met. | arsenicum metallicum |
| ars-n. | arsenicum nitricum |
| | arsenicum rubrum→ars-s-r. |
| | arsenicum stibiatum→ant-ar. |
| ars-pyr. | arseno pyrite |
| ars-s-f. | arsenicum sulphuratum flavum |
| ars-s-r. | arsenicum sulphuratum rubrum |
| ars. | arsenicum album |
| | arsenicum tri-iodatum→ars-i. |
| | arsenicum tri-oxidum →ars. |
| | artanthe elongata→mati. |
| | artemisia abrotanum→abrot. |
| | artemisia absinthium→absin. |
| | artemisia cina→cina |
| | artemisia contra→cina |
| art-d. | artemisia dracunculus |
| | artemisia judaica→cina |
| | artemisia maritima→cina |
| art-m. | arternisia mutellina |
| | artemisia selengensis→art-v. |
| art-v. | artemisia vulgaris |
| arum-dru. | arum dracunculus |
| arum-d. | arum dracontium |
| arum-i. | arum italicum |
| arum-m. | arum maculatum |
| | arum seguinum→calad. |
| arum-t. | arum triphyllum |
| | arundo communis→arund-p. |
| arund-d. | arundo donax |
| arund-p. | arundo phragmites |
| arund. | arundo mauritanica |
| asaf. | asa foetida sabad. |
| | asagraea officinalis→sabad. |
| asar-c. | asarum canadense |
| asar-o. | asaram officinale |
| asar. | asarum europaeum |
| | asarum rotundifolium→asar. |
| ascar-1. | ascaris lumbricoides |
| ascor-ac. | ascorbicum acidum |
| asc-cf. | asclepias cordifolia |
| asc-cu. | asclepias currassavica |
| asc-c. | asclepias cornuti |
| | asclepias decumbens→asc-t. |
| | arclepias gigantea→calo. |
| asc-i. | asclepias incarnata |
| | asclepias syriaca→asc-c. |
| asc-t. | asclepias tuberosa |
| | asclepias vincetoxicum→ vince. |
| | ascophyllum nodosum→fuc-n. |
| | ashoka→joan. |
| asim. | asimina triloba |
| ask. | askalabotes laevigatus |
| asparin. | asparaginum |
| aspart-ac. | L-asparticum acidum |
| aspar. | asparagus officinalis |
| | asparticum acidum→aspart-ac. |
| | aspergillus bronchialis→ asperg-fu. |

| | |
|---|---|
| asperg-fl. | aspergillus flavus |
| asperg-fu. | aspergillusfumigatus |
| asperg-n. | aspergillus niger |
| asper. | asperula odorata |
| aspho. | asphodelus albus |
| | aspidium→fil. |
| | aspidium filix mas→fil. |
| | aspidium panna→pann. |
| | aspidosperma quebracho→ queb. |
| | aspirinum→acetyls-ac. |
| aspl-a. | asplenium adiantum nigrum |
| | assaku - hura |
| astac. | astacus fluviatilis |
| astat. | astatinum |
| | asteriacanthion rubens→aster. |
| aster. | asterias rubens |
| astra-ca. | astragalus campestris |
| astra-ci. | astragalus cicer |
| astra-e. | astragalus excapus |
| astra-gl. | astragalus glycyphyllos |
| astra-gu. | astragalus gummifer |
| astra-h. | astragalus Hornii |
| | astragalus Lamberti→oxyt. |
| astra-l. | astragalus legum |
| astra-mo. | astragalus mollissimus |
| astra-m. | astragalus Menziesii |
| ast-a. | aster asper |
| atha. | athamanta oreoselinum |
| atis-r. | atista radix |
| atis. | atista indica |
| atp. | adenosinum triphosphoricum acidum |
| | atp→atp. |
| atra-r. | atrax robustus |
| atri. | atriplex hortensis |
| | atropa belladona→bell. |
| | atropa mandragora→mand. |
| atro-pur. | atropinum purum |
| atro-s. | atropinum sulphuricum |
| atro. | atropinum-pur. + -s. (old abbr.) |
| auc-j. | aucuba japonica |
| aug. | augopora |
| auran. | arurantii cortex |
| | aurantiacum→ant-s-aur. |
| | aurantii cortex→cit-v. |
| | aurantium→cit-v. |
| | aurelia aurita→medus. |
| | aureobasidium→clados-m. |
| aureom. | aureomycinum |
| | aureum→ant-s-aur. |
| | aurum arsenicicum→aur-ar. |
| aur-ar. | aurum arsenicum |
| aur-br. | aurum bromatum |
| | aurum colloidale→aur. |
| aur-cy. | aurum cyanatum |
| aur-fu. | aurum fulminans |
| aur-f. | aurum fluoratum |
| | aurum foliatum→aur. |
| aur-i. | aurum iodatum |
| aur-kcy. | aurum kalicyanatum |
| aur-m-k. | aurum muriaticum kalinatum |
| aur-m-n. | aurum muriaticum natronatum |
| aur-m. | aurum muriaticum |
| | aurum natrium chloratum→ aur-m-n. |
| aur-n-f. | aurum natrum fluoricum |
| aur-n. | aurum nitricum |
| aur-p. | aurum phosphoricum |
| aur-s. | aurum sulphuratum |
| aur-ts-n. | aurum thiosulfuricum - natronatum |
| aur. | aurum metallicum |
| aven-g. | avena germinata |
| aven. | avena sativa |
| | aviaire→tub-a. |
| avic. | avicularia |
| | avocado→pers. |
| | ayahuasca→banis-c. |
| | ayhuasca→banis-c. |
| aza. | azadirachta indica |
| bacch-c. | baccharis crispa |
| bacls-10. | bacillus 10 (Paterson) |
| bacls-7. | bacillus 7 (Paterson) |
| bac-t. | bacillinum testium |
| bac. | bacillinum Burnett |
| | bacillus acidophilus→lactob. |
| | bacillus Calmette-Gu,rin→v-a-b. |
| | bacillus clostridium botulinum →botul. |
| | bacillus Friedl,,nder→mucot. |
| | bacillus leprae→lepr. |
| | bacillus seven (Paterson)→ bacls-7. |
| | bacillus ten (Paterson)→ bacls-10. |
| bad. | badiaga |
| | bahia-pulver→chrysar. |
| baj. | baja |
| ball-f. | ballota foetida |

| | |
|---|---|
| ball-l. | ballota lanata |
| | ballota nigra→ball-f. |
| | balsamodendron myrrha→ myrrha |
| | balsamodendron roxburgii→ myrrha |
| | balsamum copaivae→cop. |
| | balsamum copaivae siccum→ cop. |
| bals-p. | balsamum peruvianum |
| | balsamum toluiferum→bals-t. |
| bals-t. | balsamum tolutanum |
| bamb-a. | bambusa arundinacea |
| | bambusa vulgaris→bamb-a. |
| | banana→musa |
| banis-c. | banisteria caapi |
| bapt-c. | baptisia confusa |
| | baptisia confusa acetica→ bapt-c. |
| bapt. | baptisia tinctoria |
| barbit. | barbital |
| barbr-vg. | barbarea vulgaris |
| | barbiflora→orthos-s. |
| barbu-s. | barbula squarrosa |
| barb. | barbae cyprini ova |
| | barii sulphas→bar-s. |
| | barium aceticum→bar-act. |
| | barium arsenicosum→bar-ar. |
| | barium bromatum→bar-br. |
| | barium calcinatum→bar-cn. |
| | barium carbonicum→bar-c. |
| | barium chloratum→bar-m. |
| | barium fluoricum→bar-f. |
| | barium gluconicum→bar-gl. |
| | barium iodatum→bar-i. |
| | barium nitricum→bar-n. |
| | barium oxydatum→bar-o. |
| | barium phosphoricum→bar-p. |
| | barium sulfuricum→bar-s. |
| | barosma crenata→baros. |
| baros. | barosma crenulatum |
| bart. | Bartfelder aqua |
| bar-act. | baryta acetica |
| bar-ar. | baryta arsenicosa |
| bar-br. | baryta bromata |
| bar-cn. | baryta calcinata |
| bar-c. | baryta carbonica |
| bar-f. | baryta fluorica |
| bar-gl. | baryta gluconica |
| bar-i. | baryta iodata |

| | |
|---|---|
| bar-met. | baryta metallicum |
| bar-m. | baryta muriatica |
| bar-n. | baryta nitrica |
| bar-o. | baryta oxydata |
| bar-p. | baryta phosphorica |
| bar-s. | baryta sulphurica |
| | basaka→just. |
| basal. | basaltic lava |
| basil. | basilicum |
| | bcg→v-a-b. |
| begon-s. | begonia semperflorens |
| | begonia tuberosa→begon-s. |
| bell-p. | bellis perennis |
| bell. | belladonna |
| | benzenum→benzol. |
| benzc. | benzocainum |
| benzl-be. | benzyl benzoicum |
| benzl-br. | benzyl bromatum |
| benzl-c. | benzyl cinnamicum |
| benzn. | benzonaphtolum |
| benzol. | benzolum |
| benzo. | benzoin oderiferum |
| benzq. | benzoquinonum |
| benz-ac. | benzoicum acidum |
| ben-d. | benzinum dinitricum |
| ben-n. | benzinum nitricum |
| ben. | benzinum |
| berbin. | berberinum |
| berb-a. | berberis aquifolium |
| berb. | berberis vulgaris |
| bers-l. | bersama lucens |
| | beryllium chloride→beryl-m. |
| beryl-f. | beryllium fluoridum |
| beryl-m. | beryllium muriaticum |
| beryl-o. | beryllium oxydatum |
| beryl. | beryllium metallicum |
| beta | beta vulgaris |
| beta-m. | beta maritima |
| | beta rapa→beta |
| betin. | betainum muriaticum |
| beto. | betonica aquatica |
| | betonica officinalis→stach. |
| | betonica stachys→stach. |
| betu-p. | betula pubescens |
| betu. | betula alba |
| | betula pendula→betu. |
| | betula verrucosa→betu. |
| bid-b. | bidens bipinnata |
| bid-p. | bidens pilosa |
| | bignonia caroba→jac-c. |

| | |
|---|---|
| | bignonia catalpa→catal. |
| | bignonia copaia→jac-c. |
| | bilinum→fel |
| bilir. | bilirubinum |
| biot. | biotinum |
| | bismithi subsalicylas→bism-sal. |
| bism-c. | bismuthum carbonicum |
| bism-gl. | bismuthum gluconicum |
| bism-i. | bismuthum iodatum |
| bism-met. | bismuthum metallicum |
| bism-m. | bismuthum muriaticum |
| bism-n. | bismuthum nitricum |
| bism-o. | bismuthum oxydatum |
| bism-sal. | bismuthum salicylicum |
| bism-sc. | bismuthum subcarbonicum |
| bism-sg. | bismuthum subgallicum |
| bism-sn. | bismuthum subnitricum |
| bism-sula. | bismuthum sulphuratum |
| bism-val. | bismuthum valerianicum |
| bism. | bismuthum-sn (+ -o.) (old abbr.) |
| | bitis arietans arietans→cloth. |
| bit-ga. | bitis gabonica |
| bix. | bixa orellana |
| blatta-a. | blatta americans |
| blatta-o. | blatta orientalis |
| blum-o. | blumea odorata |
| boerh-d. | boerhaavia diffusa |
| | boerhavia erecta→boerh-h. |
| boerh-h. | boerhavia hirsuta |
| | bofareira→ric. |
| bold. | boldo fragrans |
| bol-ed. | boletus edulis |
| | boletus esculentus→bol-ed. |
| bol-la. | boletus laricis |
| bol-lu. | boletus luridus |
| | boletus pinicola→polyp-p. |
| bol-su. | boletus suaveolens |
| bol-s. | boletus satanas |
| | bolus alba→alum-sil. |
| bomb-chr. | bombyx chrysorrhea |
| | bombyx mori→bomb-chr. |
| bomb-pr. | bombyx processionea |
| bomh. | bomhenia |
| bond. | Bondonneau aqua |
| bop-sc. | bopusia scabra |
| | boracicum acidum→bor-ac. |
| | borago officinalis→borra-o. |
| borra-o. | borrago officinalis |

| | |
|---|---|
| borx. | borax veneta |
| bor-ac. | boricum acidum |
| bor-met. | borium metallicum |
| bosw-c. | boswellia carterii |
| both-a. | bothrops alternatus |
| | bothrops jacara→both. |
| both. | bothrops lanceolatus |
| | bothrops urutu→both. |
| botul. | botulinum |
| | bougainvillea→bougv. |
| bougv. | bougenville |
| | bougmanica→dat-a. |
| | bounafa→ferul. |
| | bovista gigantea→bov. |
| bov. | bovista lycoperdon |
| brach. | brachyglottis repens |
| brad-tact. | bradykinine triacetate |
| brahmi | brahmi |
| bran. | branca ursina |
| | brassica alba→sin-a. |
| brass-c. | brassica campestris |
| brass-e. | brassica eruca |
| brass-n-o. | brassica napus oleifera |
| | brassica nigra→sin-n. |
| brass-o-r. | brassica oleracea rubra |
| brass-o. | brassica oleracea |
| brass-r. | brassica rapa |
| brass. | brassica napus oleifera (old abbr.) |
| | brauneria pallida→echi. |
| | brayera anthelminica→kou. |
| brid-at. | bridelia atroviridis |
| brid-fr. | bridelia ferruginea |
| bril-p. | brillantaisia patula |
| briz-m. | briza media |
| brod-e. | brodiaea elegans |
| bromaz. | bromazepam |
| bromof. | bromoformium |
| brom-ac. | bromium acidum |
| brom-hac. | bromhydricum acidum |
| brom-i. | bromium iodatum |
| brom. | bromium |
| bro-m. | bromus mollis |
| bro-r. | bromus ramosus |
| brucel. | brucella melitensis |
| brucin-n. | brucinum nitricum |
| brucin. | brucinum |
| bruc. | brucea antidysenterica |
| | brugmansia candida→dat-a. |
| brun-vg. | brunella vulgaris |

| | |
|---|---|
| | brunfelsia hopeana→franc. |
| | brunfelsia uniflora→franc. |
| bryo-p. | bryophyllum proliferum |
| bry. | bryonia alba |
| | bryonia dioica→bry. |
| | bryonia laciniosa→baj. |
| | bryophyllum calycinum→kal. |
| | bryophyllum pinnatum→kal. |
| | buchu→baros. |
| bufo | bufo rana |
| bufo-s. | bufo sahytiensis |
| | bufo sahytiensis Mure→bufo-s. |
| | bufo vulgaris→bufo |
| | bufonis saliva→bufo |
| | buku→diosm. |
| bunga-c. | bungarus candidus |
| bung. | bungurus fasciatus |
| buni-e. | bunias erucago |
| buni-o. | bunias orientalis |
| | bunium carvi→caru. |
| bupiv. | bupivacaine |
| bupl-f. | buplevrum falcatum |
| | Burren limestone→limest-b. |
| | bursa pastoris→thlas. |
| buth-af. | buthus afer |
| buth-a. | buthus australis |
| buth-oc. | buthus occitanus |
| but-ac. | butyricum acidum |
| | butyl chloralhydratum→crot-chlol. |
| bux. | buxus sempervirens |
| b-end. | beta endorphine |
| cactin-m. | cactinum mexicanum |
| | cachou→catechu |
| cact. | cactus grandiflorus |
| cac. | cacao |
| | cactus bonplandii→cere-b. |
| | cactus opuntia→opun-v. |
| | cactus selenicereus grandiflorus →cact. |
| | cactus serpentinus→cere-s. |
| cadm-act. | cadmium aceticum |
| cadm-ar. | cadmium arsenicosum |
| cadm-bi. | cadmium bichromatum |
| cadm-br. | cadmium bromatum |
| cadm-calc-f. | cadmium calcarea fluoricum |
| cadm-chl. | cadmium chloratum |
| cadm-chr. | cadmium chromatum |
| cadm-c. | cadmium carbonicum |
| cadm-f. | cadmium fluoratum |
| cadm-gl. | cadmium gluconicum |
| cadm-i. | cadmium iodatum |
| cadm-met. | cadmium metallicum |
| cadm-m. | cadmium muriaticum |
| cadm-n. | cadmium nitricum |
| cadm-o. | cadmium oxydatum |
| cadm-p. | cadmium phosphoricum |
| cadm-sel. | cadn-dum selenicosum |
| cadm-s. | cadmium sulphuratum |
| cael. | caela zacatechichi |
| caesal-b. | caesalpinia bonducella |
| | caesalpinia pulcherrima→poinc-p. |
| caes-m. | caesum chloratum |
| caes. | caesium metallicum |
| | caesum muriaticum→caes-m. |
| | caffeinum→coffin. |
| | cahinca→cain. |
| | cahinca racemosa→cain. |
| cain. | cainca |
| cajan. | cajanus cajan |
| caj. | cajuputum |
| cak-m. | cakile maritima |
| | calabar→phys. |
| calad. | caladium seguinum |
| calag. | calaguala |
| calami-a. | calamintha acinos |
| calami-ch. | calamintha chenopodii |
| calami-cl. | calamintha clinopodium |
| calami-g. | calamintha grandiflora |
| calami-o. | calamintha officinalis |
| calam. | calamus aromaticus |
| calc-act. | calcarea acetica |
| calc-ar. | calcarea arsenicosa |
| | calcarea biliaris→cal-bil. |
| calc-br. | calcarea bromata |
| | calcarea carbonica Hahnemanni →calc. |
| | calcarea carbonica ostrearum →calc. |
| calc-caust. | calcarea caustica |
| calc-chln. | calcarea chlorinata |
| | calcarea caustica segini→calc-caust. |
| calc-cit. | calcarea citrica |
| calc-cn. | calcarea calcinata |
| | calcarea fluorata→calc-f. |
| calc-form. | calcarea formicum |
| calc-f. | calcarea fluorica |
| | calcarea fluosilicata→lap-a. |

calc-glp. calcarea glycerophosphorica
calc-glt. calcarea glutamica
calc-gl. calcarea gluconica
calc-hi. calcarea hydriodica
calc-hox. calcarea hydroxidum
calc-hp. calcarea hypophosphorosa
calc-hs. calcarea hyposulfurosa
calc-i. calcarea iodata
calc-lac. calcarea lactica
calc-ln. calcarea lactica natronata
calcarea lactica phosphorica→calc-lp.
calc-1p. calcarea lactophosphorica
calc-met. calcarea metallicum
calc-m. calcarea muriatica
calc-n. calcarea nitrica
calcarea ostrearum→calc.
calc-ox. calcarea oxalica
calc-o-t. calcarea ovi testae
calc-o. calcarea oyxdata
calc-perm. calcarea permanganica
calc-pic. calcarea picrica
calc-pt. calcarea pantothenica
calc-py. calcarea pyrophosphorica
calc-p. calcarea phosphorica
calcarea renalis→cal-ren.
calcarea renalis praeparata→cal-ren.
calc-sil. calcarea silicata
calcarea silicica→calc-sil.
calcarea silico-fluorica→lap-a.
calc-st-s. calcarea stibiato-sulphurata
calc-s. calcarea sulphurica
calcarea sulphurata hahnemanni→hep.
calcarea sulphurata stibiata→calc-st-s.
calc-v. calcarea versaillis
calc. calcarea carbonica
calcii arsenias→calc-ar.
calcii bromidum→calc-br.
calcii chloridum→calc-caust.
calcii lactas→calc-lac.
calcium aceticum→calc-act.
calcium arsenicusum→calc-ar.
calcium bromatum→calc-br.
calcium carbonicum→calc.
calcium causticum→calc-caust.
calcium chloratum→calc-m.
calcium chlorinatum→calc-chln.
calcium citricum→calc-cit.
calcium fluoricum→calc-f.
calcium formicum→calc-form.
calcium glutamicum→calc-glt.
calcium hypophosphoricum→calc-hp.
calcium iodatum→calc-i.
calcium lacticum→calc-lac.
calcium metallicum→calc-met.
calcium ovi testae→calc-o-t.
calcium oxalicum→calc-ox.
calcium oxydatum→calc-o.
calcium phosphoricum→calc-p.
calcium picricum→calc-pic.
calcium silicatum→calc-sil.
calcium stibiato-sulphuratum→calc-st-s.
calcium sulphuricum→calc-s.
calculus urinae→cal-ren.
calen-a. calendula arvensis
calendula cerate→calen.
calen. calendula officinalis
calic. calici virus
calla lily→zant.
callil-1. callilepis laureola
calli-al. calliandra alternans
calli-h. calliandra houstoni
calluna vulgaris→eric-vg.
calocd-d. calocedrus decurrens
caloct-a. calochortus albus
calomel→merc-d.
calo-1. calotropis lactum
calo-p. calotropis procera
calo. calotropis gigantea
calth. caltha palustris
calyc-o. calycanthus occidentalis
calyp-u. calyptridium umbellatum
calys-s. calystegia sepium
cal-bil. calculus biliari
cal-ren-p. calculus renalis phosphorus
cal-ren-u. calculus renalis uricus
cal-ren. calculus renalis
cal-sal. calculus salivarii
camel-j. camelia japonica
camellia sinensis→thea
campan-ra. campanula rapunculus
campan-ro. campanula rotundifolia
campan-t. campanula trachelium

| | |
|---|---|
| campho-m. | camphorosma monspeliaca |
| | camphora monobromata→camph-br. |
| camph-ac. | camphoricum acidum |
| camph-br. | camphora bromata |
| camph-mbr. | camphora monobromata |
| camph. | camphora officinalis |
| | cancer astacus→astac. |
| | cancer fluviatilis→astac. |
| | cancerinum→carc. |
| canch. | canchalagua |
| | candida albicans→moni. |
| cand. | candida parapsilosis |
| canna | canna angustifolia |
| cann-i. | cannabis indica |
| cann-s. | cannabis sativa |
| canthin. | cantharidinum |
| canth. | cantharis vesicatoria |
| cany-d. | canyon dudleya |
| capp-crc. | capparis coriaccea |
| capp-crm. | capparis corymbifera |
| capp-g. | capparis gueinzii |
| | capsella bursa pastoris→thlas. |
| caps-f. | capsicum frutescens |
| caps. | capsicum annuum |
| cara-p. | carapa procera |
| carbam. | carbamazepine |
| | carbamidum→urea-n. |
| | carbo ligni→carb-v. |
| carbmc. | carboxymethylcellulosum |
| carbn-chl. | carboneum chloratum |
| carbn-h. | carboneum hydrogenisatum |
| carbn-o. | carboneum oxygenisatum |
| carbn-s. | carboneum sulphuratum |
| carbn-tm. | carboneum tetramuriaticum |
| carbn. | carboneum |
| carb-ac. | carbolicum acidum |
| carb-an. | carbo animalis |
| | carboneum tetrachloridum→carbn-tm. |
| carb-v. | carbo vegetabilis |
| carc-bl-adp. | carcinosinum bladder adeno papillar |
| | carcinosinum burnett→carc. |
| carc-col-adp. | carcinosinum colon adeno papillar |
| carc-col-ad. | carcinosinum colon adeno |
| | carcinosinum foubister→carc. |
| carc-in. | carcinosinum intestines co. |
| carc-lu-ads. | carcinosinum lung adeno squamous |
| | carcinosinum mammae scirrhus →scir. |
| carc-mel-met. | carconisum melanoma metastitic |
| carc-rec-ad. | carcinosinum rectum adeno |
| carc-st-ad. | carcinosinum stomach adeno |
| carc-st-sc. | carcinosinum stomach scirrhus |
| carc-st. | carcinosinum stomach |
| carc-ut-ad. | carcinosinum uterus adeno |
| carc-ut-p. | carcinosinum uterus papillar |
| carc. | carcinosinum |
| cardamo. | cardamomum |
| cardam-a. | cardamine amara |
| cardam. | cardamine pratensis |
| cardios-h. | cardiospermum halicacabum |
| card-b. | carduus benedictus |
| card-m. | carduus marianus |
| carex-a. | carex arenaria |
| | caria papaya→asim. |
| | carica papaya→asim. |
| carli-a. | carlina acaulis |
| carli-vg. | carlina vulgaris |
| carl. | Carlsbad aqua |
| carnin-m. | carnitinum muriaticum |
| carnin. | carnitinum |
| | caroba→jac-c. |
| caroten. | carotenum |
| carp-b. | carpinus betulus |
| | carthamnus ceriferus→myric. |
| cartl-s. | cartilago suis |
| caru. | carum carvi |
| caryo. | caryophyllus aromaticus |
| cary. | carya alba |
| car. | carissa schimperi |
| | cascara→cas-s. |
| casc. | cascarilla |
| casein. | caseinum |
| | cassia acutifolia→senn. |
| cassia-a. | cassia alata |
| | cassia angustifolia→senn. |
| cassia-f. | cassia fistula |
| cassia-l. | cassia laevigata |
| cassia-m. | cassia medica |
| cassia-o. | cassia occidentalis |
| cassia-s. | cassia sophera |
| cass. | cassada |
| | cassia senna→senn. |
| | cassia sophera→senn. |
| | castalia pudica→nymph. |

| | |
|---|---|
| | castalia speciosa→nymph-a. |
| | castanea sativa→castn-v. |
| caste. | castella texana |
| | castanea vulgaris→castn-v. |
| castm. | castoreum canadense |
| castn-v. | castanea vesca |
| castor-eq. | castor equi |
| cas-s. | cascara sagrada |
| | castoreum muscovitum→castm. |
| | castoreum sibericum→castm. |
| | castoreum sibinicum→castm. |
| catal. | catalpa bignonoides |
| catar. | cataria nepeta |
| catechu | catechu |
| | catharanthus roseus→vinc-r. |
| cauc-l. | caucalis latifolia |
| caul. | caulophyllum thalictroides |
| caust. | causticum |
| | causticum hahnemanni→caust. |
| | Cayenne pepper→caps. |
| | cayratia debilis→cissu-d. |
| cean-tr. | ceanothus thrysiflorus |
| cean. | ceanothus americanus |
| cecr-o. | cecropia obtusa |
| cecr. | cecropia mexicana |
| | cedar incense→calocd-d. |
| cedrus-d. | cedrus deodara |
| cedrus-l. | cedrus libani |
| cedr. | cedron |
| cefur. | cefuroxim |
| celo-t. | celosia trigyna |
| celt. | celtis occidentalis |
| cem. | cement |
| cench. | cenchris contortrix |
| centr-r. | centranthus ruber |
| cent-ca. | centaurea calcitrada |
| cent-cy. | centaurea cyanus |
| cent-j. | centaurea jacea |
| cent-n. | centaurea nigra |
| cent-u. | centaurea umbellate |
| cent. | centaurea tagana |
| | centaurium→canch. |
| | centaurium erythraea→canch. |
| | centella asiatica→hydrc. |
| | cepa→all-c. |
| | cepa vulgaris→all-c. |
| | cephaelis ipecacuanha→ip. |
| cephd-i. | cephalandra indica |
| ceph. | cephalanthus occidentalis |
| cerast-a. | cerastium aquaticum |
| | cerasus padus→prun-p. |
| | cerasus virginia→prun-v. |
| | cerasus vulgaris→prun-cs. |
| | cerato→cerstig-w. |
| cerc-o. | cercis occidentalis |
| cerc-s. | cercis siliquastrum |
| ceref-s. | cerefolium sativum |
| cerev-lg. | cerevisia lager |
| cere-b. | cereus bonplandii |
| cere-s. | cereus serpentinus |
| cerstig-w. | ceratostigma willmottigma |
| | cereus grandiflorus→cact. |
| certhec-t. | ceratotheca triloba |
| cerv. | cervus brasilicus |
| cer-met. | cerium metallicum |
| cer-m. | cerium muriaticum |
| cer-ox. | cerium oxalicum |
| cer-o. | cerium oxydatum |
| cer-s. | cerium sulfuricum |
| | cervus brasilicus campestris→cerv. |
| ces-br. | cesium bromatum |
| ces-hox. | cesium hydroxydum |
| ces-m. | cesium muriaticum |
| ceter-o. | ceterach officinarum |
| ceto. | cetonia aurata |
| cetr. | cetraria islandica |
| | chaerophyllum sativum→ceref-s. |
| chaero-t. | chaerophyllum temolum |
| | chamaecyparis lawsonia→cupre-l. |
| chamae. | chamaedrys |
| | chamaelirium→helon. |
| | chamaelirium carolinianum→helon. |
| | chamaelirium luteum→helon. |
| | chamaerops serrulata→sabal |
| cham. | chamomilla |
| | chamomilla romana→anth. |
| chap. | chaparro amargoso |
| chasm-p. | chasmanthera palmata |
| chaul. | chaulmoogra |
| cheir. | cheiranthus cheiri |
| chelin. | chelidoninum |
| chelo. | chelone glabra |
| chel-g. | chelidonium glaucum |
| chel. | chelidonium majus |

| | |
|---|---|
| chenod-ac. | chenodesoxycholicum acidum |
| | chenopodii glauci aphis→aphis |
| chen-al. | chenopodium album |
| | chenopodium ambrosioides→ chen-a. |
| chen-a. | chenopodium anthelminticum |
| chen-bh. | chenopodium bonus henricus |
| chen-bt. | chenopodium botrys |
| chen-g. | chenopodium glaucum |
| | chenopodium olidum→chen-v. |
| chen-o. | chenopodium opulifolium |
| | chenopodium ugandae→chen-o. |
| chen-vg. | chenopodium vulgare |
| chen-v. | chenopodium vulvaria |
| chim-m. | chimaphila maculata |
| chim-rot. | chimaphila rotundifolia |
| chim. | chimaphila umbellate |
| | China clay→alum-sil. |
| chinid. | chinidinum hydrochloricum |
| chinin-ar. | chininum arsenicosum |
| chinin-brh. | chininum bromhydricum |
| chinin-br. | chininum bromaticum |
| chinin-fcit. | chininum ferri citricum |
| chinin-hcy. | chininum hydrocyanicum |
| chinin-m. | chininum muriaticum |
| chinin-pur. | chininum purum |
| chinin-p. | chininum phosphoricum |
| chinin-sal. | chininum salicylicum |
| chinin-s. | chininum sulphuricum |
| chinin-val. | chininum valerianicum |
| chin-b. | china boliviana |
| chin. | china officinalis |
| | chiococca densifolia→cain. |
| | chiococca racemosa→cain. |
| | chionanthus americans→chion. |
| | chionanthus latifolia→chion. |
| chion. | chionanthus virginica |
| chivx. | chivonex |
| chlam. | chlamydinum |
| | chlora perfoliata→gent-pe. |
| chlf. | chloroformium |
| chlg-p. | chlorogalum pumeriadianum |
| chlol. | chloralum hydratum |
| chlorals. | chloralosum |
| chloramb. | chlorambucil |
| chlorami. | chloraminum |
| chloram. | chloramphenicolum |
| | chlornitrosum acidum → nit-m-ac. |
| chlordia. | chlordiazepoxide |
| chlorns-ac. | chlornitrosum acidum |
| chloroc-w. | chlorocodon whiteii |
| | chloromycetinum→chloram. |
| chlorox. | chloroxylenum |
| chlorpr. | chlorpromazinum |
| chlort. | chlortetracycline |
| chlor. | chlorum |
| chlp. | chlorophyllum |
| choc. | chocolate |
| cholcalc. | cholecalciferolum |
| cholin. | cholinum |
| chol. | cholesterinum |
| chondr-c. | chondrus crispus |
| | chondodendron tomentosa→ pareir. |
| | chondodendron tormentosum→ pareir. |
| chopn. | chopheenee |
| cho. | cholas terrapina |
| | chromium kali sulphuratum→ kali-s-chr. |
| | chromium kaliumsulfuricum→ kali-s-chr. |
| | chrysanthellum indicum→ chrystl. |
| | chrysanthemum→chrysan-m. |
| chrysan-b. | chrysanthemum balsamita |
| chrysan-ci. | chrysanthemum cinerariaefolium |
| chrysan-co. | chrysanthemum coronarium |
| chrysan-m. | chrysanthemum morifolium |
| chrysan. | chrysanthemum leucanthemum |
| chrysar. | chrysarobinum |
| chrystl. | chrysanthellum americanum |
| chrys-ac. | chrysophanicum acidum |
| chr-act. | chromicum aceticum |
| chr-ac. | chromicum acidum |
| chr-ah. | chroniicum anhydridum |
| chr-gl. | chromium gluconicum |
| chr-hox. | chromium hydroxydum |
| chr-met. | chromium metallicum |
| chr-m. | chromium muriaticum |
| chr-o. | chromium oxydatum |
| chr-p. | chromium phosphoricum |
| | chrysanthemum vulgare→ tanac. |
| | chrysanthemum parthenium→ pyre-p. |
| chr-s. | chromium sulphuricum |
| | chrysosporium pannorum→ aleur-1. |

| | |
|---|---|
| cibot-b. | cibotium balantium |
| cice. | cicer arietinum |
| cich. | cichorium intybus |
| cic-m. | cicuta maculata |
| cic. | cicuta virosa |
| cimic. | cimicifuga racemosa |
| cimx. | cimex lectularius |
| cina | cina maritima |
| | cinchona boliviana→chin-b. |
| | cinchona calisaya→chin. |
| | cinchona flava→chin. |
| | cinchona officinalis→chin. |
| | cinchona regia→chin. |
| | cinchona succirubra→chin. |
| cinchop. | cinchophenum |
| cinch. | cinchoninum sulphuricum |
| cine. | cineraria maritima |
| cinnb. | cinnabaris |
| cinnmd-c. | cinnamodendron corticosum |
| cinnm. | cinnamomum ceylanicum |
| cinn-ac. | cinnamicum acidum |
| | cinnamomum camphora→camph. |
| | cinnamomum zeylancium→cinnm. |
| circ-l. | circaea lutetiana |
| cirs-ac. | cirsium acaule |
| cirs-ar. | cirsium arvense |
| cirs-l. | cirsium lanceolatum |
| cisplat. | cisplatina |
| cissa-t. | cissampelos torulosa |
| cissu-c. | cissus cuneifolia |
| cissu-d. | cissus debilis |
| cist. | cistus canadensis |
| citl-vg. | citrullus vulgaris |
| cit-ac. | citricum acidum |
| | citrullus colocynthis→coloc. |
| | citrullus lanatus→cuc-c. |
| | citrus aurantium→cit-v. |
| cit-b. | citrus bergamia |
| | citrus canadensis→cist. |
| cit-d. | citrus decumana |
| cit-l. | citrus limonum |
| | citrus medica→cit-l. |
| cit-p. | citrus paradisi |
| cit-s. | citrus sinensis |
| cit-v. | citrus vulgaris |
| cladon. | cladonia pyxidata |
| cladop. | cladophora rupestris |
| clados-l. | cladosporium lugdunense |

| | |
|---|---|
| clados-m. | cladosporium metanigrum |
| claus-an. | clausena anisata |
| claus-in. | clausena inaequalis |
| | claviceps purpurea→sec. |
| | clematis recta→clem. |
| clem-sax | clematis saxicola |
| clem-vir. | clematis virginiana |
| clem-vit. | clematis vitalba |
| clem. | clematis erecta |
| cleom-g. | cleome gynandra |
| clerod-g. | clerodendron glabrum |
| clerod-i. | clerodendron infortunatum |
| clobaz. | clobazam |
| clomip. | clomipramine |
| | clostridium botulinum→botul. |
| cloth. | clotho arietans |
| cnic-ar. | cnicus arvensis |
| | cnicus benedictus→card-b. |
| coalt. | coaltarum |
| cob-act. | cobaltum aceticum |
| | cobaltum chloratum→cob-m. |
| | cobaltum chloridum→cob-m. |
| cob-col. | cobaltum colloidale |
| cob-f. | cobaltum fluoratum |
| cob-gl. | cobaltum gluconicum |
| cob-i. | cobaltum iodatum |
| cob-m. | cobaltum muriaticum |
| cob-n. | cobaltum nitricum |
| cob-o. | cobaltum oxydatum |
| cob-p. | cobaltum phosphoricum |
| cob-sil. | cobaltum silicatum |
| cob-sula. | cobaltum sulphuratum |
| cob-s. | cobaltum sulfuricum |
| cob. | cobaltum metallicum |
| | cobra corallinus→elaps |
| | cobra nigricolis→naja-n. |
| coca | coca |
| cocain. | cocainum hydrochloricum |
| cocarb. | cocarboxylase |
| coca-c. | coca cola |
| coccal | bacillus Coccal co. (Paterson) |
| | cocainum muriaticum→cocain. |
| | coccal compound (paterson) coccal |
| | coccal co. (paterson)→coccal |
| cocci-i. | coccinia indica |
| cocc-s. | coccinella septempunctata |
| cocc. | cocculus indicus |
| | cocculus platyphylla→pareir. |
| coch-o. | cochlearia officinalis |

| | |
|---|---|
| | cochenille cactus→opun-c. |
| | cochlearia armoracea→coch. |
| coch. | cochlearia armoracia |
| coc-c. | coccus cacti |
| | cochlearia pyrenaica→coch-o. |
| | cochlearia rusticana→coch. |
| codeth. | codethylinum |
| cod-p. | codeinum phosphoricum |
| cod-s. | codeinum sulfuricum |
| cod. | codeinum |
| | coffea arabica→coff. |
| coffin. | coffeinum |
| coff-t. | coffea tosta |
| coff. | coffea cruda |
| | cola acuminata→kola |
| | cola nitida→kola |
| | cola vera→kola |
| colchin. | colchicinum |
| colch. | colchicum aavtumnale |
| coleus-a. | coleus aromaticus |
| coli. | colibacillinum |
| collarg. | collargolum |
| collod. | collodion |
| coll. | collinsonia canadensis |
| colocin. | colocynthinum |
| coloc. | colocynthis |
| | colocynthis citrullus→coloc. |
| | colombo→chasm-p. |
| colos. | colostrum |
| | colubrina→nux-v. |
| | columbine→aqui. |
| colut-a. | colutea arborescens |
| col-met. | columbium metallicum |
| | columbium niobium→niob-met. |
| | columbo→chasm-p. |
| comar-p. | comarum palustre |
| combr-r. | combretum raimbaultii |
| com. | comocladia dentata |
| | conchae praeparatae→calc. |
| conch. | conchiolinum |
| | condurango→cund. |
| cones-bh. | conessinum bromhydricum |
| cones. | conessinum |
| congo-r. | congo red |
| conin-br. | coniinum bromatum |
| conin. | coniinum |
| | coninum→conin. |
| | coninum bromhydricum→conin-br. |
| conr-m. | cornus mas |
| consol-r. | consolida regalis |
| convlm. | convallamarinum |
| convo-a. | convolvulus arvensis |
| convo-d. | convolvulus duartinus |
| | convolvulus purga→jal. |
| | convolvulus scammonia→scam. |
| convo-se. | convolvulus sepium |
| convo-s. | convolvulus stans |
| conv. | convallaria majalis |
| | convolvulus turpenthum→oper. |
| | conyza canadensis→erig. |
| conyz-sm. | conyza sumatrensis |
| conyz-vg. | conyza vulgaris |
| con. | conium maculatum |
| | copahu→cop. |
| | copaifera langdorfii→cop. |
| | copaifera officinalis→cop. |
| coprah | coprah |
| cop. | copaiva officinalis |
| | coqueluchinum→pert. |
| corh. | corallorhiza odontorhiza |
| | cordelistris syphilitica→jac-c. |
| corian-s. | coriandrum sativum |
| cori-m. | coriaria myrtifolia |
| cori-r. | coriaria ruscifolia |
| corla-o. | corallina officinalis |
| corn-a. | cornus alternifolia |
| corn-f. | cornus florida |
| corn-sa. | cornus sanguinea |
| corn-s. | cornus sericea |
| corn. | cornus circinata |
| coron-v. | coronilla varia |
| | corpus luteum→lutin. |
| | cortex gland. adrenalis→adr-ctx. |
| | cortex peruvians→chin. |
| cortico. | corticotropinum |
| cortiso. | cortisonum |
| coryl-a. | corylus avellana |
| cory-b. | corydalis bulbosa |
| cory-c. | corydalis cava |
| cory. | corydalis formosa |
| cor-r. | corallium rubrum |
| | corynanthe yohimbe→yohim. |
| cost-s. | costus spicatus |
| coto | coto |
| cotrim. | cotrimoxazol |

| | | | |
|---|---|---|---|
| cot. | cotyledon umbilicus | cupr-ar. | cuprum arsenicosum |
| | coumarinum→cumin. | cupr-be. | cuprum benzoicum |
| crasp-v. | craspidospermum verticellatum | cupr-br. | cuprum bromatum |
| crass-o. | crassula obliqua | cupr-cy. | cuprum cyanatum |
| crass-r. | crassula rubicunda | cupr-c. | cuprum carbonicum |
| | crataegus laevigata→crat. | cupr-form. | cuprum formicum |
| | crataegus monogyna→crat. | cupr-f. | cuprum fluoratum |
| crats-ce. | craterispermum cerinanthum | cupr-gl. | cuprum gluconicum |
| crat. | crataegus oxyacantha | cupr-hdr. | cuprum hydrargyrum |
| creat-p. | creatinum phosphoricum | cupr-hox. | cuprum hydroxydum |
| creat. | creatinum | cupr-i. | cuprum iodatum |
| | cresolum→kres. | cupr-m. | cuprum muriaticum |
| | cresylolum→kres. | cupr-n. | cuprum nitricum |
| crith-m. | crithmum maritimum | cupr-ox. | cuprum oxalicum |
| croc. | crocus sativus | cupr-o. | cuprum oxydatum nigrum |
| | crocus stigmates→croc. | cupr-pi. | cuprum protoidatum |
| crot-chlol. | croton chloralum | cupr-p. | cuprum phosphoricum |
| crot-c. | crotalus cascavella | cupr-sil. | cuprum silicatum |
| | crotalus durissus→crot-h. | cupr-sula. | cuprum sulphuratum |
| | crotalus terrificus→crot-c. | cupr-s. | cuprum sulphuricum |
| | croton cascarilla→casc. | cupr. | cuprum metallicum |
| | croton chloralhydratum→crot-chlol. | curc-x. | curcuma xanthorrhiza |
| | | curc-z. | curcuma zedoaria |
| crot-f. | croton fulvum | curc. | curcuma javanensis |
| crot-h. | crotalus horridus | | curcuma longa→curc-x. |
| | croton eluteria→casc. | cur. | curare |
| crot-t. | croton tiglium | | cuscus→anan. |
| cryptc. | cryptococcinum | cusc-a. | cuscuta americana |
| cryp. | cryptopinum | cusc-ep. | cuscuta epithymum |
| cten-c. | ctenocephalides canis | cusc-eu. | cuscuta europaea |
| cub. | cubeba officinalis | | cuscuta minor→cusc-ep. |
| | cucumis colocynthis→coloc. | | cusparia febrifuga→ang. |
| cucum-h. | cucumis hirsutus | | cyanhydricum acidum→hydr-ac. |
| cucum-m. | cucumis melo | | |
| cuc-c. | cucurbita citrullus | cyanoc. | cyanocobalaminum |
| cuc-m. | cucurbita maxima | cyath. | cyathula |
| cuc-p. | cucurbita pepo | | cyclamen purpurascens→cycl. |
| culx-p. | culex pipiens | cyclop. | cyclophosphamide |
| culx. | culex musca | cyclosp. | cyclosporinum |
| cumin. | cumarinum | cyclos. | cycloserinum |
| cumn-c. | cuminum cyminum | cycl-n. | cyclamen napolitanum |
| cund. | cundurango | cycl. | cyclamen europaeum |
| | cunila pulegioides→hedeo. | cyd. | cydonia vulgaris |
| cuph. | cuphea viscosissima | cymbop-ci. | cymbopogon citratus |
| cupre-au. | cupressus australis | cymbop-n. | cymbopogon nardus |
| cupre-l. | cupressus lawsoniana | cymin. | cymarinum |
| cupre-n. | cupressus niger | | cynanchum→vince. |
| cupre-s. | cupressus sempervirens | cyna-c. | cynara cardunculus |
| cupr-act. | cuprum aceticum | cyna. | cynara scolymos |
| cupr-am-s. | cuprum ammoniae sulphuricum | cynor. | cynorrhodon |

| | |
|---|---|
| cyno. | cynoglossum officinale |
| cyn-d. | cynodon dactylon |
| | cynosbati→ros-ca. |
| cyper-l. | cyperus longus |
| cyper-o. | cyperus olivaris |
| | cyperus rotundus→cyper-o. |
| cypr. | cypripedium pubescens |
| cyrtop-p. | cyrtopodium punctatum |
| cystein-m. | cysteinum muriaticum |
| cystein. | cysteinum |
| | cystisus laburnum→cyt-l. |
| cysto-f. | cystoseira fibrosa |
| cytid. | cytidinum |
| cytin. | cytisinum |
| cyt-l. | cytisus laburnum |
| | cytisus scoparius→saroth. |
| | daboia→vip-d. |
| dact-g. | dactylis glomerata |
| | dactylopius coccus→coc-c. |
| dam. | damiana |
| | damiana aphrodisiaca→dam. |
| danaz. | danazol |
| daph-l. | daphne laureola |
| daph. | daphne indica |
| | daphne mezereum→mez. |
| | daphne odora→daph. |
| | daphne odorata→daph. |
| datin. | daturinum |
| datis. | datisca cannabina |
| dat-a. | datura arborea |
| dat-f. | datura ferox |
| dat-m. | datura metel |
| dat-s. | datura sanguinea |
| | datura stramonium→stram. |
| dauc-c. | daucus carota |
| | dedleya cymposa→cany-d. |
| delphin-n. | delphinium nudicaule |
| delphin. | delphininum staphysagria |
| | delphinium staphysagria→staph. |
| | delphinum consolida→consol-r. |
| del. | delphinus amazonicus |
| | deltacortisone→predn. |
| dema. | dematium petraeum |
| | denys→tub-d. |
| derm-f. | dermatophagoides farinae |
| derm-p. | dermatophagoides - pteronyssinus |
| der. | derris pinnata |
| desch-f. | deschampsia flexuosa |
| desm-g. | desmodium gangeticum |
| des-ac. | desoxyribonucleicum acidum |
| deut-o. | deuterium oxydatum |
| dexam. | dexamethason |
| dextr. | dextrinum |
| de-s-oestr. | diethylstilboestrolum |
| dhchol-ac. | dehydrocholicum acidum |
| dhcort. | deltahydrocortisone |
| | dextrum lacticum acidum→sarcolac. |
| | diabolus metallorum→stann. |
| | diadema aranea→aran. |
| dh-strept. | dihydrostreptomycine sulfate |
| dianthe-p. | dianthera pectoralis |
| dianthu-c. | dianthus caryophyllus |
| | dianthus superbus→dianthu-f. |
| | diastase→amyls. |
| dianthu-f. | dianthus fimbriatus |
| | dicentra canadensis→cory. |
| diaz. | diazepam |
| | dicentra formosa→cory. |
| dicen-c. | dicentra cucullaria |
| dicha. | dichapetalum |
| diclof. | diclofenac |
| | dictamnus→orig-d. |
| dicoum. | dicoumarolum |
| | dictamus fraxinella→dict. |
| | dieffenbachia seguinum→calad. |
| dict. | dictamnus albus |
| digin. | digitalinum |
| digox. | digitoxinum |
| dig-la. | digitalis lanata |
| dig-lu. | digitalis lutea |
| dig. | digitalis purpurea |
| | dikalii carbonas→kali-c. |
| | dikalii phosphas→kali-p. |
| | dikalii sulphas→kali-s. |
| | dinatrii tartras→nat-tar. |
| | dioscorea paniculata→dios. |
| diosgin. | diosgeninum |
| diosm. | diosma lincaris |
| dios. | dioscorea villosa |
| | diosma crenata→baros. |
| diphtox. | diphterotoxinum |
| diph-b. | bacillus diphteriae |
| | diphteriae bacillus→diph-b. |
| diph-t-tpt. | diphthero-tetano-typho-paratyphoidi |
| diph. | diphtherinum |

| | |
|---|---|
| diplo-t. | diplotaxis tenuifolia |
| dips-s. | dipsacus silvestris |
| dip. | dipodium punctatum |
| | dipterix odorata→tong. |
| dirc. | dirca palustris |
| diss-i. | dissotis incana |
| dithyr. | di-iodo-thyroxinum |
| | dissotis rotundifolia→hetrt-r. |
| ditin. | ditainum |
| docort-act. | deoxycorticosteroni acetas |
| | di-ammonii phospas→am-p. |
| | di-ammonii sulfas→am-s. |
| | dna→des-ac. |
| dol. | dolichos pruriens |
| dopa | dopa |
| dopam-chl. | dopamine chlorhydrate |
| | dorema ammoniacum→ammc. |
| doron-p. | doronicum pardalianches |
| dor. | doryphora decemlineata |
| | doryphora leptinotarsa→dor. |
| dovy-r. | dovyalis rhamnoides |
| doxoc. | doxycycline |
| doxor. | doxorubicine |
| | draconitum foetidum→ictod. |
| | dracunculus vulgaris→arum-dru. |
| drim-g. | drimys granatensis |
| dros-l. | drosera longifolia |
| dros. | drosera rotundifolia |
| drym-cor. | drymaria cordata |
| | drymis winteri→cinnmd-c. |
| | dryopteris filix mas→fil. |
| dryop-i. | dryopteris inaequalis |
| dryop-p. | dryopteris pentheri |
| | DTTAB→diph-t-tpt. |
| | dt-tab.→diph-t-tpt. |
| duboin. | duboisinum |
| dubo-h. | duboisia hopwoodi |
| dubo-m. | duboisia myoporoides |
| dub. | duboisinum + dubo-m. (old abbr.) |
| dudl-c. | dudleya cymposa |
| dulc. | dulcamara |
| durb. | durbital |
| dyspr-met. | dysprosium metallicum |
| | dysenteriae compound (bach) →dys. |
| | dysenteriae (bach)→dys. |
| dyspr-o. | dysprosium oxydatum |
| dys. | bacillus dysenteriae (Bach) |

| | |
|---|---|
| | dys. co. (bach)→dys. |
| eaux | Eaux Bonnes aqua |
| eberth. | eberthinum |
| | ecballium elaterium→elat. |
| echinc. | echinococcinum |
| echinp. | echinops spinosus |
| echit. | echites suberecta |
| echium | echium vulgare |
| echi-p. | echinacea purpurea |
| | echitaminum→ditin. |
| echi. | echinacea angustifolia |
| | eel serum→ser-ang. |
| eich-c. | eichornia crassipes |
| | either→aether |
| eke-me. | ekebergia meyeri |
| elaeo-v. | elaeodendron velutinum |
| elae. | elaeis guineensis |
| elaps | elaps corallinus |
| elat. | elaterium |
| elec. | electricitas |
| elem. | elemuy gauteria |
| eleph-b. | elephantorhiza burchelli |
| | elettaria cardamomum→cardamo. |
| eleut. | eleutherococcus |
| emblc. | embelica officinalis |
| emb-k. | embelia kraussii |
| emb-r. | embelia ribes |
| emb-sc. | embelia schimperi |
| | emeticus→ant-t. |
| emetin-m. | emetinum muriaticum |
| emetin. | emetinum |
| end-s. | endiva sativa |
| | endymion nutans→agra. |
| | entamoeba dysenterica→amoeb-h. |
| | entamoeba hystolytica→amoeb-h. |
| enteroc. | enterococcinum |
| | enterotoxinum→enteroc. |
| eos. | eosinum |
| ephe. | ephedra vulgaris |
| ephin-m. | ephedrinum muriatium |
| | epigaea repens→epig. |
| epig. | epigea repens |
| epih. | epihysterinum |
| epil-a. | epilobium angustifolium |
| epil-h. | epilobium hirsutum |
| epil-s. | epilobium spicatum |
| epil-t. | epilobium tetragonum |

| | | | |
|---|---|---|---|
| epil. | epilobium palustre | ery-a. | eryngium aquaticum |
| | epinephrinum→adren. | ery-c. | eryngium campestre |
| | epiphegus americanus→epiph. | ery-f. | eryngium foetidum |
| epiph. | epiphegus virginiana | ery-m. | eryngium maritimum |
| | epiphysis cerebri→pineal. | | erythroxylon coca→coca |
| epit. | epithalia syphilitica | | escherichia coli→coli. |
| eppa-an. | eppalage anemonaefolia | esch. | eschscholtzia californica |
| equis-a. | equisetum arvense | | escoba amargo→parth. |
| equis-h. | equisetum hyemale | esin-sal. | eserinum salicylicum |
| equis-p. | equisetum palustre | esin. | eserinum |
| equis-v. | equisetum variegatum | esp-g. | espeletia grandiflora |
| eran. | eranthis hymnalis | | esponjilla→luf-op. |
| erb-met. | erbium metallicum | | estrone→foll. |
| erb-o. | erbium oxydatum | | etherum→aether |
| erech. | erechthites hieracifolia | | ethylene-ethenyl-diamine→ lysd. |
| ergocalc. | ergocalciferolum | | ethylicum→aethyl. |
| ergotam-t. | ergotamini tartras | | ethylicum aceticum→aethyl-act. |
| ergotam. | ergotaminum | | ethylicum muriaticum→ aethyl-m. |
| ergot. | ergotinum | | ethylicum nitricum→aethyl-n. |
| eric-ca. | erica carnea | | ethylicum sulfuricum→aethyl-s. |
| eric-ci. | erica cinerea | | ethylicum sulfuricum dichloratum →aethyl-s-d. |
| eric-vg. | erica vulgaris | eucal-r. | eucalyptus rostrata |
| erig-a. | erigeron acris | eucal-t. | eucalyptus tereticorti |
| erig. | erigeron canadense | eucal. | eucalyptus globulus |
| | erinus lobelia→lob-e. | eucl-l. | euclea lanceolata |
| | eriodictyon californicum→ erio. | eucl-n. | euclea natalensis |
| eriog-u. | eriogonum umbellatum | eucol. | eucalyptolum |
| | eriodyction glutinosum→erio. | | eugenia carophyllata→caryo. |
| erios-co. | eriosema cordatum | | eugenia cheken→myrt-ch. |
| erio. | eriodyction californicum | | eugenia jambolana→syzyg. |
| erlan-c. | erlangea cordifolia | eug. | eugenia jambos |
| erod. | erodium cicutarium | | eugenia vulgaris→eug. |
| | eruca alba→sin-a. | | euginia chequen→myrt-ch. |
| | eruca sativa→brass-e. | euonin. | euonyminum |
| erv-e. | ervum ervilia | euon-a. | euonymus atropurpurea |
| erv-l. | ervum lens | euon. | euonymus europaea |
| eryhtrom. | erythromycinum | | euonymus vulgaris→euon. |
| erys-a. | erysimum alliaria | | eupatorium aya-pana→eup-a. |
| | erysimum barbarea→barbr-vg. | | eupatorium satureiaefolium→ gua. |
| erys-c. | erysimum capitatum | | eupatorium triplinerve→eup-a. |
| erys-o. | erysimum officinale | | eupatorium verticullatum→ eup-pur. |
| | erythraea centaurium→canch. | euphr. | euphrasia officinalis |
| | erythraea chilensis→canch. | euph-a. | euphorbia amygdaloides |
| | erythrina corallodendron→ pisc. | euph-cy. | euphorbia cyparissias |
| erythron-p. | erythronium purpurascens | | |
| erythr-ca. | erythrina caffra | | |
| eryth. | erythrinus | | |
| eryt-j. | erythrophlaeum judiciale | | |

| | | | |
|---|---|---|---|
| euph-c. | euphorbia corollate | ferr-am-s. | ferrum ammonium sulfuricum |
| euph-e. | euphorbia esula | | ferrum arsenicicum→ferr-ar. |
| euph-he. | euphorbia heterodoxa | ferr-ar. | ferrum arsenicosum |
| euph-hi. | euphorbia hirta | ferr-br. | ferrum bromatum |
| euph-hl. | euphorbia helioscopa | | ferrum chloratum→ferr-m. |
| euph-hy. | euphorbia hypericifolia | ferr-cit. | ferrum citricum |
| euph-ip. | euphorbia ipecacuanhae | ferr-coll. | ferrum colloidal |
| euph-1. | euphorbia lathyris | ferr-cy. | ferrum cyanatum |
| eilph-m. | euphorbia marginate | ferr-c. | ferrum carbonicum |
| euph-pa. | euphorbia palustris | ferr-form. | ferrum formicum |
| euph-pe. | euphorbia peplus | ferr-f. | ferrum fluoratum |
| euph-pis. | euphorbia pilosa | ferr-gl. | ferrum gluconicum |
| euph-pi. | euphorbia pilulifera | ferr-gp. | ferrum glycero phosphoricum |
| euph-po. | euphorbia polycarpa | ferr-i. | ferrum iodatum |
| euph-pr. | euphorbia prostata | ferr-lac. | ferrum lacticum |
| euph-pu. | euphorbia pulcherrima | ferr-ma. | ferrum magneticum |
| euph-re. | euphorbia resinifera | ferr-m. | ferrum muriaticum |
| euph-sp. | euphorbia splendida | ferr-n. | ferrum nitricum |
| | euphorbia sylvatica→euph-a. | ferr-ox. | ferrum oxalicum |
| euph. | euphorbium officinarum | ferr-o-r. | ferrum oxydatum rubrum |
| eupi. | eupionum | ferr-pern. | ferrum pernitricum |
| eup-a. | eupatorium aromaticum | ferr-pic. | ferrum picricum |
| eup-c. | eupatorium cannabinum | ferr-pm. | ferrum pomatum |
| eup-per. | eupatorium perfoliatum | ferr-prox. | ferrum protoxalatum |
| eup-pur. | eupatorium purpureum | ferr-py. | ferrum pyrophosphoricum |
| | euphrasia rostkoviana→euphr. | ferr-p-h. | ferrum phosphoricum hydricum |
| eur-o. | europium oxydatum | ferr-p. | ferrum phosphoricum |
| | euryangium sumbul→sumb. | ferr-r. | ferrum reductum |
| | euscorpius italicus→scor. | | ferrum sesquichloratum→ferr-m. |
| | euspongia officinalis→spong. | | |
| | evonymus atropurpureus→euon-a. | ferr-sil. | ferrum silicicum |
| | | ferr-si. | ferrum sidereum |
| | evonymus europeus→euon. | ferr-s. | ferrum sulphuricum |
| | evonymus vulgaris→euon. | ferr-t. | ferrum tartaricum |
| | exalginum→metald. | ferr-va | ferrum valerianicum |
| | exogonium purga→jal. | ferr. | ferrum metallicum |
| eys. | eysenhardtia polystachia | | ferula asa foetida→asaf. |
| faba-vg. | faba vulgaris | | ferula communis→ferul. |
| fab. | fabiana imbricata | ferul. | ferula glauca |
| faec. | bacillus Faecalis (Bach) | | ferula moschata→sumb. |
| | faecalis (bach)→faec. | | ferula narthex→asaf. |
| fago. | fagopyrum esculentum | | ferula rubicaulis→ferru-g. |
| fagu. | fagus sylvatica | | ferula scorodosma→asaf. |
| | farfara→tus-fa. | | ferula sumbul→sumb. |
| fasci-h. | fasciola hepatica | fest-e. | festuca elatior |
| fel | fel tauri | fest-r. | festuca rubra |
| fel-s. | fel sui | fibr. | fibrinum |
| | fel tauri depuratum→nat-ch. | | ficaria ranunculoides→ran-fi. |
| ferru-g. | ferrula galbanum | | ficaria verna→ran-fi. |
| ferr-act. | ferrum aceticum | fic-c. | ficus carica |

| | |
|---|---|
| | ficus indica→opun-f. |
| | ficus opuntia→opun-f. |
| fic-r. | ficus religiosa |
| fic-v. | ficus venosa |
| | fiel di piedra→flor-p. |
| fila-1. | filaria loa |
| | filipendula ulmaria→spirae. |
| fil. | filix mas |
| fisc-1. | fiscum laxum |
| | flaveinum→lutin. |
| flav. | flavus |
| fleum-p. | fleum pratense |
| flf. | fluoroformium |
| flor-p. | flor de piedra |
| flos-sol. | flos solis |
| flunit. | flunitrazepam |
| fl-ac. | fluoricum acidum |
| fl-pur. | fluor purum |
| fl-sil-ac. | fluosilicum acidum |
| foenm-g. | foenum graecum |
| foen-an. | foeniculum anethum |
| foen-d. | foeniculum dulce |
| foen. | foeniculum sativum |
| | foeniculum vulgare→foen-an. |
| foll. | folliculinum |
| fol-ac. | folicum acidum |
| formal-. | formalinum |
| form-ac. | formicicum acidum |
| form-n. | formica nigra |
| form. | formica rufa |
| | fragaria elatior→frag. |
| frag. | fragaria vesca |
| fram. | framboesinum |
| | franciscaea uniflora→franc. |
| francm. | francium |
| franc. | franciscea uniflora |
| | frangula→rham-f. |
| franz. | Franzensbad aqua |
| frax-e. | fraxinus excelsior |
| frax-o. | fraxinus ornus |
| frax. | fraxinus americana |
| fruct-f. | fructus fructicosus |
| fruc-m-s. | fructi mixtus sucus |
| | fructus phytolaccae→phyt-b. |
| fuch. | fuchsinum |
| fuc-c. | fucus crispus |
| fuc-n. | fucus nodosus |
| fuc-p. | fucus platycarpus |
| fuc-s. | fucus serratus |
| fuc. | fucus vesiculosus |
| fuli. | fuligo ligni |
| fuma-ac. | fumaricum acidum |
| fum. | fumaria officinalis |
| furf-i. | furfur iritici |
| fus. | fusarium oxysporum |
| gaba | gamma-aminobutyricum acidum |
| gab. | gabbro |
| | gabro→gab. |
| gado-ox. | gadolinium oxalicum |
| gado-o. | gadolinium oxydatum |
| gad. | gadus morrhua |
| gaert. | bacillus Gaertner (Bach) |
| | gaertner (bach)→gaert. |
| galact. | galactosum |
| galan. | galanga |
| gala. | galanthus nivalis |
| | galbanum→ferru-g. |
| galeg. | galega officinalis |
| galeob-lu. | galeobdolon luteum |
| | galeopsis dubia→galeo. |
| | galeopsis grandiflora→galeo. |
| galeo-la. | galeopsis ladanum |
| galeo-n. | galeopsis nodosa |
| galeo. | galeopsis ochroleuca |
| | galeopsis tetrahit→galeo-n. |
| galin. | galinsoga parviflora |
| | galipea cusparia→ang. |
| gali-al. | galium album |
| gali-c. | galium cruciata |
| gali-e. | galium erectum |
| gali-l. | galium luteum |
| | galium mollugo→gali-al. |
| gali-pa. | galium palustre |
| gali-po. | galium porrigens |
| gali. | galium aparine |
| | galium verum→gali-l. |
| galla-q. | galla quercina |
| galla-ti. | galla tinctora |
| galla-tu. | galla turcica |
| galph. | galphimia glauca |
| galv. | galvanismus |
| gal-ac. | gallicum acidum |
| gal-f. | gallium fluoratum |
| gal-met. | gallium metallicum |
| gal-m. | gallium muriaticum |
| gal-o. | gallium oxydatum |
| gal-p. | gallium phosphoricum |
| gal-s. | gallium sulphuricum |
| gamb. | gambogia |

| | |
|---|---|
| | garcinia hanburyi→gamb. |
| | garcinia mortella→gamb. |
| | gardenalum→phenob. |
| gard-t. | gardenia ternifolia |
| | garlic→all-s. |
| gast | Gastein aqua |
| | gaultheria humilis→gaul. |
| gaul. | gaultheria procumbens |
| | gaultheria repens→gaul. |
| geb-k. | gebera kraussii |
| gels. | gelsemium sempervirens |
| | genista scoparia→saroth. |
| genist. | genista tinctoria |
| gent-ac. | gentiana acaulis |
| gent-am. | gentiana amarella |
| gent-ch. | gentiana chirata |
| gent-c. | gentiana cruciata |
| gent-l. | gentiana lutea |
| gent-pe. | gentiana perfoliata |
| gent-pn. | gentiana pneumonanthe |
| gent-pu. | gentiana purpurea |
| | gentiana quinqueflora→gent-q. |
| gent-q. | gentiana quinquefolia |
| | geoffroya inermis→geo. |
| geom. | geomycine |
| geo. | geoffroya vermifuga |
| gerin. | geraninum |
| germ-met. | germanium metallicum |
| ger-i. | geranium inodorum |
| ger-o. | geranium odoratissimum |
| | geranium pusillum→ger. |
| | geranium robertianum→ger-i. |
| ger-r. | geranium rotundifolium |
| ger-s. | geranium sanguineum |
| ger. | geranium maculatum |
| get. | Gettysburg aqua |
| geum | geum rivale |
| geum-m. | geum montanum |
| geum-u. | geum urbanum |
| gilia-c. | gilia capitata |
| gink-b. | ginkgo biloba |
| gins. | ginseng quinquefolium |
| glad-c. | gladiolus communis |
| | glanderinum→hippoz. |
| | glandula adrenalis cortex→adr-ctx. |
| | glandula parathyroidea→parathyr. |
| | glandula parotis→parot. |
| | glandula pinealis→pineal. |

| | |
|---|---|
| | glandula suprarenalis→suprar. |
| | glandula thymus→thym-gl. |
| | glandula thyreoidea→thyr. |
| glam-ch. | glucosamine chlorhydrate |
| glech. | glechoma hederacea |
| | glinicum→med. |
| glob-a. | globularia alypum |
| glon. | glonoinum |
| glor-si. | gloriosa simplex |
| glor-su. | gloriosa superba |
| gluca. | glucagon |
| | glucinium metallicum→beryl. |
| | glucinium muriaticum→beryl-m. |
| | glucinium oxydatum→beryl-o. |
| gluco. | glucosum |
| glucrl. | glucochloral |
| glutam. | glutaminum |
| glutat. | glutathion |
| gluta-ac. | glutamicum acidum |
| gluten | gluten |
| glyco. | glycocollum |
| | glycinum→glyco. |
| glycyr-g. | glycyrrhiza glabra |
| glyc. | glycerinum |
| | glycosmis pentaphylla→atis. |
| | glynicum→med. |
| | gnaphalium dioicum→gnaph. |
| gnaph-l. | gnaphalium leontopodium |
| gnaph-o. | gnaphalium obtusifolium |
| gnaph. | gnaphalium polycephalum |
| | golondrina→euph-po. |
| gomph-f. | gomphocarpus fructicosus |
| | gonococcinum→med. |
| | gonolubus cundurango→cund. |
| gonotox. | gonotoxinum |
| goss-a. | gossypium arboreum |
| goss-h. | gossypium hirsutum |
| goss. | gossypium herbaceum |
| gou-l. | gouania longispicata |
| granit-m. | granitum murvey |
| gran. | granatum |
| | granite murvey→granit-m. |
| graph. | graphites |
| | graphites naturalis→graph. |
| grat. | gratiola officinalis |
| grew-oc. | grewia occidentalis |
| grin-sa. | grindelia subalpina |
| grin. | grindelia robusta |
| | grindelia squarrosa→grin. |

| | |
|---|---|
| gryl-c. | gryllus campestris |
| | guaiacum officinale→guaj. |
| guajol. | guajacolum |
| guaj. | guajacum officinale |
| | guako→gua. |
| guanin-m. | guanidinum muriaticum |
| guanin-n. | guanidinum nitricum |
| guan. | guano australis |
| | guao→com. |
| guare-ce. | guarea cedrata |
| | guaraninum→coffin. |
| guare. | guarea trichiloides |
| guar. | guarana |
| | guarea guidonia→guare. |
| guat-l. | guatteria longifolia |
| guat. | guatteria guameri |
| gua. | guaco |
| | guilandina dioica→gymno. |
| guips. | guipsine |
| guiz-sc. | guizotia scabra |
| | gummi guttae→gamb. |
| | gummi gutti→gamb. |
| gum-l. | gummi laccae |
| gum-t. | gummi tragacanthae |
| gunn-p. | gunnera perpensa |
| gunp. | gunpowder |
| | gutenbergia cordifolia→erlan-c. |
| gymne. | gymnema sylvestre |
| gymno. | gymnocladus canadensis |
| | gymnocladus dioicus→gymno. |
| | gymnocladus distica→gymno. |
| | gynandropsis gynandra→cleom-g. |
| | gynocardia odorata→chaul. |
| gynu-ce. | gynura cernua |
| | gyrotheca tinctoria→lachn. |
| haem. | haematoxylon campechianum |
| haff. | haffkine |
| hafn-met. | hafnium metallicum |
| | hagenia abyssinica→kou. |
| haliae-lc. | haliaeetus leucocephalus |
| hall | Hall aqua |
| halo. | haloperidolum |
| ham. | hamamelis virginiana |
| | hamamelis virginica→ham. |
| haplo-b. | haplopappus bailahuen |
| haro-ma. | haronga madagascariensis |
| haro-pa. | haronga paniculata |
| harp. | harpagophytum procumbens |
| haru-ma. | harungana madagascariensis |

| | |
|---|---|
| hecla | Hecla lava |
| hedeo. | hedeoma pulegioides |
| hedyos-a. | hedyosmum arborescens |
| hedy. | hedysarum ildefonsianum |
| hed. | hedera helix |
| | hedysarum capitatum→onob-s. |
| hein-cr. | heinsia crinita |
| | helianthemum canadense→cist. |
| | helianthemum vulgare→flos-sol. |
| helia-t. | helianthus tuberosus |
| helia. | helianthus annuus |
| helich-s. | helichrysum staechas |
| | helios→sol |
| helin. | heloninum |
| helio-eu. | heliotropium europaeum |
| helio-i. | heliotropium indicum |
| helio. | heliotropium peruvianum |
| helium | helium |
| heli-n. | helianthemum nummularium |
| hell-f. | helleborus foetidus |
| hell-o. | helleborus orientalis |
| hell-t. | helleborus trifolius |
| hell-v. | helleborus viridis |
| hell. | helleborus niger |
| helmi-e. | helminthia echioides |
| helm. | helminthochortos |
| heln-ov. | helinus ovata |
| helon. | helonias dioica |
| helo-h. | heloderma horridum |
| helo-s. | heloderma suspectum |
| helo. | heloderma-h. + -s. (old abbr.) |
| helx-p. | helix pomatia |
| helx. | helix tosta |
| | helonias viridis→verat-v. |
| hemidsm. | hemidesmus indica |
| henna | henna |
| heparin. | heparinum |
| | hepar sulphuris→hep. |
| | hepar sulphuris calcareum→hep. |
| | hepar sulphuris kalinum→kali-sula. |
| hepat. | hepatica triloba |
| hep. | hepar sulphur |
| | hepatica nobilis→hepat. |
| hera. | heracleum sphondylium |
| herna-p. | hernandia pellata |
| hern-g. | herniaria glabra |

| | |
|---|---|
| hesp-m. | hesperis matronalis |
| hetrt-r. | heterotis rotundifolia |
| heuch. | heuchera americana |
| hev-b. | hevea brasiliensis |
| hexachl. | hexachlorophenum |
| | hibiscus abelmoschus→abel. |
| hf-sil-ac. | hydrofluo-silicicum acidum |
| hib-a. | hibiscus arboreus |
| hib-sa. | hibiscus sabdariffa |
| hib-su. | hibiscus surattensis |
| hier-p. | hieracium pilosella |
| hier-u. | hieracium umbellatum |
| hippea-e. | hippeastrum equestre |
| | hippomane mancinella→manc. |
| hippop-r. | hippophae rhamnoides |
| hippoz. | hippozaeninum |
| hipp. | hippomanes |
| hip-ac. | hippuricum acidum |
| hir. | hirudo medicinalis |
| histid-m. | histidinum muriaticum |
| histid. | histidinum |
| hist-m. | histaminum muriaticum |
| hist. | histaminum |
| | histrix prehensilis→sphing. |
| | histrix subspinosum→sphing. |
| | hoang-nan→strych-g. |
| hoit. | hoitzia coccinea |
| | holarrhena antidysenterica→kurch. |
| holc-l. | holcus lanatus |
| holm-met. | holmium metallicum |
| holm-o. | holmium oxydatum |
| home. | homeria collina |
| hom-g. | homarus gammarus |
| hom. | homarus |
| | hoorali→cur. |
| hordeum-g. | hordeum semen germinatum |
| hordeum-m. | hordeum murinum |
| hordeum-vg. | hordeum vulgare |
| hordin-s. | hordeninum sulfuricum |
| | hormoflaveinum→progest. |
| hott-p. | hottonia palustris |
| | hubertia ambavilla→senec-abv. |
| | humulus lupulus→lup. |
| hphos-ac. | hypophosphorum acidum |
| hume. | humea elegans |
| hura | hura brasiliensis |

| | |
|---|---|
| hura-c. | hura crepitans |
| hyalur. | hyaluronidase |
| hydn-r. | hydnum repandum |
| | hydrangea frutescens→hydrang. |
| | hydrargyri bichloridum→merc-c. |
| | hydrargyri bijodidum→merc-i-r. |
| | hydrargyri cyanidum→merc-cy. |
| | hydrargyri lactas→merc-lac. |
| | hydrargyri oxycyanidum→merc-o-cy. |
| | hydrargyri oxydum flavum→merc-o-f. |
| | hydrargyri oxydum rubrum→merc-pr-r. |
| | hydrargyri oxydum subsulphuricum→merc-sul. |
| | hydrargyri subchloridum mite→ merc-d. |
| | hydrargyrum bijodatum rubrum →merc-i-r. |
| | hydrargyrum depuratum→merc. |
| | hydrargyrum lacticum→merc-lac. |
| | hydrargyrum sulfuratum→aethi-m. |
| | hydrargyrum sulphuratum nigrum→aethi-m. |
| | hydratum→am-caust. |
| hydrang. | hydrangea arborescens |
| | hydrochloricum→amylam. |
| hydraz-m. | hydrazinum muriaticum |
| hydrc. | hydrocotyle asiatica |
| hydrinin-m. | hydrastininum muriaticum |
| hydrinin-s. | hydrastininum sulphuricum |
| hydrin-m. | hydrastinum muriaticum |
| hydrin-pur. | hydrastinum purum |
| hydrin-s. | hydrastinum sulphuricum |
| hydrobr-ac. | hydrobromicum acidum |
| hydrochl-ac. | hydrochloridum acidum |
| | hydrofluoricum acidum→fl-ac. |
| hydrocort. | hydrocortisone |
| hydrog. | hydrogenium |
| hydroph. | hydrophis cyanocinctus |
| | hydrophobinum→lyss. |
| | hydrophyllum virginianum→hydro-v. |

| | |
|---|---|
| | hydropiper→polyg-h. |
| hydroq. | hydroquinone |
| hydroxp. | hydroxyproline |
| hydroxq. | hydroxyquinoleine |
| hydro-v. | hydrophyllum virginicum |
| hydr-ac. | hydrocyanicum acidum |
| hydr. | hydrastis canadensis |
| | hygrophila spinosa→hygroph-s. |
| hygroph-aur. | hygrophilia auriculata |
| hygroph-s. | hygrophilia sphinosa |
| hymen-ac. | hymenocardia acida |
| hymos. | hymosa |
| hyosin-hbr. | hyosciaminum hydrobromatum |
| hyosin-s. | hyosciaminum sulphatum |
| hyosin. | hyosciaminum-s. + -hbr. (old abbr.) |
| | hyosciamus niger → hyos. |
| | hyoscinum bromatum→scopin. |
| | hyoscinum bromhydricum scopin-hbr. |
| | hyoscyaminum hydrobromatum →hyosin-hbr. |
| | hyoscyaminum sulphatum→hyosin-s. |
| hyos. | hyoscyamus niger |
| hyper-ac. | hypericum acutum |
| hyper-aet. | hypericum aethiopicum |
| hyper-m. | hypericum maculatum |
| hyper-pu. | hypericum pulchrum |
| hyper-q. | hypericum quadrangulum |
| hyper. | hypericum perforatum |
| | hypericum tetrapterum→hyper-ac. |
| hypoes-t. | hypoestes triflora |
| hypop-m. | hypopitis multiflora |
| | hypophysinum→pituin. |
| | hypophysis anterior→pitu-a. |
| | hypophysis cerebri→pitu-gl. |
| | hypophysis glandula→pitu-gl. |
| | hypophysis posterior→pitu-p. |
| hypoth. | hypothalamus |
| hypo. | hypophyllum sanguineum |
| | hypothalamus of the ox→hypoth. |
| hypt-p. | hyptis pectinata |
| hypt-s. | hyptis suaveolens |
| hyss-o. | hyssopus officinalis |
| iber. | iberis amara |
| ibo. | iboga |
| | iboza riparia→tetrad-r. |
| ibupr. | ibuprofen |
| | ichthyolammonium→ichth. |
| ichth. | ichthyolum |
| | ichthyotoxinum→ser-ang. |
| ictod. | ictodes foetida |
| ign. | ignatia amara |
| | ikshugandha→trib. |
| ihydr-ac. | iodhydricum acidum |
| ille. | illecebrum verticillatum |
| ilx-a. | ilex aquifolium |
| | ilex cassine→ilx-c. |
| | ilex paraguariensis→mate |
| ilx-c. | ilex casseine |
| ilx-v. | ilex vomitoria |
| | illicium anisatum→anis. |
| | illicium stellatum→anis. |
| | illicium verum→anis. |
| impa-b. | impatiens balsamina |
| impa-g. | impatiens glandulifera |
| impa-n. | impatiens noli tangere |
| | impatiens pendulifera→impa-n. |
| imp. | imperatoria ostruthium |
| | imperatoria peucedanum→imp. |
| indgf-a. | indigofera atriceps |
| indg. | indigo tinctoria |
| | indigofera tinctoria→indg. |
| indol. | indolum |
| indom. | indometacine |
| ind. | indium metallicum |
| influ. | influenzinum |
| ing. | ingluvin |
| inos. | inositol |
| ins. | insulinum |
| interf. | interferon alpha leucocytaire |
| | inula conyza→conyz-vg. |
| inulin. | inulinum |
| inul-d. | inula dysenterica |
| inul-g. | inula graveolens |
| | inula squarrosa→conyz-vg. |
| inul-p. | inula pulicaria |
| inul-v. | inula viscosa |
| inul. | inula helenium |
| iodof. | iodoformium |
| iod-act. | iodium aceticum |

| | |
|---|---|
| iod-br. | iodium bromatum |
| iod-h. | iodium hydrogenisatum |
| iod-m. | iodium muriaticum |
| iod. | iodium |
| | iodium purum→iod. |
| | iodoformum→iodof. |
| | iodothyrinum→thyroiod. |
| ipat. | ipatropium |
| | ipeca→ip. |
| ipom-f. | ipomoea ficifolia |
| | ipomea purga→jal. |
| | ipomea turpenthum→oper. |
| | ipomoea bona-nox→convo-d. |
| ipom-p. | ipomoea purpurea |
| ip. | ipecacuanha |
| | ipomoea stans→convo-s. |
| irid-met. | iridium metallicum |
| irid-m. | iridium muriaticum |
| iris | iris versicolor |
| irisin. | irisinum |
| iris-fa. | iris factissima |
| iris-fl. | iris florentina |
| iris-foe. | iris foetidissima |
| iris-g. | iris germanica |
| | iris minor→iris-t. |
| iris-h. | iris harwegii |
| iris-ps. | iris pseudacorus |
| iris-pu. | iris pumila |
| iris-t. | iris tenax |
| ison. | isoniazide |
| isop. | isoprenaline |
| itu | itu |
| ix. | ixodes |
| jab. | jaborandi |
| | jacaranda braziliensis→jac-c. |
| jac-c. | jacaranda caroba |
| jac-g. | jacaranda gualandai |
| | jacaranda procera→jac-c. |
| | jacea→viol-t. |
| jal. | jalapa |
| | jambos eugenia→eug. |
| | jambosa vulgaris→eug. |
| | janosia→joan. |
| | jararaca→both. |
| | jararacussu→both. |
| jasm. | jasminum officinale |
| | jateorrhiza palmata→chasm-p. |
| jatr-c. | jatropha curcas |

| | |
|---|---|
| jatr-g. | jatropha gossypifolia |
| | jatropha manihot→cass. |
| jatr-u. | jatropha urens |
| | jatrorrhiza palmata→chasm-p. |
| | jenosia ashoka→joan. |
| | jequirity→abr. |
| joan. | joanesia asoca |
| | jodium→iod. |
| | jonosia asoka→joan. |
| jugin. | juglandin |
| | juglans cathartica→jug-c. |
| jug-c. | juglans cinerea |
| jug-r. | juglans regia |
| | juncus communis→junc-e. |
| junc-e. | juncus effusus |
| junc-p. | juncus pilosus |
| juni-c. | juniperus communis |
| juni-o. | juniperus oxycedrus |
| juni-p. | juniperus phoenicea |
| | juniperus sabina→sabin. |
| juni-v. | juniperus virginiana |
| | juniperus virginianus→juni-v. |
| just-r. | justicia rubrum |
| just. | justicia adhatoda |
| | justicia cydoniifolia→just. |
| | justicia paniculata→androg-p. |
| kalag. | kalagua |
| | kali hydriodicum→kali-i. |
| | kali silicatum→kali-sil. |
| | kalii acetas→kali-act. |
| | kalii antimoniotartras→ant-t. |
| | kalii bichromas→kali-bi. |
| | kalii chromas→kali-chr. |
| | kalii nitras→kali-n. |
| | kalii permangas→kali-perm. |
| kalium-ns. | kalium nitrosum |
| kali-act. | kalium aceticum |
| kali-ar. | kalium arsenicosum |
| kali-asp. | kalium asparticum |
| kali-aur-cy. | kalium auro-cyanatum |
| kali-biox. | kalium bioxalicum |
| kali-bit. | kalium bitartaricum |
| kali-bi. | kalium bichromicum |
| kali-br. | kalium bromatum |
| kali-b-t. | kalium borotartaricum |
| kali-caust. | kalium causticum |
| kali-chls. | kalium chlorosum |
| kali-chl. | kalium chloricum |

| | |
|---|---|
| kali-chr. | kalium chromicum |
| | kalium chromicum sulphuricum →kali-s-chr. |
| kali-cit. | kalium citricum |
| kali-cy. | kalium cyanatum |
| kali-c. | kalium carbonicum |
| kali-fcy. | kalium ferrocyanatum |
| kali-form. | kalium formicum |
| kali-f. | kalium fluoratum |
| kali-gl. | kalium gluconicum |
| kali-hox. | kalium hydroxydum |
| | kalium hypermanganicum→ kali-perm. |
| kali-hp. | kalium hypophosphoricum |
| kali-i. | kalium iodatum |
| | kalium iodicum→kali-i. |
| kali-l. | kalium lacticum |
| | kalium manganicum→kali-perm. |
| kali-met. | kalium metallicum |
| kali-m. | kalium muriaticum |
| kali-nat-t. | kalium natrum tartaricum |
| kali-n. | kalium nitricum |
| kali-ox. | kalium oxalicum |
| kali-o. | kalium oxydatum |
| kali-perchl. | kaliurn perchloricum |
| kali-perm. | kalium permanganatum |
| kali-picn. | kalium picronitricum |
| kali-pic. | kalium picricum |
| kali-p. | kalium phosphoricum |
| kali-sal. | kalium salicylicum |
| kali-sil. | kalium silicicum |
| kali-sula. | kaliurn sulphuratum |
| kali-sulo. | kalium sulphurosum |
| kali-s-chr. | kalium sulphuricum chromicum |
| kali-s-cy. | kalium sulfocyanicum |
| kali-s. | kalium sulphuricum |
| kali-tcy. | kalium thiocyanatum |
| kali-tel. | kalium telluricum |
| kali-t. | kalium tartaricum |
| kali-x. | kalium xanthogenicum |
| kalm. | kalmia latifolia |
| kal. | kalanchoe pinnatum |
| kam. | kamala |
| | kaolinum→alum-sil. |
| kara | karaka |
| | karlsbad aqua→carl. |
| karw-h. | karwinskia humboldtiana |

| | |
|---|---|
| | katipo→lat-k. |
| kaur. | kauri australis |
| | kava-kava→pip-m. |
| | kell→khell. |
| kerose. | kerosenum |
| keroso. | kerosolenum |
| ketogl-ac. | ketoglutaricum acidum |
| khaya-s. | khaya senegalensis |
| khell. | khellin |
| | khilte→khell. |
| | kinkeliba→combr-r. |
| | kino australiense→ango. |
| kino | kino pterocarpi |
| kino-m. | kino malabar |
| kiss. | Kissingen aqua |
| | Klebsiella pneumoniae→ mucot. |
| | kobra→naja |
| kola | kola |
| | koso→kou. |
| kou. | kousso |
| | krameria triandra→rat. |
| krent-1. | krentophyllum lanatum |
| kreos. | kreosotum |
| kres. | kresolum |
| kronth. | Kronthal aqua |
| krypt. | krypton |
| kurch. | kurchi |
| | laburnum anagyroides→cyt-1. |
| | lac defloratum→lac-d. |
| | lac delphinum→lac-dol. |
| | lac equie→lac-e. |
| | lac leonis→lac-leo. |
| | lac vaccini flos→lac-v-f. |
| lacer. | lacerta agilis |
| | lachesis alternatus→both-a. |
| | lachesis lanceolatus→both. |
| lachn. | lachnanthes tinctoria |
| lach. | lachesis mutus |
| lacta-d. | lactarius deliciosus |
| | lacticum acidum dextrum→ sarcoflac. |
| | lactis acidum→lac-ac. |
| | lactis vaccini flos→lac-v-f. |
| lactob. | lactobacillus |
| lactof. | lactoflavinum |
| lactrm. | lactucarium thridace |
| lact-e. | lactuca elongata |

| | |
|---|---|
| lact-sa. | lactuca sativa |
| lact-sc. | lactuca scariola |
| | lactuca silvestris→lact-v. |
| lact-v. | lactuca virosa |
| lact. | lactuca virosa (old abbr.) |
| lac-ac. | lacticum acidum |
| lac-cp-m. | lac caprinum masculinum |
| lac-cp. | lac caprinum |
| lac-c. | lac caninum |
| lac-dol. | lac dolphinum |
| lac-d. | lac vaccinum defloratum |
| lac-e. | lac equinum |
| lac-f. | lac felinum |
| lac-h. | lac humanum |
| lac-leo. | lac leoninum |
| lac-o. | lac ovis |
| lac-pr. | lac primatum |
| lac-sui. | lac suillinum |
| lac-urs. | lac ursinum |
| lac-v-b. | lac vaccinum butyricum |
| lac-v-c. | lac vaccinum coagulatum |
| lac-v-f. | lac vaccinum flos |
| lac-v. | lac vaccinum |
| | Lager beer→cerev-1g. |
| lamin-d. | laminaria digitata |
| | laminaria flexicaulis→lamin-d. |
| lampr-m. | lampranthus multiradiatus |
| | lamium galeobdolon→galeob-lu. |
| lamps-c. | lampsana communis |
| lam-am. | lamium amplexicaule |
| lam-m. | lamium maculatum |
| lam-p. | lamium purpureum |
| lam. | lamium album |
| land. | Landeck aqua |
| lang. | langebrucken aqua |
| lanol. | lanolinum |
| | lantana spinosa→lant-c. |
| lanth-met. | lanthanum metallicum |
| lanth-n. | lanthanum nitricum |
| lanth-o. | lanthanum oxydatum |
| lanth-s. | lanthanum sulfuricum |
| lant-c. | lantana camara |
| lant-t. | lantana trifolia |
| lapa. | lapathum acutum |
| | lapathum sylvestre→lapa. |
| lappa | lappa arctium |
| | lapis granites murvey→granit-m. |
| | lapis marmoreus Connemara→marb-w. |
| | lapis renalis→cal-ren. |
| laps. | lapsana communis |
| lap-a. | lapis albus |
| | lappa major→lappa |
| | lappa minor→lappa |
| | lappa tomentosa→lappa |
| lar-d. | larix decidua |
| lar-e. | larix europaea |
| | lasidora cubana→mygal. |
| | lathyrus cicera→lath. |
| lath-l. | lathyrus latifolius |
| | lathyrus odoratus→lath. |
| lath-sy. | lathyrus sylvestris |
| lath. | lathyrus sativus |
| | latrodectus curassavicus→ther. |
| lat-h. | latrodectus hasselti |
| lat-k. | latrodectus katipo |
| lat-m. | latrodectus mactans |
| lauru-n. | laurus nobilis |
| | laurus benzoin→benzo. |
| | laurus camphora→camph. |
| lauru-p. | laurus persea |
| laur. | laurocerasus |
| | laurus sassafras→sass. |
| | laurustinus→vib-t. |
| | lava heclae→hecla |
| | lava scoriae→hecla |
| lavand-a. | lavandula angustifolia |
| lavand-l. | lavandula latifolia |
| lavand-o. | lavandula officinalis |
| | lavandula spica→lavand-l. |
| | lavandula vera→lavand-a. |
| | lawsonia inermis→henna |
| lec. | lecithinum |
| led. | ledum palustre |
| lem-g. | lemna gibba |
| lem-m. | lemna minor |
| | lens esculenta→erv-l. |
| leont-l. | leonotis leonurus |
| leont-o. | leonotis ovata |
| | leontice thalictroides→caul. |
| | leontopodium alpinum→gnaph-l. |
| leon. | leonurus cardiaca |
| lepi-i. | lepidium iberis |

| | |
|---|---|
| lepi-s. | lepidium sativum |
| | lepidium bonariense |
| lepr. | leprominium |
| leptol-e. | leptolobium elegans |
| | leptilon canadense→erig. |
| leptos-ih. | leptospira ictero-hemorrhagica |
| lept. | leptandra virginica |
| lesp-c. | lespedeza capitata |
| lesp-s. | lespedeza sieboldii |
| leucas-a. | leucas aspera |
| leuca-g. | leucaena glauca |
| | leucantha→bid-b. |
| | leucanthemum parthenium→ pyre-p. |
| | leucanthemum vulgare→ chrysan. |
| leucop. | leucophyllus |
| leuc-d. | leucanthemum discoidum |
| levist. | levisticum officinale |
| levo. | levomepromazinum |
| lev. | Levico aqua |
| liat. | liatris spicata |
| | lichen islandicus→cetr. |
| lich-i. | lichtensteinia interrupta |
| | lignum vitae→guaj. |
| lig-vg. | ligustrum vulgare |
| | Lilium africanum→agap. |
| lil-a. | lilium album |
| | lilium candidum→lil-a. |
| lil-l. | lilium longiflorum |
| lil-m. | lilium martagon |
| lil-s. | lilium superbum |
| lil-t. | lilium tigrinum |
| limest-b. | limestone Burren |
| limx. | limex ater |
| lim. | limulus cyclops |
| lina-e. | linaria elatine |
| lina-sp. | linaria spuria |
| lina-st. | linaria striata |
| lina. | linaria vulgaris |
| lincom. | lincomycine |
| linda. | lindane |
| | lindera benzoin→benzo. |
| | lingusticum levisticum→ levist. |
| linol-ac. | linoleicum acidum |
| linu-c. | linum catharticum |
| linu-u. | linum usitatissimum |
| lipp. | Lippspringe aqua |
| lip-as. | lippia asperifolia |
| lip-c. | lippia citriodora |
| lip. | lippia mexicana |
| | liquor ammoni caustici→am-caust. |
| lir-o. | liriosma ovata |
| | lithii benzoas→lith-be. |
| | lithii carbonas→lith-c. |
| lithosp-a. | lithospermum arvense |
| lith-be. | lithium benzoicum |
| lith-br. | lithium bromatum |
| lith-cit. | lithium citricum |
| lith-c, | lithium carbonicum |
| lith-f. | lithium fluoratum |
| lith-gl. | lithium gluconicum |
| lith-i. | lithium iodatum |
| lith-lac. | lithium lacticum |
| lith-met. | lithium metallicum |
| lith-m. | lithium muriaticum |
| lith-o. | lithium oxydatum |
| lith-p. | lithium phosphoricum |
| lith-sal. | lithium salicylicum |
| lith-s. | lithium sulfuricum |
| | lithospermum officinale→mil-s |
| | lithospermum virginicum→ onos. |
| loa. | loasa tricolor |
| | loa-loa→fila-1. |
| | lobaria pulmonaria→stict. |
| | lobelia coerulea→lob-s. |
| | lobelia glandulosa→lob-s. |
| lobin-m. | lobelinum muriaticum |
| lobin-s. | lobelinum sulfuricum |
| lobin. | lobelinum |
| lobl-m. | lobularia maritima |
| lob-a. | lobelia acetum |
| lob-c. | lobelia cardinalis |
| lob-d. | lobelia dortmanna |
| lob-e. | lobelia erinus |
| lob-p. | lobelia purpurascens |
| lob-s. | lobelia syphilitica |
| lob-u. | lobelia urens |
| lob. | lobelia inflata |
| lol. | loleum temulentum |
| | lolium temulentum→lol. |
| lon-c. | lonicera caprifolium |
| lon-e. | lonicera etrusca |

| | |
|---|---|
| lon-n. | lonicera nigra |
| | lonicera ochroleuca→lon-x. |
| lon-p. | lonicera periclymenum |
| lon-x. | lonicera xylosteum |
| | lophophora williamsii→anh. |
| | lophophytum leandri→flor-p. |
| | lophophytum mirabile→flor-p. |
| | lophophytum spectabile→flor-p. |
| loraz. | lorazepam |
| lormet. | lormetazepam |
| lot-c. | lotus corniculatus |
| loxoc. | loxosceles |
| luc-g. | lucuma glycyphlocum |
| | luesinum→syph. |
| | lueticum→syph. |
| luf-act. | luffa actangula |
| luf-am. | luffa amara |
| luf-b. | luffa bindal |
| luf-op. | luffa operculata |
| luf-s. | luffa sphaerica |
| lumbr-t. | lumbricus terrestris |
| | luminal→phenob. |
| luna | luna |
| lupin. | lupulinum |
| lups-a. | lupinus-albus |
| lup. | lupulus humulus |
| lute-ox. | lutetium oxydatum |
| lutin. | luteinum |
| | luzula pilosa→junc-p. |
| | luzula vernalis→junc-p. |
| | lychnis githago→agro. |
| lyci-b. | lycium barbarum |
| | lycoperdon bovista→bov. |
| lycpr. | lycopersicum esculentum |
| lycps-eu. | lycopus europaeus |
| lycps-v. | lycopus virginicus |
| lycs-ar. | lycopsis arvensis |
| | lycopus aqauticus→lycps-eu. |
| lyc. | lycopodium clavatum |
| | lycosa fasciiventris→tarent. |
| | lycosa tarantula→tarent. |
| lysd-dnp. | lysidinum dinitrophenatum |
| lysd. | lysidinum |
| lysi-r. | lysimachia ruhmeriana |
| lysi-vg. | lysimachia vulgaris |
| lysi. | lysimachia nummularia |
| lyss. | lyssinum |
| lys-m. | lysinum muriaticum |

| | |
|---|---|
| lys. | lysinum |
| | lythrum salicaria→salic-p. |
| | lytta vesicatoria → canth. |
| | 1-dopa→dopa |
| macroz. | macroziama spiralis |
| macro. | macrotinum |
| | macrotys racemosa→cimic. |
| | madar→calo. |
| | madura album→calo. |
| maesa-l. | maesa lanceolata |
| maesa-t. | maesa trichophlebia |
| maeso-f. | maesobotrya floribunda |
| | magenta→fuch. |
| | magistery of bismuth→bism-sn. |
| | magnes artificialis→m-ambo. |
| | magnesia→mag-o. |
| | magnesii citras→mag-cit. |
| | magnesii oxydum→mag-o. |
| | magnesii sulfas→mag-s. |
| magn-gl. | magnolia glauca |
| magn-gr. | magnolia grandiflora |
| mag-act. | magnesium aceticum |
| mag-art. | magnesium artificialis |
| mag-ar. | magnesium arsenicicum |
| mag-bcit. | magnesium borocitricum |
| | magnesium calcinatum→mag-o. |
| mag-br. | magnesium bromatum |
| mag-chl. | magnesium chloricum |
| mag-cit. | magnesium citricum |
| | magnesium fluorosilicatum→ mag-sil-f. |
| mag-c. | magnesium carbonicum |
| mag-form. | magnesium formicum |
| mag-f. | magnesium fluoratum |
| mag-gl. | magnesium gluconicum |
| mag-gp. | magnesium glycerophosphoricum |
| mag-hox. | magnesium hydroxydum |
| mag-hp. | magnesium hypophosphorosum |
| mag-hs. | magnesium hyposulfurosum |
| mag-i. | magnesium iodatum |
| mag-lac. | magnesium lacticum |
| mag-met. | magnesium metallicum |
| mag-m. | magnesium muriaticum |
| mag-n. | magnesium nitricum |
| mag-o. | magnesium oxydatum |
| mag-pox. | magnesium peroxydatum |

| | |
|---|---|
| mag-p. | magnesium phosphoricum |
| mag-sal. | magnesium salicylicum |
| mag-sil-f. | magnesium silicofluoratum |
| mag-sil. | magnesium silicatum |
| mag-s. | magnesium sulphuricum |
| mag-u. | magnesia usta |
| | mahonia aquifolium→berb-a. |
| mah-p. | mahonia palustris |
| | mais→stigm. |
| | majalis→meloe-m. |
| | majeptilum→thiop. |
| | malachite→cupr-c. |
| | malachium aquaticum→ cerast-a. |
| maland. | malandrinum |
| malar. | malaria officinalis |
| malath. | malathion |
| malatox. | malariatoxinum |
| | malleinum→hippoz. |
| | mallotus philippinensis→kam. |
| malus-c. | malus communis |
| malus-d. | malus domestica |
| malus-f. | malus fusca |
| malus-p. | malus pumila |
| malvav-a. | malvaviscus arboreus |
| malva-a. | malva alcea |
| malva-m. | malva moschata |
| malva-p. | malva parviflora |
| malva-s. | malva sylvestris |
| mal-ac. | malicum acidum |
| mamm. | glandula mammalis |
| | mamma glandula→mamm. |
| | manaca→franc. |
| manc. | mancinella |
| mande-ac. | mandelicum acidum |
| mand. | mandragora officinarum |
| | mangana sulfas→mang-s. |
| mangi. | mangifera indica |
| mang-act. | manganum aceticum |
| mang-be. | manganum benzoicum |
| mang-coll. | manganum colloidale |
| mang-c. | manganum carbonicum |
| | manganum dioxydum→ mang-o. |
| mang-f. | manganum fluoratum |
| mang-gl. | manganum gluconicum |
| mang-gp. | manganum glycero phosphoricum |
| mang-i. | manganum iodatum |
| mang-lact. | manganum lacticum |
| mang-met. | manganum metallicum |
| mang-m. | manganurn muriaticum |
| mang-n. | manganum nitricum |
| mang-o. | manganum oxydatum |
| | manganum oxydatum nativum →mang-o. |
| | manganum peroxydum→ mang-o. |
| mang-p. | manganum phosphoricum |
| mang-sil-f. | manganum silicofluoratum |
| mang-sil. | manganum silicicum |
| mang-s. | manganum sulphuricum |
| mang. | manganum-act. + -c. (old abbr.) |
| | manihot utilissima→cass. |
| | manioc→cass. |
| manni. | mannitol |
| mannohep. | mannoheptulose |
| mant-r. | mantis religiosa |
| manz. | manzanita |
| mapr. | maprotiline |
| | mapato→rat. |
| | marble, white→marb-w. |
| | marigoldin→calen. |
| marb-w. | white marble |
| markh-l. | markhamia lutea |
| marr-vg. | marrubium vulgare |
| marr. | marrubium album |
| | marsdenia cundurango→cund. |
| | marum verum→teucr. |
| mate | mate |
| | mater perlarum→conch. |
| mati. | matico |
| | matricaria chamomilla→cham. |
| matr-d. | matricaria discoidea |
| matr-i. | matricaria inodora |
| | matricaria suaveolens→matr-d. |
| matth. | matthiola graeca |
| | mauritanica→arund-d. |
| mec. | meconinum |
| medic-l. | medicago lupulina |
| | medicago sativa→alf. |
| medus. | medusa |
| med. | medorrhinum |
| mein-p. | Meinberg Pyrmont aqua |
| mel | mel |

| | |
|---|---|
| melal. | melaleuca hypericifolia |
| | melaleuca leucodendron→caj. |
| melam-a. | melampyrum arvense |
| melan. | melaninum |
| mela. | melastoma Ackermanni |
| | melia azadirachta→aza. |
| | melia azadirachta indica→aza. |
| | melia grandiflora→guare. |
| melin. | melitine |
| melis. | melissa officinalis |
| melit. | melitagrinum |
| meli-alt. | melilotus altissima |
| meli-a. | melilotus alba |
| meli-xyz. | melilotus off. + -a. |
| meli. | melilotus officinalis |
| | melitococcinum→brucel. |
| | melitotoxinum→brucel. |
| meloe-m. | meloe majalis |
| melo. | melolontha vulgaris |
| meltis-g. | melittis grandiflora |
| | melittis melissophyllum→ meltis-g. |
| mel-c-s. | mel cum sale |
| | meloe vesicatoris→canth. |
| menad. | menadion |
| meningoc. | meningococcinum |
| menis. | menispermum canadense |
| | menispermum cocculus→cocc. |
| mentho. | mentholum |
| menth-aq. | mentha aquatica |
| menth-ar. | mentha arvensis |
| menth-pu. | mentha pulegium |
| menth-r. | mentha rotundifolia |
| menth-s. | mentha sylvestris |
| menth-v. | mentha viridis |
| menth. | mentha piperita |
| meny. | menyanthes trifoliata |
| mepacr-chl. | mepacrine chlorhydrate |
| meph. | mephitis putorius |
| meprob. | meprobamate |
| mercs-n. | mercuresceinum natricum |
| merc-act. | mercurius aceticus |
| merc-ar. | mercurius arsenicicus |
| merc-aur. | mercurius auratus |
| | mercurius biniodatus→merc-i-r. |
| | mercurius bi-iodatus→merc-i-r. |
| merc-br. | mercurius bromatus |
| merc-bs. | mercurius bi-sulfuricus |
| merc-chli. | mercurius chloroiodatus |
| merc-cy. | mercurius cyanatus |
| merc-c. | mercurius corrosivus |
| | mercurius cum kali→aethi-m. |
| merc-d. | mercurius dulcis |
| | mercurius flavus→merc-o-f. |
| merc-f. | mercurius fluoratum |
| merc-i-f. | mercurius iodatus flavus |
| merc-i-r. | mercurius iodatus ruber |
| merc-k-i. | mercurius biniodatus cum kali iodat |
| merc-lac. | mercurius lacticus |
| merc-meth. | mercurius methylenus |
| merc-ns. | mercurius nitrosus |
| merc-n. | mercurius nitricus |
| | mercurius nitricus oxydulatus →merc-ns. |
| | mercurius oxydatulus niger→ merc. |
| | mercurius oxydatus→merc-pr-r. |
| merc-o-cy. | mercurius oxy-cyanatus |
| merc-o-f. | mercurius oxydatus flavus |
| merc-pn. | mercurius proto-nitricus |
| merc-pr-a. | mercurius praecipitatus albus |
| merc-pr-f. | mercurius praecipitatus flavus |
| merc-pr-r. | mercurius praecipitatus ruber |
| merc-p. | mercurius phosphoricus |
| | mercurius proto-iodatus→ merc-i-f. |
| merc-r. | mercurius rhodanatus |
| | mercurius solubilis hahnemanni →merc. |
| | mercurius sublimatus→merc-c. |
| merc-sul. | mercurius sulphuricus |
| merc-s-cy. | mercurius sulphocyanatus |
| merc-tn. | mercurius tannicus |
| merc. | mercurius solubilis |
| merl-a. | mercurialis annua |
| | mercurius sulphuratus niger→ aethi-m. |
| | mercurius sulphuratus ruber→ cinnb. |
| merl. | mercurialis perennis |
| | mercurius vivus→merc. |
| | mesembrianthemum cristall-inum→mese-c. |
| mese-c. | mesembryanthemum cristall-inum |

| | |
|---|---|
| mesp. | mespillus germanica |
| | metacetaldehydum→metald. |
| metald. | metaldehydum |
| | metallum album→ars. |
| | metallum iodatum→ars-i. |
| | metastatic melanoma→carc-mel-met. |
| methan. | methanol |
| methion. | methioninum |
| | methylacetanilidum→metald. |
| | methylene blue→methyl. |
| methyl. | methylenum coeruleum |
| methys. | methysergidum |
| | methylglycoxalidine→lysd. |
| meth-ae-ae. | methylium aethyloaethereum |
| meth-bchl. | methylenum bichloratum |
| meth-sal. | methylium salicylicum |
| | metrosideros costatus→ango. |
| meum-a. | meum athamanticum |
| mez. | mezereum |
| mica | mica |
| | microccuccus catarrhalis→mucot. |
| | microccuccus tetragenius→mucot. |
| microc. | micrococcinum |
| | micrococcus melitensis→brucel. |
| microg-p. | microglossa pyrifolia |
| micr. | micromeria douglasii |
| | microphyllus pennatifolius→jab. |
| | micrurus fulvius→elaps |
| mik-c. | mikania cordata |
| | mikania guaco→gua. |
| mill. | millefolium |
| mil-s. | milium solis |
| | millipedes→onis. |
| miml-g. | mimulus guttiatus |
| mim-h. | mimosa humilis |
| mim-p. | mimosa pudica |
| mir-j. | mirabilis jalapa |
| | mispickel→ars-pyr. |
| miss. | Mississquoi aqua |
| mitom. | mitomycine |
| mitot. | mitotane |
| mitra-st. | mitragyna stipulosa |
| mit. | mitchella repens |

| | |
|---|---|
| mnng. | n-methyl-n'-nitro-n-nitrosog-uanidin |
| molin-c. | molinia coerulea |
| | molybdaenum metallicum→moly-met. |
| moly-ac. | molybdenicum acidum |
| moly-met. | molybdenium metallicum |
| moly-m. | molybdenium muriaticum |
| mom-b. | momordica balsamica |
| | momordica balsamina→mom-b. |
| mom-ch. | momordica charantia |
| | momordica elaterium→elat. |
| mom-f. | momordica foetida |
| mom-in. | momordica involucrata |
| monar. | monarda didyma |
| moni-c. | monilia coerula |
| moni. | monilia albicans |
| mono-h. | monotropa hypopitis |
| mono. | monotropa uniflora |
| monst-p. | monstera pertusa |
| mons. | monsonia ovata |
| morb. | morbillinum |
| morg-g. | bacillus Morgan-Gaertner (Paterson) |
| morg-p. | bacillus Morgan pure (Paterson) |
| morg. | bacillus Morgan (Bach) |
| | morgan pure (paterson)→morg-p. |
| | morgan (bach)→morg. |
| | morgan-gaertner (paterson)→morg-g. |
| morind-l. | morinda lucida |
| morind-m. | morinda morindoides |
| moring-p. | moringa pterygosperma |
| | morphini hydrochloridum→morph-m. |
| morph-act. | morphinum aceticum |
| morph-m. | morphinum muriaticum |
| morph-pur. | morphinum purum |
| morph-s. | morphinum sulphuricum |
| morph. | morphinum and salts (old abbr.) |
| morus-n. | morus nigra |
| moscho-r. | moschosma riparia |
| mosch. | moschus |
| | moschus moschiferus→mosch. |
| mucoc. | mucococcinum |

| | |
|---|---|
| mucor | mucor mucedo· |
| mucor-a-p. | mucor cum aspergillus cum penicilli |
| mucot. | mucotoxinum |
| mucs-nas. | mucosa nasalis |
| muc-u. | mucuna urens |
| mukul | balsamodendron mukul |
| | mucuna pruriens→dol. |
| | mudar→calo. |
| | muira puama→lir-o. |
| mum-l. | mumulus lewisii |
| muru. | murure leite |
| murx. | murex purpurea |
| mur-ac. | muriaticum acidum |
| musa | musa sapientum |
| musan-c. | musanga cecropioides |
| musa-p. | musa paradisiaca |
| muscin. | muscarinum |
| mut. | bacillus Mutabile (Bach) |
| | mustela foetida→meph. |
| | mutabile (Bach)→mut. |
| | mygale avicularia→mygal. |
| mygal. | mygale lasiodora |
| myos-a. | myosotis arvensis |
| | myosotis avicularia→myos-a. |
| | myosotis intermedia→myos-a. |
| myos-sv. | myosotis sylvatica |
| myos-s. | myosotis symphytifolia |
| myric-g. | myrica gale |
| myric. | myrica cerifera |
| | myristica officinalis→nux-m. |
| myris. | myristica sebifera |
| | myrmexin→form. |
| | myrobalanum chebula→term-c. |
| myroc-p. | myrocylon peruvianum |
| | myrospermum pereirae→bals-p. |
| | myroxylon pereira→bals-p. |
| | myroxylon peruvianum→bals-p. |
| myrox-t. | myroxylon toluiferum |
| myrrha | myrrha |
| myrrhis-o. | myrrhis odorata |
| | myrtillocactus→cact. |
| myrtic-g. | myrtillocactus geometrizan |
| | myrtillus→vacc-m. |
| myrt-ch. | myrtus cheken |
| myrt-c. | myrtus communis |
| myrt-p. | myrtus pimenta |
| mytil. | mytilus edulis |

| | |
|---|---|
| m-ambo. | magnetis poli ambo |
| m-arct. | magnetis polus arcticus |
| | myrtus jambos→eug. |
| | myrtus pimenta→pime. |
| m-aust. | magnetis polus australis |
| | myxoedema parotitis→ourl. |
| nabal. | nabalus serpentarius |
| nack. | nackelia |
| | naj naja→naja |
| naja | naja tripudians |
| naja-n. | naja nigricolis |
| nalox. | naloxon |
| | naloxone→nalox. |
| | napellus→acon. |
| naphtaz-m. | naphthazolinum muriaticum |
| naphtaz-n. | naphthazolinum nitricum |
| naphtin. | naphthalinum |
| napht. | naphtha |
| narcin. | narceinum |
| narcot-act. | narcotinum aceticum |
| narcot-m. | narcotinum muriaticum |
| narcot. | narcotinum |
| narc-po. | narcissus poeticus |
| narc-ps. | narcissus pseudonarcissus |
| narz. | Narzan aqua |
| nast-o. | nasturtium officinale |
| nast. | nasturtium aquaticum |
| | natrii acetas→nat-act. |
| | natrii benzoas→nat-be. |
| | natrii bromidum→nat-br. |
| | natrii hydroxydum→nat-caust. |
| | natrii hypophosphis→nat-hp. |
| | natrii nitras→nat-n. |
| | natrii nitris→nat-ns. |
| | natrii oxalas→nat-ox. |
| | natrii phosphas→nat-p. |
| | natrii salicylas→nat-sal. |
| nat-act. | natrium aceticum |
| nat-ae-s. | natrium aethylosulphuricum |
| nat-ar. | natrium arsenicosum |
| nat-be. | natrium benzoicum |
| | natrium biboracicum→borx. |
| nat-bic. | natrium bicarbonicum |
| bat-bis. | natrium bisulfurosum |
| bat-bi. | natrium bichromicum |
| bat-bor. | natrium boricum |
| nat-br. | natrium bromatum |
| nat-cac. | natrium cacodylicum |

| | |
|---|---|
| nat-caust. | natrium causticum |
| | natrium chloratum→nat-m. |
| | natrium chloricum→nat-m. |
| nat-chor. | natrium chloricum |
| nat-chr. | natrium chromicum |
| nat-ch. | natrium choleinicum |
| nat-cit. | natrium citricum |
| nat-cy. | natrium cyanatum |
| nat-c. | natrium carbonicum |
| nat-form. | natrium formicum |
| nat-f. | natrium fluoratum |
| nat-gchol. | natrium glycocholicum |
| nat-gent. | natrium gentisatum |
| nat-gl. | natrium gluconicum |
| nat-gp. | natrium glycerophosphoricum |
| nat-hchls. | natrium hypochlorosum |
| nat-hmp. | natrium hexa-meta-phosphoricum |
| nat-hox. | natrium hydroxydum |
| nat-hp. | natrium hypophosphorum |
| nat-hsulo. | natrium hyposulphurosum |
| nat-i. | natrium iodatum |
| nat-lac. | natrium lacticum |
| nat-mar. | natrium marinum |
| nat-meth-ar. | natrium methylarsinicum |
| nat-meth. | natrium methylate |
| nat-met. | natrium metallicum |
| nat-mlb. | natrium molybdicum |
| nat-mvan. | natrium metavanadicum |
| nat-m. | natrium muriaticum |
| nat-nic. | natrium nicotinicum |
| nat-ns. | natrium nitrosum |
| nat-n. | natrium nitricum |
| nat-ol. | natrium oleicum |
| | natrium oxalaceticum→nat-ox. |
| nat-ox. | natrium oxalicum |
| nat-o. | natrium oxydatum |
| nat-perm. | natrium permanganicum |
| nat-prop. | natrium propionicum |
| nat-p. | natrium phosphoricum |
| nat-sal. | natrium salicylicum |
| nat-sel. | natrium selenicum |
| | natrium silicatum→nat-sil. |
| nat-sil-f. | natrium silicofluoricum |
| nat-sil. | natrium silicicum |
| nat-stann. | natrium stannicum |
| nat-suc. | natrium succinicum |
| nat-sula. | natrium sulphuratum |
| | natrium sulphorinicum→nat-ae-s. |
| nat-sulo. | natrium sulphurosum |
| nat-s-c. | natrium sulphocarbolicum |
| nat-s. | natrium sulphuricum |
| nat-tar. | natrium tartaricum |
| nat-taur. | natrium taurocholicum |
| nat-tel. | natrium telluricum |
| nat-tmcy. | natrium thiosinaminum cyanatum |
| nat-val. | natrium valerianicum |
| nat-van. | natrium vanadicum |
| nauc-l. | nauclea latifolia |
| nectrin. | nectrianinum |
| | nectandra cymbarum→nect. |
| nect-p. | nectandra pichury major |
| nect. | nectandra amara |
| nego-a. | negundo aceroides |
| nego-f. | negundo fraxinifolium |
| neg. | negundium americanum |
| | neisseria flava→flav. |
| nemo-m. | nemophila menziesii |
| neod-met. | neodymium metallicum |
| neod-n. | neodymium nitricum |
| neod-o. | neodymium oxydatum |
| neod-s. | neodymium sulfuricum |
| neom. | neomycine |
| neon | neon |
| neor-m. | neorautanenia mitis |
| neos-ms. | neostigmine methyl sulfate |
| neot-n-a. | neottia nidus avis |
| nepet. | nepeta cataria |
| neph-l. | nephelium litchi |
| nep. | nepenthes distillatoria |
| | nerium odorum→olnd. |
| ner-od. | nerium odorum |
| | nerium oleander→olnd. |
| neur. | neurinum |
| | neurohypophysis→pitu-p. |
| | niacinamidum→nicotam. |
| | niacinum→nicot-ac. |
| nicc-be. | niccolum benzoicum |
| | niccolum bromatum→nicc-br. |
| nicc-br. | niccolum bromidum |
| nicc-c. | niccolum carbonicum |
| nicc-f. | niccolum fluoratum |
| nicc-gl. | niccolum gluconicum |
| nicc-met. | niccolum metallicum |

nicc-m. niccolum muriaticum
nicc-o. niccolum oxydatum
nicc-sil. niccolum siticatum
nicc-s. niccolum sulphuricum
nicc. niccolum-met. + -c. (old abbr.)
nickterina→mir-j.
nicotiana tabacum→tab.
nicotam. nicotinamidum
nicot-ac. nicotinic acidum
nicotinicum amidum→ nicotam.
nicot. nicotinum
nid. nidus edulis
nigr-a. nigritella angustifolia
nig-d. nigella damascene
nig-s. nigella sativa
ninhy. ninhydrine
niob-met. niobium metallicum
niob-m. niobium muriaticum
nitraz. nitrazepam
nitri acidum→nit-ac.
nitrobenzenum→nitrob.
nitrob. nitrobenzolum
nitroph. nitrophenolum
nitro-o. nitrogenium oxygenatum
nit-ac. nitricum acidum
nitrogenum oxygenatum→ nitro-o.
nitroglycerinum→glon.
nit-m-ac. nitromuriaticum acidum
nit-s-d. nitri spiritus dulcis
nitroso-muriaticum acidum→ nit-m-ac.
nitrum→kali-n.
noc-a. nocardia asteroides
nocardia lutea→actin-1.
nopalea coccinellifera→opun-c.
noradr. noradrenalinum
norepi. norepinephrine
norleuc. norleucine
nosc. noscapinum
novoc. novocainum
nucl-ac. nucleinicum acidum
nuph-p. nuphar pumilum
nuph. nuphar luteum
nux-a. nux absurda
nux colae→kola
nux juglans→jug-r.

nux-m. nux moschata
nux-v. nux vomica
nyckterinia capensis→zant.
nyct. nyctanthes arbor tristis
nycterinia capensis→zant.
nymph-a. nymphaea alba
nymphaea lutea→nuph.
nymph. nymphaea odorata
nymphea alba→nymph-a.
nymphea odorata→nymph.
nyst. nystatine
ochn-a. ochna atropurpurea
ocimum basilicum→basil.
oci-car. ocimum caryophyllatum
ici-g. ocimum gratissimum
oci-m. ocimum micranthum
oci-sa. ocimum sanctum
oci-su. ocimum suave
oci. ocimum canum
oct-mac. octopus maculata
oenanthe aquaticum→phel.
oena-f. oenanthe fistulosa
oena. oenanthe crocata
oenanthe phellandrium→phel.
oeno. oenothera biennis
oestrd-be. oestradiol benzoas
oestrd. oestradiol
oestronum→foll.
oest. oestrus cameli
officinalis polyporus→bol-la.
oidium albicans→moni.
okou. okoubaka aubrevillei
olden-d. oldenlandia decubens
olden-h. oldenlandia herbacea
olea europea→ol-eur.
olnd. oleander
ol-ac. oleicum acidum
oleum animae aetherum dippeli →ol-an.
ol-an. oleum animale aethereum
oleum cajuputi→caj.
ol-car. oleum caryophyllatum
oleum chaulmoogra→chaul.
oleum dippeli→ol-an.
oleum elaeis→elae.
ol-eucal. oleum eucalyptus
ol-eur. oleum europaeum

| | |
|---|---|
| ol-ha. | oleum haarlem |
| ol-hc. | oleum hydnocarpi |
| ol-hi. | oleum hippoglossi |
| ol-j. | oleum jecoris aselli |
| | oleum jecoris morrhuae→ol-j. |
| ol-lav. | oleum lavandulae |
| | oleum morrhuae→ol-j. |
| ol-mo. | oleum morrhuae |
| | oleum mulleini→verb-ol. |
| ol-myr. | oleum myristicae |
| ol-pat. | oleum patchouli |
| | oleum patchouly→ol-pat. |
| | oleum petrae→petr. |
| | oleum pogostemon patchouli →ol-pat. |
| | oleum ricini→ric. |
| | oleum ricinus→ric. |
| ol-sant. | oleum santali |
| ol-suc. | oleum succinum |
| | oleum terebinthinae→ter. |
| | oleum verbasci→verb-ol. |
| | oleum wittnebianum→caj. |
| | olibanum→bosw-c. |
| onis. | oniscus asellus |
| onob-s. | onobrychis sativa |
| | ononis arvensis→onon. |
| onon-n. | ononis natrix |
| onon-r. | ononis repens |
| onon. | ononis spinosa |
| onop. | onopordon acanthium |
| onos. | onosmodium virginianum |
| | onosmodium virginicum→ onos. |
| | oophorinum→ov. |
| | oorari→cur. |
| oper. | operculina turpenthum |
| | operculina turpethum→oper. |
| | ophelia chirata→gent-ch. |
| | opianyl→mec. |
| opl. | oplia farinosa |
| opop. | opopanax chironium |
| opun-a. | opuntia aciculata |
| opun-c. | opuntia coccinellifera |
| opun-f. | opuntia ficus |
| opun-s. | opuntia spina alba |
| opun-v. | opuntia vulgaris |
| opun-xyz. | opun-xyz |
| op. | opium |

| | |
|---|---|
| orch. | orchitinum |
| orcin. | orcinolum |
| oreo. | oreodaphne californica |
| orig-cr. | origanum creticum |
| orig-d. | origanum dictamnus |
| | origanum hortensis→orig. |
| orig-v. | origanum vulgare |
| orig. | origanum majorana |
| ornith-chl. | ornithine chlorhydrate |
| | ornithogalum nutans→agra. |
| orni-p. | ornithogalum pyrenaicum |
| orni. | ornithogalum umbellatum |
| orob-m. | orobanche major |
| | orobanche virginiana→epiph. |
| orot-ac. | oroticum acidum |
| | orteaga→eys. |
| | ortho acidum→amibe-ac. |
| orthambe-ac. | orthoaminobenzoicum acidum |
| orthos-s. | orthosiphon stamineus |
| oryz-s. | oryza sativa |
| oscilloc. | oscillococcinum |
| osmu-r. | osmunda regalis |
| osm-ac. | osmicum acidum |
| osm-met. | osmium metallicum |
| osm-o. | osmium oxydatum |
| osm. | osmium met. + -ac. (old abbr.) |
| | osteo arthritic nosode→osteo-a. |
| osteos-n. | osteospermum nervatum |
| osteo-a. | osteo-arthriticum |
| | ostrea edulis→calc. |
| ost. | ostrya virginica |
| osyr-a. | osysris alba |
| othon-n. | othonna natalensis |
| ouabin. | ouabainum |
| ourl. | ourlianum |
| | ova tosta→ovi-p. |
| ovar. | ovaries |
| ovi-p. | ovi gallinae pellicula |
| | ovi gallinae testa→calc-o-t. |
| | ovi testa→calc-o-t. |
| ovi-v. | ovi vitellus |
| ov. | ovininum |
| oxal-a. | oxalis acetosella |
| oxal-c. | oxalis corniculata |
| oxal-s. | oxalis semiloba |
| oxat. | oxatomide |
| oxaz. | oxazepam |
| oxeod. | oxeodaphne |

| | |
|---|---|
| oxpren. | oxprenololum |
| oxyd. | oxydendron arboreum |
| oxyg. | oxygenium |
| oxyq-m. | oxyquinoleinum muriaticum |
| oxyte-chl. | oxytetracycline chlorhydrate |
| oxyt-c. | oxytropis campestris |
| oxyt. | oxytropis Lamberti |
| oxy-v. | oxyurus vermicularis |
| ox-ac. | oxalicum acidum |
| ozone | ozone |
| | padus avium→prun-p. |
| paeon. | paeonia officinalis |
| | paico→chen-a. |
| | pakur→fic-r. |
| pali-a. | paliurus aculeatus |
| | paliurus australis→pali-a. |
| | paliurus spina christi→pali-a. |
| pall-f. | palladium fluoratum |
| pall-m. | palladium muriaticum |
| pall-o. | palladium oxydatum |
| pall. | palladium metallicum |
| palm-ac. | palmiticum acidum |
| palo. | paloondo |
| | pambotano→calli-h. |
| pambt. | pambotano |
| pana. | panacea arvensis |
| | panax ginseng→gins. |
| | panax quinquefolia→gins. |
| pancr. | pancreatinum |
| pann. | panna |
| pant-ac. | pantothenicum acidum |
| papain. | papainum |
| papin-m. | papaverinum muriaticum |
| | papaver somniferum→op. |
| | papaverini hydrochloridum→papin-m. |
| papin. | papaverinum |
| pap-r. | papaver rhoeas |
| | papaya vulgaris→asim. |
| paraf. | paraffinum |
| paraph. | paraphenylendiaminum |
| | parathormonum→parathyr. |
| parathyr. | parathyreoidinum |
| parat-b. | parathyphoidinum B |
| | parathyreoid glands→parathyr. |
| parat. | paratyphoidinum |
| | paratyphoidinum a→parat. |
| pareir. | pareira brava |
| pariet. | parietaria officinalis |
| parit-t. | paritium tiliaceum |
| parn-p. | parnassia palustris |
| parot. | parotidinum |
| paro-i. | paronychia illecebrum |
| parth. | parthenium hysterophorus |
| par. | paris quadrifolia |
| | parthenium hysterophorus lynn→parth. |
| | parthenocissus→ampe-qu. |
| passi-c. | passiflora coerulea |
| passi. | passiflora incarnata |
| past-u. | pastinaca urens |
| past. | pastinaca sativa |
| paull. | paullinia pinnata |
| | paullinia sorbilis→guar. |
| pectin. | pectinum |
| pect. | pecten jacobaeus |
| pedclr. | pedicularis canadensis |
| ped. | pediculus capitis |
| pelarg-o. | pelargonium odoratissimum |
| pelarg. | pelargonium reniforme |
| | pelias berus→vip. |
| pellin. | pelletierinum |
| | penghawar djambi→cibot-b. |
| penic-cm. | penicillium camemberti |
| | penicillium candidum→penic-cm. |
| | penicillium caseicolum→penic-cm. |
| | penicillium cyclopium→penic-cy. |
| penic-cy. | penicillium cyclopodium |
| penic-e. | penicillium expansum |
| | penicillium giordanoi→penic-e. |
| | penicillium glaucum→penic-e. |
| penic-g. | penicillium griseum |
| penic-n. | penicillium notatum |
| penic-p. | penicillium piceum |
| penic. | penicillinum |
| pentac-m. | pentaclethra macrophylla |
| pentad-b. | pentadiplandra brazzeana |
| pentaz. | pentazocine |
| pen. | penthorum sedoides |
| peps. | pepsinum |
| perchlet. | perchlorethylene |
| perhydr. | perhydrol |
| perh-mal. | perhexilinum maleatum |

| | |
|---|---|
| perh. | perhexilinum |
| perid-b. | perideridia bolanderi |
| perill-f. | perilla frutescens |
| perill-o. | perilla ocymoides |
| peri. | periploca graeca |
| | perlarum mater→conch. |
| pern-c. | pernus canaliculus |
| perob. | perobinha |
| pers. | persea americana |
| | persea gratissima→lauru-p. |
| | persica amygdalus→amgd-p. |
| | persica vulgaris→amgd-p. |
| | persicaria acris→polyg-h. |
| | persicaria urens→polyg-pe. |
| pert. | pertussinum |
| pest. | pestinum |
| petan-v. | petanisia variabilis |
| | petasites fragrans→tus-fr. |
| | petasites officinalis→tus-p. |
| | petasites vulgaris→tus-p. |
| peti-a. | petiveria alliacea |
| peti. | petiveria tetandra |
| petros-c. | petroselinum crispum |
| petros. | petroselinum sativum |
| petr. | petroleum |
| | peucedanum graveolens→anetho-g. |
| peuc-o. | peucedanum officinale |
| | peucedanum oreoselo→atha. |
| | peucedanum ostruthium→imp. |
| | peumus boldo→bold. |
| | pexid→perh-mal. |
| | peyotl→anh. |
| | phenolum→carb-ac. |
| | phenylglycolicum acidum→mande-ac. |
| | phosphorus muriaticus→phos-pchl. |
| | phragmites communis→ arund -p. |
| | phyllitis scolopendrium→scolo-v. |
| | physostigminum→esin. |
| | phytolacca tetandra→peti. |
| | picea nigra→abies-n. |
| | pichi-pichi→fab. |
| | picraena excelsa→quas. |
| | picronitricum acidum→pic-ac. |
| | pili-pili→caps. |
| | pilocarpus jaborandi→jab. |
| | pilocarpus microphyllus→jab. |
| | pilocarpus pennatifolius→jab. |
| | pilosella→hier-p. |
| | pimpinella alba→pimp. |
| | pinus canadensis→abies-c. |
| | pinus maritima→pin-pi. |
| | pinus murrayana→pin-s. |
| | pinus uncinata→pin-mo. |
| | piper angustifolium→mati. |
| | piper angustifolium elongatum →mati. |
| | piper cubeba→cub. |
| | piper elongatum→mati. |
| | pirus malus→malus-c. |
| | pituitaria cerebri→pitu-gl. |
| | pituitarium anteriorum→pitu-a. |
| | pituitarium posteriorum→pitu-p. |
| | piturinum→dubo-h. |
| | planifolia→vanil. |
| | platanus acerifolia→platan-or. |
| | platan. old→platan-oc. + -or.→platan. |
| | platina→plat. |
| | platonium chloratum→plat-m. |
| | plumbii acetas→plb-act. |
| | pneumococcus→pneu. |
| | pollen→poll. |
| | poly bowel compound (bach) →poly-bow. |
| | polygala senega→seneg. |
| | polygonum acre→polyg-h. |
| | polygonum fagopyrum→fago. |
| | polygonum hydropiper→polyg-pe. |
| | polygonum punctatum→polyg-h. |
| | polypodium calaguala→calag. |
| | polypodium leucotomos→calag. |
| | polyporus officinalis→bol-la. |
| | populus alba→pop-c. |
| | populus balsamifera→pop-c. |
| | populus tremula→pop. |
| | portulacca oleracea→all-a. |
| | potamobius astacus→astac. |

| | |
|---|---|
| | potassium xantate→kali-x. |
| | potentilla recta→pot-e. |
| | pothos foetidus→ictod. |
| | prednisolon→prednl. |
| | prenanthes serpentaria→nabal. |
| | primula obconca→prim-o. |
| | primula officinalis→prim-v. |
| | prionurus australis→buth-a. |
| | procaini hydrochloridum→ proc-m. |
| pg-a1ta1. | prostaglandinum a1 tromboxane a1 |
| pg-a2ta2. | prostaglandinum a2 tromboxane a2 |
| pg-all. | prostaglandinum all types |
| pg-e1. | prostaglandinum e1 |
| pg-e2. | prostaglandinum e2 |
| pg-f2a. | prostaglandinum f2 alpha |
| phal. | phallus impudicus |
| phase-1. | phaseolus lunatus |
| phase-vg. | phaseolus vulgaris |
| phase-xyz. | phase-xyz |
| phase. | phaseolus nanus |
| phel. | phellandrium aquaticum |
| phenac. | phenacetinum |
| phenan. | phenanthrenum |
| phenerg. | phenergan |
| phenob. | phenobarbitalum |
| phenolpht. | phenolphtaleinum |
| phenoth. | phenothiazinum |
| phenylal. | phenylalanine |
| phenylbe. | phenylbenzene |
| phenylbu. | phenylbutazone |
| phenylhy. | phenylhydrazinum |
| phila. | philadelphus coronarius |
| phill-a. | phillyrea angustifolia |
| phill-1. | phillyrea latifolia |
| philo-p. | philodendron pertusum |
| phle. | phleum pratense |
| phlor. | phlorizinum |
| phoen-d. | phoenix dactylifera |
| phor-t. | phormium tenax |
| phos-h. | phosphorus hydrogenatus |
| phos-m. | phosphorus muriaticus |
| phos-pbr. | phosphorus pentabromatus |
| phos-pchl. | phosphorus pentachloratus |
| phos-ps. | phosphorus pentasulfuratus |
| phos-tbr. | phosphorus tribromatus |
| phos-ti. | phosphorus triiodatus |
| phos. | phosphorus |
| phyld-b. | phyllodoce breweri |
| phyll-c. | phyllanthus casticum |
| phyll-n. | phyllanthus niruri |
| physala-p. | physalia pelagica |
| physal-al. | physalis alkekengi |
| physal-an. | physalis angulata |
| physal-p. | physalis peruviana |
| physin-sal. | physostigminum salicylicum |
| phys. | physostigma venenosum |
| phyt-b. | phytolacca berry |
| phyt. | phytolacca decandra |
| ph-ac. | phosphoricum acidum |
| picea-e. | picea excelsa |
| picea-p. | picea pungens |
| picror. | picrorhiza |
| picro-ac. | picrotoxinum acidum |
| picro. | picrotoxinum |
| pic-ac. | picricum acidum |
| pilios-t. | piliostigma thonningii |
| pilo-m. | pilocarpinum muriaticum |
| pilo-n. | pilocarpinum nitricum |
| pilo-pur. | pilocarpinum purum |
| pilo. | pilocarpinum + salts (old abbr.) |
| pime. | pimenta officinalis |
| pimp-a. | pimpinella anisum |
| pimp. | pimpinella saxifraga |
| pineal. | pinealis |
| ping-vg. | pinguicula vulgaris |
| pin-c. | pinus cupressus |
| pin-1. | pinus lambertiana |
| pin-mo. | pinus montana |
| pin-pa. | pinus palustris |
| pin-pi. | pinus pinaster |
| pin-s. | pinus silvestris |
| pipe. | piperazinum |
| pip-g. | piper guineense |
| pip-m. | piper methysticum |
| pip-n. | piper nigrum |
| pirox. | piroxicam |
| pir-c. | pirus communis |
| pisc. | piscidia erythrina |
| pist-1. | pistacia lentiscus |
| pis-s. | pisum sativum |
| pitto-v. | pittosporus viridiflorum |
| pituin. | pituitrinum |

| | | | |
|---|---|---|---|
| pitu-a. | pituitaria anterior | plume. | plumeria celinus |
| pitu-gl. | pituitaria glandula | plut-met. | plutonium metallicum |
| pitu-p. | pituitaria posterior | plut-n. | plutonium nitricum |
| pitu. | pituitaria posterior (old abbr.) | pneu. | pneumococcinum |
| pityr-o. | pityrosporum orbiculare | poa-p. | poa pratensis |
| pix | pix liquida | podoin. | podophyllinum |
| plac-s. | placenta suis | podo. | podophyllum peltatum |
| plac. | placenta humana | poinc-p. | poinciana pulcherrima |
| plan-c. | plantago coronopus | pole. | polemonium coeruleum |
| plan-l. | plantago lanceolata | polio | polio |
| plan-mi. | plantago minor | poll. | pollantinum |
| plan-p. | plantago psyllium | polon-met. | polonium metallicum |
| plan. | plantago major | polygl-a. | polygala amara |
| plast. | plastic | polygl-o. | polygala oppostifolia |
| platan-oc. | platanus occidentalis | polygl-vg. | polygala vulgaris |
| platan-or. | platanus orientalis | polygn-vg. | polygonatum vulgare |
| platan. | platan. species (old abbr.) | polyg-am. | polygonum amphibium |
| plat-col. | platinum colloidale | polyg-a. | polygonum aviculare |
| plat-f. | platinum fluoratum | polyg-bta. | polygonum bistorta |
| plat-m-n. | platinum muriaticum natronatum | polyg-btd. | polygonum bistortoides |
| | | polyg-h. | polygonum hydropiperoides |
| plat-m. | platinum muriaticum | polyg-m. | polygonum maritimum |
| plat. | platinum metallicum | polyg-pe. | polygonum persicaria |
| plb-act. | plumbum aceticum | polyg-s. | polygonum sagittatum |
| plb-ar. | plumbum arsenicicum | polyg-xyz. | polygonum h. + -pe. + ? |
| plb-br. | plumbum bromatum | polym. | polymnia uvedalia |
| plb-chr. | plumbum chromicum | polypd-vg. | polypodium vulgare |
| plb-c. | plumbum carbonicum | polyp-p. | polyporus pinicola |
| plb-f. | plumbum fluoratum | polytr-c. | polytrichum commune |
| plb-gl. | plumbum gluconicum | polytr. | polytrichum juniperinum |
| plb-i. | plumbum iodatum | polyv. | polyvinyle chlorure |
| plb-m. | plumbum muriaticum | poly-bow. | poly bowel co. (Bach) |
| plb-n. | plumbum nitricum | pop-c. | populus candicans |
| plb-o-f. | plumbum oxydatum flavum | pop-n. | populus nigra |
| plb-o-r. | plumbum oxydatum rubrum | pop. | populus tremuloides |
| plb-o. | plumbum oxydatum | portal-p. | portulacca pilosa |
| plb-p. | plumbum phosphoricum | pota. | potamogeton natans |
| plb-sact. | plumbum subaceticum | poter-sp. | poterium spinosum |
| plb-s. | plumbum sulfuratum | poter-s. | poterium sanguisorba |
| plb-tae. | plumbum tetra-aethylicum | pot-arg. | potentilla argentea |
| plb-xyz. | plumbum met. + -act. + -c. | pot-au. | potentilla aurea |
| plb. | plumbum metallicum | pot-a. | potentilla anserina |
| plect-b. | plectranthus barbatus | pot-e. | potentilla erecta |
| plect-v. | plectronia ventosa | pot-gl. | potentilla glandulosa |
| plect. | plectranthus fruticosus | pot-r. | potenfilla reptans |
| plumbg-eu. | plumbago europaea | pot-t. | potentilla tormentilla |
| plumbg. | plumbago littoralis | pras-met. | praseodymium metallicum |
| plume-a. | plumeria alba | pras-m. | praseodymium muriaticum |

| | |
|---|---|
| pras-o. | praseodymium oxydatum |
| pras-s. | praseodymium sulfuricum |
| prednl. | prednisolone acetate |
| predn. | prednison |
| pregnan. | pregnandiolum |
| pren-a. | prenanthes alba |
| prim-a. | primula auricula |
| prim-f. | primula farinosa |
| prim-o. | primula obconica |
| prim-vl. | primula vulgaris |
| prim-v. | primula veris |
| prin. | prinos verticillatus |
| priva-l. | priva leptostachya |
| proc-m. | procainum muriaticum |
| progest. | progesteron |
| prolac. | prolactine |
| proli. | proline |
| prom-chl. | promethazine chlorhydrate |
| prom. | promethazine |
| propl. | propolis |
| propr-chl. | propranololum chlorhydratum |
| propr. | propranololum |
| propyl. | propylene glycol |
| prop. | propylaminum |
| proq. | proquantil |
| prostin. | prostatinum |
| prost. | prostate gland |
| protg. | protargol |
| protin. | proteinum |
| prots-m. | proteus mirabilis |
| prots-v. | proteus vulgaris |
| prot. | bacillus Proteus (Bach) |
| | proteus (bach)→prot. |
| prune. | prunella vulgaris |
| prun-am. | prunus amygdalus |
| prun-ar. | prunus armeniaca |
| prun-av. | prunus avium |
| prun-cf. | prunus cerasifera |
| prun-cs. | prunus cerasus |
| prun-d. | prunus domestica |
| | prunus laurocerasus→laur. |
| prun-m. | prunus mahaleb |
| prun-pe. | prunus persica |
| prun-p. | prunus padus |
| prun-v. | prunus virginiana |
| prun. | prunus spinosa |
| | psalliota bispora→agar-cps. |
| | psalliota hortensis→agar-cps. |
| | pseudognaphalium obtusifolium →gnaph. |
| pseud. | pseudomonas aeruginosa |
| pseuts-m. | pseudotsuga menziesii |
| psid. | psidium guayava |
| psil. | psilocybe caerulescens |
| psoral-c. | psoralea corylifolia |
| psoral-p. | psoralea pinnata |
| psoral. | psoralea bituminosa |
| | psoricum→psor. |
| psor. | psorinum |
| | psychotria ipecacuanha→ip. |
| | psychotria viridis→banis-c. |
| | psyllium→plan-p. |
| ptel. | ptelea trifoliata |
| ptergl-ac. | pteroylglutamicum acidum |
| | pteraema excelsa→quas. |
| pteri-a. | pteris aquilina |
| ptraz. | pentetrazolum |
| | pterocarpus erinaceus→kino |
| | pterocarpus marsupium→kino |
| | ptetrocarpus santalinus→ santal. |
| pulic-d. | pulicaria dysenterica |
| pull-g. | pullus gallinaceus |
| pulmon-a. | pulmonaria angustifolia |
| pulmon-o. | pulmonaria officinalis |
| pulmon-t. | pulmonaria tuberosa |
| pulmon. | pulmonaria vulgaris |
| pulm-a. | pulmo anaphylacticus |
| pulm-v. | pulmo vulpis |
| puls-m. | pulsatilla montana |
| | pulsatilla nigricans→puls. |
| puls-n. | pulsatilla nuttaliana |
| puls-vg. | pulsatilla vulgaris |
| puls. | pulsatilla pratensis |
| pulx-c | pulex canis |
| pulx. | pulex irritans |
| | punica granatum→gran. |
| putrin-m. | putrescinum muriaticum |
| putrin. | putrescinum |
| pycno-e. | pycnostachys eminii |
| pyocyin. | pyocyanotoxinum |
| pyocy. | pyocyaninum |
| pyrar. | pyrarara |
| pyren-sc. | pyrenacantha scandens |
| pyre-o. | pyrethrum officinarum |
| pyre-p. | pyrethrum parthenium |

pyre-r. pyrethrum roseum e floribus
pyrid. pyridoxinum
pyrim. pyrimethamine
pyrogall. pyrogallol
pyrogal-ac. pyrogallicum acidum
pyrog. pyrogenium
pyrol-m. pyrola minor
pyrol. pyrola rotundifolia
pyrola umbellate→chim.
pyro-ac. pyrolignosum acidum
pyrus pyrus americana
pyrus-c. pyrus communis
pyru-ac. pyruvicum acidum
p-ambes-ac. para-aminobenzoicumsulfamidum acid
p-ambe-ac. para-aminobenzoicum acidum
p-amsal-ac. para-aminosalicylicum acidum
p-dchlbe. paradichlorobenzolum
quasin. quassinum
quas. quassia amara
queb. quebracho
querc-l. quercus lobata
quercus fructus→querc.
quercus glandium→querc.
querc-pu. quercus pubescens
querc. quercus e glandibus
quercus pedoncolata→quer-r.
quer-r. quercus robur
quercus sessilifera→quer-r.
quill. quillaya saponaria
quillaya smegmaderma→quill.
quinid-m. quinidinum muriaticum
quinid-s. quinidinum sulfuricum
quinid. quinidinum
quinol. quinoleinum
quin-chl. quinacrine chlorhydrate
Rademacher's solution→zinc-act.
rado. radon
rad-br. radium bromatum
rad-chl. radium chloratum
rad-met. radium metallicum
radix angelicae sinensis→ange-s.
raja-s. rajania subsamarata
rana bufo→bufo
ran-a. ranunculus acris
ran-b. ranunculus bulbosus
ran-fi. ranunculus ficaria
ran-fl. ranunculus flammula
ran-g. ranunculus glacialis
ran-p. ranunculus pinnatus
ran-r. ranunculus repens
ran-s. ranunculus sceleratus
raphani. raphanistrum arvense
raphis-g. raphispermum gerardioides
raph. raphanus sativus
rat. ratanhia peruviana
rauw. rauwolfia serpentine
rein. Reinerz aqua
ren. kidneys
realgar→ars-s-r.
red acarus of the fly→trom.
rescue rescue remedy
reser. reserpinum
resina cimifugae→macro.
resina itu→itu
res. resorcinum
retin-ac. retinoicum acidum
retin. retinol
rham-cal. rhamnus californica
rham-cath. rhamnus cathartica
rham-f. rhamnus frangula
rham-pr. rhamnus prinoides
rhamnus purshiana→cas-s.
rhen-met. rhenium metallicum
rhen-o. rhenium oxydatum
rheum officinale→rheum
rheum rheum palmatum
rheum-r. rheum rhaponticum
rhiz. rhizopus niger
rhizopus nigricans→rhiz.
rhodallinum→thiosin.
rhodi-o-n. rhodium oxydatum nitricum
rhodi. rhodium metallicum
rhod-f. rhododendron ferrugineum
rhod. rhododendron chrysanthum
rhus-a. rhus aromatics
rhus canadensis→rhus-a.
rhus-c. rhus cotinus
rhus-d. rhus diversiloba
rhus-g. rhus glabra
rhus-l. rhus laurina
rhus-r. rhus radicans
rhus-s. rhus succedanea
rhus-t. rhus toxicodendron

| | |
|---|---|
| rhus-ver. | rhus vernix |
| rhus-v. | rhus venenata |
| | rhus vernix→rhus-v. |
| ribes-n. | ribes nigrum |
| ribes-r. | ribes rubrum |
| ribo. | riboflavinum |
| rib-ac. | ribonucleicum acidum |
| ricino-h. | ricinodendron heudelotii |
| ric. | ricinus communis |
| rmd01 | User defined 1 |
| rmd02 | User defined 2 |
| rmd03 | User defined 3 |
| rmd04 | User defined 4 |
| rmd05 | User defined 5 |
| rmd06 | User defined 6 |
| rmd07 | User defined 7 |
| rmd08 | User defined 8 |
| rmd09 | User defined 9 |
| rmd10 | User defined 10 |
| rmd11 | User defined 11 |
| rmd12 | User defined 12 |
| rmd13 | User defined 13 |
| rmd14 | User defined 14 |
| rmd15 | User defined 15 |
| rmd16 | User defined 16 |
| rmd17 | User defined 17 |
| rmd18 | User defined 18 |
| rmd19 | User defined 19 |
| rmd20 | User defined 20 |
| rmd21 | User defined 21 |
| rmd22 | User defined 22 |
| rmd23 | User defined 23 |
| rmd24 | User defined 24 |
| rmd25 | User defined 25 |
| rmd26 | User defined 26 |
| rmd27 | User defined 27 |
| rmd28 | User defined 28 |
| rmd29 | User defined 29 |
| rmd30 | User defined 30 |
| rmd31 | User defined 31 |
| rmd32 | User defined 32 |
| rmd33 | User defined 33 |
| rmd34 | User defined 34 |
| rmd35 | User defined 35 |
| rmd36 | User defined 36 |
| rmd37 | User defined 37 |
| rmd38 | User defined 38 |
| rmd39 | User defined 39 |
| rmd40 | User defined 40 |
| rmd41 | User defined 41 |
| rmd42 | User defined 42 |
| rmd43 | User defined 43 |
| rmd44 | User defined 44 |
| rmd45 | User defined 45 |
| rmd46 | User defined 46 |
| rmd47 | User defined 47 |
| rmd48 | User defined 48 |
| rmd49 | User defined 49 |
| rmd50 | User defined 50 |
| rmd51 | User defined 51 |
| rmd52 | User defined 52 |
| rmd53 | User defined 53 |
| rmd54 | User defined 54 |
| rmd55 | User defined 55 |
| rmd56 | User defined 56 |
| rmd57 | User defined 57 |
| rmd58 | User defined 58 |
| rmd59 | User defined 59 |
| rmd60 | User defined 60 |
| rmd61 | User defined 61 |
| rmd62 | User defined 62 |
| rmd63 | User defined 63 |
| rmd64 | User defined 64 |
| rmd65 | User defined 65 |
| rmd66 | User defined 66 |
| rmd67 | User defined 67 |
| rmd68 | User defined 68 |
| rmd69 | User defined 69 |
| rmd70 | User defined 70 |
| rmd71 | User defined 71 |
| rmd72 | User defined 72 |
| rmd73 | User defined 73 |
| rmd74 | User defined 74 |
| rmd75 | User defined 75 |
| rmd76 | User defined 76 |
| rmd77 | User defined 77 |
| rmd78 | User defined 78 |
| rmd79 | User defined 79 |
| rmd80 | User defined 80 |
| rmd81 | User defined 81 |
| rmd82 | User defined 82 |
| rmd83 | User defined 83 |
| rmd84 | User defined 84 |
| rmd85 | User defined 85 |
| rmd86 | User defined 86 |
| rmd87 | User defined 87 |

rmd88 User defined 88
rmd89 User defined 89
rmd90 User defined 90
rmd9l User defined 91
rmd92 User defined 92
rmd93 User defined 93
rmd94 User defined 94
rmd95 User defined 95
rmd96 User defined 96
rmd97 User defined 97
rmd98 User defined 98
rna→rib-ac.
rmd99 User defined 99
rob. robinia pseudacacia
rosm. rosmarinus officinalis
ros-ca. rosa canina
ros-ce. rosa centifolia
ros-d. rosa damascene
ros-g. rosa gallica
ros-r. rosa rubra
rovam. rovamycine
roye-1. royena lucida
roye-v. royena villosa
rubia tinctoria→rub-t.
rubd-br. rubidium bromatum
rubd-c. rubidium carbonicum
rubd-met. rubidium metallicum
rubd-m. rubidium muriaticum
rubus chamaemorus→rubu-c.
rubu-c. rubus chamaerosus
rubu-i. rubus idaeus
rubu-r. rubus rigidus
rubu. rubus villosus
rub-c. rubia cordifolia
rub-t. rubia tinctorum
rudbeckia angustifolia→echi.
rudb-h. rudbeckia hirta
rudbeckia purpurea→echi-p.
ruizia fragrans→bold.
rumx-ab. rumex abyssinicus
rumx-acl. rumex acetosella
rumx-act. rumex acetosa
rumx-al. rumex alpinus
rumx-aq. rumex aquaticus
rumx-p. rumex patientia
rumx. rumex crispus
rumex obtusifolius→lapa.
rusc-a. ruscus aculeatus
russula emetica→agar-em.
russ. russula foetens
ruta ruta graveolens
ruta-a. ruta angustifolia
ruth-met. ruthenium metallicum
rutin. rutinum
sabad. sabadilla
sabal sabal serrulata
sabb. sabbatia angularis
sabdariffa→hib-sa.
sabin. sabina
sacchin. saccharinum
sacch-1. saccharum lactis
saccharomyces cerevisiae→tor.
saccharomyces ceru→tor.
sacch. saccharum officinale
sacmy-a. saccharomyces apiculata
sag-s. sagittaria sagittaefolia
sal amarum→mag-s.
sal glauberi→nat-s.
salam. salamandra maculata
salamandra maculosa→salam.
salbut. salbutamol
salic-p. salicaria purpurea
salin. salicinum
salisburia adiantifolia→gink-b.
salix nigricans→sal-p.
salix vitellina→sal-1.
salmon-e. salmonella enteridis
salmonella parathyphoidea→parat.
salmonella schotmullieri→parat-b.
salol. salolum
salv-p. salvia pratensis
salv-sc. salvia sclarea
salv-so. salvia sonomensis
salv-vb. salvia verbenaca
salv-vt. salvia verticillata
salv. salvia officinalis
sal-ac. salicylicum acidum
sal-al. salix alba
sal-am. salix americana
sal-1. salix lasiolepis
sal-ma. salix madagascariensis
sal-mo. salix mollissima
sal-n. salix nigra

| | |
|---|---|
| sal-p. | salix purpurea |
| samars. | samarsite |
| samb-c. | sambucus canadensis |
| samb-e. | sambucus ebulus |
| samb-r. | sambucus racemosa |
| | sambucus humilis→samb-e. |
| samb. | sambucus nigra |
| sam-ac. | samarium oxydatum |
| sangin-act. | sanguinarinum aceticum |
| sangin-n. | sanguinarinum nitricum |
| sangin-pur. | sanguinarinum purum |
| sangin-t. | sanguinarinum tartaricum |
| sanguiso-m. | sanguisorba minor |
| sanguiso. | sanguisorba officinalis |
| sang. | sanguinaria canadensis |
| | sanguisuga officinalis→hir. |
| sanic-eu. | sanicula europaea |
| sanic. | Sanicula aqua |
| sanochr. | sanochrysine |
| santal. | santalinus |
| | santalum→ol-sant. |
| santa. | santalum album |
| santin. | santoninum |
| santol. | santolina chamaecyparissus |
| | sapium sylvaticum→still. |
| sapin. | saponinum |
| sapot-a. | sapota achras |
| sapo. | saponaria officinalis |
| sap-o. | sapindus oblongifolius |
| sap-s. | sapindus saponaria |
| | saraca indica→joan. |
| sarcol-ac. | sarcolacticum acidum |
| saroth. | sarothamnus scoparius |
| sarr. | sarracenia purpurea |
| sars. | sarsaparilla officinalis |
| sass. | sassafras officinalis |
| sat-h. | satureia hortensis |
| sat-m. | satureia montanta |
| saur. | saururus cernuus |
| saxitox. | saxitoxinum |
| saxi. | saxifraga granulata |
| saxon. | saxonitum |
| scab-c. | scabiosa columbaria |
| scab-s. | scabiosa succisa |
| scam. | scammonium |
| scand-met. | scandium metallicum |
| scand-o. | scandium oxydatum |
| | scarabaeus melolontha→melo. |

| | |
|---|---|
| | scarlatininum→scarl. |
| scarl. | scarlatinum |
| scat. | scatolum |
| schin. | schinus molle |
| | schoenocaulon officinale→sabad. |
| schot-b. | schotia brachypetala |
| | scilla bifolia→squil-b. |
| | scilla maritima→squil. |
| | scilla-non-scripta→agra. |
| scirp-p. | scirpus paludicola |
| scir. | scirrhinum |
| sclero-c. | sclerocarya caffra |
| scler. | scleranthus annuus |
| scolo-v. | scolopendrium vulgare |
| scol. | scolopendra morsitans |
| | scolopendrium officinale→scolo-v. |
| scopar. | scoparius genista |
| scopin-hbr. | scopolaminum bromhydricum |
| scopin. | scopolaminum bromatum |
| scopla. | scopola |
| scop. | scopolia carniolica |
| | scorodosma foetida→asaf. |
| | scorpio australis→buth-a. |
| scor. | scorpio europaeus |
| | scorpionida→scor. |
| scroph-aq. | scrophularia aquatica |
| scroph-m. | scrophularia marylandica |
| scroph-n. | scrophularia nodosa |
| scroph-xyz. | scroph-xyz |
| scut-g. | scutellaria galericulata |
| | scutellaria lateriflora→scut. |
| scut. | scutellaria laterifolia |
| secret. | secretinum |
| secu-l. | securidaca longipedonculata |
| sec-ce. | secale cereale |
| sec. | secale cornutum |
| sedi. | sedinha |
| sed-ac. | sedum acre |
| sed-al. | sedum album |
| | sedum alpestre→sed-r. |
| sed-c. | sedum cepaea |
| | sedum purpureum→sed-t. |
| sed-rf. | sedum reflexum |
| sed-ru. | sedum rubens |
| sed-r. | sedum repens |
| sed-t. | sedum telephium |

| | |
|---|---|
| sela. | selaginella apus |
| | selenicereus grandiflorus→cact. |
| | selenicereus spinulosus→cact. |
| seli. | selinum carvifolium |
| sel-col. | selenium colloidale |
| sel-o. | selenium oxydatum |
| sel. | selenium metallicum |
| | semecarpus anacardium→anac. |
| | semen contra→cina |
| semp-a. | sempervivum arachnoideum |
| semp. | sempervivum tectorum |
| sem-t. | semen tiglii |
| seneb-c. | senebiera coronopus |
| | senebiera pinnatifida→lepi. |
| senecin. | senecinum |
| senec-abv. | senecio ambavilla |
| senec-ad. | senecio adonidifolius |
| senec-atc. | senecio aurantiacus |
| | senecio cineraria→cine. |
| senec-c. | senecio cordatus |
| | senecio cordifolius→senec-c. |
| senec-d. | senecio doronicum |
| senec-fa. | senecio faniasioides |
| senec-fu. | senecio fuschii |
| | senecio gragglis→senec. |
| senec-i. | senecio incanus |
| senec-j. | senecio jacobaea |
| senec-ma. | senecio mannii |
| senec-sa. | senecio sarracenicus |
| senec-sp. | senecio speciosus |
| senec-sy. | senecio sylvaticus |
| senec. | senecio aureus |
| | senecio vulgaris→senec. |
| seneg. | senega |
| senn. | senna |
| | senna occidentalis→cassia-o. |
| | senticosus eleutherococcus→eleut. |
| septi. | septicaeminum |
| sep. | sepia officinalis |
| | sepia succus→sep. |
| | sepsinum→pyrog. |
| seq-g. | sequoia gigantea |
| seq-s. | sequoia sempervirens |
| | serenoa serrulata→sabal |
| serot-cs. | serotoninum creatininum sulfuricum |
| serp. | serpentaria aristolochia |
| | serratula tinctoria→liat. |
| ser-ang. | serum anguillae |
| ser-a-c. | serum anti colibacillum |
| ser-eq. | serum equi |
| | seven (Paterson)→bacls-7. |
| shig-f. | shigella flexneri |
| sida-rh. | sida rhombifolia |
| sieg. | siegesbeckia orientalis |
| | sierra iris→iris-h. |
| | sigillum salomonis→polygn-vg. |
| sile-i. | silene inflata |
| silpho. | silphion cyrenaicum |
| silphu. | silphium lacinatum |
| sil-mar. | silica marina |
| sil-met. | silicium metallicum |
| sil. | silicea terra |
| | silphium laciniatum→silphu. |
| | silybum marianum→card-m. |
| | simaba cedron→cedr. |
| sima-g. | simaruba glauca |
| | simaruba cedron→cedr. |
| | simaruba ferroginea→cedr. |
| sima-v. | simaruba versicolor |
| sima. | simaruba amara |
| | simaruba officinalis→cedr. |
| simul. | simuliidae |
| sinus. | sinusitisinum |
| sin-a. | sinapis alba |
| | sinapis arvensis→brass-c. |
| sin-n. | sinapis nigra |
| | sison podagraria→aegop-p. |
| | sisymbrium alliaria→alliar-o. |
| | sisymbrium officinale→erys-o. |
| sisym-s. | sisymbrium Sophia |
| sisy. | sisyrinchium galaxoides |
| sium | sium latifolium |
| sium-a. | sium angustifolium |
| | sium podagraria→aegop-p. |
| skat. | skatolum |
| skook. | Skookum Chuck aqua |
| slag | slag silica |
| smilcin. | smilacinum |
| smil-a. | smilax aspera |
| smil-c. | smilax china |
| | smilax offinialis→sars. |

| | |
|---|---|
| | smilax sarsaparilla→sars. |
| soja-h. | soja hispida |
| sol | sol |
| solid-n. | solidago nemoralis |
| solid. | solidago virgaurea |
| solin-act. | solaninum aceticum |
| solin-pur. | solaninum purum |
| solin. | solaninum pur. + -act. (old abbr.) |
| sol-a. | solanum arrebenta |
| sol-br. | sol britannicus |
| sol-cp. | solanum capense |
| | solanum dulcamara→dulc. |
| | solanum lycopersicum→lycpr. |
| | solanum oleaceum→sol-o. |
| | solanum vesicarium→physal-al. |
| sol-crl. | solanum carolinense |
| sol-ecl. | solar eclips |
| sol-er. | solanum erythracantum |
| sol-in. | solanum integri |
| sol-mlg. | solanum melongena |
| sol-mm. | solanum mammosum |
| sol-mx. | solanum malacoxylon |
| sol-ni. | solanum nigrum |
| sol-no. | solanum nodiflorum |
| sol-o. | solanum oleraceum |
| sol-ps. | solanum pseudocapsicum |
| sol-so. | solanum sodomoeum |
| sol-t-ae. | solanum tuberosum aegrotans |
| sol-t. | solanum tuberosum |
| sol-v. | solanum villosum |
| sol-x. | solanum xanthocarpum |
| | solidago virga avrea→solid. |
| somatot. | somatotrophine |
| soph. | sophora japonica |
| sorbit. | sorbitolum |
| | sorbus americans→pyrus |
| sorb-a. | sorbus aucuparia |
| sorb-d. | sorbus domestica |
| sorg-vg. | sorghum vulgare |
| sor-ac. | sorbicum acidum |
| sparg-r. | sparganium ramosum |
| spartin-s. | sparteinum sulfuricum |
| spartin. | sparteinum |
| | spartini sulfas→spartin-s. |
| spart-j. | spartium junceum |
| | spartium scoparium→saroth. |
| sperl-r. | spergularia rubra |
| spermc-n. | spermacoce natalensis |
| sper-a. | spergula arvensis |
| | sperminum→orch. |
| | sphaerococcus helminthochortos→helm. |
| sphang-s. | sphagnum squarosum |
| sphing. | sphingurus martini |
| spig-m. | spigelia marylandica |
| spig. | spigelia anthelmia |
| | spigelia anthelmintica→spig. |
| | spiggurus martini→sphing. |
| spil. | spilanthes oleracea |
| spin-o. | spinacia oleracea |
| spirae-f. | spiraea filipendula |
| spirae. | spiraea ulmaria |
| spiram. | spiramycine |
| spira. | spiranthes autumnalis |
| spiron. | spironolacton |
| | spiritus aetheris nitrosi→nit-s-d. |
| | spiritus dulcis nitri→nit-s-d. |
| | spiritus glandium quercus→spir-q-g. |
| spirul. | spirulina |
| spir-aeth-c. | spiritus aetheris compositus |
| | spiritus nitrico-aethereus→nit-s-d. |
| spir-n-d. | spiritus nitri dulcis |
| spir-q-g. | spiritus quercus glandium |
| spir-sula. | spiritus sulphuratus |
| | spongia fluvialitis→bad. |
| | spongia officinalis→spong. |
| spong. | spongia tosta |
| | spongilla fluvialitis→bad. |
| sporg. | sporgon |
| sporob-r. | sporobolomyces roseus |
| sporob-s. | sporobolomyces salmonicolor |
| sporot. | sporothrix schenckii |
| | sporotricum beurmanni→sporot. |
| squil-b. | squilla bifolia |
| squil. | squilla maritima |
| stach-a. | stachys arvensis |
| stach-p. | stachys palustris |
| stach-s. | stachys sylvatica |
| stach. | stachys betonica |
| stann-i. | stannum iodatum |
| stann-m. | stannum muriaticum |
| stann-o. | stannum oxydatum |

| | |
|---|---|
| stann-pchl. | stannum perchloratum |
| stann-pox. | stannum peroxydatum |
| stann-s. | stannum sulfuratum |
| stann. | stannum metallicum |
| | staphylocinum→staphycoc. |
| staphycoc. | staphylococcinum |
| staphytox. | staphylotoxinum |
| staph. | staphysagria |
| stapl-g. | stapelia gigantea |
| stear-ac. | stearicum acidum |
| | stellaria aquatica→cerast-a. |
| stel. | stellaria media |
| | sterculia acuminata→kola |
| ster-c. | sterigmatocystis candidum |
| | sth→somatot. |
| | stibio-kali tartaricum→ant-t. |
| | stibium acidum→ant-ac. |
| | stibium arsenicosum→ant-ar. |
| | stibium chloridum→ant-m. |
| | stibium crudum→ant-c. |
| | stibium iodatum→ant-i. |
| | stibium metallicum→ant-met. |
| | stibium muriaticum→ant-m. |
| | stibium oxydatum→ant-o. |
| | stibium sulfuratum nigrum→ant-c. |
| | stibium sulfuratum rubrum→ant-s-r. |
| | stibium sulphuratum auratum →ant-s-aur. |
| | stibium tartaricum→ant-t. |
| stict. | sticta pulmonaria |
| stigm. | stigmata maydis |
| stilboest. | stilboestrolum |
| still. | stillingia silvatica |
| | stizolobium pruriens→dol. |
| | stovaine→amyloc-m. |
| | stovarsol→acetars. |
| stram. | stramonium |
| strepta-g. | streptanthus glandulosus |
| streptoc. | streptococcinum |
| streptom-s. | streptomycinum sulphatum |
| | streptomyces albus→actin-a. |
| | streptomyces citreus→actin-c. |
| | streptomyces griseus→actin-g. |
| streptom. | streptomycinum |
| strept-ent. | bacillus strepto-enterococcus |
| stront-ar. | strontium arsenicicum |
| stront-br. | strontium bromatum |
| stront-c. | strontium carbonicum |
| stront-gl. | strontium gluconicum |
| stront-i. | strontium iodatum |
| stront-lac. | strontium lacticum |
| stront-met. | strontium metallicum |
| stront-m. | strontium muriaticum |
| stront-n. | strontium nitricum |
| stront-o. | strontium oxydatum |
| stront-s. | strontium sulfuricum |
| strophin. | strophanthinum |
| stroph-h. | strophanthus hispidus |
| stroph-s. | strophanthus sarmentosus |
| | strychnine et ferri citras→stry-af-cit. |
| strych-g. | strychnos gaultheriana |
| strych-h. | strychnos henningsii |
| strych-s. | strychnos spinosa |
| stryph. | stryphnodendron barbatimam |
| stry-af-cit. | strychninum citricum cum ammoniofer |
| stry-ar. | strychninum arsenicosum |
| stry-n. | strychninum nitricum |
| stry-p. | strychninum phosphoricum |
| stry-s. | strychninum sulphuricum |
| | strychnos ignatii→ign. |
| | strychnos nux vomica→nux-v. |
| stry-val. | strychninum valerianicum |
| stry-xyz. | stry-xyz |
| stry. | strychninum purum |
| | strychnos tieut→upa. |
| subt. | bacillus subtilis |
| succ-ac. | succinicum acidum |
| succ. | succinum |
| sulfag. | sulfaguanidinum |
| sulfamrz. | sulfamerazine |
| sulfamtz. | sulfamethizol |
| sulfap. | sulfapyridinum |
| sulfatz. | sulfathiazolum |
| sulfa. | sulfanilamidum |
| sulfonam. | sulfonamidum |
| sulfon. | sulfonalum |
| | sulfur→sulph. |
| sulo-ac. | sulphurosum acidum |
| sulph. | sulphur |
| | sulphur lotum→sulph. |
| | sulphur sublimatum→sulph. |

| | |
|---|---|
| sulpi. | sulpiride |
| sul-ac-ar. | sulphuricum acidum aromaticum |
| sul-ac. | sulphuricum acidum |
| sul-h. | sulphur hydrogenisatum |
| sul-i. | sulphur iodatum |
| sul-s-1. | sulphur sublimatum lavum |
| | sulphuricum aromaticum acidum→sul-ac-ar. |
| sul-ter. | sulphur terebinthinatum |
| sumb. | sumbulus moschatus |
| | sumbul ferula→sumb. |
| suprar. | suprarenalis |
| syc. | bacillus Sycoccus (Paterson) |
| | sunoma sage→salv-so. |
| | suprarenalis glandula→suprar. |
| | surukuku→lach. |
| | swertia chirata→gent-ch. |
| | sycoccus bacillus (paterson)→syc. |
| | sycoccus (paterson)→syc. |
| | sycotic compound (paterson)→syc. |
| | sycotic co. (paterson)→syc. |
| symph. | symphytum officinale |
| sym-r. | symphoricarpus racemosus |
| | symphoricarpus rivularis→sym-r. |
| | symplocarpus foetidum→ictod. |
| synad-g. | synadenium grantii |
| syph. | syphilinum |
| | syriaca→asc-c. |
| syr. | syringa vulgaris |
| | syzygium aromaticum→caryo. |
| | syzygium cumini→syzyg. |
| syzyg. | syzygium jambolanum |
| | syzygium jambos→eug. |
| tabern-s. | tabernaemontana stapfiana |
| taber-i. | tabernanthe iboga |
| tab. | tabacum |
| tama-c. | tamarix cinariensis |
| tama. | tamarix germanica |
| | tamarix gallica→tama-c. |
| tamox. | tamoxifen |
| tamrnd. | tamarindus indica |
| tam. | tamus communis |
| tanac-b. | tanacetum balsamita |

| | |
|---|---|
| tanac-er. | tanacetum erectum |
| tanac. | tanacetum vulgare |
| tang. | tanghinia venenifera |
| tann-ac. | tannicum acidum |
| | tanninum→tann-ac. |
| tant-f. | tantalum fluoratum |
| tant-met. | tantalum metallicum |
| taper. | taperiba |
| | taraktogenos→chaul. |
| | taraktogenos kurzii→chaul. |
| | tarantula cubensis→tarent-c. |
| | tarantula hispanica→tarent. |
| | taraxacum dens leonis→tarax. |
| tarax. | taraxacum officinale |
| tarent-c. | tarantula cubensis |
| tarent. | tarantula hispanica |
| tartr. | tartrazine |
| tart-ac. | tartaricum acidum |
| | tartarus depuratus→kali-bit. |
| | tartarus emeticus→ant-t. |
| | tartarus stibiatus→ant-t. |
| tax-br. | taxus brevifolia |
| tax. | taxus baccata |
| techn. | technetium |
| tec-p. | tecoma pentaphylla |
| | tecoma radicans→tec-p. |
| tein. | Teinach aqua |
| tela | tela araneae |
| | tela aranearum→tela |
| | teleamethylthioninum chloridum→methyl. |
| tell-ac. | telluricum acidum |
| tell. | tellurium metallicum |
| | ten (Paterson)→bacls-10. |
| teph-k. | tephrosia kraussiana |
| teph-v. | tephrosia vogelii |
| tep. | Teplitz aqua |
| terb-o. | terbium oxydatum |
| terebe. | terebenum |
| tere-ch. | terebinthina chios |
| term-a. | terminalia arjuna |
| term-c. | terminalia chebula |
| terp-h. | terpini hydras |
| ter. | terebinthiniae oleum |
| | terra silicea→sil. |
| | testa praeparata→calc-o-t. |
| testis | testicles |
| test-act. | testosterone acetate |

| | |
|---|---|
| test-pr. | testosterone propionate |
| test. | testosterone base |
| tetan. | tetanosinum |
| tetox. | tetanotoxinum |
| | tetrabromfluoresceinum→eos. |
| tetrachl. | tetrachloroethylene |
| tetrac-m. | tetracyclinum muriaticum |
| tetrac. | tetracyclinum |
| tetrad-f. | tetradenia fructicosa |
| tetrad-r. | tetradenia riparia |
| tet. | tetradymitum |
| | tetramethylaminum→prop. |
| teucr-b. | teucrium botrys |
| | teucrium chamaedrys→chamae. |
| teucr-sdm. | teucrium scordium |
| teucr-s. | teucrium scorodonia |
| teucr. | teucrium marum verum |
| thala. | thalamus |
| thalic-r. | thalictrum rhynchocarpum |
| thal-act. | thallium aceticum |
| thal-ar. | thallium arsenicosum |
| thal-c. | thallium carbonicum |
| thal-f. | thallium fluoratum |
| thal-met. | thallium metallicum |
| thal-m. | thallium muriaticum |
| thal-n. | thallium nitricum |
| thal-o. | thallium oxydatum |
| thal-s. | thallium sulphuricum |
| thal. | thallium met. + -act. (old abbr.) |
| thap-g. | thapsia garganica |
| thaum-p. | thaumetopoea processionnea |
| thea | thea chinensis |
| | thea sinensis→thea |
| | theba<cum→op. |
| thebin. | thebainum |
| thein. | theinum |
| | theobroma cacao→cac. |
| theob. | theobrominum |
| theoph. | theophyllinum |
| ther. | theridion curassavicum |
| thev. | thevetia nerifolia |
| thiam. | thiaminum hydrochloridum |
| thioc-ac. | thiocticum acidum |
| thiop. | thioproperazinum |
| thiosin. | thiosinaminum |
| thlas. | thlaspi bursa pastoris |

| | |
|---|---|
| thom-h. | thomandersia hensii |
| thor-act. | thorium aceticum |
| thor-met. | thorium metallicum |
| thor-m. | thorium muriaticum |
| thor-n. | thorium nitricum |
| thor-o. | thorium oxydatum |
| thuj-g. | thuja gigantea |
| thuj-l. | thuja lobii |
| thuj. | thuja occidentalis |
| thyam. | thyamine |
| thycho-d. | thychosanthes dioica |
| | thymine→thyam. |
| thymi-ac. | thyminicum acidum |
| | thymoidinum→thym-gl. |
| thymol. | thymolum |
| | thymonucleicum acidum→des-ac. |
| thymul. | thymuline |
| thymum. | thymum |
| thymu-vg. | thymus vulgaris |
| | thymus→thym-gl. |
| thymu. | thymus serpyllum |
| thym-gl. | thymi glandulae extractum |
| | thypha latifolia→typh. |
| thyreotr. | thyreotropinum |
| | thyreostimulinum→thyreotr. |
| thyroiod. | thyro-iodinum |
| thyr. | thyreoidinum |
| | thyroid→thyr. |
| | thyroidinum→thyr. |
| | thyroxinum biiodatum→dithyr. |
| til-al. | tilia alburnum |
| til-ar. | tilia argentea |
| | tilia cordata→til. |
| til-p. | tilia platyphyllos |
| til-t. | tilia tomentosa |
| til. | tilia europaea |
| | tilia silvestris→til. |
| timol. | timolol |
| | tinctura sine kali→caust. |
| tinas. | tinospora cordifolia |
| tip. | tipida aqua |
| titan-ac. | titanicum acidum |
| titan-cy. | titanium cyanatum |
| titan-m. | titanium muriaticum |
| titan-n. | titanium nitridum |
| titan-o. | titanium oxydatum |

| | |
|---|---|
| titan-s. | titanium sulfuricum |
| titan-xyz. | titan-xyz |
| titan. | titanium metallicum |
| tocoph. | tocopherolum |
| tod-a. | toddalia aculeata |
| toen-s. | toenia saginata |
| toluen. | toluene |
| tol. | toluidinum |
| | toluiferum→bals-t. |
| | tonca→tong. |
| tong. | tongo odorata |
| tonsi. | tonsilinum |
| | tonsils→tonsi. |
| | tormentilla→pot-t. |
| torm. | tormentilla erecta |
| tor. | torula cerevisiae |
| | toxicodendron quercifolium vernix →rhus-t. |
| | toxicodendron vernix→rhus-v. |
| toxi. | toxicophis pugnax |
| toxo-g. | toxoplasma gondii |
| tox-th. | toxicophloea thunbergi |
| | toxoplasms gondi→toxo-g. |
| trachsp-j. | trachelospermum jasminoides |
| trach-v. | trachinus vipera |
| trach-xyz. | trach-xyz |
| trach. | trachinus draco |
| trad. | tradescantia diuretica |
| trag-p. | tragopogon pratensis |
| | trametes suaveolens→bol-su. |
| trem-g. | trema grisea |
| | trema guineensis→trem-or. |
| trem-or. | trema orientalis |
| triaetam. | triaethanolamine |
| triamc. | triamcinolon |
| | triatema→triat. |
| triat. | triatoma |
| trib. | tribulus terrestris |
| trichil-e. | trichilia emetica |
| trichlact-ac. | trichloroaceticum acidum |
| trichlae. | trichloraethylene |
| trichom. | trichomonas vaginalis |
| trichoph-d. | trichophyton depressum |
| trichoph-p. | trichophyton persearum |
| | trichophyton persicolor→trichoph-p. |
| trichoph-r. | trichophyton rubrum |
| trichr. | trichuris trichurius |

| | |
|---|---|
| trich. | trichosanthes amara |
| | trichosanthes dioica→trich. |
| triclis-g. | triclisia gilletii |
| trif-al. | trifolium alpinum |
| trif-ar. | trifolium arvense |
| trif-d. | trifolium dubium |
| trif-e. | trifolium elegans |
| trif-p. | trifolium pratense |
| trif-r. | trifolium repens |
| | trigonella foenum graecum→foenm-g. |
| | trigonocephalus lachesis→lach. |
| tril-c. | trillium cernuum |
| | trillium erectum→tril-p. |
| tril-p. | trillium pendulum |
| trimer-a. | trimeria alnifolia |
| trimeth. | trimethadione |
| trim. | trimeresurus wagleri |
| | trimethylaminum→prop. |
| | trimethylxanthin→coffin. |
| | trinatrii citras→nat-cit. |
| | trinitrophenolum→pic-ac. |
| trinit. | trinitrotoluenum |
| trion. | trional |
| trios. | triosteum perfoliatum |
| tritic-g. | triticum germinatum |
| tritic-vg. | triticum vulgare |
| tritic. | triticum repens |
| trito | trito |
| trium-r. | triumfetta rhomboidea |
| trom. | trombidium muscae domesticae |
| trop. | tropaeolum majus |
| trychs. | trychosanthes |
| trych-t. | trychophyton tonsurans |
| tryps. | trypsinum |
| trypt. | tryptophanum |
| | tsuga canadensis→abies-c. |
| | tuberculinum aviaire→tub-a. |
| tub-a. | tuberculinum avis |
| tub-d. | tuberculinum Denys |
| tub-k. | tuberculinum Koch |
| tub-m. | tuberculinum Marmoreck |
| tub-ro. | tuberculinum Rosenbach |
| tub-r. | tuberculinum residuum Koch |
| tub-sp. | tuberculinum Spengler |
| tub. | tuberculinum bovinum Kent |

| | |
|---|---|
| | tubiporus edulis→bol-ed. |
| tul. | tulipa |
| tung-met. | tungstenium metallicum |
| | turnera aphrodisiacs→dam. |
| | turnera diffusa→dam. |
| | turpethum minerale→merc-sul. |
| tur-f. | turraea floribunda |
| tur-o. | turraea obtusifolia |
| tus-fa. | tussilago farfara |
| tus-fr. | tussilago fragrans |
| tus-p. | tussilago petasites |
| tyl-i. | tylophora indica |
| typh. | typha latifolia |
| tyram. | tyramine |
| tyros. | L-tyrosinum |
| | typhobacillinum→eberth. |
| | tyrosinum→tyros. |
| tyrothr. | tyrothricinum |
| ulm-c. | ulmus campestris |
| ulm-m. | ulmus montana |
| | ulmus fulva→ulm-c. |
| ulm-pra. | ulmus procera |
| ulx-eu. | ulex europaeus |
| | ulmus pyramidalis→ulm-m. |
| | umbilicus pendulinus→cot. |
| undec-ac. | undecylenicum acidum |
| une-e. | unedo edulis |
| upa-a. | upas antiaris |
| upa. | upas tieut, |
| | uragoga ipecacuanha→ip. |
| uranoth. | uranothorium |
| uran-act. | uranium aceticum |
| uran-ar. | uranium arsenicicum |
| uran-met. | uranium metallicum |
| uran-m. | uranium muriaticum |
| uran-n. | uranium nitricum |
| uran-o. | uranium oxydatum |
| urea | urea pura |
| urea-n. | urea nitrica |
| ureth. | urethane |
| | urginea maritima→squil. |
| | urine→urin. |
| urin-d. | urinum diabeticum |
| urin. | urinum |
| urotrop. | urotropinum |
| ursin-t. | ursinia tenuiloba |
| urt-c. | urtica crenulata |
| urt-d. | urtica dioica |
| urt-g. | urtica gigas |
| urt-u. | urtica urens |
| ur-ac. | uricum acidum |
| usn. | usnea barbata |
| ust. | ustilago maydis |
| uva | uva ursi |
| uvar. | uvaria triloba |
| uza. | uzara |
| | Vaccin of Haffkine→pest. |
| vacc-m. | vaccinium myrtillus |
| vacc-v. | vaccinium vitis idaea |
| vac. | vaccininum |
| | vaccinotoxinum→vac. |
| valerl-o. | valerianella olitoria |
| valer-ac. | valerianicum acidum |
| valer. | valeriana officinalis |
| vanad-m. | vanadium muriaticum |
| vanad-o. | vanadium oxydatum |
| vanad-s. | vanadium sulphuricum |
| vanad. | vanadium metallicum |
| vang-e. | vangueria emirnensis |
| vang-1. | vangueria lasiantha |
| vanilin. | vanillinum |
| vanil. | vanilla aromatica |
| | vanilla planifolia→vanil. |
| | varech→fuc. |
| varic. | varicellinum |
| vario. | variolinum |
| vasop. | vasopressine |
| vauc-s. | vaucheria sessilis |
| | velome de mato→crot-f. |
| ven-m. | venus mercenaria |
| verat-n. | veratrum nigrum |
| | veratrum luteum→helon. |
| verat-v. | veratrum viride |
| verat. | veratrum album |
| | verbascum thapsiforme→verb. |
| verbe-h. | verbena hastata |
| verbe-o. | verbena officinalis |
| verbe-u. | verbena urticaefolia |
| verb-f. | verbascum floccosum |
| verb-n. | verbascum nigrum |
| verb-ol. | verbasci oleum |
| verb. | verbascum thapsus |
| verin. | veratrinum |
| vern-am. | vernonia amygdalina |
| vern-a. | vernonia anthelmintica |

| | |
|---|---|
| vern-co. | vernonia corymbosa |
| vern-w. | vernonia wooddii |
| | veronal→barbit. |
| | veronastricum virginicum→ lept. |
| vero-ab. | veronica abyssinica |
| vero-b. | veronica beccabunga |
| vero-c. | veronica chamaedrys |
| vero-o. | veronica officinalis |
| vero-p. | veronica persica |
| vero-t. | veronica teucrium |
| | veronica virginica→lept. |
| verr. | verrucinum |
| vesi. | vesicaria communis |
| vesp-m. | vespa maculata |
| vesp-vg. | vespa vulgaris |
| vesp-xyz. | vespa crabro + -m. + -vg. |
| vesp. | vespa crabro |
| | vetiver→anan. |
| | vetiveria zizanioides→anan. |
| vibh. | vibhuti |
| vib-1. | viburnum lantana |
| vib-od. | viburnum oderatissinum |
| vib-p. | vibumum prunifolium |
| vib-t. | viburnum tinus |
| vib. | viburnum opulus |
| vichy-g. | Vichy aqua Grande Grille |
| vichy-h. | Vichy aqua H"pital |
| | vicia ervilia→erv-e. |
| | vicia faba→faba-vg. |
| vince. | vincetoxicum officinale |
| vinc-ma. | vinca major |
| vinc-r. | vinca rosea |
| vinc. | vinca minor |
| viol-c. | viola canina |
| viol-o. | viola odorata |
| viol-s. | viola sudetica |
| viol-t. | viola tricolor |
| vip-a. | vipera aspis |
| | vipera communis→vip. |
| vip-d. | vipera daboia |
| vip-l-f. | vipera lachesis fel |
| vip-r. | vipera redi |
| vip-t. | vipera torva |
| vip. | vipera berus |
| | vipera russelli→vip-d. |
| virl. | virillium |
| | virola sebifera→myric. |
| | virus poliomyelitis→polio |
| visc-ab. | viscum abietis |
| visc-ar. | viscum armeniacae |
| visc-cr. | viscum crataegi |
| visc-1. | viscum laxum |
| visc-m. | viscum mali |
| | viscum pini→visc-1. |
| visc-pi. | viscum piri |
| visc-po. | viscum populi |
| visc-pr. | viscum pruni |
| visc-q. | viscum quercinum |
| visc-r. | viscum robiniae |
| visc-s. | viscum salicis |
| visc-t. | viscum tiliae |
| visc. | viscum album |
| | vitamin a acid→retin-ac. |
| | vitamin a alcohol→retin. |
| | vitamin bl→thiam. |
| | vitamin bl2→cyanoc. |
| | vitamin b2→ribo. |
| | vitamin b3→nicotam. |
| | vitamin b4→adenin. |
| | vitamin b5→pant-ac. |
| | vitamin b6→pyrid. |
| | vitamin b7→inos. |
| | vitamin b8→adenyl-ac. |
| | vitamin c→ascor-ac. |
| | vitamin d2→ergocalc. |
| | vitamin d3→cholcalc. |
| | vitamin e→tocoph. |
| | vitamin f→linol-ac. |
| | vitamin g→lactof. |
| | vitamin h2→amibe-ac. |
| | vitamin k→menad. |
| | vitamin pp→nicot-ac. |
| | vitamine hl→biot. |
| | vitex agnus castus→agn. |
| | vitis alba→bry. |
| | vitis quinquefolia→ampe-qu. |
| | vitis rubra→ampe-qu. |
| vitis-v. | vitis vinifera |
| vitr-an. | vitrum antimonii |
| vitr-cor. | vitrum coroni |
| vit. | vitex trifolia |
| voac-af. | voacanga africana |
| voes. | Voeslau aqua |
| v-a-b. | vaccin att,nu, bili, |
| | vulpis pulmo→pulm-v. |

| | |
|---|---|
| wede-n. | wedelia natalensis |
| weilb. | Weilbach aqua |
| wies. | Wiesbaden aqua |
| | wigardia californica→erio. |
| wildb. | Wildbad aqua |
| wildu. | Wildungen aqua |
| wist-s. | wisteria sinensis |
| with-s. | withania somnifera |
| | wood alcohol→methan. |
| | woorali→cur. |
| | woorara→cur. |
| | wrightia antidysenterica→kurch. |
| | wrightia tincto→kurch. |
| | wyethia→wye. |
| wye. | wyethia helenoides |
| xanrhi. | xanthorrhiza apifolia |
| xanrhoe. | xanthorrhoea arborea |
| xanthin. | xanthinum |
| xanth-mc. | xanthium macrocarpum |
| xanth-st. | xanthium strumarium |
| xanth. | xanthium spinosum |
| | xantoxylum americanum→xan. |
| xan. | xantoxylum fraxineum |
| xen. | xenon |
| xero. | xerophyllum |
| xime-c. | ximenia caffra |
| | xiphosura→lim. |
| xiph. | xiphosura americana |
| xyloc. | xylocaine |
| xylop-a. | xylopia aethiopica |
| xyma-m. | xymalos monospora |
| x-ray | x-ray |
| yers. | serum yersiniae |
| | yampah→perid-b. |
| | yaupon→ilx-v. |
| | yerba buena→micr. |
| | yerba mansa→anemps. |
| | yerba santa→erio. |
| | Yersin→yers. |
| | yohimbehe→yohim. |
| yohim-m. | yohimbinum muriaticum |
| yohim. | yohimbinum |
| yttrb-o. | ytterbium oxydatum |
| yttr-met. | yttrium metallicum |
| yttr-ox. | yttrium oxalicum |

| | |
|---|---|
| yttr-o. | yttrium oxydatum |
| yuc. | yucca filamentosa |
| | zaluzianskya capensis→zant. |
| zanthox-c. | zanthoxylum capense |
| zant. | zantedeschia |
| | zanthoxylum fraxineum→zant. |
| zea-i. | zea italica |
| | zea maydis→stigm. |
| | zinci sulphas→zinc-s. |
| zinc-act. | zincum aceticum |
| zinc-ar. | zincum arsenicosum |
| zinc-be. | zincum benzoicum |
| zinc-br. | zincum bromatum |
| zinc-chl. | zincum chloricum |
| | zincum chromatum→zinc-chr. |
| zinc-chr. | zincum chromicum |
| zinc-col. | zincum colloidale |
| zinc-cy. | zincum cyanatum |
| zinc-c. | zincum carbonicum |
| zinc-fcy. | zincum ferrocyanatum |
| zinc-form. | zincum formicum |
| zinc-f. | zincum fluoratum |
| zinc-gl. | zincum gluconicum |
| zinc-i. | zincum iodatum |
| zinc-m. | zincum muriaticum |
| zinc-n. | zincum nitricum |
| zinc-ox. | zincum oxalicum |
| zinc-o. | zincum oxydatum |
| zinc-pic. | zincum picricum |
| zinc-pox. | zincum peroxydatum |
| zinc-p. | zincum phosphoricum |
| zinc-s. | zincum sulphuricum |
| zinc-val. | zincum valerianicum |
| zinc. | zincum metallicum |
| | zingiber→zing. |
| zing. | zingiber officinale |
| zirc-met. | zirconium metallicum |
| zirc-m. | zirconium muriaticum |
| zirc-n. | zirconium nitricum |
| zirc-o. | zirconium oxydatum |
| | zisyphus paliurus→pali-a. |
| zizyp-j. | zizyphus jujuba |
| zizyp-m. | zizyphus mucronata |
| ziz. | zizia aurea |

# Homoeopathic Pharmacy Hahnemann's Way

*MASTER HAHNEMANN was a person who envisioned an entire system of medicine and then fully developed it into a powerful and practical tool within the span of a single life. This system of medicine he named it as Homoeopathy. In his books at various places he tells us about the various important facts and his observations which he found were important and gave us the cardinal principles of homoeopathy.*

**§ 1 Mission of Physician**

The physician's high and only mission is to restore the sick to health, to cure, as it is termed[1].

[1] His mission is not, however to construct so-called systems, by interweaving empty speculations and hypotheses concerning the internal essential nature of the vital processes and the mode in which disease originate in.

**§ 3 Knowledge of Physician**

If the physician clearly perceives what is to be cured in diseases, that is to say, in every individual case of disease *(knowledge of disease, indication)*, if he clearly perceives what is curative in medicines, that is to say, in each individual medicine *(knowledge of medicinal powers)*, and if he knows how to adapt, according to clearly defined principles, what is curative in medicine to what he has discovered to be undoubtedly morbid in the patient, so that the recovery must ensure - to adapt it, as well in respect to the suitability of the medicine most appropriate according to its mode of action to the case before him *(choice of the remedy, the medicine indicated)*, as also in respect to the exact mode of preparation and quantity of a required *(proper dose)*, and the proper period for repeating the dose; - if, finally, he knows the obstacles to recovery in each case and is aware how to remove them, so that the restoration may be permanent, *then he understands how to treat judiciously and nationally, and he is a true practitioner of the healing art.* [(4)]

**§ 4 Physician as Preserver of health**

He is likewise a preserver of health if he knows the things that derange health and cause disease, and how to remove them from persons in health.[(a)]

**§ 6 Unprejudiced observed**

The unprejudiced observer - well aware of the futility of transcendental speculations which can receive no confirmation from experience - be his powers of penetration ever so great, takes note of nothing in every individual disease, except the changes in the health of the body and of the mind *(morbid phenomena, accidents, symptoms)* which can be perceived externally by means of the senses; that is to say, he notices only the deviations from

# Doctor Hahnemann's say on Mother Tincture and Dilutions

**§ 123 Unadulterated Herbs**

Each of these medicines must be taken in a perfectly simple, unadulterated form; the indigenous plants in the form of freshly expressed juice, mixed with a little alcohol to prevent it spoiling; exotic vegetable substances, however, in the form of powder, or

**B. Jain assures herbs from original source of cultivation or reliable vendors.**

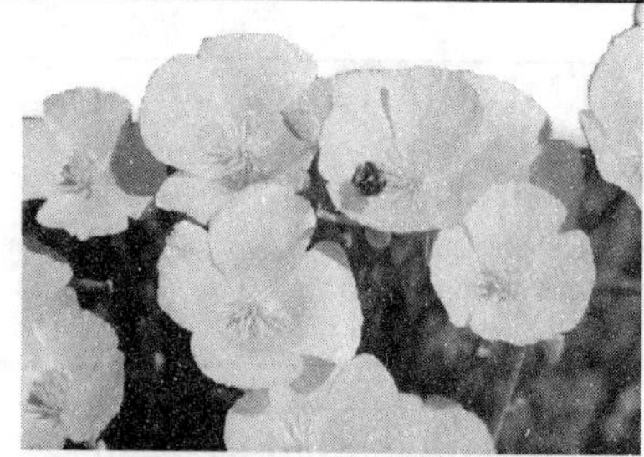

**§ 264 Genuine Medicine**

The true physician must be provided with *genuine medicines of unimpaired strength,* so that he may be able to rely upon their therapeutic powers; he must be able, himself, to judge of their genuineness.

**At B.Jain we guarantee accurate herb and thus 100% accurate & pure Mother Tincture.**

**§ 268 Quality control to check genuinity of herb**

The other exotic plants, barks, seeds and roots that cannot be obtained in the fresh state the sensible practitioner will never take in the pulverized form on trust, but will first convince himself of their genuineness in their crude, entire state before making any medicinal employment of them.[1]

[1] In order to preserve them in the form of powder, a precaution is requisite that has hitherto been usually neglected by druggists, and hence powders

**B.Jain QC Department checks various parameters like TLC, UV, Infrared assuring genuinity of herbs and 100% accurate Mother Tincture.**

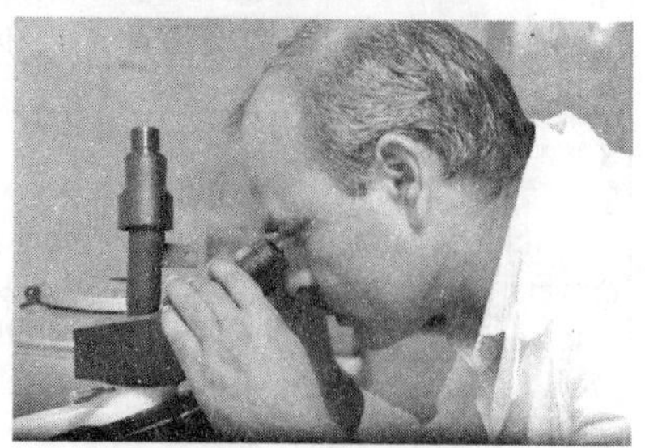